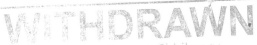

THE EPIDEMIOLOGY of DIABETES MELLITUS

Second Edition

THE EPIDEMIOLOGY of DIABETES MELLITUS

Second Edition

Edited by

Jean-Marie Ekoé *Endocrinologie, Métabolisme et Nutrition, Centre de Recherche CHUM, Montreal, Canada*
Marian Rewers *Barbara Davis Center for Childhood Diabetes, Colorado, USA*
Rhys Williams *Clinical Epidemiology at the School of Medicine, University of Swansea, Swansea, UK*
Paul Zimmet *International Diabetes Institute, Caulfield, Australia*

⟨W⟩WILEY-BLACKWELL

This edition first published 2008 © 2008, John Wiley & Sons Ltd

Wiley-Blackwell is an imprint of John Wiley & Sons, formed by the merger of Wiley's global Scientific, Technical and Medical business with Blackwell Publishing.

Registered office: John Wiley & Sons Ltd, The Atrium, Southern Gate, Chichester, West Sussex, PO19 8SQ, UK

Other Editorial Offices:
9600 Garsington Road, Oxford, OX4 2DQ, UK
111 River Street, Hoboken, NJ 07030-5774, USA

For details of our global editorial offices, for customer services and for information about how to apply for permission to reuse the copyright material in this book please see our website at www.wiley.com/wiley-blackwell

Library of Congress Cataloging-in-Publication Data:
The epidemiology of diabetes mellitus / edited by Jean-Marie Ekoé . . . [et al.].—2nd ed.
      p. ; cm.
 Includes bibliographical references and index.
 ISBN 978-0-470-01727-2 (alk. paper)
1. Diabetes—Epidemiology. I. Ekoé, J.-M.
 [DNLM: 1. Diabetes Mellitus—epidemiology. 2. Diabetes
Complications—epidemiology. WK 810 E641 2008]
 RA645.D5E654 2008
 614.5'9462–dc22
                        2008029103

ISBN 978-0-470-01727-2

A catalogue record for this book is available from the British Library.

Set in 10/12 Times New Roman by Laserwords Private Ltd, Chennai, India.
Printed in Great Britain by Antony Rowe Ltd, Chippenham, Wiltshire.

First Impression   2008

Contents

About the Editors

Jean-Marie Ekoé is Professor of Medicine, Endocrinology, Metabolism and Nutrition, Faculty of Medicine, University of Montreal, Quebec, Canada. He is a member of the Epidemiology Research Unit, Research Centre of the Centre Hospitalier Universitaire de Montréal (CHUM). He was the first recipient of the World Health Organization and International Diabetes Federation Kelly West Memorial Lilly Award in 1983. His major clinical and research interests are in the epidemiology of diabetes, diabetic foot problems and other long-term complications of diabetes mellitus.

Dr Ekoé is or has been principal investigator, co-investigator and collaborator of numerous clinical trials and projects involving epidemiology and management of diabetes and its late complications among Caucasian, Native and other populations in Canada and elsewhere. He received the 2004 Annual Award of Specialized Medicine of L'Association des Médecins de Langue Française du Canada and the Sir Alister McIntyre Distinguished Award for the year 2007 from the University of the West Indies Outreach Programme (UDOP). He has served as the Diabète Québec, Canada, Professional Council Chairman since 2006.

Marian Rewers' primary research has been in the area of epidemiology/etiology of type 1 diabetes, as well as insulin resistance and cardiovascular complications of both type 1 and type 2 diabetes. Dr Rewers is the principal investigator of five large active National Institutes of Health-funded projects: the Diabetes Autoimmunity Study in the Young (National Institute of Diabetes and Digestive and Kidney (NIDDK)/National Institute of Allergy and Infectious Diseases), The Environmental Determinants of Diabetes in the Young, the Coronary Artery Calcification in Type 1 Study (National Heart, Lung, and Blood Institute (NHLBI)), the Determinants of Premature Atherosclerosis in Type 1 Diabetes Study (NHLBI), and the Genetic and Environmental Causes of Celiac Disease (NIDDK). In the past, he has directed two additional large NHLBI-funded projects: The Insulin Resistance Atherosclerosis Study (IRAS) and The IRAS Family Study. He serves as the Clinical Investigation & Bioinformatics Core director for the University of Colorado at Denver and Health Sciences Center Diabetes Endocrinology Research Center (DERC). He is a co-investigator on additional multiyear projects in the area of diabetes and autoimmunity.

Dr Rewers is directing one of the studies that have been instrumental in learning the causes and risks of diabetes, the Diabetes Autoimmunity Study in the Young (DAISY). In 2000, Dr Rewers initiated a study of early detection of heart disease in 1400 adult patients with type 1 diabetes and their spouses/partners. The study is pioneering the use of electron beam computed tomography in detecting microscopical calcification of coronary arteries.

In addition to his research endeavors, Dr Rewers is directing a clinical team of 16 physicians and over 50 ancillary staff serving a population of nearly 6000 patients with type 1 diabetes. He received American Diabetes Association (ADA) Michaela Modan Memorial Award and served as the ADA Council on Epidemiology & Statistics Program Chair and Chair from 1996 to 2001. Currently, Dr Rewers serves as the Associate Editor of *Diabetes Care*.

Rhys Williams is Dean of Medicine and Professor of Clinical Epidemiology at the School of Medicine, Swansea University. He is the Head of Learning and Teaching at the School and the chair of the Centre for Information, Research and Evaluation. His main research interests relate to diabetes epidemiology and health care, metabolic syndrome and childhood obesity. He is Chair of Diabetes UK's Wales Advisory Council and, until recently, was a Vice President of the International Diabetes Federation (IDF), chair of the IDF's Task Force on Diabetes Awareness and Editor-in-Chief of IDF's in-house magazine *Diabetes Voice*. He is a member of the IDF's Prevention Task Force and of the *Diabetes Atlas* Editorial Board. He is also a visiting consultant to the World Health Organization, Geneva.

Paul Zimmet is Director of the International Diabetes Institute and Hon. Professor at Monash University in Australia. He co-chairs the International Diabetes Federation Task Force on Epidemiology and Prevention. He designed and leads the team carrying out the 'AusDiab Study,' the first national diabetes and obesity study in Australia. He is widely recognized for his studies in Indian and Pacific Ocean populations, which have provided new insights into the genetic and environmental contribution to type 2 diabetes and obesity as well as the role of socio-cultural change. He has received numerous international awards for his research, including the 2007 international Novartis Award for accomplishments in research that have had a major impact in diabetes. He received the national award of Officer of the Order of Australia for distinguished services to medicine, nutrition and the biotechnology industry.

Contributors

ROBERT C. ATKINS

Department of Epidemiology and Preventive Medicine
Monash University
Alfred Hospital
Melbourne
Australia

MARY A. BANERJI

SUNY Health Science Center
New York, NY
USA

ELIZABETH L. M. BARR

International Diabetes Institute
Caulfield, Victoria
Australia

ELIZABETH BARRETT-CONNOR

Division of Epidemiology/Department of Family and Preventive Medicine
University of California, San Diego
La Jolla, CA
USA

JUDITH BAXTER

Colorado School of Public Health
University of Colorado Denver
Aurora, CO
USA

ANDREW J. M. BOULTON

Department of Medicine
Manchester Royal Infirmary
Manchester
UK

EDWARD J. BOYKO

Department of Medicine
University of Washington School of Medicine
Epidemiologic Research and Information Center
VA Puget Sound Health Care System
Seattle, WA
USA

ADRIAN CAMERON

International Diabetes Institute
Caulfield, Victoria
Australia

IAN D. CATERSON

The George Institute and the Human Nutrition Unit
University of Sydney
Sydney, New South Wales
Australia

JULIANA C.N. CHAN

Department of Medicine & Therapeutics
The Chinese University of Hong Kong
The Prince of Wales Hospital
Shatin
Hong Kong

DON J. CHISHOLM

Diabetes and Obesity Program
Garvan Institute of Medical Research
Darlinghurst, New South Wales
Australia

CLIVE S. COCKRAM

Department of Medicine & Therapeutics
The Chinese University of Hong Kong
The Prince of Wales Hospital
Shatin
Hong Kong

RUTH COLAGIURI

Diabetes Unit, Australian Health Policy Unit
Sydney University
Sydney, New South Wales
Australia

STEPHEN COLAGIURI

Department of Endocrinology, Diabetes and
Metabolism
Prince of Wales Hospital
Randwick
Australia

BARBARA CURRIE

Division of Endocrinology
QEII Health Sciences Centre
Halifax, Nova Scotia
Canada

DANA M. DABELEA

University of Colorado School of Medicine
Denver, CO
USA

JEAN-MARIE EKOÉ

Endocrinologie, Métabolisme et Nutrition, Cen-
tre de Recherche du CHUM
Montreal
Canada

IMAD M. EL-KEBBI

Division of Endocrinology, Metabolism and
Lipids
Emory University School of Medicine
Atlanta, GA
USA

MICHAEL M. ENGELGAU

Division of Diabetes Translation
National Center for Chronic Disease Prevention
and Health Promotion,
Centers for Disease Control and Prevention
Atlanta, GA
USA

SANDRA R. G. FERREIRA

School of Public Health—University of São
Paulo
Paulo-SP
Brazil

LAÉRCIO J. FRANCO

Faculty of Medicine of Ribeirão
Preto—University of São Paulo
Ribeirão Preto-SP
Brazil

WILFRED Y. FUJIMOTO

University of Washington Department of
Medicine
Seattle, WA
USA

LINDA S. GEISS

Division of Diabetes Translation
Centers for Disease Control and Prevention
Atlanta, GA
USA

ANDERS GREEN

Department of Research and Applied
Health Technology Assessment, Odense
University Hospital and
Epidemiology
Institute of Public Health
University of Southern Denmark
Odense, Denmark

EDWARD W. GREGG

Department of Epidemiology
Graduate School of Public Health
University of Pittsburgh
Pittsburgh, PA
USA

LEIF GROOP

Department of Clinical Sciences/Diabetes &
Endocrinology
and Lund University Diabetes Centre
Lund University
University Hospital Malmö
Malmö
Sweden

RICHARD F. HAMMAN

Colorado School of Public Health
University of Colorado Denver
Aurora, CO
USA

ROBERT L. HANSON

National Institute of Diabetes and Digestive and
Kidney Diseases
Phoenix, AZ
USA

ZAFIML HUSSAIN

Department of Endocrinology, Diabetes and
Metabolism
Prince of Wales Hospital
Randwick
Australia

RACHEL HUXLEY

The George Institute and the Human Nutrition
Unit
University of Sydney
Sydney, New South Wales,
Australia

HARRY KEEN

Unit for Metabolic Medicine
Guy's Hospital Campus, King's College London
London
UK

RON KLEIN

Department of Ophthamology and Visual Sci-
ences
University of Wisconsin School of Medicine and
Public Health
Madison, WI
USA

WILLIAM C. KNOWLER

National Institute of Diabetes and Digestive and
Kidney Diseases
Phoenix, AZ
USA

ANDREA M. KRISKA

Department of Epidemiology
Graduate School of Public Health
University of Pittsburgh
Pittsburgh, PA
USA

KIRSTEN O. KYVIK

Institute of Regional Health Services Research
and Epidemiology
Institute of Public Health
University of Southern Denmark
Odense
Denmark

HAROLD LEBOVITZ

SUNY Health Science Center
New York, NY
USA

CHARLOTTE LING

Department of Clinical Sciences/Diabetes &
Endocrinology
and Lund University Diabetes Centre
Lund University
University Hospital Malmö
Malmö
Sweden

REBECCA B. LIPTON

Section of Pediatric Endocrinology and Depart-
ment of Health Studies
University of Chicago
Chicago, IL
USA

GILBERT L'ITALIEN

Global Epidemiology and Outcomes Research
Bristol Myers Squibb
Pharmaceutical Research Institute;
Yale University Medical School
New Haven, CT
USA

VALERIYA LYSSENKO

Department of Clinical Sciences/Diabetes &
Endocrinology
and Lund University Diabetes Centre
Lund University
University Hospital Malmö
Malmö
Sweden

DIANNA J. MAGLIANO

International Diabetes Institute
Caulfield, Victoria
Australia

JIM MANN

Department of Human Nutrition
University of Otago
Dunedin
New Zealand

MARGUERITE J. MCNEELY

University of Washington Department of
Medicine
Seattle, WA
USA

ERROL MORRISON

Departments of Biochemistry &
Endocrinology
The University of the West Indies
Mona Campus, Jamaica

AYESHA A. MOTALA

Department of Diabetes and Endocrinology
Division of Medicine
Nelson R Mandela School of Medicine
Faculty of Health Sciences
University of KwaZulu-Natal
Durban
South Africa

K. M. VENKAT NARAYAN

National Center for Chronic Disease
Prevention and Health Promotion
Centers for Disease Control and Prevention
Atlanta, GA
USA

ROBERT G. NELSON

National Institute of Diabetes and Digestive
and Kidney Diseases
Phoenix, AZ
USA

JOHN NEWCOMER

Department of Psychiatry
Washington University School of Medicine
St Louis, MO
USA

MAHOMED A.K. OMAR

Department of Diabetes and Endocrinology
Division of Medicine
Nelson R Mandela School of Medicine
Faculty of Health Sciences
University of KwaZulu-Natal
Durban
South Africa

ABDULLAH OMARI

The George Institute and the Human Nutrition
Unit
University of Sydney
Sydney, New South Wales
Australia

MARJU ORHO-MELANDER

Department of Clinical Sciences/Diabetes &
Endocrinology
and Lund University Diabetes Centre
Lund University
University Hospital Malmö
Malmö
Sweden

TANIELA PALU

Diabetes Centre
Vaiola Hospital
Nulu'alofa
Tonga

MEDA E. PAVKOV

National Institute of Diabetes and Digestive and
Kidney Diseases
Phoenix, AZ
USA

FRASER J. PIRIE

Department of Diabetes and Endocrinology
Division of Medicine
Nelson R Mandela School of Medicine
Faculty of Health Sciences
University of KwaZulu-Natal
Durban
South Africa

LOUISE PRENTICE
Department of Epidemiology and Preventive Medicine
Monash University
Alfred Hospital
Melbourne
Australia

DALIP RAGOOBIRSINGH
Departments of Biochemistry and Diabetology
The University of the West Indies
Mona Campus
Jamaica

AMBADY RAMACHANDRAN
India Diabetes Research Foundation
Dr. A. Ramachandran's Diabetes Hospitals
Chennai
India

THOMAS RANSOM
Division of Endocrinology
QEII Health Sciences Centre
Halifax, Nova Scotia
Canada

ANNE T. REUTENS
Department of Epidemiology and Preventive Medicine
Monash University
Alfred Hospital
Melbourne
Australia

ARLETA B. REWERS
Department of Pediatrics
University of Colorado at Denver and Health Sciences Center
Denver, CO
USA

MARIAN REWERS
Barbara Davis Center for Childhood Diabetes
University of Colorado School of Medicine
Aurora, CO
USA

KATHY SAMARAS
Diabetes and Obesity Program
Garvan Institute of Medical Research
Darlinghurst, New South Wales
Australia

ANDRÉ J. SCHEEN
Division of Diabetes, Nutrition and Metabolic Disorders
Department of Medicine
CHU Sart Tilman
University of Liège, Liège
Belgium

JONATHAN E. SHAW
Baker IDI, Heart & Diabetes Institute
Caulfield, Victoria
Australia

NALINI SINGH
Healthcare Partners
Arcadia, CA
USA

CHAMUKUTTAN SNEHALATHA
Department of Biochemistry
India Diabetes Research Foundation
Dr. A. Ramachandran's Diabetes Hospitals
Chennai
India

THOMAS J. SONGER
Department of Epidemiology
University of Pittsburgh
Pittsburgh, PA
USA

LARS C. STENE
Division of Epidemiology
Norwegian Institute of Public Health
Oslo
Norway

KRISTI L. STORTI

Department of Epidemiology
Graduate School of Public Health
University of Pittsburgh
Pittsburgh, PA
USA

NAOKO TAJIMA

Division of Diabetes,Metabolism and
Endocrinology
Department of Medicine
Jikei University School of Medicine
Tokyo
Japan

MONIKA TOELLER

German Diabetes Center
University of Dusseldorf
Dusseldorf
Germany

JAAKKO TUOMILEHTO

Department of Epidemiology and Health Pro-
motion
National Public Health Institute
Helsinki
Finland

EHUD UR

Division of Endocrinology
QEII Health Sciences Centre
Halifax, Nova Scotia
Canada

SATUPAITEA VIALI

Oceania Medical School
Apia
Samoa

JING WANG

Division of Diabetes Translation
Centers for Disease Control and Prevention
Atlanta, GA
USA

STEPHANIE WHEELER

University of Washington School of Medicine
VA Puget Sound Health Care System
Seattle, WA
USA

RHYS WILLIAMS

Clinical Epidemiology at the School of
Medicine
University of Swansea
Swansea
UK

TIEN Y. WONG

Centre for Eye Research Australia
University of Melbourne
Melbourne
Victoria
Australia

JEAN-FRANCOIS YALE

McGill Nutrition and Food Science Centre
Department of Medicine
McGill University
Montreal
Quebec
Canada

PAUL Z. ZIMMET

International Diabetes Institute
Caulfield, Victoria
Australia

Foreword

The epidemiology of diabetes has become a growth industry over the past 25 years—since WHO and NDDG revised the criteria for the classification and diagnosis of diabetes. This occurred shortly after the unique observations of very high prevalence rates of type 2 diabetes in Pacific islanders and Amerindians and the pioneering international comparative studies by Kelly West. Epidemiology as a discipline has matured and become much more refined over the same period. Diagnostic criteria for diabetes and the classification have been updated as knowledge has increased—and intermediate degrees of hyperglycaemia introduced as risk states for diabetes. The first edition of this book broke new ground as the definitive text focusing on the epidemiology of diabetes. At that time it was obvious that an epidemic of diabetes—particularly type 2—was in progress & much of the focus of the book was to discuss the reasons for this and tactics needed for primary prevention. Do we need a further edition—the answer is a resounding yes! Knowledge has increased greatly over the intervening years, our knowledge of the prevalence and incidence of both type 2 and type 1 diabetes has increased, and more knowledge is available on prevention. We also have better information on the complications of diabetes, the emergence of the Metabolic Syndrome as a risk state and awareness of the increasing occurrence of type 2 diabetes in young people and children.

Type 1 diabetes has perhaps received less attention than type 2 over the past decade—primarily because people with this sort of diabetes are far outnumbered by those with type 2. Nonetheless, numbers are increasing almost everywhere with Finland and Newfoundland for example now reporting alarming rates. This has massive consequences for healthcare—and for affected individuals. Knowledge on genetic aspects of type 1 and ethnic differences has increased although we are still frustratingly far from realistic preventive or curative strategies. Up to date accounts of these areas are presented in this volume.

Type 2 diabetes now presents as one of the great pandemics of the 21st Century. In some populations more than half of adults either already have the disease or are at high risk with evidence of IGT, IFG or metabolic syndrome. It affects all peoples but particularly some of our rapidly developing groups. South Asians appear to have a particular predisposition to diabetes—and the Indian subcontinent will have nearly one-third of the world's type 2 diabetic people. The disorder is however emerging as a massive threat to health everywhere. In particular diabetes increases the risk of developing macrovascular disease and is now one of the major factors behind the resurgence of heart disease and stroke world-wide—and in particular their increase in the developing world. They also of course carry the risk of the microvascular complications, particularly when glycaemic control is inadequate.

The only real solution is prevention. The results of prevention trials were beginning to emerge at the time of the last edition of this volume with much hope engendered by the large trials in the USA and Finland. Several further trials have now reported & it seems clear that by focussing on high risk people (those with IGT or IFG or both) the development of tp2 diabetes can be delayed in more than 50% with lifestyle adjustment and or metformin & even more with glitazones. Obviously this now needs testing formally in whole communities and in ''real life''—and also the thorny question of the safe long term use of drugs with potential side effects has to be tackled.

Prevention of development of the long-term complications is of course vital for those who have already developed diabetes. New drug entities are appearing which will help—as will improving blood glucose control. Here patient and professional education become all important and there is a massive task ahead if we are to get at everyone with diabetes—and all their carers.

The epidemiological background to these problems—and others—is presented exhaustively in this volume. There is an excellent introduction on the clinical syndrome and on current views on classification and diagnosis. Broad chapters on type 2 diabetes and obesity, physical activity and nutrition then provide the backdrop against which detailed accounts are given of type 2 diabetes in all the major continents and many individual countries. Type 1 diabetes then follows with separate chapters thereafter on each of the complications. There are then informative essays on mortality and economics.

Undoubtedly this book will provide a *vade mecum* for all those interested in not just diabetic epidemiology but diabetes in general.

Professor Sir George Alberti
Imperial College
London
UK
June 2008

Acknowledgements

Many people, from all corners of the globe, have been involved in this second edition, the most important of whom are the 80 authors—many new contributors as well as old friends from the first edition—all of whom have graciously helped to ensure the timely publication of this book. The editors gratefully acknowledge their contributions to this revised and expanded edition. There is no doubt in our minds that this book is their achievement as well as ours.

Once again, the team at John Wiley and Sons has been very supportive and tolerant. It's been a joy to work with all the members of the team throughout the last seven years. Particular thanks to Joan Marsh, Kate Pamphilon, Fiona Woods, Robyn Lyons and Deirdre Barry for keeping us alert and posted. Another special word of gratitude to Jon Peacock, Peter Lewis and Deepthi Unni and collaborators for their professional assistance and editorial expertise. The fine quality of their work is greatly appreciated.

And last but not least, we must thank our families for providing us, once again, with support, time and understanding. We owe them a lot.

Jean-Marie Ekoé, Marian Rewers
Rhys Williams, Paul Zimmet
Montreal, Denver
Swansea, Melbourne
June 2008

1

Introduction

Jean-Marie Ekoé,[1] Marian Rewers,[2] Rhys Williams[3] and Paul Z. Zimmet[4]

[1]Endocrinologie, Métabolisme et Nutrition, Centre de Recherche du CHUM, Montreal, Canada
[2]Barbara Davis Center for Childhood Diabetes, University of Colorado School of Medicine, Aurora, CO, USA
[3]Clinical Epidemiology at the School of Medicine, University of Swansea, Swansea, UK
[4]International Diabetes Institute, Caulfield, Victoria, Australia

1.1 INTRODUCTION TO THE SECOND EDITION

It has been seven years since the first edition of *The Epidemiology of Diabetes Mellitus. An International Perspective* appeared. The volume was generally saluted as an excellent initiative: '. . . an extremely welcome, timely and important compilation. . . ' (*Diabetes/Metabolism*, July/August 2002); '. . . a welcome and innovative addition to the lamentably few texts available on the subject. . . ' (*International Journal of Epidemiology*, vol. 31, No. 4, 2002); '. . . a good primer for clinicians and researchers. . . ' (*Trends in Endocrinology and Metabolism*); '. . . This book provides an excellent update on aetiological aspects in type 1 as well as type 2 diabetes . . . the editors have done a very good job. . . ' (*Diabetologia*, January 2003). The reviews went on hoping that '. . . . this book will contribute to change our attitude. . . ' (*Acta Cardiologica*, October 2002) and that '. . . it was just the first edition of what will become the definitive textbook in the field (of Diabetes Epidemiology). . . ' (*British Medical Journal*, 6 April 2002).

Our objective with the first edition was to bridge the two decades that had passed since Dr Kelly's West landmark monograph on *Epidemiology of Diabetes and Its Vascular Complications* and to give a broader review of recent epidemiological studies spanning the globe, different nations and cultures.

It is now clear that the bulk of the pandemic of diabetes sweeping the world (as a result of increasing obesity, physical inactivity, other environmental determinants, including intrauterine influences as well as increased longevity) will emerge in non-Europid populations. By considering diabetes in relation to different ethnic groups, cultures and geographical settings, much can be learned about the natural history, the risks, the manifestations and the complications of diabetes itself. We attempted to address these issues in the first edition.

Encouraged by the response to the first edition, we have now embarked on this second edition. This edition does not simply represent an update of the previous volume. We have also been attentive to various criticisms and suggestions in an attempt to enhance the previous edition. Therefore, several new chapters have been added, a new coeditor, Marian Rewers, introduced and many new authors asked to contribute.

In the first edition, insufficient attention was given to research exploring the effect of early life influences (such as poor growth *in utero* and childhood velocities) in determining the risk of diabetes and its associated vascular complications. This issue is discussed in this volume.

The Epidemiology of Diabetes Mellitus, second edition Edited by Jean-Marie Ekoé, Marian Rewers, Rhys Williams and Paul Zimmet
© 2008 John Wiley & Sons, Ltd

The global pandemic of diabetes is already a worldwide public health catastrophe. Action is needed at various levels. A new section in this edition focuses on screening and prevention of diabetes. This second edition, which might as well be entitled as *New Trends in Diabetes Epidemiology and Prevention*, has been extensively reorganized, with seven major subdivisions.

1. Definitions, classification and risk factors for diabetes, including the epidemiology of the metabolic syndrome or cardiometabolic risk, the epidemiology of obesity and diabetes, nutrition and diabetes, physical activity and diabetes, as well as the genetic epidemiology of type 2 diabetes.
2. Type 2 diabetes around the world. Recent data worldwide (different continents and populations) have been incorporated in this section. A specific chapter deals with the epidemiology of type 2 diabetes in children and adolescents.
3. Type 1 diabetes around the world. Global epidemiology of type 1 diabetes is presented in this section, as well as ethnic differences and genetic epidemiological components of type 1 diabetes.
4. New evidence for screening and prevention of diabetes. This section encompasses chapters on new approaches to screening and the prevention of type 1 diabetes, as well as chapters on nonpharmacological and pharmacological approaches for prevention of type 2 diabetes.
5. Epidemiology of complications. The epidemiological aspects of both acute and long-term complications of diabetes are discussed in this section in seven chapters.
6. Implications. This section deals with the diabetes economic burden from a worldwide perspective. A new chapter on the daily fight against diabetes presents clinical guidelines worldwide designed to obtain the best glycemic control.
7. New challenges. In this final section, new challenges such as antipsychotic treatment, the human immunodeficiency virus (HIV) and coexisting problems of glucose tolerance abnormalities are discussed.

Three chapters have been replaced. The chapter on 'Epidemiology of Diabetes in Mexico' is now part of Chapter 12. The chapter on 'Diabetes Field Surveys: Theory and Practical Aspects' has been omitted, although it remains important for those willing to conduct field surveys. This information can easily be retrieved if needed (from G.K. Dowse's Chapter 24 (pp. 399–423) in the first edition of the book). The chapter on 'Malnutrition-Related Diabetes Mellitus: Myth or Reality' has also been omitted this time due to the lack of additional compelling new data since 2001. The 'enigma' has not yet been resolved.

We expect that this new edition will be of great interest for professionals engaged in diabetic medicine, be they epidemiologists, physicians, nurses, nutritionists, dietitians, psychologists, physiologists, social scientists or economists. Its multi-author approach and detailed sections should also be of interest to the research scientist, public health specialists and other health care providers.

1.2   INTRODUCTION TO THE FIRST EDITION

Twenty-three years ago Dr Kelly West published the first volume on the epidemiology of diabetes and its vascular complications [1]. He left his own unique memorial in a book that critically reviewed more than 2000 papers. This outstanding review gathered most of the contributions, clinical and population based, on the subject of diabetes epidemiology and highlighted the many gaps in our diabetes epidemiology knowledge at that time.

Much has happened in the last two decades. The present volume bridges the more than twenty years that have elapsed since Dr Kelly West's milestone monograph and we hope that it will provide a stimulating 'state-of-the-art' review of recent epidemiological studies spanning the globe.

The book presents and discusses the new diagnostic criteria and classification of diabetes. At the end of the 1970s confusion reigned both with regard to the classification of diabetes and to the appropriate diagnostic tests and their interpretation. Enormous variation in diagnostic cutoff values, in size of the glucose load and clear definition of types of diabetes prevailed. In 1979 and 1980 the National Diabetes Data Group (NDDG) in the United States [2] and the World Health Organization (WHO) Second Expert Committee on Diabetes [3] brought some order. Further revisions have resulted in new recent classification and diagnostic criteria that seem to be more consistent and less controversial [4, 5]. One of the major changes in the provisional WHO consultation report is the disappearance of the malnutrition-related diabetes mellitus (MRDM) as a major category [4]. While the protein-deficient pancreatic diabetes (PDPD) variant of MRDM has been dropped, the former fibrocalculous pancreatic diabetes (FCPD) variant is now part of the other types category which include all those types where etiology is more clear. A chapter discusses this issue. One major difference remains in gestational diabetes mellitus (GDM). The American Diabetes Association (ADA) has not changed its testing and criteria, whereas the WHO includes both impaired glucose tolerance (IGT) and new diabetes in pregnancy under the banner of GDM [4, 5]. Compared with what was reigning in the 1970s, this is 'order out of chaos'. However, there is still room for improvement.

The available diagnostic criteria and classification have been widely used since the early 1980s in numerous epidemiological studies, allowing comparisons between countries, regions and different populations worldwide. The results of these studies suggest that the prevalence of diabetes will increase dramatically in the next quarter of this century, both in developed and the developing countries. The WHO [6] suggests an increase worldwide of the prevalence of diabetes in adults of 35% and an increase in the number of people with diabetes of 122%. Developing countries will face an increase of 48% in the prevalence of diabetes and an increase of 170% in the number of people with diabetes, compared with an increase in the prevalence of diabetes of 27% in developed countries and an increase of 42% in the number of people with diabetes.

Although caution should be expressed regarding these figures due to the lack of suitable survey data, and extrapolations in some places and countries, the epidemic nature of diabetes in the world is supported by studies summarized in this book.

The likely burden of diabetes during the first years of the twenty-first century should not be overlooked: Figures of 135 million adults with diabetes in 1995 rising to probably 300 million in year 2025 are not far from reality and may even underestimate the magnitude of this major public health problem. Application of new diagnostic criteria will probably add another 2% in the prevalence of diabetes. The greater longevity of women likely explains the fact that there are more women than men with diabetes in many countries. The increasing concentration of diabetes in urban areas of developing countries is notorious and clearly emerges from the reported surveys.

There is now considerable evidence that type 2 diabetes is lifestyle related. Given the dramatic change of lifestyle in many developing nations, researchers have had great opportunities to study the genetic and environmental determinants of type 2 diabetes through both cross-sectional and longitudinal studies. The book presents an extensive overview of these studies and focuses on evidence for prevention of diabetes.

In the last 20 years, dramatic changes in the management of type 1 diabetes have positively modified the natural history of this disorder. The benefits of tight metabolic control have been demonstrated in numerous studies, and most conclusively in the Diabetes Control and Complications Trial (DCCT) for type 1 diabetes [7] and in the United Kingdom Prevention Diabetes Survey (UKPDS) for type 2 diabetes [8–11]. An upsurge of interest in diabetes epidemiology that started in the early 1980s was immensely reinforced. Although incidence and prevalence data have added only limited information to our further understanding of the etiology of diabetes, their importance in adding to our knowledge of the public health implications of this disease is considerable. Evidence for prevention is surely emerging and is thoroughly discussed in this volume.

Following the euphoria of the discovery of insulin in the 1920s appeared the recognition of most of the disorders due to diabetic complications. The natural progression of the disease to nephropathy and retinopathy led to renal failure and blindness. The consequences of cardiovascular disease and neuropathy resulted in early cardiovascular death, foot disease and amputations. Although it is now possible to reduce the incidence of complications, or, when they occur, retard their progression, their prevalence and incidence remain unacceptably high. The book addresses the magnitude of diabetic complications, time trends and geographical variations.

Proper care of diabetes in the 2000s implies identification of all patients with diabetes and early detection of complications which will enable care providers to take the steps needed to combat the disease. This may not be possible at all in the absence of epidemiological data. This book, therefore, will be a very useful tool for diabetes care providers, researchers and public health experts. It provides a global picture of the characteristics of the epidemic nature of diabetes and its complications. It is hoped that those of all disciplines involved in diabetes, regardless of their fields of expertise, will find both interest and practical help from its content.

References

1. West, K.M. (1978) Epidemiology of Diabetes and its Vascular Lesions, Elsevier, New York.

2. National Diabetes Data Group (1979) Classification and diagnosis of diabetes mellitus and other categories of glucose intolerance. *Diabetes*, **28**, 1039–57.

3. World Health Organization (1980) WHO Expert Committee on Diabetes Mellitus. 2nd report, Tech. Rep. Ser. 646, WHO, Geneva.

4. Alberti, K.G.M.M. and Zimmet, P. (1998) Definition, diagnosis and classification of diabetes mellitus and its complications. Part 1: diagnosis and classification of diabetes mellitus—provisional report of a WHO Consultation. *Diabetic Medicine*, **15**, 539–53.

5. The Expert Committee on the Diagnosis and Classification of Diabetes Mellitus (2000) Report of the Expert Committee on the Diagnosis and Classification of Diabetes Mellitus. *Diabetes Care*, **23** (Suppl 1), S4–19.

6. King, H., Aubert, R.E. and Herman, W.H. (1998) Global burden of diabetes, 1995–2005: prevalence, numerical estimates and projections. *Diabetes Care*, **21** (9), 1414–31.

7. The Diabetes Control and Complications Trial Research Group (1993) The effect of intensive treatment of diabetes on the development and progression of long-term complications in insulin-dependent diabetes mellitus. *New England Journal of Medicine*, **329**, 977–86.

8. UK Prospective Diabetes Study (UKPDS) Group (1998) Intensive blood-glucose control with sulphonylureas or insulin compared with conventional treatment and risk of complications in patients with type 2 diabetes: UKPDS 33. *Lancet*, **352**, 837–53.

9. UK Prospective Diabetes Study (UKPDS) Group (1998) Effect of intensive blood-glucose control with metformin on complications in overweight patients with type 2 diabetes: UKPDS 34. *Lancet*, **352**, 854–65.

10. UK Prospective Diabetes Study (UKPDS) Group (1998) Tight blood pressure control and risk of macrovascular and microvascular complications in type 2 diabetes: UKPDS 38. *British Medical Journal*, **317**, 703–13.

11. UK Prospective Diabetes Study (UKPDS) Group (1998) Efficacy of atenolol and captopril in reducing risk of macrovascular and microvascular complications in type 2 diabetes: UKPDS 39. *British Medical Journal*, **317**, 713–20.

2

The Clinical Syndrome and the Biochemical Definition

Jean-Marie Ekoé,[1] Paul Z. Zimmet[2] and Jean-Francois Yale[3]

[1]Endocrinologie, Métabolisme et Nutrition, Centre de Recherche du CHUM, Montreal, Canada
[2]International Diabetes Institute, Caulfield, Victoria, Australia
[3]McGill Nutrition and Food Science Centre, Department of Medicine, McGill University, Montreal, Quebec, Canada

2.1 DEFINITION OF THE DIABETIC STATE

Diabetes mellitus is a disease that was recognized in antiquity. Polyuric states resembling diabetes mellitus were described as early as 1550 BC in the ancient Egyptian papyrus discovered by George Ebers [1]. The term *diabetes*, which is from the Ionian Greek meaning 'to pass through,' was first used by Aretaeus of Cappadocia in the second century AD as a generic description of conditions causing increased urine output [2]. The association of polyuria with a sweet-tasting substance in the urine was noted in the fifth to sixth centuries AD by two Indian physicians, Susruta and Charuka [1, 2]. The urine of certain polyuric patients was described as tasting like honey, sticky to the touch and attracting ants. Two forms of diabetes could be distinguished in the Indians' descriptions: one affected older, fatter people and the other thin people who did not survive long; this strongly reminds us of the present clinical descriptions of type 2 and type 1 diabetes.

The term *diabetes mellitus*, an allusion to the honeyed taste of the urine, was first used in the late eighteenth century by John Rollo [3] to distinguish it from other polyuric states in which the urine was tasteless. The concept that diabetes was a systemic disease arising in the blood was elaborated a century before (in the seventeenth century) by Matthew Dobson, a physician in Liverpool (England) who published a series of experiments showing that the serum of a patient with diabetes, as well as the urine, contained a sweet-tasting substance, namely sugar [4].

The nineteenth century is the key century that has greatly contributed to the understanding of diabetes. Claude Bernard made numerous discoveries in the field of metabolism and diabetes. He described the storage of glucose in the liver as a glycogen and the acute hyperglycemia that followed experimental damage of the medulla oblongata known as 'piqûre' diabetes [5]. Oskar Minkowski and Josef Von Mering noted that total pancreatectomy produced diabetes in dogs [6]. The pancreatic islets were named after Paul Langerhans by Edouard Lafresse. Langerhans had suggested that pancreatic islets produced a glucose-lowering substance. This substance was named insulin by Jean de Meyer in 1909, almost a decade before insulin was discovered [7]. Although diabetes mellitus has been recognized for many centuries and major advances have been accomplished since the discovery of insulin in the understanding of diabetes and metabolism, there was no clear or widely accepted definition of the diabetic state until the early 1980s.

In 1980, the World Health Organization (WHO) Expert Committee on diabetes mellitus [8] defined the diabetic state as a state of chronic hyperglycemia which may result from many environmental and

The Epidemiology of Diabetes Mellitus, second edition Edited by Jean-Marie Ekoé, Marian Rewers, Rhys Williams and Paul Zimmet
© 2008 John Wiley & Sons, Ltd

genetic factors often acting jointly. Hyperglycemia is due to defects in insulin secretion, insulin action or both. This imbalance leads to disturbances of carbohydrate, fat and protein metabolism. The major effects of diabetes mellitus include long-term damage, dysfunction and failure of various organs. Diabetes mellitus may present with characteristic symptoms: thirst, polyuria, polydipsia, blurring of vision, weight loss and infections. In its most severe forms, ketoacidosis or a nonketotic hyperosmolar state may develop and lead to stupor, coma and, in absence of effective treatment, death. Most of the time, symptoms are not severe, or may be absent; consequently, hyperglycemia of sufficient degree to cause pathological and functional changes may be present for a long time before the diagnosis is made. The long-term complications of diabetes mellitus include progressive development of disease of the capillaries of the kidney and retina, damage to the peripheral nerves and excessive atherosclerosis. The clinical manifestations of these complications, therefore, include nephropathy that may lead to renal failure, retinopathy with potential blindness, neuropathy with risk of foot ulcers, amputation, Charcot joints and features of autonomic dysfunction, including sexual dysfunction. People with diabetes are at increased risk of cardiovascular, peripheral vascular and cerebrovascular disease. Diabetes mellitus is thus defined as a set of abnormalities characterized by a state of sustained hyperglycemia. It is a clinical description with a chemical definition. Pathogenic mechanisms and various explanations, to be found, lie behind the sustained hyperglycemia. Processes which destroy the beta-cells of the pancreas, with consequent insulin deficiency, and others that result in resistance to insulin action are part of a possible group of processes involved in the development of diabetes.

2.2 THE CLINICAL SYNDROME

The usual clinical symptoms of diabetes mellitus, polyuria and polydipsia, are the direct result of the high blood glucose concentration. Weight loss in spite of polyphagia, ketoacidosis, visual changes, skin infections, sepsis and pruritus belong to the same list of symptoms. With mild hyperglycemia, these cardinal symptoms are lacking. The description of a clear clinical syndrome bears a very low

incidence (1 per 10 000 per year) and prevalence [9]. It is not surprising that few studies have systematically determined the frequency of various symptoms and their relationship to factors such as age, sex and degree of glycemia. The frequency of most symptoms is quite different in previously undiscovered diabetes, as contrasted with people with diabetes who have been under treatment for months or years. Other factors, such as intensity of treatment, degree of acceptance of recommended therapy and age of onset, do affect the frequency of the different symptoms [9]. The description of a clear clinical syndrome which encompasses different and probably nonspecific symptoms seems to be a poor definition criterion [10]. Responses recorded from approximately 1700 diabetics in Bauer's study [10] pertaining to symptoms presented in the beginning of or during the disease showed no specificity for diabetes. Almost 52% of the patients had none of these 'diabetic symptoms.' No data were gathered in this study on the frequency of these symptoms in the general population or in people without diabetes. The Welborn *et al.* study [11] was a controlled study. The authors compared rates of symptoms in known subjects with diabetes and in those found to be either affected or nonaffected with diabetes in a survey. An increase of thirst was reported by 12% of the new 'screenees' with diabetes, 13% of known people with diabetes and 5% of people without diabetes. Polyuria was reported by 28% of new cases, 13% of known people with diabetes and 11% of people without diabetes. Visual deterioration was reported by 35% of newly diagnosed cases, 31% of known individuals with diabetes and 25% of people without the disease. A history of pruritus vulvae was reported by 29% of both groups of women with diabetes and 15% of nonaffected women.

In the Bedford survey [12], symptoms of diabetes were only slightly more common in those with 2 h blood glucose levels over $6.7 \, \text{mmol} \, l^{-1}$ (120 mg dl^{-1}) than in those with lower values. In several other studies, classical diabetes symptoms are lacking in more than 25% of newly diagnosed diabetics [9].

The clinical recognition of glycosuria as the sole marker of diabetes is also unreliable. Quite a few patients with high renal thresholds or mild hyperglycemia may be missed. Furthermore, the number of false positives is not minimized by this procedure in certain conditions. Therefore, the prevalence of diabetes will be underestimated when one restricts oneself to the classical syndrome. The use of blood glucose estimation (population screening) greatly raises the prevalence of diabetes when it is used instead of glycosuria determination. West, Keen and others have estimated that, between the classical historical phase of ascertainment and the clinical/glycosuric phase, diabetes rates increased at least 10-fold. They increased 10-fold again with the epidemiological blood glucose screening phase [9, 13].

2.3 THE BIOCHEMICAL DEFINITION

2.3.1 Hyperglycemia: the Common Factor

The epidemiological attempt to study the natural history and pathogenesis of diabetes as a whole can only rely on one common and stable factor, high blood glucose, despite the wide variation in clinical manifestations and various contributing factors. However, high blood glucose alone does not answer all the questions. Over the past 30 years, evidence has accumulated that numerous and etiologically different mechanisms (genetic, environmental or immunologic processes) may play an important role in the pathogenesis, the clinical course and the emergence of complications of the 'diabetic state' [9, 14]. Does correction of hyperglycemia prevent all of the various pathologic changes observed with diabetes? There is some evidence that people with diabetes who are not treated develop more complications than well-controlled patients [9, 15, 16]. Randomized controlled trials have proven that improving glucose control can reduce the microvascular complications in type 1 and type 2 diabetes [17, 18]. Currently, the evidence suggesting that macrovascular complications can also be reduced by improved glucose control is mostly epidemiological [18, 19]. However, there are few instances in which characteristic complications of diabetes have been described before hyperglycemia was observed. This indicates the vast heterogeneity of diabetes and illustrates the fact that it is not yet clear to what extent the long-term classical diabetic complications are the result of hyperglycemia, the

generally accepted and fundamental factor for diabetes, or related factors such as, for instance, insulin deficiency, plasma or tissue osmolality changes, glycated proteins and lipid abnormalities. Despite these questions, hyperglycemia remains the most important factor required for the diagnosis of diabetes.

2.4 SIGNIFICANCE OF BLOOD GLUCOSE IN A POPULATION

In different populations, the distribution of blood glucose may vary greatly. In one of the early studies of diabetes epidemiology performed in the United States and based on medical history, urine glucose tolerance in a defined community, Wilkerson and Krall reported a large variation in the distribution of blood glucose values within the eight screenee age-groups [17]. One pertinent fact was observed: higher levels of blood glucose were apparent with aging. In the 75–79 years age-group, 50% of subjects had high blood glucose. This has been confirmed in other health surveys [18]. Where does diabetes start? In most populations, the degrees of hyperglycemia used for diagnosis of diabetes are based upon the findings in large, normal population samples and validated by prospective observations on outcome [13]. However, there are still, to some extent, arbitrary lines across a continuous distribution of values in most populations (e.g. distribution of capillary blood glucose). Most unselected Caucasian populations display a unimodal distribution of glycemia: 80–85% of people have normal blood glucose; 2–4% are in the diabetes range. Between these two extremes remains a third category of people neither frankly diabetic nor nondiabetic. These people with impaired fasting glucose and/or glucose intolerance are at increased risk of future development of diabetes, and are also at increased risk of cardiovascular disease. Of concern is the high prevalence of these abnormalities in adolescents in some countries [22].

Epidemiological observations of Pacific Islanders [9, 19, 20], Arizona Pima Indians [21] and Tamil-speaking South African East Indians [22] and other non-Caucasian populations have brought to light new patterns of blood glucose distribution. They have shown that blood glucose values are bimodally distributed. In the Pima and Nauru population studies, a 100 g glucose load was used. The 2 h plasma glucose values were bimodally distributed. When the 2 h plasma glucose was related to the rate of microvascular disease, it became evident that, from about 11 mmol l^{-1} (180–200 mg dl^{-1}) of blood glucose, microvascular disease (retinopathy) increased significantly. This remains the basis for the definition of diabetes. However, it is also clear that the presence of impaired glucose tolerance increases the risk of macrovascular disease from 2 h plasma glucose levels of 7.8 mmol l^{-1}.

In conclusion, the study of the distribution of blood glucose in a population seems to be a prerequisite to any study of diabetes in that population. It has been a common observation that, in populations with a high prevalence rate of diabetes, blood glucose values are bimodally distributed in those populations with a cut-off point around 11.1 mmol l^{-1} (200 mg dl^{-1}).

It has also been assumed that, in a general population, low levels of circulating insulin were apparent when blood glucose was around 11.1 mmol l^{-1} (200 mg dl^{-1}) [9, 13, 19, 21]. Mild, long-standing hyperglycemia might be a marker of a silent ongoing process resulting in damage of key organs.

References

1. McFarlane, I.A., Bliss, M., Jackson, J.G.L. and Williams, G. (1997) The history of diabetes mellitus, in Textbook of Diabetes, 2nd edn (eds J. Pickup and G. Williams), Blackwell Science, London, pp. 1.1–1.21.
2. Papaspyros, N.S. (1964) The History of Diabetes Mellitus, 2nd edn, Thieme Medical and Scientific Publishers, Stuttgart.
3. Rollo, J. (1797) An Account of Two Cases of Diabetes Mellitus with Remarks as they Arose During the Progress of the Cure, C. Dilly, London.
4. Dobson, M. (1776) Experiments and observations on the urine in diabetes. Medical Observations and Inquiries, 5, 298–316.
5. Bernard, C. (1855) Leçons de Physiologie, Baillière, Paris, pp. 289, 296–313.
6. Von Mering, J. and Minkowski, O. (1890) Diabetes mellitus nach Pankreasertirpation. Archives of the Experts in Pathology and Pharmacology, 26, 371–87.
7. De Meyer, J. (1940) Sur la signification physiologique de la sécrétion interne du pancréas. Zentralblatt für Physiologie, 18, S826.
8. WHO Study Group on Diabetes Mellitus (1985) Diabetes mellitus: report of a WHO study group, Tech. Rep. Ser. 727, World Health Organization, Geneva.
9. West, K.M. (1978) Epidemiology of Diabetes and its Vascular Lesions, Elsevier Science, New York.
10. Bauer, M.L. (1967) Characteristics of Persons with Diabetes, Vital and Health Statistics, Series 10, No. 40, US National Center for Health Statistics.
11. Welborn, T.A., Curnow, D.H., Wearne, J.T. et al. (1966) Diabetes detected by blood sugar measurement after glucose load: report from the Busselton survey. The Medical Journal of Australia, 2, 778–83.
12. Keen, H. (1964) The Bedford survey: a critique of methods and findings. Proceedings of the Royal Society of Medicine, 57, 196–202.
13. Keen, H. (1983) Criteria and classification of diabetes mellitus, in Diabetes in Epidemiological Perspective (eds J.I. Mann, K. Pyörälä and A. Teuscher), Churchill Livingstone, Edinburgh, pp. 167–82.
14. Fajans, S.S., Cloutier, M.C. and Crowther, R.L. (1978) Clinical and etiologic heterogeneity of idiopathic diabetes. Diabetes, 28, 1112–25.
15. Pirart, J. (1978) Diabetes mellitus and its degenerative complications: a prospective study of 4400 patients observed between 1947 and 1973. Diabetes Care, 1, 168–88.
16. Skyler, J.S. (1979) Complications of diabetes mellitus relationship to metabolic dysfunction. Diabetes Care, 2, 499–509.
17. The Diabetes Control and Complications Trial Research Group (1993) The effect of intensive treatment of diabetes on the development and progression of long-term complications in insulin-dependent diabetes mellitus. New England Journal of Medicine, 329, 977–86.
18. UK Prospective Diabetes Study (UKPDS) Group (1998) Intensive blood-glucose control with sulphonylureas or insulin compared with conventional treatment and risk of complications in patients with type 2 diabetes (UKPDS33). Lancet, 352, 837–53.
19. The Diabetes Control and Complications Trial/ Epidemiology of Diabetes Interventions and Complications (DCCT/EDIC) Study Research Group

(2005) Intensive diabetes treatment and cardio-vascular disease in patients with type 1 diabetes. *New England Journal of Medicine*, **353**, 2643–53.

20. Zimmet, P. and Taft, P. (1978) The high prevalence of diabetes mellitus in Nauru, a central Pacific island. *Advances in Metabolic Disorders*, **9**, 225–40.

21. Bennett, P.H., Burch, T.A. and Miller, M. (1971) Diabetes in American (Pima) Indians. *Lancet*, **ii**, 125–8.

22. Duncan, G.E. (2006) Prevalence of diabetes and impaired fasting glucose levels among US adolescents. National Health and Nutrition Examination Survey 1999–2002. *Archives of Pediatrics & Adolescent Medicine*, **160**, 523–8.

3

Diagnosis and Classification

Jean-Marie. Ekoé[1] and Paul Z. Zimmet[2]

[1]Endocrinologie, Métabolisme et Nutrition, Centre de Recherche du CHUM, Montreal, Canada

[2]International Diabetes Institute, Caulfield, Victoria, Australia

3.1 DIAGNOSIS AND DIAGNOSTIC CRITERIA

Diabetes mellitus may present with clear and classical symptoms (thirst, polyuria or ketoacidosis) or may be accompanied by specific complications. The lack of sensitivity and specificity of some of these 'diabetic symptoms' has already been discussed (see Chapter 2).However, when the symptoms and/or specific complications are present, the diagnosis of diabetes is confirmed by a single, unequivocally elevated blood glucose measurement, as shown in **Figure 3.1** [1]. Severe hyperglycemia found under conditions of acute infective, traumatic or other stress may be transitory and should not in itself be regarded as diagnostic of diabetes. If a diagnosis of diabetes is made, then one must feel confident that the diagnosis is fully established, since the consequences for the individual are considerable and life long [2]. For asymptomatic persons, at least one additional plasma/blood glucose test result with a value in the diabetic range is essential, either fasting, from a random (casual) sample or from the oral glucose tolerance test (OGTT). Levels of blood glucose below which a diagnosis of diabetes is virtually excluded also have been defined (**Figure 3.1**). If different samples fail to confirm the diagnosis of diabetes mellitus, then the person should be reassessed and retested until the diagnostic situation becomes clear. Additional factors, such as family history, age, ethnicity, adiposity and concomitant disorders, should be considered before deciding on a diagnostic or therapeutic course of action [2]. A single abnormal blood glucose value should never be used as the sole basis of diagnosis of diabetes in an asymptomatic subject. An alternative to the single blood-glucose estimation or OGTT has long been sought for to simplify the diagnosis of diabetes. Glycated hemoglobin reflecting average glycemia over a period of weeks was thought to provide such a test. In certain cases, it gives equal or almost equal sensitivity and specificity to glucose measurement. However, lack of standardization and its unavailability in many parts of the world make it difficult to recommend as a good alternative at this time [2, 3].

In a collaborative study involving nine British towns over 2 years of 254 newly diagnosed cases of diabetes aged 18–50 years, 81% were diagnosed on one single random/casual blood glucose measurement of 11.1 mmol l^{-1} (200 mg dl^{-1}) or more [4]. Furthermore, a diagnosis of diabetes was established from casual blood glucose estimation without any glucose tolerance test in 800 patients (90%) attending the Diabetic Clinic at King's College Hospital in London [5].

When symptoms are lacking and blood glucose levels are less markedly elevated (e.g. glucose concentration in a casual or random blood sample between 4.4 and 10.0 mmol l^{-1} for venous whole blood), measurements made after fasting or after a glucose load may be necessary to confirm or refute the diagnosis of diabetes. An entire investigation is needed if symptoms are questionable. In the case of a medical, obstetrical or family history of diabetes, a single elevated blood glucose measurement may or may not be decisive. An OGTT is indicated

The Epidemiology of Diabetes Mellitus, second edition   Edited by Jean-Marie Ekoé, Marian Rewers, Rhys Williams and Paul Zimmet

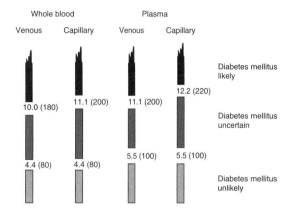

Figure 3.1 Unstandardized (casual, random) blood glucose values in the diagnosis of diabetes in mmol l^{-1} (mg dl^{-1}). (Reproduced from the 1985 WHO Study Group Report [1].)

in this situation (**Table 3.1**). **Table 3.2** shows the diagnostic values of OGTT for diabetes mellitus and other categories of glucose-tolerance abnormalities.

Collecting and interpreting epidemiologic data implies a complete understanding of diagnostic methods and the criteria applied. Therefore, it is appropriate to review briefly the indications of one

Table 3.1 Indications for oral glucose tolerance test (OGTT).

1. When a 'random' blood glucose is equivocal, e.g:
   – fasting blood glucose^a:
       $\geq$6.1–7.0 mmol l^{-1} < (IFG)
   – postprandial blood glucose^a:
       $\geq$7.8–11.0 mmol l^{-1} <

2. As part of special clinical investigation, e.g:
   – fasting glycosuria in pregnancy
   – data collection in certain endocrine or other diseases

3. For experimental and epidemiological purposes

4. To exclude diabetes mellitus or impaired glucose tolerance

IFG, impaired fasting glycemia.
^{a}Venous plasma values.

of the most widely used and misused methods of diagnosis, namely the OGTT.

3.2 THE DEMONSTRATION OF AN ABNORMAL BLOOD GLUCOSE LEVEL USING AN ORAL GLUCOSE TOLERANCE TEST

No marker other than a high blood glucose level has been discovered to identify the diabetic state. The diagnosis depends heavily on the demonstration of abnormal blood glucose levels. Symptoms and signs of diabetes and urine glucose tests are nonspecific tests for diabetes, although they should be taken into account when present.

Before performing the OGTT, it has been assumed that a random (or casual) blood glucose levels should be obtained (**Figure 3.1**). Plasma venous glucose levels greater than 11.1 mmol l^{-1} (200 mg dl^{-1}) are usually diagnostic irrespective of time of day or status of fasting, provided the elevated blood glucose values are confirmed.

3.3 THE ORAL GLUCOSE TOLERANCE TEST

Conn and Fajans believed that the diagnosis of diabetes in a completely asymptomatic patient could be made only on the basis of a carefully performed glucose tolerance test [6, 7]. Ten years earlier, Soskin believed that the OGTT was 'practically worthless as it was used and interpreted' [8]. These conflicting statements illustrate the fact that, as a clinical diagnostic tool, the OGTT has been grossly overemphasized and misused. It is now apparent that the OGTT is useful in clearly defined situations, as summarized in **Table 3.1**. For instance, the OGTT has been of prime importance in many epidemiological surveys of diabetes and is still one of the best instruments in such studies.

However, from a clinical viewpoint, the OGTT may be performed in specific circumstances. An equivocal random or casual blood glucose level (the diabetes mellitus uncertain zone as defined by the 1985 World Health Organization (WHO) Study Group on Diabetes Mellitus; **Figure 3.1**) deserves an OGTT. The establishment of a diagnosis is highly necessary in this situation. The OGTT might also be included as part of a special clinical investigation,

Table 3.2 Values for diagnosis of diabetes mellitus and other categories of hyperglycemia.

| | Glucose concentration mmol l^{-1} (mg dl^{-1}) | | | |
| | Whole blood | | Plasma | |
	Venous	Capillary	Venous	Capillary
Diabetes mellitus (DM):				
Fasting	$\geq$6.1 ($\geq$110)	$\geq$6.1 ($\geq$110)	$\geq$7.0 ($\geq$126)	$\geq$7.0 ($\geq$126)
or				
2 h post-glucose load	$\geq$10.0 ($\geq$180)	$\geq$11.1 ($\geq$200)	$\geq$11.1 ($\geq$200)	$\geq$12.2 ($\geq$220)
or both				
Impaired glucose tolerance (IGT):				
Fasting concentration (if measured) and	<6.1 (<110)	<6.1 (<110)	<7.0 (<126)	<7.0 (<126)
2 h post-glucose load	$\geq$6.7 ($\geq$120) and <10.0 (<180)	$\geq$7.8 ($\geq$140) and <11.1 (<200)	$\geq$7.8 ($\geq$140) and <11.1 (<200)	$\geq$8.9 ($\geq$160) and <12.2 (<220)
Impaired fasting glycemia (IFG):				
Fasting	$\geq$5.6 ($\geq$100) and <6.1 (110)	$\geq$5.6 ($\geq$100) and <6.1 (100)	$\geq$6.1 ($\geq$110) and <7.0 (126)	$\geq$6.1 ($\geq$110) and <7.0 (126)
2 h (if measured)	<6.7 (<120)	<7.8 (<140)	<7.8 (<140)	<8.9 (<160)

For epidemiological or population screening purposes, the fasting of 2 h value after 75 g oral glucose may be used alone. Glucose concentrations should not be determined on serum unless red cells are immediately removed, otherwise glycolysis will result in an unpredictable underestimation of the true concentrations. Glucose preservatives do not totally prevent glycolysis. If whole-blood glucose is used, the sample should be kept at 0–4°C or centrifuged immediately, or assayed immediately.

or needed for medicolegal reasons. If an OGTT is performed, then it is sufficient to measure the blood glucose values while fasting and at 2 h after a 75 g oral glucose load (Appendixes 1 and 2) [2]. For children the oral glucose load is related to body weight: 1.75 g kg^{-1}.

Diabetes in children usually presents with severe symptoms, very high blood glucose levels, marked glycosuria and ketonuria. In most children the diagnosis is confirmed without delay by blood glucose measurements and treatment (insulin injections) is initiated immediately. A small proportion of children and adolescents, however, present with less severe symptoms and may require a fasting blood glucose (FBG) and/or an OGTT for diagnosis. Diagnostic interpretations of the fasting and 2 h postload concentrations in nonpregnant subjects are shown in **Table 3.2**. The diagnostic criteria in children are the same as for adults, but, in practice,

an OGTT is rarely required to make a diagnosis of type 1 diabetes.

3.4 NEW CRITERIA IN DIAGNOSTIC VALUE FOR FASTING PLASMA BLOOD GLUCOSE CONCENTRATIONS

The main change in the diagnostic criteria for diabetes mellitus proposed by both the American Diabetes Association (ADA) and the WHO from their previous identical recommendations is the lowering of the diagnostic value of the fasting plasma glucose (FPG) concentration to 7.0 mmol l^{-1} (120 mg dl^{-1}) from the former level of 7.8 mmol l^{-1} (140 mg dl^{-1}) and above. For whole blood, the proposed new level is 6.1 mmol l^{-1} (110 mg dl^{-1}) and above from the former 6.7 mmol l^{-1} (120 mg dl^{-1}).

The recommended criteria in **Table 3.2** allow a diagnosis of diabetes mellitus on the basis of an elevation of the 2-hour blood glucose (2-h BG) (alone or with the fasting value in the 'true' overnight fasting state) provided that there is confirmation. When the FBG meets the diagnostic criteria for diabetes mellitus, it is unusual for the 2-h BG to fail to do so [9]. However, the converse is not true. Several investigators have found that a large number of subjects meeting the 2-h BG criterion had a normal FBG [10]. The new fasting criterion is chosen to represent a value which, in most persons, is of approximately equal diagnostic significance to that of the 2 h postload concentration, which remains the same.

This equivalence has been established from several population-based studies [4, 11–13] and it also represents an optimal cutoff point to separate the components of bimodal frequency distributions of FPG concentrations seen in several populations. Furthermore, several studies have shown increased risk of microvascular disease in persons with FPG concentrations of 7.0 mmol l^{-1} (126 mg dl^{-1}) and over [12] and of macrovascular disease in persons with such fasting concentrations, even in those with 2 h values of 7.8 mmol l^{-1} (140 mg dl^{-1}) [14].

Both FBG and 2 h postload show relative advantages and are complementary when true fasting can be assured.

3.5   EPIDEMIOLOGICAL STUDIES

For the purpose of diabetes epidemiology studies, a single 2 h load glucose value after a 75 g oral glucose load after an overnight fast is often adequate, since true fasting cannot be assured in certain conditions; and because of the strong correlation between fasting and 2 h values, epidemiological studies or diagnostic screening have in the past been restricted to the 2 h values only (**Table 3.2**).

OGTT may be difficult to perform for various reasons (e.g. logistic, economic). In that case, FPG alone can be used for epidemiological purposes. However, it should be known that some of the individuals identified by fasting values may be different from those identified by the 2 h values and that overall prevalence may be somewhat different [15], although not always [11, 16]. Both the 2 h and fasting values should be used if possible.

3.6   CLASSIFICATION OF THE DIABETES MELLITUS SYNDROME AND OTHER CATEGORIES OF GLUCOSE INTOLERANCE

3.6.1   Previous Classifications

In 1965, a WHO Expert Committee on Diabetes Mellitus published the first WHO report containing a classification of patients according to age of recognized onset [17]. Since that time, several pathogenic mechanisms have been described and long-term studies have shown different courses and outcomes of different types of diabetes. Many of the reclassifications proposed attempted to take into account various aspects of diabetes which, in fact, sometimes reflected the specific interests of particular investigators. A great deal of confusion arose from this and it became quite difficult to construct a simple classification that met all interests. In order to overcome these setbacks and establish a new classification that included all possible forms of diabetes mellitus and glucose intolerance, a revised classification of diabetes mellitus has been formulated by the National Diabetes Data Group (NDDG) [18]. This was reviewed, amended and adopted in the second report of the WHO Expert Committee in 1980 [19] and in a modified from in 1985. The 1980 and 1985 [1] classifications of diabetes mellitus and allied categories of glucose intolerance included clinical classes and two statistical risk classes [1, 19]. The 1980 Expert Committee proposed two major classes of diabetes mellitus and named them insulin-dependent diabetes mellitus (IDDM), or type 1, and noninsulin-dependent diabetes mellitus (NIDDM), or type 2 [19]. In the 1985 Study Group report the terms type 1 and type 2 were omitted, but the classes IDDM and NIDDM were retained and a new class of malnutrition-related diabetes mellitus (MRDM) was introduced [1]. The 1985 WHO classification was essentially based on clinical descriptions (e.g. insulin-dependent, noninsulin-dependent, gestational) and did not include terms that might indicate etiological mechanisms (such as type 1 or type 2). The question of whether certain clinical forms of diabetes (such as the so-called tropical diabetes) were given adequate priority to correct hierarchic order that was raised many years before probably led to the introduction of MRDM, although more precise epidemiological data and a better assessment were needed and called for.

Both the 1980 and 1985 reports included other types of diabetes and impaired glucose tolerance (IGT), as well as gestational diabetes mellitus (GDM). The 1985 classification was widely accepted, is used internationally, and represents a compromise between clinical and etiological classifications. Furthermore, it allows classification of individual subjects and patients in a clinically useful manner even when the specific cause of etiology is unknown. The newly proposed WHO and ADA classifications or staging of diabetes still include clinical descriptive criteria, but a complementary classification according to etiology is not recommended by both organizations [1, 3].

3.6.2 New Classifications

The ADA classification and the proposed WHO classification encompass both *clinical stages, etiological types* of diabetes mellitus and *other categories* of hyperglycemia (**Table 3.3**). Diabetes may progress through several clinical stages during its natural history regardless of its etiology. The clinical staging reflects this specific aspect. Moreover, individual subjects may move from stage to stage in either direction (**Figure 3.2**). Even in the absence of information concerning the underlying etiology, persons with diabetes or those who are developing the disease can be categorized by stage according to clinical characteristics. The classification by etiological type results from improved understanding of the cases of diabetes mellitus.

The new classification takes into account the various degrees of hyperglycemia in individual subjects with any of the disease processes which may lead to diabetes. These are glycemic stages ranging *normoglycemia* (normal glucose tolerance) to *hyperglycemia* (established diabetes mellitus where insulin is requested for survival). All individuals with the disease can be categorized according to clinical stage and this is achievable in all circumstances [2]. The stage of glycemia may change over time depending on the extent of the underlying disease processes (**Figure 3.2**). As shown in **Figure 3.2**, a disease process may be present but may not have progressed far enough to cause hyperglycemia. The etiological classification reflects the fact that the defect or process which may lead to a manifest disease, diabetes, may be

identifiable at any stage in the development of diabetes even at the stage of normoglycemia. For instance, the presence of islet cell antibodies in a normoglycemic individual makes it likely that individual has the type 1 autoimmune process. For type 2 diabetes, there are not many good highly specific indicators. Future research will probably reveal some of them. The same disease process can cause various degrees of 'dysglycemia,' such as impaired fasting glycemia (IFG) and/or IGT without fulfilling the criteria for the diagnosis of diabetes mellitus [2]. Weight reduction, exercise and/or oral agents treatment can result in adequate glycemic control in some persons with diabetes. These persons, therefore, do not require insulin. Other persons require insulin for adequate glycemic control but can survive without it. By definition these persons have some residual insulin secretion. Patients with extensive β-cell destruction (no residual insulin secretion) do require insulin for survival. The severity of the metabolic abnormality can *regress* (e.g. with weight reduction), *progress* (e.g. with weight gain) or *stay the same*.

3.7 CHANGES IN TERMINOLOGY

Both ADA and the proposed WHO classification have eliminated the terms *insulin-dependent diabetes mellitus* and *noninsulin-dependent diabetes mellitus* and their acronyms 'IDDM' and 'NIDDM' on the basis that these terms have been confusing and frequently resulted in misclassification, patients being classified on treatment rather than on pathogenesis (**Table 3.3**). The terms *type 1* and *type 2* are retained (using Arabic rather than Roman numerals). People with any form of diabetes may require insulin treatment at some stage of their disease.

The etiological type named type 1 encompasses the majority of cases which are primarily due to *pancreatic islet β-cell destruction* and are prone to ketoacidosis. Type 1 includes those cases attributable to an autoimmune process, as well as those with β-cell destruction and who are prone to ketoacidosis for which neither an etiology nor a pathogenesis is known (idiopathic). Those forms of β-cell destruction or failure to which specific causes can be assigned are not included in this type of diabetes (e.g. cystic fibrosis, mitochondrial defects).

Table 3.3 Etiologic and classification of diabetes mellitus[a].

I.   Type 1 diabetes[b] (β-cell destruction, usually leading to absolute insulin deficiency)
    A. Immune-mediated
    B. Idiopathic

II.   Type 2 diabetes[b] (may range from predominantly insulin resistance with relative insulin deficiency to a predominantly secretory defect with insulin resistance)

III. Other specific types
    A. Genetic defects of β-cell function
        1. Chromosome 20, HNF-4α (MODY1)
        2. Chromosome 7, glucokinase (MODY2)
        3. Chromosome 12, HNF-1α (MODY3)
        4. Chromosome 13, IPF-1 (MODY4)
        5. Mitochondrial DNA 3243 mutation
        6. Others
    B. Genetic defects in insulin action
        1. Type A insulin resistance
        2. Leprechaunism
        3. Rabson–Mendenhall syndrome
        4. Lipoatrophic diabetes
        5. Others
    C. Diseases of the exocrine pancreas
        1. Fibrocalculous pancreatopathy
        2. Pancreatitis
        3. Trauma/pancreatectomy
        4. Neoplasia
        5. Cystic fibrosis
        6. Hemochromatosis
        7. Others
    D. Endocrinopathies
        1. Cushing's syndrome
        2. Acromegaly
        3. Pheochromocytoma
        4. Glucagonoma
        5. Hyperthyroidism
        6. Somatostatinoma
        7. Aldosteronoma
        8. Others
    E. Drug- or chemical-induced
        1. Nicotinic acid
        2. Glucocorticoids
        3. Thyroid hormone
        4. α-Adrenergic agonists
        5. β-Adrenergic agonists
        6. Thiazides
        7. Dilantin
        8. Pentamidine
        9. Vacor
       10. α-Interferon therapy
       11. Diazoxide
       12. Others

Table 3.3 (*continued*)

F.	Infections
	1. Congenital rubella
	2. Cytomegalovirus
	3. Others
G.	Uncommon forms of immune-mediated diabetes
	1. Insulin autoimmune syndrome (antibodies to insulin)
	2. Anti-insulin receptor antibodies
	3. 'Stiff-man' syndrome
	4. Others
H.	Other genetic syndromes sometimes associated with diabetes
	1. Down's syndrome
	2. Klinefelter's syndrome
	3. Turner's syndrome
	4. Wolfram's syndrome
	5. Friedreich's ataxia
	6. Huntington's chorea
	7. Laurence–Moon–Biedl syndrome
	8. Myotonic dystrophy
	9. Porphyria
	10. Prader–Willi syndrome
	11. Others
IV.	Gestational diabetes mellitus (GDM)

[a]HNF, hepatocyte nuclear factor; MODY, maturity-onset diabetes of the young; IPF, insulin promoter factor.
[b]Patients with any form of diabetes may require insulin treatment at some stage of their disease. Such use of insulin does not, of itself, classify the patient.

The form named type 2 includes the common major form of diabetes which results from defect(s) in insulin secretion, almost always with a major contribution form insulin resistance. The class MRDM has been deleted in the proposed WHO classification. The former subtype of MRDM, namely protein-deficient pancreatic diabetes (PDPD) or protein-deficient diabetes mellitus (PDDM), needs more studies for a better definition. The other former subtype of MRDM, fibrocalculous pancreatic diabetes (FCPD), is now classified as a disease of the exocrine pancreas, fibrocalculous pancreatopathy, which may lead to diabetes. Chapter 1824Cc18 on MRDM discussed this issue extensively in the first edition of this book [20]. No additional and strong data have been published in the last 5 years to really establish MRDM as a precisely coined diabetes entity.

The class IGT is reclassified as a stage of impaired glucose regulation (**Table 3.4**), since it can be observed in any hyperglycemic disorder and is itself not diabetes.

Gestational diabetes is retained, but now encompasses the groups formerly classified as gestational impaired glucose tolerance (GIGT) and GDM according to the new proposed WHO criteria [2].

3.8 CLINICAL CLASSIFICATION OF DIABETES MELLITUS AND OTHER CATEGORIES OF GLUCOSE TOLERANCE

Table 3.3 summarizes the etiological classification of diabetes mellitus. Etiological and clinical stages are presented in **Figure 3.2**.

The concepts for new staging/etiological classification were proposed by Kuzuya and Matsuda [21]. Their proposals sought to separate clearly the criteria related to etiology and those related to degree of deficiency of insulin or insulin action and to define each patient on the basis of these two criteria.

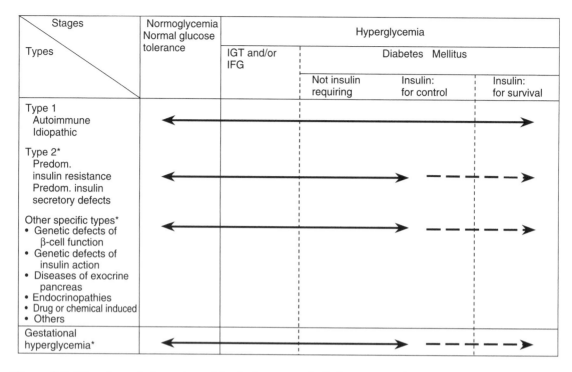

Figure 3.2 Disorders of glycemia: etiological types and clinical stages. *In rare instances, patients in these categories (e.g. Vacor toxicity, type 1 presenting in pregnancy) may require insulin for survival.

Table 3.4 Glucose levels for diagnosis of glucose tolerance abnormalities.

Category	FPG^a		PG^a (mmol l^{-1}) [mg dl^{-1}]	
	(mmol l^{-1})	(mg dl^{-1})	After 1 h	After 2 h
Impaired fasting glycemia (IFG)	5.6–6.9	10–124	N/A	N/A
Impaired glucose tolerance (IGT)	<7.0	<126	N/A	≥7.8 [≥140]
Diabetes mellitus (DM)	≥7.0	≥126	N/A	≥11.1 [≥200]
Gestational diabetes^b (GM)	≥5.3	≥95.4	≥10.6 [≥191]	≥8.9 [≥160]

^{a}FPG, fasting plasma glucose; PG, plasma glucose (75 g glucose load); N/A, not applicable.
^{b}A diagnosis of gestational diabetes mellitus requires two abnormal values among the three measurements according to the American Diabetes Association and the Canadian Diabetes Association.

The newly suggested WHO classification and the new ADA classification bring in both clinical stages of hyperglycemia as well as etiological types (**Figure 3.2** and **Table 3.3**). The classification by etiological type results from new knowledge to the causes of hyperglycemia including diabetes. The actual staging proposed reflects that any etiological type of diabetes can pass or progress through several clinical phases (both asymptomatic and symptomatic) during its natural history. Moreover, individuals may move (in either direction), from stage to stage (**Figure 3.2**).

3.9   THE NEWLY PROPOSED STAGING CLASSIFICATION

The new classification proposes that hyperglycemia, regardless of the underlying cause can be subcategorized as follows.

3.9.1 Diabetes Mellitus

Diabetes mellitus, regardless of underlying cause, is subdivided into:

insulin requiring for survival: (corresponding to the former clinical class of 'IDDM') C-peptide deficient, for example;

insulin requiring for control: that is, for metabolic control, rather than for survival. For example, some endogenous insulin secretion but insufficient to achieve normoglycemia without added exogenous insulin and not insulin requiring; that is, those who may be treated and controlled satisfactorily by nonpharmacological methods or drugs other than insulin.

These two categories, correspond to the former 'NIDDM.'

3.9.2 Impaired Glucose Regulation (Prediabetes)

3.9.2.1 Impaired Glucose Tolerance and Impaired Fasting Glycemia (Nondiabetic Fasting Hyperglycemia)

IGT was considered a class in the previous WHO classification but is now categorized as a stage in the natural history of disordered carbohydrate metabolism. A stage called *impaired fasting hyperglycemia*, or IFG or *nondiabetic fasting hyperglycemia*, is now recognized, as these people also appear to be at greater risk for progression to diabetes and macrovascular disease, although prospective data are sparse and early data suggest a lower risk of progression than IGT [22]. IFG refers to fasting glucose concentrations which are lower than those required to diagnose diabetes mellitus but higher than the 'normal' reference range.

Patients with IFG and/or IGT are now referred to as having 'prediabetes,' indicating the relatively high risk for development of diabetes in these patients.

IGT and IFG are not clinical entities in their own right (mostly in the absence of pregnancy), but rather are risk categories for future diabetes and/or cardiovascular disease [23, 24]. IGT and IFG represent impaired glucose regulation, which refers to a metabolic intermediate between normal glucose homeostasis and diabetes (prediabetes).

Individuals who meet criteria for IGT or IFG may be euglycemic in their daily lives, as shown by normal or near-normal glycated hemoglobin levels [2]. IGT is often associated with the metabolic syndrome (insulin resistance syndrome) [25]. An individual with an FPG concentration of 6.1 mmol l^{-1} (110 mg dl^{-1}) or greater (whole blood 5.6 mmol l^{-1}; 100 mg dl^{-1}) but less than 7.0 mmol l^{-1} (126 mg dl^{-1}) (whole blood 6.1 mmol l^{-1}; 110 mg dl^{-1}) is considered to have *IFG*. If an OGTT is performed, then some individuals with IFG will have IGT. Some may have diabetes, but this cannot be determined without an OGTT. If resources allow, then it is recommended that those with IFG have an OGTT to exclude diabetes [2].

3.9.3 Normoglycemia

A fasting venous plasma glucose concentration of less than 6.1 mmol l^{-1} (110 mg dl^{-1}) has been chosen as 'normal' (**Table 3.2**). These values are observed in people with normal glucose tolerance and values above this are associated with progressively greater risks of developing micro- and macro-vascular complications [13, 14, 24, 25].

The etiological processes which often lead to diabetes mellitus begin, and may be recognizable, in some subjects who have normal glucose tolerance. Recognition of the pathological process at an early stage may be useful if progression to more advanced stages can be prevented. The proposed classification includes a stage of normoglycemia in which persons who have evidence of the pathological processes that may lead to diabetes mellitus or in whom a reversal of the hyperglycemia has occurred are classified (**Figure 3.2**, **Table 3.3**).

3.10 THE NEWLY PROPOSED ETIOLOGICAL TYPES

The etiological types listed represent processes, or disorders, which may result in diabetes mellitus.

3.10.1 Type 1

Type 1 indicates the processes of β-cell destruction that may ultimately lead to diabetes in which 'insulin is required for survival' in order to prevent the development of ketoacidosis, coma and death. While the type 1 process is characterized by the presence of autoantibodies to glutamic acid decarboxylase (GAD, islet cells, insulin or the protein tyrosine phosphatase-like protein (ICA512), which identify the autoimmune process associated with β-cell destruction, in some cases there is no evidence of antibodies present and these are classified as 'type 1 idiopathic.'

3.10.2 Type 2

Type 2 is the commonest form of diabetes and is characterized by disorders of insulin resistance and insulin secretion, either of which may be a predominant feature. Both are usually present at the time that the diabetes is clinically manifest. The specific reasons for the development of these are not yet known. Genetic components are highly suspected to be involved.

3.10.3 Other Specific Types

The other specific types (**Table 3.3**) are less common, but are those in which the underlying defect or disease process can be identified in a relatively specific manner, particularly those where a monogenic defect has been identified, in maturity-onset diabetes of the young (MODY) for example.

3.10.3.1 Type 1 Diabetes (β-cell Destruction, Usually Leading to Absolute Insulin Deficiency)
This category is composed of the following:

(a) **Immune-mediated diabetes mellitus:** This form of diabetes, previously encompassed by the terms insulin-dependent diabetes, type 1 diabetes, or juvenile-onset diabetes, results from a cellular-mediated autoimmune destruction of the β cells of the pancreas. The rate of destruction is quite variable. It can be rapid in children, but a slowly progressive form, previously known as latent autoimmune diabetes in adults (LADA), is well described in adults [26, 27].

Markers of immune destruction, including islet cell antibodies, and/or insulin autoantibodies, autoantibodies to GAD_{65} and ICA512, are present in 85–90% of individuals when fasting hyperglycemia is initially detected, and often many years before [28]. The peak incidence of this form of type 1 diabetes occurs in childhood and adolescence, but the onset may occur at any age ranging from childhood to the ninth decade of life [29]. Patients are rarely obese when they present with this type of diabetes. However, the presence of obesity is not incompatible with the diagnosis. Other autoimmune disorders such as Graves' disease, Hashimoto's thyroiditis and Addison's disease may be associated with type 1 diabetes mellitus [30].

(b) **Idiopathic:** There are some forms of type 1 diabetes which have no known etiologies. Some of these patients have permanent insulinopenia and are prone to ketoacidosis, but have no evidence of autoimmunity [31]. This form is more common among individuals of African and Asian origin [32]. In another form found in Africans, an absolute requirement for insulin replacement therapy in affected patients may fluctuate with time, and come and go, and patients periodically develop ketoacidosis [32].

3.10.3.2 Type 2 Diabetes (Ranging from Predominantly Insulin Resistance with Relative Insulin Deficiency to Predominantly an Insulin Secretory Defect with/without Insulin Resistance)
This form of diabetes mellitus, previously referred to as *NIDDM* or *adult-onset diabetes*, is a term used for individuals who have relative (rather than absolute) insulin deficiency. People with type 2 diabetes frequently are resistant to the action of insulin [33, 34]. At least initially, and often throughout their lifetime, these individuals do not need insulin treatment to survive. Type 2 diabetes is frequently undiagnosed for many years because the hyperglycemia is often not severe enough to provoke noticeable symptoms of diabetes. Nevertheless, such patients are at increased risk of developing macrovascular and microvascular complications. There are probably many different causes of this form of diabetes, and it is likely that the number of patients in this category will decrease in the future as identification of specific pathogenic processes and genetic defects permit better differentiation and a more definitive classification. Although the specific etiologies of this form of diabetes are not known, autoimmune destruction of the pancreas does not occur and

patients do not have any other known causes of diabetes as listed in **Table 3.2**.

Most patients with this form of diabetes are obese, and obesity itself causes insulin resistance [35, 36]. Many of those not obese by traditional criteria, body mass index (BMI) for example, may have an increased percentage of body fat distributed predominantly in the abdominal region [36, 37]. Ketoacidosis seldom occurs in type 2 diabetes, and when seen it usually arises in association with the stress of another illness such as infection [38, 39].

Often, insulin secretion is defective in these patients and insufficient to compensate for the insulin resistance. On the other hand, insulin action is essentially normal in some individuals, but insulin secretion is markedly impaired. Insulin resistance may improve with weight reduction, increased physical activity and/or pharmacologic treatment of hyperglycemia, but it is not restored to normal [40, 41].

The risk of developing type 2 diabetes increases with age, obesity and lack of physical activity [42, 43]. It occurs more frequently in women with prior GDM, in those with hypertension or dyslipidemia, and its frequency varies in different ethnic subgroups [42–45]. Type 2 diabetes is often associated with strong familial, likely genetic, predisposition [44–46]. The genetics of type 2 diabetes are quite complex and not clearly defined. Some patients who present a clinical picture consistent of type 2 diabetes have been shown to have autoantibodies similar to those found in type 1 diabetes. This form of diabetes may masquerade type 2 diabetes if antibody determinations are not made. Patients who are not obese or who have relatives with type 1 diabetes and are Caucasian (northern European origin) may be suspected of having late-onset type 1 diabetes [2].

3.10.3.3   Other Specific Types

These include identified *genetic*, *exocrine pancreatic*, *endocrine* and *drug-induced* causes. A more comprehensive breakdown is provided in **Table 3.3**.

3.11   GENETIC DEFECTS OF β-CELL FUNCTION

The diabetic state may be associated with monogenetic defects in β-cell function. These forms are characterized by onset of mild hyperglycemia at an early age (generally <25 years). They are inherited in an autosomal dominant pattern. Patients with these forms of diabetes, formerly referred to as MODY, have impaired insulin secretion with minimal or no defect in insulin action [47, 48]. Abnormalities at three genetic loci on different chromosomes have been identified to date. The most common form is associated with mutations on chromosome 12 in a hepatic transcription factor referred to as *hepatocyte nuclear factor* (HNF)-1alpha [49]. A second form is associated with mutations in the glucokinase gene on chromosome 7 p [50, 51] and results in a defective glucokinase molecule. Glucokinase converts glucose to glucose-6-phosphate, the metabolism of which in turn stimulates insulin secretion by the β cell. Thus, glucokinase serves as the 'glucose sensor' for the β cell. Owing to defects in the glucokinase gene, increased levels of glucose are necessary to elicit normal levels of insulin secretion. A mutation in the *HNF-4* alpha gene on chromosome 20 q characterizes the third form [52]. HNF-4 alpha is a transcription factor which is involved in the regulation of the expression of HNF-12. A fourth variant has recently been described to mutations in another transcription factor gene, *1PF-1*, which in its homozygous form leads to total pancreatic agenesis [53]. Specific genetic defects in other individuals who have a similar clinical presentation are currently being investigated.

In addition, point mutations in mitochondrial DNA have been found to be associated with deafness [54]. The most common mutation occurs at position 3243 in the tRNA leucine gene leading to an A to G substitution. An identical lesion occurs in mitochondrial myopathy, encephalopathy, lactic acidosis and stroke-like (MELAS) syndrome. However, diabetes is not part of this syndrome, suggesting different phenotypic expressions of this genetic lesion [55].

Genetic abnormalities that result in the inability to convert proinsulin to insulin have been identified in a few families. Usually, such traits are inherited in an autosomal dominant pattern [56, 57] and the resultant carbohydrate intolerance is mild. Mutant insulin molecules with impaired receptor binding have also been identified in a few families. These are also associated with autosomal inheritance and either normal or only mildly impaired carbohydrate metabolism [58, 59].

3.12   GENETIC DEFECTS IN INSULIN ACTION

These causes of diabetes are unusual and result from genetically determined abnormalities of insulin action. The metabolic abnormalities' associated mutations of the insulin receptor may range from hyperinsulinemia and modest hyperglycemia to severe symptomatic diabetes [60, 61]. Acanthosis nigricans may be present in some of these individuals. Women may have virilization and have enlarged cystic ovaries. This syndrome was termed *type A insulin resistance* in the past [60]. Two pediatric syndromes that have mutations in the insulin receptor gene with subsequent alterations in insulin receptor function and extreme insulin resistance are called *leprechaunism* and *Rabson–Mendenhall syndrome* [61]. Leprechaunism has characteristic facial features, whereas Rabson–Mendenhall syndrome is associated with abnormalities of teeth, nails and pineal gland hyperplasia. In patients with insulin-resistant lipoatrophic diabetes, alterations in the structure and function of the insulin receptor cannot be demonstrated. Therefore, it is assumed that the lesion(s) must reside in the postreceptor signal transduction pathways.

3.13   DISEASES OF THE EXOCRINE PANCREAS

Pancreatitis, trauma, infection, pancreatic carcinoma and pancreatectomy are some of the acquired processes of the pancreas that can cause diabetes. Any process that diffusely injures the pancreas may cause diabetes [62, 63]. With the exception of cancer, damage to the pancreas must be extensive for diabetes to occur. However, adenocarcinomas that involve only a small portion of the pancreas have been associated with diabetes. This implies a mechanism other than single reduction in β-cell mass [64]. Depending on their extent, cystic fibrosis and hemochromatosis will also damage β-cell and impair insulin secretion [64, 65]. Fibrocalculous pancreatopathy may be accompanied by abdominal pain radiating to the back and pancreatic calcification on X-ray and ductal dilatation [20]. Pancreatic fibrosis and calcified stones in the exocrine ducts are found at autopsy [20, 66].

3.14   ENDOCRINOPATHIES

Insulin action can be antagonized by several hormones (e.g. growth hormone, cortisol, glucagon and epinephrine). Diseases associated with excess secretion of these hormones can cause diabetes (e.g. acromegaly, Cushing's syndrome, glucagonoma and pheochromocytoma) [67]. These forms of hyperglycemia resolve when the hormone excess is removed. Somatostinoma and aldosteronoma-induced hypokalemia can cause diabetes at least in part by inhibiting insulin secretion [68, 69]. Hyperglycemia generally resolves following successful removal of the tumor.

3.15   DRUG- OR CHEMICAL-INDUCED DIABETES

Insulin secretion may be impaired by many drugs. They may not, by themselves, cause diabetes, but they may precipitate diabetes in persons with insulin resistance [70, 71]. Classification is ambiguous in such cases, as the primacy of β-cell destruction or insulin resistance is unknown. Pancreatic β-cell destruction may occur with the use of certain toxins or drugs such as Vacor (a rat prison) and pentamidine [72–74]. There are also many drugs and hormones which can impair insulin action. The list shown in **Table 3.3** is not all-inclusive, but reflects the more commonly recognized drug-, hormone- or toxin-induced forms of diabetes and hyperglycemia.

3.16   INFECTIONS

Certain viruses have been associated with β-cell destruction. Diabetes occurs in some patients with congenital rubella [75]. Coxsackie B, cytomegalovirus and other viruses (e.g. adenovirus and mumps) have been implicated in inducing diabetes [76–78].

3.17   UNCOMMON BUT SPECIFIC FORMS OF IMMUNE-MEDIATED DIABETES MELLITUS

Diabetes may be associated with several immunological diseases with a pathogenesis or etiology different from that which leads to the type 1 diabetes process. Postprandial hyperglycemia of a severity sufficient to fulfill the criteria for diabetes has been reported in rare individuals who spontaneously develop insulin autoantibodies. However, these individuals generally present with symptoms of hypoglycemia rather than hyperglycemia. The 'stiff-man syndrome' is an autoimmune disorder of the central nervous system, characterized by stiffness of the axial muscles with painful spasms. Affected people usually have high titers of the GAD autoantibodies and approximately one-third to one-half will develop diabetes [2, 3]. Patients receiving interferon alpha have been reported to develop diabetes associated with islet cell autoantibodies and, in certain instances, severe insulin deficiency [79].

Anti-insulin receptor antibodies can cause diabetes by binding to the insulin receptor thereby reducing the binding of insulin to target tissues [80]. However, these antibodies also can act as an insulin agonist after binding to the receptor and can thereby cause hypoglycemia [81]. Anti-insulin receptor antibodies are occasionally found in patients with systemic lupus erythematosus and other autoimmune diseases [82]. As in other states of extreme insulin resistance, patients with anti-insulin receptor antibodies often have acanthosis nigricans. In the past, this syndrome was termed *type B insulin resistance*.

3.18 OTHER GENETIC SYNDROMES ASSOCIATED WITH DIABETES

Many genetic syndromes are accompanied by an increased incidence of diabetes mellitus. These include the chromosomal abnormalities of Down's syndrome, Klinefelter's syndrome and Turner's syndrome. Wolfram's syndrome is an autosomal recessive disorder characterized by insulin-deficient diabetes and the absence of β cells at autopsy [83]. Additional manifestations include diabetes insipidus, hypogonadism, optic atrophy and neural deafness. These and other similar disorders are listed in **Table 3.3**.

3.19 GESTATIONAL DIABETES MELLITUS

Gestational diabetes is carbohydrate intolerance resulting in hyperglycemia of variable severity with onset or first recognition during pregnancy. The definition applies irrespective of whether or not insulin is used for treatment or the condition persists after pregnancy. It does not exclude the possibility that the glucose intolerance may antedate pregnancy but has been previously unrecognized [2, 3].

Women who become pregnant and who are known to have diabetes mellitus which antedates pregnancy do not have gestational diabetes but have 'diabetes mellitus and pregnancy' and should be treated accordingly before, during and after the pregnancy [2, 3].

Fasting and postprandial glucose concentrations are normally lower in the early part of pregnancy (e.g. first trimester and first half of second trimester) than in normal, nonpregnant women. Elevated fasting or postprandial plasma glucose levels at this time in pregnancy may well reflect the presence of diabetes which has antedated pregnancy, but criteria for designating abnormally high glucose concentrations at this time have not yet been established. The occurrence of higher than normal plasma glucose levels at this time in pregnancy mandates careful management and may be an indication for carrying out an OGTT (**Table 3.5** and Appendix 1). Nevertheless, normal glucose tolerance in the early part of pregnancy does not itself establish that gestational diabetes may not develop later.

Individuals at high risk for gestational diabetes include older women for pregnancy (>25 years of age), those with abnormal body weight, those with previous history of abnormal glucose metabolism (IFG and IGT) or family history of diabetes, those with a history of large for gestational-age babies, women from certain high-risk ethnic groups (e.g. Hispanic American, Native American, Asian American, African American, Pacific Islander) and any pregnant woman who has elevated fasting, or casual, blood glucose levels [2, 3]. It may be appropriate to screen pregnant women belonging to high-risk populations during the first trimester of pregnancy in order to detect previously undiagnosed diabetes mellitus. If they are found not to have GDM at that initial screening, they should be retested between 24 and 28 weeks of gestation. Formal systematic testing for gestational diabetes is usually done between 24 and 28 weeks of gestation.

Table 3.5 Diagnosis of gestational diabetes mellitus (GDM) with a 100 or 75 g glucose load according to the american diabetes association.

	Glucose threshold value	
	mmol l^{-1}	mg dl^{-1}
100 g glucose load		
Fasting	5.3	95
1 h	10.0	180
2 h	8.6	155
3 h	7.8	140
75 g glucose load		
Fasting	5.3	95
1 h	10.0	180
2 h	8.6	155

Two or more of the venous plasma concentrations must be met or exceeded for a positive diagnosis. The test should be done in the morning after an overnight fast of between 8 and 14 h and after at least 3 days of unrestricted diet (≥ 150 g carbohydrate per day) and unlimited physical activity. The subject should remain seated and should not smoke throughout the test (see Appendix 1).

3.20 DIAGNOSIS OF GESTATIONAL DIABETES

To determine if gestational diabetes is present in pregnant women, a standard OGTT should be performed after overnight fasting (8–14 h) by giving 75 g anhydrous glucose in 250–300 ml water (Appendix 1). Plasma glucose is measured fasting and after 2 h. Pregnant women who meet WHO criteria for diabetes mellitus or IGT are classified as having GDM. After the pregnancy ends, the woman should be reclassified as having either diabetes mellitus (or IGT) or normal glucose tolerance based on the results of a 75 g OGTT 6 weeks or more after delivery [3]. It should be emphasized that such women, regardless of the 6-week postpregnancy result, are at increased risk of subsequently developing diabetes. The significance of IFG in pregnancy remains to be established. Any woman with IFG, however, should have a 75 g OGTT. An FPG load >7.0 mml l^{-1} (126 mg dl^{-1}) or a casual plasma glucose >11.1 mmol l^{-1} (200 mg dl^{-1}) meets the threshold for the diagnosis

of diabetes, if confirmed on a subsequent day, and precludes the need for any glucose challenge. In the absence of this degree of hyperglycemia, according to the ADA, evaluation for GDM in women with average or high-risk characteristics should follow one of the two approaches [3].

One-step approach: Perform a diagnostic OGTT without prior plasma or serum glucose screening. This approach may be cost-effective in high-risk patients or populations.

Two-step approach: Perform an initial screening by measuring the plasma or serum glucose concentration 1 h after a 50 g oral glucose load (glucose challenge test (GCT)) and perform a diagnostic OGTT on that subset of women exceeding the glucose threshold value on the GCT. When the two-step approach is applied, a glucose threshold value >7.8 mmol l^{-1} (140 mg dl^{-1}) identifies approximately 80% of women with GDM and the yield is further increased to 90% by using a cutoff of >7.2 mmol l^{-1} (130 mg dl^{-1}). With either approach, the diagnosis of GDM is based on OGTT. Loads of 100 or 75 g and the glucose threshold values listed for fasting, 1 and 2 h (**Table 3.5**).

The prevalence in the United States of GDM may range from 1 to 14% of pregnancies [3]. It may complicate about 4% of all pregnancies, resulting in 135 000 cases annually. GDM represents nearly 90% of all pregnancies complicated by diabetes [3].

The criteria cited above for abnormal glucose tolerance in pregnancy which are widely used in the United States were proposed by O'Sullivan and Mahan in 1964 [83]. In 1979, the NDDG revised the O'Sullivan and Mahan criteria converting whole-blood values to plasma values. Carpenter and Coustan suggested that the NDDG conversion of the O'Sullivan and Mahan values from the original Somogyi–Nelson determinations may have resulted in values that are too high. They proposed cutoff values for plasma glucose that appear to represent more accurately the original O'Sullivan and Mahan determinations [84]. The 75 g OGTT provides values for plasma glucose concentrations that are similar to the Carpenter–Coustan extrapolations of the 100 g OGTT [3].

Recommendations from the ADA Fourth International Workshop Conference on Gestational

Diabetes Mellitus in 1997 support the use of the Carpenter–Coustan diagnostic criteria as well as the alternative use of a diagnostic 75 g, 2 h OGTT (**Table 3.5**). The 75 g is probably more practical.

3.21 CONCLUSIONS

The most substantive change in diagnostic criteria for glucose intolerance is that the FPG concentration for the diagnosis of diabetes has been lowered from 7.8 mmol 1^{-1} (140 mg dl^{-1}) to 7 mmol 1^{-1} (126 mg dl^{-1}).

A new category of impaired FPG of 5.6–7.0 mmol 1^{-1} (111–126 mg dl^{-1}) has been created, as the ADA recommended abolition of the OGTT. This suggestion has not been supported by the 1998 WHO report [2].

The OGTT is not used very often to diagnose diabetes in a clinical setting and has been mainly used for clinical research and epidemiological studies. Diabetes can usually be diagnosed without an OGTT, but this is not the case for IGT. While in many settings, the logistics and costs of measuring glycated hemoglobin are less than those of obtaining fasting blood or performing an OGTT, the current disadvantage of glycated hemoglobin is the lack of standardization of methodology and the fact there is no universal reference standard for interlaboratory calibration [2]. In addition, there are fewer outcome data available than for the OGTT. However, these limitations may be overcome in the near future, so that further evaluation of the properties of HbA_{1c} measurements for screening and diagnosis could justify postponing a change in screening recommendations.

There are several arguments for abolishing the OGTT as a routine screening test for type 2 diabetes. The complexity of the current diagnostic criteria reflect both the difficulty in distinguishing diabetic from nondiabetic patients on the basis of a single measurement and the considerable test/retest variability of the OGTT.

However, a major argument for continuing the OGTT relates to the identification of high-risk subjects, namely those with IGT for clinical trials of type 2 diabetes prevention. In addition, the 2-h plasma glucose (2-h PG) value from the OGTT was in particular recommended by the WHO for epidemiological studies, to overcome uncertainties about whether study subjects were fasting or not.

Blood glucose is a continuum; therefore, the choice of a distinct cutpoint will always be somewhat arbitrary. The determination of diagnostic cutpoints which gave rise to the NDDG and WHO recommendations was based on studies performed which evaluated the association between 2-h PG and the subsequent development of the microvascular complications of diabetes.

The diagnostic cutpoint of 11.1 mmol 1^{-1} for the 2-h PG concentration was originally adopted for two reasons. First, the bimodality of glucose distributions in populations with high prevalence of diabetes suggested that 11.1 mmol 1^{-1} represented the cutpoint separating the two components of the bimodal frequency distributions. Second, when the prevalence of microvascular complications was plotted against the 2-h PG value it became obvious that the former sharply increased at about 11.1 mmol 1^{-1}.

Using the WHO cutpoint values to define type 2 diabetes, it became apparent that FPG and 2-h PG detect different sectors of the hyperglycemic state. The 1985 WHO FPG criterion for diabetes (7.8 mmol 1^{-1} or 140 mg dl^{-1}) represents a greater degree of hyperglycemia than the 2-h PG criterion for diabetes (11.1 mmol 1^{-1} or 200 mg dl^{-1}). The effect of the change will have variable, but not great, consequences on diabetes prevalence in most populations.

The new WHO/ADA recommendations will be welcomed as a basis on which to build. They are based on the accumulated research of many researchers. The rapid advances in molecular biology in the last decade have provided the means to extend our knowledge of the basis for the metabolic and clinical heterogeneity of diabetes. The classification should provide a more rational platform for phenotyping and choosing appropriate therapies for persons with diabetes. Inevitably, the classification and criteria will need to be revised in future years as new evidence-based data emerge.

APPENDIX 1 THE ORAL GLUCOSE TOLERANCE

The OGTT is principally used for diagnosis when blood glucose levels are equivocal, during pregnancy or in an epidemiological setting to screen for diabetes and IGT.

The OGTT should be administered in the morning after at least 3 days of unrestricted diet (greater than 150 g of carbohydrate daily) and usual physical activity. The test should be preceded by an overnight fast of 8–14 h, during which water may be drunk. Smoking is not permitted during the test. The presence of factors that influence interpretation of the results of the test must be recorded (e.g. medications, inactivity, infection).

After collection of the fasting blood sample, the subject should drink 75 g of anhydrous glucose (or partial hydrolysates of starch of the equivalent carbohydrate content) in 250–300 ml of water over the course of 5 min. For children, the test load should be 1.75 g of glucose per kilogram of body weight up to a total of 75 g of glucose. Blood samples must be collected 2 h after the test load.

Unless the glucose concentration can be determined immediately, the blood sample should be collected in a tube containing sodium fluoride (6 mg ml^{-1} whole blood) and immediately centrifuged to separate the plasma; the plasma should be frozen until the glucose concentration can be estimated. For interpretation of results, refer to **Tables 2.2** and **3.5**)

APPENDIX 2 METHODS FOR MEASURING SUBSTANCES IN BLOOD AND URINE

Measurement of Glucose in Blood

Reductiometric methods (the Somogyi–Nelson, the ferricyanide and neocuprine autoanalyzer methods) are still in use for blood glucose measurement. The *o*-toluidine method also remains in use, but enzyme-based methods are widely available, for both laboratory and near-patient use. Highly accurate and rapid (1–2 min) devices are now available based on immobilized glucose oxidase electrodes. Hexokinase and glucose dehydrogenase methods are used for reference.

Whole blood samples preserved with fluoride show an initial rapid fall in glucose of up to 10% at room temperature, but subsequent decline is slow; centrifugation prevents the initial fall. Whole-blood glucose values are 15% lower than corresponding plasma values in patients with a normal hematocrit reading, and arterial values are about 7% higher than corresponding venous values.

The use of reagent-strip glucose oxidase methods has made bedside estimation of blood glucose very popular. However, the cost of the reagent strips remains high. Some methods still require a punctilious technique, accurate timing and storage of strips in airtight containers. Reasonably quantitative results can be obtained even with visual color-matching techniques. Electrochemical and reflectance meters can give coefficients of variation of well under 5%. Reagent-strip methods have been validated under tropical conditions, but are sensitive to extreme climatic conditions. Diabetes may be strongly suspected from the results of reagent-strip glucose estimation, but the diagnosis cannot be confidently excluded by the use of this method. Confirmation of diagnosis requires estimation by laboratory methods.

Patients can easily collect small blood samples themselves (either in specially prepared plastic or glass capillary tubes or on filter paper), and self-monitoring using glucose reagent-strips with direct color matching or meters is now widely practiced. Patients should be properly trained in the appropriate techniques to avoid inaccurate or misleading results.

The insulin-treated patient is commonly requested to build up a 'glycemic profile' by self-measurement of blood glucose at specific times of the day (and night). A 'seven-point profile' is useful, with samples taken before and 90 min after breakfast, before and 90 min after lunch, before and 90 min after an evening meal, and just before going to bed. Occasionally, patients may arrange to wake at 3 a.m. to collect and measure a nocturnal sample. The complete profile rarely needs to be collected within a single 24 h period, and it may be compiled from samples collected at different times over several days.

Measurement of Glucose in Urine

Insulin-treated patients who do not have access to facilities for self-measurement of blood glucose should test urine samples passed after rising, before main meals, and before going to bed. Patients with type 2 diabetes do not need to monitor their urine so frequently. Urine tests are of somewhat limited value, however, because of the great variation in urine glucose concentration for given levels of blood glucose. The correlation between blood and urine glucose may be improved a little by collecting short-term fractions (15–30 min) or the urine output. Benedict's quantitative solution or self-boiling, caustic soda/copper sulfate tablets may be used, or the more convenient, but costly, semiquantitative enzyme-based test strips.

Ketone Bodies in Urine and Blood

The appearance of persistent ketonuria associated with hyperglycemia or high levels of glycosuria in the diabetic patient points to an unacceptably severe level of metabolic disturbance and indicates an urgent need for corrective action. The patient should be advised to test for ketone bodies (acetone and aceto-acetic acid) when tests for glucose are repeatedly positive, or when there is substantial disturbance of health, particularly with infections. Rothera's sodium nitroprusside test may be used or, alternatively, reagent-strips that are sensitive to ketones. In emergency situations, such as diabetic ketoacidosis, a greatly raised concentration of plasma ketones can be detected with a reagent strip and roughly quantified by serial 1-in-2 dilution of plasma with water.

References

1. World Health Organization (1985) Diabetes mellitus: report of a WHO study group, Tech. Rep. Ser. 727, WHO, Geneva.
2. Alberti, K.G.M.M. and Zimmet, P. (1998) Definition, diagnosis and classification of diabetes mellitus and its complications part 1: diagnosis and classification of diabetes mellitus—provisional report of a WHO consultation. *Diabetic Medicine*, **15**, 539–53.
3. American Diabetes Association (2006) Diagnosis and classification of diabetes mellitus. *Diabetes Care*, **29**, (Suppl 1), S43–8.
4. Barker, D.J.P., Gardner, M.J. and Power, C. (1982) Incidence of diabetes amongst people aged 18-50 years in nine British towns: a collaborative study. *Diabetologia*, **22**, 421–5.
5. Watkins, P.J. (1979) A new look at diagnostic criteria. *Diabetologia*, **17**, 127–8.
6. Conn, J.W. (1940) Interpretation of the glucose tolerance test: the necessity of a standard preparatory diet. *American Journal of the Medical Sciences*, **199**, 555–64.
7. Conn, J.W. and Fajans, S.S. (1961) The prediabetic state. *American Journal of Medicine*, **31**, 839–50.
8. Soskin, S. (1951) Use and abuse of the dextrose tolerance test. *Postgraduate Medicine*, **10**, 108–16.
9. Sayetta, R.B. and Murphy, R.S. (1979) Summary of current diabetes related data from the National Center for Health Statistics. *Diabetes Care*, **2**, 105–19.
10. Sasaki, A. (1981) Assessment of the new criteria for diabetes mellitus according to 10 year relative survival rates. *Diabetologia*, **20**, 195–8.
11. Finch, C.F., Zimmet, P.Z. and Alberti, K.G.M.M. (1990) Determining diabetes prevalence: a rational basis for the use of fasting plasma glucose concentrations? *Diabetic Medicine*, **7**, 603–10.
12. McCance, D.R., Hanson, R.L., Charles, M.A. *et al.* (1994) Comparison of tests for glycated haemoglobin and fasting and two hour plasma glucose concentrations as diagnostic methods for diabetes. *British Medical Journal*, **308**, 1323–28.
13. Engelgau, M.M., Thompson, T.J., Herman, W.H. *et al.* (1997) Comparison of fasting and 2-hour glucose and HbA_{1c} levels for diagnosing diabetes: diagnostic criteria and performance revisited. *Diabetes Care*, **20**, 785–91.
14. Charles, M.A., Balkau, B., Vauzelle-Kervoeden, F. *et al.* (1996) Revision of diagnostic criteria for diabetes (Letter). *Lancet*, **348**, 1657–8.
15. Harris, M.I., Eastman, R.C., Cowie, C.C. *et al.* (1997) Comparison of diabetes diagnostic categories in the US population according to 1997 American Diabetes Association and 1980–1985 World Health Organization diagnostic criteria. *Diabetes Care*, **20**, 1859–62.
16. Ramachandran, A., Snehalatha, C., Latha, E. and Vijay V. (1998) Evaluation of the use of fasting plasma glucose as a new diagnostic criterion for diabetes in Asian Indian population (Letter). *Diabetes Care*, **21**, 666–7.
17. WHO Expert Committee (1965) Diabetes mellitus. 1st report, Tech. Rep. Ser. 310, WHO, Geneva.
18. National Diabetes Data Group (1979) Classification and diagnosis of diabetes mellitus and other categories of glucose intolerance. *Diabetes*, **28**, 1039–57.
19. WHO Expert Committee (1980) WHO Expert Committee on Diabetes Mellitus . 2nd report, Tech. Rep. Ser. 646, WHO, Geneva.
20. Ekoé, J.M. and Shipp, J. (2001) Malnutrition-related diabetes mellitus. Myth or reality, in The Epidemiology of Diabetes Mellitus. An International Perspective, 1st edn (eds J.M. Ekoé, P. Zimmet and R. Williams), John Wiley & Sons, Ltd, Chichester, pp. 263–72.
21. Kuzuya, T. and Matsuda, A. (1997) Classification of diabetes on the basis of etiologies versus degree of insulin deficiency. *Diabetes Care*, **20**, 1185–97.
22. Shaw, J.E., Zimmet, P.Z., de Courten, M. *et al.* (1999) Impaired fasting glucose or impaired glucose

tolerance. What best predicts future diabetes in Mauritius? *Diabetes Care*, **22** (3), 399–402.

23. Fuller, J.H., Shipley, M.J., Rose, G. *et al.* (1980) Coronary heart disease risk and impaired glucose tolerance: the Whitehall Study. *Lancet*, **i**, 1373–6.

24. Alberti, K.G.M.M. (1996) The clinical implications of impaired glucose tolerance. *Diabetic Medicine*, **13**, 927–37.

25. Reaven, G.M. (1988) Role of insulin resistance in human disease. *Diabetes*, **37**, 1595–607.

26. Zimmet, P.Z., Tuomi, T., Mackay, R. *et al.* (1994) Latent autoimmune diabetes mellitus in adults (LADA): the role of antibodies to glutamic acid decarboxylase in diagnosis and prediction of insulin dependency. *Diabetic Medicine*, **11**, 299–303.

27. Humphrey, A.R.G., McCarty, D.J., Mackay, I.R. *et al.* (1998) Autoantibodies to glutamic acid decarboxylase and phenotypic features associated with early insulin treatment in individuals with adult-onset diabetes mellitus. *Diabetic Medicine*, **15**, 113–19.

28. Verge, C.F., Gianani, R., Kawasaki, E., *et al.* (1996) Predicting type 1 diabetes in first-degree relatives using a combination of insulin, GAD, and ICA512bdc/IA-2 autoantibodies. *Diabetes*, **45**, 926–33.

29. Molbak, A.G., Christau, B., Marner, B. *et al.* (1994) Incidence of insulin-dependent diabetes mellitus in age groups over 30 years in Denmark. *Diabetic Medicine*, **11**, 650–5.

30. Betterle, C., Zanette, F., Pedini, B. *et al.* (1983) Clinical and subclinical organ-specific autoimmune manifestations in type 1 (insulin-dependent) diabetic patients and their first-degree relatives. *Diabetologia*, **26**, 431–6.

31. McLarty, D.G., Athaide, I., Bottazzo, G.F. *et al.* (1990) Islet cell antibodies are not specifically associated with insulin-dependent diabetes in rural Tanzanian Africans. *Diabetes Research and Clinical Practice*, **9**, 219–24.

32. Ahrén, B. and Corrigan, C.B. (1984) Intermittent need for insulin in a subgroup of diabetic patients in Tanzania. *Diabetic Medicine*, **2**, 262–4.

33. DeFronzo, R.A., Bonadonna, R.C. and Ferrannini, E. (1997) Pathogenesis of NIDDM, in International Textbook of Diabetes Mellitus, 2nd edn (eds K.G.M.M. Alberti, P. Zimmet and R.A. De Fronzo), John Wiley & Sons, Ltd, Chichester, pp. 635–712.

34. Lillioja, S., Mott, D.M., Spraul, M. *et al.* (1993) Insulin resistance and insulin secretory dysfunction as precursors of non-insulin-dependent diabetes. Prospective study of Pima Indians. *The New England Journal of Medicine*, **329**, 1988–92.

35. Campbell, P.J. and Carlson, M.G. (1993) Impact of obesity on insulin action in NIDDM. *Diabetes*, **42**, 405–10.

36. Bogardus, C., Lillioja, S., Mott, D.M. *et al.* (1985) Relationship between degree of obesity and in vivo insulin action in man. *The American Journal of Physiology*, **248**, E286–91.

37. Kissebah, A.H., Vydelingum, N., Murray, R. *et al.* (1982) Relationship of body fat distribution to metabolic complications of obesity. *The Journal of Clinical Endocrinology and Metabolism*, **54**, 254–60.

38. Banerji, M.A., Chaiken, R.I., Huey, H. *et al.* (1994) GAD antibody negative NIDDM in adult black subjects with diabetic ketoacidosis and increased frequency of human leukocyte antigen DR3 and DR4: flatbush diabetes. *Diabetes*, **43**, 741–5.

39. Umpierrez, G.E., Casals, M.M.C., Gebhardt, S.S.P. *et al.* (1995) Diabetic ketoacidosis in obese African-Americans. *Diabetes*, **44**, 790–5.

40. Simonson, D.C., Ferrannini, E., Bevilacqua, S. *et al.* (1984) Mechanism of improvement in glucose metabolism after chronic glyburide therapy. *Diabetes*, **33**, 838–45.

41. Wing, R.R., Blair, E.H., Bononi, P. *et al.* (1994) Caloric restriction per se is a significant factor in improvements in glycemic control and insulin sensitivity during weight loss in obese NIDDM patients. *Diabetes Care*, **17**, 30–6.

42. Zimmet, P.Z. (1992) Kelly West Lecture 1991: challenges in diabetes epidemiology: from West to the rest. *Diabetes Care*, **15**, 232–52.

43. Harris, M.I., Cowie, C.C., Stern, M.P. *et al.* (eds) (1995). Diabetes in America, 2nd edn, NIH Publ. No. 95-1468 , US Government Printing Office, Washington, DC.

44. Valle, T., Tuomilehto, J. and Eriksson, J. (1997) Epidemiology of NIDDM in Europids, in International Textbook of Diabetes Mellitus, 2nd edn (eds K.G.M.M. Alberti, P. Zimmet and R.A. De Fronzo), John Wiley & Sons, Ltd, Chichester, pp. 125–42.

45. De Courten, M., Bennett, P.H., Tuomilehto, J. and Zimmet, P. (1997) Epidemiology of NIDDM in non-Europids, in International Textbook of Diabetes Mellitus, 2nd edn (eds K.G.M.M. Alberti, P. Zimmet and R.A. De Fronzo), John Wiley & Sons, Ltd, Chichester, pp. 143–70.

46. Knowler, W.C., Nelson, R.G., Saad, M., *et al.* (1943) Determinants of diabetes mellitus in the Pima Indians. *Diabetes Care*, **16**, 216–27.

47. Byrne, M.M., Sturis, J., Menzel, S. *et al.* (1996) Altered insulin secretory response to glucose in diabetic and nondiabetic subjects with mutations in the diabetes susceptibility gene MODY 3 on chromosome 20. *Diabetes*, **45**, 1503–10.

48. Clement, K., Pueyo, M.E., Vaxillaire, M. *et al.* (1996) Assessment of insulin sensitivity in glucokinase-deficient subjects. *Diabetologia*, **39**, 82–90.

49. Yamagata, K., Oda, N., Kaisaki, P.J. *et al.* (1996) Mutations in the hepatocyte nuclear factor-1α gene in maturity-onset diabetes of the young (MODY 3). *Nature*, **384**, 455–8.

50. Froguel, P., Vaxillaire, M., Sun, F. *et al.* (1992) Close linkage of glucokinase locus on chromosome 7p to early-onset non-insulin-dependent diabetes. *Nature*, **356**, 162–4.

51. Vionnet, N., Stoffel, M., Takeda, J. *et al.* (1992) Nonsense mutation in the glucokinase gene causes early-onset non-insulin-dependent diabetes. *Nature*, **356**, 721–2.

52. Yamagata, K., Furuta, H., Oda, N. *et al.* (1996) Mutations in the hepatocyte nuclear factor-4α gene in maturity-onset diabetes of the young (MODY 1). *Nature*, **384**, 458–60.

53. Stoffers, D.A., Ferrer, J., Clarke, W.L. *et al.* (1997) Early-onset type-II diabetes mellitus (MODY4) linked to IPF1. *Nature Genetics*, **117**, 138–9.

54. Walker, M. and Turnbull, D.M. (1997) Mitochondrial related diabetes: a clinical perspective. *Diabetic Medicine*, **14**, 1007–9.

55. Johns, D.R. (1995) Mitochondrial DNA and disease. *The New England Journal of Medicine*, **333**, 638–44.

56. Gruppuso, P.A., Gorden, P., Kahn, C.R. *et al.* (1984) Familial hyperproinsulinemia due to a proposed defect in conversion of proinsulin to insulin. *The New England Journal of Medicine*, **311**, 629–34.

57. Robbins, D.C., Shoelson, S.E., Rubenstein, A.H. *et al.* (1984) Familial hyperproinsulinemia: two cohorts secreting indistinguishable type II intermediates of proinsulin conversion. *Journal of Clinical Investigation*, **73**, 714–19.

58. Haneda, M., Polonsky, K.S., Bergenstal, R.M. *et al.* (1984) Familial hyperinsulinemia due to a structurally abnormal insulin. Definition of an emerging new clinical syndrome. *The New England Journal of Medicine*, **310**, 1288–94.

59. Sanz, N., Karam, J.H., Horita, S. *et al.* (1986) Prevalence of insulin-gene mutations in non-insulin-dependent diabetes mellitus. *The New England Journal of Medicine*, **314**, 1322–3.

60. Kahn, C.R., Flier, J.S., Bar, R.S. *et al.* (1976) The syndromes of insulin resistance and acanthosis nigricans. *The New England Journal of Medicine*, **294**, 739–45.

61. Taylor, S.I. (1992) Lilly Lecture: molecular mechanisms of insulin resistance: lessons from patients with mutations in the insulin-receptor gene. *Diabetes*, **41**, 1473–90.

62. Gullo L., Pezzilli, R., and Morselli-Labate A.M. (1994) Diabetes and the risk of pancreatic cancer. *The New England Journal of Medicine*, **331**, 81–4.

63. Larsen, S., Hilsted, J., Tronier, B. *et al.* (1987) Metabolic control and B cell function in patients with insulin-dependent diabetes mellitus secondary to chronic pancreatitis. *Metabolism*, **36**, 964–7.

64. Moran, A., Pyzdrowski, K.L., Weinreb, J. *et al.* (1994) Insulin sensitivity in cystic fibrosis. *Diabetes*, **43**, 1020–6.

65. Phelps, G., Chapman, I., Hall, P. *et al.* (1989) Prevalence of genetic haemochromatosis among diabetic patients. *Lancet*, **ii**, 233–4.

66. Yajnik, C.S., Shelgikar, K.M., Naik, S.S. *et al.* (1992) The ketoacidosis-resistance in fibro-calculous-pancreatic-diabetes. *Diabetes Research and Clinical Practice*, **15**, 149–56.

67. MacFarlane, I.A. (1997) Endocrine diseases and diabetes mellitus, in Textbook of Diabetes, 2nd edn (eds J.C. Pickup and G. Williams), Blackwell Science, Oxford, pp. 64.1–20.

68. Krejs, G.J., Orci, L., Conlon, J.M. *et al.* (1979) Somatostatinoma syndrome. *The New England Journal of Medicine*, **301**, 285–92.

69. Conn, J.W. (1965) Hypertension, the potassium ion and impaired carbohydrate tolerance. *The New England Journal of Medicine*, **273**, 1135–43.

70. Pandit, M.K., Burke, J., Gustafson, A.B. *et al.* (1993) Drug-induced disorders of glucose tolerance. *Annals of Internal Medicine*, **118**, 529–40.

71. O'Byrne, S. and Feely, J. (1990) Effects of drugs on glucose tolerance in non-insulin-dependent diabetes (parts I and II). *Drugs*, **40**, 203–19.

72. Gallanosa, A.G., Spyker, D.A. and Curnow, R.T. (1981) Diabetes mellitus associated with autonomic and peripheral neuropathy after Vacor poisoning: a review. *Clinical Toxicology*, **18**, 441–9

73. Esposti, M.D., Ngo, A. and Myers, M.A. (1996) Inhibition of mitochondrial complex 1 may account for IDDM induced by intoxication with rodenticide Vacor. *Diabetes*, **45**, 1531–4.

74. Assan, R., Perronne, C., Assan, D. *et al.* (1995) Pentamidine-induced derangements of glucose homeostasis. *Diabetes Care*, **18**, 47–55.

75. Forrest, J.A., Menser, M.A. and Burgess, J.A. (1971) High frequency of diabetes mellitus in young patients with congenital rubella. *Lancet*, **ii**, 332–4.

76. King, M.L., Bidwell, D., Shaikh, A. *et al.* (1983) Coxsackie-B-virus-specific IgM responses in children with insulin-dependent (juvenile-onset; type 1) diabetes mellitus. *Lancet*, **i**, 1397–9.

77. Karjalainen, J., Knip, M., Hyoty, H. *et al.* (1988) Relationship between serum insulin antibodies, islet cell antibodies and Coxsackie-B4 and mumps virus-specific antibodies at the clinical manifestation of type 1 (insulin-dependent) diabetes. *Diabetologia*, **31**, 146–52.

78. Pak, C.Y., Eun, H., McArthur, R.G. *et al.* (1988) Association of cytomegalovirus infection with autoimmune type 1 diabetes. *Lancet*, **ii**, 1–4.

79. Fabris, P., Betterle, C., Floreani, A. *et al.* (1992) Development of type 1 diabetes mellitus during interferon alfa therapy for chronic HCV hepatitis (Letter). *Lancet*, **340**, 548.

80. Flier, J.S. (1992) Lilly Lecture: syndromes of insulin resistance: from patient to gene and back again. *Diabetes*, **41**, 1207–19.

81. Khan, C.R., Baird, K.L., Flier, J.S. *et al.* (1977) Effects of autoantibodies to the insulin receptor on isolated adipocytes. *Journal of Clinical Investigation*, **60**, 1094–106.

82. Tsokos, G.C., Gorden, P., Antonovych, T. *et al.* (1985) Lupus nephritis and other autoimmune features in patients with diabetes mellitus due to autoantibody to insulin receptors. *Annals of Internal Medicine*, **102**, 176–81.

83. Barrett, T.G., Bundey, S.E. and Macleod, A.F. (1995) Neurodegeneration and diabetes: UK nationwide study of Wolfram (DIDMOAD) syndrome. *Lancet*, **346**, 1458–63.

84. Carpenter, M.W. and Coustan, D.R. (1982) Criteria for screening tests for gestational diabetes. *American Journal of Obstetrics and Gynecology*, **144**, 768–73.

Further Reading

Bodansky, H.J., Grant, P.J., Dean, B.M. *et al.* (1986) Islet-cell antibodies and insulin autoantibodies in association with common viral infections. *Lancet*, **ii**, 1351–3.

Hirata, Y., Ishizu, H., Ouchi, N. *et al.* (1970) Insulin autoimmunity in a case of spontaneous hypoglycaemia. *The Journal of the Japan Diabetes Society*, **13**, 312–20.

McCance, D.R., Hanson, R.L., Pettitt, D.J. *et al.* (1997) Diagnosing diabetes mellitus—do we need new criteria? *Diabetologia*, **40**, 247–55.

O'Sullivan, J.B. and Mahan, C.M. (1964) Criteria for the oral glucose tolerance test in pregnancy. *Diabetes*, **13**, 278.

Permert, J., Larsson, J., Westermark, G.T. *et al.* (1994) Islet amyloid polypeptide in patients with pancreatic cancer and diabetes. *The New England Journal of Medicine*, **330**, 313–18.

Solimena, M. and De Camilli, P. (1991) Autoimmunity to glutamic acid decarboxylase (GAD) in stiff-man syndrome and insulin-dependent diabetes mellitus. *Trends in Neurosciences*, **14**, 452–7.

4

Epidemiology of Metabolic Syndrome

Dianna J. Magliano, Adrian Cameron, Jonathan E. Shaw and Paul Z. Zimmet

International Diabetes Institute, Caulfield, Victoria, Australia

4.1 INTRODUCTION

Metabolic syndrome (MetS), also previously known by a variety of other names, including insulin resistance syndrome and the *deadly quartet*, is characterized by clustering of abdominal (visceral and retroperitoneal) obesity and other cardiovascular risk factors, including impaired glucose regulation, raised triglycerides, decreased high-density lipoprotein cholesterol (HDL-C), elevated blood pressure (BP).

Associated with increased risk of both type 2 diabetes and cardiovascular disease (CVD), MetS is believed to be a contributor to the modern-day epidemics of diabetes and CVD and has become a major public health challenge around the world [1]. Currently, there are five different sets of criteria which have been developed to characterize the syndrome. These definitions differ in the components included and the cut-points used for each component. The prevalence of MetS in the westernized world is significant (10–50%) and believed to be increasing over time. The pathophysiology of the syndrome is unclear, but it is thought that obesity and/or insulin resistance are key underlying components. Genetics, lifestyle and environment factors are also important causes of MetS.

This chapter provides:

- a historical overview of the evolution of MetS;
- a summary of the value of the different definitions used to characterize the syndrome;
- a summary of the underlying pathophysiology, the causes and other important risk factors of MetS;
- a summary of the evidence describing the association of MetS with CVD and diabetes;
- a summary of the prevalence of MetS using the various definitions in different countries.

4.2 WHAT IS METABOLIC SYNDROME?

MetS can be described as a constellation of metabolic abnormalities, including centrally distributed obesity, decreased HDL-C, elevated triglycerides, elevated BP and hyperglycemia, which cluster together to a greater degree than expected by chance.

4.3 HISTORICAL OVERVIEW

Although MetS has received a considerable amount of attention as a new syndrome in recent years, the concept of MetS can be dated back several hundred years. In the 1600s, a prominent physician, Nicolaes Tulp, linked hypertriglyceridemia and the ingestion of saturated fatty acids, obesity and bleeding tendency in the documentation of the first case report of a syndrome that he called 'hypertriglyceridemia syndrome' [2]. In the mid 1700s, Morgagni noted the association between visceral obesity, hypertension, atherosclerosis and obstructive sleep apnea [3]. About 80 years ago, a Swedish physician, Kylin, described a clustering of hypertension, hyperglycemia and gout [4]. Two decades later, in 1947, Vague [5] observed that a particular obesity phenotype, upper body, android or male-type obesity, was associated with the metabolic abnormalities often

The Epidemiology of Diabetes Mellitus, second edition Edited by Jean-Marie Ekoé, Marian Rewers, Rhys Williams and Paul Zimmet
© 2008 John Wiley & Sons, Ltd

seen with type 2 diabetes and with CVD. The frequency of the co-occurrence of metabolic risk factors in individuals who were also at high coronary risk was reported by Avogaro *et al.* [6] in 1965; later, in 1977, Haller [7] noted the association of the syndrome with atherosclerosis, coining the term *metabolic syndrome*. In the next decade, Vague *et al.* [8] further emphasized the importance of visceral fat in the upper part of the body being associated with diabetes and atherosclerosis, and Reaven described the clinical importance of the syndrome as a cluster of metabolic abnormalities with insulin resistance as the central pathophysiological feature, labeling it *syndrome X* [9]. Interestingly, despite Vague's descriptions of the importance of central obesity to MetS and the risk of diabetes and CVD that was associated with it, Reaven did not include obesity in his pivotal report about MetS. Several years later, and consistent with Reaven's theory about MetS, Ferrannini *et al.* [10] suggested that this clinical entity characterized by abnormal metabolic factors could be attributed to insulin resistance and introduced the term *insulin resistance syndrome*.

4.4 ETIOLOGY OF METABOLIC SYNDROME

The pathogenesis of MetS is poorly understood, and likely to be complex and multifactorial. Insulin resistance and abdominal obesity have received the most attention as the putative underlying features explaining the frequently observed clustering of the other components. Of these features, insulin resistance (primarily in skeletal muscle and liver) and hyperinsulinemia were first postulated to be the unifying pathophysiology underlying the syndrome [1, 9, 11]. This was supported by the fact that, for the majority of components in the definition, there are studies which implicate insulin resistance as contributing to their pathophysiology [9, 11], in that insulin resistance induces the abnormality via more than one biological pathway, that most subjects with the syndrome had one or the other abnormality and that insulin resistance is a consistent early abnormality of diabetes. However, critics argue that not all those with MetS are insulin resistant and some components of the syndrome are not directly related to insulin resistance. For example, in factor analysis, hypertension does not usually cluster

with insulin resistance [12]. There are also some methodological issues with the measurement of insulin resistance (such as lack of standardization) which have made interpretation of the data about insulin resistance difficult. For example, the ability of fasting plasma insulin levels (often used as a surrogate for insulin resistance) to predict insulin resistance is modest.

Instead, the link between obesity, particularly central adiposity, and the other components is very strong and the syndrome may well be best viewed as the metabolic consequences of central visceral obesity. This theory suggests that adipose tissue, in particular visceral adipose tissue, expresses various factors which are involved in the regulation of a variety of metabolic parameters, including insulin in skeletal muscle cells. One such factor, adiponectin, has been found to have antidiabetic, antiatherosclerotic and anti-inflammatory functions [13, 14]. Reduced production of adiponectin is associated with excessive intra-abdominal adipose tissue and insulin resistance [15]. Furthermore, a study by Carr *et al.* [16] examining the association of the insulin sensitivity index and intra-abdominal fat (IAF) showed that, while central body fat and insulin resistance were both associated with the MetS syndrome, IAF was independently associated with all of the criteria of the Adult Treatment Panel III (ATPIII) definition, suggesting that it may have a pathophysiological role in the development of MetS [16].

Another concept underpinning the MetS, which may be related in some way to the 'central obesity theory' is one based on leptin resistance. Leptin is a hormone produced by adipose tissue which acts on a specific receptor in the hypothalamus to decrease appetite and increase energy expenditure [17]. Although leptin-deficient persons (a very rare genetic disorder) are clinically obese, most obese people have increases in leptin levels, indicating that obesity is associated with leptin resistance [17]. With regard to MetS, it has been postulated that conditions in which leptin deficiency or resistance are present are associated with triglyceride accumulation in non-adipose tissue (e.g. liver, muscle and pancreatic islet cells). In this state, the deposition of triglycerides could relate to the downregulation of sterol response proteins by leptin [18] and/or the inability of leptin to inactivate AMP kinase in muscle [19]. In other studies, leptin has also been associated with lower insulin secretion [20], but may also contribute to hyperinsulinemia that develops in MetS prior to the defects in insulin secretion that lead to the development of diabetes [21].

In light of the controversy, factor analysis has been used to show that there are several dominant, independent factors/components which underpin MetS. This work by Hanson *et al.* [22] suggests that insulin resistance, body mass index (BMI)/waist circumference, BP and lipid factors (triglycerides/HDL-C) are important factors in MetS. Similar analyses by Wang *et al.* [23] suggested that insulin resistance and BMI and waist:hip ratio (WHR) are very closely related. It has also been suggested by others that obesity has only been placed as a central feature of MetS because it decreases insulin-mediated glucose disposal. The argument is that excess abdominal adiposity is not a consequence of insulin resistance but a factor which modifies insulin resistance [24]. In addition, some authors note that not all insulin-resistant individuals are obese or vice versa [12]. In terms of MetS, it is suggested that obesity is best viewed as contributing to insulin resistance and hyperinsulinemia, rather than being consequence of abnormal insulin metabolism. It also must be borne in mind that the methods of factor analysis are not well standardized and that the interpretation of any results from this technique can be problematic.

Such controversy over which components are the most important is not limited to insulin resistance and abdominal obesity. Some argue that a definition should not have diabetes as a component if it is also considered to be an outcome of the syndrome [12]. However, since the links between hyperglycemia and each of the other components are very clear, it is hard to justify the exclusion of diabetes simply because many researchers choose to attempt to predict one component of the syndrome using the other components.

Further research is required to determine which factors are central to the development of this syndrome. Whatever the pathophysiological mechanism underlying MetS is, it seems highly likely that a sedentary lifestyle and dietary and genetic factors contribute to its development.

The diverse history of the evolving concept of MetS clearly illustrates how complex and heterogeneous the condition is. In recent times, there has been a distinct lack of agreement as to what

MetS is, and this confusion appears set to continue. What is agreed by researcher and physicians alike is that there is a need for some consensus in the thinking around the syndrome and an easy way to define it.

The benefits of deriving a clear, consistent definition for MetS are obvious. The establishment of a cohesive definition of MetS will allow the identification of individuals at high risk for prevention and treatment purposes, and the ability to compare the prevalence of MetS among populations and over time.

4.5 APPROACHES TO DEFINING METABOLIC SYNDROME

Efforts to understand and characterize MetS have led to several differing conceptual approaches when defining this syndrome, all of which begin from the simple observation of clustering of the key components. In one paradigm, an underlying feature (e.g. abdominal obesity or insulin resistance) is apparently clear, and any definition is derived from, and can be tested against, the association of potential components (and the proposed overall syndrome) with the identified underlying feature (**Figure 4.1a**). In a second paradigm, no assumptions are made about etiology, but components are simply selected by the statistical strength of their association with other components, and investigation of these associations may then lead to insights into the underlying causes (**Figure 4.1b**). The tensions between these competing approaches are readily apparent and are neatly illustrated by two recent papers. Both publications examined the associations between insulin resistance and the components of MetS, as defined by ATPIII, and found that the associations were not universally strong [16, 25]. One group concluded, therefore, that the ATPIII definition was flawed, since it failed to identify those with insulin resistance adequately [25]. In contrast, the other group suggested that since visceral fat was strongly related to all other components, it, rather than insulin resistance, was the underlying cause [16].

Superimposed on the two approaches noted above is the desire for clinical and public health relevance, which demands that any clinical decision (e.g. diagnosing MetS) is demonstrably valuable. This usually means that outcomes can be predicted

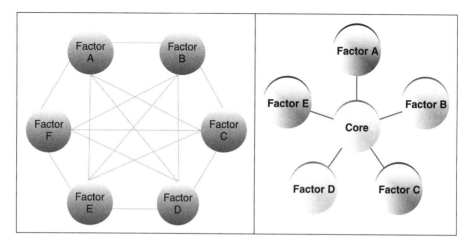

Figure 4.1 The two most common conceptual frameworks used to describe MetS. (a) MetS is represented by a set of factors which cluster with each other and no factor is known to be at the etiological core. (b) There is a presumed underlying feature which is related to and causes the other factors.

and preventative measures then taken. In the context of MetS, this means that it can be shown to be a good predictor of new cases of type 2 diabetes and CVD. However, since age, sex, smoking status and family history are not included in any definition of MetS (as they do not feature in the observed clusters), it is likely that MetS will never be the best predictor of either CVD or diabetes. Nevertheless, while risk prediction is a valuable asset, it may not be the single most important feature of any definition, even though it may dictate the extent to which the disorder is used in clinical practice. For example, in the general population, rheumatoid arthritis is unlikely to be useful as a predictor of joint replacements (most of which are due to osteoarthritis), but that does not mean that definitions of rheumatoid arthritis are without value.

Finally, there is a practical need to maintain simplicity. Thus, for example, it is desirable to have the cut-points used to define hyperglycemia and high BP in MetS the same as those used elsewhere to define states of abnormal glucose metabolism and hypertension. This can limit the freedom of *definition committees* in their selection of cut-points of the various components. The need for practicality also means that definitions that include insulin resistance, and perhaps even the oral glucose tolerance test (OGTT), will be of limited value, as measurement of insulin resistance is fraught with difficulties and the OGTT is often inconvenient and impractical.

4.6 CURRENT WORKING DEFINITIONS OF METABOLIC SYNDROME

In recent years, several working sets of criteria/definitions and/or statements have been developed for MetS, the most widely recognized of which are from the World Health Organization (WHO) [26], National Cholesterol Education Program Expert Panel on Detection, Evaluation and Treatment of High Blood Cholesterol in Adults (ATPIII) [27], the European Group for the Study of Insulin Resistance (EGIR) [28], the American College of Endocrinology (ACE) Task Force on the Insulin Resistance Syndrome [11] and more recently the International Diabetes Federation (IDF) [29, 30] (**Tables 4.1 and 4.2**).

Before such definitions were available, those characterizing this condition applied their own constructs which varied considerably in the number and weighting of the components, and the thresholds used for the various abnormalities. This approach and the fact that there were at least five available definitions of MetS led to a range of prevalences of MetS reported in the literature based on differing components and cut-points.

The first official definition of MetS developed was by a WHO consultative group [26] in 1998, which was later modified in 1999. This had glucose as a central theme, such that those with insulin resistance (measured using a euglycemic

Table 4.1 Current definitions of MetS.

WHO 1999	EGIR 1999	ATPIII 2001	IDF 2005
Diabetes or impaired glucose tolerance or insulin resistance[a]	Insulin resistance[b] or hyperinsulinemia (only nondiabetic subjects)		Central obesity: waist circumference (ethnicity specific)[c]
Plus two or more of the following:	Plus two or more of the following:	Three or more of the following:	Plus any two of the following:
1. Obesity: BMI > 30 kg m^{-2} or WHR > 0.9 (M) >0.85 (F)	1. Central obesity: waist circumference ≥ 94 cm (M), ≥ 80 cm (F)	1. Central obesity: waist circumference >102 cm (M), >88 cm (F)	1. Raised triglycerides ≥ 150 mg dl^{-1} (1.7 mmol l^{-1}) or specific treatment for this abnormality
2. Dyslipidemia: triglycerides ≥ 150 mg dl^{-1} (1.7 mmol l^{-1}) or HDL-C <35 mg dl^{-1} (0.9 mmol l^{-1}) (M) <39 g dl^{-1} (1.0 mmol l^{-1}) (F)	2. Dyslipidemia: triglycerides >177 mg dl^{-1} (2.0 mmol l^{-1}) or HDL-C <40 mg dl^{-1} (1.0 mmol l^{-1})	2. Hypertriglyceridemia: triglycerides ≥ 150 mg dl^{-1} (1.7 mmol l^{-1})	2. Reduced HDL-C <40 mg dl^{-1} (1.03 mmol l^{-1}) (M) <50 mg dl^{-1} (1.29 mmol l^{-1}) (F) or specific treatment for this abnormality
3. Hypertension: blood pressure $\geq 140/90$ mmHg or medication	3. Hypertension: blood pressure $\geq 140/90$ mmHg or medication	3. Low HDL-C: <40 mg dl^{-1} (1.03 mmol l^{-1}) (M), <50 mg dl^{-1} (1.29 mmol l^{-1}) (F)	3. Hypertension: 130/85 mmHg or medication
4. Microalbuminuria: albumin excretion ≥ 20 μg min^{-1} or albumin : creatinine ratio ≥ 30 mg g^{-1}	4. Fasting plasma glucose ≥ 110 mg dl^{-1} (6.1 mmol l^{-1})	4. Hypertension: blood pressure $\geq 130/85$ mmHg or medication	4. Fasting plasma glucose ≥ 100 mg dl^{-1} (5.6 mmol l^{-1}) or previously diagnosed type 2 diabetes[d]
		5. Fasting plasma glucose ≥ 110 mg dl^{-1} (6.1 mmol l^{-1})	

[a] Defined under hyperinsulinemic euglycemic conditions, glucose uptake below lowest quartile for background population.

[b] Defined as the top quartile of fasting insulin in the nondiabetic population.

[c] For guidelines on how to measure waist circumference accurately, see Table 4.3. If BMI is >30 kg m^{-2}, then central obesity can be assumed and waist circumference does not need to be measured.

[d] In clinical practice, IGT is also acceptable, but all reports of the prevalence of MetS should use only the fasting plasma glucose and presence of previously diagnosed diabetes to assess these criteria. If fasting plasma glucose is above 5.6 mmol l^{-1}, then OGTT is strongly recommended but is not necessary to define the presence of the syndrome.

Table 4.2 'Identifying abnormalities' according to the ACE position statement on the insulin resistance syndrome [11].

Identifying abnormality	Cut-point
1. Triglycerides	>150 mg dl^{-1} (1.7 mmol l^{-1})
2. HDL cholesterol	
Men	<40 mg dl^{-1} (1.03 mmol l^{-1})
Women	<50 mg dl^{-1} (1.29 mmol l^{-1})
3. Blood pressure	$>130/85$ mmHg
4. Glucose	
Fasting	110–125 mg dl^{-1} (6.1 mmol l^{-1})
2-h post glucose challenge	140–200 mg dl^{-1} (7.8-11.1 mmol l^{-1})

clamp), impaired glucose tolerance (IGT) or diabetes, together with at least two of raised BP, hypertriglyceridemia and/or low HDL-C, obesity, as measured by WHR or BMI, and microalbuminuria are classified as having the syndrome. This definition also highlighted several other factors that have been associated with MetS but which are not necessary for recognition of the syndrome. These include inflammatory or hemostatic factors such as hyperuricemia, coagulation disorders and raised plasminogen activating inhibitor. The crux of the WHO definition was the biological and physiological description of insulin resistance. Its main focus was to detect cases with insulin resistance and then its associated comorbidities. However, it must be borne in mind that this definition was initially promoted as a working model, with the authors acknowledging that it should be improved on as new data came to light [28].

Critics of the WHO definition identified several limitations, of which the most important relate to the use of the euglycemic clamp to measure insulin sensitivity, making the definition almost impossible to use in either clinical practice or epidemiological studies. They also contended that microalbuminuria was not a key metabolic component, though it may be an important consequence of the syndrome. Other weaknesses of this definition relate to the use of BMI and WHR as measures of obesity. Studies has indicated that BMI is not a good measure of obesity in the elderly due to the changes in height with advancing age and to the different ratio of lean and fat mass compared with younger adults [31]. It has also been shown that, for any given BMI, individuals in the highest waist tertile have a worse risk profile than those individuals with the same BMI but with a lower waist circumference measure [31]. Further, the use of WHR as a measure of central obesity may have some limitations, as it is an index of the relative accumulation of abdominal over peripheral fat rather than an absolute measure of visceral adiposity.

Recognizing that the WHO criteria were too complex to apply in many settings, and relied heavily on insulin resistance, the EGIR released a modification of the WHO criteria which would be easier to use as it relied on fasting insulin levels, instead of the euglycemic clamp, to measure insulin resistance [28]. This definition still retained insulin resistance as an essential component, arguing that this was a rational decision since much of the evidence to date suggested that insulin resistance was the underlying cause of MetS. This, in turn, meant that their modified definition had to be restricted to those in whom insulin resistance could be easily and reliably measured, and so the criteria were restricted to those without diabetes (as the addition of significant beta-cell dysfunction, which occurs in diabetes, to insulin resistance can make estimates of insulin sensitivity unreliable). However, the inclusion of fasting insulin in the EGIR definition is problematic, as insulin measurement is not well standardized [25]. The EGIR definition attempts to overcome this by defining insulin resistance as being in the top quartile of insulin measurements for the background population, but this is rarely known in clinical settings and could easily be biased in epidemiological studies (e.g. is it reasonable to use this definition if the population studied is all over the age of 50?). This definition also introduced waist circumference as the measure of adiposity, used modified cut-points for the other components and neither IGT or microalbuminuria were included as features.

Several years later, the ATPIII definition of MetS was developed [27]. The authors wanted to develop criteria which would be simple and hoped that its widespread use would ultimately lead to prevention of CVD and type 2 diabetes. Designed to have clinical utility, this definition did not include a specific measure of insulin sensitivity and also adopted a less *glucocentric* approach by treating all components with equal importance. Notably, it retained waist circumference as the measure of obesity (though with higher cut-points than EGIR). This definition has been noted for its simplicity, in that its components are easily and routinely measured in most settings, but studies have shown that it fails to identify all those with insulin resistance [32], which has led to some criticism.

A modification of the ATPIII definition was also developed by the American College of Clinical Endocrinology [11], and was based on the belief that insulin resistance was the core feature, and aimed to identify individuals with insulin resistance. The statement, deliberately labeled as such to allow the diagnosis to rely strongly on clinical judgment rather than satisfying specific criteria, lists four factors as 'identifying abnormalities' of the MetS. These were elevated triglycerides, reduced HDL-C, elevated BP and elevated fasting and postload glucose. Factors such as obesity, diagnosis of hypertension, gestational diabetes or CVD or family history of diabetes, hypertension, non European ancestry or age greater than 40 years and a sedentary lifestyle, are classified as factors which increase the likelihood of the syndrome rather than as key identifying abnormalities. While similar to the ATPIII definition, in that it excludes hyperinsulinemia, it also differs as it excludes obesity as a component, since abdominal obesity is viewed as a contributory factor in the development of insulin resistance rather than as a consequence of insulin resistance. The authors rationalize this approach on the basis that insulin assays are not standardized and the evidence implicating elevated plasma insulin as an independent risk factor for CVD is limited [33]. Omission of abdominal obesity as an identifying component in this statement has

evoked much criticism, especially in light of the growing evidence that central obesity is a major risk factor for type 2 diabetes and CVD [34, 35].

Since the initial release of the WHO and ATPIII definitions, there has also been much controversy about how best to measure obesity. It is generally accepted that BMI, though widely used, is not sufficiently sensitive to detect abdominal obesity in different ethnic groups. For example, South Asians have higher upper body and visceral fat for a given BMI when compared with Europids (people of white European origin). Furthermore, an elevated risk of type 2 diabetes [36] and CVD [37] for those with the MetS in this ethnic group is apparent at much lower levels of adiposity than in Europids. The likely inappropriateness of the ATPIII waist circumference cut-points for non-Europid populations is exemplified by the applying the ATPIII definition to an Asian population. This resulted in a very low prevalence of MetS, which seems out of keeping with the high prevalence of diabetes in such populations [36, 38]. This issue has been partly addressed by the recommendation by the WHO and others [39] that a lower BMI (BMI > 23 kg m^{-2}) should be used to classify South Asians as obese. Unfortunately, it has been argued that this modification only serves to add more confusion to already murky waters.

In light of the controversy over the various limitations in the current definitions, the IDF decided that a more practical definition that would be applicable globally for the identification of people at high risk of CVD, and diabetes, was urgently required [1, 29]. A consensus group was formed comprising members of the IDF from all regions and representatives from organizations, including those who had contributed to the previous definitions. The primary aim of this group was to develop a new set of criteria which would be clinically useful, particularly in a primary health care setting, and which would facilitate the comparison of data on MetS across countries and populations and highlight areas where more research was needed.

Recognizing that abdominal obesity is an important determinant in the causative pathway of MetS and that there is a strong association between waist circumference, CVD and other components of MetS, central obesity was placed in a central position of the construct. This has the further public

Table 4.3 Country/Ethnic specific values for waist circumference [30].

Country/ethnic group[a]	Waist circumference[b] (as measure of central obesity)		
Europids	Male	$\geq$94 cm	
	Female	$\geq$80 cm	
South, Southeast Asians, Japanese	Male	$\geq$90 cm	
	Female	$\geq$80 cm	
Ethnic South and Central Americans	Use Asian recommendations until more specific data are available		
Sub-Saharan Africans and Eastern Mediterranean and Middle East (Arab) populations	Use European recommendations until more specific data are available		

[a]Ethnicity should be the basis for classification, not the country of residence.
[b]In the United States the ATP III values (102 cm male; 88 cm female) are likely to continue to be used for clinical purposes.

health advantage of highlighting the importance of obesity, as the definition can be viewed as encompassing the key metabolic consequences of central obesity.

The consensus group also placed particular emphasis on developing criteria for obesity which were appropriate for a wider variety of populations. Using all the ethnic-specific body composition data available, they derived cut-points for abdominal obesity based on waist circumference that were applicable to individual ethnic groups (**Table 4.3**). It was also decided that the definition should be less *glucocentric* and, therefore, relegated diabetes status to a noncentral position. Moreover, it was recognized that since there are practical difficulties in accurately measuring insulin resistance, it was omitted as a component. This was thought to be reasonable, given that other components included (such as waist circumference and triglycerides) were so highly correlated with insulin resistance [35] that few of those with insulin resistance would be missed. The position and thresholds of other components were similar to those used in the ATPIII definition, except for glucose, where the cutoff of 100 mg dl^{-1} (5.6 mmol l^{-1}) recently recommended by the American Diabetes Association [40] was adopted for impaired fasting glucose.

In line with the WHO definition, the IDF definition also describes several other components which are sometimes associated with the syndrome but whose evidence is not sufficient as yet for inclusion in the definition. These include markers

of body composition, inflammatory markers, thrombotic markers, additional lipid-based factors, insulin resistance and others. It was recommended that these additional variables should be included in future research studies of MetS so that, when sufficient data concerning these additional markers does accumulate, the presence or absence of these factors may allow refinement of the definition of MetS, especially in different ethnic groups.

4.7 METABOLIC SYNDROME AND OTHER DISEASES

Clearly, the development of these definitions over the years has led to considerable confusion, an inability to compare prevalences of MetS between populations accurately and has hampered the progress of research into the area. To a large extent, the approach with each definition reflects different conceptual frameworks underlying each construct. For those who see MetS as a collection of components which reflect the clinical manifestations of insulin resistance, the WHO and EGIR definitions are the most appropriate. For others that believe MetS to be the consequence of abdominal obesity, a constellation of risk factors which predict CVD risk or merely a statistical phenomenon, the ATPIII definition may be more relevant. Not surprisingly, the choice of definition does matter, as each definition categorizes a distinct group of people [33]. The choice of the most suitable definition for MetS, therefore, depends on first deciding on what we are trying to achieve by having a definition for MetS. Among the many competing criteria a definition should meet, the highest priority may be the identification of those at risk of diabetes, CVD and all-cause mortality.

Many studies have examined the association of MetS with all-cause mortality, CVD and diabetes (reviewed in [41]). A summary of the evidence supporting the relationship between CVD, all-cause mortality and diabetes is featured below.

4.8 ALL-CAUSE MORTALITY

Of the many cohorts studies [42–51] examining the association of MetS and all-cause mortality, several studies showed a positive association. The San Antonio Heart Study [43] showed that meeting the MetS criteria by the ATPIII was associated with a 50% increased risk of mortality (hazard ratio (HR) of 1.5 (1.1–1.9) after adjustment for age, sex and race), while the Kuopio Ischemic Heart Study [42] using the WHO definition reported an adjusted relative risk (RR) of all-cause mortality of 1.8 (1.1–2.9), and the second National Health and Nutrition Examination Survey (NHANES) [51] reported an HR of mortality of 1.4 (1.2–1.7) for those defined by the ATP definition. The Aerobic Center Longitudinal Study (ACLS) showed using 10.2 years of follow-up and the ATP definition that MetS does predict all-cause mortality after adjustment for conventional risk factors, but this association was attenuated with the addition of physical activity. In later analyses using the same data, but longer follow-up, MetS defined by IDF (HR = 1.3 (1.1–1.5) or ATPIII (HR = 1.4 (1.1–1.6)) adjusted for smoking alcohol, history of CVD was associated with an increased risk of mortality.

More recently, a cohort study [50] from Sweden, with 32 years of follow-up showed that the WHO definition, but not the ATPIII definition, was associated with an increased risk of all-cause mortality after adjustment for conventional risk factors (HR = 1.4 (1.0–1.8)). The Diabetes Epidemiology: Collaborative Analysis of Diagnostic Criteria in Europe (DECODE) study [46], based on 11 prospective European cohort studies, also showed that participants with MetS defined by a modified version of the WHO criteria had increased all-cause mortality (HR = 1.4 (1.2–1.8)). In contrast, the National Health and Nutrition Examination

Survey II Mortality Study [44], the Health, Aging, and Body Composition (Health ABC) study [49], the Hoorn study [45], and patients with type 2 diabetes in the Casale Monferrato Study [47] failed to show that meeting the MetS criteria by ATPIII or WHO increased risk of all-cause mortality.

In a recent meta-analysis combining the data from only three of the above studies, the summary estimate for all-cause mortality was 1.3, indicating that any association between MetS and all-cause mortality is modest at best [41].

4.8.1 Cardiovascular Disease

The relationship between MetS and CVD has been well documented in many observational studies [52, 53]. Studies comparing the ability of MetS to predict coronary heart disease (CHD) and stroke with traditional means of CVD risk prediction, such as the Framingham risk score, have shown that while MetS is a significant predictor of CHD, it is does not predict as well as the Framingham risk score [54, 55]. Given that the MetS definition does not include smoking status or age, which are strong drivers of CVD risk, these results are not surprising. However, there was also no advantage gained in risk assessment by adding the component of MetS to the Framingham risk score [56].

The large preponderance of evidence describing the ability of MetS to predict 'hard CVD events' suggests that MetS is an independent predictor of CVD, regardless of the definition used [41]. Of the many studies [42–44, 49, 50, 57–63] examining this association prospectively, using the ATPIII definition or a modification of it, the vast majority of studies have shown MetS to be an independent predictor of CVD or CHD or composite CVD outcome, of an approximate magnitude ranging from 1.6 to 1.8. The notable exceptions to this are the Strong Heart Study (SHS) [49], which examined heart disease and diabetes in American Indians, and the ACLS [49]. In the SHS, ATPIII-defined MetS only predicted CVD in diabetic patients. The reasons why MetS did not predict CVD in the SHS are unclear, but the authors suggest that most of the CVD risk from MetS is mediated through the development of diabetes and that they may have had too few incident cases of diabetes as the possible explanations. In the ACLS, MetS was a predictor for CVD mortality after adjustment for conventional risk factors; but, similar to all-cause mortality, with further adjustment for cardiovascular fitness the association became nonsignificant, indicating that cardiovascular fitness attenuates the mortality risk associated with the syndrome [49].

Similar to the ATPIII-defined MetS, WHO-defined MetS significantly predicts incident CVD or CVD mortality in the vast majority of prospective studies [42, 45, 46, 50, 52]. However, since the WHO definition mandates the use of a euglycemic clamp to measure insulin resistance, there is considerably more heterogeneity in the actual WHO definitions used in each study. Early reports from the Botnia study showed that, using a modified version of the WHO definition, individuals with MetS were at increased risk of CVD mortality (HR = 1.8 (1.2–2.7)) [52]. Interestingly, a study in Sweden using both the modified and the *exact* WHO definitions showed that while both definitions predicted CVD, the exact WHO-defined individuals were at lower risk than those classified by the modified WHO definition [50]. In a Finnish study, the Kuopio Ischemic Heart Disease Study, with 11.4 years of follow-up, it was reported that CVD mortality was increased 2.6-fold in middle-aged men with WHO-defined MetS [42].

In the DECODE study, WHO-defined MetS was highly predictive of CVD mortality with an HR of 2.3 (1.6–3.2) for men and 2.8 (1.6–4.9) for women after adjustment for other risk factors [46]. In older patients from the Cardiovascular Health Study [64], the WHO-defined MetS was not an independent predictor of CVD events.

Using patients with diabetes, who had neither ATPIII- nor WHO-defined MetS as the reference group, in 2 years of follow-up, it was observed that WHO-defined MetS, but not ATPIII-defined MetS, had the highest mortality, adjusted for sex [38]. In contrast, patients with diabetes in the Casale Monferrato Study defined as having MetS using the WHO definition were not at increased risk of CVD mortality [47].

Most, but not all, of the current evidence suggests that the WHO definition of MetS is better able to predict those at risk of CVD than the ATPIII or the IDF definitions (although many more of prospective studies used the ATPIII definition of MetS to predict the CVD than the WHO definition, and only one for the IDF definition). This finding has been attributed mainly to the central position of insulin resistance in the WHO construct. In a

study by Lakka *et al*. [42], when insulin resistance was added to the ATPIII definition it performed similarly to the WHO definition. For this reason, many favor the inclusion of insulin resistance in the definition; but because the measurement of insulin resistance is problematic, the inclusion of insulin resistance as a component in any definition can also represent a weakness. It has also been suggested that the better predictive value of the WHO over the ATPIII definition of MetS for prediction of CVD may be due to the inclusion of microalbuminuria in the WHO definition [38].

However, a recent meta-analysis, which considered in subgroup analyses, only those studies which used both definitions, reported a summary estimate for CVD based on the ATPIII-defined MetS of 2.7 (1.9–3.8). In the same study, using a modified version of the WHO definition, the summary relative risk for CVD was 1.9 (1.3–2.6). The Cardiovascular Health Study, which also used both definitions in the prediction of CVD, was excluded as the patient population was considerably older at 65 years or greater. In this study, the MetS defined by the ATPIII, but not the WHO criteria, was an independent predictor of coronary or CVD events. Consideration of these findings must be tempered by the fact that there are very few studies using both definitions and many of the studies used a modified version of the WHO definition.

There are very few studies examining the association of the more recent IDF-defined MetS and CVD. In a population-based cross-sectional study of an urban sample of 2334 participants from Beijing, China, aged 60–95, there was an increased CVD risk for those defined by the ATPIII (odds ratio (OR) = 1.5 (1.3–1.8)), and for those defined by the IDF (OR = 1.7 (1.5–2.1)) definitions of MetS [65]. In a Greek population, IDF-defined MetS individuals had much lower risk of vascular events when compared with their ATPIII-defined counterparts [66]. The only prospective studies which have examined whether IDF-defined MetS is associated with CVD were conducted in Hispanic men from the Health ABC study and women from the British Women's Heart and Health Study. In the former study, the RR values for CVD mortality for ATPIII- and IDF-defined MetS were 1.8 (1.4–2.4) and 1.7 (1.3–2.2) respectively, indicating little difference between the two definitions in their ability to predict CVD mortality [67]. In the British Women's Heart and Health Study, IDF-, ATP- and WHO-defined MetS predicted incident CHD of similar magnitude (1.3 versus 1.5 versus 1.4), although the latter two were of borderline significance [68]. Since there are limited prospective data examining the relationship between the IDF-defined MetS and CVD disease, the true value of the IDF definition in the prediction of CVD cannot be fully clarified.

4.8.2   Diabetes

Several studies have shown that MetS is associated with diabetes using either the ATPIII or the WHO definition [55, 60, 61, 69–73]. Among those studies which used the ATPII definition to define the syndrome, the magnitude of risk associated with MetS varied from three- to six-fold [41]. In a meta-analysis of five prospective studies using the ATPIII or a modified version of the ATPIII to define MetS, the estimate was 3.0 (2.2–4.4) [41]. Prospective studies which used a modified WHO definition to show that the MetS is associated with incident diabetes are limited to only a few [55, 72]. In meta-analyses of the findings of two of these studies, the summary estimate of risk associated with MetS was 6.0 (4.8–7.8) [41]. In a recent study, MetS defined by the five definitions (ATPIII, IDF, WHO, EGIR and ACE) was associated with a 1.9–3.0 times higher risk for incident diabetes [73]. A comparison of the predictive ability of the ATPIII and WHO definitions to predict diabetes with conventional diabetes-prediction tools, such as the diabetes predicting model [55], showed that both of the MetS definitions were inferior to the diabetes-predicting model in the prediction of diabetes [55]. Since impaired glucose tolerance (IGT) is a predictor of type 2 diabetes, it is not surprising that WHO-defined MetS is a better predictor of diabetes than the ATPII-defined MetS. In studies where IGT was excluded from the WHO definition, MetS defined by the ATPIII and WHO definitions predicted incident diabetes at a similar magnitude [55].

4.9   RISK FACTORS FOR METABOLIC SYNDROME

Given the rising prevalence of MetS, determining who is at risk of developing the condition has become very important. Although, obesity has

been reported to be a risk factor for MetS in cross-sectional and prospective studies [74–76], health behaviors and dietary composition (other modifiable risk factors) have been identified as risk factors for the development of MetS. In the Coronary Artery Risk Development in Young Adults (CARDIA) Study, high BMI, no alcohol intake, male sex, higher intake of carbohydrates, low intake of crude fiber and low education levels were also independent risk factors for MetS after adjustment for age, sex and race [76]. In this study, regular physical activity over low physical activity was protective against MetS. The Insulin Resistance Atherosclerosis Study showed that proinsulin, HDL-C, and waist circumference were also predictors of incident MetS in those without diabetes after adjustment for age, sex, ethnicity and IGT [75]. Prevention strategies for MetS should focus on lifestyle modification specifically, weight loss, increased physical levels and modification to dietary intake of carbohydrate.

4.10   PREVALENCE OF METABOLIC SYNDROME

4.10.1   Prevalence of Metabolic Syndrome in Adults

Since the introduction of classification systems to define MetS, there have been many reports in the medical literature of the prevalence of the condition in various populations. A summary of the current worldwide prevalence data of MetS is detailed in **Table 4.4**, but this is by no means exhaustive. The studies included vary with respect to study design, the definition of MetS that is used, sample selection, the year the study was conducted, and the age and sex structure of the population. For these reasons, the prevalence varies considerably and it is difficult to draw global conclusions. If any general comments can be made, then it can be said that East Asians (Koreans, Chinese and Japanese) have a lower prevalence of MetS even when obesity cut-points appropriate for Asians are used. The prevalence of MetS appears high in indigenous populations [77, 78], consistent with the high risk of type 2 diabetes and CVD often found in these populations. In the studies that have compared IDF-defined MetS with ATPIII-defined MetS, the prevalence of the IDF-defined MetS is almost always higher than that estimated by

Table 4.4 A summary of the studies estimating prevalence of the metabolic syndrome using various definitions.

Reference	Country, city	Year	Diagnostic criteria	Sample size N	Age (years)	Prevalence (%)
Abdul-Rahim et al. [79]	Kobar & Ramallah; occupied Palestinian Territories	1996–1998	WHO (modified)	992 (500 rural, 492 urban)	30–65	Rural: 17 Urban: 17
Adams et al. [80]	South Australia, Australia	2005[a]	IDF ATPIII	4060	≥18	ATPIII Total: 15 Male: 19 Female: 14 IDF Total: 23 Male: 26 Female: 16
Alexander et al. [81] Al-Lawati et al. [82, 83]	USA Nizwa, Oman	2003[a] 2001	ATPIII ATPIII	3510 1419	≥50 ≥20	ATPIII: 44 Total: 21[c] Male: 20[c] Female: 23[c]
Araneta et al. [84]	San Diego, USA	1992–1999	ATPIII	294 Filipino 379 Caucasian	50–69	Filipina women: 34 Caucasian women: 13
Athyros et al. [66]	Greece	2003	ATPIII	N1: 4513 N2: 300 N3: 300	N1: mean age 47 N2: mean age 55 N3: mean age 37	N1: 24[c] N2: 35[c] N3: 9[c]
Athyros et al. [85]	Greece	2005[a]	IDF ATP	9669	≥18	IDF: 43[c] ATPIII: 25[c]
Azizi et al. [86]	Tehran, Islamic Republic of Iran	1999–2001	ATPIII	9846	>20	Total: 30 Male: 42 Female: 24
Balkau et al. [87]	England	1992	EGIR WHO (modified)	1115	40–65	WHO Male: 45 Female: 34 EGIR Male: 18 Female: 14
Balkau and co-workers [87, 88]	France	1996	EGIR WHO (modified)	4779	30–65	WHO Males: 24 Females: 10 EGIR Males:16 Females:10
Bo et al. [89]	Asti, Italy	2005[a]	ATPIII	1658	45–64	Total: 23 Male: 24 Female: 22

Reference	Location	Year	Criteria	N	Age	Prevalence
Boronat et al. [90]	Telde, Gran Canaria Islands	1998	ATPIII WHO (modified) EGIR	1030	≥30	WHO Male: 33[c] Female: 24[c] ATPIII Male: 22[c] Female: 24[c] EGIR Male: 17[c] Female: 15[c]
Cameron et al. [91]	Mauritius	1987	WHO ATPIII EGIR (modified)	3171	>24	WHO Total: 19 Male: 21 Female: 18 ATPIII Total: 13 Male: 11 Female: 15 EGIR Total: 10 Male: 9.0 Female: 10
Deepa et al. [92]	Chennai, India	2002[a]	EGIR (modified)	1070	>20	EGIR Total: 11 Male: 13 Female: 10
Deepa et al. [93]	Chennai, India	2002–2004	IDF ATPIII WHO	2350	≥20	IDF: 26 ATPIII: 18 WHO: 23
Drivsholm and co-workers [94]	Denmark	1997	WHO EGIR	678	60	WHO Male: 38 Female: 22 EGIR Male: 22 Female: 16
Balkau et al. [87] Ford [95]	USA	1999–2002	IDF ATPIII	3601	≥20	IDF Total: 39[c] Male: 41[c] Female: 38[c] ATPIII Total: 35[c] Male: 35[c] Female: 35[c]
Gu et al. [96]	China	2000–2001	ATPIII (modified)	15540	35–74	Male: 10[c], Female: 8[c]
Guerrero-Romero and Rodriguez-Moran [97]	Durango City, Mexico	2005[a]	IDF ATPIII WHO	700	30–64	IDF: 22 ATPIII: 23 WHO: 15
Gutpa et al. [98]	Jaipur, India	2003[a]	ATPIII	1091	>20	Total: 13 Male: 8 Female: 18

(continued)

Table 4.4 (*continued*)

Reference	Country, city	Year	Diagnostic criteria	Sample size N	Age (years)	Prevalence (%)
He et al. [65]	Beijing, China	2001–2002	ATPIII (modified) IDF	2334	>60	ATPIII Total: 31, Male: 18, Female: 39; IDF Total: 46, Male: 35, Female: 54
Hedblad et al. [99] Balkau et al. [87]	Sweden	1994	EGIR (modified) WHO (modified)	5296	46–68	WHO Male: 43, Female: 26; EGIR Male: 24, Female: 14
Hu et al. [46]	DECODE study – 11 European prospective studies	2005	WHO	11512	30–89	WHO Male: 16[c], Female: 14[c]
Ilanne-Parikka et al. [100]	Finland	1992	WHO (modified)	2049	45–94	WHO Male: 39, Female: 22
Ko et al. [101]	Hong Kong	2005[a]	WHO EGIR ATPIII (modified)	1513	18–66	ATPIII Total: 10, Male: 11, Female: 8; EGIR Total: 9, Male: 9, Female: 10; WHO Total: 13, Male: 15, Female: 11
Laaksonen et al. [72]	Kuopio, Finland	1988–1989	EGIR (modified) ATPIII (modified)	1005	42, 48, 54 or 60	EGIR (WHR > 0.90): 25, EGIR (WC ≥ 94 cm): 21, ATPIII (WC ≥ 102 cm): 14, ATPIII (WC ≥ 94 cm): 21
Lawlor et al. [68]	England	1999–2001	IDF ATPIII WHO	3589	60–79	IDF: 48, ATPIII: 30, WHO: 21
Lean et al. [102] Balkau et al. [87]	Netherlands	1995	EGIR (modified) WHO (modified)	1378	20–60	WHO Male:19, Female:8; EGIR Male: 13, Female: 8

Reference	Location	Year	Criteria	Sample	Age	Prevalence
Lorenzo et al. [67]	South America	2006	ATPIII, IDF	San Antonio – Mexicans, San Antonio – NH whites, Mexico City, Spain, Peru	Mean age: 49.0, Mean age: 49.5, Mean age: 46.6, Mean age: 48.5, Mean age: 47.5	ATPIII: Male: 33. Female: 36 / Male: 29. Female: 26 / Male: 33. Female: 56 / Male: 22. Female: 31 / Male: 12. Female: 26. IDF: Male: 46. Female: 41 / Male: 38. Female: 29 / Male: 54. Female: 61 / Male: 28. Female: 34 / Male: 26. Female: 28
Lorenzo et al. [103], Balkau et al. [87]	Spain	1996	EGIR, WHO (modified)	2025	35–64	WHO: Male: 26, Female: 20. EGIR: Male: 16, Female: 15
Marques-Vidal et al. [104]	Haute Garonne, southwestern France	1994–1997	WHO (modified)	1153	35–64	WHO: Total: 17, Male: 23, Female: 12
Meigs et al. [105]	Framingham, USA; San Antonio, USA	2003[a]	ATPIII, WHO	3224 Framingham Study; 2737 San Antonio Heart Study:	30–79	ATPIII: Framingham-ATPIII Male: 27[c]. Female: 21[c]; San Antonio-ATPIII Mexican Male: 29[c] Female: 33[c] Non-Hispanic whites Male: 25[c]. Female: 21[c]. WHO: Males: 32[c]. Females: 20[c]
Mohamed-Ali et al. [106], Balkau et al. [87]	England	1991	EGIR (modified), WHO (modified)	887	40–75	WHO: Male: 13, Female: 13. EGIR: Male: 5, Female: 4
Oh et al. [107]	Mokdong, South Korea	1997	ATPIII (modified)	774	30–80	ATPIII: Male: 29, Female: 17
Onat et al. [57]	Turkey	2000	ATPIII	2296	≥31	ATPIII: Male: 27, Female: 39
Pollex et al. [77]	Ontario, Canada	1993–1995	ATPIII	515	≥18	ATPIII: Total: 30, Male: 25, Female: 34
Ramachandran et al. [108]	Chennai, India	1995	ATPIII (modified)	475	20–75	ATPIII: Total: 41, Male: 36, Female: 47
Resnick et al. [60]	USA	1989–1992	ATPIII	2283	45–74	ATPIII: 35
Satter et al. [61]	Scotland	1989–1995	ATPIII (modified)	6447	45–64	ATPIII: 26

(continued)

Table 4.4 (*continued*)

Reference	Country, city	Year	Diagnostic criteria	Sample size N	Age (years)	Prevalence (%)	
Scuteri et al. [64]	USA	1989–1990	ATPIII WHO (modified)	2175	40–79	ATPIII Total: 35 Male: 32 Female: 37	WHO Total: 28 Male: 32 Female: 24
Shiwaku et al. [109]	Japan, Korea and Mongolia	1999–2003	ATPIII (modified)	752	30–60	ATPIII (BMI ≥ 25) Japanese: 12 Koreans: 13 Mongolians: 16	ATPIII (BMI ≥ 30) Japanese: 7 Koreans: 7 Mongolians: 12
Simmons and Thompson [78]	Auckland, New Zealand	2004[a]	ATPIII	1592	≥40	ATPIII Ages: 40–59 *European* Male: 25 Female: 13 *Maori* Male: 53 Female: 52 *Pacific Islander* Male: 49 Female: 46	ATPIII Ages: 60–79 *European* Male: 22 Female: 31 *Maori* Male: 67 Female: 45 *Pacific Islander* Male: 40 Female: 44
Son et al. [110]	Ho Chi Minh City, Vietnam	2005[a]	ATPIII (modified)	611	≥20	12[d]	
Song et al. [111]	Ansan, South Korea	1999–2001	ATPIII (modified)	1798	25–74	Total: 32 Male: 35 Female: 29	
Thomas et al. [112]	Hong Kong	1994–1996	ATPIII (modified)	2843	18–84	ATPIII (Asian specific waist) Total: 25[d] Male: 21[d] Female: 29[d]	ATPIII (WHO waist) Total: 22[d] Male: 20[d] Female: 24[d]

Study	Location	Date	Criteria	Sample size	Age	Prevalence (%)
Tillin et al. [113]	London, England	1988–1991	ATPIII WHO	2346 European Asians 803 Afro-Caribbeans	40–69	ATPIII — South Asian Male: 29[c], Female: 32[c]; European Male: 18[c], Female: 14[c]; Africans-Caribbean Male: 14[c], Female: 23[c]. WHO — South Asian Male: 46[c], Female: 31[c]; Europeans Male: 9[c], Female: 9[c]; Africans-Caribbean Male: 27[c], Female: 26[c]
Unpublished[b]	Australia	1999–2000	ATPIII EGIR WHO (modified)	7982	>35	ATPIII — Total: 18, Male: 20, Female: 17. EGIR — Total: 16, Male: 19, Female: 13. WHO — Total: 21, Male: 25, Female: 17
Villegas et al. [114]	Ireland	2003[a]	WHO ATPIII	1018	50–69	WHO — Total: 21, Male: 25, Female: 18. ATPIII — Total: 21, Male: 22, Female: 22
Vozarova de Courten et al. [115]	Zate Klasy, southern Slovakia	1998	WHO (modified)	501 Non-gypsies 156 Gypsies	≥30	Non-gypsies: 20, Gypsies: 4
Zavoroni et al. [116] Balkau et al. [87]	Italy	1981	EGIR WHO (modified)	729	22–73 (men) 22–55 (women)	EGIR — Male: 12, Female: 5. WHO — Male: 9, Female: 2
Zavoroni et al. [116] Balkau et al. [87]	Italy	1995	EGIR WHO (modified)	375	40–81 (men) 40–55 (women)	EGIR — Male: 25, Female: 14. WHO — Male: 35, Female: 18

[a] Indicates date of publication, rather than the date the study was conducted.
[b] Unpublished work from the International Diabetes Institute, Melbourne, Australia, presented at the Australian Diabetes Society meeting in Melbourne, 2003.
[c] Age standardized prevalence.
[d] Age and sex standardized prevalence. Prevalence estimates have been rounded to one decimal place.

the ATPIII definition. Furthermore, the prevalence of MetS increased with age irrespective of the definitions used.

Studies describing the change in prevalence over time of MetS have shown that the prevalence of MetS is increasing. In the San Antonio Heart Study, an increase in the prevalence of MetS was observed in most age groups studied. The increase was also apparent in Mexican Americans, non-Hispanic whites, and in diabetic and nondiabetic individuals [117]. Also, in this study, worsening obesity was associated with a rising prevalence of MetS. An increase in the prevalence of MetS was also shown in cross-sectional surveys conducted between 1988 and 1994 and 1999–2000 in the United States, although this increase was only statistically significant in women. Interestingly, an increase in waist circumference over the two surveys was reported in both sexes in this study [118].

4.10.2 Prevalence of Metabolic Syndrome in Children and Adolescents

There are several studies which have reported the prevalence of MetS in children and adolescents using various definitions [77, 119–124]. A study by Csabi et al. [119] conducted in obese and normal-weight Hungarian children, aged 8–18 years, identified those with MetS by the presence of hyperinsulinemia, hypertension, IGT and dyslipidemia. Using this definition, 8.9% of obese children and 0.4% of controls were classified as being MetS positive. However, in that study, the controls did not have an OGTT. Two studies from the American NHANES study have produced interesting results. One group studying a representative sample of 2430 children, aged 12–19, from NHANES (1988–1992), using the ATPIII definition with modified cut-points, reported a prevalence of 4.2% overall and 28.7% in overweight adolescents [123]. The other group studied a sample of 991, aged 12–19, from NHANES (1999–2000) and using the ATPIII definition modified for age showed that the overall prevalence had increased to 6.4% and to 32.1% in overweight adolescents [124]. A smaller study of 126 obese Hispanic children, aged 8–13, also from the United States (defining the syndrome as at least three of abdominal obesity, low HDL cholesterol, hypertriglyceridemia, hypertension and/or IGT), reported a prevalence of 30% [125]. In adolescent aboriginal Canadians, the crude

prevalence using the ATPIII definition was found to be not dissimilar to other ethnic groups at 5.4% [77]. More recently, Invitti et al. [120] derived a modified WHO-based definition of MetS with child-specific criteria based on age and sex. Using this definition on Caucasian children, and ethnically matched controls, the prevalence of MetS was 23.0% in the overall group and 23.3% in the subgroup of obese children. Perhaps even more interesting is that this work also showed that nontraditional CVD risk factors, such as plasminogen activator inhibitor type 1, uric acid and microalbuminuria, are associated with MetS in children, suggesting further reasons why these children may be at a heightened risk of CVD.

It is difficult to ascertain whether the variation in the prevalence of MetS in children and adolescents is due to the use of very different definitions of MetS or some other factors; thus, there is a greater degree of uncertainty surrounding the prevalence of MetS in these populations. What is abundantly clear is that MetS is certainly present in young people, highlighting the need to derive a standardized definition for adolescents and children.

4.11 GENETICS OF METABOLIC SYNDROME

With a condition such as the MetS, environmental factors (namely obesity and sedentary lifestyles) are obvious significant determinants of the disease [126]. There is, however, a growing body of evidence to suggest that there may be a genetic basis to this condition. Family studies have shown that clusters of metabolic risk factors, such as insulin resistance and BP may be inherited [127, 128], and twin studies suggest a higher concordance of components of MetS among monozygotic twins compared with dizygotic twins. Furthermore, heritabilities of key qualifying components of MetS, such as waist circumference and WHR, are reasonably high, at around 60%. Heritability also influences other components of the syndrome, such as hypertension [129], triglycerides and HDL-C [130] and microalbuminuria [131]. Traits of MetS have also been linked to loci on chromosomes 1, 3, 6, 7, 17 and 18, although the significance of these loci is unknown. Family studies have shown that common sets of genes may determine fasting insulin, lipid and obesity traits of MetS [132]. More recently conducted family studies have shown that MetS strongly predicts cardiac morbidity and mortality in healthy patients with a family background of coronary artery disease (CAD) at a much higher rate than those without a family history of CAD [133].

Several single nucleotide polymorphisms or combinations of them (haplotypes) have been identified in individuals with MetS in genes encoding $\beta2$ and $\beta3$ adrenergic receptor, calpain 10, peroxisome proliferator-activated receptor γ, skeletal muscle glycogen synthase (GYS1) and adiponectin, all of which may increase risk for MetS. However, it must be understood that each of these genes contributes only a small portion to the individual and population risk for MetS and the contribution of each, not surprisingly, varies with ethnicity.

The thrifty gene hypothesis has also been implicated to be associated with MetS. This hypothesis, proposed first by Neel [134], suggests that individuals living in harsh environments with unstable food supply would maximize their probability of survival if they could maximize storage rather than oxidation of surplus energy. Therefore, in times of famine, those with this genotype would be naturally selected to survive. While this theory initially received much attention as a possible explanation for type 2 diabetes and MetS, the actual genes responsible for it have remained elusive. More recently, a somewhat related, but distinct, phenomenon coined the 'thrifty phenotype' has been described. The thrifty phenotype hypothesis proposes that the epidemiological associations between poor fetal and infant growth and the subsequent development of type 2 diabetes and MetS result from the effects of poor nutrition in early life, which produces permanent changes in glucose–insulin metabolism. In this theory, poor fetal and early postnatal malnutrition impose mechanisms of nutritional thrift upon the growing individual by leading to an immature pancreas and low birth weight, which in turn leads to insulin resistance and increased risk of MetS later in life; small birthweight babies and insulin resistance later in life being the phenotype for the thrifty gene [135]. Some support for this work can be found in family studies showing that the risk of small birthweight babies is increased in families with MetS, indicating that small birthweight is a phenotype for the thrifty gene [136]. Furthermore, children with a glucokinase defect (and accompanying decrease in insulin) have a low birthweight [137].

4.12 SUMMARY AND CONCLUSION

MetS is a constellation of metabolic abnormalities, including centrally distributed obesity, decreased HDL-C, elevated triglycerides, elevated blood pressure, and hyperglycemia and insulin resistance/hyperinsulinemia, which cluster together to a greater degree than expected by chance. An important feature of MetS is its association with type 2 diabetes and atherosclerotic CVD. Obesity and/or insulin resistance have been described as the key underlying components of the syndrome, but the exact etiology and pathogenesis of the condition is still unclear. While lifestyle and environment factors contribute to MetS, there is also a genetic basis for the condition, which is an area that requires more research. The prevalence of MetS worldwide ranges from 10 to 50%, is highly age dependent [33] and is increasing primarily due to the pandemic of obesity and diabetes experienced by both developed and developing worlds. Past attempts to characterize and define this condition have led to confusion. The recent development of new criteria from the IDF does in part find some compromises between the WHO and the ATPIII definitions, and also begins to address ethnic differences between populations. It may not, however, completely resolve all of the confusion and inconsistencies in defining MetS.

Perhaps of greatest significance is the fact that, in concert with an aging population and the rising prevalence of glucose intolerance and obesity [138], the burden imposed by MetS, which is already large, is set to increase. The scope for prevention of CVD and diabetes for those with MetS is indeed vast and poses a great challenge for the next decade.

References

1. Eckel, R.H., Grundy, S.M. and Zimmet, P.Z. (2005) The metabolic syndrome. *Lancet*, **365**, 1415–28.

2. Beijer, T., Bosman-Jelgersema, H.A., Dudok van Heel, S.A.C. *et al.* (1991) *Nicolaes Tulp*, Six Art Promotions BV, Amsterdam.

3. Morgagni, J.B. (1765/1975) *The Seats and Causes of Diseases Investigated by Anatomy (De Sedibus et Causis Morborum per Anatomen Indagata)*, Remondini, Padova.

4. Kylin, E. (1923) Studien uber das Hypertonie-Hyperglyka 'mie-Hyperurika' miesyndrom. *Zentralblatt fuer Innere Medizin*, **44**, 105–27.

5. Vague, J. (1947) La differenciation sexuelle, factuer determinant des formes de l'obesite. *Presse Medicale*, **30**, 339–40.

6. Avogaro, P., Crepaldi, G., Enzi, G. and Tiengo, A. (1965) Metabolic aspects of essential obesity. *Epatologia*, **11**, 226–38.

7. Haller, H. (1977) Epidemiology and associated risk factors of hyperlipoproteinemia. *Zeitschrift für die Gesamte innere Medizin und ihre Grenzgebiete*, **32**, 124–8.

8. Vague, P., Juhan-Vague, I., Chabert, V. *et al.* (1989) Fat distribution and plasminogen activator inhibitor activity in nondiabetic obese women. *Metabolism*, **38**, 913–15.

9. Reaven, G. (1988) Role of insulin resistance in human disease. *Diabetes*, **37**, 1595–607.

10. Ferrannini, E., Haffner, S., Mitchell, B. *et al.* (1991) Hyperinsulinaemia: the key feature of a cardiovascular and metabolic syndrome. *Diabetologia*, **34**, 416–22.

11. American College of Endocrinology Task Force on the Insulin Resistance Syndrome (2003) American College of Endocrinology position statement on the insulin resistance syndrome. *Endocrine Practice*, **9**, 236–52.

12. Aguilar-Salinas, C.A., Rojas, R., Gomez-Perez, F.J. *et al.* (2005) The metabolic syndrome: a concept hard to define. *Archives of Medical Research*, **36**, 223–31.

13. Matsuda, M., Shimomura, I., Sata, M. *et al.* (2002) Role of adiponectin in preventing vascular stenosis. The missing link of adipo-vascular axis. *The Journal of Biological Chemistry*, **277**, 37487–91.

14. Stefan, N. and Stumvoll, M. (2002) Adiponectin – its role in metabolism and beyond. *Hormone and Metabolic Research*, **34**, 469–74.

15. Gil-Campos, M., Canete, R.R. and Gil, A. (2004) Adiponectin, the missing link in insulin resistance and obesity. *Clinical Nutrition*, **23**, 963–74.

16. Carr, D.B., Utzschneider, K.M., Hull, R.L. *et al.* (2004) Intra-abdominal fat is a major determinant of the National Cholesterol Education Program Adult Treatment Panel III criteria for the metabolic syndrome. *Diabetes*, **53**, 2087–94.

17. Mantzoros, C.S. (1999) The role of leptin in human obesity and disease: a review of current evidence. *Annals of Internal Medicine*, **130**, 671–80.

18. Kakuma, T., Lee, Y., Higa, M. *et al.* (2000) Leptin, troglitazone, and the expression of sterol regulatory element binding proteins in liver and pancreatic islets. *Proceedings of the National Academy of Sciences of the United States of America*, **97**, 8536–41.

19. Minokoshi, Y. and Kahn, B.B. (2003) Role of AMP-activated protein kinase in leptin-induced fatty acid oxidation in muscle. *Biochemical Society Transactions*, **31**, 196–201.

20. Cases, J.A., Gabriely, I., Ma, X.H. *et al.* (2001) Physiological increase in plasma leptin markedly inhibits insulin secretion in vivo. *Diabetes*, **50**, 348–52.

21. Seufert, J. (2004) Leptin effects on pancreatic beta-cell gene expression and function. *Diabetes*, **53** (Suppl 1), S152–8.

22. Hanson, R.L., Imperatore, G., Bennett, P.H. and Knowler, W.C. (2002) Components of the 'metabolic syndrome' and incidence of type 2 diabetes. *Diabetes*, **51**, 3120–7.

23. Wang, J.J., Qiao, Q., Miettinen, M.E. *et al.* (2004) The metabolic syndrome defined by factor analysis and incident type 2 diabetes in a Chinese population with high postprandial glucose. *Diabetes Care*, **27**, 2429–37.

24. American Association of Clinical Endocrinology (2003) American Association of Clinical Endocrinology position statement on insulin resistance syndrome. *Endocrine Practice*, **9**, 237–52.

25. Cheal, K.L., Abbasi, F., Lamendola, C. *et al.* (2004) Relationship to insulin resistance of the Adult Treatment Panel III diagnostic criteria for identification of the metabolic syndrome. *Diabetes*, **53**, 1195–200.

26. World Health Organisation (1999) *Definition, Diagnosis and Classification of Diabetes Mellitus and Its Complications. Part 1: Diagnosis and Classification of Diabetes Mellitus*, Department of Non-communicable Diseases Surveillance, World Health Organization, Geneva.

27. Expert Panel on Detection, Evaluation, and Treatment of High Blood Cholesterol in Adults (2001) Executive summary of the third report of The National Cholesterol Education Program (NCEP) Expert Panel on Detection, Evaluation, and Treatment of High Blood Cholesterol in Adults (Adult Treatment Panel III). *Journal of the American Medical Association*, **285**, 2486–97.

28. Balkau, B. and Charles, M.A. (1999) Comment on the provisional report from the WHO consultation. European Group for the Study of Insulin Resistance (EGIR). *Diabetic Medicine*, **16**, 442–3.

29. Zimmet, P., Alberti, G. and Shaw, J. (2005) Mainstreaming the metabolic syndrome: a definitive definition. *The Medical Journal of Australia*, **183**, 175–6.

30. Alberti, K.G., Zimmet, P. and Shaw, J. (2006) Metabolic syndrome – a new world-wide definition. A consensus statement from the International Diabetes Federation. *Diabetic Medicine*, **23**, 469–80.

31. Després, J.-P., Nadeau, A., Tremblay, A. *et al.* (1989) Role of deep abdominal fat in the association between regional adipose tissue distribution and glucose tolerance in obese women. *Diabetes*, **38**, 304–9.

32. Liao, Y., Kwon, S., Shaughnessy, S. *et al.* (2004) Critical evaluation of Adult Treatment Panel III criteria in identifying insulin resistance with dyslipidemia. *Diabetes Care*, **27**, 978–83.

33. Cameron, A.J., Shaw, J.E. and Zimmet, P.Z. (2004) The metabolic syndrome: prevalence in worldwide populations. *Endocrinology and Metabolism Clinics of North America*, **33**, 351–76.

34. Zimmet, P., Alberti, K.G. and Shaw, J. (2001) Global and societal implications of the diabetes epidemic. *Nature*, **414**, 782–7.

35. Lemieux, I., Pascot, A., Couillard, C. *et al.* (2000) Hypertriglyceridemic waist: a marker of the atherogenic metabolic triad (hyperinsulinemia; hyperapolipoprotein B; small, dense LDL) in men? *Circulation*, **102**, 179–84.

36. Tan, C.E., Ma, S., Wai, D. *et al.* (2004) Can we apply the National Cholesterol Education Program Adult Treatment Panel definition of the metabolic syndrome to Asians? *Diabetes Care*, **27**, 1182–6.

37. Lackland, D., Orchard, T. and Keil, J. (1992) Are race differences in the prevalence of hypertension explained by body mass and fat distribution? A survey in a biracial population. *International Journal of Epidemiology*, **21**, 236–45.

38. Ko, G.T., Chan, J.C., Cockram, C.S. and Woo, J. (1999) Prediction of hypertension, diabetes, dyslipidaemia or albuminuria using simple anthropometric indexes in Hong Kong Chinese. *International Journal of Obesity and Related Metabolic Disorders*, **23**, 1136–42.

39. Inoue, S., Zimmet, P., Caterson, I. *et al.* (2000) *The Asia-Pacific Perspective: Redefining Obesity and Its Treatment*, International Diabetes Institute, Melbourne, pp. 1–56.

40. Genuth, S. (2003) Lowering the criterion for impaired fasting glucose is in order. *Diabetes Care*, **26**, 3331–2.

41. Ford, E.S. (2005) Risks for all-cause mortality, cardiovascular disease, and diabetes associated with the metabolic syndrome: a summary of the evidence. *Diabetes Care*, **28**, 1769–78.

42. Lakka, H.M., Laaksonen, D.E., Lakka, T.A. *et al.* (2002) The metabolic syndrome and total and cardiovascular disease mortality in middle-aged men. *Journal of the American Medical Association*, **288**, 2709–16.

43. Hunt, K.J., Resendez, R.G., Williams, K. *et al.* (2004) National Cholesterol Education Program versus World Health Organization metabolic syndrome in relation to all-cause and cardiovascular mortality in the San Antonio Heart Study. *Circulation*, **110**, 1251–7.

44. Ford, E.S. (2004) The metabolic syndrome and mortality from cardiovascular disease and all-causes: findings from the National Health and Nutrition Examination Survey II Mortality Study. *Atherosclerosis*, **173**, 309–14.

45. Dekker, J.M., Girman, C., Rhodes, T. *et al.* (2005) Metabolic syndrome and 10-year cardiovascular disease risk in the Hoorn Study. *Circulation*, **112**, 666–73.

46. Hu, G., Qiao, Q., Tuomilehto, J. *et al.* (2004) Prevalence of the metabolic syndrome and its relation to all-cause and cardiovascular mortality in nondiabetic European men and women. *Archives of Internal Medicine*, **164**, 1066–76.

47. Bruno, G., Merletti, F., Biggeri, A. *et al.* (2004) Metabolic syndrome as a predictor of all-cause and cardiovascular mortality in type 2 diabetes: the Casale Monferrato Study. *Diabetes Care*, **27**, 2689–94.

48. Butler, J., Rodondi, N., Zhu, Y. *et al.* (2006) Metabolic syndrome and the risk of cardiovascular disease in older adults. *Journal of the American College of Cardiology*, **47**, 1595–602.

49. Katzmarzyk, P.T., Church, T.S. and Blair, S.N. (2004) Cardiorespiratory fitness attenuates the effects of the metabolic syndrome on all-cause and cardiovascular disease mortality in men. *Archives of Internal Medicine*, **164**, 1092–7.

50. Sundstrom, J., Riserus, U., Byberg, L. *et al.* (2006) Clinical value of the metabolic syndrome for long term prediction of total and cardiovascular mortality: prospective, population based cohort study. *British Medical Journal*, **332**, 878–82.

51. Malik, S., Wong, N.D., Franklin, S.S. *et al.* (2004) Impact of the metabolic syndrome on mortality from coronary heart disease, cardiovascular disease, and all causes in United States adults. *Circulation*, **110**, 1245–50.

52. Isomaa, B., Almgren, P., Tuomi, T. *et al.* (2001) Cardiovascular morbidity and mortality associated with the metabolic syndrome. *Diabetes Care*, **24**, 683–9.

53. Trevisan, M., Liu, J., Bahsas, F.B. and Menotti, A. (1998) Syndrome X and mortality: a population-based study. Risk Factor and Life Expectancy

Research Group. *American Journal of Epidemiology*, **148**, 958–66.

54. Wannamethee, S.G., Lowe, G.D., Shaper, A.G. *et al.* (2005) The metabolic syndrome and insulin resistance: relationship to haemostatic and inflammatory markers in older non-diabetic men. *Atherosclerosis*, **181**, 101–8.

55. Stern, M.P., Williams, K., Gonzalez-Villalpando, C. *et al.* (2004) Does the metabolic syndrome improve identification of individuals at risk of type 2 diabetes and/or cardiovascular disease? *Diabetes Care*, **27**, 2676–81.

56. Grundy, S.M. (2006) Metabolic syndrome: connecting and reconciling cardiovascular and diabetes worlds. *Journal of the American College of Cardiology*, **47**, 1093–100.

57. Onat, A., Ceyhan, K., Basar, O. *et al.* (2002) Metabolic syndrome: major impact on coronary risk in a population with low cholesterol levels – a prospective and cross-sectional evaluation. *Atherosclerosis*, **165**, 285–92.

58. Bonora, E., Targher, G., Formentini, G. *et al.* (2004) The metabolic syndrome is an independent predictor of cardiovascular disease in type 2 diabetic subjects. Prospective data from the Verona Diabetes Complications Study. *Diabetic Medicine*, **21**, 52–8.

59. McNeill, A.M., Rosamond, W.D., Girman, C.J. *et al.* (2005) The metabolic syndrome and 11-year risk of incident cardiovascular disease in the atherosclerosis risk in communities study. *Diabetes Care*, **28**, 385–90.

60. Resnick, H.E., Jones, K., Ruotolo, G. *et al.* (2003) Insulin resistance, the metabolic syndrome, and risk of incident cardiovascular disease in nondiabetic American Indians: the Strong Heart Study. *Diabetes Care*, **26**, 861–7.

61. Sattar, N., Gaw, A., Scherbakova, O. *et al.* (2003) Metabolic syndrome with and without C-reactive protein as a predictor of coronary heart disease and diabetes in the West of Scotland Coronary Prevention Study. *Circulation*, **108**, 414–19.

62. Girman, C.J., Rhodes, T., Mercuri, M. *et al.* (2004) The metabolic syndrome and risk of major coronary events in the Scandinavian Simvastatin Survival Study (4S) and the Air Force/Texas Coronary Atherosclerosis Prevention Study (AFCAPS/TexCAPS). *The American Journal of Cardiology*, **93**, 136–41.

63. Ridker, P.M., Buring, J.E., Cook, N.R. and Rifai, N. (2003) C-reactive protein, the metabolic syndrome, and risk of incident cardiovascular events: an 8-year follow-up of 14 719 initially healthy American women. *Circulation*, **107**, 391–7.

64. Scuteri, A., Najjar, S.S., Morrell, C.H. and Lakkatta, E.G. (2005) The metabolic syndrome in older individuals: prevalence and prediction of cardiovascular events: the Cardiovascular Health Study. *Diabetes Care*, **28**, 882–7.

65. He, Y., Jiang, B., Wang, J. *et al.* (2006) Prevalence of the metabolic syndrome and its relation to cardiovascular disease in an elderly Chinese population. *Journal of the American College of Cardiology*, **47**, 1588–94.

66. Athyros, V.G., Mikhailidis, D.P., Papageorgiou, A.A. *et al.* (2004) Prevalence of atherosclerotic vascular disease among subjects with the metabolic syndrome with or without diabetes mellitus: the METS-GREECE Multicentre Study. *Current Medical Research and Opinion*, **20**, 1691–701.

67. Lorenzo, C., Serrano-Rios, M., Martinez-Larrad, M.T. *et al.* (2006) Geographic variations of the International Diabetes Federation and the National Cholesterol Education Program – Adult Treatment Panel III definitions of the metabolic syndrome in nondiabetic subjects. *Diabetes Care*, **29**, 685–91.

68. Lawlor, D.A., Smith, G.D. and Ebrahim, S. (2006) Does the new International Diabetes Federation definition of the metabolic syndrome predict CHD any more strongly than older definitions? Findings from the British Women's Heart and Health Study. *Diabetologia*, **49**, 41–8.

69. Klein, B.E., Klein, R. and Lee, K.E. (2002) Components of the metabolic syndrome and risk of cardiovascular disease and diabetes in Beaver Dam. *Diabetes Care*, **25**, 1790–4.

70. Schmidt, M.I., Duncan, B.B., Bang, H. *et al.* (2005) Identifying individuals at high risk for diabetes: The Atherosclerosis Risk in Communities Study. *Diabetes Care*, **28**, 2013–18.

71. Lorenzo, C., Okoloise, M., Williams, K. *et al.* (2003) The metabolic syndrome as predictor of type 2 diabetes: the San Antonio Heart Study. *Diabetes Care*, **26**, 3153–9.

72. Laaksonen, D.E., Lakka, H.M., Niskanen, L.K. *et al.* (2002) Metabolic syndrome and development of diabetes mellitus: application and validation of recently suggested definitions of the metabolic syndrome in a prospective cohort study. *American Journal of Epidemiology*, **156**, 1070–7.

73. Wang, J.J., Li, H.B., Kinnunen, L. *et al.* (2006) How well does the metabolic syndrome defined by five definitions predict incident diabetes and incident coronary heart disease in a Chinese population? *Atherosclerosis*, **192** (1), 161–8.

74. McKeown, N.M., Meigs, J.B., Liu, S. *et al.* (2004) Carbohydrate nutrition, insulin resistance, and the

prevalence of the metabolic syndrome in the Framingham Offspring Cohort. *Diabetes Care*, **27**, 538–46.

75. Palaniappan, L., Carnethon, M.R., Wang, Y. *et al.* (2004) Predictors of the incident metabolic syndrome in adults: the Insulin Resistance Atherosclerosis Study. *Diabetes Care*, **27**, 788–93.

76. Carnethon, M.R., Loria, C.M., Hill, J.O. *et al.* (2004) Risk factors for the metabolic syndrome: the Coronary Artery Risk Development in Young Adults (CARDIA) study, 1985–2001. *Diabetes Care*, **27**, 2707–15.

77. Pollex, R.L., Hanley, A.J.G., Zinman, B. *et al.* (2006) Metabolic syndrome in aboriginal Canadians: prevalence and genetic associations. *Atherosclerosis*, **184**, 121–9.

78. Simmons, D. and Thompson, C.F. (2004) Prevalence of the metabolic syndrome among adult New Zealanders of Polynesian and European descent. *Diabetes Care*, **27**, 3002–4.

79. Abdul-Rahim, H.F., Husseini, A., Bjertness, E. *et al.* (2001) The metabolic syndrome in the West Bank population: an urban–rural comparison. *Diabetes Care*, **24**, 275–9.

80. Adams, R.J., Appleton, S., Wilson, D.H. *et al.* (2005) Population comparison of two clinical approaches to the metabolic syndrome: implications of the new International Diabetes Federation consensus definition. *Diabetes Care*, **28**, 2777–9.

81. Alexander, C.M., Landsman, P.B., Teutsch, S.M. and Haffer, S.M. (2003) Third National Health and Nutrition Examination Survey, National Cholesterol Education Program. NCEP-defined metabolic syndrome, diabetes, and prevalence of coronary heart disease among NHANES III participants age 50 years and older. *Diabetes*, **52**, 1210–14.

82. Al-Lawati, J.A., Al Riyami, A.M., Mohammed, A.J. and Jousilahti, P. (2002) Increasing prevalence of diabetes mellitus in Oman. *Diabetic Medicine*, **19**, 954–7.

83. Al-Lawati, J.A., Mohammed, A.J., Al-Hinai, H.Q. and Jousilahti, P. (2003) Prevalence of the metabolic syndrome among Omani adults. *Diabetes Care*, **26**, 1781–5.

84. Araneta, M.R., Wingard, D.L. and Barrett-Connor, E. (2002) Type 2 diabetes and metabolic syndrome in Filipina-American women: a high-risk nonobese population. *Diabetes Care*, **25**, 494–9.

85. Athyros, V.G., Ganotakis, E.S., Elisaf, M. and Makhailidis, D.P. (2005) The prevalence of the metabolic syndrome using the National Cholesterol Educational Program and International Diabetes Federation definitions. *Current Medical Research and Opinion*, **21**, 1157–9.

86. Azizi, F., Salehi, P., Etemadi, A. and Zahedi-Asl, S. (2003) Prevalence of metabolic syndrome in an urban population: Tehran Lipid and Glucose Study. *Diabetes Research and Clinical Practice*, **61**, 29–37.

87. Balkau, B., Charles, M.A., Drivsholm, T. *et al.* (2002) Frequency of the WHO metabolic syndrome in European cohorts, and an alternative definition of an insulin resistance syndrome. *Diabetes and Metabolism*, **28**, 364–76.

88. Balkau, B., Eschwege, E., Tichet, J. *et al.* (1997) Proposed criteria for the diagnosis of diabetes: evidence from a French epidemiological study (D.E.S.I.R). *Diabetes and Metabolism*, **23**, 428–34.

89. Bo, S., Gentile, L., Ciccone, G. *et al.* (2005) The metabolic syndrome and high C-reactive protein: prevalence and differences by sex in a southern-European population-based cohort. *Diabetes-Metabolism Research and Reviews*, **21**, 515–24.

90. Boronat, M., Chirino, R., Varillas, V.F. *et al.* (2005) Prevalence of the metabolic syndrome in the island of Gran Canaria: comparison of three major diagnostic proposals. *Diabetic Medicine*, **22**, 1751–6.

91. Cameron, A.J., Shaw, J.E., Zimmet, P.Z. *et al.* (2003) Comparison of WHO and NCEP metabolic syndrome definitions over 5 years in Mauritius. *Diabetologia*, **46**, A3068.

92. Deepa, R., Shanthirani, C.S., Premalatha, G. *et al.* (2002) Prevalence of insulin resistance syndrome in a selected south Indian population – the Chennai Urban Population Study-7 [CUPS-7]. *Indian Journal of Medical Research*, **115**, 118–27.

93. Deepa, M., Farooq, S., Datta, M. *et al.* (2006) Prevalence of metabolic syndrome using WHO, ATPIII and IDF definitions in Asian Indians: the Chennai Urban Rural Epidemiology Study. *Diabetes/Metabolism Research and Reviews*, **23**, 127–34

94. Drivsholm, T., Ibsen, H., Schroll, M. *et al.* (2001) Increasing prevalence of diabetes mellitus and impaired glucose tolerance among 60-year-old Danes. *Diabetic Medicine*, **18**, 126–32.

95. Ford, E.S. (2005) Prevalence of the metabolic syndrome defined by the International Diabetes Federation among adults in the U.S. *Diabetes Care*, **28**, 2745–9.

96. Gu, D., Reynolds, K., Wu, X. *et al.* (2005) Prevalence of the metabolic syndrome and overweight among adults in China. *Lancet*, **365**, 1398–405.

97. Guerrero-Romero, F. and Rodriguez-Moran, M. (2005) Concordance between the 2005 International Diabetes Federation definition for

diagnosing metabolic syndrome with the National Cholesterol Education Program Adult Treatment Panel III and the World Health Organization definitions. *Diabetes Care*, **28**, 2588–9.

98. Gupta, A., Gupta, R., Sarna, M. *et al.* (2003) Prevalence of diabetes, impaired fasting glucose and insulin resistance syndrome in an urban Indian population. *Diabetes Research and Clinical Practice*, **61**, 69–76.

99. Hedblad, B., Nilsson, P., Janzon, L. and Berglund, G. (2000) Relation between insulin resistance and carotid intima-media thickness and stenosis in non-diabetic subjects. Results from a cross-sectional study in Malmo, Sweden. *Diabetic Medicine*, **17**, 299–307.

100. Ilanne-Parikka, P., Eriksson, J.G., Lindstrom, J. *et al.* (2004) Prevalence of the metabolic syndrome and its components: findings from a Finnish general population sample and the Diabetes Prevention Study cohort. *Diabetes Care*, **27**, 2135–40.

101. Ko, G.T.-C., Cockram, C.S., Chow, C.-C. *et al.* (2005) High prevalence of metabolic syndrome in Hong Kong Chinese – comparison of three diagnostic criteria. *Diabetes Research and Clinical Practice*, **69**, 160–8.

102. Lean, M.E., Han, T.S. and Seidell, J.C. (1998) Impairment of health and quality of life in people with large waist circumference. *Lancet*, **351**, 853–6.

103. Lorenzo, C., Serrano-Rios, M., Martinez-Larrad, M.T. *et al.* (2001) Was the historic contribution of Spain to the Mexican gene pool partially responsible for the higher prevalence of type 2 diabetes in Mexican-origin populations? The Spanish Insulin Resistance Study Group, the San Antonio Heart Study, and the Mexico City Diabetes Study. *Diabetes Care*, **24**, 2059–64.

104. Marques-Vidal, P., Mazoyer, E., Bongard, V. *et al.* (2002) Prevalence of insulin resistance syndrome in southwestern France and its relationship with inflammatory and hemostatic markers. *Diabetes Care*, **25**, 1371–7.

105. Meigs, J.B., Wilson, P.W., Nathan, D.M. *et al.* (2003) Prevalence and characteristics of the metabolic syndrome in the San Antonio Heart and Framingham Offspring Studies. *Diabetes*, **52**, 2160–7.

106. Mohamed-Ali, V., Gould, M.M., Gillies, S. *et al.* (1995) Association of proinsulin-like molecules with lipids and fibrinogen in non-diabetic subjects – evidence against a modulating role for insulin. *Diabetologia*, **38**, 1110–16.

107. Oh, J.-Y., Hong, Y.S., Sung, Y.-A. and Barrett-Connor, E. (2004) Prevalence and factor analysis of metabolic syndrome in an urban Korean population. *Diabetes Care*, **27**, 2027–32.

108. Ramachandran, A., Snehalatha, C., Satyavani, K. *et al.* (2003) Metabolic syndrome in urban Asian Indian adults – a population study using modified ATP III criteria. *Diabetes Research and Clinical Practice*, **60**, 199–204.

109. Shiwaku, K., Nogi, A., Kitajima, K. *et al.* (2005) Prevalence of the metabolic syndrome using the modified ATP III definitions for workers in Japan, Korea and Mongolia. *Journal of Occupational Health*, **47**, 126–35.

110. Son, L.N.T.D., Kunii, D., Hung, N.T.K. *et al.* (2005) The metabolic syndrome: prevalence and risk factors in the urban population of Ho Chi Minh City. *Diabetes Research and Clinical Practice*, **67**, 243–50.

111. Song, J., Kim, E., Shin, C. *et al.* (2004) Prevalence of the metabolic syndrome among South Korean adults: the Ansan study [see comment]. *Diabetic Medicine*, **21**, 1154–5.

112. Thomas, G.N., Ho, S.-Y., Janus, E.D. *et al.* (2005) The US National Cholesterol Education Programme Adult Treatment Panel III (NCEP ATP III) prevalence of the metabolic syndrome in a Chinese population. *Diabetes Research and Clinical Practice*, **67**, 251–7.

113. Tillin, T., Forouhi, N., Johnston, D.G. *et al.* (2005) Metabolic syndrome and coronary heart disease in South Asians, African-Caribbeans and white Europeans: a UK population-based cross-sectional study. *Diabetologia*, **48**, 649–56.

114. Villegas, R., Perry, I.J., Creagh, D. *et al.* (2003) Prevalence of the metabolic syndrome in middle-aged men and women. *Diabetes Care*, **26**, 3198–9.

115. Vozarova de Courten, B., de Courten, M., Hanson, R.L. *et al.* (2003) Higher prevalence of type 2 diabetes, metabolic syndrome and cardiovascular diseases in gypsies than in non-gypsies in Slovakia. *Diabetes Research and Clinical Practice*, **62**, 95–103.

116. Zavaroni, I., Bonini, L., Gasparini, P. *et al.* (1999) Hyperinsulinemia in a normal population as a predictor of non-insulin-dependent diabetes mellitus, hypertension, and coronary heart disease: the Barilla factory revisited. *Metabolism*, **48**, 989–94.

117. Lorenzo, C., Williams, K., Hunt, K.J. and Haffner, S.M. (2006) Trend in the prevalence of the metabolic syndrome and its impact on cardiovascular disease incidence: the San Antonio Heart Study. *Diabetes Care*, **29**, 625–30.

118. Ford, E.S. (2004) Prevalence of the metabolic syndrome in US populations. *Endocrinology and Metabolism Clinics of North America*, **33**, 333–50.

119. Csabi, G., Torok, K., Jeges, S. and Molnar, D. (2000) Presence of metabolic cardiovascular syndrome in obese children. *European Journal of Pediatrics*, **159**, 91–4.

120. Invitti, C., Maffeis, C., Gilardini, L. *et al.* (2006) Metabolic syndrome in obese Caucasian children: prevalence using WHO-derived criteria and association with nontraditional cardiovascular risk factors. *International Journal of Obesity (London)*, **30**, 627–33.

121. Cruz, M.L. and Goran, M.I. (2004) The metabolic syndrome in children and adolescents. *Current Diabetes Reports*, **4**, 53–62.

122. Csabi, G., Kozari, A., Farid, G. and Molnar, D. (1995) Multi-metabolic syndrome in obese children. *Orvosi Hetilap*, **136**, 595–7.

123. Cook, S., Weitzman, M., Auinger, P. *et al.* (2003) Prevalence of a metabolic syndrome phenotype in adolescents: findings from the third National Health and Nutrition Examination Survey, 1988–1994. *Archives of Pediatrics and Adolescent Medicine*, **157**, 821–7.

124. Duncan, G.E., Li, S.M. and Zhou, X.-H. (2004) Prevalence and trends of a metabolic syndrome phenotype among U.S. adolescents, 1999–2000. *Diabetes Care*, **27**, 2438–43.

125. Goodman, E., Daniels, S.R., Morrison, J.A. *et al.* (2004) Contrasting prevalence of and demographic disparities in the World Health Organization and National Cholesterol Education Program Adult Treatment Panel III definitions of metabolic syndrome among adolescents [see comment]. *The Journal of Pediatrics*, **145**, 445–51.

126. Hu, F.B., Manson, J.E., Stampfer, M.J. *et al.* (2001) Diet, lifestyle, and the risk of type 2 diabetes mellitus in women. *The New England Journal of Medicine*, **345**, 790–7.

127. Liese, A.D., Mayer-Davis, E.J., Tyroler, H.A. *et al.* (1997) Familial components of the multiple metabolic syndrome: the ARIC study. *Diabetologia*, **40**, 963–70.

128. Xiang, A.H., Azen, S.P., Raffel, L.J. *et al.* (2001) Evidence for joint genetic control of insulin sensitivity and systolic blood pressure in Hispanic families with a hypertensive proband. *Circulation*, **103**, 78–83.

129. DeStefano, A.L., Larson, M.G., Mitchell, G.F. *et al.* (2004) Genome-wide scan for pulse pressure in the National Heart, Lung and Blood Institute's Framingham Heart Study. *Hypertension*, **44**, 152–5.

130. Snieder, H., van Doornen, L.J. and Boomsma, D.I. (1999) Dissecting the genetic architecture of lipids, lipoproteins, and apolipoproteins: lessons from twin studies. *Arteriosclerosis, Thrombosis, and Vascular Biology*, **19**, 2826–34.

131. Forsblom, C.M., Kanninen, T., Lehtovirta, M. *et al.* (1999) Heritability of albumin excretion rate in families of patients with type II diabetes. *Diabetologia*, **42**, 1359–66.

132. Mitchell, B.D., Kammerer, C.M., Mahaney, M.C. *et al.* (1996) Genetic analysis of the IRS. Pleiotropic effects of genes influencing insulin levels on lipoprotein and obesity measures. *Arteriosclerosis, Thrombosis, and Vascular Biology*, **16**, 281–8.

133. Reinhard, W., Holmer, S.R., Fischer, M. *et al.* (2006) Association of the metabolic syndrome with early coronary disease in families with frequent myocardial infarction. *The American Journal of Cardiology*, **97**, 964–7.

134. Neel, J.V. (1962) Diabetes mellitus: a 'thrifty' genotype rendered detrimental by 'progress'? *American Journal of Human Genetics*, **14**, 353–62.

135. Zimmet, P., McCarty, D. and de Courten, M. (1997) The global epidemiology of non-insulin dependent diabetes mellitus and the metabolic syndrome. *Journal of Diabetes and Its Complications*, **11**, 60–8.

136. Melander, O., Mattiasson, I., Marsal, K. *et al.* (1999) Heredity for hypertension influences intrauterine growth and the relation between fetal growth and adult blood pressure. *Journal of Hypertension*, **17**, 1557–61.

137. Hattersley, A.T., Beards, F., Ballantyne, E. *et al.* (1998) Mutations in the glucokinase gene of the fetus result in reduced birth weight. *Nature Genetics*, **19**, 268–70.

138. Zimmet, P., Boyko, E., Collier, G. and de Courten, M. (1999) The etiology of the metabolic syndrome – potential role of insulin resistance, leptin resistance and other players, in *The Metabolic Syndrome X*, (eds B. Hansen, J. Saye and L. Wennogle), New York Academy of Sciences, New York, pp. 25–44.

5

Obesity and Diabetes

Rachel Huxley, Abdullah Omari and Ian D. Caterson

The George Institute and the Human Nutrition Unit, University of Sydney, Sydney,
New South Wales, Australia

5.1 INTRODUCTION: DEFINING OBESITY

In epidemiological studies, the most widely used method to estimate the degree of obesity is the body mass index (BMI), (body weight measured in kilograms divided by the height in meters squared (kg m^{-2}) [1]. BMI is highly correlated with adiposity in large populations ($r = 0.8$) [2] and has been shown to be continuously associated with cardiovascular risk in a range of populations [3].

Although the relationship between BMI and cardiovascular risk is continuous (at least down to a BMI of 18 kg m^{-2}), BMI is frequently dichotomized to provide cut-points that signify theoretical points at which overweight or obesity is a clinical problem. For example, the World Health Organization (WHO) in 2000 state that a 'healthy' adult range of BMI is regarded as between 18.5 and 24.9 kg m^{-2}, with BMIs in excess of 25 kg m^{-2} being overweight or preobese. Recent guidelines issued by the WHO [4] define overweight and obesity using BMI as follows:

- overweight (preobese): 25.0–29.9 kg m^{-2};
- obesity grade 1: 30.0–34.9 kg m^{-2};
- obesity grade: 2 35.0–39.9 kg m^{-2};
- obesity grade: 3 $\geq$40.0 kg m^{-2}.

These cut-points are based on morbidity and mortality data chiefly obtained from European, or predominantly Caucasian, populations and reflect the risk associated with the development of type 2 diabetes and cardiovascular disease (CVD) and of premature death.

As these cut-points were largely derived using predominantly Caucasian studies, it is unknown whether they are applicable to non-Caucasian populations [5], but there is accumulating evidence to suggest that BMI cut-points should be lowered for Asians, which will be discussed later in the chapter.

A further limitation of the use of BMI (other than in population studies) is that it is a relatively crude measure, as it provides no information regarding the distribution of body fat, nor does it take into account the extremes of musculature, aging or growth phases. Measures of central obesity such as waist circumference and waist:hip ratio have been suggested to be better predictors of cardiovascular risk [6–8]. However, despite the limitations of using BMI, the reasonable correlation between BMI and body fat, and its ease of measurement, has ensured its widespread use at determining the prevalence of obesity in populations.

5.2 EPIDEMIOLOGICAL TRENDS IN OBESITY

There are vast differences in the worldwide prevalence of obesity. This is illustrated by **Table 5.1**, which shows the obesity prevalence of selected countries using data from the WHO. Recently, the Department of Nutrition for Health and Development at the WHO has established the online Global Database on Body Mass Index to monitor the change in prevalence rates of obesity among adults between countries (http://www.who.int/bmi/index.jsp).

The Epidemiology of Diabetes Mellitus, second edition   Edited by Jean-Marie Ekoé, Marian Rewers, Rhys Williams and Paul Zimmet
© 2008 John Wiley & Sons, Ltd

Table 5.1 Prevalence (%) of adult obesity (BMI > 30 kg m^{-2}) in selected countries.

Country	Period	Age range (years)	Men	Women
Europe				
Germany	1998	18–79	19	22
France	1995–1996	35–65	8	7
Ireland	1997–1999	18–64	20	16
Latvia	1997	19–64	10	17
Norway	1994	16–79	5	6
Sweden	1996–1997	16–84	7	7
United Kingdom	1997	16+	17	19
North America				
United States	2001–2002	>20	31.1	33.2
Canada	2000–2001	20–64	16	14
Asia				
China	1990–2000	>20	2	4
India	1998	>18	0.3	0.5
Japan	2001	>15	3	3
Singapore	1998	18–69	5	7
Pacific Islands				
Fiji	1993	>18	7	21
Nauru	1994	25–69	80	79
Vanuatu	1998	>20	12	20
Middle East				
Bahrain	1998–1999	>19	23	34
Egypt	1998–1999	18–60	13	33
Iran	1999	>15	6	14
Saudi Arabia	1995	>18	13	20
Africa				
Ghana	1987–1989	20–65	1	6
Morocco	1998–1999	>18	4	16
South Africa	1998	>15	9	30

Using the WHO criteria for overweight (BMI > 25 kg m^{-2}) and obesity (BMI > 30 kg m^{-2}), the highest levels are observed among Pacific Islanders, with rates as high as 79% of the adult population affected [9]. It is interesting to note that, in the Pacific Islands, large body size is often associated with power, beauty and affluence [10], which may in part account for the very high prevalence of the condition. By contrast, the lowest rates of obesity occur in Asia, where typically less than 10% of the adult population is classified as obese. However,

given the rapid escalation of the prevalence of obesity witnessed in many parts of Asia over the past decade, including China, where over 200 million individuals are overweight and a further 30 million are obese, this intimates that such low estimates may be more indicative of the past than the present [11].

By comparison, the United States and most European countries generally have a relatively high prevalence of obesity. For example, 2004 survey data indicate that nearly one-third of adult men and women in the United States are obese [12]. Countries of the Middle East show variable rates of obesity, with countries such as Iran with less than 10% of the adult population obese compared with 29% in Bahrain and more than 30% in Lebanon. Only countries in sub-Saharan Africa remain relatively unaffected by the pandemic, with most of these countries having an obesity prevalence typically <5% [13]. For example, Ghana has an obesity prevalence of only 3% compared with the more developed South Africa with a prevalence of 21%.

5.3 OBESITY AND DIABETES ARE CAUSALLY LINKED

Numerous large epidemiological studies from the United States, Europe and Asia have clearly indicated the direct and continuous associations between BMI and diabetes. The magnitude of the association between obesity (BMI $\geq$ 30 kg m^{-2}) and subsequent risk of diabetes has varied in published reports, with excess risks ranging between 10 and 20 times that of individuals of normal body weight (BMI < 25 kg m^{-2}). For example, in the Nurses Health Study, the risk of diabetes among obese women (BMI > 30 kg m^{-2}) was approximately 20 times higher [14, 15] than women with BMI < 23 kg m^{-2}. By comparison, data from the US Male Health Professionals Study suggested a smaller (approximately 10 times), but still significantly elevated risk of diabetes among obese men [15].

The discrepancies in the strength of the reported associations are due, in part, to different populations and study methodology. Both the Nurses Health Study and the Health Professionals studies used self-reported measures of weight, height and diabetic status. It is known from epidemiological studies that weight and height are often under- and over-estimated, particularly among heavier and shorter individuals respectively. Hence, BMI based on self-reported anthropometric data will tend to be biased downwards, which would in effect create an artificially steep slope of the relation between BMI and the risk of diabetes. Consequently, the association between the two variables will be overestimated, dependent upon the level of under- or over-reporting of weight and height in the study. Similarly, if incorrect self-reporting of positive diabetic status was directly associated with BMI,

this too would generate an artificially steep slope of the relationship, resulting in an overestimation of the association between BMI and diabetes.

5.4 ATTRIBUTABLE BURDEN OF DIABETES DUE TO EXCESS WEIGHT

Nevertheless, despite such discrepant findings in the reported magnitude of the relationship between obesity and diabetes, there remains little doubt as to its strong, direct and continuous nature. This is further evidenced from a recent study from the Asia-Pacific Cohort Studies Collaboration, a large-scale meta-analysis of prospective cohort studies in the region, including information on over 150 000 individuals [16]. Rather than categorizing individuals as obese and nonobese, the authors examined the relationship between BMI and diabetes as a continuum. Furthermore, the analyses were largely based on reported measures rather than self-report. In this study, a 2 kg m^{-2} reduction in BMI (which is roughly equivalent to a 5–6 kg reduction in body weight) was associated with an approximate 25% lower risk of diabete and, more importantly, this association was apparent down to a baseline BMI of at least 21 kg m^{-2} (**Figure 5.1**).

This finding is in agreement with recent analyses from the International Obesity Task Force for the WHO's Global Burden of Disease Study, which attributed 58% of the global burden of type 2 diabetes to BMI of above 21 kg m^{-2}, but with substantial regional variation [17]. For example, in North America, 90% of the attributable burden of diabetes is due to weight gain compared with only 50% in Southeast Asia and Africa.

5.5 AGE AND REGIONAL VARIATION IN THE ASSOCIATION BETWEEN OBESITY AND DIABETES

In the Asia-Pacific Cohort Studies Collaboration, the association between BMI and diabetes was also observed to be age dependent, with stronger proportional associations in younger individuals [16]. For example, for every 2 kg m^{-2} lower BMI, the risk of diabetes was significantly reduced by 31% and 19% among individuals less than 60 years of age compared with those aged more than 70 years respectively (**Figure 5.2**). There is also some

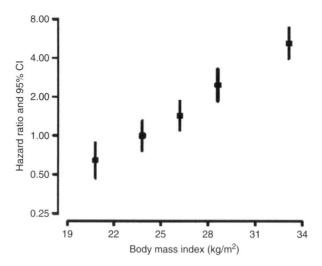

Figure 5.1 BMI and risk of diabetes. The hazard ratios for total diabetes event adjusted for age, sex, cohort and smoking habit are plotted on a log scale against BMI for each of the five groups defined by baseline BMI (<22.5, 22.5–24.9, 25.0–27.4, 27.5–29.9 and $>30 \, \text{kg m}^{-2}$). The x-axis coordinate for each group is the mean baseline BMI. The 95% confidence intervals for the y-axis coordinate, hazard ratios are calculated as floating absolute risks with the BMI group 22.5–24.9 kg m^{-2} [16]. (Reproduced by permission of *Asia Pacific Journal of Clinical Nutrition*.)

suggestion that the association between BMI with diabetes is stronger among Asians than in Caucasian populations. In this study, a $2 \, \text{kg m}^{-2}$ decrement in BMI was associated with a reduction in the risk of diabetes of 37% in the Asian cohorts compared with a 25% risk reduction in populations from Australia and New Zealand, implying that, for a given BMI,

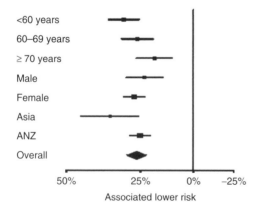

Figure 5.2 Associations of $2 \, \text{kg m}^{-2}$ lower BMI and risk of diabetes by age, sex and region from the Asia Pacific Cohort Studies Collaboration [16]. (Reproduced by permission of *Asia Pacific Journal of Clinical Nutrition*.)

the risk of diabetes is significantly higher among Asian individuals than Caucasian individuals.

The finding of a regional difference in the strength of the association is supported by previous studies which have suggested that, for any given BMI, Asian populations have a greater percentage of body fat than Caucasians [19]. Moreover, there is evidence to suggest that within Asian populations there is significant variation in the association between adiposity and BMI. For example, Hong Kong Chinese, Indonesians, Singaporeans and urban Thai have been shown to have lower BMIs at any given percentage of body fat than Europeans do.

5.6 CENTRAL OBESITY VERSUS BMI AS A PREDICTOR OF DIABETES

There is also a growing body of evidence to suggest that other measures of body anthropometry that better reflect central adiposity, such as waist circumference and waist:hip ratio, may be better predictors of obesity-related risk than BMI [6–8]. Central adiposity is suggested to be more strongly associated with CVD risk and it has been highlighted as a growing problem, particularly in countries of the

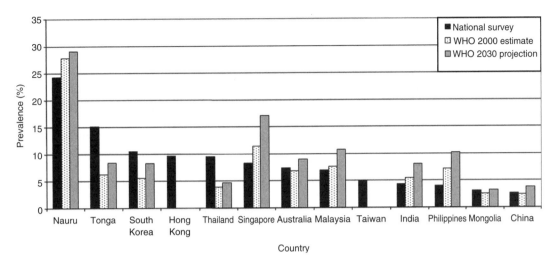

Figure 5.3 Prevalence of diabetes from national surveys, WHO 2000 estimate and 2030 projection. (Reproduced with permission of the World Health Organization, from Lee *et al.* [18].)

Asia-Pacific region, where individuals may exhibit a relatively normal BMI (i.e. $<25\,\mathrm{kg\,m}^{-2}$) but have a disproportionately large waist circumference [20, 21]. It also supports the finding that, despite having a substantially lower mean population BMI, the prevalence of diabetes in some Asian countries is on *a par* with, or even exceeds, those levels found in the West. For example, in a recent review, the prevalence of diabetes in some Asian countries, most noticeably Singapore, Thailand and Hong Kong, was higher than that of Australia, despite these countries having significantly lower population mean levels of BMI than Australia (**Figure 5.3**) [18].

5.7 PHYSIOLOGICAL MECHANISMS MEDIATING EXCESS WEIGHT WITH DIABETES

Obesity, most of which results from an energy imbalance (food intake versus physical activity), though there are some underlying genetic factors, is widely acknowledged to be one of the major causal determinants of diabetes. The mechanisms that mediate the association between excess body weight and diabetes operate through several mechanisms. Increased levels of body fat, particularly visceral adiposity, due to increased food intake or lower levels of physical activity, are major determinants of insulin resistance (**Figure 5.4**). Insulin resistance is

a state resulting from impairment in the responsiveness of muscle, liver and adipose tissue to insulin, which, as a result, causes a rise in the levels of blood glucose and triglycerides with a lowering in HDL cholesterol. Prolonged raised levels of blood glucose can lead to overt manifestation of type 2 diabetes.

The relationship between BMI and fasting insulin is continuous and linear, such that a unit increase in BMI is associated with a $1\,\mathrm{U\,ml}^{-1}$ increase in fasting insulin concentration [23]. There is also

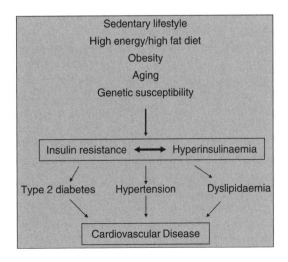

Figure 5.4 Causes and consequences of insulin resistance.

accumulating evidence that intra-abdominal (visceral) fat is more strongly associated with the development of insulin resistance [24, 25]. Epidemiological studies have shown that modest weight loss, particularly of intra-abdominal fat, improves insulin sensitivity [26, 27] and, conversely, that subsequent weight regain is frequently accompanied by impaired insulin action.

A lack of physical activity, irrespective of its role in weight gain, has been shown by numerous studies to be independently associated with the development of insulin resistance [28, 29]. Regular physical aerobic exercise has been observed in cross-sectional studies to be positively associated with insulin sensitivity and among diabetic patients physical fitness is inversely related to small, but significant, changes in levels of glycosylated hemoglobin and glucose tolerance [30].

There are several mechanisms hypothesized to mediate the effects of physical activity on insulin sensitivity aside from causing a reduction in body fat stores. Randomized controlled trials have shown that regular aerobic exercise (at least three times a week for a duration of between 6 and 10 months), in the absence of any reduction in body weight, improves insulin action possibly by reducing intramuscular stores of triglycerides, or by increasing the capacity of skeletal muscle to metabolize, or store, glucose. An example, of such a trial is the Chinese Da Qing Study [31], a randomized trial that examined the impact of dietary modification and physical activity on the development of type 2 diabetes in individuals with impaired glucose tolerance (IGT). IGT patients were randomized to one of four groups: one group was provided with generic health advice and served as the control, two groups were given advice on how to either modify their diet or their activity levels and the fourth group was given advice on both diet and exercise. All groups were followed for 6 years, after which time each of the intervention groups recorded a 40% lower incidence of diabetes compared with the control group. Of note, the effectiveness of the interventions was not confined to overweight individuals (BMI > 25 kg m^{-2}) but was also apparent among individuals within the 'normal' BMI range (i.e. BMI < 25 kg m^{-2}). It is of note, however, that, although both dietary modification and physical activity improve measures of insulin sensitivity, independent of each other, most studies have shown that their individual effects are outweighed by the combined impact of diet and exercise [32].

5.8 OTHER KEY RISK FACTORS FOR OBESITY AND DIABETES

Aside from high-fat, high-energy diets in conjunction with relatively low levels of physical activity, there are several other important risk factors that are associated either with both obesity and diabetes or solely with obesity, and hence indirectly with diabetes, including age, female gender and low socioeconomic position.

Of these, age is perhaps the most important non-modifiable risk factor that is positively associated with both obesity and diabetes. In a large European survey of 15 000 adults, the risk of obesity was shown to rise steeply with increasing age up to 45–64 years, particularly among individuals of low socioeconomic status, and declined among those over 65 years for all social classes [33]. Similar findings were observed in cross-sectional analyses from the Asia Pacific Cohort Studies Collaboration, where mean levels of BMI tended to increase with age, peaking at around 50 years in Asians and 60 years in Caucasians, and then declined thereafter with each successive decade of age [22]. Similarly, the prevalence of diabetes increased linearly with each decade of life in both men and women, and in both Asian and the predominantly Caucasian populations of Australia and New Zealand (**Figure 5.5**).

Twin studies have identified a genetic component to obesity, with some studies suggesting that the heritable component of obesity is between 25 and 40% [34]. Although several gene mutations have been identified that induce obesity in humans, it is highly unlikely that genetic mutations contribute much to the global pandemic given the multifactorial origins of obesity and the relatively short space of time over which the obesity pandemic has emerged [35].

5.9 IMPACT OF SOCIAL CLASS ON OBESITY

As alluded to in the previous section, a low social class is also associated with a greater risk of obesity, although the relationship is complex, it often differs

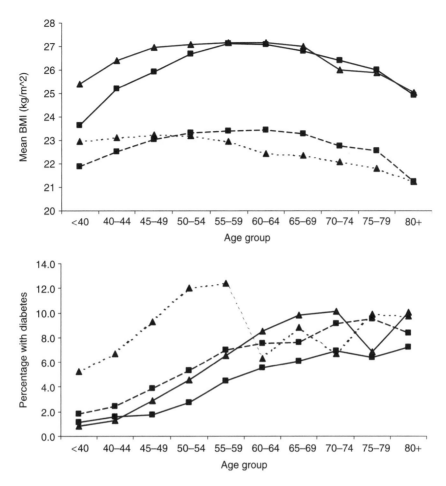

Figure 5.5 Mean levels of diabetes and BMI by 10-year age interval group in men and women from Asia and ANZ. Block lines and squares: females ANZ; block lines and triangles: males ANZ; dashed lines and squares: females Asia; dashed lines and triangles: males Asia. (Each graph was based on data from the number of individuals as shown in Table 5.2.) (Reproduced from Huxley _et al._ [22], by permission of Oxford University Press.)

by sex and is dependent in large part upon the level of economic and nutritional development of the population. One of the most recent, and comprehensive, analyses of the association between obesity and socioeconomic position comes from the MONICA Project, a large cross-sectional study conducted in 26 countries that was repeated at an interval of 10 years [36]. The study indicated that, among women, there was a statistically significant inverse association between educational level and BMI in almost all of the 26 populations, with the difference between the highest and the lowest educational tertiles ranging from −3.1 to 0.4 kg

m^{-2} in the initial survey and from −3.3 to 0.6 kg m^{-2} in the final survey.

Among men, the difference in BMI between the educational tertiles was less marked than among women, ranging from −1.2 to 2.2 kg m^{-2} and from −1.5 to 1.2 kg m^{-2} in the two surveys respectively. Interestingly, there was no discernible geographical pattern among women, but among men there was a positive association between the level of education and BMI, particularly in the transitional economies of several eastern and central European countries and in China. Moreover, in those countries with a low prevalence of obesity, the risk of becoming overweight was positively associated with BMI;

conversely, in countries with a high prevalence of obesity, BMI was negatively associated with the prevalence of obesity.

In Western countries, particularly in women, there is a strong educational gradient with the risk of obesity, such that the prevalence of obesity is greatest among those with low education than with the more highly educated groups. In many countries, including Sweden and Denmark, a high level of education seems to confer some protection against obesity, whereas obesity among men is increasing across the entire educational spectrum [37, 38]. Interestingly, this pattern is beginning to emerge in several developing countries such as Brazil, where a decrease in the prevalence of obesity has occurred among urban women [39].

By comparison with developed countries, the relationship between the prevalence of obesity and the level of education attained is dependent on the overall prevalence of obesity in countries of sub-Saharan Africa. For example, in those countries where the prevalence of obesity is low, obesity rates are much higher among the more highly educated women than those with a lower level of education

(**Figure 5.6**). However, when the prevalence of obesity is relatively high, as in Zimbabwe, level of education appears to offer no barrier to the risk of becoming obese.

5.10 EARLY LIFE ENVIRONMENT AND THE 'PROGRAMMING' HYPOTHESIS

Over the past two decades a hypothesis has emerged that suggested new possibilities as to the origins of chronic disease. The hypothesis, originally termed the *fetal-origins* hypothesis, suggests that impaired fetal growth as a consequence of an adverse intrauterine environment can increase the individual's susceptibility for developing a wide range of chronic conditions in later life [40]. Most of the evidence for the hypothesis has come from historical cohort and other observational studies which have related some index of fetal growth, such as birth weight, birth length or ponderal index (birth length/height^3), with subsequent health outcomes. For example, associations between low birth weight, or thinness at birth, and raised blood

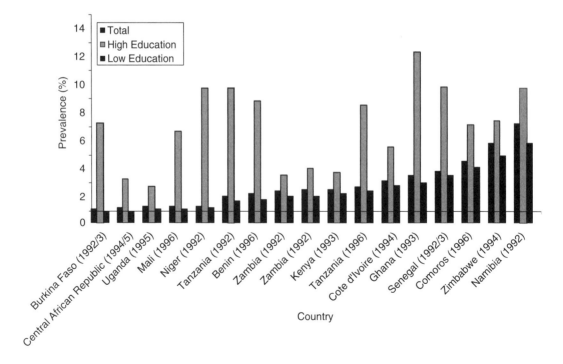

Figure 5.6 Prevalence of obesity (%) among women (15–49 years) in countries of sub-Saharan Africa by educational status (low versus high).

pressure, diabetes and CVD have been widely reported in the literature–otherwise known as the *thrifty phenotype* hypothesis [40–44]. However, it remains unclear to what extent these associations are causal or governed by some underlying, and unmeasured, factors that are related both to birth weight and to disease risk in later life (e.g. socioeconomic status) [45].

Data from the Dutch Famine Study [46] was among the first to suggest a possible association between poor fetal nutrition and increased susceptibility toward the development of obesity and diabetes in adult life, although these findings have received inconsistent support from the literature. In contrast, most studies have observed a *positive* association between birth weight and BMI in childhood and adult life of the magnitude that a 1 kg higher increment in birth weight is associated with a 0.5–0.7 kg m^{-2} higher BMI in later life [47]. However, the possibility that low birth weight is a precursor to central obesity has been reported by some, but not all, studies. By comparison, there appears to be stronger support from the literature for an association between small size at birth and subsequent risk of diabetes. A recent qualitative review of 48 observational studies concluded that individuals who were light at birth were more susceptible to disturbances in glucose and insulin metabolism and were more prone to developing insulin resistance than individuals of 'normal' birth weight [48].

Some commentators contend that the possible associations between size at birth and subsequent disease risk, including diabetes, are mediated more through growth trajectories in early childhood and adolescence, rather than through fetal growth per se. Low birth-weight infants often experience rapid 'catch-up' growth in childhood that persists into adulthood, and it is this crossing of BMI centiles which is considered to be particularly hazardous for later health. In prospective cohort of singleton births, Ong *et al.* [49] reported that catch-up growth was related to intrauterine growth restraint and that children who 'caught up' in the first 2 years of life were fatter and had a greater deposition of abdominal fat at the age of 5 years than other children did. This particular patterning of fat deposition in early life may underlie the reported association between catch-up growth and risk of diabetes. For example, in a large British birth cohort followed since 1958 there was no excess risk

of diabetes among individuals born small without excessive weight gain throughout childhood and adult life [50].

This concept, that undernutrition in early life followed by relative overabundance postnatally, may be of particular relevance to developing countries that are experiencing rapid economic and nutritional transformations, such as India and China [51]. The hypothesis has been used to explain the growing epidemic of diabetes in these countries, particularly in India, which has a higher number of individuals with diabetes than any other country and where, by 2025, one in five people with diabetes will live [52].

Currently, there is no universal agreement as to the potential mechanisms governing the associations between changes in body size in early and postnatal life and subsequent diabetes risk. Moreover, the potential implications for obesity and diabetes prevention, at both the individual and population level, remain unclear. However, given the strong and direct association between excess weight and diabetes, the primary prevention of obesity among all individuals, irrespective of their size at birth, should remain a primary focus for diabetes prevention programs (DPPs).

5.11 THE INCREASING GLOBAL BURDEN OF DIABETES AND OBESITY

It has been widely reported that the global prevalence of both obesity and diabetes has increased substantially over the past 30 years in both developed and developing countries. Recent projections from the Global Burden of Disease Study suggest that these trends are set to continue well into the first half of the twenty-first century. Recently, the WHO estimated that the number of individuals who are overweight, of which there are approximately 1 billion, now exceeds those who are underweight, currently estimated at 800 million. Indeed, even this estimate for the number of overweight is thought to be an underestimate of the real figure, which has been suggested to be as high as 1.7 billion depending on the BMI criteria used for defining overweight and obesity. For diabetes, the expected number of affected individuals is expected to double in the next 20 years from 171 million in 2002 to 366 million in 2030 [53].

5.12 GLOBAL BURDEN
OF DIABETES

In 1985, the WHO had estimated the prevalence of
diabetes as 30 million individuals, but by 2000 this
figure had increased to over 170 million affected
individuals. In the same year, the excess global
mortality attributable to diabetes was estimated
to be 2.9 million deaths or approximately 5% of
global mortality [54]. Using data compiled from
representative and national surveys, Wild *et al.*
estimated the number of individuals worldwide
affected by the disorder. By 2030, the worldwide
prevalence of diabetes is expected to double, with
recent projections putting the figure at 360 million
individuals living with diabetes. However, this
might significantly underestimate the true burden
of the disease, as a recent review conducted using
nationally representative data from the Asia-Pacific
region reported that for several countries in the
region the current prevalence already exceeded the
WHO 2030 projection (**Figure 5.3**) [18].

Most of the increase in the prevalence of diabetes
will occur in lower- and middle-income countries,
especially those of the Asia-Pacific region. For
example, China and India currently have the highest
number of affected individuals (52 million), which
is expected to more than double to over 120 million
in 2030 (**Table 5.2**). By 2025, it is estimated that
three out of four individuals with diabetes will be
from the developing world [52]. The magnitude of

the diabetes epidemic affecting countries such as
India really becomes apparent when examining the
changing prevalence of diabetes over a relatively
short time interval. For example, between the 1970s
and 2000, the prevalence of diabetes among Indian
adults living in urban areas has been estimated to
have more than quadrupled to 12%, with a similar
number of individuals having IGT [20].

King *et al.*'s projections [52] take into consideration various sociodemographic factors, including
population growth, population aging and increased
urbanization. The latter is particularly pertinent
to lower- and middle-income countries, many of
which are undergoing massive nutritional and economic transformations that are often characterized
by the move away from traditional rural existences
toward more urban lifestyles and the associated
factors that accompany it, such as increased sedentariness and high-fat diets. The result is significantly
higher levels of overweight and obesity in urban
compared with rural areas in developing countries.

Another major difference in the pattern of diabetes, between developed and developing countries
is the age at which diabetes becomes manifest. In
higher income countries, such as the United States,
United Kingdom and continental Europe, over 50%
of individuals with diabetes are over 65 years of
age. By comparison, in lower- and middle-income
countries, more than three-quarters of individuals
with diabetes are less than 65 years of age and 25%

**Table 5.2 The top 10 countries with the greatest current and projected burden of diabetes [53].
(Copyright © 2004 American Diabetes Association, from *Diabetes Care*®,Vol.27, 2004; 1047-1053,
reprinted with permission from The American Diabetes Association.)**

Rank	2000		2030	
	Country	People with diabetes (millions)	Country	People with diabetes (millions)
1	India	31.7	India	79.4
2	China	20.8	China	42.3
3	United States	17.7	United States	30.3
4	Indonesia	8.4	Indonesia	21.3
5	Japan	6.8	Pakistan	13.9
6	Pakistan	5.2	Brazil	11.3
7	Russian Federation	4.6	Bangladesh	11.1
8	Brazil	4.6	Japan	8.9
9	Italy	4.3	Philippines	7.8
10	Bangladesh	3.2	Egypt	6.7

of all cases occur in people younger than 44 years [52]. Needless to say, aside from the massive health consequences that this entails, the economic implications of having a significant proportion of the workforce affected by diabetes in their most productive years is potentially catastrophic for these countries.

5.13 DOES WEIGHT LOSS IMPROVE DIABETIC OUTCOMES? EVIDENCE FROM RANDOMIZED TRIALS

As previously described, observational data illustrate a strong and continuous association between BMI and both plasma glucose levels and the risk of diabetes, down to a baseline of at least 20 kg m^{-2}. A logical progression from this, therefore, is that weight loss would be associated with improved insulin resistance and the prevention of new-onset diabetes. Indeed, evidence from several randomized trials of either surgical or nonsurgical (diet, exercise or orlistat) [55–61], interventions among overweight populations has demonstrated a significant reduction in the risk of diabetes associated with weight loss. Surgical interventions were the most effective at reducing the risk of diabetes, largely because the subsequent weight loss (often exceeding 50 kg) resulting from surgery is far greater than that achieved through modification of lifestyle (approximately 4–7 kg). However, neither surgery nor pharmacotherapy are ethical or practical solutions for the epidemics of obesity and diabetes that we are currently experiencing.

Fortunately, convincing evidence that changing our eating and physical activity patterns can significantly reduce the incidence of diabetes has been recently demonstrated by the DPPs. There have been a number of these interventions, in countries as diverse as China [31], Finland [59] and the United States [62]. In these trials, lifestyle interventions have prevented the development of diabetes in those at high risk of developing the disorder.

The Finnish Diabetes Prevention Study (DPS) was one of the first randomized controlled studies to show that diabetes is preventable with appropriate lifestyle interventions. In the DPS, there was a focus on community involvement and five major goals were set for those at risk of developing diabetes. These goals were: lose weight, reduce total fat intake to less than 30% of total energy intake,

reduce saturated fat to <10% energy, more fiber in the diet (>15 g day^{-1}) and 30 min of physical activity a day. In the intervention group, these measures reduced the incidence of diabetes by 58%. Those who achieved four or five of the goals did not develop diabetes, those who lost more weight and those who were older did better, and when the subjects were followed up 7 years later there was a lasting benefit of the intervention [59].

The US DPP differed slightly from the Finnish study primarily because it was not designed for use in a primary care setting. In addition to examining the impact of diet and exercise on the risk of diabetes, DPP tested whether the diabetes drug metformin could also prevent or delay the onset of type 2 diabetes in people with IGT. Over 3000 overweight individuals with IGT were randomized to either the control or one of two of the intervention groups. Individuals randomized to the first intervention group received intensive training in diet, exercise and behavior modification, whereas the second intervention group received metformin in addition to intensive training. The third group received placebo pills instead of metformin and received standard advice about healthy eating. At 4 years, there was essentially no weight loss in the control group, about a 1 kg loss in those treated with metformin and about 4.5 kg loss in those on the lifestyle program. Though not seeming much of a weight loss, this amount of loss reduced diabetes incidence by 58%. Of note, the behavioral intervention was significantly more effective than metformin at reducing the risk of diabetes: 31% with metformin versus 58% with diet and physical activity [62].

In a long-term trial (4 years) using the weight-loss drug orlistat (the Xenical in the prevention of diabetes in obese subjects (XENDOS) trial) [63], the maintained weight loss in the lifestyle treatment (placebo) group was 4.1 kg, while in the active treatment group (lifestyle plus orlistat) the maintained loss was 6.9 kg. Diabetes incidence in the placebo group was reduced to a similar extent as in the DPP, while the extra 2.8 kg in the active treatment group produced a further reduction in diabetes incidence, in essence a reduction of 80%.

Obesity, particularly abdominal obesity, and type 2 diabetes are closely linked. Given the results of these prevention programs, it would seem sensible to target prediabetes and those at high risk of diabetes, provide them with an active lifestyle intervention and prevent or delay diabetes. More emphasis needs to be placed on this effective strategy, which could be run in the community, in workplaces and in a health care setting. Introduction of such an approach would prevent diabetes, reduce suffering and reduce costs to the individual and health care system. This is the challenge of the next 20 years to reduce obesity and prevent diabetes.

References

1. Garrow, J.S. and Webber, J. (1985) Quetelet's index (W/H^2) as a measure of fatness. *International Journal of Obesity and Related Metabolic Disorders*, **9**, 147–53.

2. Heitmann, B.L. (1990) Evaluation of body fat estimated from body mass index, skinfolds and impedance. A comparative study. *European Journal of Clinical Nutrition*, **44**, 831–7.

3. WHO/NUT/NCD (1998) Obesity: preventing and managing the global epidemic. Report of a WHO consultation in obesity, WHO, Geneva.

4. World Health Organisation, International Association for the Study of Obesity, International Obesity Task Force (2000) *The Asia-Pacific Perspective: Redefining Obesity and its Treatment*. Sydney Health Communications.

5. WHO Expert Consultation (2004) Appropriate body-mass index for Asian populations and its implications for policy and intervention strategies. *Lancet*, **363**, 157–63.

6. Janssen, I., Katzmarzyk, P.T. and Ross, R. (2004) Waist circumference and not body mass index explains obesity-related health risk. *American Journal of Clinical Nutrition*, **79**, 379–84.

7. Zhu, S.K., Wang, Z.M., Heshka, S. *et al.* (2002) Waist circumference and obesity-associated risk factors among whites in the Third National Health and Nutrition Examination Survey: clinical action thresholds. *American Journal of Clinical Nutrition*, **76**, 743–9.

8. Reddy, K.S., Prabhakaran, D., Shah, P. and Shah, B. (2002) Differences in body mass index and waist:hip ratios in north Indian rural and urban populations. *Obesity Reviews*, **3**, 197–202.

9. Lee, C.M.Y., Martiniuk, A.L.C., Woodward, M. *et al.* (2007) The burden of overweight and obesity in the Asia-Pacific region. *Obesity Reviews*, **8**, 191–6.

10. Brewis, A.A., McGarvey, S.T. and Tu'u'au-Potoi, N. (1998) Structure of family planning in Samoa. *Australian and New Zealand Journal of Public Health*, **22**, 424–7.

11. Wu, Y. (2006) Overweight and obesity in China. *British Medical Journal*, **333**, 362–3.

12. Ogden, C.L., Carroll, M.D., Curtin, L.R. *et al.* (2006) Prevalence of overweight and obesity in the United States, 1999–2004. *Journal of the American Medical Association*, **295**, 1549–55.

13. Martorell, R., Khan, L.K., Hughes, M.L. *et al.* (2000) Obesity in women from developing countries. *European Journal of Clinical Nutrition*, **54**, 247–52.

14. Hu, F.B., Manson, J.E., Stampfer, M.J. *et al.* (2001) Diet, lifestyle and the risk of type-2 diabetes mellitus in women. *New England Journal of Medicine*, **345**, 790–7.

15. Chan, J.M., Rimm, E.B., Colditz, G.A. *et al.* (1994) Obesity, fat distribution, and weight gain as risk factors for clinical diabetes in men. *Diabetes Care*, **17**, 961–9.

16. Asia Pacific Cohort Studies Collaboration (2006) Body mass index and risk of diabetes mellitus in the Asia-Pacific Region. *Asia Pacific Journal of Clinical Nutrition*, **15**, 127–33.

17. World Health Organisation (2002) World Health Report 2002, World Health Organisation, Geneva.

18. Lee, C.M.Y., Huxley R., Lam, T.H. *et al.* (2007) Prevalence of diabetes mellitus and population attributable fractions for coronary heart disease and stroke mortality in the WHO South-East Asia and Western Pacific regions. *Asia-Pacific Journal of Clinical Nutrition*, **16**, 187–92.

19. Deurenberg, P., Deurenberg-Yap, M. and Guricci, S. (2002) Asians are different from Caucasians and from each other in their body mass index/body fat per cent relationship. *Obesity Reviews*, **3**, 141–6.

20. Reddy, K.S. (1993) Cardiovascular diseases in India. *World Health Statistics Quarterly—Rapport Trimestriel de Statistiques Sanitaires Mondiales*, **46**, 101–7.

21. Li, G., Chen, Y., Jang, Y. *et al.* (2002) Obesity, coronary heart disease risk factors and diabetes in Chinese: an approach to the criteria of obesity in the Chinese population. *Obesity Reviews*, **3**, 167–72.

22. Huxley, R., Barzi, F., Lam, T.H. *et al.* (2006) The impact of cardiovascular risk factors on the age-related excess risk of coronary heart disease. *International Journal of Epidemiology*, **35** (4), 1025–33.

23. Strain, G., Zumoff, B., Rosner, W. *et al.* (1994) The relationship between serum levels of insulin and sex hormone-binding globulin in men: the effect of

weight loss. *Journal of Clinical Endocrinology and Metabolism*, **79**, 1173–6.

24. Ivandic, A., Prpic-Krizevac, I., Sucic, M. *et al.* (1998) Hyperinsulinemia and sex hormones in healthy premenopausal women: relative contribution of obesity, obesity type, and duration of obesity. *Metabolism: Clinical and Experimental*, **47**, 13–19.

25. Haffner, S.M. (2000) Sex hormones, obesity, fat distribution, type 2 diabetes and insulin resistance: epidemiological and clinical correlation. *International Journal of Obesity and Related Metabolic Disorders: Journal of the International Association for the Study of Obesity*, **24** (Suppl 2), S56–8.

26. Fogelholm, M., Kukkonen-Harjula, K., Nenonen, A. *et al.* (2000) Effects of walking training on weight maintenance after a very-low-energy diet in premenopausal obese women: a randomized controlled trial. *Archives of Internal Medicine*, **160**, 2177–84.

27. Ross, R., Dagnone, D., Jones, P.J. *et al.* (2000) Reduction in obesity and related comorbid conditions after diet-induced weight loss or exercise-induced weight loss in men. A randomized, controlled trial. *Annals of Internal Medicine*, **133**, 92–103.

28. Raastad, T., Bjoro, T. and Hallen, J. (2000) Hormonal responses to high- and moderate-intensity strength exercise. *European Journal of Applied Physiology*, **82**, 121–8.

29. Bonen, A. and Shaw, S.M. (1995) Recreational exercise participation and aerobic fitness in men and women: analysis of data from a national survey. *Journal of Sports Sciences*, **13**, 297–303.

30. Albright, A., Franz, M., Hornsby, G. *et al.* (2000) American College of Sports Medicine position stand. Exercise and type 2 diabetes. *Medicine and Science in Sports and Exercise*, **32**, 1345–60.

31. Pan, X.R., Li, G.W., Hu, Y.H. *et al.* (1997) Effects of diet and exercise in preventing NIDDM in people with impaired glucose tolerance. The Da Qing IGT and Diabetes Study. *Diabetes Care*, **20**, 537–44.

32. Dengel, D.R., Pratley, R.E., Hagberg, J.M. *et al.* (1996) Distinct effects of aerobic exercise training and weight loss on glucose homeostasis in obese sedentary men. *Journal of Applied Physiology*, **81**, 318–25.

33. Martinez, J.A., Kearney, J.M., Kafatos, A. *et al.* (1999) Variables independently associated with self-reported obesity in the European Union. *Public Health Nutrition*, **2** (1A), 125–33.

34. Bouchard, C. (1995) Genetics of obesity: an update on molecular markers. *International Journal of Obesity Related Metabolic Disorders*, **19** (Suppl 3), S10–13.

35. Chagnon, Y.C., Perusse, L., Weisnagel, S.J. *et al.* (2000) The human obesity gene map: the 1999 update. *Obesity Research*, **8**, 89–117.

36. Molarius, A., Seidell, J.C., Sans, S. *et al.* (2000) Educational level, relative body weight, and changes in their association over 10 years: an international perspective from the WHO MONICA Project. *American Journal of Public Health*, **90**, 1260–8.

37. Peltonen, M., Huhtasaari, F., Stegmayr, B. *et al.* (1998) Secular trends in social patterning of cardiovascular risk factor levels in Sweden. The Northern Sweden MONICA Study 1986–1994. Multinational monitoring of trends and determinants in cardiovascular disease. *Journal of Internal Medicine*, **244**, 1–9.

38. Heitmann, B.L. (2000) Ten-year trends in overweight and obesity among Danish men and women aged 30–60 years. *International Journal of Obesity and Related Metabolic Disorders: Journal of the International Association for the Study of Obesity*, **24**, 1347–52.

39. Monteiro, C.A., Benicio, M.H.D'A., Conde, W.L. *et al.* (2000) Shifting obesity trends in Brazil. *European Journal of Clinical Nutrition*, **54**, 342–6.

40. Barker, D.J.P. (1998) Mothers, Babies and Disease in Later Life, BMJ, London.

41. Barker, D.J., Winter, P.D., Osmond, C. *et al.* (1989) Weight in infancy and death from ischaemic heart disease. *Lancet*, **2**, 577–80.

42. Barker, D.J.P., Osmond, C., Simmonds, S.J. and Wield, G.A. (1993) The relation of small head circumference and thinness at birth to death from cardiovascular disease in adult life. *British Medical Journal*, **306**, 422–6.

43. Leon, D.A., Lithell, H.O., Vagero, D. *et al.* (1998) Reduced fetal growth rate and increased risk of death from ischaemic heart disease: cohort study of 15 000 Swedish men and women born 1915–29. *British Medical Journal*, **317**, 241–5.

44. Stein, C.E., Fall, C.H., Kumaran, K. *et al.* (1996) Fetal growth and coronary heart disease in south India. *Lancet*, **348**, 1269–73.

45. Huxley, R., Neil, A. and Collins, R. (2002) Unravelling the fetal origins hypothesis: is there really an inverse association between birthweight and subsequent blood pressure? *Lancet*, **360**, 659–65.

46. Ravelli, G.P., Stein, Z.A. and Susser, M.W. (1976) Obesity in young men after famine exposure *in utero* and early infancy. *New England Journal of Medicine*, **295**, 349–53.

47. Sorensen, H.T., Sabroe, S., Rothman, K.J. *et al.* (1997) Relation between weight and length at birth

and body mass index in young adulthood. *British Medical Journal*, **315**, 1137.

48. Newsome, C.A., Shiell, A.W., Fall, C.H. *et al.* (2003) Is birth weight related to later glucose and insulin metabolism? A systematic review. *Diabetic Medicine*, **20**, 339–48.

49. Ong, K.K., Ahmed, M.L., Emmett, P.M. *et al.* (2000) Association between postnatal catch-up growth and obesity in childhood. *British Medical Journal*, **320**, 967–71.

50. Hypponen, E., Power, C. and Smith, G.D. (2003) Prenatal growth, BMI, and risk of type 2 diabetes by early midlife. *Diabetes Care*, **26**, 2512–17.

51. Yajnik, C.S. (2004) Obesity epidemic in India: intrauterine origins? *Proceedings of the Nutrition Society*, **63**, 387–96.

52. King, H., Aubert, R.E. and Herman, W.H. (1998) Global burden of diabetes, 1995–2025: prevalence, numerical estimates, and projections. [See comment.] *Diabetes Care*, **21**, 1414–31.

53. Wild, S., Roglic, G., Green, A. *et al.* (2004) Global prevalence of diabetes: estimates for the year 2000 and projections for 2030. [See comment.] *Diabetes Care*, **27**, 1047–53.

54. Roglic, G., Unwin, N., Bennett, P.H. *et al.* (2005) The burden of mortality attributable to diabetes: realistic estimates for the year 2000. [See comment.] *Diabetes Care*, **28**, 2130–5.

55. Rossner, S., Sjostrom, L., Noack, R. *et al.* (2000) Weight loss, weight maintenance, and improved cardiovascular risk factors after 2 years treatment with orlistat for obesity. European Orlistat Obesity Study Group. *Obesity Research*, **8**, 49–61.

56. Davidson, M.H., Hauptman, J., DiGirolamo, M. *et al.* (1999) Weight control and risk factor re-duction in obese subjects treated for 2 years with orlistat: a randomized controlled trial. *Journal of the American Medical Association*, **281**, 235–42.

57. Foryet, J.P. (1997) A 2-year multicenter study of the effects of orlistat (Xenical) on weight loss and disease risk factors. *Obesity Research*, **5** (Suppl 1), 53S.

58. Eriksson, J., Lindstrom, J., Valle, T. *et al.* (1999) Prevention of type II diabetes in subjects with impaired glucose tolerance: the Diabetes Prevention Study (DPS) in Finland. Study design and 1-year interim report on the feasibility of the lifestyle intervention programme. *Diabetologia*, **42**, 793–801.

59. Tuomilehto, J., Lindstrom, J. and Eriksson, J. (2001) Prevention of type 2 diabetes mellitus by changes in lifestyle among subjects with impaired glucose tolerance. *New England Journal of Medicine*, **344**, 13243–50.

60. Hess, D.S. and Hess, D.W. (1998) Biliopancreatic diversion with a duodenal switch. *Obesity Surgery*, **8**, 267–82.

61. Pories, W.J., MacDonald, K.G. Jr, Flickinger, E.G. *et al.* (1992) Is type II diabetes mellitus (NIDDM) a surgical disease? *Annals of Surgery*, **215**, 633–43.

62. Knowler, W.C., Barrett-Connor, E., Fowler, S.E. *et al.* (2002) Reduction in the incidence of type 2 diabetes with lifestyle intervention or metformin. *New England Journal of Medicine*, **346**, 393–403.

63. Torgerson, J.S., Hauptman, J., Boldrin, M.N. *et al.* (2004) XENical in the prevention of diabetes in obese subjects (XENDOS) study: a randomized study of orlistat as an adjunct to lifestyle changes for the prevention of type 2 diabetes in obese patients. *Diabetes Care*, **27**, 155–61.

6

Methodology for Physical Activity Assessment

Kristi L. Storti, Edward W. Gregg and Andrea M. Kriska

Department of Epidemiology, Graduate School of Public Health,
University of Pittsburgh, Pittsburgh, PA, USA

6.1 INTRODUCTION

It is generally accepted that an active lifestyle is beneficial in the fight to prevent or delay the development of type 2 diabetes. This has been supported by extensive physiological and epidemiological literature. Active individuals have better insulin and glucose profiles than their inactive counterparts, whereas complete physical inactivity, with detraining and bed rest, results in a deterioration of these metabolic parameters. Likewise, training studies have found that exercise improves insulin action or, in other words, decreases insulin resistance. Physical activity has also been shown to be inversely related to obesity and central fat distribution, particularly visceral obesity. In summary, it appears that physical activity may reduce the risk for type 2 diabetes both directly, by improving insulin sensitivity, and indirectly, by producing beneficial changes in body mass and body composition [1–3]; see also the *Handbook of Exercise in Diabetes* [4].

The epidemiologic literature, from observational studies to the more powerful randomized clinical trials, mirrors the physiology literature suggesting that physical activity can be an important risk factor in the prevention or delay of type 2 diabetes development (for reviews of the epidemiology literature in the area of physical activity and diabetes prevention, see [5, 6]). Lifestyle intervention, of which physical activity was an integral part, was shown to reduce the incidence of type 2 diabetes

by 31–63% in four intervention studies (three of which were randomized clinical trials). In these studies, a decreased progression to type 2 diabetes development, due to lifestyle intervention, was observed at follow-up in adult Swedish men and US, Chinese and Finnish men and women with impaired glucose intolerance at baseline [7–10]. The physical activity goals of the various trials were largely similar to the recommendations with in *Physical Activity & Health: A Report by the Surgeon General* [11]. These public health recommendations also suggested that it is the daily accumulation of physical activity bouts that is important (therefore, activity can be split up over the course of the day) and that activity may come from sources other than leisure and sporting activities.

The flexibility of this public health activity goal appears to have contributed to the successful adherence of the physical activity intervention in these clinical trials of diabetes prevention [6], but it makes for a more challenging measurement issue. It is much easier to measure structured, higher intensity activity than to attempt to quantify lower intensity activities accumulated throughout the day. Yet, public health interventionists need to be able to rely on physical activity assessment to identify subgroups that are the most inactive (and would most benefit from an activity intervention) and need to be able to monitor the progress of intervention efforts. Both researchers and interventionists would like to be able to identify the specific levels

The Epidemiology of Diabetes Mellitus, second edition   Edited by Jean-Marie Ekoé, Marian Rewers, Rhys Williams and Paul Zimmet
© 2008 John Wiley & Sons, Ltd

of physical activity likely to provide the most protection. For all of these issues, physical activity measurement is a crucial link and sometimes a lingering hurdle.

6.2   WHAT IS PHYSICAL ACTIVITY?

Physical activity has been defined by Caspersen *et al.* [12] as 'any bodily movement produced by skeletal muscles that results in energy expenditure'. Components of total energy expenditure in a sedentary individual include basal metabolic rate, which typically encompasses 50–70% of total energy, and the thermic effect of food, which accounts for another 7–10% [13]. The remaining 20–43% is composed of energy expended through some type of 'physical activity,' which can then be subdivided (see **Figure 6.1**) into energy expended in general activities of daily living (such as bathing, feeding and grooming), occupation activity, sporting and other leisure activities, transportation activity and household and caretaking activities (including home repair). The relative contribution of each of these components can vary considerably both within and among individuals and populations.

Measurement of physical activity is further complicated by the fact that there are several health-related dimensions of physical activity [14]. For example, in addition to quantifying physical activity based on the amount of energy expended, physical activity can be quantified based on the *manner* in which energy is expended. Physical activity can be measured according to its effects on different systems of the body by assessing attributes such as aerobic intensity, muscular resistance, degree of weight-bearing and range of motion or flexibility involved. These qualitative differences in physical activity may have implications for the prevention of specific diseases. For example, 100 cal burned swimming may be particularly beneficial to cardiovascular health, but 100 cal expended through weight training may have a more favorable effect on bone mass or osteoporosis risk.

6.3   HOW HAS PHYSICAL ACTIVITY BEEN MEASURED?

Physical activity assessment tools have been used to measure many dimensions and attributes of

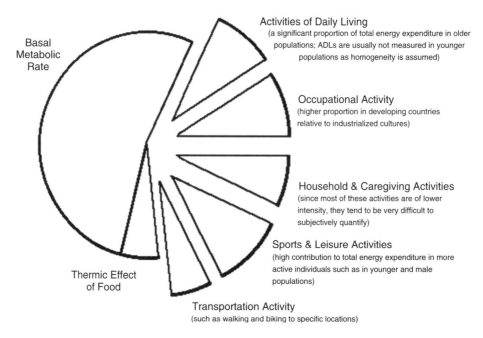

Figure 6.1 Schematic representation of components of total energy expenditure.

physical activity. These tools can be categorized into objective and subjective approaches.

Objective approaches include:

- Measures of energy expenditure, such as the respiratory chamber or the doubly labeled water (DLW) technique.
- Movement monitors, such as pedometers and accelerometers.
- Measures of the physiological responses to physical activity, including heart rate monitoring and fitness testing.

Subjective measures include:

- An array of questionnaires and surveys which require the individual to *recall* their past activity behavior. These tools vary in their ability to quantify the type, frequency, duration and intensity of various occupational, sports and leisure, transportation and household activities over a variety of time frames.
- Activity logs and diaries for recording specific activities as they occur.

Each approach has advantages and disadvantages that can vary based upon the population being studied and the research objectives. In epidemiological research, subjective measures have typically been used for the practical assessment of physical activity in populations, and objective measures have often been utilized to validate these subjective activity measures.

6.3.1 Description of Some of the Popular Objective Approaches

6.3.1.1 Direct Calorimetry

Direct calometry involves the measurement of body heat production and is the most precise estimate of energy expenditure [15–18]. Direct calorimetry is characteristically performed under laboratory conditions with the individual in an airtight chamber, known as a *room calorimeter*. Room calorimeters measure the heat produced by an individual at rest or during exercise by circulating water through pipes in the insulated chamber, and carefully measuring, at frequent intervals, the temperature of the ingoing and outgoing water and the water flow. Measurements are usually made over a 24 h period and follow a 10–12 h fast, so that resting metabolic rate (RMR) can be accurately assessed. Room calorimeters are typically small and confined and are not practical for assessing activity-related energy expenditure for a variety of free-living activity patterns. Therefore, they restrict the type and pattern of physical activity that can be studied. Moreover, while providing highly precise measures of energy expenditure, the cost and technical limitations make direct calorimetry generally impractical for assessing activity-related energy expenditure in large epidemiological studies.

6.3.1.2 Indirect Calorimetry

Indirect calometry does not directly measure heat production; instead, energy expenditure is estimated from VO_2 consumption and VCO_2 production. The heat energy released from substrate oxidation during physical activity can be estimated from measured O_2. Energy expenditure estimates are based on assumed relations between VO_2 and the caloric cost of substrate oxidation [16, 19, 20]. Individuals are confined to a metabolic chamber for the duration of the assessment. Similar to the room calorimeter (see Section 6.3.1.1), the respiratory chamber is an airtight, insulated, temperature–humidity-controlled room [15, 16, 18, 21]. Specific concentrations of O_2 and CO_2 are introduced to the room at a controlled rate of airflow. Fractional concentrations of O_2 and CO_2 are measured as the air leaves the system. Based on the gas concentrations and flow rate of expired air, VO_2 and VCO_2 can be determined. This technique is used for validation of other physical activity measures in both children [22] and adults [23, 24].

Methods for performing oxygen-uptake-based indirect calorimetry outside the chamber have been developed. These techniques utilize an integrated measurement system comprised of an O_2 and CO_2 analyzer, a ventilation flow-volume meter and a microcomputer to process expired air collected through a fitted hood, face mask, or mouthpiece [25]. Typically, these techniques are used to assess task-specific activities, such as housework, yardwork and particular occupational activities [26].

6.3.1.3 DLW Technique

The DLW technique is the best estimate of free-living, total energy expenditure and is currently used as a gold standard of energy expenditure in validation studies. It involves the ingestion of isotopically labeled water, from which the amount of labeled hydrogen (^2H_2O) and oxygen ($H_2^{18}O$) eliminated can be measured over a set period of time, usually 1–2 weeks. The difference in hydrogen and oxygen turnover rates provides an estimate of metabolic carbon dioxide production and, thus, an estimate of total energy expenditure [13, 18, 27, 28]. By subtracting the resting energy expenditure, which is typically determined using standard laboratory procedures of indirect calorimetry, an estimate of energy expended during physical activity is obtained.

DLW provides precise estimates of energy expenditure in free-living populations, with no influence on behavior and no constraints on the time or setting of physical activity. The fact that it is nonreactive and does not likely result in an alteration of the participant's behavior is an important advantage over some other measures of physical activity, such as activity diaries. Unfortunately, the higher cost makes it less practical for use in many epidemiologic studies. DLW is also only relevant for studying total energy expended and provides no information about the intensity of or the specific type of activity performed during the sample time frame. Therefore, physical activity patterns must be measured using other assessment techniques. Furthermore, it is not applicable for the evaluation of physical activity energy expenditure for more than a 1–2 week period unless repeat assessments are made.

6.3.1.4 Activity Monitors

Activity monitors have been used to estimate physical activity levels and, more often, to help validate subjective measures of activity. Some of the most popular activity monitors utilized for physical activity assessment are pedometers and accelerometers.

Pedometers have gained widespread popularity in research and intervention efforts to quantify ambulatory physical activity in terms of accumulated steps in free-living settings. Pedometers are small, inexpensive, battery-operated devices. They are most often worn at the waist and estimate general trunkal movement. Pedometers are reasonably precise and are used in research and clinical settings where walking and related movement are

the primary types of physical activity. Moreover, their ease of administration makes them a practical assessment tool for individuals encompassing most age groups [29–33]. Lastly, pedometers have the ability to promote behavior change and have been increasingly used in intervention settings as an intervention tool.

There are some limitations to pedometers, in that they do not provide information relating to activity type, duration, or intensity. Therefore, accurate quantification of activity-related energy expenditure and patterns of activity (e.g. time spent in type- or intensity-specific activities, short versus continuous bouts) cannot be assessed. Similar to other movement monitors, pedometers are unable to account for upper body movements, such as arm work, water activities and uphill walking [34], and have difficulty accurately assessing activity levels in individuals at slower gait speed [35, 36].

Accelerometers are small, noninvasive, battery-operated devices often worn on the waist, arm or ankle. They detect not only the frequency of movement, but also the acceleration and deceleration of movement in a single and/or multiple planes. Microcomputer technology integrates and sums the absolute value and frequency of acceleration forces over a defined observation period (e.g. every minute) and physical activity data is expressed in the form of an activity 'count.' Regression equations have been developed from controlled laboratory experiments to allow for the estimation of activity-related energy expenditure from these activity counts [37, 38].

Accelerometers are more advanced than pedometers, in that they provide information about the frequency, duration, intensity and patterns of physical activity and have the capability to record and store information over long periods of time. Unfortunately, information regarding the specific type of physical activity (i.e. gardening versus walking) is not captured. In addition, like pedometers, accelerometers are limited in their ability to quantify energy expenditure due to upper body involvement, water activities or uphill walking [39].

In short, accelerometers and pedometers have been used successfully in both children [29, 30, 40–43] and adults [44–48] and have been shown to be significantly correlated with other measures of physical activity, such as questionnaires [23, 49–52] and DLW [53, 54]. Since activity monitors were originally designed to quantify walking and running activity, they become less accurate in the measurement of activities that are not similar to walking or running. They can also be affected by passive movement, such as car or bus rides on bumpy roads, and cannot be used in water, limiting the full scope of activity assessment.

6.3.1.5 Heart Rate Monitoring

Heart rate monitoring has been used in both clinical and research settings to estimate activity-related energy expenditure based upon the assumption of a linear relationship between heart rate and oxygen consumption (VO_2) [55]. Because the heart rate–VO_2 relationship is somewhat attenuated during low and very high intensity activities [56], and because of considerable between person and day-to-day heart rate–VO_2 variability [57, 58], individual heart rate–VO_2 calibration curves [59] are necessary for estimation of activity-related energy expenditure. While the calibration technique is somewhat cumbersome, the actual heart rate monitoring itself is easy and quick to administer and can be utilized in either a laboratory or free-living setting. It is modestly accurate in the assessment of physical activity intensity and has been utilized in both children [60] and adults [26, 61]. Unfortunately, there is the potential for heart rate monitoring to cause an alteration in activity behavior and, like the DLW technique, heart rate monitoring is usually limited to a short time frame. Lastly, body temperature, size of the active muscle mass (e.g. upper versus lower body), type of exercise (static versus dynamic), stress and medication influence heart rate, which may result in an imprecise estimation of activity-related energy expenditure [18, 56].

6.3.1.6 Physical Fitness

Physical fitness is a set of attributes, such as cardiorespiratory fitness, that people have or can achieve that relate to the ability to carry out physical activity participation [12]; therefore, it has been used as a surrogate measure for physical activity. The rationale for using fitness as a method to assess physical activity extends from the consistent findings that aerobic activity improves cardiorespiratory fitness [62]. Fitness provides an objective way of comparing individuals in the population and of evaluating progress in exercise interventions.

Like physical activity, higher levels of physical fitness have been shown to be protective against cardiovascular disease and all-cause mortality [63–65]. However, it appears that physical fitness has a strong genetic component [66].

There are two types of testing most often used to assess physical fitness, maximal oxygen uptake (VO_2 max) and submaximal oxygen uptake. VO_2 max can be defined as the highest level of oxygen consumption that is utilized by the body during peak physical exertion [67]. However, in instances where VO_2 max testing is not practical, cardiovascular fitness can be measured indirectly using submaximal VO_2. Submaximal VO_2 tests use heart rate to predict the oxygen consumption that would have occurred during maximal workloads (VO_2 max). Submaximal VO_2 tests are able to predict VO_2 max because of the linear relationship that exists between heart rate and exercise workload/intensity (i.e. as work and intensity increases, heart rate increases) [67]. Examples of submaximal VO_2 tests include the YMCA Cycle ergometer test and McArdle step test. Field tests are also used to estimate submax VO_2 by using established prediction equations that take into consideration the distance that is covered or the amount of time it took to cover a particular distance [67]. Examples of field tests include the Rockport walking test, the 1.5-mile run test, and the long-distance corridor walk.

6.3.2 Subjective Measures

Physical activity questionnaires have emerged as the tool of choice for activity assessment. This is primarily because of practical considerations, but also because they can estimate patterns of physical activity such as frequency, duration and intensity. Physical activity surveys likely do not alter an individual's behavior, but are subject to recall biases. These tools vary considerably in their complexity, from self-administered single questions to comprehensive interviewer-administered surveys. Single-item questionnaires have been used which ask an individual whether or not they are more active than others their age and sex or whether they exercise long enough to break in to a sweat [68, 69]. More complex questionnaires, such as recall questionnaires, attempt to survey a wide range of popular activities over a selected time frame, such as over a lifetime. Lastly, diaries are often used to record activities in 'real time' over a short time frame such as a few days.

6.3.2.1   Time Frame

Physical activity questionnaires and diaries are further distinguished by the time frame that they cover. Diaries and logs may require the participant to record activities over 1 day, 3 days or the past week. Past-week-recall surveys query the frequency and duration of participation in activities performed over the past week, with examples that include the Harvard alumni questionnaire, the Baecke physical activity questionnaire, and the 7-day physical activity recall questionnaire [68, 70, 71]. Surveys with a shorter time frame, such as the past day or week, are less vulnerable to recall bias and are more practical to validate with objective tools than are questionnaires of a longer time frame. However, since physical activity may vary with season, or as a result of an acute illness or time commitment, assessment over a short time period is less likely to reflect 'usual' behavior [72].

Questionnaires of a longer time frame, such as 1 year, may be more likely to represent usual activity patterns and have been used extensively in epidemiologic studies. Past-year physical activity has been assessed by questionnaires such as the Minnesota leisure-time physical activity questionnaire (MLTPQ), the modifiable physical activity questionnaire or MAQ (modified version of the Pima activity questionnaire) and the Harvard alumni questionnaire [68, 72, 73]. All of these questionnaires result in a summary estimate of physical activity expended per week averaged over the past year. Although the potential for recall bias is greater when measuring long-term activity patterns, these assessments are less likely to be influenced by acute changes in activity levels than questionnaires with a shorter time frame. To account for these methodological issues, some studies include physical activity assessment over both short and long time periods in order to obtain the best overall estimate of an individual's typical activity levels [74].

6.3.2.2   Lifetime Physical Activity

A few studies have attempted to assess a lifetime or portion of a lifetime of physical activity. Since chronic diseases such as osteoporosis and cancer tend to have a long developmental period, it is potentially the long-term chronic exposure to physical inactivity that increases risk for disease. In addition, historical physical activity assessment has the advantage of being feasible to use in case-control studies of rare diseases and avoiding the expense and time of longitudinal studies.

Early measures of historical physical activity categorized people according to employment history [75–77]. This approach made assumptions about the activity level associated with specific job titles and ignored any contribution of leisure physical activity. Other lifetime assessments have grouped subjects according to participation in high school or intercollegiate athletics [78–82]. This approach disregarded the contribution of physical activity outside of organized sports.

More recent physical activity surveys have assessed historical physical activity in a more comprehensive manner, evaluating the extent to which physical activities (mostly leisure) were performed during specific age periods [75, 83–85]. Studies utilizing these historical physical activity questionnaires have demonstrated that people who participated in less leisure physical activity over their lifetime had lower bone mass, more hip fractures and are more likely to develop noninsulin-dependent diabetes mellitus and certain types of cancer [83, 86–92]. Historical physical activity assessment is obviously limited by problems with recall and the difficulty in validation. One study by Winters-Hart *et al.* [85] was able to validate their historical measure by comparing the historical physical activity recall with physical activity levels assessed by questionnaire at four previous time points over a 17-year period in postmenopausal women. The findings of this study noted statistically significant correlations between historical physical activity recall and the original questionnaires, concluding that historical recall of leisure physical activity can be reasonably estimated. While an ideal study design would collect lifetime physical activity prospectively, the use of historical physical activity questionnaires as described above has enabled examination of factors that would otherwise require many years of study, thousands of participants and high expense to conduct.

6.3.2.3 Types of Physical Activity Assessed

It is imperative that the activities queried are both comprehensive and representative of the population and culture being studied. Physical activity questionnaires vary according to the types of physical activity they assess. Early studies in physical activity epidemiology estimated physical activity performed at work [93, 94]. Using a classification scheme such as the *US Dictionary of Occupational Titles*, created and published by the Department of Labor [95–99], individuals were categorized into groups of 'sedentary, light, medium, heavy or heavy work' [77]. Job classification has the advantage of being relatively objective and less vulnerable to recall bias. However, misclassification of individuals is likely due to assumptions about the amount of activity expended in a given occupation and the fact that activity levels of a given occupation can vary across regions. Relatively more recent occupational physical activity questionnaires have been developed which query the frequency, duration and intensity of physical activities within a job rather than simply inquiring about the job title itself [74, 100–102].

However, most contemporary physical activity surveys only assess leisure activities. Owing to the decline in physical activity levels within occupations in most industrialized countries [103], the assessment of leisure physical activity may provide the best representation of population-wise variance in physical activity. Leisure-time and sporting activities are more distinctive behaviors with more specific starting and ending times, making recall by the participant more precise and definition and quantification easier for the researcher. It is assumed that the activities of daily living, such as bathing or feeding, are similar among most individuals within the population and that differences in these activities are less likely to contribute substantially to energy expenditure in a population.

Although this focus on leisure and sporting physical activity may be valid for younger and healthier populations, some have suggested that differences in activities of daily living or other low-level leisure activities may be the most important determinant of energy expenditure and physical activity in an older or sick population [104]. Therefore, questionnaires have been developed to assess physical activity at the lower end of the physical activity spectrum. The physical activity scale for the elderly (PASE), the Yale physical activity survey (YPAS) and the modified Baecke questionnaire all query these lower-level leisure activities [49, 105, 106].

6.3.2.4 Intensity of Physical Activity Assessed

It is well known that lower intensity unstructured activities tend to be difficult to recall and have been shown to be less reproducible when assessed subjectively than higher intensity activities, such as many of the organized sports [71, 74]. Examples of physical activities of low intensity include general activities of daily living, such as bathing, feeding and grooming. Across this spectrum of activity (see **Figure 6.2**) are physical activities that vary in intensity, including sports and leisure activities, household activities, care taking, transportation and occupation activities. Since they are difficult to recall, measurement of these lower intensity activities, for the most part, may require the use of objective measures, such as activity monitors.

6.3.3 An Example of a Comprehensive Physical Activity Survey

The most popular survey approaches measure the type, frequency (e.g. number of times per given time frame), duration (e.g. number of minutes or hours per session) and estimate the intensity (e.g. degree of vigor or estimated metabolic cost) of physical activities performed during a particular time period. It is this comprehensive assessment of physical activity that has allowed for a more sensitive discrimination between individuals of different activity levels and lends itself to subanalyses based on type, duration and intensity of activity. This approach has served as the basis for much of the epidemiologic research relating physical activity to the prevention of diabetes, cardiovascular and other diseases. Examples of questionnaires that use this approach are the modifiable activity questionnaire and the MLTPQ [73, 74].

As described in **Figure 6.3**, the data obtained from a more extensive questionnaire format give the researcher options to analyze data at several different levels. Multiplying the number of times per week of participation by the number of hours per time leads to an estimate of total duration of

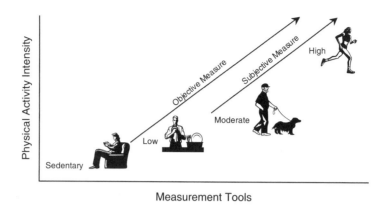

Figure 6.2 Spectrum of physical activity.

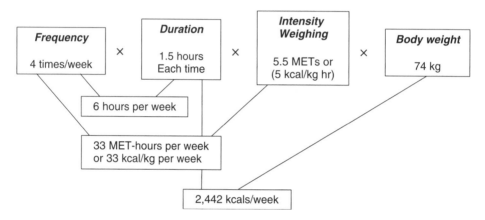

Figure 6.3 Steps in the computation of the summary estimates with a past week physical activity questionnaire as an example.

physical activity within a specific time frame (the past week in this example). Comparisons can be made at this step in this process by comparing individuals based on the total time (frequency and duration) spent participating in physical activities. If possible, time spent in each activity can then be multiplied by an estimate of the relative intensity of that activity. These intensity estimates are obtained from the literature and correspond to how vigorous the specific activity is and how intense the individual thought they performed the activity. All of the activities are then summed and expressed in metabolic equivalent '(MET)-hours per week' (or kcal kg^{-1} week^{-1}), which can be converted to kilocalories per week if one knows the body weight of the individual. However, this last calculation involves making an assumption about the weight

of the individual throughout the time frame that is being assessed.

Rather than weighting each specific activity by its relative intensity as described above, some questionnaires group activities and then assign intensity weights to each group. The Harvard alumni questionnaire, for example, assigns 5.0 kcal min^{-1} to a group of activities deemed to be of low cardiovascular intensity (e.g. gardening, bowling), 7.5 kcal min^{-1} to moderate-intensity activities (e.g. dancing) and 10 kcal min^{-1} for high-intensity activities (e.g. running) [68].

Lists of MET values for most activities are available in the literature. Regardless of the intensity-weighting list used, several assumptions are made by the researcher when incorporating intensity into the analysis process. When obtaining an MET or kcal value from a list, the value provided is assumed to be representative of the manner in which the activity was performed by the individual. Since skill level varies for sporting activities and a wide range of paces may be selected for activities like cycling, walking, jogging, there may be considerable variation in the actual energy expenditure across subjects. Weighting physical activities by intensity also assume that body weight is proportional to resting metabolic rate and that the relative increase in metabolic cost of a specific activity above resting is constant from person to person regardless of body weight.

Because of the assumptions made with physical activity questionnaires, estimates of physical activity obtained from them give a relatively crude and incomplete assessment of 'absolute' energy expenditure. However, since physical activity represents the most variable component of total energy expenditure, they are valuable in 'relative' terms and can be used to rank individuals or groups of subjects within a population from the least to the most active. This relative distribution of individuals based on their reported levels of physical activity can then be examined according to its relationship to physiological parameters and disease outcomes, such as the existence of or development of diabetes.

6.4 APPLICATION OF PHYSICAL ACTIVITY ASSESSMENT: POPULATION AND OUTCOME CONSIDERATIONS

Considering the wide variety of approaches for assessing physical activity, the researcher is frequently left in a quandary when designing a specific study. Since physical activity can be defined in several ways, no single standard exists by which to measure physical activity. Characteristics of the population being studied and the outcome of interest emerge as important factors in the choice of a physical activity assessment tool. Time considerations often require the researcher to choose a survey that is a brief but efficient measure of the most common physical activities of a population.

When choosing the best way to assess physical activity, it is important that the assessment tool (i) accurately represents physical activity of the study population and (ii) focuses on the component of energy expenditure that encompasses the

greatest proportion of total energy expenditure for that population. For these reasons, it is important to consider the culture, gender and age ranges of the population of interest. In industrialized, developed countries, recent surveys have focused on leisure activity because of the general decline in physical activity in most occupations. The focus on leisure physical activity in these countries differentiates active from inactive people more effectively than would an occupational physical activity questionnaire. However, occupational activity probably remains of greater importance in developing counties, where much of the population have physically demanding occupations. Therefore, some questionnaires have included both leisure and occupational physical activity assessment. As an example, physical activity levels were assessed with the modifiable activity questionnaire in two populations located almost halfway around the world from each other: Pima Indian men and women from Arizona and residents from Mauritius, located in the Indian Ocean [107]. In contrast to the Pima Indians, in which leisure activity was the largest contributor to activity levels for most age/sex groups, occupational physical activity was the largest contributor to total physical activity levels for both men and women in Mauritius. In fact, over 90% of the total physical activity was due to occupational activity in Mauritius men. Omitting the leisure section of the activity questionnaire would have resulted in an underestimation of activity levels in the Pima Indian sample, whereas omitting the occupation section would have resulted in an incorrect picture of activity levels in men from the country of Mauritius.

Physical activity patterns have traditionally differed between men and women. Perhaps due to the historic tendency to conduct epidemiological research on men rather than women, physical activity questionnaires have been more oriented around the types of leisure and occupational activities typically performed by men. In addition, women tend to engage in lower intensity activities, such as childcare and household activities, all of which are relatively more difficult to assess and may result in invalid estimates of activity if subjectively determined by questionnaire.

Since different dimensions of physical activity, such as frequency, duration, intensity and type, could conceivably have different influences on risk factors for disease and disease outcomes, the choice of a physical activity assessment tool may be determined, in part, by the disease endpoint being studied. While the majority of health benefits seem to be linked principally to the total amount of activity performed, physical activity assessment could focus on other dimensions, including aerobic intensity, resistance to the muscular system and weight-bearing, any of which could affect specific diseases or health outcomes.

Whether activity intensity can influence risk for disease outcomes independent of the total amount of activity expended is controversial and difficult to determine in population-based studies because subjects who participate in vigorous activities usually tend to be more physically active in general. Yet, in many cases, stronger relationships between physical activity and diseases or risk factors for disease have often been observed when physical activity is weighted by intensity. While this could be due to a true relationship between the intensity of activity and the risk factor and/or disease of interest, it may also be because higher intensity activities are easier to recall and may be more reliably measured [74].

6.5 CONCLUDING REMARKS

The evaluation of the relationship between physical activity and type 2 diabetes risk is complicated by the fact that type 2 diabetes is a multifaceted disease with a variety of risk factors and disease endpoints, including obesity, insulin resistance and sensitivity, glucose intolerance, diabetes incidence and glycemic control. Evidence exists from experimental, intervention and/or population-based studies that physical activity may have beneficial effects in most of these steps [1–3]; see also the *Handbook of Exercise in Diabetes* [4].

Recent national physical activity recommendations and summary statements suggest that the majority of overall health benefits from physical activity seem to be gained by performing activities that are not necessarily of high intensity [108]. Whether or not this holds for type 2 diabetes specifically is currently not known. However, in examining some of the prospective data, the largest and most consistent difference in risk of type 2 diabetes appears to occur between those individuals who report relatively no activity and those who report some activity. For example, when examining the association

between frequency of reported vigorous activity per week in both nurses and physicians, most of the difference in incidence of type 2 diabetes occurred between those who reported less than one time per week of activity compared with those who were active a minimum of once per week [109, 110].

The benefit of moderate-intensity activity in diabetes prevention was suggested in examination of the four intervention studies of diabetes prevention in which a decreased progression to type 2 diabetes development was observed at follow-up in adult Swedish men and in US, Chinese and Finnish men and women with impaired glucose intolerance at baseline [7–10]. For the most part, the physical activity goals of these four clinical trials were similar to the public health recommendations as described in [11], which call for an increase in moderate-intensity levels of physical activity, such as walking for about 30 min on most days (see Table 6.1). The activity intensity and type recommended was, in general, moderate-intensity activity (walking) and was basically aerobic (although the Finnish study also incorporated some strength training in the regimen). With regard to the weekly activity goal, all but the Finnish trial recommended a weekly goal of between 120 and 150 min per week. The Finnish Diabetes Prevention Study, in contrast, recommended 30 min per day (which is 210 min per week), although the actual weekly minutes performed by the participants in this trial are not known. Since all of these studies demonstrated a significant decrease in the incidence of type 2 diabetes in the lifestyle intervention groups (which included activity), their results would suggest that the activity goal for the general public is a reasonable goal to start with in attempting to reduce the risk of developing diabetes (and/or to increase weight loss that, in turn, results in the decreased risk of diabetes developing) in those overweight individuals that are at high risk for diabetes.

Individuals who are obese and/or sedentary are at the highest risk for type 2 diabetes and obviously, are the best targets for physical activity interventions. Since intense exercise is not likely to be feasible or popular in these individuals, interventions appear to be more successful if they focus on lower intensity activities. Yet, of course, lower intensity physical activities are the most difficult to measure.

Table 6.1 Summary of the physical activity goals from four intervention studies of diabetes prevention in comparison to the 1996 US Surgeon General's Recommendations.

	Activity type	Activity intensity	Average physical activity weekly goal	
US Surgeon General's Report [11]	Aerobic	Moderate intensity (similar to a brisk walk)	Moderate intensity levels of physical activity similar to a brisk walk for 30 min on most days or about 150–180 min per week	
Clinical trials in diabetes prevention				
US Diabetes Prevention Program (3-year study) [10]	Aerobic— brisk walking	Moderate intensity	150 min: (minimum of 10 min/time, spread out over ≥3 days per week)	~150 min of moderate intensity activity per week
Finnish Diabetes Prevention Study (4-year study) [9]	Aerobic (also some resistance training)	Moderate to somewhat vigorous intensity	30 min/day	~210 min of moderate to vigorous intensity activity per week
Da Qing Study (6-year study) [8]	Aerobic—ranging from slow walking to running, swimming and basketball	Ranged from mild to very strenuous (although most chose moderate walking)	20 min of brisk walking daily	~140 min of walking per week
Malmö Feasibility Study (6-year study) [7]	Aerobic—walk-jog, soccer, calisthenics and badminton	Moderate intensity (more intensive activity was only performed late in the training)	Two weekly 60 min sessions	~120 min or moderate intensity activity per week

The specific components of physical activity that we have focused on, as well as our definition of inactivity, have changed over these years. The challenge has been to modify the assessment tools to reflect these changes. Initial interest in the field focused on higher intensity, well-defined sports and recreational activities and/or occupational activities. The assessment of physical activity at that point in time was determined primarily with questionnaires, which were found to be relatively accurate for assessment of those higher intensity activities. However, more recently, our focus has evolved to that of total activity and overall movement. Technological advances, such as cars, elevators and remote controls, have decreased the amount of movement necessary to get us through a day, causing us to redefine what it means to be 'inactive'. It is no longer the absence of a significant amount of intense activity in an occupation or in leisure time that is considered 'inactive,' but more so the lack of substantial movement during the course of a day or week. To measure this level of physical activity, which would encompass both low- and high-intensity activities, we may need to include objective measures of physical activity in our repertoire of tools. Because of the contribution of physical activity assessment tools, physical activity is now regarded as one of the fundamental behaviors necessary for a healthy lifestyle. It is likely that any improvement in the accuracy of these tools will only enhance the ability to observe true relationships between physical activity, health and disease, serving as an incentive and challenge for future researchers.

References

1. Hawley, J.A. (2004) Exercise as a therapeutic intervention for the prevention and treatment of insulin resistance. *Diabetes Metabolism Research and Reviews*, **20** (5), 383–93.
2. Albright, A., Franz, M., Hornsby, G. *et al.* (2000) ACSM position stand: exercise and type 2 diabetes. *Medicine and Science in Sports and Exercise*, **32**, 1345–60.
3. Ivy, J.L., Zderic, T.W. and Fogt, D.L. (1999) The prevention and treatment of non-insulin-dependent diabetes mellitus. *Exercise and Sport Sciences Reviews*, **27**, 1–35.
4. Ruderman, N. (2002) Handbook of Exercise in Diabetes, American Diabetes Association, Alexandria, VA.
5. Kriska, A. and Horton, E. (2002) Physical activity in the prevention of type 2 diabetes: the epidemiological evidence across ethnicity and race, in Handbook of Exercise in Diabetes (eds N. Ruderman, J.T. Devlin, S.H. Schneider and A. Kriska), American Diabetes Association, Alexandria, VA, pp. 145–54.
6. Kriska, A. (2003) Can a physically active lifestyle prevent type 2 diabetes? *Exercise and Sport Sciences Reviews*, **31**, 132–7.
7. Eriksson, K.F. and Lindgärde, F. (1991) Prevention of type 2 (non-insulin-dependent) diabetes mellitus by diet and physical exercise. The 6-year Malmö feasibility study. *Diabetologia*, **34**, 891–8.
8. Pan, X.R., Li, G.W., Hu, Y.H. *et al.* (1997) Effects of diet and exercise in preventing NIDDM in people with impaired glucose tolerance: the Da Qing IGT and diabetes study. *Diabetes Care*, **20**, 537–44.
9. Tuomilehto, J., Lindstrom, J., Eriksson, J.G. *et al.* (2001) Prevention of type 2 diabetes mellitus by changes in lifestyle among subjects with impaired glucose tolerance. *The New England Journal of Medicine*, **344**, 1343–50.
10. Diabetes Prevention Program Research Group (2002) Reduction in the incidence of type 2 diabetes with lifestyle intervention or metformin. *The New England Journal of Medicine*, **346**, 393–403.
11. US Department of Health and Human Services (1996) Surgeon General's Report on Physical Activity and Health. From the Centers for Disease Control and Prevention. US Government Printing Office, Washington, DC.
12. Caspersen, C.J., Powell, K.E. and Christenson, G.M. (1985) Physical activity, exercise and physical fitness: definitions and distinctions for health-related research. *Public Health Reports*, **100**, 126–31.
13. Ravussin, E. and Rising, R. (1992) Daily energy expenditure in humans: measurement in a respiratory chamber and by doubly labeled water, in Energy Metabolism: Tissue Determinants and Cellular Corollaries (eds J.M. Kinney and H.N. Tucker), Raven Press, New York, pp. 81–96.
14. Caspersen, C.J. (1989) Physical activity epidemiology: concepts, methods, and applications to exercise science. *Exercise and Sport Sciences Reviews*, **17**, 423–73.
15. Brooks, G.A., Fahey, T.D. and White, T.P. (1996) Exercise Physiology. Human Bioenergetics and Its Applications, 2nd edn, Mayfield, Mountain View, CA.

16. Jequier, E., Acheson, K. and Schutz, Y. (1987) Assessment of energy expenditure and fuel utilization in man. *Annual Review of Nutrition*, **7**, 187–208.

17. Horton, E.S. (1983) An overview of the assessment and regulation of energy balance in humans. *The American Journal of Clinical Nutrition*, **38**, 972–7.

18. Montoye, H.J., Kemper, H.C.G., Saris, W.H.M. and Washburn, R.A. (1996) Measuring Physical Activity and Energy Expenditure, Human Kinetics, Champaign, IL.

19. Ferrannini, E. (1988) The theoretical bases of indirect calorimetry. *Metabolism*, **37**, 287–301.

20. Ravussin, E., Lillioja, S., Anderson, T.E. *et al.* (1986) Determinants of 24-hour energy expenditure in man. Methods and results using a respiratory chamber. *Journal of Clinical Investigation*, **78** (6), 1568–78.

21. Jequier, E. and Schutz, Y. (1983) Long-term measurements of energy expenditure in humans using a respiratory chamber. *The American Journal of Clinical Nutrition*, **38**, 989–98.

22. Ventham, J.C. and Reilly, J.J. (1999) Reproducibility of resting metabolic rate measurement in children. *The British Journal of Nutrition*, **81**, 435–7.

23. Strath, S.J., Bassett, D.R. and Swartz, A.M. (2003) Comparison of MTI accelerometer cut-points for predicting time spent in physical activity. *International Journal of Sports Medicine*, **24**, 298–303.

24. Starling, R.D., Mathews, D.E., Ades, P.A. and Poehlman, E.T. (1999) Assessment of physical activity in older individuals: a doubly labeled water study. *Journal of Applied Physics*, **86**, 2090–6.

25. Davis, J.A. (1996) Direct determination of aerobic power, in Physiological Assessment of Human Fitness (eds P.J. Maud and C. Foster), Human Kinetics, Champaign, IL, pp. 9–17.

26. Strath, S.J., Bassett, D.R., Thompson, D.L. and Swartz, A.M. (2002) Validity of the simultaneous heart rate-motion sensor technique for measuring energy expenditure. *Medicine and Science in Sports and Exercise*, **34**, 888–94.

27. Schoeller, D.A. and van Santen, E. (1982) Measurement of energy expenditure in humans by doubly labeled water method. *Journal of Applied Physiology: Respiratory, Environmental and Exercise Physiology*, **53**, 955–9.

28. Schoeller, D.A., Leitch, C.A. and Brown, C. (1986) Doubly labeled water method: in vivo oxygen and hydrogen isotope fractionation. *The American Journal of Physiology*, **251**, R1137–43.

29. Scruggs, P.W., Beveridge, S.K., Eisenman, P.A. *et al.* (2003) Quantifying physical activity via pedometry in elementary physical education. *Medicine and Science in Sports and Exercise*, **35**, 1065–71.

30. Scruggs, P.W., Beveridge, S.K., Watson, D.L. and Clocksin, B.D. (2005) Quantifying physical activity in first- through fourth-grade physical education via pedometry. *Research Quarterly for Exercise and Sport*, **76**, 166–75.

31. Bassett, D.R., Cureton, A.L. and Ainsworth, B.E. (2000) Measurement of daily walking distance—questionnaire versus pedometer. *Medicine and Science in Sports and Exercise*, **32**, 1018–23.

32. Coleman, K.L., Smith, D.G., Boone, D.A. *et al.* (1999) Step activity monitor: long-term, continuous recoding of ambulatory function. *Journal of Rehabilitation Research and Development*, **36**, 8–18.

33. Macko, R.F., Haeuber, E., Shaughnessy, M. *et al.* (2002) Microprocessor-based ambulatory activity monitoring in stroke patients. *Medicine and Science in Sports and Exercise*, **34**, 394–9.

34. Tudor-Locke, C.E. and Myers, A.M. (2001) Methodological considerations for researchers and practitioners using pedometers to measure physical (ambulatory) activity. *Research Quarterly for Exercise and Sport*, **71**, 1–12.

35. Storti, K.L., Pettee, K.K., Brach, J.S. *et al.* (2005) Gait Speed and Step-Count Monitor Accuracy in Community Dwelling Older Adults. *Medicine & Science in Sports and Exercise*, **40**(1), 59–64.

36. Bassett, D.R., Ainsworth, B.E., Leggett, S.R. *et al.* (1996) Accuracy of five electronic pedometers for measuring distance walked. *Medicine and Science in Sports and Exercise*, **28**, 1071–7.

37. Freedson, P.S., Melanson, E. and Sirard, J. (1998) Calibration of the Computer Science and Applications, Inc. accelerometer. *Medicine and Science in Sports and Exercise*, **30**, 772–81.

38. Melanson, E.L. and Freedson, P.S. (1995) Validity of Computer Science and Applications, Inc. (CSA) activity monitor. *Medicine and Science in Sports and Exercise*, **27**, 934–40.

39. Ainsworth, B.E., Bassett, D.R., Strath, S.J. *et al.* (2000) Comparison of three methods for measuring the time spent in physical activity. *Medicine and Science in Sports and Exercise*, **32** (9 Suppl), S457.

40. Trost, S.G., Pate, R.R., Sallis, J.F. *et al.* (2002) Age and gender differences in objectively measured physical activity in youth. *Medicine and Science in Sports and Exercise*, **34**, 350–5.

41. Eston, R.G., Rowlands, A.V. and Ingledew, D.K. (1998) Validity of heart rate, pedometry, and accelerometry for predicting the energy cost of children's activities. *Journal of Applied Physiology*, **84**, 362.

42. Rodriguez, G., Beghin, L. and Michaud, L. *et al.* (2002) Comparison of the TriTrac-R3D accelerometer and a self report activity diary with heart-rate monitoring for the assessment of energy expenditure in children. *The British Journal of Nutrition*, **87**, 623–31.

43. Beets, M.W., Patton, M.M. and Edwards, S. (2005) The accuracy of pedometer steps and time during walking in children. *Medicine and Science in Sports and Exercise*, **37**, 513–20.

44. Bassett, D.R., Schneider, P.L. and Huntington, G.E. (2004) Physical activity in an Old Order Amish community. *Medicine and Science in Sports and Exercise*, **36**, 79–85.

45. Bennett, G.G., Wolin, K.Y., Puleo, E. and Emmons, K.M. (2006) Pedometer-determined physical activity among multiethnic low-income housing residents. *Medicine and Science in Sports and Exercise*, **38**, 768–73.

46. LeMasurier, G.C. and Tudor-Locke, C. (2003) Comparison of pedometer and accelerometer accuracy under controlled conditions. *Medicine and Science in Sports and Exercise*, **35**, 867–71.

47. Leenders, N.Y.J.M., Sherman, W.M. and Nagaraja, H.N. (2000) Comparisons of four methods of estimating physical activity in adult women. *Medicine and Science in Sports and Exercise*, **32**, 1320–6.

48. Campbell, K.L., Crocker, P.R.E. and McKenzie, D.C. (2002) Field evaluation of energy expenditure in women using Tritrac accelerometers. *Medicine and Science in Sports and Exercise*, **34**, 1667–74.

49. Washburn, R.A., Smith, K.W., Jette, A.M. and Janney, C.A. (1993) The physical activity scale for the elderly (PASE): development and evaluation. *Journal of Clinical Epidemiology*, **46**, 153–62.

50. Matthews, C.E. and Freedson, P.S. (1995) Field trial of a three-dimensional activity monitor: comparison with self-report. *Medicine and Science in Sports and Exercise*, **27**, 1071–8.

51. Matthews, C.E., Ainsworth, B.E., Hanby, C. *et al.* (2005) Development and testing of a short physical activity recall questionnaire. *Medicine and Science in Sports and Exercise*, **37**, 986–94.

52. Bassett, D.R., Ainsworth, B.E., Swartz, A.M. *et al.* (2001) Validity of four motion sensors in measuring moderate intensity physical activity. *Medicine and Science in Sports and Exercise*, **32** (9 Suppl), S471–80.

53. Ekelund, U., Sjostrom, M., Yngve, A. *et al.* (2001) Physical activity assessed by activity monitor and doubly labeled water in children. *Medicine and Science in Sports and Exercise*, **33** (2), 275–81.

54. Leenders, N.Y., Sherman, W.M., Nagaraja, H.N. and Kien, C.L. (2001) Evaluation of methods to assess physical activity in free-living conditions. *Medicine and Science in Sports and Exercise*, **33** (7), 1233–40.

55. Wilmore, J.H. and Haskell, W.L. (1971) Use of the heart rate–energy expenditure relationship in the individualized prescription of exercise. *The American Journal of Clinical Nutrition*, **24**, 1186–92.

56. Acheson, K.J., Campbell, I.T., Edholm, O.G. *et al.* (1980) The measurement of daily energy expenditure – an evaluation of some techniques. *The American Journal of Clinical Nutrition*, **33**, 1155–64.

57. Li, R., Deurenberg, P. and Hautvast, J.G.A.J. (1993) A critical evaluation of heart rate monitoring to assess energy expenditure in individuals. *The American Journal of Clinical Nutrition*, **58**, 602–7.

58. McCroy, M.A., Mole, P.A., Nommsen-Rivers, L.A. and Dewey, K.G. (1997) Between-day and within-day variability in the relation between heart rate and oxygen consumption: effect on the estimation of energy expenditure by heart rate monitoring. *The American Journal of Clinical Nutrition*, **66**, 18–25.

59. Haskell, W.L., Yee, M.C., Evans, A. *et al.* (1993) Simultaneous measurement of heart rate and body motion to quantitate physical activity. *Medicine and Science in Sports and Exercise*, **25**, 109–15.

60. Beghin, L., Michaud, L. and Guimber, D. *et al.* (2002) Assessing sleeping energy expenditure in children using heart-rate monitoring calibrated against open circuit indirect calorimetry: a pilot study. *The British Journal of Nutrition*, **88**, 533–43.

61. Kashiwazaki, H., Inaoka, T., Suzuki, T. and Kondo, Y. (1986) Correlations of pedometer readings with energy expenditure in workers during free-living daily activities. *European Journal of Applied Physiology*, **54**, 585–90.

62. American College of Sports Medicine (1990) The recommended quantity and quality of exercise for developing and maintaining cardiorespiratory and muscular fitness in healthy adults. *Medicine and Science in Sports and Exercise*, **22**, 265–74.

63. Ekelund, L.G., Haskell, W.L., Johnson, J.L. *et al.* (1988) Physical fitness as a prevention of cardiovascular mortality in asymptomatic North

American men. *The New England Journal of Medicine*, **319**, 1379–84.

64. Blair, S.N., Kohl, H.W., Paffenbarger, R.S. *et al.* (1989) Physical fitness and all-cause mortality: a prospective study of healthy men and women. *The Journal of the American Medical Association*, **262**, 2395–401.

65. Lakka, T.A., Venalainen, J.M., Rauramaa, R. *et al.* (1994) Relation of leisure physical activity and cardiorespiratory fitness to the risk of acute myocardial infarction in men. *The New England Journal of Medicine*, **330**, 1549–54.

66. Bouchard, C., Dionne, F.T., Simoneau, J. and Boulay, M.R. (1992) Genetics of aerobic and anaerobic performances. *Exercise and Sport Sciences Reviews*, **20**, 27–58.

67. American College of Sports Medicine (2000) ACSM's Guidelines for Exercise Testing and Prescription, 6th edn, Lippincott Williams & Wilkins, Baltimore, MD.

68. Paffenbarger, R.S., Wing, A.L. and Hyde, R.T. (1978) Physical activity as an index of heart attack risk in college alumni. *American Journal of Epidemiology*, **108**, 161–75.

69. Washburn, R.A., Goldfield, S.R., Smith, K.W. and McKinlay, J.B. (1990) The validity of self-reported exercise-induced sweating as a measure of physical activity. *American Journal of Epidemiology*, **132**, 107–31.

70. Baecke, J.A.H., Burema, J. and Frijters, J.E.R. (1982) A short questionnaire for the measurement of habitual physical activity in epidemiological studies. *The American Journal of Clinical Nutrition*, **36**, 936–42.

71. Sallis, J.J.F., Haskell, W.L. and Wood, P.D. (1985) Physical activity assessment methodology in the five-city project. *American Journal of Epidemiology*, **121**, 91–106.

72. Kriska, A.M. and Caspersen, C.J. (1997) Introduction to the collection of physical activity questionnaires in a collection of physical activity questionnaires for health-related research. Centers for Disease Control and Prevention. *Medicine and Science in Sports and Exercise*, **29** (Suppl), S5–9.

73. Taylor, H.L., Jacobs, D.R., Schucker, B. *et al.* (1978) A questionnaire for the assessment of leisure time physical activities. *Journal of Chronic Diseases*, **31**, 741–55.

74. Kriska, A.M., Knowler, W.C., LaPorte, R.E. *et al.* (1990) Development of a questionnaire to examine the relationship of physical activity and diabetes in the Pima Indians. *Diabetes Care*, **13**, 401–11.

75. Housley, E., Leng, G.C., Donnan, P.T. and Fowkes, F.G. (1993) Physical activity and risk of peripheral arterial disease in the general population: Edinburgh Artery Study. *Journal of Epidemiology and Community Health*, **47** (6), 475–80.

76. Vena, J.E., Graham, S., Zielezny, M. *et al.* (1985) Lifetime occupational exercise and colon cancer. *American Journal of Epidemiology*, **122**, 357–65.

77. Vena, J.E., Graham, S., Zielezny, M. *et al.* (1987) Occupational exercise and risk of cancer. *American Journal of Clinical Nutrition*, **45**, 318–27.

78. Sarna, S., Sahi, T., Koskenvuo, M. and Kaprio, J. (1993) Increased life expectancy of world-class male athletes. *Medicine and Science in Sports and Exercise*, **25**, 237–44.

79. Marti, B., Suter, E., Riesen, W.F. *et al.* (1990) Effects of long-term, self-monitored exercise on the serum lipoprotein and apolipoprotein profile in middle-aged men. *Atherosclerosis*, **81** (1), 19–31.

80. Fogleholm, M., Kaprio, J. and Sarna, S. (1994) Healthy lifestyles of former Finnish world class athletes. *Medicine and Science in Sports and Exercise*, **26** (2), 224–9.

81. Sunman, M.L., Hoerr, S.L., Prague, H. *et al.* (1991) Lifestyle variables as predictors of survival in former college men. *Nutrition Research*, **11**, 141–8.

82. Frisch, R.E., Wyshak, G., Albright, T.E. *et al.* (1986) Lower prevalence of diabetes in female former college athletes compared with nonathletes. *Diabetes*, **35**, 1101–5.

83. Kriska, A.M., Sandler, R.B., Cauley, J.A. *et al.* (1988) The assessment of historical physical activity and its relation to adult bone parameters. *American Journal of Epidemiology*, **127**, 1053–63.

84. Halioua, L. and Anderson, J.J.B. (1989) Lifetime calcium intake and physical activity habits: independent and combined effects on the radial bone of healthy premenopausal women. *The American Journal of Clinical Nutrition*, **49**, 534–41.

85. Winters-Hart, C.S., Brach, J.S., Storti, K.L. *et al.* (2004) Validity of a questionnaire to assess historical physical activity in older women. *Medicine and Science in Sports and Exercise*, **36**, 2082–7.

86. Kriska, A., LaPorte, R., Pettitt, D. *et al.* (1993) The association of physical activity with obesity, fat distribution and glucose intolerance in Pima Indians. *Diabetologia*, **36**, 863–9.

87. Jaglal, S.B., Kreiger, S.B. and Darlington, G. (1993) Past and recent physical activity and risk of hip fracture. *American Journal of Epidemiology*, **138**, 107–18.

88. Greendale, G.A., Barrett-Connor, E., Edelstein, S. *et al.* (1995) Lifetime leisure exercise and osteoporosis. *American Journal of Epidemiology*, **141**, 951–9.
89. Friedenreich, C.M., McGregor, S.E., Courneya, K.S. *et al.* (2004) Case-control study of lifetime total physical activity and prostate cancer risk. *American Journal of Epidemiology*, **159** (8), 740–9.
90. Kolbe-Alexander, T.L., Charlton, K.E. and Lambert, E.V. (2004) Lifetime physical activity and determinants of estimated bone mineral density using calcaneal ultrasound in older South African adults. *The Journal of Nutrition, Health and Aging*, **8** (6), 521–30.
91. Pierotti, B., Altieri, A., Talamini, R. *et al.* (2005) Lifetime physical activity and prostate cancer risk. *International Journal of Cancer*, **114** (4), 639–42.
92. Matthews, C.E., Shu, X.O., Jin, F. *et al.* (2001) Lifetime physical activity and breast cancer risk in the Shanghai Breast Cancer Study. *British Journal of Cancer*, **84** (7), 994–1001.
93. Morris, N.H., Heady, J.A., Raffle, P.A. *et al.* (1953) Coronary heart disease and physical activity of work. *Lancet*, **2**, 1053–7, 1111–20.
94. Paffenbarger, R.S. and Hale, W.E. (1975) Work activity and coronary heart mortality. *The New England Journal of Medicine*, **292**, 545–50.
95. US Department of Labor (1949) *Dictionary of Occupational Titles*, vol. **1**, 2nd edn, US Government Printing Office, Washington, DC.
96. US Department of Labor (1965) *Dictionary of Occupational Titles*, vol. **1**, 3rd edn, US Government Printing Office, Washington, DC.
97. US Department of Labor (1979) *Dictionary of Occupational Titles*, 4th edn, US Government Printing Office, Washington, DC.
98. US Department of Labor, Employment Service, Bureau of Employment Security (1956) *Estimates of Worker Trait Requirements for 4000 Jobs as Defined in the Dictionary of Occupational Titles*, US Government Printing Office, Washington, DC.
99. Vena, J.E., Graham, S., Zielezny, M. *et al.* (1987) Occupational exercise and risk of cancer. *American Journal of Clinical Nutrition*, **45**, 318–27.
100. Yore, M.M., Ham, S.A., Ainsworth, B.E. *et al.* (2005) Occupational physical activity: reliability and comparison of activity levels. *Journal of Physical Activity Health*, **2** (3), 358–65.
101. Ainsworth, B.E., Richardson, M.T., Jacobs, D.R. *et al.* (1999) Evaluation of occupational activity surveys. *Journal of Clinical Epidemiology*, **52**, 219–27.
102. Montoye, H.J. (1971) Estimation of habitual physical activity by questionnaire and interview. *The American Journal of Clinical Nutrition*, **24**, 1113–18.
103. Powell, K.E., Thompson, P.D., Caspersen, C.J. and Kendrick, J.S. (1987) Physical activity and the incidence of coronary heart disease. *Annual Review of Public Health*, **8**, 253–87.
104. LaPorte, R.E., Adams, L.L., Savage, D.D. *et al.* (1984) The spectrum of physical activity, cardiovascular disease and health: an epidemiologic perspective. *American Journal of Epidemiology*, **120**, 507–17.
105. Voorrips, L.E., Ravelli, A.C.J., Dongelmans, P.C.A. *et al.* (1991) A physical activity questionnaire for the elderly. *Medicine and Science in Sports and Exercise*, **23**, 974–9.
106. Dipietro, L., Caspersen, C.J., Ostfeld, A.M. and Nadel, E.R. (1993) A survey for assessing physical activity among older adults. *Medicine and Science in Sports and Exercise*, **25**, 628–42.
107. Kriska, A.M., Pereira, M.A., Hanson, R.L. *et al.* (2001) Association of physical activity and insulin concentrations in two populations at high risk for type 2 diabetes but differing by body mass index. *Diabetes Care*, **24**, 1175–80.
108. Pate, R.R. (1995) Physical activity and health: dose–response issues. *Research Quarterly for Exercise and Sport*, **66**, 313–17.
109. Manson, J.E., Rimm, E.B., Stampfer, M.J. *et al.* (1991) Physical activity and incidence of non-insulin-dependent diabetes mellitus in women. *Lancet*, **338**, 774–8.
110. Manson, J.E., Nathan, D.M., Krolewski, A.S. *et al.* (1992) A prospective study of exercise and incidence of diabetes among US male physicians. *Journal of the American Medical Association*, **268**, 63–7.

7

Epidemiology of Nutrition and Diabetes Mellitus: Etiology and Environmental Factors

Jim Mann[1] and Monika Toeller[2]

[1]Department of Human Nutrition, University of Otago, Dunedin, New Zealand
[2]German Diabetes Center, University of Dusseldorf, Germany

7.1 INTRODUCTION

The first evidence for an environmental factor in the etiology of type 2 diabetes was described in the sixth century during the Brahman period of Hindu medicine by the three physicians Charaka, Susrut and Vagbhata. They wrote of diabetes:

> It is the disease of the rich and one that is brought about by the gluttonous overindulgence in oil, flour and sugar.

In about 400 BC in China, Neijing described diabetes, its complications and its relationship to overnutrition. Over 1000 years later, dietary factors were implicated as a major factor in the occurrence of type 2 diabetes by Thomas Willis:

> Diabetes was so rare among the ancients that many famous physicians made no mention of it and Galen knew only two sick of it. But in our age given to food fellowship and gushing down chiefly of unalloyed wine, we meet examples and instance enough, I may say daily, of this disease.

In contrast, war-related deprivations have been associated with marked reductions in rates of death from diabetes. An impressive decline in diabetes death rates during the World Wars I and II has been reported in different places [1]. In Berlin, for instance, the diabetes mortality rate declined from 23.1 per 100 000 in 1914 to 10.9 per 100 000

in 1919. The same trends were found in other European countries in populations that were short of food.

No changes in diabetes mortality were described in places where there was no food shortage during the World War I, such as Japan and North America [2].

The probable influence of caloric consumption on risk of diabetes has been further demonstrated in many places. At a time when food consumption per caput was rising sharply in Japan [3], in Taiwan [4] and, more recently, in some Pacific islands [5] there was a sharp rise in the prevalence of diabetes. In 1969, Charles and Medard [6] published an instructive report on the relationship of diabetes to nutrition in Haiti, one of the poorest developing countries in the world. Poor people in Haiti consumed 980–1500 kcal per person per day compared with more than 3000 kcal per person per day consumed by rich people during the study period. Diabetes rates were about 100 times as great in the rich. Although food consumption and diabetes rates have usually been quite low in rural villages in many developing countries, both urbanization and/or severe undernutrition (less than 1000 kcal and less than 50 g of protein consumed per day per caput) may enhance rates of diabetes. Traditionally living populations seem more or less 'protected' from diabetes; but severe deprivation of protein and calories may

The Epidemiology of Diabetes Mellitus, second edition   Edited by Jean-Marie Ekoé, Marian Rewers, Rhys Williams and Paul Zimmet
© 2008 John Wiley & Sons, Ltd

cause diabetes [7]. This issue will be discussed in the section on malnutrition-related diabetes mellitus.

There is now a considerable amount of evidence to suggest that rapid acculturation is associated with increased rates of type 2 diabetes [8]. There are clearly several characteristics of the Western way of life which predispose to the development of obesity. It may simply be that the increase in obesity resulting from an aggregation of these factors (especially physical inactivity and increased intake of energy-dense foods leading to energy intake in excess of requirements) explains the increasing rates of type 2 diabetes, particularly in individuals or populations with an appropriate genetic predisposition. The roles of obesity and genetic factors are considered in Chapter 19.Energy intake is impossible to assess adequately in epidemiological studies even when the best instruments presently available for assessing dietary intake are employed, since it has now been clearly demonstrated that overweight and obese individuals underestimate their intake.

On the other hand, energy output can be accurately measured [9] but the techniques are not suited for use in large-scale epidemiological studies. This chapter, therefore, will describe the role of individual nutrients and other possible environmental factors in the etiology of type 2 diabetes. It is important to emphasize that there are major difficulties in assessing nutritional etiologies of any chronic disease. The pros and cons of the various dietary instruments (diet records, 24 h recalls and food frequency questionnaires) and problems inherent in the various epidemiological approaches are discussed elsewhere [10].

7.2   CARBOHYDRATE AND DIETARY FIBER

The suggestion that refined carbohydrates, and sugars in particular, might be involved in the etiology of type 2 diabetes dates back to the writings of early Indian physicians. However, in the 1960s, Yudkin [11] resurrected the suggestion that high intakes of sucrose may be particularly important in the etiology of type 2 diabetes when he drew attention to the positive correlation between intakes of sucrose and diabetes prevalence in 22 countries. But it has subsequently become clear that the

correlations were heavily dependent upon which countries were selected for inclusion and that such geographic correlations do no more than provide clues for further research; they certainly do not imply causality. Over 40 studies have examined the role of sugars in the etiology of type 2 diabetes, with about half suggesting a positive association and a comparable number suggesting no association. Some have even suggested an inverse association between diabetes incidence and sucrose intake [12]. Poor assessment of dietary intake, inability to disentangle dietary and other confounding factors, and overinterpretation of data derived from observational studies characterize many of these studies. Further evidence to suggest that sucrose is not an important contributing factor in the etiology of type 2 diabetes comes from carefully controlled studies in people with type 2 diabetes [13].

Isoenergetic substitution of moderate amounts of sucrose in the diets of individuals participating in a randomized crossover experiment did not result in deterioration in glycemic control. Despite the lack of direct evidence incriminating sucrose in the etiology of type 2 diabetes it is probably inappropriate to totally exonerate sucrose. A recent epidemiological prospective study in school children has shown a clear relationship between the difference in measures of obesity over a 19-month period and change in consumption of sugar-sweetened drinks. For each additional serving of sugar-sweetened drinks, both body mass index (BMI) (mean $0.24 \, kg/m^2$) and frequency of obesity (odds ratio 1.6) increased after adjustment for anthropometric, demographic, dietary and lifestyle variables [14]. If excessive sucrose does predispose to obesity, then it is clearly an indirect predisposing factor to type 2 diabetes. Recent data suggest an association between high fructose corn syrup (HFCS) intake, which has been immensely increased in the United States during the last decade, and obesity as well as an increased risk of type 2 diabetes [15, 16].

On the other hand, there is rather more support for the suggestion that foods rich in slowly digested or resistant starch or high in dietary fiber (nonstarch polysaccharide) might be protective. Countries with high intakes of these foods have low rates of diabetes, and Trowell [17] drew attention to the fact that the reduced mortality rates for diabetes during and after World War II paralleled the increased intake of dietary fiber during that period. These observations on their own provide no more evidence for a protective role for these foods than do comparable studies suggesting a causal role of sucrose. However, there is some corroborative evidence for a protective role of dietary fiber (nonstarch polysaccharide), and slowly absorbed or resistant starch and low glycemic index foods which may be rich in these nutrients.

In a cross-sectional study of normoglycemic men, intake of pectin (a soluble form of dietary fiber) was shown to be inversely associated with postload blood glucose levels, independently of energy intake and BMI, which could potentially have confounded the association [18].

Although the study was a cross-sectional one, participants were unaware of their state of glucose tolerance, so that dietary recall could not have been influenced thereby. In a prospective study involving over 65 000 US women aged 40–65 years, diets low in cereal fiber and with a high glycemic load (i.e. rich in high glycemic index foods) were associated with an increased risk of type 2 diabetes. Comparing the highest with the lowest quintile of intake of cereal fiber, the relative risk of developing diabetes was 1.37 and for glycemic load 1.47 (p for trend was 0.005 and 0.003), after adjusting for other important risk factors for diabetes [19]. Experimental studies provide further confirmation. In controlled experiments, diets high in soluble fiber-rich foods [20] or foods with a low glycemic index are associated with improved diurnal blood glucose profiles and long-term overall improvement in glycemic control, as evidenced by reduced levels of glycated hemoglobin [21]. At first glance there appears to be some inconsistency in these observations, in that the epidemiological data suggest a protective effect of cereal (insoluble) fiber, whereas most of the experimental data suggest that soluble fiber has a more profound effect on glycemic control. However, the methodologies for distinguishing between different types of dietary fiber are not well developed and the protective effect is most appropriately attributed to the entire group of carbohydrates classified as nonstarch polysaccharides or dietary fiber.

Some other studies provide indirect support for this hypothesis. Diabetes risk appears to be lower in Seventh-Day Adventists who are vegetarians than

in those who are not strict vegetarians [22]. The diet of vegetarians is characterized by a high intake of dietary fiber, but differs in other ways from that of nonvegetarians.

In addition to not eating meat and animal products, vegetarians also have less saturated fat, more polyunsaturated fat and a diet which differs in micronutrient composition when compared with nonvegetarians.

7.3 DIETARY FATS

More than 60 years ago, Himsworth [23] suggested that high intakes of fat increased the risk of diabetes in populations and individuals. West and Kalbfleisch [24] confirmed these observations, but these studies are subject to similar biases to those already described for cross-sectional and case–control studies. Furthermore, diets which are high in carbohydrate are likely to be low in fat, so that it may be impossible to disentangle the consequences of increased intakes of the former and low intakes of the latter. Nevertheless, it is noteworthy that prospective studies have found associations between intake of fat and subsequent risk of developing type 2 diabetes. In the San Luis Valley Diabetes Study, a high fat intake was associated with an increased risk of type 2 diabetes and impaired glucose tolerance (IGT) [25]; in a follow-up, 1 to 3 years later, fat consumption predicted progression to type 2 diabetes in those with IGT [26]. On the other hand, no association was found between fat intake and risk of type 2 diabetes in a 12-year follow-up of women in Gothenburg, Sweden [27].

The type of dietary fat may also be relevant [28]. Saturated fatty acids were positively related to fasting and postprandial glucose levels in normoglycemic Dutch men, the effect being independent of energy intake and obesity. In a recent Italian study, intake of butter (rich in palmitic and myristic acids) was positively associated with fasting glucose levels, and the use of olive oil (high in oleic acid) was inversely associated with fasting glucose levels [29]. In women in the United States, the relative risk of developing diabetes was significantly reduced amongst those with the highest intake of vegetable fats [30].

In a small group of Japanese Americans with IGT, intake of animal fat was related to progression of

IGT to diabetes [31]. A high intake of saturated fat is also associated with high fasting and postprandial insulin levels and high insulin levels during an oral glucose tolerance test [32, 33]. Polyunsaturated fatty acids are inversely associated with insulin levels [34].

The relationship between nature of dietary fat and type 2 diabetes has also been studied using more sophisticated laboratory measurements. Finnish subjects with IGT and undiagnosed type 2 diabetes were reported to have higher proportions of saturated fatty acids in serum cholesterol esters than subjects with normal glucose tolerance, and the ratio of polyunsaturated to saturated fatty acids in serum phospholipids has been shown to be inversely associated with insulin secretion and positively associated with insulin action [35]. Experimental studies confirm the role of fatty acids as determinants of insulin function [36]. Saturated fatty acids induce insulin resistance in isolated rat adipocytes [37]. A controlled dietary intervention study in humans performed under isoenergetic conditions indicates that an exchange of saturated fatty acids with unsaturated fatty acids significantly improves insulin sensitivity [38]. Monounsaturated fatty acids may be associated with improved insulin action when compared with complex carbohydrates which are not also rich in nonstarch polysaccharides [39].

A suggestion that n-3 polyunsaturated fatty acids may also have an important role in the development of diabetes first came from the study of populations consuming large amounts of fatty fish, which are rich in these long-chain unsaturated fatty acids. Greenland and Alaskan Eskimos and Alaskan Indians have low rates of diabetes [40, 41]. In a recent prospective study of elderly men and women, habitual fish eaters were shown to have a 50% lower risk of developing glucose intolerance than those who are not regular fish eaters over a 4-year follow-up period [42]. The n-3 polysaturated fatty acids have a wide range of metabolic effects and, of particular relevance, influence the production of eicosanoids, which in turn may have an appreciable effect on pancreatic β-cell function [43].

However, the extent by which n-3 polyunsaturated fatty acids protect against diabetes remains to be established with certainty. One study has suggested that the addition of these fatty acids to the diet of healthy volunteers resulted in a significant increase in insulin sensitivity, but the KANWU

Study found no change when a diet relatively high in n-3 polyunsaturated fatty acids replaced monounsaturated fatty acids [38].

Thus, it appears that the effects of the various fatty acids on diabetes risk and measures of glycemic control and insulin resistance are similar to their effects on lipoprotein-mediated risk of coronary heart disease. Saturated fatty acids are associated with a deleterious effect, whereas monounsaturated fatty acids and n-3 and n-6 polyunsaturated fatty acids are associated with potentially beneficial effects. Modifying the intake of dietary fats may reduce the risk of developing type 2 diabetes, as well as reduce the risk of cardiovascular disease amongst those suffering from the condition.

7.4   PROTEIN

There are no firm epidemiological data concerning the role of protein intake in the etiology of type 2 diabetes, though the fact that meat-eating Seventh-Day Adventists have higher rates than those who do not eat meat has been taken to suggest a possible deleterious effect of animal protein [22]. The strong positive associations between animal protein and saturated fatty acids and vegetable protein and dietary fiber mean that it is almost impossible to disentangle separate effects in epidemiological studies. Some amino acids (e.g. arginine, leucine and phenylalanine) can influence β-cell function, but the epidemiological approach clearly does not readily lend itself to examining further the role of individual amino acids. High intakes of proteins, especially animal protein, appear to be associated with an increased risk of nephropathy in type 1 diabetes [44], so restriction of protein may help to delay progression of microalbuminuria to clinical nephropathy [45].

7.5   ALCOHOL

The relationship between alcohol and other dietary variables similarly complicates attempts to evaluate a potential etiological role for alcohol. Furthermore, confounding by obesity, distribution of adipose tissue and smoking result in difficulties in interpreting the epidemiological data.

In a French prospective study, abnormal liver function tests used as an indicator of alcohol excess formed an independent predictor of 4-year diabetes risk in middle-aged men [46]. In the Rancho Bernardo study, increasing intakes of alcohol in obese men were associated with an increased risk of diabetes [47]. However, a light to moderate intake of alcohol is associated with enhanced insulin sensitivity [48].

7.6 OTHER DIETARY FACTORS AND SMOKING

Several micronutrients, most notably chromium, zinc, magnesium and vitamin E, have been implicated in the pathogenesis of type 2 diabetes and/or been shown to be associated with improved glycemic control. However, no epidemiological studies have provided convincing support for the role of any of these nutrients in the etiology of the disease. There is, perhaps, rather more support for the suggestion vitamin D deficiency may be important. Vitamin D deficiency impairs insulin release, followed, if prolonged, by impairment of insulin secretion and reduction of glucose tolerance which progresses to irreversible diabetes. Asians living in East London have a reduction in insulin secretion associated with vitamin D deficiency which is improved after treatment with vitamin D [49]. There has been much recent interest in the observation that babies with a low birthweight and infants with a low weight at 1 year are at increased risk of developing IGT and type 2 diabetes later in life. The precise role of maternal malnutrition in determining this phenomenon of 'programming' remains to be established [50]. The role of smoking as a risk factor for type 2 diabetes has received relatively little attention. Smoking induces insulin resistance [51], and cigarette smokers have been shown to be relatively glucose intolerant and dyslipidemic [52].

Thus, smokers might be expected to be at considerably increased risk of type 2 diabetes. A negative association has been reported between coffee consumption and risk of type 2 diabetes [53].

7.7 PHYSICAL INACTIVITY

In 1972, Björntorp and colleagues suggested that physical training resulted in lower plasma insulin levels and improved insulin sensitivity. This has been convincingly confirmed in many subsequent experiments. In cross-sectional epidemiological studies, type 2 diabetes rates have been shown to be lower amongst physically active individuals than amongst those not having regular physical activity [54]. The protective effect of physical activity against type 2 diabetes has been confirmed in several prospective studies. For example, in the Nurses' Health Study, women who engaged in vigorous exercise at least once a week had an age-adjusted relative risk of type 2 diabetes of 0.67 compared with women who exercised less frequently than weekly [55]. The relative risk was reduced after adjustments for BMI, but remained highly statistically significant. A similar graded reduction in risk of subsequently developing type 2 diabetes associated with a graded increase in physical activity was observed amongst men participating in the Physicians' Health Study [56]. This inverse association was particularly strong in men who were overweight and was not confounded by the presence of obesity. Furthermore, controlling for smoking, hypertension and other coronary risk factors did not materially alter the association.

7.8 POTENTIAL FOR INTERVENTION

The ultimate aim of identifying environmental risk factors for type 2 diabetes lies in the hope of preventing the disease or of stopping, or at very least delaying, the progression of IGT to type 2 diabetes. Studies aimed at such primary or secondary prevention are important not only from the point of view of assessing the potential value of intervention programs, but also because they can, at least in theory, provide definitive proof of causality of particular environmental factors in the etiology of the disease.

No controlled trials have examined the potential of modifying environmental factors in the primary prevention of type 2 diabetes. Clearly, this could only be undertaken in the context of national dietary intervention programs. However, some studies have been undertaken to determine the role of lifestyle modification programs in reducing the risk of progression of IGT to type 2 diabetes. The early and less definitive studies were reviewed in detail some time ago [57]. Since then the results of three major controlled intervention trials have been published: the Da Qing study carried out in China and the Finnish and United States Intervention Trials [58–60]. In these studies, diet and exercise programs were associated with an appreciable reduction (nearly 60%) in the risk of progression of IGT to type 2 diabetes. Diets restricted in saturated fatty acids and with increased fiber content seemed to be particularly successful in this context.

Unfortunately, from the point of view of disentangling potential causal factors, a multifactorial approach involving all putative lifestyle factors (including recommendations to increase physical activity) has been adopted so that no conclusions can be drawn concerning individual components of the programs. Furthermore, weight loss appears to be the major determinant of benefit, leading to the conclusion that any or all lifestyle factors which promote obesity may be involved in the etiology of the disease. However, the Finnish Diabetes Prevention Study recently showed that dietary fat and fiber intake are significant predictors of sustained weight reduction and progression to type 2 diabetes in high-risk subjects, even after adjustment for other risk factors [61].

7.9   CONCLUSIONS

Studies utilizing a variety of epidemiological approaches have implicated a range of lifestyle-related environmental factors in the etiology of type 2 diabetes. The limitations inherent in ecological studies, case–control and prospective studies, the difficulties of accurately assessing nutrient intake and the close associations between different dietary characteristics mean that it is almost impossible to disentangle separate effects in observational studies.

The difficulties are compounded by the fact that many of the lifestyle-related factors are linked with the development of obesity, which in turn, besides genetic factors, is a major determinant of the risk of developing type 2 diabetes in individuals and populations. Intervention studies do, in theory, provide the means of studying individual putative factors, but there are unlikely ever to be any such studies because, for obvious pragmatic reasons, intervention studies focus on 'best bet' programs, which will include a range of lifestyle manipulations. For these reasons, the best evidence concerning the etiological role of individual factors is likely to come from relatively

small carefully controlled studies using metabolic rather than clinical endpoints. In such studies, it is possible to control for potential confounding by alterations in energy intake and body weight. Studies of this kind which are presently available suggest that the nature of dietary fat (saturated fatty acids being deleterious and certain polyunsaturated fatty acids being protective) and carbohydrate (fiber-rich and low glycemic index foods being beneficial) and physical inactivity may be directly related to the development of type 2 diabetes, as well as via their role in increasing the risk of obesity. It is difficult to envisage the epidemiological or, indeed, even the experimental study which will finally resolve this issue.

References

1. Himsworth, H.P. (1935) The influence of diet on the sugar tolerance of healthy men and its reference to certain extrinsic factors. *Clinical Science*, **2**, 67–94.
2. Mann, J.I. and Houston, A.C. (1983) The aetiology of non-insulin-dependent diabetes mellitus, in *Diabetes in Epidemiological Perspective* (eds J.I. Mann, K. Pyörälä and A. Teuscher), Churchill Livingstone, Edinburgh, pp. 122–64.
3. Oiso, T. (1970) Recent annual changes in nutrition in Japan, in *Diabetes Mellitus in Asia* (eds S. Tsuji and M. Wada), Excerpta Medica, Amsterdam, pp. 234–42.
4. Tsai, S. (1971) Epidemiology of diabetes in Taiwan. *Journal of Japan Diabetic Society*, **14**, 33–5.
5. Zimmet, P. and King, H. (1982) Epidemiological studies of diabetes mellitus in Pacific populations: a review, in *Diabetes Mellitus. Primary Health Care, Prevention and Control* (eds J. Tuomilehto, P. Zimmet, H. King and M. Pressley), IDF, Ames Division Miles Laboratories, Australia, pp. 8–21.
6. Charles, R.W. and Medard, F. (1969) Relation of diabetes to nutrition in Haiti (abstracts). *Diabetes*, **18** (Suppl 1), 349.
7. Harsha Rao, R. (1984) The role of undernutrition in the pathogenesis of diabetes mellitus. *Diabetes Care*, **7**, 595–601.
8. Zimmet, P., Dowse, G., Finch, C. *et al.* (1990) The epidemiology and natural history of NIDDM; lessons from the South Pacific. *Diabetes/Metabolism Reviews*, **6**, 91–124.
9. Prentice, A.M., Black, A.E., Coward, W.A. *et al.* (1986) High levels of energy expenditure in obese women. *British Medical Journal*, **292**, 983–7.
10. Willett, W. (1990) Nutritional Epidemiology, Oxford University Press, New York.

11. Yudkin, J. (1964) Dietary fat and dietary sugar in relation to ischemic heart disease and diabetes. *Lancet*, **1**, 4–5.

12. West, K.M. (1978) Epidemiology of Diabetes and its Vascular Lesions, Elsevier, New York.

13. Peterson, D.B., Lambert, J., Gerring, S. *et al.* (1986) Sucrose in the diet of diabetic patients – just another carbohydrate? *Diabetologia*, **29**, 216–20.

14. Ludwig, D.S., Peterson, K.E. and Gortmaker, S.L. (2001) Relation between consumption of sugar-sweetened drinks and childhood obesity: a prospective, observational analysis. *Lancet*, **357**, 505–8.

15. Bray, G.A., Nielsen, S.J. and Popkin, B.M. (2004) Consumption of high-fructose corn syrup in beverages may play a role in the epidemic of obesity. *The American Journal of Clinical Nutrition*, **79**, 537–43.

16. Schulze, M.B., Manson, J.E., Ludwig, D.S. *et al.* (2004) Sugar-sweetened beverages, weight gain and incidence of type 2 diabetes in young and middle-aged women. *Journal of the American Medical Association*, **292**, 927–34.

17. Trowell, H.C. (1975) Dietary-fibre hypothesis of the etiology of diabetes mellitus. *Diabetes*, **24**, 762–5.

18. Feskens, E.J.M. and Kromhout, D. (1990) Habitual dietary intake and glucose tolerance in middle-aged euglycaemic men. The Zutphen Study. *International Journal of Epidemiology*, **19**, 953–9.

19. Salmerón, J., Manson, J.E., Stampfer, M.J. *et al.* (1997) Dietary fiber, glycemic load, and risk of non- insulin-dependent diabetes mellitus in women. *Journal of the American Medical Association*, **277**, 472–7.

20. Mann, J.I. (1984) Lines to legumes: changing concepts of diabetic diets. *Diabetic Medicine*, **1**, 191–8.

21. Brand, J.C., Colagiuri, S., Crossman, S. *et al.* (1991) Low-glycemic index foods improve long-term glycemic control in NIDDM. *Diabetes Care*, **14**, 95–101.

22. Snowdon, D.A. and Phillips, R.L. (1985) Does a vegetarian diet reduce the occurrence of diabetes? *American Journal of Public Health*, **75**, 507–12.

23. Himsworth, P.H. (1935) Diet and the incidence of diabetes mellitus. *Clinical Science*, **2**, 117–48.

24. West, K.M. and Kalbfleisch, J.M. (1971) Influence of nutritional factors on prevalence of diabetes. *Diabetes*, **20**, 99–108.

25. Marshall, J.A., Hamman, R.F. and Baxter, J. (1991) High-fat, low-carbohydrate diet and the etiology of non-insulin-dependent diabetes mellitus: the San Luis Valley Diabetes Study. *American Journal of Epidemiology*, **134**, 590–603.

26. Marshall, J.A., Shetterly, S., Hoag, S. and Hamman, R.F. (1994) Dietary fat predicts conversion from impaired glucose tolerance to NIDDM. *Diabetes Care*, **17**, 50–6.

27. Lundgren, H., Bengtsson, C., Biohmé, G. *et al.* (1989) Dietary habits and incidence of non-insulin-dependent diabetes mellitus in a population study of women on Gothenburg, Sweden. *The American Journal of Clinical Nutrition*, **49**, 708–12.

28. Kinsell, L.W., Walker, G., Michels, G.D. *et al.* (1959) Dietary fats and the diabetic patient. *The New England Journal of Medicine*, **261**, 431–4.

29. Trevisan, M., Krogh, V., Freudenheim, J. *et al.* (1990) Consumption of olive oil, butter and vegetable oils and coronary heart disease risk factors. *Journal of the American Medical Association*, **263**, 688–92.

30. Colditz, G.A., Manson, J.E., Stampfer, M.J. *et al.* (1992) Diet and risk of clinical diabetes in women. *The American Journal of Clinical Nutrition*, **55**, 1018–23.

31. Tsunehara, C.H., Leonetti, D.L. and Fujimoto, W.Y. (1991) Animal fat and cholesterol intake is high in men with IGT progressing to NIDDM. *Diabetes*, **40**, 427A.

32. Maron, D.J., Fair, J.M., Haskel, W.L. *et al.* (1991) Saturated fat intake and insulin resistance in men with coronary artery disease. *Circulation*, **84**, 2020–7.

33. Parker, D.R., Weiss, S.T., Troisi, R. *et al.* (1993) Relationship of dietary saturated fatty acids and body habitus to serum insulin concentrations: the Normative Aging Study. *The American Journal of Clinical Nutrition*, **58**, 129–36.

34. Houtsmuller, A.J. (1975) The role of fat in the treatment of diabetes mellitus, in *The Role of Fats in Human Nutrition* (ed. A.J. Vergrocsen), Academic Press, New York, pp. 231–302.

35. Salomaa, V., Ahola, I., Tuomilehto, J. *et al.* (1990) Fatty acid composition of serum cholesterol esters in different degrees of glucose intolerance; a population-based study. *Metabolism*, **39**, 1285–91.

36. Vessby, B., Tengblad, S. and Lithell, H. (1994) Insulin sensitivity is related to the fatty acid composition of serum lipids and skeletal muscle phospholipids in 70-year-old men. *Diabetologia*, **37**, 1044–50.

37. Hunnicutt, J.W., Hardy, R.W., Williford, J. and Mc-Donald, J.M. (1994) Saturated fatty acid-induced insulin resistance in rat adipocytes. *Diabetes*, **43**, 540–5.

38. Vessby, B., Uusitupa, M., Hermansen, K. *et al.* (2001) Substituting dietary saturated fat with monounsaturated fat impairs insulin sensitivity in

healthy men and women: the KANWU Study. *Diabetologia*, **44**, 312–19.

39. Garg, A., Bonamone, A., Grundy, S.M. *et al.* (1988) Comparison of a high-carbohydrate diet with a high-monounsaturated-fat diet in patients with non-insulin-dependent diabetes mellitus. *The New England Journal of Medicine*, **319**, 829–34.

40. Kromann, N. and Green, A. (1980) Epidemiological studies in the Upernavik district, Greenland. *Acta Medica Scandinavica*, **208**, 401–6.

41. Mouratoff, G.J., Carrol, N.V. and Scot, E.M. (1969) Diabetes mellitus in Athabaskan Indians in Alaska. *Diabetes*, **18**, 29–32.

42. Feskens, E.J.M., Bowles, C.H. and Kromhout, D. (1991) Inverse association between fish intake and risk of glucose intolerance in normoglycemic elderly men and women. *Diabetes Care*, **14**, 935–41.

43. Robertson, R.P. (1988) Eicosanoids as pluripotential modulators of pancreatic islet function. *Diabetes*, **37**, 367–70.

44. Toeller, M., Buyken, A., Heitkamp, G. *et al.* (1997) Protein intake and urinary albumin excretion rates in the EURODIAB Complications Study. *Diabetologia*, **40**, 1219–26.

45. Wiseman, M., Viberti, G., Mackintosh, D. *et al.* (1984) Glycaemia, arterial pressure and microalbuminuria in type 1 (insulin dependent) diabetes mellitus. *Diabetologia*, **26**, 401–5.

46. Popoz, L., Eschwege, E., Warnet, J.-M. *et al.* (1982) Incidence and risk factors of diabetes in the Paris Protective Study (GREA), in *Advances in Diabetes Epidemiology* (ed. E. Eschwège), Elsevier, Amsterdam, pp. 113–22.

47. Holbrook, T.L., Barrett-Connor, E. and Wingard, D.L. (1990) A prospective population-based study of alcohol use and non-insulin-dependent diabetes mellitus. *American Journal of Epidemiology*, **132**, 902–9.

48. Facchini, F., Chen, J. and Reaven, G.M. (1994) Light to moderate alcohol intake is associated with enhanced insulin sensitivity. *Diabetes Care*, **17**, 115–19.

49. Boucher, B.J. (1995) Strategies for reduction in the prevalence of NIDDM. *Diabetologia*, **38**, 1125–29.

50. Hales, C.N., Barker, D.J.P., Clark, P.M.S. *et al.* (1991) Fetal and infant growth and impaired glucose tolerance at age 64. *British Medical Journal*, **303**, 1019–22.

51. Atvall, S., Fowelin, J., Lager, I. *et al.* (1993) Smoking induces insulin resistance–a potential link with the insulin resistance syndrome. *Journal of Internal Medicine*, **233**, 327–32.

52. Zavaroni, I., Bonini, L., Gaspirino, P. *et al.* (1994) Cigarette smokers are relatively glucose intolerant, hyperinsulinemic and dyslipidemic. *The American Journal of Cardiology*, **73**, 904–5.

53. Van Dam, R.M. and Feskens, E.J. (2002) Coffee consumption and risk of type 2 diabetes mellitus. *Lancet*, **360**, 1477–8.

54. Björntorp, P., de Jounge, K., Sjöström, L. and Sullivan, L. (1973) Physical training in human obesity. II. Effects of plasma insulin in glucose-intolerant subjects without marked hyperinsulinemia. *Scandinavian Journal of Clinical and Laboratory Investigation*, **32**, 41–5.

55. Manson, J.E., Rimm, E.B., Stampfer, M.J. *et al.* (1991) Physical activity and incidence of non-insulin-dependent diabetes mellitus in women. *Lancet*, **338**, 774–8.

56. Manson, J.E., Nathan, D.M., Krolewski, A.S. *et al.* (1992) A prospective study of exercise and incidence of diabetes among US male physicians. *Journal of the American Medical Association*, **268**, 63–7.

57. Bourn, D.M. (1996) The potential for lifestyle change to influence the progression of impaired glucose tolerance to non-insulin dependent diabetes mellitus. *Diabetic Medicine*, **13**, 938–45.

58. Pan, X.-R., Li, G.-W., Hu, Y.-H. *et al.* (1997) Effects of diet and exercise in preventing NIDDM in people with impaired glucose tolerance. The Da Qing IGT and Diabetes Study. *Diabetes Care*, **20**, 537–44.

59. Tuomilehto, J., Lindstrom, J., Eriksson, J.G. *et al.* (2001) Prevention of type 2 diabetes by changes in lifestyle among subjects with impaired glucose tolerance. *The New England Journal of Medicine*, **344**, 1343–50.

60. Knowler, W.C., Barrett-Connor, E., Fowler, S.E. *et al.* (2002) Reduction in the incidence of type 2 diabetes with lifestyle intervention or metformin. *The New England Journal of Medicine*, **346**, 393–403.

61. Lindström, J., Peltonen, M., Eriksson, J.G. *et al.* (2006) High fibre, low-fat diets predicts long-term weight loss and decreased type 2 diabetes risk: the Finnish Diabetes Prevention Study. *Diabetologia*, **49**, 912–20.

8

Genetic Epidemiology of Type 2 Diabetes

Leif Groop, Valeriya Lyssenko, Charlotte Ling and Marju Orho-Melander

Department of Clinical Sciences/Diabetes & Endocrinology and Lund University Diabetes Centre,
Lund University, University Hospital Malmö, Malmö, Sweden

8.1 INTRODUCTION

A disease can be inherited or acquired, or both. Wheras cystic fibrosis is an example of an inherited disease, most infectious diseases are acquired. But susceptibility to an infectious disease can also be influenced by genetic factors. Heterozygous carriers of the mutation causing sickle cell anemia are resistant against malaria [1]. A 32-bp deletion in the gene encoding for the lymphoblastoid chemokine receptor (CCR5) was introduced in Europe during the plague by *Yersina pestis* in the fourteenth century [2]. Carriers of this deletion are today less susceptible to HIV infections.

Cystic fibrosis is caused by mutations in one gene, namely *CFTR*, and represents a monogenic disorder with early onset of symptoms, usually from birth. The segregation of the disease follows a clear Mendelian recessive inheritance; in Europe, 1 in 2000 children is affected. Similarly, maturity-onset diabetes in the young (MODY) 3 is also a monogenic disease caused by mutations in the hepatocyte nuclear factor 1 alpha (*HNF1α*) gene [3]; although onset is 'early,' it is clearly later than in cystic fibrosis, usually during puberty or pregnancy. In contrast, a polygenic disease like type 2 diabetes is caused by common variations with modest effects in several genes, it shows a late onset and it does not follow a clear Mendelian mode of inheritance. A polygenic disease is also referred to as *complex* because of its complex inheritance pattern. A complex disease often appears to be acquired; the development of obesity and type 2 diabetes is triggered by environmental factors like intake of dense caloric food and lack of exercise in genetically susceptible individuals. However, not all obese individuals develop diabetes; genetic susceptibility is a prerequisite. Given the complex interplay between genetic and environmental factors, a complex polygenic disease is also referred to as *multifactorial*.

8.2 GENETIC RISK

The *relative genetic risk* λ_R of an inherited disease is defined as the recurrence risk for a relative of an affected person divided by the risk for the general population; it can either be risk to a sibling (λ_S) or to an offspring (λ_O). The higher the λ_S, the easier it is to find (map) the genetic cause of the disease: the λ_S value for cystic fibrosis is approximately 500, for MODY 50, and for type 2 diabetes it is 3. Therefore, it is not surprising that cystic fibrosis was the first disease to be mapped by positional cloning or linkage analysis [4], whereas success for type 2 diabetes has been limited until now [4] and mostly restricted to the identification of the underlying genetic causes for different forms of MODY [5–7]. It may seem paradoxical that λ_S is higher for type 1 diabetes than for type 2 diabetes ($\lambda_S \approx 15$ versus $\lambda_S \approx 3$), as familial clustering (more than one affected member in the family) is stronger for type 2 diabetes than for type 1 diabetes (40% versus 10%). The lower λ_S for type 2 diabetes is due to the much higher frequency of type 2 diabetes than of type 1 diabetes in the population. In polygenic diseases, it can be estimated how much of the λ_S value the different genes account for: in the case of type 1 diabetes, concordance at the *HLA* locus on the short arm of chromosome 6 explains about

The Epidemiology of Diabetes Mellitus, second edition   Edited by Jean-Marie Ekoé, Marian Rewers, Rhys Williams and Paul Zimmet

half of the λ_S value of 15. For type 2 diabetes, no genetic factor has been shown to explain more than a few percent of the individual risk of the disease.

The relative genetic risk should not be mixed up with the *population attributable risk* (PAR). The PAR is important from a public health perspective, but it does not tell us anything about the individual risk. Instead, it describes the fraction of a disease that would be eliminated if the genetic risk factor was removed from the population. The PAR is high if the risk allele is common in the population, but it is low for rare alleles in complex diseases. This is illustrated by the role of the Apo $\varepsilon4$ allele in Alzheimer's disease and of the Pro12Ala polymorphism in the PPARγ gene in type 2 diabetes: the PAR for Apo $\varepsilon4$ in Alzheimer's disease is 20% because of the high frequency of the Apo $\varepsilon4$ allele in the population (16%), whereas the PAR for the Pro12Ala polymorphism in the PPARγ gene is even higher (25%), as about 80% of the general population carries the risk allele Pro [8].

8.3   EVIDENCE THAT TYPE 2 DIABETES IS INHERITED

There is ample evidence that type 2 diabetes has a strong genetic component. The concordance of type 2 diabetes in monozygotic twins is approximately 70%, compared with 20–30% in dizygotic twins [9, 10]. Given the age-dependent penetrance of the disease, it is clear that the longer the follow-up is, the higher is the concordance rate [9]. Type 2 diabetes also clusters in families. The lifetime risk of developing type 2 diabetes is about 40% in offspring of one parent with type 2 diabetes [11]; the risk approaches 70% if both parents have diabetes. Intriguingly, the risk in the offspring seems to be greater if the mother rather than the father has type 2 diabetes [12]. Translated into a λ_S value, it means that a first-degree relative of a patient with type 2 diabetes has a threefold increased risk of developing the disease [13]. Large ethnic differences in the prevalence of type 2 diabetes have also been ascribed to a genetic component. The prevalence of type 2 diabetes is higher in full-blooded Nauruans than in Nauruans with foreign admixture [14]. Furthermore, there is higher prevalence of type 2 diabetes in full-blooded North Dakota Indians than in Indians with less than one half of Indian heritage [15].

In Sweden, type 2 diabetes is two- to three-fold more common in immigrants from the Far East than in native Swedes (Haghanifar, F. unpublished observation). Although this could be a consequence of the new Western environment, the prevalence of type 2 diabetes is significantly higher in countries in the Far East than in Sweden.

It is clear that the change in the environment toward a more affluent Western life style plays a key role in the epidemic increase in the prevalence of type 2 diabetes worldwide. This change has occurred during the last 50 years, during which period our genes have not changed. This does not exclude an important role for genes in the rapid increase in type 2 diabetes, since genes or variation in them explain how we respond to the environment.

8.4   THRIFTY GENOTYPES OR PHENOTYPES?

A plausible explanation for this interaction between genes and environment comes from the thrifty gene hypothesis. Neel [16] proposed that individuals living in an environment with unstable food supply (as for hunters and nomads) would maximize their probability of survival if they could maximize storage of energy. Genetic selection would thus favor energy-conserving genotypes in such environments. Storage of energy as fat, especially as intra-abdominal fat, is a more efficient way of storing energy than as glycogen in muscle and liver. Metabolically, this is seen as an insulin-resistant phenotype. This could explain the finding that offspring of patients with type 2 diabetes show early accumulation of abdominal fat [12]. Support for this hypothesis comes from studies in the ob/ob and db/db mice [17]. Heterozygous animals matched for body weight with the wild-type animal survived longer during total fasting than the wild-type animal. The sand rat is another example of such an insulin-resistant thrifty genotype with a metabolism aimed at ensuring survival during long periods of fasting in the desert.

An alternative explanation has been proposed by which these changes can be the consequence of intrauterine programming, the so-called thrifty phenotype hypothesis [18]. According to this hypothesis, intrauterine malnutrition would lead to a low birthweight and an increased risk of metabolic syndrome (clustering of cardiovascular risk factors, like abdominal obesity, dyslipidemia, hypertension and glucose intolerance) later in life. Although these findings have been replicated in several studies, it has also been shown that the risk of a small birthweight is increased in families with metabolic syndrome [19], suggesting that a small birthweight could be a phenotype for a thrifty gene. In support of this, children with a glucokinase defect, and thereby a decrease in insulin secretion, have a low birthweight [20]. This was particularly apparent in children of diabetic mothers, since these children would be expected to have a high birthweight as a consequence of high glucose concentrations passing the placenta and thereby stimulating the fetal pancreas to produce increasing amounts of anabolic insulin.

8.5   PREDICTION OF FUTURE TYPE 2 DIABETES

Risk factors for type 2 diabetes seem to differ between different ethnic populations. Consistent to all of them is that a family history of diabetes confers an increased risk of future type 2 diabetes [13], but its relative effect decreases with increasing frequency of type 2 diabetes in the population. Its predictive value is also relatively poor in young subjects whose parents have not yet developed the disease. A low level of physical activity, abdominal obesity and the presence of metabolic syndrome [21, 22] also confer an increased risk of type 2 diabetes. In addition, elevated glucose concentrations per se are strong predictors of future type 2 diabetes [13, 23]. In a prospective study of 2115 nondiabetic individuals followed for 6 years within the Botnia study we showed that individuals with a family history of type 2 diabetes, with a body mass index BMI $\geq$ 30 and a fasting plasma glucose concentration $\geq$5.5 mmol l^{-1}, had a 16-fold increased risk of developing type 2 diabetes (**Figure 8.1**). In the Botnia study, the presence of a family history of type 2 diabetes was confirmed by oral glucose tolerance tests in the parents. In general practice this is rarely the case and the value of a family history of type 2 diabetes in predicting future diabetes is attenuated. Whether a family history of diabetes can be replaced by genetic testing in the prediction of type 2 diabetes will be discussed later.

8.6   GENETIC VARIABILITY

Mapping of an inherited disease requires the identification of the genetic variability contributing to the disease. Such variability can be deletions, insertions, copy number repeats or changes in a single nucleotide in the genome, single nucleotide polymorphism (SNP). If an SNP results in a change in the amino acid sequence it is called a *nonsynonymous SNP*. There are about 10 million SNPs in the 3 billion base-pair human genome, which means one SNP at about 300 bp intervals. SNPs in coding sequences (exons) are seen at 1250 bp intervals. Microsatellites are short tandem repeats of nucleotide sequences (e.g. CA) found at about 5000 bp intervals. Whereas SNPs are frequently biallelic, microsatellites have multiple alleles and are thus much more polymorphic than SNPs. Several public databases provide information on SNPs in human and other genomes (e.g. http://www.ncbi.nlm.nih.gov/sites/entrez).

An SNP can either be the cause of the disease (causative SNP) or it can be a marker of the disease. This occurs when the disease susceptibility allele and the marker allele are so close to each other that they are inherited together, a situation called *linkage disequilibrium* (LD or *allelic association*). Such a combination of tightly linked alleles on a discrete chromosome is called a *haplotype*. While this region is characterized by little or no recombination (haplotype block), regions with high recombination rate usually separate haplotype blocks. LD thus describes the nonrandom correlation between alleles at a pair of SNPs; it is usually defined by D' or r^2 values. $D' = 1$ indicates that the two alleles are in complete LD, whereas values below 0.5 indicate low LD and a high recombination rate. LD extends over longer distances in isolated populations but is also seen in European compared with African populations. (This is considered to reflect a population bottleneck at the time when humans first left Africa.)

An international joint effort to create a genome-wide map of LD and haplotype blocks is called the *HapMap project* (http://www.hapmap.org/groups. html). The hope is that, by knowing the haplotype block structure of the genome, one could capture the genetic variability of the genome by genotyping a much smaller number of SNPs that describe the haplotype block (haplotype tag or htg SNPs).

More recently, it has become clear that copy number variations (CNVs) can contribute to disease

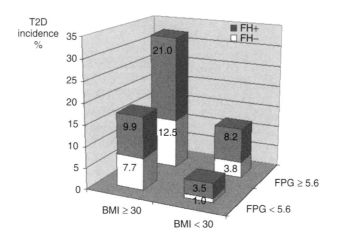

Figure 8.1 The effect of the combination of risk factors for the development of type 2 diabetes (T2D). Incident diabetes was estimated as the number of subjects who developed diabetes during the 7-year follow-up period [13]. (Copyright © 2005, American Diabetes Association, from *Diabetes*®,Vol.54, 2005; 166-174,. Reprinted with permission from The American Diabetes Association.)

susceptibility. CNVs are DNA segments of 1 kb or longer which present at variable copy number; they can include deletions, insertions, duplications or complex structural variations. CNVs are thought to affect 12% of the human genome [24–26].

8.7 MAPPING GENETIC VARIABILITY

Profiling genetic variation aims to correlate biological variation (phenotype) with variation in DNA sequences (genotype). The ultimate goal of mapping genetic variability is to identify the SNP causing a monogenic disease or the SNPs increasing susceptibility to a polygenic disease. The most straightforward approach would be to sequence the whole genome in affected and unaffected individuals, but practical reasons this is for not yet possible. The situation may change rapidly with the introduction of new large-scale sequencing tools like Solexa sequencing. Many indirect methods have been developed to achieve the goal, like linkage and association approaches.

8.8 LINKAGE

The traditional way of mapping a disease gene has been to search for linkage between a chromosomal region and a disease by genotyping a large number (about 400–500) of polymorphic markers

(microsatellites) in affected family members. If the affected family members were to share an allele more often than expected by nonrandom Mendelian inheritance, then there is evidence of excess allele sharing. The most likely explanation for excess allele sharing is that a disease-causing gene is in close proximity to the genotyped marker. Ideally, such a genome-wide scan would be carried out in large pedigrees where mode of inheritance and penetrance were known. Since these parameters are not known and parents are rarely available in a complex disease with late onset, most genome-wide scans are performed in affected siblings with no assumptions on mode of inheritance and penetrance (nonparametric linkage).

The logarithm of odds (LOD) score defines the strength of linkage. This takes into account the recombination fraction θ, which is the likelihood that a parent will produce a recombinant in an offspring. If the parental genotype is intact in the offspring, then the recombination fraction is zero (loci are linked); for completely unlinked loci it approaches 0.5. The probability test of linkage is called the *LOD score*. Two loci are considered linked when the probability of linkage as opposed to the probability against linkage is equal to or greater than the ratio 1/1000. An LOD = 3 corresponds to an odds ratio (OR) of 1/1000 ($p < 10^{-4}$). In a study of affected sib pairs a nonparametric LOD (NPL) score is presented. Although this threshold was developed for linkage mapping of monogenic disorders with complete information of genotype and phenotype, the situation for mapping complex disorders is much more complex. Lander and Kruglyak [27] have proposed that the LOD threshold for *significant genome-wide linkage* should be raised to 3.6 ($p < 2 \times 10^{-5}$), whereas that for *suggestive linkage* (would occur one time at random in a genome-wide scan) can be set at 2.2 ($p < 7 \times 2^{-4}$). In addition, they suggest reporting all nominal p-values <0.5 without any claim for linkage. In reality, each data set will have different thresholds based upon information on affection status, marker density, marker informativeness and so on. Therefore, these thresholds should be simulated using the existing data set before any claims of linkage can be made.

Accuracy of genotyping and exclusion of Mendel errors are important for the success, but also the careful definition, of affection status. This may not always be easy for diseases like asthma, schizophrenia or systematic lupus erythematosus (SLE). Even for diabetes the definition is based upon man-made cutoffs of plasma glucose. Dichotomizing variables may result in loss of power. One alternative, therefore, is to search for linkage to a qualitative trait, such as blood glucose, blood pressure or BMI, instead of diabetes, hypertension and obesity. Heritability h^2 is often used as a measure of the genetic component of a quantitative trait. The higher the heritability, the more likely it is that the genetic factors affecting the trait can be identified. Several statistical programs have been developed to support genome-wide scans of quantitative trait loci (QTL), like the variance component models SOLAR (http://www.sfbr.org/solar/) and Merlin (www.sph. umich.edu/csg/abecasis/Merlin/tour). Linkage will only identify relatively large chromosomal regions often corresponding to >20 cM (around 10–30 million base pairs) with more than 100 genes. Fine mapping with additional markers can narrow the region further, but at the end the causative SNP or an SNP in LD with the causative SNP has to be identified by large-scale association studies. Several approaches have been described to estimate whether an observed association can account for linkage [28]. Without functional support, it is not always possible to know whether linkage and association represent the genetic cause of the disease. For many complex disorders this can require a cumbersome sequence

of in vitro and in vivo studies. Therefore, the success of identifying type 2 diabetes susceptibility genes by linkage has been limited and restricted to the story of calpain 10.

8.9 CALPAIN 10 AND TYPE 2 DIABETES

In the first successful genome-wide scan of a complex disease like type 2 diabetes, Graeme Bell and coworkers [29] in 1996 reported significant linkage (LOD $= 4.1$; $p < 10^{-4}$) of type 2 diabetes in Mexican American sib pairs to a locus on chromosome 2q37, called *NIDDM1*. Still, this region was quite large (12 cM), encompassing a large number of putative genes. A reexamination of the data suggested an interaction (*epistasis*) with another locus on chromosome 15 (with a nominal LOD $= 1.5$) [30].

This enabled the researchers to narrow the region down to 7 cM. Luckily, because it is telomeric with a high recombination rate, the 7 cM genetic map only represents 1.7 megabases of physical DNA. To clone the underlying gene they genotyped 21 SNPs in this 7 cM interval and identified a three-marker haplotype which was nominally associated with type 2 diabetes. At the end, three intronic SNPs (43, 44 and 63) in the gene encoding for calpain 10 (*CAPN10*) could explain most of the linkage [31]. Calpain 10, a cystein protease with largely unknown functions in glucose metabolism, was no obvious candidate gene for type 2 diabetes. Despite a number of subsequent negative studies, several meta-analyses have shown consistent association of SNPs 43 and 44 with type 2 diabetes [33]. Neither was it easy to understand how intronic variation in this gene could increase risk for type 2 diabetes. Carriers of the G allele of SNP43 are associated with decreased expression of the gene in skeletal muscle and insulin resistance [32]. How this translates into increased risk of type 2 diabetes is not known and will require further functional studies.

8.10 ASSOCIATION STUDIES AND CANDIDATE GENES FOR TYPE 2 DIABETES

If there is a prior strong candidate gene for the disease, then the best approach is to search for association between SNPs in the gene and the disease [32]. This can either be a case-control or nested cohort study. In a case-control study, the inclusion criteria for the cases are predefined and thereafter matched individual controls are searched for (or selected), representing the same ethnic group as the cases. In a cohort study, affected and unaffected groups (not individuals) are matched. Ideally, cohorts are population based, but they often represent consecutive patients from an outpatient clinic. It is preferable that controls are older than cases to exclude the possibility that they will still develop the disease. The question of matching is crucial for the results: matching for a parameter influenced by the genetic variant (e.g. BMI) might influence its effect on a disease like type 2 diabetes. If cases and controls are not drawn from the same ethnic group, then a spurious association can be detected due to ethnic stratification.

One way to circumvent this problem is to perform a family-based association study. Distorted transmission of alleles from parents to affected offspring would indicate that the allele showing excess transmission is associated with the disease. The untransmitted alleles serve as control. This transmission disequilibrium test (TDT) represents the most unbiased association study approach, but it suffers from the drawback of low power as only transmissions from heterozygous parents are informative. The prerequisite of DNA from parents usually enrich for individuals with an earlier onset of the disease.

It is still debated as to whether common or rare variants are the cause of common complex diseases. The haplotype approach would work for common but not for rare variants. The common variant–common disease hypothesis assumes that relatively ancient common variants increase susceptibility to common diseases like obesity, hypertension, type 2 diabetes and so on. These variants would be enriched in the population, as they have been associated with survival advantage during the evolution, the so-called thrifty genes [16]. Storage of surplus energy during periods of famine may have been beneficial for survival, while in the Westernized society we rather need genetic variants which would waste energy.

One way to reduce the number of SNPs to be genotyped is to perform the initial screening in a reference panel, preferentially parent–offspring

trios, to make it easier to define which SNPs are polymorphic and thereby informative. This also allows one to create haplotypes and to identify which SNPs capture the genetic information encompassed in the haplotype. Several programs for defining haplotypes and haplotype tag single-nucleotide polymorphisms (htgSNPs) are publicly available; for example, HaploView www.broad.mit.edu/mpg/haploview/index.php. These htgSNPs (which probably represent only 30% of the initial SNPs) can then be genotyped in the case-control test panel.

8.10.1   PPARG

Even screening only one gene for SNPs can represent a huge and expensive undertaking. The PPARγ gene on the short arm of chromosome 3 spans 83 000 nucleotides with 231 SNPs in public databases; seven of them are coding SNPs. The gene encodes for a nuclear receptor, which is predominantly expressed in adipose tissue where it regulates transcription of genes involved in adipogenesis. In the 5′ untranslated end of the gene is an extra exon B that contains an SNP changing a proline in position 12 of the protein to alanine. The rare Ala allele is seen in about 15% of Europeans and in an initial study was shown to be associated with increased transcriptional activity, increased insulin sensitivity and protection against type 2 diabetes [34]. Subsequently, there were a number of studies that could not replicate the initial finding. Using the TDT approach we could show excess transmission of the Pro allele to the affected offspring [8]. We thereafter performed a meta-analysis combining the results from all published studies showing a highly significant association with type 2 diabetes. The Pro12Ala polymorphism of the PPARγ2 gene is one of the best replicated genes for type 2 diabetes ($p < 2 \times 10^{-10}$) (**Figure 8.2**). The individual risk reduction conferred by the Ala allele is moderate (about 15%); but since the risk allele Pro is so common, it translates into a PAR of 25%.

8.10.2   KCNJ 11

The ATP-sensitive potassium channel Kir 6.2 (*KCNJ11*) forms together with the sulfonylurea receptor SUR1 (*ABCC8*) an octamer protein that regulates transmembrane potential and thereby

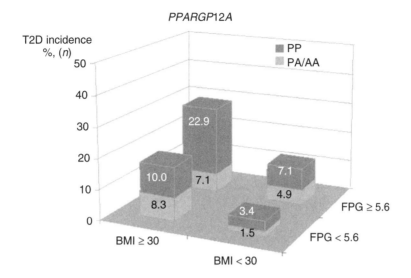

Figure 8.2 The effect of risk genotypes (/PP) of the *PPARG* P12A polymorphism together with fasting plasma glucose (FPG) and BMI for the risk of developing type 2 diabetes (T2D). (Lyssenko, V., Anevski, D., Almgren, P. *et al.* (2005) Genetic prediction of type 2 diabetes. *PloS Medicine*, 2, 1299–308.)

glucose-stimulated insulin secretion in pancreatic beta cells. Closure of the potassium channel is a prerequisite for insulin secretion. A Glu23Lys polymorphism (*E23K*) has been associated with type 2 diabetes and a modest impairment in insulin secretion [35, 36]. In addition, an activating mutation in the gene causes a severe form of neonatal diabetes [37]. Whereas these neonatal mutations result in a 10-fold activation of the ATP-dependent potassium channel, the *E23K* variant results in only a twofold increase in activity [38].

8.10.3 TCF 7 L 2

By far the strongest association with type 2 diabetes is seen for SNPs in the gene encoding for the transcription factor-7-like 2 (*TCF7L2*) [39]. *TCF7L2* encodes for a transcription factor involved in Wnt signaling. Heterodimerization of *TCF7L2* with β-catenin induces transcription of a number of genes including intestinal proglucagon. It is clear that risk variants in *TCF7L2* are associated with impaired insulin secretion, possibly due to an impaired incretin effect; that is, impaired stimulatory effect of incretin hormones like GLP-1 and GIP on insulin secretion [40] (**Figures 8.3** and **8.4**). It is also possible that the gene is involved in proliferation of β cells in response to increased demands. At onset of diabetes, type 2 diabetes

patients show a fivefold increased expression of *TCF7L2* in their islets, this being higher the more copies of the risk allele there are (**Figure 8.5**). Since overexpression of *TCF7L2* in human islets resulted in impaired insulin secretion, it is unlikely that the increased expression is a consequence of a defect in the downstream pathway; rather, it reflects a defect in transcription or translation of *TCF7L2* itself. It will be one of the greatest challenges to identify these mechanisms, as *TCF7L2* is undoubtedly an exciting novel drug target in type 2 diabetes.

8.10.4 WFS 1

Recently, 1536 SNPs in 84 candidate genes were studied for association with type 2 diabetes [41]. Only one of these genes was associated with type 2 diabetes, namely *WFS1*. The result was then replicated in 9533 cases and 11 389 controls. *WFS1* encodes for wolframin, a protein, which is defective in individuals with the Wolfram syndrome. This syndrome is characterized by diabetes insipidus, juvenile diabetes, optic atrophy and deafness. *WFS1* can thereby be considered the fourth candidate gene for type 2 diabetes. The study also highlights some of the difficulties of candidate gene studies. We are limited by our own imagination and only one out of 84 candidate genes gave a positive result!

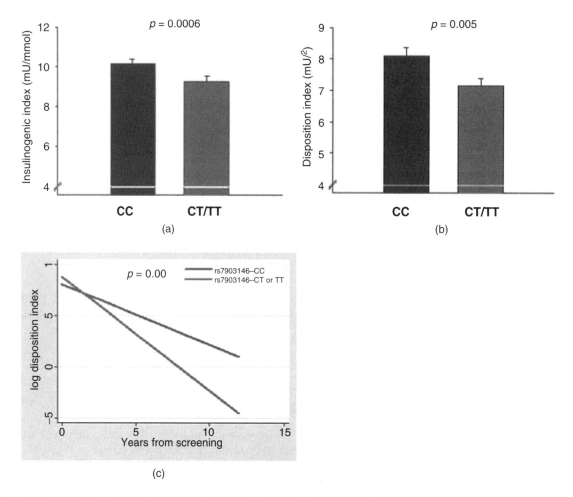

Figure 8.3 Insulin secretion according to different *TCF7L2* rs 7903146 genotypes. (a) Insulinogenic index; that is, incremental insulin response to oral glucose. (b) Disposition index represents the insulinogenic index adjusted for insulin sensitivity. (c) Change in insulin secretion (disposition index) over time in subjects who converted to type 2 diabetes in the Botnia cohort [40]. (Reproduced with permission from The American Society for Clinical Investigation.)

8.11   COMMON VARIANTS IN MODY GENES

There are at least six forms of MODY which are caused by mutations in a distinct gene. Apart from MODY that is caused by mutations in the glucokinase gene, most other forms of MODY are caused by mutations in different transcription factors, like HNF4α (MODY1), HNF1α (MODY3), IPF-1 (MODY4), HNF1β (MODY5) and NeuroD

(MODY6). Common to all of them is that they result in impaired insulin secretion and usually show strong allelic heterogeneity; that is, different mutations cause the disease in different families. It was logical, therefore, to study whether more 'mild' variations in these genes could contribute to late-onset type 2 diabetes. This turned out to be the case, at least for common variants in HNF1α and HNF4α [42]. However, it was not easy to detect these subtle effects, which seem to be stronger in

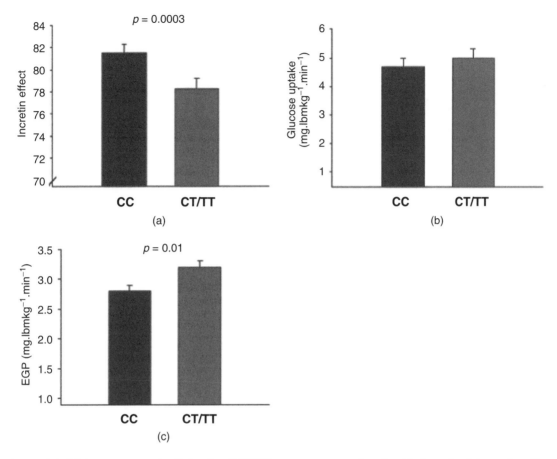

Figure 8.4 Risk genotypes (red) in the *TCF7L2* gene are associated with impaired incretin effect, I insulin response to oral compared with intravenous glucose (a) t normal peripheral insulin sensitivity (b) but impaired hepatic insulin sensitivity, that is, enhanced rate of endogenous glucose production [40]. (Reproduced with permission from The American Society for Clinical Investigation.)

insulin-resistant obese elderly individuals. These studies not only emphasized the need for a large sample size, but also the need to consider BMI and age in the statistical analysis—genes causing subtle defects in insulin secretion are more likely to be unmasked in individuals with increased insulin needs; that is, in insulin-resistant individuals [43].

8.12 GENETIC PREDICTION OF TYPE 2 DIABETES

There are only a few studies which have tried to use genetic variants to predict future type 2 diabetes. Lyssenko *et al.* [44] showed that the Pro12Pro genotype in *PPARG* predicted future type 2 diabetes in individuals with BMI $\geq$ 30 and fasting plasma glucose >5.5 mmol l^{-1} with an OR = 1.7. The risk TT genotype of SNP44 in the *CAPN10* gene increased this risk in an additive manner to an OR = 2.7 (**Figure 8.6**). More recently we showed that risk genotype carriers of *TCF7L2* had a 1.5-fold increased risk of developing future type 2 diabetes in two independent studies (**Figure 8.7**). Combining the risk variants in *TCF7L2* with those in *PPARG* and *KCJN11* increased the OR to 3 (Lyssenko, V. *et al.* unpublished observations). In keeping with this observation, Weedon *et al.* [45] showed in a cross-sectional study that each risk allele

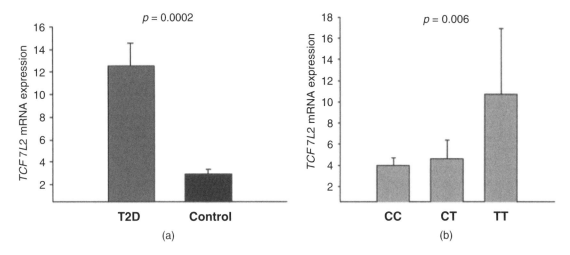

Figure 8.5 Expression of *TCF7L2* in human pancreatic islets was markedly increased in patients with type 2 diabetes (A), especially in carriers of risk genotypes in the *TCF7L2* gene [40]. (Reproduced with permission from The American Society for Clinical Investigation.)

of these three genes increased the OR by 1.28, yielding an additive OR of 5.78. It can be expected that cross-sectional studies will give higher risk estimates than prospective studies, as they tend to include more severe cases of type 2 diabetes.

8.13 WHY IS IT DIFFICULT TO REPLICATE A FINDING OF AN ASSOCIATION WITH A COMPLEX DISEASE?

The literature on the genetics of complex diseases has been enriched with papers not being able to replicate the initial findings. There are several reasons for this. There is a clear tendency that the first study reports the strongest association, as researchers and editors prefer strong positive findings ('winners curse'). False positive findings are unfortunately common. In an analysis of 301 published studies covering 25 different reported associations, only half showed significant replication in a meta-analysis [46]. The most important reason is lack of power. The OR for a complex disease is often below 1.5. The sample size is dependent not only upon the OR, but also on the frequency of the at-risk genetic variant. For an OR = 1.3 and a frequency of the at-risk allele of 20%, at least 1000 cases and controls are required.

The genetic power calculator is a useful tool for power calculations in genetic association studies (http://ibgwww.colorado.edu/ pshaun/gpc/) [47].

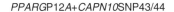

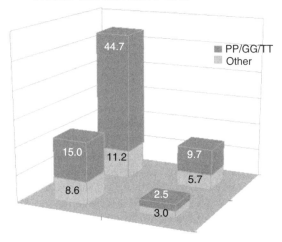

Figure 8.6 The effect of the combination of risk genotypes (/PP) of the *PPARG* P12A polymorphism and calpain 10 (*CAPN10*, SNPs 43 or 44) together with fasting plasma glucose (FPG) and BMI for the risk of developing type 2 diabetes. (Lyssenko, V., Anevski, D., Almgren, P. *et al.* (2005) Genetic prediction of type 2 diabetes. *PloS Medicine*, 2, 1299–308.)

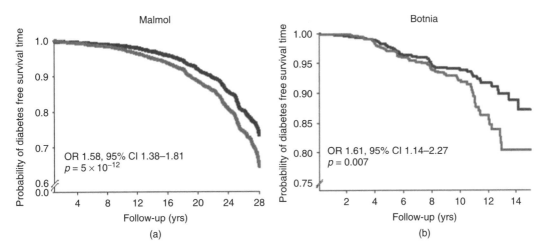

Figure 8.7 Diabetes free survival (Kaplan Meier curves) in carriers of different *TCF7L2* rs 7903146 genotypes, (a) the Malmö Preventive Project cohort (*n* = 6913) and (b) the Botnia cohort (*n* = 2651). (Lyssenko, V., Anevski, D., Almgren, P. *et al*. (2005) Genetic prediction of type 2 diabetes. *PloS Medicine*, 2, 1299–308.)

8.14 WHY DO NOT LINKAGE STUDIES DETECT ALL ASSOCIATIONS?

Despite initial linkage, it has often been difficult to identify the underlying genetic variation. This is particularly difficult if the disease-causing allele has a high frequency in the population. Under those circumstances many individuals will be homozygous for the disease allele, in which case one will not observe linkage between the disease allele and an allele at a nearby locus, because either of the homologous chromosomes can be transmitted to an affected offspring. This was the case for the Pro12Ala polymorphism in the PPARγ gene. No linkage has been observed between type 2 diabetes and the region for PPARγ on chromosome 3p, since the Pro allele will typically be transmitted from both parents. A simulation indicated that 3 million sib pairs would be required to detect such a linkage [8].

8.15 WHOLE-GENOME ASSOCIATION STUDIES

Given the limited success with linkage studies and candidate gene studies, researchers turned their hope toward new tools. The rapid improvement in high-throughput technology for SNP genotyping, and thereby decreasing costs per genotype (in 10 years the cost has decreased by a factor of 10), has opened up new possibilities for both linkage and association studies. The Hap Map provided another important tool, showing that genotyping approximately 500 000 SNPs in the entire genome would cover about 75% of all common variants in the genome. The year 2007 has brought about a real breakthrough in the genetics of type 2 diabetes. The reason was that several so-called whole-genome association studies (WGASs) using DNA chips with >500 000 SNPs in a large number of patients with type 2 diabetes and controls have been performed and published [48–53]. In our collaborative study with the Broad Institute and Novartis (Diabetes Genetic Initiative, DGI) we performed a WGAS in 1464 patients with type 2 diabetes and 1467 nondiabetic control subjects from Finland and Sweden. Prior to publication we shared the results with researchers from the Finnish–USA Study of NIDDM (FUSION) and the Wellcome Trust Case Control Consortium (WTCCC) groups [50]. We only considered positive results that were seen and replicated in all three studies; that is, together with replication samples, the results were based upon DNA from 32 000 individuals! Two other WGASs [49, 53] in type 2 diabetes have been published in the past year, supporting and complementing our results.

Together, these studies have identified at least six novel genes/loci for type 2 diabetes in addition to

Table 8.1 Gene variants increasing risk of type 2 diabetes.

Gene	Chromosome	OR	Risk allele (%)
TCF7L2	10	1.38	0.30
IGFBP2 (IMP2)	3	1.17	0.32
CDKN2A/ CDKN2B	9	1.20	0.86
CDKAL1	6	1.12	0.32
HHEX	10	1.14	0.54
KNCJ11	11	1.15	0.47
PPARG	3	1.20	0.84
SLC30A8	8	1.12	0.65
FTO	16	1.23	0.40

TCF7L2, PPARG, KCJN11 and WFS1 (**Table 8.1**). Notably, TCF7L2 was on top of each WGAS with a joint p value in the three scans of 10^{-50}. Several of the new genes seem to influence cell proliferation by interfering with the cell cycle; for example, CDKAL1 and CDKN2A/CDKN2B on chromosome 9. Intriguingly, the same region on chromosome 9 that showed association with type 2 diabetes was associated with increased risk of myocardial infarction in three independent WGASs [54–56]. However, there are most likely different SNPs operative for type 2 diabetes and myocardial infarction. FTO is an obesity gene that increases the risk of type 2 diabetes through obesity [57, 58]. Therefore, it is not surprising that FTO was not detected as associated with type 2 diabetes in the WGAS which matched for BMI.

We can assume that these 10 type 2 diabetes genes only represents the tip of the iceberg, and more refined analyses will certainly yield more genes associated with type 2 diabetes.

8.16 GENETIC INFLUENCES ON AGE-RELATED DECLINE IN MITOCHONDRIAL DYSFUNCTION

Since genes are transcribed to RNA, and since RNA is translated into proteins, and since defects

in proteins cause disease, the ultimate goal would be to carry out a random search of expressed proteins in target tissues. This may not yet be completely feasible, but the study of large-scale transcript profiles is. This approach has been successful in defining prognosis of cancers, but for complex diseases affecting many target tissues it may not be that simple. Also, defining what is differentially expressed among more than 20 000 gene transcripts on a chip is a statistical challenge. Despite these problems, analysis of gene expression in skeletal muscle of patients with type 2 diabetes and prediabetic individuals has provided new insights into the pathogenesis of the disease. However, it required the analysis of coordinated gene expression in metabolic pathways rather than of individual genes. This is based upon the assumption that if one member of the pathway shows altered expression, this will also be translated into the whole pathway [58]. Genes regulating oxidative phosphorylation in mitochondria showed a 20% coordinated downregulation in muscle from prediabetic and diabetic individuals [58, 59]. Furthermore, a similar downregulation of the gene encoding for a master regulator of oxidative phosphorylation, the PPARγ coactivator PGC-1α, was observed. This pathway has thus merged as central in the pathogenesis of type 2 diabetes and suggests that impaired mitochondrial function and impaired oxidation of fat may predispose to type 2 diabetes through a 'thrifty gene' mechanism (see below). By studying young and elderly twins we could also demonstrate that elderly carriers of a Gly482Ser polymorphism in the PGC-1α gene had decreased expression of the PGC-1α gene in skeletal muscle, suggesting that genetic variants determine age-related decline in expression of key genes regulating oxidative phosphorylation [60] (**Figure 8.8**). This study gives an example of how genetic factors, in combination with nongenetic factors, can influence gene expression, which subsequently affects glucose and fat metabolism.

Furthermore, the interaction between genetic and nongenetic factors may be even more complex and involve epigenetic factors, such as DNA methylation and histone modifications. So far, the influence of epigenetic factors on the pathogenesis of type 2 diabetes remains limited.

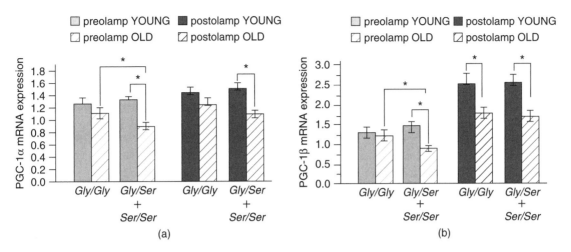

Figure 8.8 **The effect of age on the association between skeletal muscle PGC-1α mRNA expression and the PGC-1α Gly482Ser polymorphism. (Reproduced from [60]. Copyright © 2004, The American Society for Clinical Investigation.)**

8.17 GENE–ENVIRONMENT INTERACTIONS

It is obvious that the rapid increase in type 2 diabetes during the past 50 years must be ascribed to changes in the environment rather than to genes, as the genetic background has not changed during this period. But the genetic background determines how we respond to the environment.

The PPARγ receptor is a good example for an interaction between genes and the environment. *PPARG* activators have become a major new type of antidiabetic drug (thiazolidinediones) and dietary long-chain polyunsaturated fatty acids are supposedly natural ligands for *PPARG*. The importance of the genetic variation in *PPARG* as a significant modulator of physiological responses to dietary fat in humans has been demonstrated in several studies [61–63]. The different genotype carriers show different associations between intake of total fat, fat subtypes and obesity. There are also data to suggest that the protective effect of the Ala allele is influenced by the degree of saturation of ingested fat [61–63]. This may not be too surprising, as free fatty acids have been proposed as natural ligands for PPARγ.

8.18 PHARMACOGENETICS

An important goal of genetics is to use the information to improve treatment; that is, to identify individuals who are more likely than others to respond to a specific therapy. This has been beautifully shown in neonatal diabetic patients with the *KCJN11* mutation [63]. When the patients were switched from insulin to sulfonylurea their symptoms markedly improved. This was especially dramatic for the severe neurological symptoms often associated with the disease.

Patients with MODY 3 (*HNF1α*) mutations are supersensitive to treatment with sulfonylureas, whereas they respond poorly to treatment with metformin [64].

It has also recently been shown that individuals with the risk genotype in *TCF7L2* respond poorly to treatment with sulfonylureas, eventually as a consequence of their more severe impairment in β-cell function [65].

8.19 FUTURE DIRECTIONS

Genetics of type 2 diabetes is still complicated, but no longer the nightmare once proposed. The year 2007 has brought about a real breakthrough. We can now list at least 10 genes which consistently increase risk of type 2 diabetes, and we are likely to see a doubling of this number within the next 1 to 2 years. However, these 10 genes explain only a small proportion ($\sim$0.3) of the individual risk of type 2 diabetes ($\lambda_S = 3$). Although we now seem to cover approximately 75% of the genetic map of type 2 diabetes, the genetic variants detected most likely represent so-called low hanging fruits or common variants. It is still possible that there are more rare variants with stronger effects not detected with current methods. These rare variants are most likely seen in patients with early-onset forms of diabetes or in individuals with a marked β-cell dysfunction. It is unlikely that genotyping using high-density DNA arrays can detect these rare variants. Rather, their detection will require sequencing. Sequencing of the whole genome was once a dream, but with the new technology this dream may become true in the very near future.

Also, the role of CNV in the pathogenesis of disease has been highlighted in recent years, but the tools to detect these CNVs have been limited. This problem may be solved with the introduction of new DNA chips with a much better coverage of CNVs.

Lastly, we are only now beginning to realize that epigenetic changes (DNA methylation, histone acetylation and deacetylation) can introduce epigenetic changes during a lifetime. Such changes may influence age-related changes in gene expression and thereby contribute to age-related diseases. Until now, DNA methylation was studied by laborious bisulfite sequencing of single genes. In the future, the possibility of whole-genome DNA methylation studies may shed new light on the extent of these epigenetic effects.

Dissection of the genetic complexity of type 2 diabetes may thus be possible after all.

References

1. Miller, L.H., Mason, S.J., Dvorak, J.A. et al. (1975) Erythrocyte receptors for (*Plasmodium knowlesi*) malaria. Duffy blood group determinants. *Science*, **189**, 561–3.
2. Stephens, J.C., Reich, D.E., Goldstein, D.B. et al. (1998) Dating the origin of the CCR-5-Delta 32 AIDS resistance allele by the coalescence of haplotypes. *American Journal of Human Genetics*, **62**, 1507–15.

3. Lehto, M., Tuomi, T., Mahtani, M. et al. (1997) Characterization of the MODY3 phenotype: early-onset diabetes caused by an insulin secretion defect. *The Journal of Clinical Investigation*, **99**, 582–91.
4. Kerem, B., Rommens, J.M., Buchanan, J.A. et al. (1989) Identification of the cystic fibrosis gene: genetic analysis. *Science*, **245**, 1073–80.
5. Vionnet, N., Stoffel, M., Takeda, J. et al. (1992) Nonsense mutation in the glucokinase gene causes early-onset non-insulin-dependent diabetes mellitus. *Nature*, **356**, 721–2.
6. Yamagata, K., Oda, N., Kaisaki, P.J. et al. (1996) Mutations in the hepatocyte nuclear factor-1alpha gene in maturity-onset diabetes of the young (MODY3). *Nature*, **384**, 455–8.
7. Yamagata, K., Furuta, H., Oda, N. et al. (1996) Mutations in the hepatocyte nuclear factor-4alpha gene in maturity-onset diabetes of the young (MODY1). *Nature*, **384**, 458–60.
8. Altshuler, D., Hirschhorn, J.N., Klannemark, M. et al. (2000) The common *PPARG* Pro12Ala polymorphism is associated with decreased risk of type 2 diabetes. *Nature Genetics*, **26**, 76–80.
9. Newman, B., Selby, J.V., King, M.C. et al. (1987) Concordance for type 2 diabetes in male twins. *Diabetologia*, **30**, 763–68.
10. Kaprio, J., Tuomilehto, J., Koskenvuo, M. et al. (1992) Concordance for type 1 (insulin-dependent) and type 2 (non-insulin-dependent) diabetes mellitus in a population-based cohort of twins in Finland. *Diabetologia*, **35**, 1060–7.
11. Köbberling, J. and Tillil, H. (1982) Empirical risk figures for first-degree relatives of non-insulin dependent diabetics, in *The Genetics of Diabetes Mellitus* (eds J. Köbberling and R. Tattersall), Academic Press, London, pp. 201–9.
12. Groop, L., Forsblom, C., Lehtovirta, M. et al. (1996) Metabolic consequences of a family history of NIDDM (the Botnia Study)—evidence for sex-specific parental effects. *Diabetes*, **45**, 1585–93.
13. Lyssenko, V., Almgren, P., Anevski, D. et al. (2005) Predictors and longitudinal changes in insulin sensitivity and secretion preceding onset of type 2 diabetes. *Diabetes*, **54**, 166–174.
14. Serjeantson, S., Owerbach, D., Zimmet, P. et al. (1983) Genetics of diabetes in Nauru. Effects of foreign admixture, HLA antigens and insulin-gene linked polymorphism. *Diabetologia*, **25**, 13–17.
15. Brosseau, J., Eelkema, R., Crawford, A. and Abe, T. (1979) Diabetes among the three affiliated tribes: correlations with degree of Indian inheritance. *American Journal of Public Health*, **69**, 1277–8.

16. Neel, V. (1962) Diabetes mellitus: a "thrifty" genotype rendered detrimental by progress? *American Journal of Human Genetics*, **14**, 352–62.

17. Coleman, D. (1979) Obesity genes: beneficial effects in heterozygous mice. *Science*, **203**, 663–5.

18. Hales, C. and Barker, D. (1992) Type 2 diabetes mellitus: the thrifty phenotype hypothesis. *Diabetologia*, **35**, 595–601.

19. Melander, O., Mattiasson, I., Marsal, K. *et al.* (1999) Heredity for hypertension influences intrauterine growth and the relation between foetal growth and adult blood pressure. *Journal of Hypertension*, **17**, 1557–61.

20. Hattersley, A., Beards, F., Ballantyne, E. *et al.* (1998) Mutations in the glucokinase gene of the fetus result in reduced birth weight. *Nature Genetics*, **19**, 268–70.

21. Laaksonen, D.E., Lakka, H.M., Niskanen, L.K. *et al.* (2002) Metabolic syndrome and development of diabetes mellitus: application and validation of recently suggested definitions of the metabolic syndrome in a prospective cohort. *American Journal of Epidemiology*, **156**, 1070–7.

22. Lorenzo, C., Okolosie, M., Williams, K. *et al.* (2003) The metabolic syndrome as a predictor of type 2 diabetes: the San Antonio Heart Study. *Diabetes Care*, **26**, 3153–9.

23. Tirosh, A., Shai, I., Tekes-Manova, D. *et al.* (2005) Normal fasting plasma glucose levels and type 2 diabetes in young men. *New England Journal of Medicine*, **353**, 1454–62.

24. Sebat, J., Lakshmi, B., Troge, J. *et al.* (2004) Large-scale copy number polymorphism in the human genome. *Science*, **305**, 525–8.

25. Redon, R., Ishikawa, S., Fitch, K.R. *et al.* (2006) Global variation in copy number in the human genome. *Nature*, **444**, 444–54.

26. Beckman, J.S., Estivill, X. and Antonarakis, S.E. (2007) Copy number variants and genetic traits: closer to the resolution of phenotypic to genotypic variability. *Nature Reviews. Genetics*, **8**, 639–46.

27. Lander, E. and Kruglyak, L. (1995) Genetic dissection of complex traits: guidelines for interpreting and reporting linkage results. *Nature Genetics*, **11**, 241–7.

28. Li, C., Scott, L.J. and Boehnke, M. (2004) Assessing whether an allele can account in part for a linkage signal: the genotype-IBD sharing test (GIST). *American Journal of Human Genetics*, **74**, 418–31.

29. Hanis, C.L., Boerwinkle, E., Chakraborty, R. *et al.* (1996) A genome-wide search for human non-insulin-dependent (type 2) diabetes genes reveals a major susceptibility locus on chromosome 2. *Nature Genetics*, **13**, 161–6.

30. Cox, N.J., Frigge, M., Nicloale, D.L. *et al.* (1999) Loci on chromosomes 2 (NIDDM1) and 15 interact to increase susceptibility to diabetes in Mexican Americans. *Nature Genetics*, **2**, 213–15.

31. Oda, N., Cox, N.J., Horikawa, Y. *et al.* (2000) Genetic variation in the gene encoding calpain-10 is associated with type 2 diabetes mellitus. *Nature Genetics*, **26**, 163–75.

32. Carlsson, E., Poulsen, P., Storgaard, H. *et al.* (2005) Genetic and non-genetic regulation of *CAPN10* mRNA expression skeletal muscle. *Diabetes*, **54**, 3015–20.

33. Parikh, H. and Groop, L., (2004) Candidate genes for type 2 diabetes. *Reviews in Endocrine and Metabolic Disorders*, **5**, 151–76.

34. Deeb, S.S., Fajas, L., Nemoto, M. *et al.* (1998) A Pro12Ala substitution in *PPARG2* associated with decreased receptor activity, lower body mass index and improved insulin sensitivity. *Nature Genetics*, **20**, 284–7.

35. Gloyn, A.L., Weedon, M.N., Owen, K.R. *et al.* (2003) Large-scale association studies of variants in genes encoding the pancreatic beta-cell KATP channel subunit Kir2 (*KCNJ11*) and SUR1 (*ABCC8*) confirm that the *KCJN11* W23K variant is associated with type 2 diabetes. *Diabetes*, **52**, 568–72.

36. Florez, J.C., Burtt, N., de Bakker, P.I.W. *et al.* (2004) Haplotype structure and genotype–phenotype correlations of the sulfonylurea receptor (SUR1) and the islet ATP—sensitive potassium channel (*kir2*) gene region. *Diabetes*, **53**, 1360–8.

37. Gloyn, A.L., Pearson, E.R., Antcliff, J.F., *et al.* (2004) Activating mutations in the gene encoding the ATP-sensitive potassium channel subunit *Kir6.2* and permanent neonatal diabetes. *New England Journal of Medicine*, **350**, 1838–49.

38. Nichols, C.G. and Koster, J.C. (2002) Diabetes and insulin secretion: whiter KATP? *American Journal of Physiology. Endocrinology and Metabolism*, **283**, E403–12.

39. Grant, S.F., Thorleifsson, G., Reynisdottir, I. *et al.* (2006) Variant of transcription factor 7-like 2 (*TCF7L2*) gene confers risk of type 2 diabetes. *Nature Genetics*, **38**, 320–3.

40. Lyssenko, V., Orho-Melander, M., Sjögren, M. *et al.* (2007) Common variants in the *TCF7L2* gene increase risk of future type 2 diabetes by influencing pancreatic alpha and beta-cell function. *The Journal of Clinical Investigation*, **117**, 2155–63.

41. Sandhu, M.S., Weedon, M.N., Fawcett, K.A. *et al.* (2007) Common variants in *WFS1* confer risk of type 2 diabetes. *Nature Genetics*, **39**, 951–3.

42. Winckler, W., Weedon, M.J., Graham, R.R. *et al.* (2007) Evaluation of common variants in six known MODY genes for association with type 2 diabetes. *Diabetes*, **56**, 685–93.

43. Holmkvist, J., Cervin, C., Lyssenko, V. *et al.* (2006) Common variants in the MODY3 gene (*HNF-1α*) and risk of type 2 diabetes. *Diabetologia*, **49**, 2882–91.

44. Lyssenko, V., Anevski, D., Almgren, P. *et al.* (2005) Genetic prediction of type 2 diabetes. *PLoS Medicine*, **2**, 1299–308.

45. Weedon, M.N., McCarthy, M.I., Hitman, G. *et al.* (2006) Combining information from common type 2 diabetes risk polymorphisms improves disease prediction. *PLoS Medicine*, **3**, e374.

46. Lohmueller, K.E., Pearce, C.L., Pike, M. *et al.* (2003) Meta-analysis of genetic association studies supports a contribution of common variants to susceptibility to common disease. *Nature Genetics*, **33**, 177–82.

47. Purcell, S., Cherny, S.S. and Sham, P.C. (2003) Genetic power calculator: design of linkage and association genetic mapping studies of complex traits. *Bioinformatics*, **19**, 149–50.

48. Sladek, R., Rochelau, G., Rung, J., *et al.* (2007) A genome-wide association study identifies novel risk loci for type 2 diabetes. *Nature*, **445**, 881–5.

49. Saxena, R., Voigt, B., Lyssenko, V. *et al.* (2007) Genome wide association analysis identifies loci for type 2 diabetes and triglyceride levels. *Science*, **316**, 1331–6.

50. Zeggini, E., Weedon, M.N., Lindgren, C.M. *et al.* (2007) Replication of genome-wide association signals in UK samples reveals risk loci for type 2 diabetes. *Science*, **316**, 1336–440.

51. Scott, L., Moehlke, K., Bonnycatle, L.L. *et al.* (2007) A genome-wide association study of type 2 diabetes in Finns detects multiple susceptibility variants. *Science*, **316**, 1341–5.

52. Steinthorsdottir, V., Thorleifsson, G., Reynisdottir, I. *et al.* (2007) A variant in *CDKAL1* influences insulin response and risk of type 2 diabetes. *Nature Genetics*, **39**, 770–5.

53. McPherson, R., Pertsemilidis, A., Kavaslar, N. *et al.* (2007) A common allele on chromosome 9 associated with coronary heart disease. *Science*, **316**, 14888–91.

54. Helgadottir, A., Thorleifsson, G., Manolesco, A. *et al.* (2007) A common variant on chromosome 9p21 affects the risk of myocardial infarction. *Science*, **316**, 1491–3.

55. The Wellcome Trust Case Control Consortium (2007) Genome-wide association study of 14,000 cases of seven common diseases and 3,000 shared controls. *Nature*, **447**, 661–78.

56. Frayling, T., Timpson, Nj., Weedon, M.N. *et al.* (2007) A common variant in the *FTO* gene is associated with body mass index and predisposes to childhood and adult obesity. *Science*, **316**, 889–94.

57. Dina, C., Meyre, D., Gallina, S. *et al.* (2007) Variation in *FTO* contributes to childhood obesity and severe adult obesity. *Nature Genetics*, **39**, 724–6.

58. Mootha, V.K., Lindgren, C.M., Eriksson, K.F. *et al.* (2003) PGC-1alpha-responsive genes involved in oxidative phosphorylation are coordinately down-regulated in human diabetes. *Nature Genetics*, **34**, 267–73.

59. Patti, M.E., Butte, A.J., Crunkhorn, S. *et al.* (2003) Coordinated reduction of genes of oxidative metabolism in humans with insulin resistance and diabetes: potential role of *PGC1* and *NRF1*. *Proceedings of the National Academy of Science*, **100**, 8466–71.

60. Ling, C., Poulsen, P., Carlsson, E. *et al.* (2004) Multiple environmental and genetic factors influence skeletal muscle PGC-1α and PGC-1β gene expression in twins. *Journal of Clinical Investigation*, **114**, 1518–26.

61. Luan, J., Browne, P.O., Harding, A.H. *et al.* (2001) Evidence for gene-nutrient interaction at the *PPARG* locus. *Diabetes*, **50**, 686–9.

62. Memisoglu, A., Hu, F.B., Hankinson, S.E. *et al.* (2003) Interaction between a peroxisome proliferator-activated receptor gamma gene polymorphism and dietary fat intake in relation to body mass. *Human Molecular Genetics*, **12**, 2923–9.

63. Ylönen, K., Salminen, I., Lyssenko, V. *et al.* (2007) The Pro12Ala polymorphism of the PPAR-γ2 gene affects associations of fish intake and marine n-3 fatty acids with glucose metabolism. *European Journal of Clinical Nutrition*, advance online publication, 15 August 2007, DOI: 10.1038/sj.ejcn.1602882.

64. Pearson, E.R., Flecthner, I., Njolstad, P.R. *et al.* (2006) Switching from insulin to oral sulfonylureas in patients with diabetes due to *Kir6.2* mutations. *New England Journal of Medicine*, **355**, 467–77.

65. Pearson, E.R., Donnelly, L.A., Kimber, C. *et al.* (2007) Variations in *TCF7L2* influences therapeutic response to sulfonylureas. A GoDARTs study. *Diabetes*, **56**, 2178–82.

9

Epidemiologic Aspects of Type 2 Diabetes Mellitus in Europe

Harry Keen

Unit for Metabolic Medicine, Guy's Hospital Campus,
King's College London, London, UK

9.1 INTRODUCTION

Observations on the incidence and prevalence of diabetes in Europe, as in any other region, should only be regarded as a contemporary 'snapshot' of what is a constantly changing scene. The distribution of diabetes and lesser degrees of glucose intolerance in the European population at the present time certainly differ from what has gone before and very probably from what will come after. Population changes in age composition, in the degree of adiposity (perhaps affecting sex or age groups differently), reduced levels of physical activity and growing migratory shifts resulting in large ethnic minority populations all impact on European diabetes risk and rates.

In different ways, these factors may affect incidence and prevalence of both major types of diabetes. It is, however, the much larger numbers of people with type 2 diabetes mellitus (T2DM), now estimated to account for 90% or more of the total diabetic population [1], that will constitute the bulk of the world's diabetic population and the rapid growth of which is now widely regarded as responsible for an epidemic rise in diabetes prevalence. There has been at least a doubling of numbers of people with diabetes in Europe since 1970 [2], almost entirely attributable to the great majority of people with type 2 diabetes. This is predicted to continue to rise in Europe well into the twenty-first century [3], though at a substantially slower rate of increase than in many other parts of the world [4].

9.2 A DIABETES EPIDEMIC?

The notion that, like the rest of the world, Europe is in the grip of a growing 'diabetes epidemic' [5] has received wide attention, from the lay and the scientific communities. The propriety of uncritical use of the term *epidemic*, particularly perhaps in the European context, has been challenged in Denmark by Green *et al.* [6]. Auditing the numbers of prescriptions for antidiabetic medications issued annually to the population of Fyn County, Denmark, over the decade 1993–2003, they noted that the annual number of new patients showed only a small increase but that annual totals rose much faster because of the progressively rising longevity of existing patients. More of the rising prevalence was due to diminishing numbers leaving the group rather than increasing numbers joining it. Diabetes prevalence data from the ongoing diabetes information system in Tayside, Scotland, however, supported the alternative explanation—that the rise in diabetes prevalence there owed more to increasing incidence rates than to decreasing diabetes mortality rates [7]. The contributions to an ever-mounting diabetes prevalence of increasing incidence, lengthening duration and rising population numbers will vary considerably from country to country and from time to time.

9.3 CHANGING PATTERNS

Diabetes prevalence within European (and other) communities is thus not a fixed quantity. An

The Epidemiology of Diabetes Mellitus, second edition   Edited by Jean-Marie Ekoé, Marian Rewers, Rhys Williams and Paul Zimmet
© 2008 John Wiley & Sons, Ltd

early pointer to changing patterns came from the observations made on the changing sex ratio of patients newly presenting with diabetes to a large diabetes clinic in Birmingham, England [8]. The middle years of the last century saw a progressive change in the sex ratio of new patients from 2 to 1 in favor of women to a small excess of men. This shift was due to a progressive slowing in the numbers of women newly presenting with diabetes with little change in the numbers of men. It was ascribed to growing popularity of feminine slimness and, perhaps equally plausibly, to a preceding dramatic national restriction in family sizes from the beginning of the twentieth century, though the role of parity as a determinant of female diabetes risk is still debated [9].

The burgeoning increase in the number of older people with T2DM was all too apparent in clinical practice over the last half century. The progressive and massive increase in numbers of people with type 2 diabetes totally changed the character and practice of most European diabetes clinics over this period and firmly established the critical importance of high-quality primary care facilities for routine care while establishing rapid referral pathways to specialist units as special needs emerge. In many countries of Europe, this reconfiguration of services for diabetes is still ongoing. Successful redeployment of clinical resources is likely to impact on survival and so to influence the epidemiology of diabetes and its complications quite profoundly in the future.

9.3.1 The Impact of Revised Diagnostic Criteria on Epidemiological Estimates

Some variation in the European epidemiological picture can also be expected to result from modifications in the glycemic criteria for the diagnosis of diabetes over the past decade [10, 11]. These changes now promote the diagnostic use of the *fasting* plasma glucose, reduce its diagnostic cutoff value from 7.8 to 7.0 mmol l^{-1} and introduce a new category of impaired fasting glucose (IFG) for concentrations between 6.1 and 6.9 mmol l^{-1}. The diagnostic cutoff values for the 2 h postload plasma glucose of 11.1 mmol l^{-1} for diabetes mellitus (DM) and of 7.8–11.0 mmol l^{-1} for impaired glucose tolerance (IGT) remain unchanged. A new category of impaired glucose regulation (IGR) includes both

IFG and IGT. One purpose of these changes, both explicit and implicit, is that use of the fasting glucose will encourage easier, earlier and so increased use of screening for undiagnosed diabetes. Although the diagnostic category predicated by the fasting value now nominally takes priority, the revised World Health Organisation (WHO) recommendations [12] reaffirm the 'gold standard' role of the 2 h value as originally agreed in the 1980 and 1985 WHO criteria [13, 14].

The potential effect of the diagnostic use of fasting blood has been explored in the European context by the DECODE Study Group [15]. Using oral glucose tolerance test data collected from 13 population-based studies in eight European countries since 1980 (when WHO diagnostic methods and glycemic criteria [13, 14] were adopted), the DECODE Study Group pointed out the substantial numbers of glucose-intolerant individuals, particularly older women, who would remain undetected were diagnosis and classification to be restricted only to consideration of the fasting blood glucose level [15, 16]. Although the 'new' 1999 fasting criteria produce around the same number of new cases as the older 1980 postload criteria, in large part, they are different people, younger, fatter and more likely to be male. The overlap between the extended IFG and IGT is even smaller. The main reason for the differences in the diagnostic yields is the fact that, unlike the fasting blood glucose, postload glucose concentrations in the population increase with age with progressively greater numbers of people who would have qualified for the diagnosis of DM or IGT on that basis. A switch to the new lone fasting criteria will inevitably affect prevalence estimates in the older European populations more than others with more youthful age compositions and produce a slowing in the rate of diagnosis of new, older people with T2DM that is more apparent than real.

9.3.2 Changing Diabetes Prevalence in Europe

Diabetes prevalence can change over the course of a few decades from being a relative rarity (usually under the primitive conditions of the hunter–gatherer/sharecropper economy) to becoming outstandingly common (usually in conditions of rapidly increasing affluence) [17]. These dramatic rises in diabetes prevalence in non-European communities have accompanied rapid transitions in the economic, nutritional and working environments and a rapidly increasing incidence of overweight and obesity affecting whole populations. Europe has seen major socioeconomic, educational, nutritional and work-life changes with progressive lengthening of years of life, all likely to have increased the prevalence of diabetes. The data are relatively scant, but scattered reports strongly suggest that diabetes prevalence in Europe has increased [17–20], though not in the almost explosive way experienced elsewhere. This may indicate a more general European ethnic resistance to diabetes or the fact that it has not been subjected to the dramatic transitions from dire poverty to relative affluence experienced by others [21]. The lesser susceptibility of Europeans to T2DM (as distinct from type 1 DM) may have a genetic basis; this may be inferred from the reduction in diabetes risk in high-risk populations which seems to be associated with admixture of European genes [21].

9.3.3 Europe in the Global Context: The IDF Analysis

The third edition of the *Diabetes Atlas* [23] provides comprehensive estimates for the year 2007 of the absolute numbers and percentage prevalence rates of DM and IGT globally and in the regions, including in Europe (**Table 9.1**) and in its constituent nation states (**Table 9.2**). Rates are expressed directly for the age/sex and rural/urban compositions of the populations considered; but, for the sake of comparability, they are also calculated after standardization to the global age/sex rural/urban composition. It also estimates predicted numbers of cases and rates for the year 2025 based on demographic trends and expected changes [24].

Total global prevalences for 2007 for DM and IGT are estimated at 6.0% and 7.5% respectively, rising to 7.3% and 8.0% respectively in 2025. Corresponding crude European region prevalences for 2007 are estimated at 8.4% and 10.3% respectively. Standardized to global age/sex population composition, these fall to 6.6 and 9.1%, with the difference reflecting the greater mean age of the European population. This

Table 9.1 Regional estimates of diabetes prevalence 2007.[a]

Region	DM prevalence (%)		IGT prevalence (%)	
	Reg'l	Comp.	Reg'l	Comp.
Africa	3.1	3.6	7.2	8.2
Eastern Mediterranean and Middle East	7.7	9.2	7	8.1
Europe	8.4	6.6	10.3	9.1
North America	9.2	8.4	6.8	5.8
South Central America	6	6.3	7.3	7.5
Southeast Asia	6	6.5	5.9	6
West Pacific	4.6	4.4	7.6	7.5
Overall		5.9		7.5

[a]Estimates of prevalence of DM and IGT by region. The regional (Reg'l) columns list the crude total population rates regardless of age/sex composition. In the comparative (Comp.) columns these are adjusted to the age/sex composition of the world population to make regions more directly comparable with each other. These rates are based on both known plus estimated undiagnosed cases and include type 1 patients who contribute at most 10% of these totals. Estimates are formed from a number of acceptable methods of case ascertainment which vary both between and within regions. Data from *Diabetes Atlas*, 3rd edn [23].

Table 9.2 European national estimates of diabetes prevalence 2007.[a]

Country	Prevalence (%)		Extrapolated states[d]
	National pop.[b]	Comp. pop.[c]	
Albania	4.8	4.5	Andorra, Austria, Azerbaijan
Cyprus	10.3	8.9	Belarus, Bosnia, Bulgaria
Denmark	7.5	5.5	Channel Islands, Croatia, Czech Republic
Finland	8.4	5.9	Estonia, Georgia, Hungary
France	8.4	5.9	Kazakhstan, Kyrgyzstan
Germany	11.8	7.9	Latvia, Lichtenstein, Luxemburg
Greece	8.6	5.9	Macedonia, Moldova, Portugal
Iceland	2	1.6	Romania, Russian Federation
Ireland	5.6	5.1	San Marino, Serbia/Montenegro
Israel	7.8	6.9	Slovakia, Slovenia, Switzerland
Italy	8.7	5.8	Tajikistan, Turkmenistan, Ukraine
Malta	9.7	6.7	Uzbekistan
Netherlands	7.3	5.2	
Norway	4.7	3.6	
Poland	9.1	7.6	
Spain	7.5	5.7	
Sweden	7.2	5.2	
Turkey	7.1	7.8	
United Kingdom	4	2.9	

[a] Data from *Diabetes Atlas*, 3rd edn [23].
[b] Crude prevalences based on current age/sex composition.
[c] Prevalences standardized to global age/sex composition.
[d] States with prevalence rates extrapolated from those of similar countries.

age effect is further illustrated when European region diabetes prevalence rates are compared with those of other world regions (**Table 9.1**). Europe's high crude ranking order falls considerably when the rates are world standardized.

The effect of increasing longevity on diabetes prevalence is likely to increase. Currently, 33% of the European population is aged 50 years or more, a proportion expected to rise to over 40% in 2025 [24]. Thus, the predicted rises of 20.5% and 9.0% respectively for absolute numbers of people with DM and IGT in Europe over that time period are largely due to further aging of the population, which, unlike other regions, is actually expected to decline in numbers. This prediction does not take account of the added impact of increasing rates of overweight and obesity, which would be expected

to boost the numbers of people developing glucose intolerance further.

9.3.4 Individual Countries of Europe

Of the 53 countries included in this European analysis, for only 19 are there relatively recent publications or collections [23]. Though these sources varied in nature, purpose, scope and methodology, they all met preset quality standards and the prevalence estimates provided are extracted from them. Estimates for the other 34 are extrapolated from those for states which they most closely resemble, adjusted for varying population distributions. Reliable recent data were not available for many of the newly independent states of eastern and central Europe; data are scanty or inadequate even for several western European countries. The contrast with the well-constructed and regularly renewed diabetes data from the

US National Health and Nutrition Survey [25] is striking. How much more effectively would data be collected if it related to some physically equally damaging disorder affecting animal livestock?

Restricting comment to the 19 countries for which reasonably up-to-date estimates were available (**Table 9.2**), national estimates for DM prevalence varied between a high of 11.8% for Germany (7.9% after age/sex standardization) and a low of 2.0% for Iceland (1.6%). Poland provided the highest national estimate for IGT at 16.4% (15.2%) and Ireland the lowest at 1.9% (1.6%). No clear pattern of distribution is evident in respect of geographical location, although the low rates for Iceland and Norway and the high rates for Cyprus, Malta, Greece and Turkey might suggest a north–south gradient. However, the high German and Polish rates do not fit well into this scheme. It is also hard to see any socioeconomic patterning to the distribution. However, the lack of agreed methodology for population sampling and diagnostic and case ascertainment call for caution before drawing any conclusions, positive or negative, from these data. Future studies might valuably include analysis of differences in ethnic sensitivity to the effect of increasing adiposity on emergence of diabetes. The prevalence of diabetes and its predicted behavior in Europe was considered briefly by Passa [26] in a review of the trends for type 1 and type 2 diabetes and their complications. His special focus on France was reinforced by the observations of Detournay et al. [27].

9.3.5   Diabetes in Ethnic Minorities in Europe

The arrival in Europe of large groups of ethnically diverse peoples has been a growing feature of the increasing mobility of human populations over the past century. Ethnic minority communities from the Indian subcontinent, of African ancestry (either from Africa or from the Caribbean), people from the Middle East and the Far East, and particularly in Germany from Turkey [28] have almost without exception emphasized their greater susceptibility to type 2 diabetes than the settled local populations. This relatively low susceptibility of peoples of European origin has also perhaps been reflected in the apparent reduction of diabetes risk in high-susceptibility peoples such as the Pima Indians by the admixture of European genes [21, 22]. Although environmental factors such as obesity

and physical activity clearly play an important role in determining the emergence of diabetes, the admixture effect suggests that there is a distinct genetic component which is contributing to the variation in ethnic susceptibility to T2DM and probably to the varying susceptibility within ethnic groups.

A survey in Manchester, United Kingdom [29], showed surprisingly high age-standardized diabetes prevalence of known and newly detected diabetes in Europeans of 20%, indistinguishable from rates in people of Afro-Caribbean origin (22%) but still exceeded by those of Pakistani ancestry (33%). The largest immigrant population in Europe is from Turkey, with large numbers of Moroccan and North African immigrants in France. In a subset of suitably collected and comparable populations from their larger meta-analysis, Uitewaal et al. [28] found that, compared with local indigenous European populations, the prevalence of diabetes was 1.3–2.8 times higher in Turks and 1.9–3.2 times higher in Moroccans. A house-to-house survey in a suburb of London [30] found two to three times higher prevalence of diabetes in residents of South Asian origin than of European origin, observations that have been confirmed repeatedly elsewhere [31–33]. Interestingly, the same high rates were found among Indian residents of a relatively affluent neighborhood of New Delhi, the Darya Ganj [34]. This dispels the notion that high diabetes risk was only visited upon members of the Indian diasporate.

9.3.6   T2DM in Children in Europe

Since 1990 there has been a rapid growth in the number of reports of type 2 diabetes in children [35–38]. Although the spread of T2DM into progressively younger people was first noted among American Indians [39], where it was associated with increasing rates of childhood obesity, the emergence of obesity-associated childhood type 2 diabetes has now been almost universally reported [40, 41]. In European children of Caucasian origin, a startlingly strong association with obesity has been demonstrated by Wiegand et al. [42].

Type 2 diabetes in children and young people is also addressed in a separate section of the third edition of the *Diabetes Atlas* [23]. Most of the published literature on T2DM and IGT in children to date has been clinic based and there is relatively little dealing with the epidemiology of the condition.

It is perhaps not surprising that it was in young US Pima Indians that the emerging phenomenon first drew major attention, since high prevalence in youth appears to run parallel with enhanced adult susceptibility, apparently displaying even at this early age their readier development of glucose intolerance in response to a given degree of adiposity [43]. Though the incidence of youthful T2DM and IGR appears to be increasing along with the progressive rise in obesity in children and young people, it remains relatively uncommon and estimates of its prevalence uncertain. Population-based epidemiological surveys will be required to distinguish this from the closely studied inherited monogenic forms of diabetes collectively known as maturity-onset diabetes of the young (MODY) [44, 45]. Misclassification may also occur with young T2DM patients presenting with onset ketonuria and assumed to be type 1 DM, or with the occasional, aketotic young type 1 DM patients.

Children of European ancestry with their greater susceptibility to type 1 DM seem to share with their seniors a relative resistance to T2DM. In Japan, 80% of all new cases of diabetes in children and adolescents are diagnosed as T2DM, compared with France, Austria and Sweden where the proportion is under 5%. Reported incidence rates of T2DM in children and adolescents are quoted as about 2 per 100 000 in England, nearly 15 per 100 000 in Japan but almost 25 per 100 000 in Montana and Wyoming among native American youngsters [45, 46]. In Europe, rates among ethnic minority young people are likely to be notably higher than in the indigenous population. In Britain, for example, many of the young people developing T2DM are emerging from the South Asian and Afro-Caribbean minorities [48]. There are several major implications to this rising tide of youthful T2DM. Diabetic complications are certainly no less prevalent among them [49], and with the prolonged exposure to hyperglycemia we already see T2DM providing the majority of people with diabetes presenting for renal dialysis and transplantation [50]. Equally, the increased risk of cardiovascular disease in South Asian people will be further intensified by the advent of the additional risk factor of glucose intolerance [51]. Energetic preventive efforts are clearly called for that are directed at obesity prevention in all children, but particularly those from ethnic minorities and those with a parental history of diabetes.

9.3.7 Genetic and Epigenetic Aspects of Diabetes Epidemiology

Any consideration of differing genetic contributions to variations in diabetes prevalence between regions or between ethnic groups within regions such as Europe will need to take environmental factors into account, both in their own right and in respect of possible differential interaction with ethnic genetic constitutions. The effects of aging, degrees of adiposity and sedentary lifestyle may vary from group to group depending on their genetic makeup, and this may also affect the expression of the diabetic state in terms of its age of appearance, rate of advance and severity of expression.

Neel's 'thrifty genotype' hypothesis [52], genetic selection driven by exposure to famine, holds a favored explanatory role for ethnic differences in the metabolic capacity to deal with nutritional adequacy or surfeit. An alternative explanation, the 'thrifty phenotype' [53], proposes that subnutrition during early development, indicated by low birthweight, sets the metabolic pattern for T2DM in adult life, though alternative explanations have been forcefully argued [54]. Recently, the possible role of epigenetic regulation [55, 56] has attracted attention as a potential explanation for T2DM and other features of the broader 'metabolic syndrome' [57, 58]

9.3.7.1 The Pima Indian Experience

A powerful example of the influence of genetic–environmental interaction is provided by diabetes in Pima Indian people. The US branch of the Pima people is now notable for its high prevalence of obesity, its relatively sedentary life style and a lifetime expectation of developing type 2 diabetes exceeding 50% [59]. As recently described [60], however, the Mexican branch of the Pima, which shares the same genetic background, is lean, physically active and has low rates of diabetes comparable to those of neighboring rural, non-Pima Mexicans. Analysis of the diabetes heritability of the two groups could come to very different conclusions. The mechanisms underlying 'obesity-linked' diabetes could well differ from those responsible for the 'wild-type' diabetes.

This major determinant role of environmental factors probably explains why, even with modern molecular techniques of whole-genome analysis, the elucidation of the complex genetic background of T2DM remains elusive [61, 62]. Of the substantial number of weak mapping linkages that have been found, few have been replicated in other studies and the gene locus identified in even fewer. Authenticity of such a linkage is often sought by observing its reproducibility in other ethnic groups, and though this strategy will identify diabetes susceptibility genes common to all populations (if they exist), it will reduce the likelihood of recognition of an ethnically specific genetic susceptibility locus.

It seems virtually certain that the genetic platform for T2DM consists of relatively large numbers of genes, each of small effect and possibly differing qualitatively from 'case' to 'case'. Some risk alleles may be very commonly involved and contribute to increased susceptibility in several or even all ethnic groups. Permutt *et al.* [61] tabulate 10 known gene locus associations that had been replicated in two or more studies at that date. Since then, the picture has changed somewhat with the description by Grant *et al.* [63] in a large Icelandic case-control study (and to something of an editorial fanfare [64]) of a relatively powerful genetic association of T2DM with a variant of the transcription factor TCF7L2. One copy of the high-risk variant allele increases the risk of T2DM by 1.45 and two copies by 2.41. Subsequent studies have confirmed the association in many diverse ethnic populations [65], including people of European, Asian, African and Indian ancestry.

There is as yet no clear evidence of the nature of the genetic contribution to *diversity* of ethnic susceptibility. Demonstration of the existence and location in the genome of ethnically specific diabetes susceptibility genes will require many large, well-designed studies of large and carefully selected populations and the type of coordinated, collaborative settings for data compilation and analysis described by Bracken [66]. If the genetic basis of ethnic susceptibility or resistance to T2DM could be better identified and understood, then it could open the way for targeted measures of treatment or prevention. Similar arguments apply to ethnic variation in the liability to the broader 'metabolic syndrome' or 'insulin resistance syndrome' [58] of which T2DM is a frequent, though

not obligatory, component. It may be the ethnic 'genetic background' that influences the expression of susceptibility genes or even possibly an epigenetic response to a major environmental change.

9.3.7.2 Epigenetic Mechanisms: Epidemiological Considerations

Interest has recently reawakened in the possible pathogenic role of epigenetic mechanisms: stable, perhaps heritable, changes in gene expression provoked by environmental influences [55, 56, 67, 68]. An epigenetic response to major transitions in the nutritional environment, by affecting the expression of the genes of metabolism, could thereby provoke sustained metabolic changes with clear relevance to glucose intolerance, diabetes and perhaps other disorders, such as those described as the metabolic syndrome. The basic epigenetic mechanisms of acetylation of chromatin protein histones and methylation of DNA cytosines effecting gene activation and repression respectively are now well described and understood [55, 56]. Exploration of these mechanisms may provide important new approaches to understanding how aging, nutritional extremes, toxic hazards or other environmental factors may impact via gene action on metabolic health and disease. Epigenetic mechanisms may explain, in part at least, the ethnic variation in susceptibility to type 2 diabetes and other features of the metabolic syndrome. The European resistance to T2DM, perhaps reflecting the relative stability of European nutritional history and the absence of exposure to severe and frequent famine, may thus be explained as much by heritable epigenetic modification of the genome as by classical Darwinian selective mechanisms.

9.4 CONCLUSION

The epidemiology of T2DM in Europe has a number of special features. Those populations 'indigenous' to Europe, often classed as Caucasoids, have relatively low susceptibility to T2DM compared with other major regional ethnic groups. Europe also hosts (and sometimes absorbs) large migrant populations, often composed of peoples who, in European surroundings, evince much higher diabetes susceptibility, providing opportunities for etiological research and application of preventive initiatives. People of European ancestry have colonized many other regions where admixture of European genes appears in some cases to reduce high indigenous diabetes susceptibility. Classical epidemiological study of the nutritional and cultural habits of such contrasting populations, now reinforced with the enormously powerful new techniques of genetic (and epigenetic) analysis, should be the source of important new hypotheses and mutual benefits bearing on patterns of health and disease in a rapidly changing world.

References

1. King, H., Aubert, R.E. and Herman, W.H. (1998) Global burden of diabetes, 1995–2025 prevalence, numerical estimates and projections. *Diabetes Care*, **21**, 1414–31.

2. Quing, Q., Williams, D.E. and Imperatore, G. (2004) Epidemiology and geography of type 2 diabetes mellitus, in *International Textbook of Diabetes Mellitus*, 3rd edn (eds R.A. De Fronzo, E. Ferrannini, H. Keen and P. Zimmet), John Wiley & Sons, Ltd, pp. 33–56.

3. King H. and Rewers M. (1993) Global estimates for prevalence of diabetes mellitus and impaired glucose tolerance in adults. *Diabetes Care*, **16**, 157–77.

4. Wild, S., Roglic, G., Green, A. *et al.* (2004) Global prevalence of diabetes. Estimates for the year 2000 and projections for 2030. *Diabetes Care*, **27**, 1047–53.

5. Zimmet, P., Alberti, K.G. and Shaw, J. (2001) Global and societal implications of the diabetes epidemic. *Nature*, **414**, 782–87.

6. Green, A., Stovring, H., Andersen, M. and Beck-Nielsen, H. (2005) The epidemic of type 2 diabetes is a statistical artefact. *Diabetologia*, **48**, 1456–8.

7. Evans, J., Barnett, K., Ogston, S. and Morris, A. (2007) Increasing prevalence of type 2 diabetes in a Scottish population: effect of increasing incidence or decreasing mortality? *Diabetologia*, **50**, 729–32.

8. Malins, J.M., Fitzgerald, M.G. and Wall, M. (1965) A change in the sex incidence of diabetes mellitus. *Diabetologia*, **1**, 121–4.

9. Manson, J.E., Rimm, E.B., Colditz, G.A. *et al.* (1992) Parity and incidence of non-insulin-dependent diabetes mellitus. *The American Journal of Medicine*, **93**, 13–18.

10. Gale, E.A. and Gillespie, K.M. (2001) Diabetes and gender. *Diabetologia*, **44**, 3–15.

11. Expert Committee on the Diagnosis and Classification of Diabetes Mellitus (1997) Report of the Expert Committee on the diagnosis and classification of diabetes mellitus. *Diabetes Care*, **20**, 1183–97.

12. World Health Organisation (1999) *Definition, Diagnosis and Classification of Diabetes Mellitus and its Complications. Report of a WHO Consultation, Part 1 Diagnosis and Classification of Diabetes Mellitus*. WHO, Geneva.

13. World Health Organisation Expert Committee (1980) Diabetes Mellitus: Second Report of the WHO Expert Committee on Diabetes Mellitus. Tech. Rep. Ser. 646, WHO, Geneva.

14. World Health Organisation (1985) Diabetes Mellitus, Report of a WHO Study Group. Tech. Rep. Ser. 727, WHO, Geneva.

15. DECODE Study Group (2003) Age- and sex-specific prevalence of diabetes and impaired glucose regulation in 13 European cohorts. *Diabetes Care*, **26**, 61–9.

16. The DECODE Study Group (1999) Is fasting glucose sufficient to define diabetes? Epidemiological data from 20 European studies. *Diabetologia*, **42**, 647–54.

17. Zimmet, P.Z. (1992) Kelly West Lecture 1991. Challenges in diabetes epidemiology–from West to the rest. *Diabetes Care*, **15**, 232–52.

18. Katsilambros, N., Aliferis, K. and Darviri, C. *et al.* (1993) Evidence for an increase in the prevalence of known diabetes in a sample of an urban population in Greece. *Diabetic Medicine: A Journal of the British Diabetic Association*, **10**, 87–90.

19. Neil, H.A., Gatling, W. and Mather, H.M. *et al.* (1987) The Oxford Community Diabetes Study: evidence for an increase in the prevalence of known diabetes in Great Britain. *Diabetic Medicine: A Journal of the British Diabetic Association*, **4**, 539–43.

20. Laakso, M., Reunanen, A. and Klaukka, T. *et al.* (1991) Changes in the prevalence and incidence of diabetes in Finnish adults, 1970–87. *American Journal of Epidemiology*, **133**, 850–7.

21. Diamond, J. (2003) The double puzzle of diabetes. *Nature*, **423**, 599–602.

22. Williams, R.C., Long, J.C., Hanson, R.L. *et al.* (2000) Individual estimates of European genetic admixture associated with lower body-mass index, plasma glucose, and prevalence of type 2 diabetes in Pima Indians. *American Journal of Human Genetics*, **66**, 527–38.

23. International Diabetes Federation (2006) *Diabetes Atlas*, 3rd edn, International Diabetes Federation, Brussels, www.idf.org.

24. United Nations Secretariat Population Division (2003) *United Nations Technical Working Group Report Long-range population projections*, Department of Economic and Social Affairs.

25. Cowie C.C., Keith F., Rust K.F. *et al.* (2006) Prevalence of diabetes and impaired fasting glucose in adults in the U.S. Population National Health and Nutrition Examination Survey 1999–2002. *Diabetes Care*, **29**, 1263–8.

26. Passa, P. (2002) Diabetes trends in Europe. *Diabetes/Metabolism Research and Reviews*, **18**, S3–8.

27. Detournay, B., Fagnani, F., Pribil, C. and Eschwege, E. (2000) Epidemiology, management and costs of type 2 diabetes in France in 1998. *Diabetes and Metabolism*, **26**, 225–31.

28. Uitewaal, P.J.M., Manna, D.R., Bruijnzeels, M.A. *et al.* (2004) Prevalence of type 2 diabetes mellitus, other cardiovascular risk factors, and cardiovascular disease in Turkish and Moroccan immigrants in north west Europe: a systematic review. *Preventive Medicine*, **39**, 1068–76.

29. Riste, L., Khan, F. and Cruickshank, K. (2001) High prevalence of type 2 diabetes in all ethnic groups, including Europeans, in a British inner city. *Diabetes Care*, **24**, 1377–83.

30. Mather, H.M. and Keen, H. (1985) The Southall Diabetes Survey: prevalence of known diabetes in Asians and Europeans. *British Medical Journal*, **291**, 1081–4.

31. Burden, A.C. (2001) Diabetes in Indo-Asian people. *The Practitioner*, **245**, 445–51.

32. Oldroyd, J., Banerjee, M., Heald, A. and Cruickshank, J.K. (2005) Diabetes and ethnic minorities. *Postgraduate Medical Journal*, **81**, 486–90.

33. Barnett, A.H., Dixon, A., Bellary, S. *et al.* (2006) Type 2 diabetes and cardiovascular risk in the UK south Asian community. *Diabetologia*, **49**, 2234–46.

34. Verma, N.P., Mehta, S.P., Madhu, S. *et al.* (1986) Prevalence of known diabetes in an urban Indian environment: the Darya Ganj diabetes survey. *British Medical Journal*, **293**, 423–4.

35. Fagot-Campagna, A., Narayan, K.M. and Imperatore, G. (2001) Type 2 diabetes in children. *British Medical Journal*, **322**, 377–8.

36. Schober, E., Holt, R.W., Grabert, M. *et al.* (2005) Diabetes mellitus type 2 in childhood and adolescence in Germany and parts of Austria. *European Journal of Pediatrics*, **164**, 705–7.

37. Feltbower, R.G., McKinney, P.A., Campbell, F.M. *et al.* (2003) Type 2 and other forms of diabetes in 0–30 year olds: a hospital based study in Leeds UK. *Archives of Disease in Childhood*, **88**, 676–9.

38. Alberti, G., Zimmet, P. and Shaw, J. *et al.* (2004) Consensus Workshop Group: type 2 diabetes in the young: the evolving epidemic: the International Diabetes Federation consensus workshop. *Diabetes Care*, **27**, 1798–811.

39. Dabelea, D., Hanson, R.L., Bennett, P.H. *et al.* (1998) Increasing prevalence of type 2 diabetes in American Indian children. *Diabetologia*, **41**, 904.

40. Pinhas-Hamiel, O. and Zeitler, P. (2005) The global spread of type 2 diabetes mellitus in children and adolescents. *The Journal of Pediatrics*, **146**, 693–700.

41. Lipton, R.B., Drum, M., Burnet, D. *et al.* (2005) Obesity at the onset of diabetes in an ethnically diverse population of children: what does it mean for epidemiologists and clinicians? *Pediatrics*, **115**, e553–60.

42. Wiegand, S., Maikowski, U., Blankenstein, O. *et al.* (2004) Type 2 diabetes and impaired glucose tolerance in European children and adolescents with obesity–a problem that is no longer restricted to minority groups. *European Journal of Endocrinology*, **151**, 199–206.

43. McAuley, K.A., Williams, S.M., Mann, J.I. *et al.* (2002) Increased risk of type 2 diabetes despite same degree of adiposity in different racial groups. *Diabetes Care*, **25**, 2360–1.

44. Hattersley, A.T. (1998) Maturity-onset diabetes of the young; clinical heterogeneity explained by genetic heterogeneity. *Diabetic Medicine: A Journal of the British Diabetic Association*, **15**, 15–24.

45. Fajans, S.S., Bell, G.I. and Polonsky, K.S. (2001) Molecular mechanisms and clinical physiopathology of maturity-onset diabetes of the young. *The New England Journal of Medicine*, **345**, 971–80.

46. Wilson, C., Susan, L., Lynch, A. *et al.* (2001) Patients with diagnosed diabetes mellitus can be accurately identified in an Indian Health Service patient registration database. *Public Health Reports*, **116**, 45–9.

47. Harwell, T.S., McDowall, J.M., Moore, K. *et al.* (2001) Establishing surveillance for diabetes in American Indian youth. *Diabetes Care*, **24**, 1029–32.

48. Ehtisham, S., Hattersley, A.T., Dunger, D.B. and Barrett, T.G. (2004) First UK survey of paediatric type 2 diabetes and MODY. *Archives of Disease in Childhood*, **89**, 526–9.

49. Pinhas-Hamiel, O. and Zeitler, P. (2007) Acute and chronic complications of type 2 diabetes mellitus in children and adolescents. *Lancet*, **369**, 1823–31.

50. Rychlik, I., Miltenberger-Miltenyi, G. and Ritz, E. (1998) The drama of the continuous increase in end-stage renal failure in patients with type II diabetes mellitus. *Nephrology, Dialysis, Transplantation*, **13** (8), 6–10.

51. Hillier, T.A. and Pedula, K.L. (2003) Complications in young adults with early-onset type 2 diabetes. *Diabetes Care*, **26**, 2999–3005.

52. Neel, J.V. (1999) The 'thrifty genotype' in 1998. *Nutrition Reviews*, **57**, S2–9.

53. Hales, C.N. and Barker, D.J. (2001) The thrifty phenotype hypothesis. *British Medical Bulletin*, **60**, 5–20.

54. Frayling, T.M. and Hattersley, A.T. (2001) The role of genetic susceptibility in the association of low birth weight with type 2 diabetes. *British Medical Bulletin*, **60**, 89–101.

55. Jaenisch, R. and Bird, A. (2003) Epigenetic regulation of gene expression: how the genome integrates intrinsic and environmental signals. *Nature Genetics Supplement*, **33**, 245–54.

56. Simmons, R.A. (2007) Developmental origins of β-cell failure in type 2 diabetes: the role of epigenetic mechanisms. *Pediatric Research*, **61**, 64R–67R.

57. Gallou-Kabani, C. and Junien, C. (2005) Nutritional epigenomics of metabolic syndrome. *Diabetes*, **54**, 1899–906.

58. Alberti, K.G., Zimmet, P. and Shaw, J. (2005) The metabolic syndrome–a new worldwide definition. *Lancet*, **366**, 1059–62.

59. Knowler, W.C., Pettit, D.J., Saad, M.F. and Bennett, P.H. (1990) Diabetes mellitus in the Pima Indians: incidence, risk factors and pathogenesis. *Diabetes/Metabolism Reviews*, **6**, 1–27.

60. Schulz, L.O., Bennett, P.H., Ravussin, E. *et al.* (2006) Effects of traditional and Western environments on prevalence of type 2 diabetes in Pima Indians in Mexico and the U.S. *Diabetes Care*, **29**, 1866–71.

61. Permutt, M.A., Wasson, J. and Cox, N. (2005) Genetic epidemiology of diabetes. *The Journal of Clinical Investigation*, **115**, 1431–9.

62. Barroso, I. (2005) Genetics of type 2 diabetes. *Diabetic Medicine: A Journal of the British Diabetic Association*, **22**, 517–35.

63. Grant, S.F., Thorleifsson, G., Reynisdottir, I. *et al.* (2006) Variant of transcription factor 7-like 2 (*TCF7L2*) gene confers risk of type 2 diabetes. *Nature Genetics*, **38**, 320–3.

64. Zeggini, E. and McCarthy, M.I. (2007) *TCF7L2*: the biggest story in diabetes genetics since HLA? *Diabetologia*, **50**, 1–4.

65. Sladek, R., Rocheleau, G., Rung, J. *et al.* (2007) A genome-wide association study identifies novel risk loci for type 2 diabetes. *Nature*, **445**, 881–5.

66. Bracken, M.B. (2005) Genomic epidemiology of complex disease: the need for an electronic evidence-based approach to research synthesis. *American Journal of Epidemiology*, **162**, 297–301.

67. Pembrey, M.E. (2002) Time to take epigenetic inheritance seriously. *European Journal of Human Genetics*, **10**, 669–71.

68. Egger, G., Liang, G., Aparicio, C. and Jones, P.A. (2004) Epigenetics in human disease and prospects for epigenetic therapy. *Nature*, **429**, 457–63.

10

The Burden of Diabetes and its Complications in the Middle East and Eastern Mediterranean Region

Imad M. El-Kebbi[1] and Michael M. Engelgau[2]

[1]Division of Endocrinology, Metabolism and Lipids, Emory University School of Medicine, Atlanta, GA, USA

[2]Division of Diabetes Translation, National Center for Chronic Disease Prevention and Health Promotion, Centers for Disease Control and Prevention, Atlanta, GA, USA

10.1 INTRODUCTION

Communicable diseases used to be the main diseases in developing countries. However, rapid economic development, urbanization and social and lifestyle changes during the past few decades have led to an enormous increase in the prevalence of chronic disorders, including diabetes, hypertension, obesity and cardiovascular disease.

Populations of the Middle East and the eastern Mediterranean are experiencing a sharp increase in diabetes mellitus (DM), approaching and in some cases exceeding levels found in developed countries. This is especially true in affluent oil-rich countries, where obesity has been increasing at a rapid rate. Predominantly rural countries are not spared, but they appear to be affected to a lesser extent. The International Diabetes Federation estimates that the prevalence rate of diabetes for the 20–79 years age group in the eastern Mediterranean region and the Middle East was 7.0% in 2003 compared with 7.8% in Europe and 7.9% in North America. These values are in contrast to a rate of 2.4% in Africa [1].

Assuming that the levels of risk factors for diabetes remain constant, it is estimated that the worldwide prevalence of diabetes will increase from 2.8% in 2000 to 4.4% in 2030 for all age groups [2]. However, this projection is likely to be an underestimate, since the prevalence and severity of risk factors are increasing rather than remaining constant. The Middle East Crescent, along with sub-Saharan Africa and India, is expected to experience the greatest relative increase in individuals with diabetes on the basis of changes in demographic numbers.

In this chapter, we review the epidemiology of type 1 and type 2 diabetes in the Middle East and eastern Mediterranean region. Unfortunately, epidemiologic data are sparse; they have been collected in the region only during the past two decades.

10.2 TYPE 1 DIABETES

Wide variations are reported in the global incidence of type 1 diabetes. Although a polar–equatorial gradient was suggested, with a high incidence in the Scandinavian countries, it now appears that the variation in regional incidence rates is more likely related to racial and ethnic differences among world populations, with a possible contribution from environmental factors that have not yet been determined.

The Epidemiology of Diabetes Mellitus, second edition   Edited by Jean-Marie Ekoé, Marian Rewers, Rhys Williams and Paul Zimmet
© 2008 John Wiley & Sons, Ltd

Data on the epidemiology of type 1 diabetes in the Middle East are scarce. However, limited information suggests that the incidence of type 1 diabetes is increasing in many countries of the region. The World Health Organization (WHO) DiaMond project [3], a worldwide effort to monitor the incidence of type 1 diabetes, has provided an opportunity to examine this disorder in a few Middle Eastern countries. **Table 10.1** shows incidence data of type 1 diabetes for several countries of the Middle East and the Eastern Mediterranean region.

Using the DiaMond protocol, a study in Kuwait that surveyed hospitals and clinics showed that the yearly incidence rate in 1992–1997 was 20.1 per 100 000 children aged 0–14 years [4]. Surprisingly, the incidence of diabetes for children younger than 5 years old was 11.6 per 100 000 and that age group accounted for 22% of newly diagnosed cases. This finding is in contrast to an earlier study from Kuwait that showed an incidence rate of only 3.96% for the 0–14 years age group in 1980–1981 [5]. There was a significant trend toward an increase in incidence during the survey period, from 15.7 in 1992 up to 25.6 in 1997.

A survey of hospitals and clinics in a southern province of Iran from 1991 to 1996 found a relatively low incidence rate for type 1 diabetes of 3.7 per 100 000 for people aged 0–29 years. The incidence was 4.37 per 100 000 for urban dwellers and 3.27 per 100 000 for residents of rural areas [6]. The peak incidence was among children aged 10–14 years.

A hospital-based study in Saudi Arabia revealed an increase in the number of children aged 0–14 years with type 1 diabetes from 1986 to 1997, with an overall age-adjusted incidence rate of 12.3 per 100 000 [7].

Another study found a surprisingly low incidence of type 1 diabetes among Jordanian children aged 0–14 years. Although the incidence was low, it was also rising from 2.8 per 100 000 in 1992 to 3.6 per 100 000 in 1996 [8].

Similarly, a population-based prospective study of children aged 0–14 years in the Sultanate of Oman revealed a low incidence of type 1 diabetes: 2.45 per 100 000 in 1993 and 2.62 per 100 000 in 1994 [9].

Ethnicity appears to influence type 1 incidence in the region. An example is the incidence of type 1 diabetes in Israel among individuals aged 0–17 years. Studies based on the country register showed that Yemenite Jews in 1990–1993 had an incidence rate of 18.5 per 100 000, Ashkenazi Jews had a rate of 10.0 per 100 000 and the rate for Israeli Arabs was 2.9 per 100 000. The overall incidence in Israel increased from 3.2 per 100 000 in 1965–1969 to 7.3 per 100 000 in 1990–1993 [10].

Using a retrospective review of records from city hospitals and clinics, researchers found an exceedingly low incidence of type 1 diabetes in Karachi, Pakistan, in 1989–1993, with a 1.02 per 100 000 per year for children aged 0–16 years. This low incidence rate is consistent with rates found in other nations in Asia [11].

Overall, few studies on the epidemiology of type 1 diabetes are published and the majority tend to be hospital based (therefore with several potential biases) or limited geographically to a specific area within the country of interest. The incidence rate of type 1 diabetes varies widely among countries in the region; however, the overall trend appears to be an increase in incidence. The reasons for this remain unclear, but a similar trend is observed worldwide [12]. The most likely explanation is that

Table 10.1 Incidence of type 1 diabetes (per 100 000, per year).

Country	Reference	Years studied	Age group studied (years)	Incidence
Kuwait	Shaltout *et al.* [4]	1997	0–14	25.6
Iran	Pishdad [6]>	1991–1996	0–29	3.7
Saudi Arabia	Kulaylat and Narchi [7]	1986–1997	0–14	12.3
Jordan	Ajlouni *et al.* [8]	1996	0–14	3.6
Oman	Soliman *et al.* [9]	1994	0–14	2.62
Israel	Shamis *et al.* [10]	1990–1993	0–17	7.3
Pakistan	Staines *et al.* [11]	1989–1993	0–16	1.02

this increase is due to changes in environmental factors that are unidentified so far.

10.3 TYPE 2 DIABETES

Similar to the situation elsewhere in the developing world, countries of the Middle East and eastern Mediterranean region are experiencing a rise in the prevalence of impaired glucose tolerance and diabetes. Data suggest great heterogeneity in the prevalence of these disorders among the countries of the region. Although some real differences may exist, many reported differences can be explained in part because published studies were done at different times and because the methods and diagnostic criteria varied. Most studies done in the 1990s used the WHO's 1985 diagnostic criteria [13] (**Table 10.2**).

To diagnose diabetes, these criteria required a fasting plasma glucose of 7.8 mmol l^{-1} (140 mg dl^{-1}) or higher, or a plasma glucose of 11.1 mmol l^{-1} (200 mg dl^{-1}) or more 2 h after a 75 g oral glucose load; impaired glucose tolerance required a plasma glucose measurement between 7.8 mmol l^{-1} (140 mg dl^{-1}) and 11.1 mmol l^{-1} (200 mg dl^{-1}) after a 75 g oral glucose load. By contrast, most studies published after 2000 used the WHO's 1999 criteria [14], which lowered the fasting plasma glucose cutoff for diabetes to 7.0 mmol l^{-1} (126 mg dl^{-1}) or higher and introduced a category called impaired fasting glucose, defined as a fasting plasma glucose measurement between 6.1 mmol l^{-1} (110 mg dl^{-1}) and 6.9 mmol l^{-1} (125 mg dl^{-1}). Although the categories of impaired fasting glucose and impaired glucose tolerance are not identical, they overlap significantly in most populations and both indicate high risk for diabetes.

In this section, we discuss published population-based data from several countries of the Middle East and eastern Mediterranean region.

High prevalences of glucose intolerance were reported in the Arabian Peninsula. A population-based study that screened Saudi Arabians aged 30–70 years for glucose intolerance [15] showed that, in 1995–2000, 26.2% of men and 21.5% of women had diabetes (based on 1999 WHO diagnostic criteria). The age-adjusted prevalence was estimated at 21.9% and diabetes was more common in urban areas (25.5%) than in rural areas (19.5%). Of those with diabetes, 27.9%

were unaware of their disease. The prevalence of impaired fasting glucose was similar for men (14.4%) and women (13.9%). A survey done in 1990–1993 using different methods, and 1985 WHO diagnostic criteria showed that the age-adjusted prevalence of diabetes was 12.0% for men and 14.0% for women in urban areas and 7.0% for men and 7.7% for women in rural areas [16]. Since then, the prevalence appears to have increased, but the use of different case definitions and methods limits a valid comparison.

A study in Oman in 2000 [17] used a cross-sectional survey and found that 11.8% of men and 11.6% of women aged 20 years or older had diabetes. Impaired fasting glucose was found in 7.1% of men and 5.1% of women. After applying the same diagnostic criteria to a 1991 survey [18], the researchers noted that, within the 30–64 years age group, 16.1% had diabetes in 2000 compared with 12.2% in 1991. Therefore, in 9 years, the prevalence of diabetes appears to have increased by approximately 32%.

A national survey of the adult population of the United Arab Emirates in 1999–2000 [19] found that 21.5% of men and 19.2% of women had diabetes. The corresponding values for impaired fasting glucose were 4.5% for men and 8% for women. For close to 41% of those with diabetes, their disease had not been previously diagnosed. When data on foreigners living in the Emirates were excluded from the analysis, the prevalence for citizens of the Emirates was 24.5% for diabetes and 8.8% for impaired fasting glucose.

Data from a cross-sectional study of 498 residents of Sana'a, Yemen, surveyed in 1999–2000 showed a relatively low prevalence of diabetes than in neighboring states [20]. Only 7.4% of men and 2.0% of women had diabetes, and the corresponding rates for impaired fasting glucose were 3.7% for men and 0.8% for women. A possible explanation for these low rates is that people in Yemen appeared to be leaner than people in other countries of the region; only 4.8% of the survey participants were obese.

A cross-sectional survey of a representative sample of Kuwaiti subjects in 1995–1996 found that 14.7% of men and 14.8% of women had diabetes and 2.6% of men and 3.3% of women had impaired glucose tolerance [21]. However, that study used WHO 1985 diagnostic criteria and subjects were screened with the fasting plasma glucose test. Only

Table 10.2 Prevalence (%) of diabetes and impaired glucose tolerance, according to WHO 1999 or 1985 diagnostic criteria.

Country	Researchers	Years studied	Age group studied (years)	DM males	DM females	IGT (or IFG) males	IGT (or IFG) females	WHO criteria
Saudi Arabia	Al-Nozha et al. [15]	1995–2000	30–70	26.2	21.5	14.4 (IFG)	13.9 (IFG)	1999
Oman	Al-Lawati et al. [17]	2000	≥20	11.8	11.3	7.1 (IFG)	5.1 (IFG)	1999
United Arab Emirates	Malik et al. [19]	1999–2000	≥20	21.5	19.2	4.5 (IFG)	8.0 (IFG)	1999
Yemen	Al-Habori et al. [20]	1999–2000	25–65	7.4	2.0	3.7 (IFG)	0.8 (IFG)	1999
Kuwait	Abdella et al. [21]	1995–1996	≥20	14.7	14.8	2.6	3.3	1985
Iran	Azizi et al. [22]	1999–2001	≥20	9.8	11.1	11.3	13.2	1985
Pakistan, urban	Shera et al. [23]	1995	≥25	11.1	10.6	6.5	14.3	1985
Pakistan, rural	Shera et al. [23]	1995	≥25	10.2	4.8	7.4	13.0	1985
Lebanon	Salti et al. [22]	1994–1995	≥30	13.1	13.2	5.6	6.4	1985
Jordan	Ajlouni et al. [23]	1997	≥25	14.9	12.5	9.0	10.3	1985
Palestinian West Bank, urban	Abdul-Rahim et al. [26]	1996–1998	30–65	7.4	14.9	4.2	7.0	1985
Palestinian West Bank, rural	Abdul-Rahim et al. [26]	1996–1998	30–65	10.0	9.6	6.2	10.3	1985
Egypt, urban, high SES	Herman et al. [27]	1991–1994	≥20	26.7	15.6	1.9	13.0	1985
Egypt, urban, low SES	Herman et al. [27]	1991–1994	≥20	10.1	17.5	3.8	7.3	1985
Egypt, rural	Herman et al. [27]	1991–1994	≥20	4.3	5.5	14.0	12.3	1985

DM, diabetes mellitus; IGT, impaired glucose tolerance; IFG, impaired fasting glucose (used instead of IGT in the first four studies); SES, socioeconomic status.

those with a fasting glucose level above or equal to 6.1 mmol l^{-1} were given the oral glucose tolerance test. This screening method may lower the prevalence estimates.

A 1999–2001 study of residents of Tehran, Iran, aged 20 years or older used WHO's 1985 diagnostic criteria and an oral glucose tolerance test to screen for diabetes [22]. The researchers reported that 9.8% of men and 11.1% of women had diabetes and 11.3% of men and 13.2% of women had impaired glucose tolerance. Interestingly, 54.0% of those with diabetes had no history of the disease. The prevalence of both diabetes and impaired glucose tolerance increased with age.

In 1995 in Pakistan, a survey was done to compare the prevalence of diabetes and impaired glucose tolerance in an urban area and a rural area [23]. Using the oral glucose tolerance test and WHO's 1985 criteria, the study reported that, among adults aged 25 years or older, the prevalence of diabetes was 10.8% in the urban area and 6.5% in the rural area. Impaired glucose intolerance was 11.9% in the urban area and 11.2% in the rural area. Interestingly, diabetes was more common than impaired glucose tolerance among men, whereas the reverse was true among women, especially in rural areas. Previously undiagnosed diabetes was found among 56.0% of women and 36.0% of men. The prevalence of abnormal glucose tolerance increased with age and with central obesity.

In 1994–1995, researchers in Lebanon used 1985 WHO criteria to survey people aged 30 years or older in three communities to learn the prevalence of abnormal glucose tolerance [24]. One community was urban and most residents were of low socioeconomic status; the second was also urban, but most residents had higher socioeconomic status than the first community; and the third community was rural. The prevalence of diabetes was 13.1% and was similar for men and women. Impaired glucose tolerance was 5.6% for men and 6.4% for women. Among those aged 30–64 years, the rate of diabetes was 17.2% and the rate of impaired glucose tolerance was 6.9% in the low socioeconomic urban area, 4.9% for diabetes and 3.0% for impaired glucose tolerance in the high socioeconomic urban area and 12.3% for diabetes and 5.9% for impaired glucose tolerance in the rural area. Those in the high socioeconomic urban group were leaner and younger than those in the other two

groups, which may explain the lower prevalence of abnormal glucose tolerance.

In 1997, researchers in Jordan used fasting and postoral glucose loading tests to evaluate the prevalences of diabetes and impaired glucose tolerance in a sample of subjects in four semiurban communities [25]. According to WHO 1985 criteria, the prevalence of diabetes among Jordanians aged 25 years or older was 14.9% for men and 12.5% for women. The prevalence of impaired glucose tolerance was 9.0% for men and 10.3% for women.

In 1996–1998, the oral glucose tolerance test and WHO 1985 diagnostic criteria were used to evaluate diabetes in the Palestinian West Bank [26]. In rural areas, the prevalence was 9.8% for diabetes and 8.6% for impaired glucose tolerance. In urban areas, the prevalence was 12.0% for diabetes and 5.9% for impaired glucose tolerance. Women had a higher prevalence than men of abnormal glucose tolerance, especially in urban areas, and a higher prevalence of obesity. Of urban subjects, 41.5% were obese compared with 28.2% of rural subjects.

No recent data are available from Egypt. However, a cross-sectional population-based survey done in 1991–1994 of people aged 20 years or older showed that, overall, the prevalence of diabetes was 9.3% and that half of the cases of diabetes were undiagnosed before the survey [27]. Diabetes was diagnosed by history, a 2 h glucose tolerance test and WHO 1985 criteria. In rural areas, 16% of those surveyed were obese and 4.9% had diabetes. In low socioeconomic urban areas, 37% were obese and 13.5% had diabetes, whereas 49% were obese and 20% had diabetes in high socioeconomic areas. Impaired glucose tolerance was diagnosed in 13.1% of people living in rural areas, 5.4% of people living low socioeconomic urban areas and 8.6% of people living in high socioeconomic urban areas.

The above studies show a relatively high prevalence of diabetes in countries of the region compared with the prevalence in developed countries such as the United States, where the prevalence of type 2 diabetes was 9.6% among people aged 20 years or older in 2005 [28]. Although large variations in diabetes prevalence are evident among these countries, comparisons between countries are not possible because of differences in survey methods and case definitions. However, the trend for diabetes prevalence shows an increase over time and diabetes appears to be more common than impaired glucose tolerance, especially in areas with a high prevalence of obesity (see later discussion on obesity data). A possible explanation is that excessive insulin resistance associated with increased body fat is causing people with impaired glucose tolerance to progress faster to diabetes in areas with a high prevalence of obesity.

10.4 RISK FACTORS FOR DIABETES IN THE MIDDLE EAST AND EASTERN MEDITERRANEAN REGION

Major factors that contribute to the rising prevalence of diabetes in the developing world include urbanization, physical inactivity and sedentary lifestyles, and increasing rates of obesity, especially central obesity. The latter appears to be related to the increase in carbohydrates and fats in the diet and to aggressive advertisements and widespread availability of fast food items [29]. Traditional local diets, which were high in fiber and low in fat, are being replaced by processed high-fat Western-style food items which are energy dense and lack nutritional value. In contrast, the consumption of fruits, vegetables and grains is declining.

In addition, populations worldwide are experiencing an increase in longevity. The increase in the number of elderly people is expected to contribute to the increase in the prevalence of diabetes. With improvement in basic health care and in prevention of communicable diseases, longevity has increased in many countries of the Middle East. Data from the WHO show that longevity or healthy life expectancy is more than 60 years in many affluent Middle Eastern countries, such as Bahrain, Kuwait, Oman, Qatar and Saudi Arabia [30].

However, with affluence comes easy access to modern modes of transportation and a tendency to physical inactivity, which is by itself a risk factor for obesity and diabetes. A study in Riyadh, Saudi Arabia, revealed that, in 1996, 53.0% of adult men were physically inactive and only 19.5% were regularly active [31].

In Egypt, a cross-sectional population-based survey of people older than 20 years showed that the prevalence of a sedentary lifestyle was 52.0% in a rural areas, 73.0% in low socioeconomic areas, and 89.0% in a high socioeconomic areas [27].

10.5 ADULT OBESITY

Obesity and weight gain are major risk factors for type 2 diabetes, and they have been blamed for or implicated in the rising prevalence of diabetes worldwide. Many countries in the Middle East are experiencing a dramatic increase in obesity. Most studies suggest (i) that overweight is more common among men, (ii) that obesity is more common among women and (iii) that prevalences of both overweight and obesity are higher in urban areas than in rural areas. A number of studies cited here used the classification criteria recommended by the WHO [32] for overweight (defined as body mass index (BMI) of $25.0-29.9 \, \text{kg m}^{-2}$) and obesity (defined as BMI of $30.0 \, \text{kg m}^{-2}$ or more).

A community-based survey in Saudi Arabia in 1995–2000 of people aged 30–70 years found that 36.9% were overweight and 35.5% were obese. Men were more likely to be overweight and women were more likely to be obese [33].

A study of Tehranians in Iran in 2001–2002 showed that the prevalences of overweight were 46.0% for men and 39.5% for women; the prevalences of obesity were 40.3% for men and 20.8% for women [34]. These rates were lower in 1998–1999: prevalence of overweight was 42.5% for men and 40% for women and obesity was 32.7% for men and 16.5% for women. In Jordan, a study based on self-reports showed a 32.0% prevalence of overweight and a 13.0% prevalence of obesity, with obesity being more common among women [35]. In Oman, the prevalence in 2000 of overweight was 32.1% for men and 27.3% for women; the prevalence of obesity was 16.7% for men and 23.8% for women [36]. A Lebanese study showed that, in 1995–1996, the prevalence of overweight was 57.7% for men and 49.9% for women and that the prevalence of obesity was 14.3% for men and 18.8% for women [37]. A study published in 2002 showed that urban residents of the Palestinian West Bank were more likely to be obese than were residents of rural areas: the prevalence of obesity was 30.6% for men and 49.1% for women in urban areas and 18.0% for men and 36.8% for women in rural areas [38].

An Israeli study found a 39.3% prevalence of overweight and a 22.9% prevalence of obesity in 1999–2001. Again, obesity was more common among women and overweight was more common among men. Israeli Arabs were more obese than Israeli Jews [39].

In Egypt, a cross-sectional population-based survey of people older than 20 years showed that the prevalence of obesity was 16.0% in a rural areas, 37% in low socioeconomic areas, and 49.0% in a high socioeconomic areas [27].

10.6 CHILDHOOD OBESITY

The sharp increase in the prevalence of overweight and obesity worldwide is not only limited to adults, but also extends to adolescents and children and even to preschool children. This increase in weight led to an increase in the incidence of type 2 diabetes in childhood, to a point that it is becoming more common than type 1 diabetes in a few countries, such as in Japan and Taiwan [40, 41]. The unchecked increase in obesity will lead to (i) an explosion in the prevalence of type 2 diabetes at an early age, especially among children at high risk for diabetes, such as overweight or obese children living in the Middle East, and (ii) a corresponding increase in diabetes complications due to the early onset of exposure to hyperglycemia.

Obese children are likely to remain obese in adulthood. Data from the WHO show that, for preschool children, Middle Eastern countries have some of the highest prevalences of overweight in the world. That prevalence was 8.6% for Egyptian children in 1995–1996, 6.8% for Qatari children in 1995, 5.7% for Jordanian children in 1990 and 5.7% for Kuwaiti children in 1996–1997 [42]. These values compare with a prevalence of 4.5% for US children in 1988–1994.

A study from the United Arab Emirates of children aged 6–16 years in the late 1990s estimated that 8.0% of boys and girls were obese and close to 17.0% were overweight [43].

In Lebanon, it was estimated that 22.5% of boys aged 3–19 years were overweight and 7.5% were obese; 16.1% of girls in the same age category were overweight and 3.2% were obese [37].

Urgent measures to limit the escalation of childhood obesity are needed. Malnutrition and micronutrient deficiencies used to be the focus of public health interventions. Now, however, efforts should focus on preventing obesity among children, especially in developing countries.

10.7 COMPLICATIONS OF DIABETES

Studies addressing the prevalence of diabetic complications in countries of the eastern Mediterranean region and the Middle East tend to be clinic or hospital based. One cross-sectional population-based study was done in Egypt in 1991–1994 [44]. That study surveyed people aged 20 years or older for microvascular complications and foot ulcers. The results showed that 42.0% of patients with diabetes had diabetic retinopathy, diagnosed by retinal photography, 22.0% had peripheral neuropathy, 0.8% had foot ulcers and 5.0% were legally blind. In addition, 25.0% of patients with diabetes and hypertension and 17.0% of patients with diabetes but no hypertension had albuminuria (defined as an albumin/creatinine ratio at or above 100 mg g^{-1}, but less than 300 mg g^{-1} creatinine) and 7% of people had clinical nephropathy (defined as an albumin to creatinine ratio at or above 300 mg g^{-1} creatinine).

The remaining studies from the eastern Mediterranean area are clinic or hospital based and reported higher overall prevalence rates of diabetic complications, possibly due to the selection bias inherent to these studies. For example, a study from a clinic in Riyadh, Saudi Arabia, reported a 13.0% prevalence of clinical proteinuria and 41.0% prevalence of microalbuminuria (defined as a 24 h urine albumin content 30–300 mg) among patients with non-insulin-dependent diabetes [45]. A hospital-based study in Riyadh, Saudi Arabia, found that 38.0% of patients with diabetes had peripheral neuropathy [46].

Another Saudi study of patients at a diabetes center reported a prevalence of retinopathy of 31.3% (42.5% for insulin-dependent and 25.3% for non-insulin-dependent patients) [47]. At a hospital in Oman, however, the prevalence of retinopathy was 14.4% [48]. Both the Saudi and Omani studies found that advanced age, duration of diabetes, poor glycemic control and presence of nephropathy were associated with retinopathy.

A multicenter clinic-based study from Pakistan found a microalbuminuria prevalence of 34.0% among patients with type 2 diabetes [49]. A survey of patients with type 2 diabetes who attended an outpatient diabetes clinic in Karachi [50] reported that 43.0% had retinopathy, 40.0% had neuropathy and 20.0% had nephropathy.

A hospital-based study from Oman [48] found that the prevalence of diabetic retinopathy was 14.4% in 2000–2001. The prevalence of background retinopathy was 8.6% and the prevalence of proliferative retinopathy was 2.7%. Again, retinopathy was correlated with diabetes of long duration, high HbA$_{1c}$, hypertension and nephropathy.

In 2001 in Jordan, 45.0% of patients at a national diabetes center in 2001 had retinopathy, 33% had microalbuminuria and 19% had impaired vibration sense [51]. In addition, 5.0% of patients had suffered some type of amputation.

At the Bengazi Diabetic Clinic in Libya, 30.5% of patients registered between 1981 and 1990 had retinopathy, 25.2% had nephropathy and 45.7% had neuropathy [52].

10.8 DIABETES PREVENTION

Mounting evidence suggests that type 2 diabetes can be prevented or that its onset can be delayed. Studies from China [53], the United States [54] and Finland [55] show that, for obese patients with glucose intolerance, a 3-year program that includes weight loss and regular physical activity can lead to close to 60% reduction in the risk of progression to diabetes. Educating the public about a healthy diet, avoidance of excessive energy intake and regular physical activity are likely to help reverse the escalating obesity pandemic.

Preventing the complications of diabetes is also a public health issue of utmost importance. Clinic-based quality improvement programs are being developed in a number of countries to enhance diabetes care and screen for its complications. A 2-year program to improve diabetes management by primary care providers in an Israeli Health Maintenance Organization led to marked improvement in the processes of care (e.g. monitoring of HbA$_{1c}$ and lipids, foot inspections, fundus examinations) and in the group of patients whose disease is poorly controlled [56]. The introduction of a diabetes miniclinic in a primary health care center in Saudi Arabia also led to an improvement in the

processes of diabetes care and in screening for diabetes complications [57].

10.9 DIABETES SURVEILLANCE

The WHO has supported countries in the region in establishing national surveillance programs based on the STEPwise approach to surveillance [58], which is a simple tool for collecting information on noncommunicable diseases (e.g. diabetes) and their risk factors (e.g. unhealthy diet, physical inactivity). The aim is to help member states to collect population-based data on a continuous basis. This will help them predict the current burden and future needs, which will, in turn, help them develop a comprehensive health policy in addition to devising interventions (e.g. promoting healthy diets and lifestyles) for the primary prevention of chronic conditions. In addition, a joint program of the WHO and the International Diabetes Foundation has been in existence for some years to support developing countries in diabetes surveillance and prevention [59]. Termed Diabetes Action Now, this initiative aims to increase awareness of diabetes and provide guidance for planning and implementing national diabetes programs.

10.10 CONCLUSIONS

Despite mounting evidence that type 2 diabetes can be prevented or delayed with lifestyle changes and weight loss, the diabetes epidemic continues worldwide, and countries of the Middle East and eastern Mediterranean region are amongst those disproportionately affected. Although prevalence estimates may vary among the countries of the region, the trend for type 2 diabetes is on the increase, especially in affluent countries. With increasing rates of childhood obesity and improved longevity, the prevalence of diabetes is expected to increase even more than projected by statistical models. Systematic and reliable surveillance data about diabetes, its risk factors and its complications are urgently needed at the national level for countries of the region. Public health efforts to introduce healthy lifestyle changes are necessary to curb the consequences of this global health problem.

References

1. International Diabetes Federation (2003) *Diabetes Atlas*, 2nd edn, International Diabetes Federation, Brussels.
2. Wild, S., Roglic, G., Green, A. *et al.* (2004) Global prevalence of diabetes: estimates for the year 2000 and projections for 2030. *Diabetes Care*, **27**, 1047–53.
3. Karvonen, M., Viik-Kajander, M., Moltchanova, E. *et al.* (2000) Incidence of childhood type 1 diabetes worldwide. Diabetes Mondiale (DiaMond) Project Group [see comment]. *Diabetes Care*, **23**, 1516–26.
4. Shaltout, A.A., Moussa, M.A., Qabazard, M. *et al.* (2002) Kuwait Diabetes Study G: further evidence for the rising incidence of childhood type 1 diabetes in Kuwait. *Diabetic Medicine: A Journal of the British Diabetic Association*, **19**, 522–5.
5. Taha, T.H., Moussa, M.A., Rashid, A.R. and Fenech, F.F. (1983) Diabetes mellitus in Kuwait. Incidence in the first 29 years of life. *Diabetologia*, **25**, 306–8.
6. Pishdad, G.R. (2005) Low incidence of type 1 diabetes in Iran. *Diabetes Care*, **28**, 927–8.
7. Kulaylat, N.A. and Narchi, H. (2000) A twelve year study of the incidence of childhood type 1 diabetes mellitus in the Eastern Province of Saudi Arabia. *The Journal of Pediatric Endocrinology*, **13**, 135–40.
8. Ajlouni, K., Qusous, Y., Khawaldeh, A.K. *et al.* (1999) Incidence of insulin-dependent diabetes mellitus in Jordanian children aged 0–14 years during 1992–1996. *Acta Paediatrica Scandinavica. Supplement*, **88**, 11–13.
9. Soliman, A.T., Al-Salmi, I.S. and Asfour, M.G. (1996) Epidemiology of childhood insulin-dependent diabetes mellitus in the Sultanate of Oman. *Diabetic Medicine: A Journal of the British Diabetic Association*, **13**, 582–6.
10. Shamis, I., Gordon, O., Albag, Y. *et al.* (1997) Ethnic differences in the incidence of childhood IDDM in Israel (1965–1993). Marked increase since 1985, especially in Yemenite Jews. *Diabetes Care*, **20**, 504–8.
11. Staines, A., Hanif, S., Ahmed, S. *et al.* (1997) Incidence of insulin dependent diabetes mellitus in Karachi, Pakistan. *Archives of Disease in Childhood*, **76**, 121–3.
12. Onkamo, P., Vaananen, S., Karvonen, M. and Tuomilehto, J. (1999) Worldwide increase in incidence of type I diabetes – the analysis of the data on published incidence trends [see comment].

Diabetologia, **42**, 1395–403; [Erratum appears in (2003) *Diabetologia*, **43** (5), 685].
13. World Health Organization (1985) Diabetes Mellitus: Report of a WHO Study Group, WHO Tech. Rep. Ser. 727, World Health Organization, Geneva.
14. WHO Consultation (1999) Definition, Diagnosis and Classification of Diabetes Mellitus and its Complications, World Health Organization, Geneva.
15. Al-Nozha, M.M., Al-Maatouq, M.A., Al-Mazrou, Y.Y. *et al.* (2004) Diabetes mellitus in Saudi Arabia. *Saudi Medical Journal*, **25**, 1603–10.
16. Al-Nuaim, A.R. (1997) Prevalence of glucose intolerance in urban and rural communities in Saudi Arabia. *Diabetic Medicine: A Journal of the British Diabetic Association*, **14**, 595–602.
17. Al-Lawati, J.A., Al-Riyami, A.M., Mohammed, A.J. and Jousilahti, P. (2002) Increasing prevalence of diabetes mellitus in Oman. *Diabetic Medicine: A Journal of the British Diabetic Association*, **19**, 954–7.
18. Asfour, M.G., Lambourne, A., Soliman, A. *et al.* (1995) High prevalence of diabetes mellitus and impaired glucose tolerance in the Sultanate of Oman: results of the 1991 national survey. *Diabetic Medicine: A Journal of the British Diabetic Association*, **12**, 1122–5.
19. Malik, M., Bakir, A., Saab, B.A. *et al.* (2005) Glucose intolerance and associated factors in the multi-ethnic population of the United Arab Emirates: results of a national survey. *Diabetes Research and Clinical Practice*, **69**, 188–95.
20. Al-Habori, M., Al-Mamari, M. and Al-Meeri, A. (2004) Type II diabetes mellitus and impaired glucose tolerance in Yemen: prevalence, associated metabolic changes and risk factors. *Diabetes Research and Clinical Practice*, **65**, 275–81.
21. Abdella, N., Al Arouj, M., Al Nakhi, A. *et al.* (1998) Non-insulin-dependent diabetes in Kuwait: prevalence rates and associated risk factors. *Diabetes Research and Clinical Practice*, **42**, 187–96.
22. Azizi, F., Rahmani, M., Emami, H. *et al.* (2002) Cardiovascular risk factors in an Iranian urban population: Tehran lipid and glucose study (phase 1). *Sozial- und Praventivmedizin*, **47**, 408–26.
23. Shera, A.S., Rafique, G., Khawaja, I.A. *et al.* (1999) Pakistan National Diabetes Survey: prevalence of glucose intolerance and associated factors in Baluchistan province. *Diabetes Research and Clinical Practice*, **44**, 49–58.
24. Salti, I.S., Khogali, M., Alam, S. *et al.* (1997) Epidemiology of diabetes mellitus in relation

to other cardiovascular risk factors in Lebanon. *Eastern Mediterranean Health Journal*, **3**, 462–71.

25. Ajlouni, K., Jaddou, H. and Batieha, A. (1998) Diabetes and impaired glucose tolerance in Jordan: prevalence and associated risk factors. *Journal of Internal Medicine*, **244**, 317–23.

26. Abdul-Rahim, H.F., Husseini, A., Bjertness, E. *et al.* (2001) The metabolic syndrome in the West Bank population: an urban–rural comparison. *Diabetes Care*, **24**, 275–9.

27. Herman, W.H., Ali, M.A., Aubert, R.E. *et al.* (1995) Diabetes mellitus in Egypt: risk factors and prevalence. *Diabetic Medicine: A Journal of the British Diabetic Association*, **12**, 1126–31.

28. Centers for Disease Control and Prevention (2005) National Diabetes Fact Sheet: General Information and National Estimates on Diabetes in the United States, 2005, US Department of Health and Human Services, Atlanta.

29. Tucker, K.L. and Buranapin, S. (2001) Nutrition and aging in developing countries. *The Journal of Nutrition*, **131**, 2417S–23S.

30. World Health Organization (2004) World Health Report 2004, Geneva, Switzerland.

31. Al-Refaee, S.A. and Al-Hazzaa, H.A. (2001) Physical activity profile of adult males in Riyadh City. *Saudi Medical Journal*, **22**, 784–9.

32. World Health Organization (1997) Obesity: Preventing and Managing the Global Epidemic. Report of a WHO Consultation on Obesity, World Health Organization, Geneva, Switzerland.

33. Al-Nozha, M.M., Al-Mazrou, Y.Y., Al-Maatouq, M.A. *et al.* (2005) Obesity in Saudi Arabia. *Saudi Medical Journal*, **26**, 824–9.

34. Fereidoun, A., Leila, A. and Parvin, M. (2005) Trends in overweight, obesity and central fat accumulation among Tehranian adults between 1998–1999 and 2001–2002: Tehran Lipid and Glucose Study. *Annals of Nutrition and Metabolism*, **49**, 3–8.

35. Shehab, F., Belbeisi, A. and Walke, H. (2003) Prevalence of selected risk factors for chronic disease – Jordan, 2002. *Morbidity and Mortality Weekly Report*, **52**, 1042.

36. Al-Lawati, J.A. and Jousilahti, P.J. (2004) Prevalence and 10-year secular trend of obesity in Oman. *Saudi Medical Journal*, **25**, 346–51.

37. Sibai, A.M., Nahla, H., Nada, A. and Boushra, R. (2003) Prevalence and covariates of obesity in Lebanon: findings from the first epidemiological study. *Obesity Research*, **11**, 1353–61.

38. Abdul-Rahim, H.F., Holmboe-Ottesen, G., Stene, L.C.M. *et al.* (2003) Obesity in a rural and an urban Palestinian West Bank population. *International Journal of Obesity*, **27**, 140–6.

39. Kaluski, D.N. and Berry, E.M. (2005) Prevalence of obesity in Israel. *Obesity Reviews*, **6**, 115–16.

40. Urakami, T., Kubota, S., Nitadori, Y. *et al.* (2005) Annual incidence and clinical characteristics of type 2 diabetes in children as detected by urine glucose screening in the Tokyo metropolitan area. *Diabetes Care*, **28**, 1876–81.

41. Wei, J.N., Sung, F.C., Lin, C.C. *et al.* (2003) National surveillance for type 2 diabetes mellitus in Taiwanese children. *The Journal of the American Medical Association*, **290**, 1345–50.

42. De Onis, M. and Blossner, M. (2000) Prevalence and trends of overweight among preschool children in developing countries. *The American Journal of Clinical Nutrition*, **72**, 1032–9.

43. Al-Haddad, F., Al-Nuaimi, Y., Little, B.B. and Thabit, M. (2000) Prevalence of obesity among school children in the United Arab Emirates. *American Journal of Human Biology*, **12**, 498–502.

44. Herman, W.H., Aubert, R.E., Engelgau, M.M. *et al.* (1998) Diabetes mellitus in Egypt: glycaemic control and microvascular and neuropathic complications. *Diabetic Medicine: A Journal of the British Diabetic Association*, **15**, 1045–51.

45. Alzaid, A.A., Sobki, S. and De Silva, V. (1994) Prevalence of microalbuminuria in Saudi Arabians with non-insulin-dependent diabetes mellitus: a clinic-based study. *Diabetes Research and Clinical Practice*, **26**, 115–20.

46. Nielsen, J.V. (1998) Peripheral neuropathy, hypertension, foot ulcers and amputations among Saudi Arabian patients with type 2 diabetes. *Diabetes Research and Clinical Practice*, **41**, 63–9.

47. El-Asrar, A.M., Al-Rubeaan, K.A., Al-Amro, S.A. *et al.* (1998) Risk factors for diabetic retinopathy among Saudi diabetics. *International Ophthalmology*, **22**, 155–61.

48. Khandekar, R., Al Lawatii, J., Mohammed, A.J. and Al Raisi, A. (2003) Diabetic retinopathy in Oman: a hospital based study. *The British Journal of Ophthalmology*, **87**, 1061–4.

49. Ahmedani, M.Y., Hydrie, M.Z., Iqbal, A. *et al.* (2005) Prevalence of microalbuminuria in type 2 diabetic patients in Karachi: Pakistan: a multi-center study. *The Journal of the Pakistan Medical Association*, **55**, 382–6; [Erratum appears in (2005) *The Journal of the Pakistan Medical Association*, **55** (12), 570].

50. Shera, A.S., Jawad, F., Maqsood, A. *et al.* (2004) Prevalence of chronic complications and associated

factors in type 2 diabetes. *The Journal of the Pakistan Medical Association*, **54**, 54–9.

51. Jbour, A.S., Jarrah, N.S., Radaideh, A.M. *et al.* (2003) Prevalence and predictors of diabetic foot syndrome in type 2 diabetes mellitus in Jordan. *Saudi Medical Journal*, **24**, 761–4.

52. Kadiki, O.A. and Roaed, R.B. (1999) Epidemiological and clinical patterns of diabetes mellitus in Benghazi, Libyan Arab Jamahiriya. *Eastern Mediterranean Health Journal*, **5**, 6–13.

53. Pan, X.R., Li, G.W., Hu, Y.H. *et al.* (1997) Effects of diet and exercise in preventing NIDDM in people with impaired glucose tolerance. The Da Qing IGT and Diabetes Study [see comment]. *Diabetes Care*, **20**, 537–44.

54. Diabetes Prevention Program Research Group (2002) Reduction in the incidence of type 2 diabetes with lifestyle intervention or metformin. *The New England Journal of Medicine*, **346**, 393–403.

55. Tuomilehto, J., Lindstrom, J., Eriksson, J. *et al.* (2001) Prevention of type 2 diabetes mellitus by changes in lifestyle among subjects with impaired glucose tolerance. *The New England Journal of Medicine*, **344**, 1343–50.

56. Goldfracht, M. and Porath, A. (2000) Nationwide program for improving the care of diabetic patients in Israeli primary care centers. *Diabetes Care*, **23**, 495–9.

57. Al-Khaldi, Y.M. and Khan, M.Y. (2002) Impact of a mini-clinic on diabetic care at a primary health care center in southern Saudi Arabia. *Saudi Medical Journal*, **23**, 51–5.

58. Bonita, R., de Courten, M., Dwyer, T. *et al.* (2001) *Surveillance of Risk Factors for Noncommunicable Diseases: the WHO Stepwise Approach. Summary*, World Health Organization, Geneva.

59. Unwin, N. and Marlin, A. (2004) Diabetes action now: WHO and IDF working together to raise awareness worldwide. *Diabetes Voice*, **29**, 27–31.

11

Epidemiology of Diabetes in Africa

Ayesha A. Motala, Mahomed A. K. Omar and Fraser J. Pirie

Department of Diabetes and Endocrinology, Division of Medicine, Nelson R Mandela School of Medicine, Faculty of Health Sciences, University of KwaZulu-Natal, Durban, South Africa

11.1 INTRODUCTION

From as early as the turn of the twentieth century and up to the early 1960s, diabetes mellitus was considered to be rare in sub-Saharan Africa (SSA) [1]. Traditionally, type 2 diabetes was regarded as a disease of urbanization and industrialization and one that is still rare or unknown in rural Africa [1]. However, over the past few decades, diabetes has emerged as an important medical problem in developing regions of the world, including Africa. Although its prevalence varies and is thought to be lower than in developed countries, diabetes is relatively frequently encountered and currently, few major African hospitals are without a diabetes clinic.

A significant advance in diabetes epidemiology was the introduction of standardized diagnostic criteria for glucose tolerance in the 1980s by the National Diabetes Data Group (NDDG) [2] and the World Health Organization (WHO) [3, 4]; such criteria allowed for assessment and comparison of current and projected estimates on a global level [5–9].

In 1993, using 1985 WHO criteria and age-standardized estimates, King et al. [5] showed that type 2 diabetes in adults is a global problem and that populations of developing countries, minority groups and disadvantaged communities in industrialized countries face the greatest risk.

From projected global estimates for the years 2000–2010, Amos et al. [6] reported that the prevalence of type 2 diabetes would increase from 115 million in 1995 to >200 million by 2010 for the world and from 7.2 million to 7.4 million for Africa. Such predictions of the epidemic nature of type 2 diabetes were confirmed by King et al. in 1998 [7], who reported that the greatest increases in prevalence and numbers could be expected to occur in developing countries, in which the prevalence was projected to increase by 48%, from 3.3% in 1995 to 4.9% in 2025, with a corresponding 170% increase in the numbers, from 84 million to 227 million. For SSA, there was an expected increase of 18% for the prevalence (from 1.1 to 1.3%) and a corresponding 185% increase in the numbers, from approximately 3 million to 8 million [7]. Other interesting points which emerged are that, for SSA, the urban/rural ratio will increase, there is and there will be a male preponderance and that the greatest numbers and increases are and will be in the two younger age groups, namely 20–44 years and 45–64 years [7].

In a more recent report on global diabetes estimates and projections for the years 2000–2030, Wild et al. [8] showed that the worldwide prevalence of diabetes for all age groups would increase from 2.8% in 2000 to 4.4% in 2030, with a corresponding 114% increase in the numbers, from 171 million to 366 million. The greatest relative increases will occur in developing regions, nmely SSA, India and the Middle Eastern Crescent. Important contributors include an increase in the urban population in developing countries and an increase in the proportion of people >65 years of age across the world.

The most recent estimates from the International Diabetes Federation (IDF) [9] indicate that for

The Epidemiology of Diabetes Mellitus, second edition   Edited by Jean-Marie Ekoé, Marian Rewers, Rhys Williams and Paul Zimmet

the years 2003 and 2025, in the 20- to 79-year age-group, the global prevalence will increase from 5% (194 million) in 2003 to 6.3% (333 million) by 2025. The largest proportional and absolute increases will occur in developing countries, where the prevalence will rise from 4.2% to 5.6%.

The American Diabetes Association (ADA) in 1997 [10] and the WHO in 1998 [11] introduced changes to criteria for the diagnosis of diabetes and other categories of glycemia. These included the lowering of the cut-point of fasting plasma glucose (FPG) for the diagnosis of diabetes and the introduction of the category of impaired fasting glucose (IFG) glycemia.

After the introduction of the 1985 WHO criteria, and especially over the last decade, data on the impact of diabetes in Africa has increased; however, it is still limited, in contrast to the wealth of epidemiology data from other continents. Yet, Africa is the second largest continent with an estimated population of 642 million living in about 50 countries and comprising 3000 ethnic groups and having over 1000 languages [12].

This is a report on the impact of type 2 diabetes mellitus in nonpregnant adults in mainly continental SSA based on population-based epidemiology studies which examined the prevalence of diabetes in different communities and the factors associated with its development.

11.2 PREVALENCE OF DIABETES

11.2.1 Early Studies

Prior to the introduction of standardized WHO criteria for glucose tolerance [3, 4] and since the early 1960s, several studies examined the prevalence of diabetes in Africa. However, those studies involved widely differing study populations, methodologies and criteria for the diagnosis of diabetes. Despite these limitations, such studies showed prevalence rates ranging between 0 and 1.0%. Only six studies reported rates >1.0%; of these, three studies were those from the same country, namely South Africa [1] (**Table 11.1**).

Table 11.1 Prevalence of diabetes mellitus in Africa: studies done before 1980/1985 WHO criteria (adapted from [1]).

Country	Author	Year	U/R[a]	Study population	Sample size	Detection method	Prevalence (%)
Ethiopia	Peters	1983	U/R	Community[b]	2381	Urine	0.3
Ghana	Dodu	1958	U	Outpatients	4000	Urine	0.4
	Dodu and de Heer	1964	U	Community[b]	5537	Urine	0.2
Ivory Coast	Zmirou	1979	U/R	Community	5000	Blood	5.7
Lesotho	Politzer et al.	1960	R	Outpatients	3000	Urine	0.2
Malawi	Davidson	1963	U/R	Outpatients	4725	Urine	0.1
Mali	Imperato et al.	1976	U/R	Community[b]	297	Blood	1.4
South Africa	Seftel and Abrams	1960	U	Outpatients	2122	Urine	1.3
	Politzer and Schneider	1962	U	Outpatients	3121	Urine	0.6
	Goldberg et al.	1969	U	Community	882	Urine/blood	2.7
	Goldberg et al.	1969	U	Community	2015	Urine	2.9
	Marine et al.	1969	U	Community	1029	Urine/blood	3.6
Uganda	Tulloch	1964	U/R	Outpatients	7164	Urine	0.2
Zambia	Davidson et al.	1969	R	Community	369	Blood	1.1
Zimbabwe	Corr and Gèlfand	1961	U	Community	107	Urine	0.1
	Wicks et al.	1973	U	Community	1078	Urine	0.3
	Guidotti and Gèlfand	1976	R	Community	5456	Urine	0.0

[a]U: urban; R: rural.

[b]Selected community. Ethiopia: schools/factories; Ghana: males >15years old; Mali: police/farmers/students.

11.2.2 Based on 1980/1985 WHO Criteria

Over the past two decades there have been several reports from West Africa [13–21], East Africa [22, 23], North Africa [24–27] and South Africa [28–30] (**Table 11.2**).

Prevalence rates range from an absence of diabetes in Togo to moderate (3–10%) rates in Cape Town in South Africa (8%) and Egypt in North Africa (9.3%), with high (>10%) diabetes prevalence in Northern Sudan (10.4%).

In SSA, the prevalence of diabetes is low (<3%) in both rural and urban communities in West African countries and in Tanzania in East Africa. By contrast, moderate rates have been reported in rural, semiurban and urban communities in South Africa.

Studies from North and North East Africa indicate moderate rates in Tunisians and in African-origin populations in Sudan (3.4–3.8%); in the Egyptian study the overall diabetes prevalence was moderate (9.3%), with high rates (13.5%, 20%) in urban communities in Cairo. In a population of mixed Egyptian ancestry in northern Sudan, there was a high prevalence of diabetes (10.4%).

Therefore, the available, albeit limited data, using 1985 WHO criteria suggest that, in SSA north of the Limpopo River, diabetes prevalence is low in both urban and rural communities. However, in South and North Africa, moderate rates are found and are comparable to rates in developed countries; and in populations of Egyptian ancestry in North East Africa, high rates are observed. There also appears to be a difference in urban and rural prevalence.

11.2.3 Based on 1997 ADA and 1998 WHO Criteria

Only a few recent studies which have been undertaken using 1997 ADA [10], 1998 WHO [11] or 2003 ADA [32] and include those from Tanzania [33], Ghana [34] and South Africa [31] (**Table 11.3**). This precludes studies in which such criteria were compared to the 1985 WHO criteria (*vide infra*).

Diabetes prevalence was low in rural communities in Tanzania (M versus F; 1.7% versus 1.1%) while moderate rates were found in rural South Africans (3.9%), urban Tanzanians (M versus F; 5.9% versus 5.7%) and urban and rural Ghanians (6.4%). Of note is that in the Tanzanian study, only fasting blood glucose (FBG) was done.

What is further highlighted is the relative paucity of information on diabetes epidemiology in Africa and the need for further studies, both urban and rural.

11.2.4 The 1997 ADA versus 1985 WHO Diagnostic Criteria

The impact on the prevalence of diabetes and other categories of glycemia using the 1997 ADA criteria was explored on data from 11 epidemiology studies from Cameroon, South Africa and Tanzania (**Figure 11.1**).

In 7 of the 10 studies which included only African-origin populations, when compared with 1985 WHO criteria, the age-standardized prevalence of diabetes was higher when the ADA criteria were applied but the absolute difference between the two systems was small (<2%); the level of agreement was *fair–good* (kappa statistic κ 0.17–0.86).

The prevalence of IFG (ADA) was lower than that for IGT (WHO) in 10 of the studies and the level of agreement was fair (κ 0.26).

11.3 INTERMEDIATE CATEGORIES OF ABNORMAL GLUCOSE TOLERANCE/GLYCEMIA; TOTAL GLUCOSE INTOLERANCE (TGI)

11.3.1 Based on 1985 WHO Criteria

Using the 1985 WHO criteria, a subject is classed as normal glucose tolerance (NGT), impaired glucose tolerance (IGT) or diabetes (*D*). The combined prevalence of *D* and IGT, namely total glucose intolerance (TGI), may serve as a useful measure of the public health impact of glucose intolerance in a given population [7, 35], because IGT may indicate a high risk of subsequent diabetes development. Moreover, it has been suggested that the percentage of TGI made up by IGT, that is, the 'epidemicity index' (EI) or the ratios IGT:*D* or IGT:TGI may have some predictive value in determining the stage of an epidemic of glucose intolerance in a given population. A high IGT prevalence in the face of a low prevalence of diabetes (high EI; high IGT:*D* ratio; high IGT:TGI ratio) may indicate an early stage of a diabetes epidemic.

Table 11.4 shows the prevalence of IGT and TGI (and the EI) in the [10] studies in which

Table 11.2 Prevalence of diabetes mellitus (D) and impaired glucose tolerance (IGT) in Africa: studies using the 1980/1985 WHO criteria.

Location	Reference	Year	Urban (U)/ rural (R)	Age group (years)	n	Prevalence (%) D	Prevalence (%) IGT
Tanzania	Ahrén and Corrigan [22]	1984	U + R	≥20	3145	0.7	—
Kahalanga			R		996	0.5	—
Ndolage			R		1141	2.5	—
Mwanza			U		1008	1.9	—
Mali	Fisch *et al.* [13]	1987	R	>15	7472	0.9	—
Togo	Teuscher *et al.* [14]	1987	R	>1	1381	0.0	—
Nigeria	Ohwovoriole *et al.* [15]	1988	U		1627	1.7	—
	Erasmus *et al.* [16]	1989	U + R		2800	1.4	—
	Cooper *et al.* [17]	1997	R	25–74	247	2.8	—
	Olatunbosun *et al.* [20]	1998	U	—	875	0.8	2.2
Tunisia	Papoz *et al.* [24]	1988		≥20	5613		
Tunis			U		3826	3.8	—
Siliana			R		1787	1.3	—
Tanzania	McLarty *et al.* [23]	1989	R	≥15	6097	0.9	7.8
						1.1[a]	8.4[a]
South Africa							
Cape Town	Levitt *et al.* [29]	1993	U	>30	729	6.3	5.9
Durban	Omar *et al.* [28]	1993	U	>15	479	4.2	6.9
Orange Free State Mangaung	Mollentze *et al.* [30]	1995	U	≥25	758	6.0[a]	12.2[a]
Qwa-Qwa			R		853	4.8[a]	10.7[a]
Ubombo	Motala *et al.* [31]	2006	R	>15	1021	4.2	6.7
						3.5[a]	4.9[a]
Egypt	Herman *et al.* [25]	1995	U + R	≥20	4620	9.3	9.6
Cairo			U-h[b]		899	20.0	8.6
			U-l[b]		1973	13.5	5.4
Kaliubia			R		1748	4.9	13.1
Mauritania	Ducorps *et al.* [18]	1996	U + R	>17	744	1.88	—
Cameroon	Mbanya *et al.* [19]	1997	U + R	24–74	1767	1.1	2.7
Yaoundé			U		1048	1.3	1.8
Evodoula			R		719	0.8	3.9
Sudan	Elbagir *et al.* [26]	1996	U + R	≥25	1284	3.4	2.9
			U		826	3.9	3.3
			R		458	2.6	2.2
	Elbagir *et al.* [27]	1998	U + R	≥25	724	8.3	7.9
						10.4[a]	9.8[a]
			U		461	9.6	8.0
			R		263	6.1	7.6
Cameroon	Mbanya *et al.* [21]	1999	U + R	25–74	679	—	—
Yaoundé			U		295	2.0[a]	—
Evodoula			R		384	0.8[a]	—

[a] Age-adjusted rates.
[b] U-h, urban, high socioeconomic status; U-l, urban, low socioeconomic status.

Table 11.3 Age-adjusted prevalence of diabetes mellitus, impaired glucose tolerance (IGT) and impaired fasting glycemia (IFG) using the 1997 ADA, 1998 WHO and 2003 ADA criteria.

Location	Reference	Urban (U)/ rural (R)	Age group (years)	Blood sample	Diagnostic criteria	n	Gender (M/F)	Prevalence (%)		
								D	IGT	IFG
Tanzania	Aspray *et al.* [33]	U + R	≥15	FCBG	1998 WHO	1698				
Dar-es-Salaam		U				332	M	5.9	—	3.6
						438	F	5.7	—	4.7
Kilimanjaro		R				401	M	1.7	—	0.8
						527	F	1.1	—	1.6
Ghana	Amoah *et al.* [34]	U + R	≥25	FPG + 2PG	1997 ADA and 1998 WHO	4733	M + F	6.4	10.7	6.0
Accra						1860	M	7.7	—	—
						2873	F	5.5	—	—
South Africa	Motala *et al.* [31]	R	>15	FPG + 2PG	1998 WHO	1021	M + F	3.9	4.8	1.5
Ubombo						210	M	3.5	4.6	4.0
						811	F	3.9	4.7	0.8
				FPG	1997 ADA		M + F	2.5	—	2.6
				FPG	2003 ADA		M + F	2.5	—	7.0

FCBG, fasting capillary whole blood glucose; FPG, fasting venous plasma glucose; 2PG, 2-h postload venous plasma glucose.

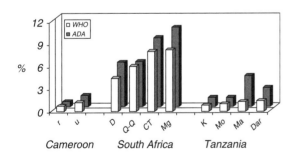

Figure 11.1 Age-adjusted prevalence of diabetes mellitus using the 1997 ADA criteria [■] and 1985 WHO criteria [□] in African-origin populations. r, rural; u, urban, D, Durban; Q–Q, Qwa–Qwa; CT, Cape Town; Mg, Mangaung; M, Mamre; K, Kilimanjaro; Mo, Morogoro; Ma, Mara; Dar, Dar-es-Salaam.

these variables were analyzed [19, 20, 23, 25–31]. The prevalence of IGT ranges from 1.8% in rural Cameroon [19] to 13.1% in rural Egypt [25], and the prevalence of TGI ranges from 3.0% in urban Nigerians [20] to 28.6% in urban Egyptians from a high socioeconomic group [25]. It is apparent that in Africa, as in the rest of the world, the IGT rates are higher where the prevalence of diabetes is low (<3%) [5], as reported in rural Tanzanians (*D* 1.1%; IGT 8.4%) [22] and Cameroonians (*D* 0.8%; IGT 3.0%) [19]. By contrast, in high diabetes prevalence (>10%) populations, the IGT rates are lower, as shown in urban Egyptians (*D* 20.0%; IGT 8.6%) [25].

The EI is found to decrease as the diabetes prevalence increases. In the low-prevalence rural

Table 11.4 Prevalence of impaired glucose tolerance (IGT), total glucose intolerance (TGI) and epidemicity index in studies using 1985 WHO criteria.

Location	Urban (U)/ rural (R)	Authors	Prevalence (%)			EI[a] (%)
			D	IGT	TGI	
Tanzania	R	McLarty *et al.* [23]	1.1	8.4	9.5	88.4
South Africa						
Orange Free State		Mollentze *et al.* [30]	4.8	10.7	15.5	69.0
Qwa-Qwa	R		6.0	12.2	18.2	67.0
Mangaung	U					
Durban	U	Omar *et al.* [28]	5.3	7.7	13.0	59.2
Cape Town	U	Levitt *et al.* [29]	8.0	7.0	15.0	46.7
Ubombo	R	Motala *et al.* [31]	4.2	6.7	10.9	61.5
Sudan[b]	U + R	Elbagir *et al.* [26]	3.4	2.9	6.3	46.0
	U		3.9	3.3	7.2	45.8
	R		2.6	2.2	4.8	45.8
	U + R	Elbagir *et al.* [27]	10.4	9.8	20.2	48.5
	U[b]		9.6	8.0	17.6	45.5
	R[b]		6.1	7.6	13.7	55.5
Egypt[b]	U + R	Herman *et al.* [25]	9.3	9.6	18.9	50.8
Kaliubia	R		4.9	13.1	18.0	72.8
Cairo[c]	U-h		20.0	8.6	28.6	30.1
	U-l		13.5	5.4	18.9	28.6
Cameroon	U + R	Mbanya *et al.* [21]	1.1	2.7	3.8	71.1
Yaounde	U		1.3	1.8	3.1	58.1
Evodoula	R		0.8	3.9	4.7	83.0
Nigeria[b]	U	Olatunbosun *et al.* [20]	0.8	2.2	3.0	73.3

[a]EI = IGT/TGI
[b]Crude rates.
[c]U-h, urban, high socioeconomic status; U-l, urban, low socioeconomic status.

Tanzanians [23] the index is 88.4%, possibly indicating an early stage of an epidemic of glucose intolerance. By contrast, a low EI of 30.1% is observed in urban Egyptians with high diabetes prevalence [25] (**Table 11.4**).

11.3.2 Based on 1997 ADA Criteria and 1998 WHO Criteria

The ADA in 1997 [10] and the WHO in 1998 [11] introduced the category of IFG ($6.1 \leq FPG < 7.0$ mmol l^{-1}) and the lowering of the cut-point of FPG for the diagnosis of diabetes (FPG ≥ 7.0 mmol l^{-1}). The difference between the two systems is that the ADA recommended the use of

FPG alone, both for clinical and epidemiological studies, whereas the WHO system retained the oral glucose tolerance test. In 2003, the ADA recommended further lowering of the cut-point of FPG for the diagnosis of IFG from ≥ 6.1 mmol l^{-1} to ≥ 5.6 mmol l^{-1} [32].

In the study which compared the 1985 WHO criteria (FBG + 2BG) with the 1997 ADA criteria (FBG only) [36], of the 10 studies that included African-origin populations in Africa, the prevalence of IFG ranged from 3.0% in urban and rural Cameroonians to 9.1% in urban Sesotho in South Africa (i.e. low to moderate rates) when using FBG only (ADA criteria).

Regarding recent studies [31, 33, 34] (**Table 11.3**), in the Tanzanian study [33], using FBG alone and based on the 1998 WHO criteria (and, therefore, the 1997 ADA criteria also), the prevalence of IFG was low in the rural community (male (M) versus (F), 0.8% versus 1.6%) and moderate in the urban community (M versus F, 3.6% versus 4.7%). In urban and rural Ghanians [34], using the 1998 WHO and 1997 ADA criteria (FPG + 2PG) the prevalence of IFG was 6.0%, IGT was 10.7% and the total disorders of glycemia was 23.1%. In the rural South African study [31], using the 1998 WHO criteria (FPG + 2PG) the prevalence of IFG was 1.5%, IGT was 4.8% and the total disorders of glycemia was 10.2%; if only FPG was used (i.e. the 1997 ADA criteria), then the prevalence of IFG was 2.6%. When the 2003 ADA [32] criteria are applied, there is a marked increase in the proportion classified as IFG, from 2.6% (using the 1997 ADA criteria) to 7.0% (using the 2003 ADA criteria) in rural South Africans [31].

11.4 URBAN–RURAL DIFFERENCES

The prevalence of diabetes in rural and urban communities in the same country has been examined in several studies (**Tables 11.2, 11.3**; **Figure 11.2**) [19, 21, 22, 25–27, 30, 33]. In all except one study [22] the rates were higher in urban communities. The difference was most striking in the Egyptian

study [25] and a recent Tanzanian [33] study; in the former, the urban prevalence (13.5%, 20%) was two- to four-fold higher than the rural rate (4.9%) and in the latter, urban rates (M versus F, 5.9% versus 5.7%) were three- to five-fold higher than rural (M versus F, 1.7% versus 1.1%).

In South Africa, Sudan and Cameroon, although diabetes prevalence was higher in urban groups, the difference was not marked. In South Africa, this is thought to be accounted for by the fact that, in recent years, urbanization and industrialization have affected even the so-called 'rural' areas; it has been estimated that, in this century, >75% of the country's population will be urbanized [30].

In the studies in which this has been examined [26, 29, 31, 33], urbanization was found to be an independent risk factor for diabetes in urban South African Xhosas [29] and urban and rural Tanzanians [33], but not in Sudanese [26] or in rural South African Zulus [31]. In urban Xhosas in Cape Town, South Africa [29], urbanization as judged by the proportion of life spent in the city (cutoff >40%) was an independent risk factor.

In a recent study in Cameroonians [37], total lifetime exposure to an urban environment (lifetime EUt) was independently associated with disorders of glycemia (IFG or diabetes) in women.

11.5 ETHNIC DIFFERENCES AND THE EFFECT OF MIGRATION

Evidence for ethnic differences in the same country comes from studies in Tanzania [23, 38, 39] and South Africa [28, 29, 40, 41]. In both countries, diabetes prevalence was lower in the indigenous African population than in the migrant Asian group (African versus Asian, 5.3% versus 13% in Durban, South Africa; 1.1% versus 9.1/7.1% in Dar-es-Salaam, Tanzania) [23, 28, 38–40] and when compared with a community of mixed ancestry (Khoi–East Indian–Europid) (African versus mixed ancestry, 8% versus 10.8% in the Cape Province, South Africa) [29, 41] (**Figure 11.3**).

The impact of environmental influences on the prevalence of diabetes in populations of similar genetic origin has been explored and confirmed in two studies [17, 21]. These studies compared native West African populations from Nigeria [17] and Cameroon [21] with populations of West African origin in the Caribbean [17, 21], United Kingdom

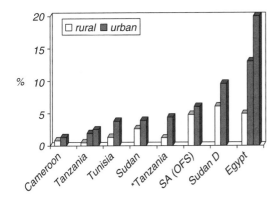

Figure 11.2 Prevalence of diabetes mellitus (D) in rural [□] and urban [■] communities in Africa: studies using the 1985 WHO criteria except for *Tanzania (Ref. [33]) which used the 1998 WHO criteria.

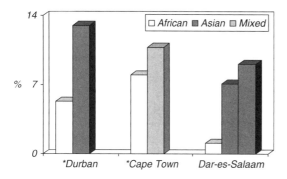

Figure 11.3 Prevalence of diabetes mellitus in indigenous African [□], migrant Asian [■] and mixed ancestry [▨] populations in *South Africa (Durban, Cape Town) and Tanzania (Dar-es-Salaam).

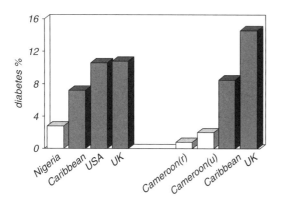

Figure 11.4 Prevalence of diabetes in native West African populations in Africa [□] and in migrant West African-origin populations living abroad [■].

[17, 21] and United States [17]. In both studies, the prevalence of diabetes was substantially higher in the African-origin populations living abroad (**Figure 11.4**).

11.6 PREVALENCE OF KNOWN DIABETES

The proportion of known and newly discovered cases of diabetes in a community may reflect the availability of health care facilities for detection and treatment [5].

From the available data (**Table 11.5, Figure 11.5**), the proportion of subjects with known diabetes is lowest in Tanzanian subjects [22, 23, 33], including earlier and recent studies which included an urban sample [22, 33]. By contrast, >50% were known to have diabetes in studies from Tunisia [24] and Egypt [25] in North Africa and in urban South Africans [28, 29] and compares with findings in developed countries [7]. In Tunisia and Egypt, this was true even for the rural populations, in which >45% were known to have the disorder. However, only 15% were known to have diabetes in a recent rural study in South Africa [31]; this is in contrast to the urban studies cited above and to earlier studies in the 1960s which reported that the proportion of African (Black) subjects with known diabetes ranged from 28 to 33% and compared with that found in the Europid population in that country [1]. Previous findings are probably accounted for by the fact that only urban communities were examined [1, 28, 29] and suggest that there is a disparity in health care access and facilities between rural and urban areas in South Africa.

11.7 GENDER DISTRIBUTION

From global estimates, it is reported that there was a male excess for SSA for 1995 and that this was likely to increase by 2025 [7]. However, from the available reports, the gender distribution varies widely both between and within populations with no obvious trend.

A male preponderance is reported from studies in rural Cameroon, rural Tanzania, Tunisia, Egypt, urban Sudan and Ghana [19, 23–25, 27, 33, 34]. A female excess was observed in Mali, Mauritania, urban Cameroon, rural Sudan and in urban and rural Zulu populations in South Africa [13, 18, 19, 27, 28, 31]. Gender distribution was equal in studies in Tanzania, Sudan and urban Xhosas in South Africa [22, 26, 29].

11.8 IMPACT OF AGE

Using age-specific rates, diabetes prevalence in Africa, as in other regions of the world, increases with age in both men and women. King *et al.* [7] report that the age range in which peak prevalence of diabetes occurs is markedly different for developed and developing countries: for the former, the peak is

Table 11.5 Prevalence of known and newly discovered subjects with diabetes mellitus from population-based studies in Africa.

Location	Urban (U)/ rural (R)	Reference	Diabetes mellitus		
			Total n	Known % (n)	Discovered % (n)
Tanzania	U + R	Ahrén and Corrigan [22]	22	4.6 (1)	95.4 (21)
	R	McLarty *et al*. [23]	53	13.2 (7)	86.8 (46)
	U + R[a]	Aspray *et al*. [33]	46	17.4 (8)	82.6 (38)
Dar-es-Salaam	U		34	20.6 (7)	79.4 (27)
Kilimanjaro	R		12	8.3 (1)	91.7 (11)
Tunisia		Papoz *et al*. [24]			
Tunis	U		144	59.7 (86)	40.3 (54)
Siliana	R		24	45.8 (11)	54.2 (13)
South Africa					
Durban	U	Omar *et al*. [28]	20	60.0 (12)	40.0 (8)
Cape Town	U	Levitt *et al*. [29]	46	52.2 (24)	47.8 (22)
Ubombo	R[a]	Motala *et al*. [31]	46	15.2 (7)	84.8 (39)
Sudan	U + R	Elbagir *et al*. [26]	44	36.4 (16)	63.6 (28)
	U		32	37.5 (12)	62.5 (20)
	R		12	33.3 (4)	66.7 (8)
	U + R	Elbagir *et al*. [27]	60	38.3 (23)	61.7 (37)
	U		44	34.1 (15)	65.9 (29)
	R		16	50.0 (8)	50.0 (8)
Egypt	U + R	Herman *et al*. [25]	648	77.9 (505)	22.1 (143)
Kaliubia	R		—	48.9 (—)	51.1 (—)
Cairo	U-h[b]		—	50.0 (—)	50.0 (—)
	U-l[b]		—	62.2 (—)	37.8 (—)
Cameroon	U + R	Mbanya *et al*. [19]	20	40.0 (8)	60.0 (12)
Yaoundé	U		14	42.9 (6)	57.1 (8)
Evodoula	R		6	33.3 (2)	66.7 (4)
Mauritania	U + R	Ducorps *et al*. [18]	14	28.6 (4)	71.4 (10)
Nigeria	U	Olatunbosun *et al*. [20]	7	28.6 (2)	71.4 (5)
Ghana	U + R[a,c]	Amoah *et al*. [34]	300	30.3 (91)	69.7 (209)

[a] 1998 WHO criteria.
[b] U-h: urban, high socioeconomic status; U-l: urban, low socioeconomic status.
[c] 1997 ADA criteria.

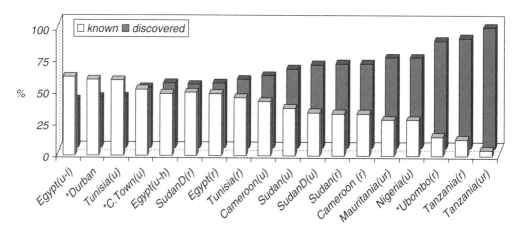

Figure 11.5 Known [□] and newly (survey) diagnosed [■] subjects with diabetes mellitus *South Africa.

in the oldest age-group (≥65 years); for developing countries, it is in the 45–64 years age group; and for SSA, the greatest numbers and increasers are (in 1995) and will be (in 2025) in the two younger age groups (20–44 years, 45–64 years). Data from 13 SSA countries [13, 17, 18, 22, 23, 26–31, 33, 34] indicate peak prevalence in the oldest age-group (≥65 years) in seven studies [13, 18, 23, 24, 29, 30, 34]; a peak in the 45–64-year group was observed in the remaining six studies [17, 22, 27, 28, 31, 33].

Age was found to be a significant risk factor for diabetes in three [26, 27, 29] of the studies in which this was examined [26, 27, 29, 31].

11.9 MEASURES OF ADIPOSITY: BODY MASS INDEX (BMI) AND WAIST CIRCUMFERENCE; WAIST: HIP RATIO (WHR)

Several studies have examined and confirmed the association between diabetes prevalence and body mass index (BMI), waist circumference and waist:hip ratio (WHR), but the lack of standardized reporting has made comparison between studies difficult.

Regarding BMI and (total body) obesity, the aspects which have been examined include BMI-specific diabetes prevalence, mean BMI and prevalence of obesity in different categories of glucose/glycemia and BMI/obesity as risk factors for diabetes. Using BMI-specific rates, it has been found that diabetes prevalence increases with BMI

in all the studies in which this has been examined [13, 17, 23, 24]. When compared with nondiabetic subjects, the mean BMI [13, 17, 23, 31] was higher in subjects with diabetes. BMI was found to be a significant independent risk factor for diabetes in all [17, 26, 27, 30, 33] but one [31] of the studies in which it was examined; obesity emerged as a risk factor in two studies [29, 33].

WHR has been examined in five studies [17, 29–31, 33]. In three studies [17, 29, 31], diabetes prevalence increased with increasing WHR. Mean WHR was higher with worsening of glucose tolerance/glycemia in the Egyptian [25] and rural South African [31] studies. When compared with nondiabetic subjects, the prevalence of abdominal (upper body) obesity was higher in Tanzanians [33] and rural South Africans [31]. Abdominal obesity was an independent risk factor for diabetes in urban Tanzanian men [33] and urban [29, 30] and semiurban [30] South Africans.

Only two recent studies [31, 33] have examined waist circumference as a variable. In the Tanzanian study [33], waist circumference was higher in urban than in rural subjects and was higher in diabetes subjects. In the rural South African study [31], the prevalence of diabetes increased with increasing waist circumference, the mean waist circumference increased with worsening of glycemia and the prevalence of abnormally increased waist circumference was higher in diabetes subjects than in those without diabetes; waist circumference was an independent risk factor for diabetes.

11.10 FAMILY HISTORY

A positive family of diabetes was more frequent in diabetes subjects and was an independent risk factor in the two Sudanese studies [26, 27] and in rural South Africans [31]; in an urban South African study [29], this variable was not an independent risk factor for diabetes.

11.11 PHYSICAL ACTIVITY

Physical activity was not found to be an independent risk factor for diabetes in the three studies in which it was examined [29, 31, 33]. In the Tanzanian study [33], physical inactivity was higher in diabetes subjects; and in rural South Africans [31], both occupational and leisure physical activity were inversely related to disorders of glycemia. The prevalence of diabetes was inversely related to physical activity in Egyptians [25].

11.12 IS THE PREVALENCE OF DIABETES INCREASING IN AFRICA?

The paucity of data from earlier studies in the same population and the changing diagnostic criteria used make it difficult to answer this question. Notwithstanding, evidence from studies in urban South Africa (extrapolation of data) [1, 29] and Tanzania [23, 33, 36] appear to support this notion.

In urban Xhosas in Cape Town, using the 1985 WHO criteria, the crude prevalence of diabetes in subjects >30 years is 6.3% and of IGT it is 5.9% (TGI 12.2%) [29]. In 1969, Marine et al. [42], using less stringent criteria, reported that the crude prevalence of diabetes in subjects >25 years was 7%; therefore, it would appear that the prevalence of abnormal glucose tolerance has almost doubled in 20 years.

Confirmatory evidence comes from urban Tanzania. Applying the 1998 WHO criteria, the crude overall prevalence of diabetes has increased from 2.3% to 4.4% between the 1980s and 1996; in the 35–54 years age group there is a threefold increase in men, from 3.3% to 9.9%, and a sevenfold increase in women, from 0.9% to 6.8% [33, 36].

11.13 OTHER BIOCHEMICAL VARIABLES

In the rural South African study [31], mean serum total cholesterol, total triglyceride (tTg) and uric acid increased with worsening of glycemia (diabetes > IGT > IFG > normoglycemia); serum tTg and total cholesterol emerged as significant independent risk factors for diabetes [31].

11.14 LONGITUDINAL STUDIES

To date, there are no published reports of longitudinal studies which have examined the incidence of diabetes or the natural history of intermediate stages of glucose intolerance (IFG, IGT) in Africa.

11.15 OTHER FACTORS

There is also a dearth of data on the impact of dietary and genetic factors and the role of insulin from population studies. Moreover, what needs to be established is the impact that HIV/AIDS will have on global estimates and projections for the prevalence of diabetes in Africa.

11.16 COMPLICATIONS

11.16.1 Mortality and Acute Complications

The natural history and clinical cause of diabetes in Africa are poorly understood, and this is due in many instances to poor follow-up [43].

From the limited evidence, mortality rates are unacceptably high and the major contributors still include preventable acute metabolic complications and infective causes. Mortality rates of 5.0–11.8% have been reported from clinic studies [43] and of 7.6–41% from outcome studies [44–47]; the major causes of death were diabetic ketoacidosis (DKA) and infection. From earlier necropsy studies [48–50], most deaths were due to DKA (34–54%), with infection the second leading cause. However, the limitations of these studies were that they included mixed cohorts of subjects with type 1 and type 2 diabetes and varying diabetes duration.

11.16.2 Chronic Complications

Previous impressions that chronic complications of diabetes are rare in Africa are likely related to the decreased survival from the disease and inadequate screening [1, 43, 51]. Several clinic-based studies have examined the prevalence of chronic complications, both macro- and micro-vascular; however, in most instances they included mixed cohorts of type 1 and type 2 diabetes and varying diabetes duration. Such studies have shown that, where examined, the prevalence of macrovascular disease is uncommon (peripheral vascular disease, 1.7–10%; angina, 0.4–10.0%), hypertension is common (19–50%) and diabetic foot disease was reported as 0.6–36.6%. Regarding microvascular compli-cations, the prevalence of retinopathy ranges from 2.9 to 57.1%, of nephropathy from 1.0 to 30.5% and of neuropathy from 5.9 to 69.6% [1, 43, 51].

The only population-based study was that which examined the prevalence of microvascular compli-cations in Egyptians with type 2 diabetes [52]; this study showed rates among subjects with known diabetes and subjects with newly (survey) diag-nosed diabetes of 41.5% and 15.7% respectively for retinopathy, of 6.7% and 6.8% respectively for nephropathy, of 21.9% and 13.6% respectively for neuropathy and of 0.8% for both groups for foot ulcers. Each of the microvascular complications was significantly associated with increased blood glucose.

Most of the data on long-duration disease in defined patient groups are from studies in type 1 diabetes; these data have shown rates of micro-vascular complications ranging from 40 to 50% for retinopathy, 20 to 40% for neuropathy and 20 to 30% for nephropathy [43]. A recent report in South African Indians and Africans (Blacks) with long-duration (>10 years) type 2 diabetes showed that retinopathy was present in 64.5%, nephropathy in 25%, treatment-requiring hypertension in 68%, abnormal serum creatinine in 25% and abnormal glomerular filtration rate in 42%. There was no significant ethnic difference for the prevalence of complications except for hypertension, which was more prevalent in Africans (84.8%) than in Indians (47.4%) [53].

Therefore, the available data indicate that, with improving survival rates and the emergence of larger African populations with long-duration diabetes, the prevalence of chronic complications will approach that seen in the developed world.

What needs to be established, though, is the apparent low frequency of macrovascular disease and the high prevalence of hypertension.

11.17 COSTS OF DIABETES CARE

There is a dearth of data on the costs of diabetes care in Africa [9]; the most recent country estimates were those for Tanzania in 1992, which confirmed that diabetes placed a severe strain on the limited resources of developing countries [54]. The report estimated that the annual cost of outpatient care was $2.7 million, of which 32.2% was for insulin; annual direct costs of inpatient care were estimated at $1.25 million; around 0.2% of the Tanzanian population aged ≥ 15 years used the equivalent of 8% of the total government health expenditure of $47 408 832.

11.18 FUTURE TRENDS

From global estimates [6–8], there is an anticipated worldwide increase in the prevalence of diabetes for all age groups, with the greatest relative increases expected to occur in developing regions, including SSA. Important contributors include an increase in the urban population and an increase in the proportion of people >65 years of age. What needs to be established is the impact that HIV/AIDS will have on global estimates and projection for the prevalence of diabetes in Africa.

References

1. McLarty, D.G., Pollitt, C. and Swai, A.B.M. (1990) Diabetes in Africa. *Diabetic Medicine: A Journal of the British Diabetic Association*, **7**, 670–84.
2. National Diabetes Data Group (1979) Classification and diagnosis of diabetes mellitus and other categories of glucose intolerance. *Diabetes*, **28**, 1039–57.
3. World Health Organization (1980) WHO Expert Committee on Diabetes Mellitus. 2nd report, WHO Tech. Rep. Ser. 626, World Health Organization, Geneva.
4. World Health Organization (1985) Diabetes Melli-tus. Report of Study Group, WHO Tech. Rep. Ser. 727, World Health Organization, Geneva.
5. King, H. and Rewers, M. (1993) Global esti-mates for prevalence of diabetes mellitus and impaired glucose tolerance in adults. WHO Ad Hoc Diabetes Reporting Group. *Diabetes Care*, **16**, 157–77.

6. Amos, A.F., McCarty, D.J. and Zimmet, P. (1997) The rising global burden of diabetes and its complications. Estimates and projections to the year 2010. *Diabetic Medicine: A Journal of the British Diabetic Association*, **14** (Suppl 5), S1–85.

7. King, H., Aubert, R.E. and Herman, W.H. (1998) Global burden of diabetes. Prevalence, numerical estimates and projections. *Diabetes Care*, **21**, 1414–31.

8. Wild, S., Roglic, G., Green, A. *et al.* (2004) Global prevalence of diabetes. Estimates for the year 2000 and projections for 2030. *Diabetes Care*, **27**, 1047–53.

9. International Diabetes Federation (2006) *Diabetes Atlas*, http://www.eatlas.idf.org (accessed February 2006).

10. The Expert Committee on the Diagnosis and Classification of Diabetes Mellitus (1997) Report of the Expert Committee on the Diagnosis and Classification of Diabetes Mellitus. *Diabetes Care*, **20**, 1183–97.

11. Alberti, K.G.M.M. and Zimmet, P.Z. (1998) Definition, diagnosis and classification of diabetes mellitus and its complications. Part 1: diagnosis and classification of diabetes mellitus. Provisional report of a WHO consultation. *Diabetic Medicine: A Journal of the British Diabetic Association*, **15**, 539–53.

12. Motala, A.A., Omar, M.A. and Pirie, F.J. (2003) Diabetes in Africa. Epidemiology of type 1 and type 2 diabetes in Africa. *Journal of Cardiovascular Risk*, **10**, 77–83.

13. Fisch, A., Pichard, E., Prazuck, T. *et al.* (1982) Prevalence and risk factors of diabetes mellitus in the rural regions of Mali (West Africa): a practical approach. *Diabetologia*, **30**, 859–62.

14. Teuscher, T., Rosman, J.B., Baillod, P. and Teuscher, A. (1987) Absence of diabetes in a rural West African population with a high carbohydrate/cassava diet. *Lancet*, **1**, 765–8.

15. Ohwovoriole, A.E., Kuti, J.A. and Kabiawu, S.I.O. (1988) Casual blood glucose levels and prevalence of undiscovered diabetes mellitus in Lagos metropolis Nigerians. *Diabetes Research and Clinical Practice*, **4**, 153–8.

16. Erasmus, R.T., Fakeye, T., Olukoga, O. *et al.* (1989) Prevalence of diabetes mellitus in a Nigerian population. *Transactions of the Royal Society of Tropical Medicine and Hygiene*, **83**, 417–18.

17. Cooper, R., Rotimi, C., Kaufman, J. *et al.* (1997) Prevalence of NIDDM among populations of the African diaspora. *Diabetes Care*, **20**, 343–8.

18. Ducorps, M., Baleynaud, S., Mayaudon, H. *et al.* (1996) A prevalence survey of diabetes in Mauritania. *Diabetes Care*, **19**, 761–3.

19. Mbanya, J.C., Ngogang, J., Salah, J.N. *et al.* (1997) Prevalence of NIDDM and impaired glucose tolerance in a rural and urban population in Cameroon. *Diabetologia*, **40**, 824–9.

20. Olatunbosun, S.T., Ojo, P.O., Fineberg, N.S. and Bella, A.F. (1998) Prevalence of diabetes mellitus and impaired glucose tolerance in a group of urban adults in Nigeria. *Journal of the National Medical Association*, **90**, 293–301.

21. Mbanya, J.C., Cruickshank, J.K., Forrester, T. *et al.* (1999) Standardized comparison of glucose intolerance in West African-origin populations of rural and urban Cameroon, Jamaica, and Caribbean migrants to Britain. *Diabetes Care*, **22**, 434–40.

22. Ahrén, B. and Corrigan, C.B. (1984) Prevalence of diabetes mellitus in northwestern Tanzania. *Diabetologia*, **26**, 333–6.

23. McLarty, D.G., Swai, A.B.M., Kitange, H.M. *et al.* (1989) Prevalence of diabetes and impaired glucose tolerance in rural Tanzania. *Lancet*, **1**, 871–5.

24. Papoz, L., Ben Khalifa, F., Eshwege, E. and Ben Ayed, H. (1988) Diabetes mellitus in Tunisia: descriptions in urban and rural populations. *International Journal of Epidemiology*, **17**, 419–22.

25. Herman, W.H., Ali, M.A., Aubert, R.E. *et al.* (1995) Diabetes mellitus in Egypt: risk factors and prevalence. *Diabetic Medicine: A Journal of the British Diabetic Association*, **12**, 1126–31.

26. Elbagir, M.N., Eltom, M.A., Elmahadi, E.M.A. *et al.* (1996) A population-based study of the prevalence of diabetes and impaired glucose tolerance in adults in northern Sudan. *Diabetes Care*, **19**, 1126–8.

27. Elbagir, M.N., Eltom, M.A., Elmahadi, E.M.A. *et al.* (1998) A high prevalence of diabetes mellitus and impaired glucose tolerance in the Danagla community in northern Sudan. *Diabetic Medicine: A Journal of the British Diabetic Association*, **15**, 164–9.

28. Omar, M.A.K., Seedat, M.A., Motala, A.A. *et al.* (1993) The prevalence of diabetes mellitus and impaired glucose tolerance in a group of urban South African Blacks. *South African Medical Journal*, **83**, 641–3.

29. Levitt, N.S., Katzenellenbogen, J.M., Bradshaw, D. *et al.* (1993) The prevalence and identification of risk factors for NIDDM in urban Africans in Cape Town, South Africa. *Diabetes Care*, **16**, 601–7.

30. Mollentze, W.F., Moore, A.J., Steyn, A.F. *et al.* (1995) Coronary heart disease risk factors in a rural and urban Orange Free State black population. *South African Medical Journal*, **85**, 90–6.

31. Motala, A.A., Esterhuizen, T., Gouws, E. *et al.* (2008) Diabetes mellitus and other disorders of

glycaemia in a rural South Africa community: prevalence and associated risk factors.. *Diabetes care*, **10.2337**, 08–0212.

32. The Expert Committee on the Diagnosis and Classification of Diabetes Mellitus (2003) Follow up report on the diagnosis of diabetes mellitus. *Diabetes Care*, **26**, 3160–7.

33. Aspray, T.J., Mugusi, F., Rashid S., *et al.* (2000) Rural and urban differences in diabetes prevalence in Tanzania: the role of obesity, physical inactivity and urban living. *Transactions of the Royal Society of Tropical Medicine and Hygiene*, **94**, 637–44.

34. Amoah, A.G., Owusu, S.K. and Adjei, S. (2002) Diabetes in Ghana: a community based prevalence study in Greater Accra. *Diabetes Research and Clinical Practice*, **56**, 197–205.

35. Dowse, G., Zimmet, P. and King, H. (1991) Relationship between prevalence of impaired glucose tolerance and NIDDM in a population. *Diabetes Care*, **14**, 968–74.

36. Levitt, N.S., Unwin, N.C., Bradshaw, D. *et al.* (2000) Application of the new ADA criteria for the diagnosis of diabetes to population studies in sub-Saharan Africa. *Diabetic Medicine: A Journal of the British Diabetic Association*, **17**, 381–5.

37. Sobngwi, E., Mbanya, J.C., Unwin, N.C. *et al.* (2004) Exposure over the life course to an urban environment and its relation with obesity, diabetes, and hypertension in rural and urban Cameroon. *International Journal of Epidemiology*, **33**, 769–76.

38. Ramaiya, K.L., Swai, A.B., McLarty, D.G. and Alberti, K.G. (1991) Impaired glucose tolerance and diabetes mellitus in Hindu Indian immigrants in Dar es Salaam. *Diabetic Medicine: A Journal of the British Diabetic Association*, **8**, 738–44.

39. Swai, A.B., McLarty, D.G., Sherrif, F. *et al.* (1990) Diabetes and impaired glucose tolerance in an Asian community in Tanzania. *Diabetes Research and Clinical Practice*, **8**, 227–34.

40. Omar, M.A.K., Seedat, M.A., Dyer, R.B. *et al.* (1994) South African Indians show a high prevalence of NIDDM and bimodality in plasma glucose distribution patterns. *Diabetes Care*, **17**, 70–3.

41. Levitt, N.S., Steyn, K., Lambert, E.V. *et al.* (1999) Modifiable risk factors for type 2 diabetes mellitus in a peri-urban community in South Africa. *Diabetic Medicine: A Journal of the British Diabetic Association*, **16**, 946–50.

42. Marine, N., Vinik, A.I., Edelstein, I. and Jackson, W.P. (1969) Diabetes, hyperglycemia and glycosuria among Indians, Malays and African (Bantu) in Cape Town, South Africa. *Diabetes*, **18**, 840–57.

43. Motala, A.A. (2002) Diabetes trends in Africa. *Diabetes/Metabolism Research and Reviews*, **18** (Suppl 3), S14–20.

44. Castle, W.M. and Wicks, A.C.B. (1980) A follow-up of 93 newly diagnosed African diabetics for 6 years. *Diabetologia*, **18**, 121–3.

45. Lester, F.T. (1983) Long-standing diabetes mellitus in Ethiopia: a survey of 105 patients. *Diabetologia*, **25**, 222–5.

46. Lester, F.T. (1991) Clinical status of Ethiopian diabetic patients after 20 years of diabetes. *Diabetic Medicine: A Journal of the British Diabetic Association*, **8**, 272–6.

47. McLarty, D.G., Kinabo, L. and Swai, A.B. (1990) Diabetes in tropical Africa: a prospective study, 1981–1987. II. Course and prognosis. *British Medical Journal*, **300**, 1107–10.

48. Parson, W., Macdonald, F.W. and Shaper, A.G. (1968) African diabetics necropsied at Mulago Hospital, Kampala, Uganda 1957–1966. *East African Medical Journal*, **45**, 89–99.

49. Adetuyibi, A. (1976) Diabetes in the Nigerian African. I. Review complications. *Tropical and Geographical Medicine*, **28** (3), 155–9.

50. Bhoola, K.D. (1976) A necropsy study of diabetes mellitus in Natal Blacks. *South African Medical Journal*, **50**, 1364–6.

51. Mbanya, J.C. and Sobngwi, E. (2003) Diabetes microvascular and macrovascular disease in Africa. *Journal of Cardiovascular Risk*, **10**, 97–102.

52. Herman, W.H., Aubert, R.E., Engelgau, M.M. *et al.* (1998) Diabetes mellitus in Egypt: glycaemic control and microvascular and neuropathic complications. *Diabetic Medicine: A Journal of the British Diabetic Association*, **15**, 1045–51.

53. Motala, A.A., Pirie, F.J., Gouws, E. *et al.* (2001) Microvascular complications in South African patients with long-duration diabetes mellitus. *South African Medical Journal*, **91**, 987–92.

54. Chale, S.S., Swai, A.B., Mujinja, P.G. and McLarty, D.G. (1992) Must diabetes be a fatal disease in Africa? Study of costs of treatment. *British Medical Journal*, **304**, 1215–18.

12

Epidemiology of Diabetes Mellitus in Latin America

Laércio J. Franco and Sandra R. G. Ferreira

[1]Faculty of Medicine of Ribeirão, Preto - University of São Paulo,
Ribeirão Preto-SP, Brazil

[2]School of Public Health - University of São Paulo, Paulo-SP,
Brazil

12.1 INTRODUCTION

Diabetes mellitus is a universally distributed syndrome which is recognized in countries and populations independently of their development status. As far type 1 diabetes is concerned, great variability in its incidence is observed world-wide [1, 2], and a role for both genetic and environmental factors has been shown. On the other hand, considering the frequency of the diabetic syndrome in populations, type 2 diabetes is beyond doubt the most frequent type, characterized by a marked heterogeneity of clinical features.

The population of Latin America is a heterogeneous group, made up of the descendants of Hispanics, Portuguese and other European Caucasians, Africans, American Indians and Asians. This admixture is quite common in many countries; such populations reflect not only great ethnic and genetic heterogeneity, but also socioeconomic and cultural diversity.

Diabetes in Latin America is an issue of great interest; type 1 and type 2 diabetes patterns in such heterogeneous populations are difficult to predict and the incidence rates of type 1 diabetes vary dramatically among them. Population-based studies on type 2 diabetes prevalence show that some populations exhibit rates comparable to those found in developed countries.

12.2 EPIDEMIOLOGY OF TYPE 1 DIABETES IN LATIN AMERICA

The lack of standardized data has made it difficult to determine the true magnitude of type 1 diabetes in Latin America. The World Health Organization (WHO) Multinational Project for Childhood Diabetes (the Diabetes Mondiale (DiaMond) Project) that started in 1990 has lessened the problem, since standardized epidemiological data are now being collected from several countries around Latin America, allowing international comparisons [2]. DiaMond participating centers are required to register all new cases diagnosed under 15 years of age. However, accurate population-based registries are still limited and little information has been published from Latin American countries. Most of the available data on type 1 diabetes incidence reviewed come from regional surveys and may not represent the whole country. Others have not validated their completeness yet and should be interpreted with caution. In the international context, studies on type 1 diabetes epidemiology among children of Spanish and Portuguese heritage are much needed as an attempt to identify determinants of type 1 diabetes throughout the world. As far as Iberian heritage populations are concerned, great variability in incidence is detected among ethnic groups. Much of the incidence variation has been attributed to the percentage of

The Epidemiology of Diabetes Mellitus, second edition   Edited by Jean-Marie Ekoé, Marian Rewers, Rhys Williams and Paul Zimmet

Table 12.1 Incidence rates (per 100 000 per year) of type 1 diabetes in some countries of Latin America.

Country and area	Study period	Age group (years)	Estimate of ascertainment (%)	Incidence per 100 000			Male-to-female ratio
				Boys	Girls	Overall	
Argentina							
Avellaneda [2, 3]	1990–1994	<15	88–97	5.6	7.5	6.5	0.7
Cordoba [3]	1991–1992	<15	88–92	6.2	7.9	7	0.8
Brazil							
São Paulo [4]	1987–1991	<15	>90	5.6	9.5	7.6	0.6
Londrina [5]	1990–1996	<15	79	—	—	12.7	0.7
Passo Fundo [6]	1996	<15	100	—	—	12	1
Chile							
Santiago [7]	1986–2003	<15	NA	—	—	4	NA
Santiago [8]	1992	<15	NA	—	—	3	NA
Colombia							
Bogota [2]	1990s	<15	NA	4.7	2.9	3.8	1.8
Mexico							
Vera Cruz [2]	1990-–1993	<15	100	—	—	1.5	NA
Paraguay [2]	1990–1994	<15	NA	1	0.8	0.9	1.3
Peru							0.9
Lima [9]	1985–1990	<15	85	0.4	0.4	0.4	
Puerto Rico [2]	1990–1994	<15	90–97	16.2	18.7	17.4	0.9

NA: not available.

Caucasians in the population. Racial admixture and local environmental factors might provide important data about the genetic–environment interaction. **Table 12.1** summarizes the available data on type 1 diabetes incidence in Latin American countries.

12.2.1 Argentina

As Argentina is located in the southern part of South America, seasons are usually well defined. The population is 95% Caucasian. Avellaneda, a suburb of the capital Buenos Aires, and the city of Cordoba are DiaMond participating centers. The primary source of ascertainment was composed of kindergarden and elementary schools, while hospitals, private clinics, diabetologists and pediatricians represented the secondary sources. The degree of ascertainment permitted validation of the studies.

The annual type 1 diabetes incidence rate reported for Avellaneda during the period 1990–1994 was 6.5 per 100 000 inhabitants under 15 years of age and 7.0 per 100 000 for Cordoba in the period 1991–1992 [2, 3]. There was a tendency for higher rates among girls (**Table 12.1**). In the international context, Argentine cities showed an intermediate level of type 1 diabetes risk, situated between that of Japan and northern European countries and near the average figures of southern Europe (except for Sardinia) [10–12].

12.2.2 Brazil

This tropical country has an area of 8.5×10^6 km^2, which represents almost half of South America. Population-based reports on type 1 diabetes started in a defined population from the state of São Paulo in

January 1987. This state is considered a developed area, located in the southern part of Brazil, crossed by the Tropic of Capricorn. Migration from Europe, Africa and Asia made the Brazilian population ethnically heterogeneous. The majority of the population is White (54%), followed by Mulatto (39%) and Black (6%); less than 1% is of Asian origin and only 0.1% is Amerindian, according to the national census. Three cities from the state of São Paulo, where the population is 75% White, mainly of Portuguese and Italian origins, 5% Black, 18% Mulatto and 0.9% Asian [13], participated in a prospective population-based study. Data of newly diagnosed type 1 diabetes patients under 15 years of age have been collected according to the methods recommended by the Diabetes Epidemiology Research International Group [14]. Reports from physicians have been considered the primary source of case identification and school surveys as the main secondary source. In the period 1985–1990, the average annual incidence of childhood type 1 diabetes was 7.6 per 100 000 inhabitants (95% confidence interval 5.6–9.7) [4] (**Table 12.1**). Such a rate has been interpreted as an intermediate type 1 diabetes risk, which is similar to that found in Argentina [3]. A tendency to female excess was noticed (male-to-female ratio 0.61). The highest rates were found in the 5–9-year-old age group for girls and 10–14-year-old age group for boys. Validation procedures showed satisfactory completeness of each source and the degree of ascertainment for the combined registry was >90%.

This study was extended to other centers with different climatic and ethnic characteristics. Data concerning the period 1991–1993 pointed to lower overall incidence rates than those previously reported (6.3 per 100 000; ascertainment rate of 71%), being similar between genders [15].

Further studies, using similar methodology, were conducted in two other locations in the southern region of Brazil. The report from Londrina, state of Parana [5], described an incidence of 12.7 per 100 000 inhabitants under 15 years of age (95% confidence interval 9.6–15.8); in Passo Fundo, state of Rio Grande do Sul, a rate of 12.0 per 100 000 inhabitants under 15 years of age was found [6]. The population of these states is characterized by a higher concentration of individuals of Italian, German, Polish and Portuguese ancestries.

12.2.3   Chile

Climatic conditions in Chile differ from other countries in Latin America because winter temperatures are markedly low for several months a year. The population is 25% Caucasian and the majority is Mestizo (Indian–European admixture). During 1986–1989, a retrospective study pointed to a low incidence rate (1.9 per 100 000 inhabitants) in the capital Santiago [8]. Since 1990, data on incidence has been collected prospectively according to DiaMond recommendations [2]. During the period 1986–2003, the overall annual incidence rate was 4.02 per 100 000 inhabitants under 15 years old (95% confidence interval 2.98–4.83) [7]. Even lower incidence rates were found in the IX Region of Chile; there was a significant difference in the incidence in Caucasian children (1.58 per 100 000; 95% confidence interval 1.11–2.04) compared with Mapuche Indians (0.42 per 100 000; 95% confidence interval 0.00–0.95), suggesting that the native population has a lower risk of developing type 1 diabetes.

12.2.4   Colombia

Colombia is located in the northwest corner of South America. Its population has experienced much genetic admixture, which started with the Spaniards mingled with the native Indians (Mestizos) and later continued with the influx of Black slaves from Africa. Data on type 1 diabetes incidence in this country are very limited. A published report from the population living in the capital Bogotá, at the beginning of 1990s, pointed to an annual incidence rate of 3.8 per 100 000 inhabitants under 15 years of age (95% confidence interval 2.9–4.9) [2].

12.2.5   Mexico

The Mexican population has a genetic admixture mainly from the native Indians mixing with the Spaniards (Mestizos). The apparent low incidence of type 1 diabetes in this country is based on data collected in Vera Cruz during the period 1990–1993 [2]. The incidence rate was 1.5 per 100 000 (95% confidence interval 0.70–2.94).

12.2.6   Paraguay

Data on the incidence of type 1 diabetes in Paraguay derived from primary source only showed an overall rate of 0.9 per 100 000 inhabitants under 15 years old (95% confidence interval 0.71–1.11). The contribution of natives for the general population of Paraguay is markedly high, supporting the idea that Amerindians are at low risk for type 1 diabetes.

12.2.7 Peru

The great majority of the Peruvian population is made up of Mestizos and only 15% are Caucasians. The type 1 diabetes incidence survey in the capital Lima was based on the diagnosis of type 1 diabetes according to the DiaMond project, before 15 years of age at the time of the diagnosis. Primary source data were obtained from 25 hospitals and the secondary source was the Peruvian Diabetes Association with 85% validation. The annual incidence observed for the period 1985–1994 was 0.4 per 100 000 inhabitants (95% confidence interval 0.32–0.49) [9]. The population under 15 years old in 1993 was 1 698 137 inhabitants. From 1985 to 1994 the degree of ascertainment ranged from 74% (1987) to 100% (1994). Such a rate represents one of the lowest incidence rates observed worldwide [2], suggesting that this Mestizo population may be genetically protected from type 1 diabetes.

12.2.8 Puerto Rico

Puerto Rico is a tropical island with a population of Hispanic descent with a lifestyle and economic resources similar to those observed in the United States. Using hospital records as the primary source and the government diabetic registry as the secondary source for the years 1990–1994, the overall type 1 diabetes incidence rate was 17.4 per 100 000 (95% confidence interval 16.2–18.6) inhabitants under 15 years [2]. The pattern of type 1 diabetes in Puerto Rico may be the result of a genetic–environmental interaction that is more similar to that from Hispanic Americans than that from the Cuban population [16].

12.2.9 Other Countries in Latin America

Recent reviews about incidence of type 1 diabetes in Latin America and the Caribbean include data from several countries using nonstandardized or poorly reported methodology [2, 17]. The rates vary considerably, ranging from 0.1 per 100 000

(95% confidence interval 0.09–0.18) in Caracas, Venezuela [18], to 8.3 per 100 000 (95% confidence interval 5.4–12.1) in Uruguay [17].

12.3 EPIDEMIOLOGY OF TYPE 2 DIABETES IN LATIN AMERICA

Since type 2 diabetes has been recognized as a major public health problem in Latin America, attempts have been made to assess its prevalence. However, the majority of the studies available nowadays are not based on standardized methods and criteria for diagnosis [19], which limit international comparisons. Also, it is well known that frequency for diseases such as diabetes is strongly age related, and age differences between populations can confound direct comparisons of crude rates. We will summarize some population-based studies conducted in Latin America. Few studies of diabetes included standardized age groups and age-adjusted rates. As far as incidence of type 2 diabetes is concerned, this rate could only be calculated by monitoring the population continuously, or by repeated cross-sectional surveys. The resources required for such studies are often considerable. Furthermore, it is well known that a substantial proportion of subjects with type 2 diabetes remain undetected in the community, and incidence estimates based upon routine data sources are much less reliable than they may be for type 1 diabetes. For these reasons, this type of study is even rarer in Latin America, and scarce data have been published. **Table 12.2** summarizes the available data on type 2 diabetes prevalence in Latin American countries.

12.3.1 Argentina

A study on prevalence of diabetes in the cities of Rosario and Santa Fe, Argentina, was carried out in 1967. The diagnosis was based on 2 h blood glucose levels after receiving a mixed meal containing at least 50 g of carbohydrate, and levels >8.3 mmol l^{-1} were considered positive for diabetes. About 5% of the population aged 20–70 years (22 351 inhabitants for Rosario and 10 148 inhabitants for Santa Fe) was included. Rates of 6.1% and 4.3% respectively were found, and at least half of the cases of diabetes were undiagnosed. Another survey was conducted in 1976 among

Table 12.2 Prevalence of type 2 diabetes in some countries of Latin America.

Location	Study period	Age group (years)	Diagnostic criteria	Glucose cut-off (mmol l^{-1})	Prevalence (%)		
					Men	Women	Overall
Argentina							
Avellaneda [21]	1976	20–69	2 h capillary glucose after 75 g oral glucose	≥8.3	—	—	8
Humboldt [22]	1976	20–69	2 h capillary glucose after 75g oral glucose	≥8.3	—	—	5.8
La Plata [23]	1987	20–74	2 h capillary glucose after 50 g oral glucose	≥8.3	—	—	5
Dean Funes, Oncativo, Venado Tuerto [24]	1995–1998	≥20	Fasting and 2 h plasma glucose	≥7.0 or ≥11.1	—	—	6.9
Bolivia							
La Paz, El Alto, Santa Cruz, Cochabamba [25]	1998	≥20	Fasting or 2 h venous glucose after 75 g oral glucose	≥7.0 or ≥11.1	7.6	7.2	6.8
Brazil							
General population, 9 cities [26]	1986–1989	30–69	2 h capillary glucose after 75 g oral glucose	≥11.1	7.4	7.4	7.4
Ribeirão Preto [27]	1997	30–69	2 h capillary glucose after 75 g oral glucose	≥11.1	12	12.1	12.1
Xingu, indigenous community [28]	1979	>15	1 h venous glucose after 100 g oral glucose	>10.8	0	0	0
Bauru, Japanese-Brazilian community [29]	1993	40–79	Fasting or 2 h venous glucose after 75 g oral glucose	≥7.0 or ≥11.1	12.4 / 21.7	11.6 / 11.4	(Issei) (Nisei)

(continued overleaf)

Table 12.2 (*continued*)

Location	Study period	Age group (years)	Diagnostic criteria	Glucose cut-off (mmol l^{-1})	Prevalence (%)		
					Men	Women	Overall
Bauru, Japanese-Brazilian community [30]	2000	≥30	Fasting or 2 h venous glucose after 75 g oral glucose	≥7.0 or ≥11.1	39.6	30.7	36.2
Chile							
Santiago, general population [31]	1979	>20	2 h venous glucose after 50 g oral glucose	≥8.3	—	—	6.5
Mapuche, indigenous community [32]	1997–1998	>20	Fasting or 2 h venous glucose after 75 g oral glucose	≥7.0 or ≥11.1	3.2	4.5	—
7th Region [33]	1999–2000	≥20	Fasting or 2 h venous glycemia after 75 g oral glucose	≥7.0 or ≥11.1	—	—	5.4
Colombia							
Bogota [34]	1988–1989	≥30	2 h venous glycemia	≥11.1	7.3	8.7	NA
Mexico							
Mexico City [35]	1992	20–90	Fasting or 2 h venous glycemia after 75g oral glucose	≥7.0 or ≥11.1	6	10.6	8.1
National Survey of Chronic Diseases [36]	1993	20–69	Casual plasma glucose ≥11.1 mmol l^{-1} or fasting or 2 h glycemia after 75 g oral glucose	≥7.0 or ≥11.1	8.7	9.2	8.9
National Health Survey [37]	2000	≥20	fasting or 2 h venous glycemia after 75 g oral glucose	≥7.0 or ≥11.1	7.7	8.4	8.2

Table 12.2 (*continued*)

Location	Study period	Age group (years)	Diagnostic criteria	Glucose cut-off (mmol l^{-1})	Prevalence (%)		
					Men	Women	Overall
Paraguay							
Asuncion [38]	1991	20–74	Fasting or 2 h venous glycemia after 75g oral glucose	≥11.1	5.5	6.5	6.5
Peru							
Lima [39]	1990s	≥18	Fasting or 2 h venous glycemia after 75 g oral glucose	≥7.0 or ≥11.1	—	—	4.8

NA: not available.

596 subjects aged 20–69 years, living in an urban area of the province of Buenos Aires (Avellaneda district), now using 75 g oral glucose load. A 2 h capillary glycemia ≥8.3 mmol l^{-1} was indicative of diabetes [20]. A prevalence rate of 8.0% was found. Using the same age group and diagnostic criteria, a lower rate (5.8%) was observed in the rural area of Humboldt (province of Santa Fe) [21]. When adjusting these results to the 1985 WHO criteria [19], the diabetes prevalence rates in the province of Buenos Aires (urban area) and Santa Fe (rural area) dropped markedly from 8.0% to 4.0% and from 5.8% and 1.8% respectively. In 1987, a prevalence of 5% was reported from La Plata City [22]. This rate may have been an underestimate, since the survey was based upon a 50 g oral glucose challenge. More recently, a study was conducted in a selected urban population living in Resistencia City [39]. The diagnosis of type 2 diabetes was self-reported and 2797 individuals were questioned. An overall prevalence rate of 3.8% was found and the male-to-female ratio was 0.67. Such a study design underestimates the true prevalence rate and the population sample studied may not be representative of the whole population. Between 1995 and 1998, a survey was conducted in three cities located in the pampas, including 1794 individuals of 20 years and over. Diabetes diagnosis

was based on the 1999 WHO criteria [40]. The rates ranged from 6.5% (95% confidence interval 4.8–8.6) in Oncativo to 7.7% (95% confidence interval 5.3–10.8) in Venado Tuerto [23].

12.3.2 Bolivia

Bolivia is an Andean South American country of some 7 900 000 inhabitants. Its population is mostly composed of aboriginal groups; people of Hispanic origin constitute only 20%. In 1998, a population-based survey was conducted in four cities (La Paz, El Alto, Santa Cruz and Cochabamba). The total sample size was 2948 persons. Diabetes was diagnosed through an oral glucose tolerance test (OGTT), 2 h after an overload of 75 g of glucose, using the 1985 WHO criteria [19]. The overall prevalence of diabetes was 7.2% (95% confidence interval 6.2–8.3), being slightly higher in women (7.6% versus 6.8%). The high frequency of overweight in the Bolivian population (60.7%) is remarkable [24].

12.3.3 Brazil

Little information was available concerning diabetes among the Brazilian population until 1986. A cross-sectional home survey was conducted from 1986 to 1988 in a random sample of 21 847 individuals aged 30–69 years in nine Brazilian cities [25]. The 1980 Brazilian census [41] provided the basic demographic data to characterize the population and to assess representativeness of the eligible samples. Besides a questionnaire, fasting capillary glycemia was determined in the screening phase. Subjects with previously diagnosed diabetes or with fasting capillary glycemia ≥ 11.1 mmol l^{-1} at screening were considered to have diabetes. All persons with fasting capillary glycemia ≥ 5.6 mmol l^{-1} and every sixth consecutive negative screenee (<5.6 mmol l^{-1}) were scheduled for an OGTT. Results from the sixth negatives were extrapolated to all negative screenees. Using the 1985 WHO criteria for diagnosis [19], the overall age-adjusted rates for diabetes and impaired glucose tolerance (IGT) were 7.4% and 7.7% respectively. Both conditions were more prevalent in the south and southeast regions, and also the most industrialized regions. The highest rate of diabetes was found in São Paulo city (9.7%), located in the most economically developed region of Brazil. Age strongly influenced diabetes prevalence, with the rate in the 60–69-year-old group (17.4%) being 6.4 times higher than that seen among people aged 30–39 years (2.7%, $p < 0.01$). For age-adjusted rates, no difference was found in diabetes prevalence between men (7.4%) and women (7.4%); however, women had a higher rate of IGT than men (8.4% versus 6.7%, $p < 0.01$). Rates of diabetes and IGT were similar in Whites and non-Whites. Almost half of the diabetic subjects in the age group studied were undiagnosed. Data obtained in this study indicated that the occurrence rates of diabetes and IGT in Brazil are similar to those found in countries such as the United States, Italy, Israel, Argentina and others [42, 43].

In 1997, another population-based study was conducted in Ribeirão Preto, located in the interior of the state of São Paulo, including 1473 individuals aged 30–69 years [26]. Such a developed city is characterized by its prosperous agrobusiness and a population of high income level. The prevalence rates were very similar in men and women (12.1% and 12.0% respectively). When compared with the national survey, these higher rates reflect changes in lifestyle of the population.

Another survey based on OGTT was carried out in a Brazilian indigenous population, living in the 'Parque Nacional do Xingu' along the Xingu River, located in the state of Mato Grosso, central Brazil [27]. Their diet included mainly manioc and fish, and the Upper Xingu Indians are well nourished. In 1979, 106 of them received a 100 g oral glucose load and venous blood sample was taken 1 h later. Considering 10.8 mmol l^{-1} as the cut-off value for diagnosis, diabetes was not found among the Upper Xingu Indians. In spite of intermittent contact with the Brazilian society, diabetes does not represent a cause of morbidity and mortality among these Brazilian Indians, contrasting with the North American Indians [44].

Also of great interest in Brazil was the study of diabetes in migrant populations. Brazil has the largest population of Japanese origin located outside Japan, the majority living in the state of São Paulo. This community differs from other migrant populations in Brazil concerning its genetic and cultural homogeneity. During 1987–1990, data regarding the prevalence of diabetes were restricted to self-reported surveys [45]. Recently, a population-based survey, using 75 g OGTT and the 1985 WHO diagnostic criteria [19], was conducted in the Japanese-Brazilian community aged 40–79 years, living in the city of Bauru, state of São Paulo [28]. These data showed high prevalence of type 2 diabetes and IGT, even higher than in the general Brazilian population [25], particularly among men. Age-adjusted rates for Issei (first-generation or Japan-born) men and women were 12.4% and 11.6% respectively; for Nisei (second-generation or Brazil-born) men the prevalence of diabetes was significantly higher than in women (21.7% versus 11.4% respectively). These findings were in accordance with those from Fujimoto et al. [46], obtained in the Japanese-American community in Seattle, USA. In 2000, a prevalence study in the same Japanese-Brazilian population over 30 years of age was carried out; this showed an alarming increase in the rates of disturbances of glucose metabolism (**Figure 12.1**) [29]. Prevalence of diabetes in the overall Japanese-Brazilian population increased from 22.6% to 36.2%. This second survey allowed one to estimate the incidence of type 2 diabetes in this specific population for the period 1993–2000 (30.9 per 1000 per year). These high rates could reflect their strong genetic susceptibility associated with unfavorable environmental conditions.

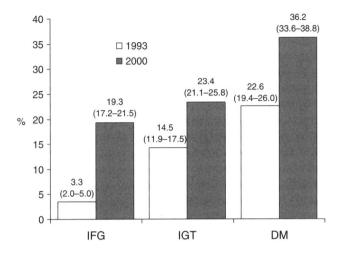

Figure 12.1 Prevalence (95% confidence interval) of disturbances of glucose metabolism observed in 1993 and 2000 in Japanese-Brazilians (IFG: impaired fasting glycemia; IGT: impaired glucose tolerance: DM: diabetes mellitus)

12.3.4   Chile

Initial prevalence rates of type 2 diabetes in Chile were based upon postprandial glycosuria, and certainly the rate of 1.2% did not reflect the true magnitude of the disease in this country [47]. In 1979, a prevalence survey was conducted in 1100 individuals of age >20 years from Santiago [30]. A 50 g oral glucose load was used, with 2 h whole venous blood for glucose determinations. A 2 h glycemia ≥ 8.3 mmol l^{-1} was indicative of diabetes. Such procedures resulted in a prevalence rate of 6.5%, which is within the range of rates found in many Western countries. Similar rates were found in both sexes and in the different socioeconomic levels. In 44% of the cases identified by the survey, the diabetic condition was undiagnosed. An estimate of the prevalence using the National Diabetes Data Group criteria [48], whose cut-off point for the 2 h whole-blood glucose is 10.0 mmol l^{-1}, resulted in a prevalence of 5.3% for the same population. Contrasting rates are observed when indigenous populations are studied. Among the Mapuche community, a prevalence rate of type 2 diabetes of 1.0% was reported in 1985 [49], in contrast to the situation found in several American Indian populations in the United States [44]. During the period 1997–1998, higher prevalence rates were found in a sample of individuals ≥ 20 years of age: 3.2% in men (95% confidence interval 0.7–9.0) and 4.5% (95%

confidence interval 2.2–8.1) [31]. This increase could be the result of accelerated socioeconomic changes and their related nutritional behaviors observed in Chile.

In 1999–2000, another survey was carried out in the VII Region of Chile, which has an estimated population of 1 million inhabitants, 37.4% of them living in rural areas. Using the 1999 WHO criteria [40], the overall prevalence of diabetes was 5.4%, being 5.8% in urban areas and 4.5% in rural areas [32].

12.3.5   Colombia

Almost 6 million Colombians live in the capital city, Santafé de Bogotá, which is located on a plateau at the altitude of 2600 m. Considering the high rate of drift in Colombia, a relatively stable urban community of medium–low socioeconomic status (named *San Isidro*, in Santafé de Bogotá) was chosen for the diabetes survey, which was carried out in 1988–1989 [33]. The study sample was representative of 70–80% of the urban population of this country with regard to Hispanic ethnicity and socioeconomic status. The age range studied was 30–80 years and more and the 1985 WHO diagnostic criteria [19] were adopted, using 2 h blood glucose values after a 75 g oral glucose challenge. Age-adjusted prevalence rates were 7.3% (95% confidence interval 3.7–10.9) and 8.7% (95% confidence interval 5.2–12.3) for men and women respectively. Less than 40% of the diabetics were aware of such a diagnosis. For IGT, age-adjusted prevalence was 3.1% for men and 7.2% for women. Rates of diabetes in urban Colombians and Brazilians are comparable to rates seen in Whites in similar settings in Europe and North America [43].

12.3.6 Mexico

A number of prevalence studies, restricted to relatively small populations, have yielded estimates in the range of 1.3–6.0% for the Mexican adult population, until the 1980s [50]. Many reports come from hospital workers or subjects seeking medical attention. Given the differences in diagnostic criteria, time interval among the surveys (they span nearly 30 years) and age structure of the populations studied (with the proportion of those aged over 30 years ranging from 25 to 65%), it is difficult to draw any confident conclusions about the national level or pattern of diabetes from these data.

A cross-sectional survey, conducted in 1992, among 805 individuals aged 20–90 years from Mexico City [51], using 75 g OGTT and the 1985 WHO criteria for diagnosis [19], reported an age-adjusted prevalence rate of type 2 diabetes of 8.1% (6.0% and 10.6% for men and women respectively). The same study compared these results with data obtained in Mexican Americans with comparable socioeconomic level (low income) living in San Antonio, Texas, where the rates were higher (17.8% for men and 23% for women). The analysis of such data suggested a role for environmental factors in the expression of the type 2 diabetes trait.

The Mexico City study is a population-based study of type 2 diabetes in six low-income neighborhoods in Mexico City. From 3326 individuals aged 35–64 years, 2813 underwent a home interview and 2282 (68.5%) completed a baseline medical examination during 1990–1992. The study included a follow-up evaluation 7 years later, which was completed by 1764 individuals. Baseline prevalence was 12.9%, and this study provided data about the incidence of obesity and other comorbidities [52].

The National Survey of Chronic Diseases (1993) is a nationwide, cross-sectional study that included individuals aged 20–69 years from 417 cities. Information was obtained from 15 607 individuals (response rate of 83%). A blood sample was requested in all cases; however, samples were

obtained after a 9–12 h fasting period only in 16% of the population (2256 individuals). Diabetes was diagnosed in known cases or if casual plasma glucose concentration was ≥ 11.1 mmol l^{-1} or the fasting plasma glucose was ≥ 7.0 mmol l^{-1}. Prevalence of diabetes was 8.9% (8.7% for men and 9.2% for women). Remarkably, 13% of the cases were <40 years of age [53]. As a result, the prolonged exposure of these individuals to the adverse effects of diabetes makes this group highly susceptible to chronic diabetic complications.

The National Health Survey (2000) is a cross-sectional study that includes information obtained from 42 886 individuals aged ≥ 20 years, from 400 cities, using a multistage sampling procedure. Diabetes was diagnosed according to the 1999 WHO criteria [40], using capillary glycemia. The age-adjusted prevalence of diabetes was 8.2% (7.7% in men and 8.4% in women). Diabetes affected 13.2% of the individuals <40 years of age [54].

In summary, the prevalence of type 2 diabetes in Mexico has increased in recent years and there is a growing concern that diabetes is an important health problem in Mexico. In fact, this disease represents one of the leading causes for hospital admissions and outpatient visits in heath care facilities and one of the main causes of death since the year 2000. The increasing prevalence of type 2 diabetes, the high proportion of cases at younger ages, the higher rates among individuals with lower income and the growing prevalence of obesity are alarming signs that the worst is still to come for the health system if preventive actions are not taken [55].

12.3.7 Paraguay

The prevalence of type 2 diabetes was studied in an urban White-Hispanic population sample from Asunción, the capital of Paraguay, consisting by 512 men and 1094 women, aged 20–74 years [34, 56]. Diagnosis of diabetes was based on fasting and on 2 h after 75 g glucose load glycemia, using the 1985 WHO diagnostic criteria [19]. An overall age-adjusted prevalence rate of 6.5% was found (5.5% in men and 6.5% in women). IGT was detected in 11.3% of the individuals, being more frequent in women (13.5% versus 7.2%). The levels of abnormalities in glycemic homeostasis (IGT and diabetes mellitus) highlight the importance of this health problem in Paraguay.

12.3.8 Peru

A prevalence survey in Peru was conducted in the adult population from Lima, including 4113 men and 4089 women. The results were presented at the VIII Latin American Diabetes Association Congress in 1992 in Mar Del Plata, Argentina [57]. Prevalence rates of type 2 diabetes and IGT were 4.4% and 4.6% respectively, with male preponderance for both conditions. No information was provided with respect to the population studied and diagnostic criteria.

A more recent survey (1997), using the 1985 WHO [19] diagnostic criteria, was carried out in individuals aged ≥18 years, living in three regions: coast, mountain and forest. The overall prevalence was 4.8% (95% confidence interval 3.2–7.0). The rates were lower in the population living at an altitude above 3000 m (1.3% in Ancash Huaraz) than at the coast (7.6% in Lima) or in the forest (3.7% in Wayku) [35]. It is interesting to note that 100% of the cases of diabetes diagnosed in one community of the forest (Wayku) did not have a previous diagnosis, denoting lack of access to medical care.

12.3.9 Other Countries in Central and South America

West and Kalbfleisch [36] were probably the first to investigate the prevalence of diabetes using standardized criteria for its diagnosis in Latin America countries. Almost all the subjects over 30 years that were enrolled in these surveys received oral glucose load (1 g per kilogram of body weight) and diagnosis was based upon 2 h venous blood glucose ≥ 8.3 mmol l^{-1}. The prevalence rates of diabetes for some countries are shown in **Table 12.3**. The differences in prevalence were likely due to the varying degree of obesity, since a marked correlation ($r = 0.89$) was found between the prevalence of diabetes and the mean percentage of standard weight of the populations studied [36, 58, 59].

More recent data from Central America and the Caribbean are available only from Costa Rica and Barbados and are restricted to self-reported diabetes. In 1992, a survey carried out in Costa Rica compared the self-reported rates of diabetes between urban (4.5%) and rural (2.7%) adult populations of Puriscal [37]. The 1998 National Household Survey in the same country reported a

Table 12.3 Reported prevalence rates of diabetes mellitus in some Latin-American countries. (Data from [60].)

Country	Prevalence rate (%)
Panama	2.5
El Salvador	3.2
Honduras	4.1
Guatemala	4.2
Nicaragua	5.0
Costa Rica	5.4
Uruguay	6.9
Venezuela	7.0

prevalence of diagnosed diabetes of 2.8% for the general population and 9.4% among those aged 40 years and over [61].

Barbados is a predominantly Black English-speaking Caribbean nation known by higher diabetes mortality rates in the region. In the Barbados Eye Study Cohort (1988–1992), 4709 individuals aged 40–84 years provided information about diagnosed diabetes. The overall prevalence of known diabetes was 17.0% and varied by ethnic group, being 17.5% in Blacks, 12.5% in mixed (Black–White) and 6.0% in the White population [38].

No published reports in the last 20 years were found concerning results based on glucose tolerance tests and WHO diagnostic criteria for Ecuador, French Guiana, Guiana, Suriname, Uruguay and Venezuela.

12.4 MORTALITY BY DIABETES

It is known that health statistics based upon death certification underestimate mortality from diabetes, since the majority of the diabetics die from complications of the disease, mainly cardiovascular events. Much of the reported variation in diabetes mortality among countries may be due to differences in certification practices and in coding procedures for assigning the underlying cause of death. It is also known that the number of deaths certified by physicians varies widely among countries.

In Latin America, there is a lack of information concerning mortality data by type of diabetes. Also, mortality data for Latin American countries are

Table 12.4 Estimated death rates (per 100 000 population) and proportional mortality (%) by diabetes as underlying cause of death in some Latin American countries, in which diabetes figures among the 10 leading causes of death, according to sex, by the year 2000. (Reproduced from [64]. Copyright © 2004, The World Health Organization.)

Country	Death rate				Proportional mortality (%)		
	Total	Men (M)	Women (W)	M/W ratio	Total	Men	Women
Argentina	25.6	27.2	24.1	1.13	3.3	3.1	3.4
Belize	31.2	22.6	36.6	0.62	5.9	3.6	8.7
Brazil	27.3	23.3	31.2	0.75	4.3	3.1	6.0
Chile	20.2	19.4	21.0	0.92	3.9	3.4	4.5
Colombia	22.0	17.3	26.6	0.65	3.7	2.6	5.5
Costa Rica	23.0	19.3	26.8	0.72	4.5	3.4	6.0
Dominican Rep.	21.8	19.4	24.4	0.79	3.9	3.2	5.4
Ecuador	22.3	19.6	25.4	0.77	5.0	3.9	6.7
El Salvador	20.7	—[a]	25.9	—[a]	3.3	—[a]	4.9
French Guiana	10.1	10.3	9.8	1.05	3.3	2.8	3.7
Guatemala	19.9	—[a]	22.0	—[a]	3.4	—[a]	4.6
Guyana	29.4	—[a]	34.1	—[a]	4.6	—[a]	6.4
Mexico	59.9	56.5	63.2	0.89	12.2	10.0	15.1
Nicaragua	28.4	23.2	33.5	0.69	5.6	4.2	7.5
Panama	32.8	27.4	38.3	0.71	6.4	4.5	8.8
Paraguay	34.8	27.4	42.4	0.65	7.3	5.4	9.8
Puerto Rico	62.9	61.7	64.1	0.96	8.6	7.2	10.5
Uruguay	22.1	—[a]	24.4	—[a]	2.3	—[a]	2.7
Venezuela	25.0	23.6	26.5	0.89	5.7	4.5	7.5

[a]Not among the 10 leading causes of death.

available only considering diabetes as underlying cause of death. The traditional method for expressing mortality rates has been number of deaths per year per 100 000 population. The age distribution among countries varies markedly; therefore, comparison of crude rates needs some caution. Despite these limitations, death registration data have been a highly useful source of information.

Table 12.4 presents death rates per 100 000 population and proportional mortality by diabetes as underlying cause of death in some Latin American countries where diabetes figures among the 10 leading causes of death, around the year 2000. It should be noted that death rates per 100 000 population ranged from as low as 10.1 in French Guiana to 62.9 in Puerto Rico or 59.9 in Mexico. On the other hand, when looking for the contribution of diabetes as the underlying cause of death for the total mortality, the proportion varies from 2.3% in Uruguay to 12.2% in Mexico or 8.6% in Puerto

Rico, highlighting the importance of diabetes as a health problem in Mexico and Puerto Rico.

The men-to-women death rates ratios are usually lower than one, except for Argentina and French Guiana, showing that there is an excess of mortality by diabetes among women.

12.5 DIABETIC COMPLICATIONS

Diabetic complications account for much of the social and financial burdens of diabetes. Diabetes is ranked among the leading causes of blindness, renal failure and lower limb amputations in many countries, while some 50% of people with diabetes die of cardiovascular disease [62].

Most of the published data about diabetic complications in Latin America came from clinic-based populations, with restrictions to be generalized for the whole country.

Few population-based data about diabetic chronic complications are available for Latin

America. The *Latin American Dialysis and Renal Transplantation Registry* collects information from 20 countries in the region and provides the frequency of diabetes as the reported cause of end-stage renal disease, which has varied from 32.9% in Colombia and 38% in Venezuela to 60% in Mexico and 62.2% in Puerto Rico, among the incident population on dialysis [63].

The QUALIDIAB study [64], carried out to evaluate the quality of the health care provided to diabetic patients in Latin America, analyzed 13 513 registries from the public and private sector from Argentina, Brazil, Chile, Colombia, Paraguay and Uruguay. From these registries it was possible to get information about the presence of diabetic complications and duration of the diagnosis; see **Table 12.5**.

Lower limb amputation is a major health problem and is associated with significant morbidity, disability and mortality. Using the capture–recapture method, the incidence of lower limb amputation in the city of Rio de Janeiro, Brazil, for the period 1992–1994 among individuals with diabetes was estimated as 186.6 per 100 000 persons-year, representing a 13 times higher risk than for individuals without diabetes, and diabetes was the cause for 27.4% of all amputations [65].

A multinational cross-sectional study of complications in type 1 diabetes (DiaComp) estimated the prevalence of reported chronic complications by duration of diabetes [66]. Argentina (Buenos Aires), Brazil (Rio de Janeiro and São Paulo) and Chile (nationwide) participated in this study for the short-duration group (5–15 years), and Argentina (Rosario) and Brazil (Rio de Janeiro) for the long-duration group (15–25 years). The prevalence of retinopathy in the short-duration group was 2.7% (95% confidence interval 0.1–14.2) in Chile, 3.1% (95% confidence interval 1.3–64) in Buenos Aires, 3.0% (95% confidence interval 1.0–6.8) in São Paulo and 9.5% (95% confidence interval 2.7–22.6) in Rio de Janeiro. In the long-duration group, the rates and 95% confidence intervals for retinopathy, neuropathy, macroangiopathy and renal disease were 62.5% (40.6–81.2), 12.5% (2.7–32.4), 20.8% (7.1–42.2) and 34.8% (16.4–57.3) respectively for Rio de Janeiro, and 35.3% (22.4–49.9), 3.9% (0.5–13.2), 1.9% (0.05–10.0) and 29.4% (11.5–44.0) respectively for Rosario.

Recently, an estimation of the direct costs of diabetes in Latin American and Caribbean countries for the year 2000 was published [67]. The estimated direct costs for diabetic complications were US$2480.4 billion, being US$1492.5 or 60.2% for South America and US$635.4 or 25.6% only for Mexico.

Despite the limitations of the data for Latin America, it is possible to realize that diabetic complications impose a high economic and social burden to individuals, society and to the health system of these countries.

12.6 CONCLUSION

The data now available on diabetes morbidity, expected population growth, increase in life

Table 12.5 Frequency (%) of diabetic chronic complications according duration of the diagnosis in some Latin American countries [65].

	Frequency (%)				p value[a]
	Duration of the diagnosis of diabetes (years)				
	0–5	6–10	11–20	>20	
Retinopathy	10.0	20.0	38.0	48.0	<0.001
Blindness	1.7	2.8	3.2	6.7	<0.001
Neuropathy	21.0	29.0	37.0	42.0	<0.001
Renal disease	0.2	0.4	0.7	1.5	<0.001
Myocardial infarction	1.5	1.8	4.3	6.7	<0.001
Stroke	2.1	3.5	2.9	3.3	<0.001
Lower limb amputation	1.0	1.4	3.6	7.3	<0.001

[a]χ^2 for tendencies.

expectancy, increase in the costs of heath care for diabetes and its complications, and the high proportion of new cases at younger ages lead to the assumption that diabetes will become an increasingly serious health problem for the Latin American countries. Diabetes prevention and control programs are urgently needed and are potentially cost-effective strategies that can reduce the huge burden of diabetes. Despite the important contribution that research can make to a better understanding of diabetes, it is the health authorities, the patients and the public who still have the major task of coping with this increasingly prevalent disease.

References

1. Diabetes Epidemiology Research International Group (1990) Secular trends in incidence of childhood IDDM in 10 countries. *Diabetes*, **39**, 858–64.

2. Karvonen, M., Viik-Kajander, M., Moltchanova, E. and Libman, I. (2000) Incidence of childhood type 1 diabetes worldwide. *Diabetes Care*, **23**, 1516–26.

3. Sereday, M., Marti, M.L., Damiano, M.M. and Moser, M.E.C. (1994) Establishment of a registry and incidence of IDDM in Avellaneda, Argentina. *Diabetes Care*, **17** (9), 1022–5.

4. Ferreira, S.R.G., Franco, L.J., Vivolo, M.A. *et al.* (1993) Population-based incidence of IDDM in the state of São Paulo, Brazil. *Diabetes Care*, **16** (5), 701–4.

5. Campos, J.J.B., Almeida, H.G.G., Iochida, L.C. and Franco, L.J. (1998) Incidência de diabetes mellitus insulino-dependente (tipo 1) na cidade de Londrina, PR–Brasil. *Arquivos Brasileiros de Endocrinologia e Metabologia*, **42** (1), 36–44.

6. Lisbôa, H.R.K., Graebin, R., Butzke, L. and Rodrigues, C.S. (1998) Incidence of diabetes mellitus in Passo Fundo, RS, Brazil. *Brazilian Journal of Medical and Biological Research*, **31** (12), 1553–6.

7. Carrasco, E., Pérez-Bravo, F., Dorman, J. *et al.* (2006) Increasing incidence of type 1 diabetes in population from Santiago of Chile: trends in a period of 18 years (1986–2003). *Diabetes-Metabolism Research and Reviews*, **22** (1), 34–7.

8. Carrasco, E., Pérez-Bravo, F., Santos, J.L., Lopes, G. (1996) One of the lowest validated incidence rates of insulin-dependent diabetes mellitus in the Américas: Santiago, Chile. *Diabetes Research and Clinical Practice*, **34** (Suppl 1), S153–7.

9. Seclen, S., Rojas, M.I., Nuñez, O. *et al.* (2000) Muy baja incidencia de diabetes mellitus tipo 1 (insulino

10. dependiente) en población infantil peruana: registro de 10 años (1985–1994) en el Proyecto DiaMond. *Reviews of ALAD*, **VIII** (3), 128–37.

11. Levy-Marchal, C., Papor, L., de Beaufort, C. *et al.* (1990) Incidence of juvenile type 1 (insulin-dependent) diabetes mellitus in France. *Diabetologia*, **33**, 465–9.

12. Serrano-Rios, M., Moy, C.S., Martin Serrano, M. *et al.* (1990) Incidence of type 1 (insulin-dependent) diabetes mellitus in subjects 0–14 years of age in Comunidad de Madrid, Spain. *Diabetologia*, **33**, 422–4.

13. Sorgini, M. and Muntoni, S. (1991) High incidence of type 1 diabetes in Sardinia. *Lancet*, **337**, 1047.

14. Fundação Instituto Brasileiro de Geografia e Estatística (1992) *IX Recenseamento Geral do Brasil–1980*, Vol. **1**, Book 4, IBGE, Rio de Janeiro, pp. 10–11.

15. Diabetes Epidemiology Research International Group (1988) Geographic patterns of childhood insulin-dependent diabetes mellitus. *Diabetes*, **37**, 1113–19.

16. Lima, L.P., Franco, L.J., Ferreira, S.R.G. and Vivolo, M.A. (1994) Estudo Brasileiro de Incidência de Diabetes: dados preliminares de 1991–93 (abstract). *Arquivos Brasileiros de Endocrinologia e Metabologia*, **38** (Suppl 2), 134.

17. Frazer de Llado, T., Hawk, B., Vasquez, J. *et al.* (1991) Incidence of youth-onset insulin-dependent diabetes mellitus in southern and western Puerto Rico (abstract). *Diabetes*, **40** (Suppl 1), 316A.

18. Barceló, A. and Rajpathak, S. (2001) Incidence and prevalence of diabetes mellitus in the Americas. *Pan American Journal of Public Health*, **10** (5), 300–8.

19. Gunczler, P., Lanes, R., Díaz, G.L. and Esaa, S. (1992) Presentation clinica y epidemiologia en el debut de la diabetes mellitus tipo I en Venezuela. *Archivos Venezoelanos Puericultura Pediatria*, **55** (1), 37–47.

20. World Health Organization (1985) *Report of WHO Study Group on Diabetes Mellitus. Diabetes Mellitus*, Technical Report Series 727, World Health Organization, Geneva.

21. Cardonnett, L.J., Nusimovich, B., Badano, H. *et al.* (1967) Epidemiologia de la diabetes: prevalencia en la poblacion urbana de la republica. *Revista Argentina de Endocrinología y Metabolismo*, **13**, 133–56.

22. Sereday, M., Di Toro, C.H., Correa, A. *et al.* (1979) Encuesta de prevalencia de diabetes: metodología y resultados. *Boletin de la Oficina Sanitaria Panamericana*, **86** (4), 293–305.

23. Hernandez, R.E., Cardonnet, L.J., Libman, C. and Gagliardino, J.J. (1987) Prevalence of diabetes

and obesity in an urban population of Argentina. *Diabetes Research and Clinical Practice*, **3**, 277–83.

23. Sereday, M.S., Gonzalez, C., Giorgini, D. *et al.* (2004) Prevalence of diabetes, obesity, hypertension and hyperlipidemia in the central area of Argentina. *Diabetes and Metabolism*, **30**, 335–9.

24. Barceló, A., Daroca, M.C., Ribera, R. *et al.* (2001) Diabetes in Bolivia. *Pan American Journal of Public Health*, **10** (5), 318–23.

25. Malerbi, D.A. and Franco, L.J. (1993) Multicenter study of the prevalence of diabetes mellitus and impaired glucose tolerance in the urban Brazilian population aged 30–69 yr. The Brazilian Cooperative Group on the Study of Diabetes Prevalence. *Diabetes Care*, **15**, 1509–15.

26. Torquato, M.T.C.G., Montenegro Junior, R.M., Viana, L.A.L. *et al.* (2003) Prevalence of diabetes mellitus and impaired glucose tolerance in the urban population aged 30–69 years in Ribeirão Preto (São Paulo), Brazil. *São Paulo Medical Journal*, **121** (6), 224–30.

27. Baruzzi, R. and Franco, L. (1981) Amerindians of Brazil, in *Western Diseases: Their Emergence and Prevention*, (eds H.C. Trowell and D.P. Burkitt), Edward Arnold, London.

28. Franco, L.J. (1994) Diabetes in Japanese-Brazilians: influence of the acculturation process. *Diabetes Research and Clinical Practice*, **24** (Suppl), S51–7.

29. Gimeno, S.G.A., Ferreira, S.R.G., Franco, L.J. *et al.* (2002) Prevalence and 7-year incidence of type 2 diabetes mellitus in a Japanese-Brazilian population: an alarming public health problem. *Diabetologia*, **45**, 1635–8.

30. Mella, I., Garcia de los Rios, M., Parker, M. and Covarrubias, A. (1983) Prevalencia de la diabetes mellitus. Una experiencia en grandes ciudades. *Boletin de la Oficina Sanitaria Panamericana*, **94** (2), 157–66.

31. Perez-Bravo, F., Carrasco, E., Santos, J.L. *et al.* (2001) Prevalence of type 2 diabetes and obesity in rural Mapuche population from Chile. *Nutrition*, **17** (3), 236–8.

32. Baechler, R., Mujica, V., Aqueveque, X. *et al.* (2002) Prevalencia de diabetes mellitus en la VII Región de Chile. *Revista Medica de Chile*, **130** (11), 1257–64.

33. Aschner, P., King, H., de Torrado, M.T. and Rodriguez, B.M. (1993) Glucose intolerance in Colombia: a population-based survey in an urban community. *Diabetes Care*, **16** (1), 90–3.

34. Jimenez, J.T., Palacios, M., Cañete, F. *et al.* (1998) Prevalence of diabetes mellitus and associated cardiovascular risk factors in an adult urban population in Paraguay. *Diabetic Medicine*, **15** (4), 334–8.

35. Seclén, S., Leey, J., Villena, A. *et al.* (1999) *Acta Medica Peruana*, **17** (1), 1–7.

36. West, K.W. and Kalbfleisch, J.M. (1966) Glucose tolerance, nutrition and diabetes in Uruguay, Venezuela, Malaysia and East Pakistan. *Diabetes*, **15**, 9–18.

37. Campos, H., Mata, L., Siles, X. *et al.* (1992) Prevalence of cardiovascular risk factors in rural and urban Costa Rica. *Circulation*, **85** (2), 648–58.

38. Hennis, A., Wu, S.Y., Nemesure, B. *et al.* (2002) Diabetes in a Caribbean population: epidemiological profile and implications. *International Journal of Epidemiology*, **31**, 234–9.

39. Sosa, M.K. and Szymula, C. (1992) Prevalencia de diabetes en poblacion urbana no seleccionada. *Revista de la Sociedad Argentina de Diabetes*, **26** (Suppl), 30.

40. WHO Consultation (1999) Definition, Diagnosis and Classification of the Diabetes Mellitus and its Complications, World Health Organization, Geneva.

41. Fundação Instituto Brasileiro de Geografia e Estatística (1985) *Anuário Estatístico do Rio de Janeiro*, Brasil.

42. King, H. and Zimmet, P. (1988) Trends in the prevalence and incidence of diabetes: non-insulin dependent diabetes mellitus. *World Health Statistics Quarterly*, **41**, 190–6.

43. King, H. and Rewers, M. (1993) Global estimates for prevalence of diabetes mellitus and impaired glucose tolerance in adults. WHO Ad Hoc Diabetes Reporting Group. *Diabetes Care*, **16** (1), 157–77.

44. Knowler, W.C., Bennett, P.H., Hamman, R.F. and Miller, M. (1978) Diabetes incidence and prevalence in Pima Indians: a 19-fold greater incidence than in Rochester, Minnesota. *American Journal of Epidemiology*, **108**, 497–505.

45. Iunes, M., Franco, L.J., Wakisaka, K. *et al.* (1994) Self-reported of non-insulin-dependent diabetes mellitus in the first and second-generation of Japanese-Brazilians over 40 years of age. *Diabetes Research and Clinical Practice*, **24** (Suppl), S53–7.

46. Fujimoto, W.Y., Leonetti, D.L., Kinyoun, J.L. *et al.* (1987) Prevalence of diabetes mellitus and impaired glucose tolerance among second generation Japanese American men. *Diabetes*, **36**, 721–9.

47. Canessa, I., Valiente, S., Jaramillo, J. *et al.* (1960) Encuesta de morbidad diabética. *Revista Medica de Chile*, **88**, 22.

48. National Diabetes Data Group (1979) Classification and diagnosis of diabetes mellitus and other categories of glucose intolerance. *Diabetes*, **28**, 1039–57.

49. Aguilar Salinas, C.A., Rojas, R., Gómez-Pérez, F.J. *et al.* (2002) Early onset type 2 diabetes in Mexico. *American Journal of Medicine*, **113**, 569–74.

50. Gonzalez Villalpando, C. (1989) Estado del arte de la diabetes en México. *Anuario Médico de la Asociacion Médica HABC*, **34** (4), 187–201.

51. Posadas-Romero, C., Yamamoto-Kimura, L., Lerman-Garber, I. *et al.* (1944) The prevalence of NIDDM and associated coronary risk factors in México City. *Diabetes Care*, **17** (12), 1441–8.

52. Meigs, J., Williams, K., Sullivan, L. *et al.* (2004) Using metabolic syndrome traits for efficient detection of impaired glucose tolerance. *Diabetes Care*, **27**, 1417–26.

53. Aguilar Salinas, C.A., Rojas, R., Gómez-Pérez, F.J. *et al.* (2002) Early onset type 2 diabetes in Mexico. *American Journal of Medicine*, **113**, 569–74.

54. Aguilar Salinas, C.A., Velasquez, M.O., Gómez-Pérez, F.J. *et al.* (2003) Characteristics of the patients with type 2 diabetes in Mexico: results from a large population-based, nation-wide survey. *Diabetes Care*, **26**, 2021–6.

55. Rull, J.A., Aguilar-Salinas, C.A., Rojas, R. *et al.* (2005) Epidemiology of type 2 diabetes in México. *Archives of Medical Research*, **36**, 188–96.

56. Jiménez, J.T., Palacios, C.M., Cañete, F. *et al.* (1992) Prevalencia de diabetes e intolerancia a la glucosa en Asuncion y area metropolitana (abstract). *Revista de la Sociedad Argentina de Diabetes*, **26**, 14.

57. Zubiate, M., Valdivia, F., Diaz, E. *et al.* (1992) Diabetes mellitus, intolerancia a la glucosa, obesidad, hipertension arterial y antecedentes familiares de diabetes en la poblacion de Lima (abstract). *Revista de la Sociedad Argentina de Diabetes*, **26**, 14.

58. Poon-King, T. and Henry, M.V. (1968) Prevalence and natural history of diabetes in Trinidad. *Lancet*, **i**, 155–63.

59. West, K.M. (1978) *Epidemiology of Diabetes and its Vascular Lesions*, Elsevier, New York.

60. Pan American Health Organization (2007) Health Statisticas from the Americas. The Leading Causes of Death in Selected Countries of the Americas, 2006 edn. Available in: http://www.paho.prg (accessed 18 May 2007).

61. Morice, A., Roselló, M., Arauz, A.G. *et al.* (1999) *Diabetes mellitus in Costa Rica*, Serie de Documentos Tecnicos, INCIENSA, San José.

62. International Diabetes Federation (2006) *Diabetes Atlas*, 3rd edn. Diabetes Atlas Committee, International Diabetes Federation, Brussels, Belgium.

63. Cusumano, A., Garcia-Garcia, G., Di Gioia, C. *et al.* (2006) End stage renal disease and its treatment in Latin-America in the twenty-first century. *Renal Failure*, **28** (8), 631–7.

64. Gagliardino, J.J., de la Hera, M., Siri, F. and QUALIDIAB Group (2001) Evaluación de la calidad de la asistencia al paciente diabético en América Latina. *Pan-American Journal of Public Health*, **10** (5), 309–17.

65. Spichler, E.R.S., Spichler, D., Lessa, I. *et al.* (2001) Capture–recapture method to estimate lower extremity amputation rates in Rio de Janeiro, Brazil. *Pan-American Journal of Public Health*, **10** (5), 334–40.

66. Walsh, M.G., Zgibor, J., Borch-Johnsen, K. and Orchard, T.J. (2006) A multinational assessment of complications in type 1 diabetes: the DiaMond substudy of complications (DiaComp) level 1. *Diabetes and Vascular Disease Research*, **3** (2), 84–92.

67. Barceló, A., Aedo, C., Rajpathak, S. and Robles, S. (2003) The cost of diabetes in Latin America and the Carribbean. *Bulletin of the World Health Organization*, **81** (1), 19–27.

Further Reading

Rewers, M., LaPorte, R., King, H. and Tuomilehto, J. Epidemiology Research International Study Group (1988) Trends in incidence of diabetes: insulin-dependent diabetes in childhood. *World Health Statistics Quarterly*, **41**, 179–89.

13

Diabetes in the Caribbean . . . an Epidemiological Review!

Errol Morrison and Dalip Ragoobirsingh

Departments of Biochemistry and Diabetology, The University of the West Indies, Mona Campus, Jamaica

13.1 INTRODUCTION

The Caribbean in this discussion will include all those island territories nestled between North and South America and whose shores are washed by the Caribbean Sea. This will embrace the French: Haiti, Martinique, Guadeloupe, St Martin; the Dutch: Aruba, the Netherlands Antilles, Suriname; the Hispanic territories of Cuba and the Dominican Republic, but not Puerto Rico; the Anglophones: Jamaica, Cayman, Belize, Bahamas, Antigua, St Kitts and Nevis, Montserrat, British Virgin Islands, Anguilla, Dominica, St Lucia, Guyana, Grenada, St Vincent and the Grenadines, Barbados, Trinidad and Tobago, Turks and Caicos. All this represents some 35 million persons, the demographics of which are as illustrated in **Table 13.1**.

Economically, these are low- to middle-income countries. The common factor linking all of these Caribbean peoples, irrespective of their lingua franca, is their miscegenation, with the predominance of the African phenotype, ranging from least of all in the Hispanic groups to a significant majority in the Anglophones.

This, then, suggests a pervading presence of the 'thrifty gene(s),' which is purported to have been life-protective during the adverse conditions and deprivations of the transatlantic passage of our forebears. The relative sufficiency of food in more recent times has thus come to haunt this population, as the once needed thriftiness in conservation of salt, sugar and water now turns to a predisposition to the chronic diseases, most notably obesity, diabetes and hypertension.

In addition, the cultural norms as reported by Henry [1] point to a lifestyle acceptance that favors development of overweight. Some selected results are as follows:

- On obesity, size was an important determinant of perceived beauty and social adequacy.
- In no country was slimness quoted as ideal, though there were individuals who aspired to attain or maintain slimness.
- Men were far less concerned about their size than women, who saw overweight as a result of childbearing, late-night eating, contraceptive usage and so on.
- Fruit and vegetable intake were restricted and not seen as best value for money. Hence, there is an increase in consumption of more energy-dense foods, leading to obesity.

The media has impacted North American norms on the Caribbean region, affecting perceptions, attitudes, values and lifestyles in both adults and youth.

The prevalences of diabetes mellitus and impaired glucose tolerance in the Caribbean are shown in **Table 13.2**.

Type 2 diabetes mellitus accounts for some 97.5% of all cases, and translates to some 1.5 million. Associated with diabetes are some 21 000 deaths annually with an estimated 70 000 years of productive life lost. (Adapted from Barcelo *et al* [2].)

The Epidemiology of Diabetes Mellitus, second edition Edited by Jean-Marie Ekoé, Marian Rewers, Rhys Williams and Paul Zimmet
© 2008 John Wiley & Sons, Ltd

Table 13.1 The demographics of diabetes mellitus in the Caribbean.

Country (20–79 years)	Population (×000s)	Ethnicity	Health expenditure per capita US$	Infant mortality per 1000 live births	Life expectancy (F/M)
French					
Haiti	4113	B	21	79	55/46
Martinique	265	B	—	—	—
Guadeloupe	289	B	—	—	—
Dutch					
Aruba	43	O	—	—	—
Netherlands Antilles	—	O	—	—	—
Suriname	251	O	—	26	71/64
Hispanic					
Cuba	7980	H	169	7	79/75
Dominican Republic	4991	H	151	41	71/64
Anglophone					
Anguilla	8	B	—	—	—
Antigua and Barbuda	41	B	179	12	74/69
Bahamas	193	B	612	13	75/69
Barbados	189	B	601	12	78/71
Belize	124	O	82	34	73/68
British Virgin Islands	13	B	—	—	—
Cayman Islands	22	B	—	—	—
Dominica (Commonwealth of)	42	B	208	14	71/64
Grenada	54	B	193	20	69/66
Guyana	457	B/I	51	54	67/61
Jamaica	1528	B	165	17	75/71
St Kitts and Nevis	23	B	408	20	73/69
St Lucia	101	B	151	17	73/70
St Vincent and the Grenadines	71	B	2	22	73/68
Trinidad and Tobago	861	B/I	204	17	73/67

Ethnicity, predominant racial characteristic: B, Black; I, East Indian; H, Hispanic; O, other.

13.2 SOME RELATED HEALTH ISSUES

In general, the epidemiological data required for an accurate description of trends in mortality and causal risk factors at a national level are not available in these poor and developing territories in the Caribbean. Thus, in an effort to surmount the paucity of information, there is an increasing tendency to pool and share resources. This works well for most of the Caribbean, given that the population in most territories is of predominantly African descent. The foods consumed and the culture are similarly influenced by the ethnic dominance. Thus, the health studies conducted in one island, very often the larger ones, such as Jamaica, Barbados and Trinidad and Tobago of the Anglophone Caribbean and Cuba of the non-Anglophone group, can be extrapolated.

In Guyana, Suriname and Trinidad, where there is a larger East Indian population, the trends would be comparable.

Prevalence of type 2 diabetes mellitus among the populations of the African diaspora has been extensively studied by Cooper *et al.* [4], Cruickshank

Table 13.2 Diabetes mellitus and impaired glucose tolerance prevalence. (Adapted from the International Diabetes Federation[2]).

Country (20–79 years)	Prevalence (%)	
	DM[a]	IGT[a]
Anguilla	5.5	11.3
Antigua and Barbuda	5.8	11.3
Aruba	9.7	11.3
Bahamas	9.0	10.7
Barbados	8.5	11.6
Belize	5.7	9.8
Bermuda	9.7	11.3
British Virgin Islands	8.3	11.3
Cayman Islands	9.7	11.3
Dominica (Commonwealth of)	8.4	11.3
Grenada	6.8	11.3
Guyana	6.0	10.2
Haiti	5.7	10.0
Jamaica	17.9	10.8
St Kitts and Nevis	6.6	11.3
St Lucia	6.2	10.7
St Vincent and the Grenadines	7.7	11.3
Trinidad and Tobago	7.9	11.1
French Departments: Martinique/Guadeloupe	6.5/6.5	12.2/11.9
Cuba	13.2	12.2
Dominican Republic	10.0	10.4
Netherlands Antilles	12.3	12.3
Suriname	8.6	7.1

[a]DM: diabetes mellitus; IGT: impaired glucose tolerance.

et al. [5] and Hennis et al. [6] and all have found similar rates.

Hypertension is also prevalent and an important risk factor for cardiovascular-related morbidity and mortality. The Jamaican study by Ragoobirsingh et al. [7] reported 31% prevalence of hypertension, and this may be due in part to the more than 95% of the population being Afro-Caribbean (i.e. predominantly African, the evident miscegenation notwithstanding). A similar finding was reported in a Cuban study [8]. Here again, Grim and Wilson [9] have postulated that the evolutionary outcome of Africans living in a salt-deprived environment while under the yoke of the many vagaries of slavery subsequently manifested itself physiologically as an enhanced genetic expression of a salt-retaining system with resulting higher propensity for developing hypertension.

In addition, Fray [10] pointed out that not only are Afro-descendants more likely to develop hypertension, but also the disorder appears at an earlier age and is more likely to be fatal compared with Caucasian counterparts.

The primacy of ethnicity and/or polygenic susceptibility is even more pronounced when looking at the data from Suriname, which has a large East Indian population alongside its Afro-descendant groups. The Qualiform project, which lasted from February 2003 to March 2006, reported that 64% of the diabetic population studied was hypertensive, 31% was obese and 42% was hypercholesterolemic; in all of the groupings, Afro-descendants predominated [11].

Cardiovascular disease is the most common cause of death in developed countries. So, too, is it in the Caribbean.

A 20-year follow-up study in the island of Tobago reported significantly higher mortality related to hypercholesterolemia, cardiomegaly, diabetes, hypertension and alcoholism [12].

Studies in Trinidad and the Bahamas on patients with acute myocardial infarction revealed 55% diabetic, 49% hypertensive, 30% smokers and 59% hyperlipidemic [12].

Cuba, the largest of the Caribbean islands, has been reporting heart disease as the leading cause of death since 1970, and the major associated risks were hypertension, hypercholesterolemia, obesity, diabetes and physical inactivity.

13.3 DIABETES AND OBESITY

Obesity is higher amongst the lower socioeconomic and educational groups. It is the single most important factor in the development of diabetes mellitus, as well as an aggravating influence on the progress of complications. It seems to be related more to the lifestyles than to any underlying genetic predisposition. The recent dramatic rises in the rates of obesity in the same genetic pool in the region suggest that it is more related to lifestyle than to biological factors. The World Health Organization (WHO) emphasizes that the obesity epidemic stems from an environment that promotes sedentary lifestyles and consumption of high-fat, energy-dense diets [10]. Socioeconomic factors are important here, as the poor eat more bread, pasta and fatty cuts of meat and less vegetables, nuts, grains and fruits. This pattern reflects a higher satisfaction with a greater satiety effect at lower costs. Studies

indicate that the higher carbohydrate and fat content reduces costs by 31.78% per food basket [1].

In addition to the eating patterns, the increase in sedentariness contributes to the overweight and obesity data. Throughout the Caribbean region, the populations are ageing more rapidly and there is increasing migration to urban areas. A definition of sedentary lifestyle has been offered by Pena and Bacallao [13], wherein this status is said to be present when individuals do not engage in continuous uninterrupted physical activity of at least 15 min duration at least twice per week. The adverse social environment, such as crime and violence, in many of these communities discourages walking, jogging, biking and other outdoor activities, further predisposing to sedentariness and consequent weight gain.

Obesity, defined as $>30 \, \text{kg m}^{-2}$ (weight/height), is noted to be on the increase in the Caribbean region, with some territories, such as Jamaica, reporting a 36.6% prevalence; and this is accompanied with high waist/hip ratios approaching >1. This is seen especially in those populations with a predominance of African heritage, where this type of fat distribution is indicative of high levels of perivisceral fat, which is correlative with increased chronic maladies such as heart disease, type 2 diabetes and hypertension.

Nutritional status will undoubtedly impact on the intrauterine growth retardation (IUGR) figures. In a report from the WHO in 2003, [3] doubts are expressed as to whether IUGR in developing countries portends similar increased outcomes for diseases such as diabetes and hypertension as it

Table 13.3 Cost (US$ $\times$ 10^6) of diabetes in year 2000.

Country	Total cost	Indirect cost	Direct cost
Anglophone			
Bahamas	148.80	138.10	10.70
Barbados	151.20	138.40	12.80
Guyana	36.30	15.90	20.40
Jamaica	409.50	273.40	136.10
Trinidad and Tobago	284.50	246.50	38.00
Other			
Cuba	1346.60	624.40	722.20
Dominican Republic	625.10	399.40	225.70
Haiti	78.70	30.70	48.00
Overall cost	3080.70	1866.80	1179.70

Table 13.4 Comparative costs of Diabetes mellitus in the Caribbean.

	Cuba/Dominican Republic/Haiti	English Caribbean	Total	
Medication				
No. of persons taking insulin ($\times 10^3$)	64.5	21.1	85.6	
No. of persons taking oral drugs ($\times 10^3$)	725.4	249.4	974.8	
Cost of insulin (US$ $\times 10^6$)	159.5	30		189.5
Cost of oral drugs (US$ $\times 10^6$)	416.4	122.9		539.3
Hospitalization				
Related to diabetes mellitus ($\times 10^3$)	93.2	22.1	115.3	
Duration of stay (days)	248 189	62 352	310 541	
Cost (US$ $\times 10^6$)	17.6	2.8		20.4
Consultations				
Related to diabetes ($\times 10^3$)	3 369.7	154.2	2 523.9	
Costs (US$ $\times 10^6$)	84.2	3.9		88.1
Complications				
No. of persons with retinopathy ($\times 10^3$)	116.0	39.7	155.7	
Cost of retinopathy (US$ $\times 10^6$)	13.8	4.9		18.7
No. of persons with cardiovascular disease ($\times 10^3$)	113.7	39.0	152.7	
Costs (US$ $\times 10^6$)	12.5	4.4		16.9
No. of persons with nephropathy ($\times 10^3$)	49.1	16.8	65.9	
Costs (US$ $\times 10^6$)	94.9	33.8		128.7
No. of persons with neuropathy ($\times 10^3$)	72.1	24.7	96.8	
Costs (US$ $\times 10^6$)	4.2	1.5		5.7
No. of persons with peripheral vascular disease ($\times 10^3$)	46.9	16.1	63.0	
Cost (US$ $\times 10^6$)	3.3	1.1		4.4
Total cost (direct) US$ $\times 10^6$				1 011.7

Adapted from Barcelo, A., *et al.*, WHO, 2003.

does in developed countries. Studies are yet to determine the data on this possible correlation for the Caribbean.

Despite the general reduction in the prevalence of protein-energy malnutrition in the region, some 11% of children under age 5 years are low in weight-for-age. Further, there is a low height-for-age, which is the frequent hallmark of nutritional deficiency [13]. These situations are associated with the development of malnutrition-related diabetes mellitus [14]. Nevertheless, diabetes is uncommon in the young, and studies still emphasize the over-15 age group. However, the increasing overweight and obesity being witnessed in the populations of the region are being paralleled by an increase in the appearance of type 2 diabetes in adolescence and the very young.

13.4 ATYPICAL DIABETES

An unusual clinical pattern of diabetes mellitus, called *J-type*, was first described in adolescents in Jamaica in 1955 by Hugh Jones [15], and was seen in severe protein-energy malnutrition. A forme frustes was further described in 1981 by Morrison [16], who pointed out that micronutrient deficiency was sufficient to predispose to its development. This clinical syndrome was characterized by hyperglycemia, aglycosuria and tolerance of very high blood sugar levels without even complaints of malaise. Further, to maintain normoglycemia, intermittent insulin administration was required. During the insulin-treated phase, high doses were necessary, which is indicative of insulin resistance. During the noninsulin-requiring phase, ketosis did not develop to any significant degree.

Abdominal pain was often reported, and ultrasound examination detected hyperechoic areas in the pancreas that were indicative of some earlier insult. These patients typically gave a history of childhood or adolescent undernutrition and had low body mass indices $<19 \, \text{kg m}^{-2}$.

This syndrome, named phasic insulin-dependent diabetes mellitus, is seen mainly in tropical countries, such as in the Caribbean, where root crops are the staple diet and bush-tea drinking a popular folklore.

An important aspect of this group, which constitutes some 13% of the patients attending the diabetes clinic at the university hospital in Kingston,

Jamaica, is that they go on quite rapidly to develop renal failure. It should be noted that end-stage renal failure is a leading cause of death in our diabetic patients, and the reported incidence is 1000 per million population per year.

13.5 THE BURDEN OF DIABETES MELLITUS IN THE CARIBBEAN

The burden of diabetes mellitus is best described as the costs, the morbidity and mortality attendant on the disease. Costs can be further categorized into direct and indirect. An estimate of costs in a few selected countries of the region is presented in **Table 13.3**.

Direct costs include those of drugs, hospitalizations, consultations and management of complications. Indirect costs relate more to human capital and include loss of earnings for diabetic persons and their support groups, absenteeism, disability and premature death. In the Caribbean region, persons with diabetes have limited access to health care, which implies that indirect costs could exceed direct health care costs in some situations.

Table 13.4 attempts to outline the burden of costs of this condition, using a sampling from the Hispanic, Haitian and some Anglophone countries.

13.6 ACKNOWLEDGMENTS

We wish to recognize the contributions from colleagues throughout the region; to name a few: Oscar Jordan, Michael Boyne, Godfrey Xuereb, James Mills and Rachel Irving.

References

1. Henry, F. (2004) *Public Policies to Control Obesity in the Caribbean, Prepared for the Caribbean Commission for Health and Development*, Caribbean Food and Nutrition Institute, PAHO, Kingston, Jamaica.
2. International Diabetes Federation (2003) *Diabetes Atlas*, 2nd edn, International Diabetes Federation, Brussels.
3. Barcelo, A., Aedo, C., Rajpathak, S. and Robles, S. (2003) The cost of diabetes in Latin America and the Caribbean. *Bulletin of the World Health Organization*, **81** (1), 19–27.
4. Cooper, R.S., Rotimi, C.N., Kaufman, J.S. *et al.* (1997) Prevalence of NIDDM among populations

of the African diaspora. *Diabetes Care*, **20** (3), 343–8.

5. Cruickshank, J., Mbanya, J., Wilks, R. *et al.* (2001) Sick genes, sick individuals, sick populations with chronic disease? The emergence of diabetes and high blood pressure in African-origin populations. *International Journal of Epidemiology*, **30**, 111–17.

6. Hennis, A., Wu, S.Y., Nemensure, B. *et al.* (2002) Diabetes in a Caribbean population; epidemiological profile and implications. *International Journal of Epidemiology*, **31**, 234–9.

7. Ragoobirsingh, D., McGrowder, D., Morrison, E. *et al.* (2002) The Jamaican hypertension prevalence study. *Journal of the National Medical Association*, **94** (7), 561–5.

8. Cooper, R.S., Ordunez, P., Ferrer, M. *et al.* (2006) Cardiovascular disease and associated risk factors in Cuba: prospects for prevention and control. *American Journal of Public Health*, **96** (1), 94–101.

9. Grim, C.E. and Wilson, T.W. (1992) Salt, slavery and survival: physiological principles underlying the evolutionary hypothesis of salt sensitivity hypertension in Western hemisphere blacks, in *Pathophysiology of Hypertension in Blacks* (eds J.C.S. Fray and J.G. Douglas), Oxford University Press, New York.

10. Fray, J.C.S. (1993) Hypertension in blacks: physiological, psychosocial, theoretical, and therapeutic challenges, in *Pathophysiology of Hypertension in Blacks* (eds J.C.S. Fray and J.G. Douglas), Oxford University Press, New York, pp. 3–32.

11. Ragoobirsingh, D. and Barcelo, A. (2006) PAHO Site Visit Report, March 16–18, Suriname.

12. Thomas, C. (2005) Coronary artery disease – the reasons, in *Health Issues in the Caribbean* (ed O. Morgan), Ian Randle Publishers, Kingston, Jamaica, pp. 128–30.

13. Pena, M. and Bacallao, J. (eds) (2000) *Obesity and Poverty, A New Public Health Challenge*, Scientific Publication No. 576. Pan American Health Organisation (PAHO), Washington, DC.

14. Morrison, E.Y.St.A., Ragoobirsingh, D., Thompson, H., *et al.* (1995) Phasic insulin dependent diabetes mellitus: manifestations and cellular mechanisms. *The Journal of Clinical Endocrinology and Metabolism*, **80** (7), 1996–2001.

15. Jones, H. (1955) Diabetes in Jamaica. *The Lancet*, **269** (6896), 891–7.

16. Morrison, E.Y.St.A. and Richards, R. (1985) Clinical profile of diabetes mellitus in Jamaica (phasic insulin dependence). *West Indian Medical Journal*, **34**, 96–7.

Further Reading

McDougall, L. (2002) Trends in diabetes mortality in the Caribbean: 1981–1995. *CAREC Survelliance Report*, **22** (2), 1–6.

Miller, G.J., Kirkwood, B.R., Beckles, G.I.A. *et al.* (1988) Adult male all-cause cardiovascular and cerebrovascular mortality in relation to ethnic group, systolic blood pressure and blood glucose concentration in Trinidad, West Indies. *International Journal of Epidemiology*, **17**, 62–9.

14

Japan

Naoko Tajima

Division of Diabetes, Metabolism and Endocrinology, Department of Medicine,
Jikei University School of Medicine, Tokyo, Japan

14.1 INTRODUCTION

A drastic change in the eating behavior, together with an imbalance in the proportion of nutrients, and the sedentary lifestyle that has occurred over the past 60 years has made the Japanese Archipelago an 'islands of diabetes'. The International Diabetes Federation has reported that the total number of individuals with diabetes in Japan was estimated to be 6.8 million and the prevalence as 6.9% in 2003 [1]. The westernized lifestyle, which the Japanese people had never experienced in the 2000 years of Japanese history, has changed the disease structure of its society.

The Japanese government considered the situation seriously, and the Ministry of Health, Labor and Welfare initiated the government project 'Healthy Japan 21' in 2000, which will be finally assessed in 2010. To take appropriate measures against diabetes is one of the top priorities in this project. The numerical targets include: (i) number of persons with diabetes: 10 million (estimated as 10.8 million); (ii) continuous treatment rate, 30–100%. Other major activities include the National Diabetes Survey (1997, 2002 and 2010), the establishment of the Committee of Antidiabetes Promotion and the Japan Diabetes Outcome Intervention Trial (J-DOIT) 1, 2, 3.

14.2 INCIDENCE AND PREVALENCE STUDY

14.2.1 Type 1 Diabetes

14.2.1.1 Overall and Age-specific Incidence

Type 1 diabetes is one of the most important chronic diseases among children, yet its nationwide incidence in Japan had not been clarified until the past decade. The Diabetes Study Group of the Ministry of Health and Welfare reported the mean incidence rate as 1.5 per 100 000 for nine areas with no discernible pattern from the north to the south [2]. The most reliable data were reported from three areas that included Hokkaido, Tokyo and Kagoshima, with a total population of 3.6 million [3]; the degree of case ascertainment was more than 95% and demonstrated that the overall incidence rates for children 0–14 years of age during 1985–1989 were 2.07, 1.65 and 1.78 per 100 000 respectively, with a peak incidence seen in the 10–14 years age group and with a predominance of developing type 1 diabetes in females (male/female ratio: 0.7).

The Hokkaido Registry demonstrated a slight, but significant, increase in incidence during 1973 and 1992 (1973–1977: 0.90 per 100 000; 1978–1982: 1.57 per 100 000; 1983–1987: 1.92 per 100 000; 1988–1992: 2.28 per 100 000) [4]. The rates are quite low compared with those in Caucasian children. There are no published data that demonstrate the secular increase of type 1 diabetes thereafter.

14.2.1.2 Prevalence

Hososako and Matsuyama [5] first reported type 1 diabetes prevalence in Japan in 1964. They conducted a survey on childhood diabetes among the families of a large industrial company in Kita-Kyushu-city and found four type 1 diabetes cases among 40 000 children aged 0–14 years. Since then, several studies have been done mainly using a questionnaire survey at schools and the prevalence

The Epidemiology of Diabetes Mellitus, second edition   Edited by Jean-Marie Ekoé, Marian Rewers, Rhys Williams and Paul Zimmet
© 2008 John Wiley & Sons, Ltd

data of type 1 diabetes have been accumulated [6, 7]. The data obtained are quite consistent with approximately 10 per 100 000 population.

The Central Registry for Free Medical Care, launched in 1974 and sponsored by the Ministry of Health and Welfare, Government of Japan, is the another good source for estimating the prevalence of type 1 diabetes, in which the number of newly diagnosed diabetic children aged 0–17 years are registered annually. Because of the nature of this system, the degree of case ascertainment is estimated to be more than 95%. Through the distribution of this system, the number of patients receiving its benefit has increased gradually, and the calculated prevalence was reported to be 2.38 per 10 000 in 1994 [8]. The prevalence rate obtained from the registry is almost twice as high as those seen in the previous studies; however, this should be treated with caution due to the possible inclusion of type 2 diabetes among children, which will be discussed later in this chapter.

14.2.1.3 Clinical Characteristics at Diagnosis of Type 1 Diabetes

Japanese children may develop type 1 diabetes gradually. It has been reported that a large number of patients have been diagnosed as having type 1 diabetes by urine glucose screening at schools without showing any distinct symptoms. At Nihon University Hospital, Tokyo, out of 88 type 1 diabetes children diagnosed during 1974–1991, 55 had an abrupt onset with severe clinical symptoms but 33 had minimal or no clinical symptoms at diagnosis. Obesity was not seen in either of the groups, but the clinical features were different. Figures for type 1 diabetes with an abrupt onset are: (i) mean onset age of 8.8 ± 4.5 years old; (ii) male/female of 28/27; (iii) HbA_{1c} level of 9.88 $\pm 3.66\%$; and (iv) a high prevalence of positive islet cell antibodies (ICAs) at onset (83%) with rapid decline. In contrast, type 1 diabetes patients with slow onset show: (i) older mean onset age of 11.9 ± 3.1 years old ($p < 0.05$); (ii) male/female of 9/24; (iii) HbA_{1c} level of $7.05 \pm 1.49\%$ ($p < 0.05$); and (iv) a lower prevalence of positive ICAs at onset (62%, $p < 0.05$) with gradual decline. Moreover, type 1 diabetes with an abrupt onset had significantly lower 2 h postprandial C-peptide levels and higher daily insulin dosage for at least 10 years after the onset [9]

The genetic background between the two is slightly different. Human leukocyte antigen (HLA) DR9 and DR4 are significantly more common in the abrupt onset group than in the slow onset group [10]. Therefore, the two different type 1 diabetes groups seen among the Japanese children cannot be explained by the different timing of diagnosis; for example, the appearance of slow onset type 1 diabetes due to early detection of type 1 diabetes by urine glucose screening at schools. A similar group of type 1 diabetes is also seen in adults, as demonstrated by Kobayashi and co-workers. According to their studies, slowly progressive type 1 diabetes is characterized by slow progression of β-cell failure with persistent positive low-titer ICA, frequent involvement of exocrine pancreas, positive family history of type 2 diabetes, association with HLA-DQAl *0301-DQBl *0401, and a lack of association with HLA-A24 [11], which indicates the complete destruction of the pancreatic β-cells [12].

14.2.1.4 Type 1 Diabetes Incidence/Prevalence in Adults

Little information is available regarding the incidence and prevalence of type 1 diabetes after the age of 20 years. An attempt to estimate the prevalence of type 1 diabetes using the capture–recapture method was first conducted in Kakogawa City with a 234 249 adult population [13]. Several independent sources, such as hospital records, lists of the diabetic patients at the local diabetes association and personal health data on the medical information network system, were used for the capture–recapture method and the accuracy of diagnosis was confirmed by physicians. The prevalence of type 1 diabetes obtained in 1994 was estimated to be 1.75 per 10 000. As the sample size is small and the data are still premature, further nationwide study is warranted.

14.2.2 Type 2 Diabetes
14.2.2.1 Prevalence
Population-based studies on type 2 diabetes prevalence have been conducted in Japan since the early 1960s. They have provided invaluable information on the extent of diabetes, however, in the early studies; people were first screened by urine glucose tests and then further evaluated by an oral glucose tolerance test (OGTT). The prevalence of type 2

diabetes in the population aged 40 years or older is reported to be 1.3–4.7% in those studies [14].

After 1985, a type 2 diabetes prevalence study using the World Health Organization (WHO) criteria became popular and the figures obtained were 6.8 ± 11.7%, which is much higher than the number seen in the earlier literature [2]. In the population-based settings, the report from Funagata-machi, Yamagata Prefecture, demonstrated that the prevalence rate among adults in 1991–1992 was 10.5% for males and 12.9% for females [15]. Similarly, the age-adjusted type 2 diabetes prevalence rates in males and females reported from Hisayama-cho, Fukuoka Prefecture, in 1988 were 12.8% and 8.4% respectively [16].

In 1997 and 2002, the National Diabetes Survey was conducted by the Ministry of Health, Labor and Welfare [17]. All of Japan has been divided by the survey units using the stratified cluster random sampling method. Approximately 500 units were randomly selected at first, and then each unit was geographically divided into 300 units. The whole households within each unit were invited to participate in the National Health and Nutrition Survey. Known diabetics on oral hypoglycemic agent (OHA)/insulin or persons with $HbA_{1c} > 6.1\%$ were classified as having 'diabetes' and those with $5.6 \leq HbA_{1c} < 6.1\%$ were classified as having 'possible diabetes' (or prediabetes).

In the 2002 survey, a total of 10 067 people aged 20 years and older had participated in the study. Of those, 5792 were subject to blood testing. The prevalence of 'diabetes' and 'possible diabetes' were 9.0% and 10.6% respectively. Under the assumption that these prevalence rates can be extrapolated to the general Japanese population, the number of people with type 2 diabetes counts approximately 7.4 million and prediabetes as 8.8 million. People with diabetes, including those who have not yet been diagnosed, increased to over 2.5 million in the previous 5 years. The respective figures were 6.9 million and 6.8 million in the 1997 survey.

14.2.2.2 Epidemiology of Type 2 Diabetes among Children

The annual change in the incidence rates of childhood type 2 diabetes for the years 1974–2002 in the Tokyo metropolitan area has been reported [9, 18]. A total of 8 812 356 school children aged 6–15 years old (primary and junior high

school) participated in the urine glucose-screening program at schools. Participation rate was almost 100% and the diagnosis of diabetes was made by OGTT (WHO criteria), which was performed on those whose urine glucose showed positive. During that period, a total of 232 school children were diagnosed as having type 2 diabetes, giving an overall incidence rate of 2.63 per 100 000. It appears that an approximately 1.6-fold increase of type 2 diabetes was observed during 1981–2002 (2.76 per 100 000) compared with 1974–1980 (1.73 per 100 000), which is associated with an increase in the prevalence of obesity among schoolchildren. The rate was significantly higher in junior high-school students than in primary-school students (0.78 per 100 000 versus 6.43 per 100 000). The data also demonstrate that 83.4% were overweight (≥20% overweight), and the degree of obesity were markedly high in boys [18]. Westernization of their diet, decrease in physical activities and the mental stress which has occurred in society appear to have influenced the disease structure of Japanese children.

14.2.2.3 Characteristics of Type 2 Diabetes Children at Onset

Owada *et al.* [19] have examined the detailed clinical features of 180 patients with type 2 diabetes detected by urine glucose screening program for the year 1974–1995 and found that 67 or 87% were diagnosed after 12 years of age. The youngest child was age 6 and had a delayed mental development. Other characteristics of type 2 diabetes can be summarized as: (i) the prevalence rate increases according to age; (ii) the male/female ratio is 0.75; (iii) obesity over ideal bodyweight of more than 140% is 68.8% in males and 34.9% in females; (iv) hyperinsulinemia; and (v) a high prevalence of family history of diabetes. As the majority of the cases with type 2 diabetes are asymptomatic, compliance was poor and resulted in a high rate of dropouts. They often returned to hospital with advanced complications. Early detection and constant care for type 2 diabetes children, therefore, is a critical problem.

14.2.2.4 Risk Factors for Developing Type 2 Diabetes

Nutritional factors are perceived as a potent risk factor playing a predominant role in the increase of type 2 diabetes in Japan. Indirect evidence has been provided by studies on the Japanese American population, where the prevalence of type 2 diabetes is almost twice as high as that seen in the Japanese in Japan [20, 21]. Hara *et al.* [21] demonstrated that the total caloric intake in these two populations was similar; however, consumption of animal fat and refined carbohydrate was at least twice as high in the Hawaiian Japanese as in the Japanese in Hiroshima. The estimated level of physical activity was significantly reduced in Hawaiian subjects when compared with their counterparts in Hiroshima. A westernized diet coupled with reduced physical activity may foster the development of obesity and insulin resistance [22] and could be partially responsible for the higher prevalence of diabetes among Japanese-nisei in the United States. Such dietary and physical factors may also operate within Japan and should be taken into account as possible causative factors implicated in the increase of type 2 diabetes in Japan.

Besides dietary factors, a family history of diabetes, a plasma glucose level of more than $180 \, mg \, dl^{-1}$ at 120 min after a 75 g oral glucose loading, the low initial response of insulin during OGTT [23, 24], the sum of insulin concentration during OGTT, serum triglycerides, body mass index, waist/hip ratio and blood pressure levels [25] are the possible risk factors for type 2 diabetes among Japanese.

14.2.2.5 *National Strategic Research Project: J-DOIT 1, 2, 3*

It can easily be assumed that the increase in type 2 diabetes patients will result in an increase in patients with macro- and micro-vascular complications and an explosion of medical care costs, leading to a burden on society. From the public health and epidemiological perspectives, an intervention in the population with impaired glucose tolerance (IGT) as well as those with type 2 diabetes is urgently needed for the prevention of diabetes and its complications. The Japanese government, therefore, has launched a large national strategic research project named J-DOIT 1, 2, 3 [26]. It is a 5-year large-scale project and is supported by the national fund of approximately ¥4 billion ($4 million) from the budget of the Ministry of Health, Labor and Welfare. The aim of J-DOIT 1 is primary prevention of type 2 diabetes. A 50%

reduction in the conversion rate from prediabetes to diabetes by intensive lifestyle modification is expected in the intervention group. J-DOIT 2 aims at a 50% reduction in the drop-out rate from regular clinic visits by providing primary care physicians with patients' data management using information technology and certified diabetes educator assistance for the intervention group. The aim of J-DOIT 3 is challenging, since 30% reduction in the development of diabetes complications by intensive lifestyle modification together with a step-by-step medication target for HbA_{1c} of less than 5.8% in the intervention group. Approximately 3000 type 2 diabetics are now being recruited from 71 medical institutions. The results will be evaluated in 2011.

14.3 MORTALITY STUDY

14.3.1 *Type 1 Diabetes*

14.3.1.1 *Long-term Mortality*

Diabetes remains a major risk factor for premature death among children. The Diabetes Epidemiology Research International (DERI) Mortality Study was initiated in 1986 to compare the type 1 diabetes mortality in four countries – Japan, United States (Allegheny County), Finland and Israel – with diverse differences in environmental surroundings and genetic backgrounds [27, 28]. The inclusion criteria for this study were (i) diagnosed as having diabetes between 1965 and 1979 and (ii) as having developed diabetes before 18 years of age. The subjects in the countries other than Japan were taken from the population-based registry that is on ongoing incidence surveys. In contrast, there was no type 1 diabetes registry in Japan; therefore, the study subjects were recruited from the two nationwide prevalence surveys conducted in 1970 and 1981. The surveys identified at least 75% of the eligible people in Japan.

The latest results of the DERI Mortality Study up to the 1995 follow-up, including a total of 1408 Japanese individuals with type 1 diabetes, in comparison with those from Finland ($n = 5126$) were reported in 2003 [29]. Overall mortality rates in Japan and Finland were 607 (97% confidence interval (CI) 510–718) and 352 (97% CI 315–393) respectively per 100 000 person-years; standardized mortality ratios (SMRs) were 12.9 (97% CI 10.8–15.3) and 3.7 (97% CI 3.3–4.1). The increased risk of death from type 1 diabetes seems to vary by sex, age at diagnosis and calendar time period of diagnosis. Stratified cumulative-predicted survival probabilities by calendar time period of diagnosis revealed a major decline in the mortality. This may be attributed to the improved total care for diabetic children, including glycemic and blood pressure controls, as well as the treatment of acute complications [30, 31].

14.3.1.2 Causes of Death

Causes of death of 90 deceased cases were determined using the standardized procedure of the DERI mortality classification committee, which consisted of five international members. On the basis of information collected through hospital records, death certificates and direct family contact, (i) the underlying cause of death and contributory conditions, (ii) pattern of death and (iii) the contribution of type 1 diabetes to the death were examined [28]. The main reason for the high death rate in Japan was the high mortality caused by diabetic renal disease and acute complications such as ketoacidosis and hypoglycemia.

14.3.1.3 Risk Factors for Premature Death

The next step in the DERI Mortality Study consisted of two components. One was to identify the risk factors for premature deaths among Japanese type 1 diabetes children by an ecological study in order to build the hypotheses regarding risk factors for death, and a case-control study to test the hypotheses. Another component was the study to clarify the reasons why Japanese with type 1 diabetes were more likely to die from diabetic renal disease compared with other counties. In the DERI ecological studies, area-specific mortality in Japan was associated with the availability of diabetologists, indicating a possible contribution of supervision by specialists to the prognosis of individuals with type 1 diabetes [32].

A case-control study for testing the hypothesis was conducted to identify the risk factors for premature deaths [33]. The study was based on 90 cases that died during follow-up and 90 living controls, selected from the rest of the cohort, who were matched for sex, birth year and year of diagnosis and duration of diabetes. Socioeconomic and behavioral statuses were surveyed through a questionnaire. Conditional logistic regression analyses revealed that the better educated patients, who retained the same physician (number of times a patient changed physician) and who attended a clinic specializing in diabetes (attendance at university hospital clinic), who injected insulin several times a day (number of insulin injections) and those who attended the clinic more frequently were at substantially lower risk of death.

To elucidate the reasons why Japanese with type 1 diabetes are more likely to die from renal disease, the DERI Mortality Study compared the incidence of end-stage renal disease (ESRD) between Japanese and the US DERI cohorts [34, 35]. It was reported that Japanese with type 1 diabetes were 2.4-fold more likely to develop ESRD. Moreover, 10 of the 36 renal-failure-related deaths in the Japanese cohort had never been treated by dialysis, whereas all renal-failure-related deaths in the US cohort had been treated by dialysis. The data suggested that a greater frequency of diabetic ESRD and reduced access/acceptance to dialysis underlie much of the excess of diabetic renal deaths in Japan. It also indicated that pubertal-onset is a risk factor for renal replacement therapy [36]. Not only better glycemic and blood pressure control [37], but also tender-loving care by the diabetes specialist in a multidisciplinary team approach appears to be associated with a marked reduction of premature death due to ESRD [38].

Recently, the high mortality in the Japanese DERI cohort has been improved to the same level as in the other three countries [30]. This is probably the result of the establishment of a medical care system, such as free access to medical care for young-onset diabetic patients. However, Japanese type 1 diabetes patients in the DERI Mortality Study are still approximately twofold more likely to die than the general population of the same age group as the patients (SMR = 2), which means that half of the deaths can potentially be prevented.

14.3.2 Type 2 Diabetes

14.3.2.1 Mortality Rate

To my knowledge, there have been no population-based follow-up studies regarding the mortality for individuals with type 2 diabetes in Japan. Two reports in a hospital-based setting have been published, demonstrating an increased risk of 1.5–1.7 of death among type 2 diabetes patients compared with that in the general population [39,

40]. Such an observation of mortality among people with type 2 diabetes is the same as that in the reports for the Caucasian population.

14.3.2.2   A Changing Pattern of Causes of Death

It is of interest, however, that the constitution of causes of death in people with type 2 diabetes differs between Japanese and Caucasians [41–43]. A report from England and Wales (1975–1977) [41] demonstrated that deaths due to disease of the heart, of the cerebrovascular system, of renal disease and of malignant neoplasm were 31.6%, 14.7%, 0.7% and 7.2% respectively, whereas in Osaka (1975–1979) the corresponding figures were 12.5%, 13.9%, 1.2% and 7.8% respectively [42]. The difference in causes of deaths between Japanese and Caucasians (i.e. the lower risk for cardiovascular deaths and higher risk for renal deaths in the Japanese with type 2 diabetes) may be attributed to genetic factors and environmental factors such as dietary characteristics. In Japan, dietary habits changed from a conventional diet including low-protein and low-fat intake, with low calories, to the westernized diet with high-fat and high-calorie rates after World War II. With this change, Japanese with type 2 diabetes have been more likely to die from coronary artery disease [43]. Only 8.9% of those who developed diabetes during 1960–1974 had died of coronary artery disease, whereas 15.3% of those who developed diabetes during 1980–1984 died of the disease [44]. As described, the characteristics of causes of death in Japan may get close to those in Europe and the United States in the near future. In terms of diabetes care, the risk factors for cardiovascular disease should be granted much more attention by doctors, as well as the Japanese patients with type 2 diabetes. Further investigation, especially a population-based follow-up study for type 2 diabetes, is essential in order to conduct an unbiased evaluation of the prognosis and its risk factors.

References

1. Sicree, R., Shaw, J.E. and Zimmet, P.Z. (2003) The global burden of diabetes, in *Diabetes Atlas*, 2nd edn (ed D. Gan), International Diabetes Federation, Brussels, pp. 15–17.

2. Akazawa, Y. (1994) Prevalence and incidence of diabetes mellitus by WHO criteria. *Diabetes Research and Clinical Practice*, **24** (Suppl), S23–7.

3. Japan IDDM Epidemiology Study Group (1993) Lack of regional variation in IDDM risk in Japan. *Diabetes Care*, **16**, 796–800.

4. Matsuura, N., Fukuda, K., Okuno, K. *et al.* (1998) Descriptive epidemiology of IDDM in Hokkaido, Japan. The Childhood IDDM Hokkaido Registry. *Diabetes Care*, **21**, 1632–6.

5. Hososako, A. and Matsuyama, T. (1966) Prevalence of IDDM among children in the family members of Yahata-Iron Company. *Journal of Japan Diabetes Society*, **9**, 160–2.

6. Matsuura, N., Fukushima, N., Fujita, H. *et al.* (1983) Epidemiologic study of juvenile-onset insulin dependent diabetes mellitus (IDDM) in Hokkaido, Japan, 1973–1981. *The Tohoku Journal of Experimental Medicine*, **141** (Suppl), 181–9.

7. Okamoto, N., Kobayashi, M., Sasaki, A. *et al.* (1989) Epidemiology of childhood IDDM in Ohsaka. *Shonika Rinsho*, **42** (Suppl), 821–5.

8. Sakurami, T., Kono, Y., Nakahara, T. and Akazawa, Y. (1995) Epidemiological Study on Childhood Diabetes in Saitama Prefecture (year 1995). Diabetes Study Group Report (1995), The Ministry of Health and Welfare, Government of Japan, pp. 66–70 (in Japanese).

9. Kitagawa, T., Owada, M., Urakami, T. and Tajima, N. (1994) Epidemiology of type 1 (insulin-dependent) and type 2 (non-insulin-dependent) diabetes mellitus in Japanese children. *Diabetes Research and Clinical Practice*, **24** (Suppl), S7–13.

10. Urakami, T., Miyamoto, Y., Fujita, H. and Kitagawa, T. (1989) Type I (insulin-dependent) diabetes in Japanese children is not a uniform disease. *Diabetologia*, **32**, 312–15.

11. Kobayashi, T., Tamemoto, K., Nakanishi, K. *et al.* (1993) Immunogenetic and clinical characterization of slowly progressive IDDM. *Diabetes Care*, **16**, 780–8.

12. Nakanishi, K., Kobayashi, T., Sugimoto, T. *et al.* (1993) Association of HLA-A24 with complete B-cell destruction in insulin-dependent diabetes mellitus. *Diabetes*, **42**, 1086–93.

13. Chinzei, T., Kawanishi, M., Maeda, Y. *et al.* (1994) Study of Diabetes Epidemiology – Efficacy of Capture–Mark–Recapture Method and Application of Local Medical Information Network System. Diabetes Study Group Report (1994), The Ministry of Health and Welfare, Government of Japan, pp. 103–5 (in Japanese).

14. Kuzuya, K., Ito, C., Sasaki, A. *et al.* (1992) Prevalence and incidence of diabetes in Japanese

people compiled from the literature – a report of the Epidemiology Data Committee, the Japan Diabetes Society. *Journal of Japan Diabetes Society*, **35**, 173–94 (in Japanese).

15. Sekikawa, A., Tominaga, M., Takahashi, K. *et al.* (1993) Prevalence of diabetes and impaired glucose tolerance in Funagata, Japan. *Diabetes Care*, **16**, 570–74.

16. Ohmura, T., Ueda, K., Kiyohara, Y. *et al.* (1993) Prevalence of type 2 (non-insulin-dependent) diabetes mellitus and impaired glucose tolerance in the Japanese general population: the Hisayama study. *Diabetologia*, **36**, 1198–203.

17. The Ministry of Health, Labor and Welfare (2002) The Report of the National Diabetes Survey in 2002 (in Japanese).

18. Urakami, T., Kubota, S., Nitadori, Y. *et al.* (2005) Annual incidence and clinical characteristics of type 2 diabetes in children as detected by urine glucose screening in the Tokyo Metropolitan Area. *Diabetes Care*, **28**, 1876–81.

19. Owada, M., Nitadori, Y. and Kitagawa, T. (1996) Present status of childhood onset NIDDM in Japan. *Shoni-Naika*, **28**, 823–8 (in Japanese).

20. Fujimoto, W.Y., Leonetti, D.L., Kinyoun, J.L. *et al.* (1987) Prevalence of diabetes mellitus and impaired glucose tolerance among second-generation Japanese-American men. *Diabetes*, **36**, 721–9.

21. Hara, H., Egusa, G., Yamakido, M. and Kawate, R. (1994) The high prevalence of diabetes mellitus and hyperinsulinemia among the Japanese-Americans living in Hawaii and Los Angeles. *Diabetes Research and Clinical Practice*, **24** (Suppl), S37–42.

22. Fujimoto, W.Y., Bergstrom, R.W., Boyko, E.J. *et al.* (1994) Diabetes and diabetes risk factors in second- and third-generation Japanese Americans in Seattle, Washington. *Diabetes Research and Clinical Practice*, **24** (Suppl), S43–52.

23. Kosaka, K., Hagura, R. and Kuzuya, T. (1977) Insulin responses in equivocal and definite diabetes with special reference to subjects who had mild glucose tolerance but later developed definite diabetes. *Diabetes*, **26**, 944–52.

24. Kadowaki, K., Miyake, Y., Hagura, R. *et al.* (1984) Risk factors for worsening to diabetes in subjects with impaired glucose tolerance. *Diabetologia*, **26**, 44–9.

25. Ohmura, T., Ueda, K., Kiyohara, Y. *et al.* (1994) The association of the insulin resistance syndrome with impaired glucose tolerance and 10 NIDDM in the Japanese general population: the Hisayama study. *Diabetologia*, **37**, 891–904.

26. Yazaki, Y. and Kadowaki, T. (2006) Combating diabetes and obesity in Japan. *Nature Medicine*, **12**, 73–4.

27. Diabetes Epidemiology Research International Mortality Study Group (1990) Mortality associated with insulin-dependent diabetes mellitus in Japan, Israel, Finland and Allegheny County, Pennsylvania (USA). *Diabetes Care*, **14**, 49–54.

28. Diabetes Epidemiology Research International Mortality Study Group (1990) Cause specific mortality and insulin-dependent diabetes mellitus. An international evaluation. *Diabetes Care*, **14**, 55–60.

29. Asao, K., Sarti, C., Forsen, T. *et al.* (2003) Long-term mortality in nationwide cohorts of childhood-onset type 1 diabetes in Japan and Finland. *Diabetes Care*, **26**, 2037–42.

30. Nishimura, R., Matsushima, M., Tajima, N. *et al.* (1996) A major improvement of in the prognosis of individuals with IDDM in the past 30 years in Japan. *Diabetes Care*, **19**, 758–60.

31. Borch-Johnsen, K., Kreiner, S. and Deckert, T. (1986) Diabetic nephropathy – susceptible to care? A cohort-study of 641 patients with type 1 (insulin-dependent) diabetes. *Diabetes Research*, **3**, 397–400.

32. Nishimura, R., Agata, T., Shimizu, H. *et al.* (1995) The relationship between medical infrastructure and IDDM mortality rate in Japan, *Journal of Japan Diabetes Society*, **38**, 689–96.

33. Matsushima, M., Shimizu, K., Maruyama, M. *et al.* (1996) Socioeconomic and behavioural risk factors for mortality of individuals with. IDDM in Japan: population based case-control study. *Diabetologia*, **39**, 710–16.

34. Patrick, S., Tajima, N., LaPorte, R. and Kitagawa, T. (1992) A comparison of renal disease mortality among individuals with insulin-dependent diabetes mellitus (IDDM) in Japan and Allegheny County, PA, the United States. *Journal of Japan Diabetes Society*, **35**, 993–1000.

35. Matsushima, M., Tajima, N., LaPorte, R.E. *et al.* (1995) Markedly increased renal disease mortality and incidence of renal replacement therapy among IDDM patients in Japan in contrast to Allegheny County, Pennsylvania, USA. *Diabetologia*, **38**, 236–43.

36. Morimoto, A., Nishimura, R., Matsudaira, T. *et al.* (2007) Is pubertal onset a risk factor for blindness and renal replacement therapy in childhood-onset type 1 diabetes in Japan? *Diabetes Care*, **30**, 2338–40.

37. Uchigata, Y., Asao, K., Matsusima, M. *et al.* (2004) Impact on mortality and incidence of end-stage renal disease of education and treatment at a diabetes center among patients with type 1 diabetes. Comparison of two subgroups in the Jananese DERI cohort. *Journal of Diabetes and its Complications*, **18**, 155–59.

38. Nishimura, R., Dorman, J.S., Bosnylak, Z. *et al.* (2003) Incidence of ESRD and survival after renal replacement therapy in patients with type 1 diabetes: a report from the Allegheny County Registry. *American Journal of Kidney Diseases*, **42**, 117–24.

39. Mihara, T., Oohashi, H. and Hirata, Y. (1988) A long-term prospective follow-up study of Japanese patients with diabetes-A 10 year follow-up study. *Journal of Japanese Life Assurance Medicine*, **86**, 419–34.

40. Sasaki, A., Horiuch, N. and Hasegawa, K. (1989) Mortality and causes of death in Type 2 diabetic patients. A long term follow-up study in Osaka district, Japan. *Diabetes Research and Clinical Practice*, **7**, 33–40.

41. Fuller, J.H., Elford, J. and Goldblatt, P. (1983) Diabetes mortality: new light on an underestimated public health problem. *Diabetologia*, **23**, 336–41.

42. Sasaki, A. (1994) Mortality and causes of death in patients with diabetes mellitus in Japan. *Diabetes Research and Clinical Practice*, **24** (Suppl), S299–306.

43. Sasaki, A. (1994) Long-Term Observation Study on the Prognosis and Causes of Death of Diabetes Mellitus. Diabetes Study Group Report (1994), Ministry of Health and Welfare, Government of Japan, pp. 110–14 (in Japanese).

44. Sasaki, A., Horiuchi, N., Hasegawa, K. and Uehara, M. (1987) Studies on the natural history of non-insulin dependent diabetic (NIDDM) patients based on long-term observation (2)-causes of death and factors related to them. *Journal of Japan Diabetes Society*, **30**, 1003–22.

15

Epidemiology of Diabetes Mellitus in China

Juliana C. N. Chan and Clive S. Cockram

Department of Medicine & Therapeutics, The Chinese University of Hong Kong,
The Prince of Wales Hospital, Shatin, Hong Kong

15.1 INTRODUCTION

China is the most populous nation on Earth with 1.3 billion people. The population contains 55 ethnic minority groups, although approximately 90% belong to the Han group. The majority of the Han people live in the coastal and midland areas of China, while many of the other ethnic minority groups live in the far western region; some still lead subsistence or nomadic lifestyles. While China was closed to the outside world between the 1950s and 1970s, overseas Chinese living in Hong Kong, Taiwan, Singapore, Mauritius and elsewhere have undergone dramatic changes in lifestyles. Since the 1980s, China has 'opened up' and has displayed rapid economic development. This chapter provides an overview of the epidemiology of diabetes and its complications in Chinese people, making frequent references to published data (in the English literature) from Hong Kong, China, Taiwan and Singapore. Other Asian populations, such as Japanese and Koreans, are also referred to for comparison purposes. Hong Kong, situated in the south of China, is one of the most cosmopolitan cities in the world. Despite its total area of just over $1000\,\mathrm{km}^2$, 80% of which is mountainous, the city is inhabited by 6.8 million Chinese, the majority of whom, or their ancestors, originated from southern China. Given the similarities in ethnicity, cultures and social values between Hong Kong and southern Chinese, data concerning epidemiology of diabetes collected in Hong Kong are pertinent to mainland China as it continues to modernize.

15.2 SOCIOECONOMIC IMPACT OF DIABETES

On a global basis, lifestyle factors such as smoking, physical inactivity and unhealthy diet have led to expansion of major chronic diseases, including cardiovascular disease (CVD) and diabetes, that collectively account for 50–60% of deaths globally [1]. In the last 2 decades, a large body of evidence has been collected in Asian countries including China confirming the disease burden of diabetes including cardio-renal complications. [2, 3]. Recently, the World Health Organization (WHO) has estimated that the excess global mortality attributable to diabetes in the year 2000 was 2.9 million deaths, equivalent to 5.2% of all deaths. Excess mortality attributable to diabetes accounted for 2–3% of deaths in the poorest countries and over 8% in the United States, Canada and the Middle East. In people 35–64 years old, 6–27% of deaths were attributable to diabetes [4].

In China alone, US$ 558 billion national income is expected to be foregone over the next 10 years as a result of premature deaths caused by heart disease, stroke and diabetes [1]. According to the International Diabetes Federation (IDF), the annual direct healthcare costs of diabetes worldwide, for people in the 20–79 age bracket, are estimated to be 153–286 billion international dollars, increasing to 213–396 billion international dollars in 2025, the international dollars being calculated using purchasing power parities, which are rates of currency conversion constructed to account for

The Epidemiology of Diabetes Mellitus, second edition   Edited by Jean-Marie Ekoé, Marian Rewers, Rhys Williams and Paul Zimmet
© 2008 John Wiley & Sons, Ltd

differences in price level between countries. This figure translates to 7–13% of the global healthcare budget, with high prevalence countries, such as Nauru, spending up to 40% of their budget. These estimations have not taken into account the indirect and intangible costs on diabetes-related diseases [5].

Compared with the West, the health care costs of diabetes are less well documented in Asia. In Taiwan, based on a national extrapolation of Bureau of National Health Insurance claims between July 1997 and July 1998, it was estimated that 11.5% of the healthcare budget was spent on diabetes treatment, which averaged 4.3 times higher than that for a person without diabetes [6]. In China, based on a survey consisting of 1111 type 2 diabetes patients recruited from 11 cities between May 2002 and January 2003, 54% had at least one complication. Overall, the annual direct medical cost of patients with complications was increased by 3.7 times compared with those without complications, with fivefold increase in the presence of cardiovascular complications, 13-fold for renal complications, twofold for microvascular complications, threefold for any macrovascular complication and ninefold for both micro- and macro-vascular complications. The total direct medical cost for treating diabetes and its complications in urban China was estimated to be 1875 billion RMB (approximately US$ 240 billion), which accounted for 3.9% of total health care expenditure in 2001, 81% of which was due to diabetic complications [7].

15.3 PREVALENCE OF HYPERGLYCEMIA AND TYPE 2 DIABETES

In a recent review article, based on literature published in the MEDLINE (January 1966–October 2005), Wong and Wang [8] summarized the findings from prevalence studies conducted in Chinese populations. A total of 35 studies published in either Chinese or English languages were included: 21 studies from mainland China (1978–2003), four studies from Hong Kong (1987–1996) and 10 studies from Taiwan (1985–2001). The consolidated prevalence rates of diabetes in China, Hong Kong and Taiwan are shown in **Figure 15.1**. Compared with their mainland counterparts, Chinese in Hong Kong and Taiwan have 1.5- and 2.0-fold increased risks of diabetes adjusted for age and diagnostic

criteria. On average, 69% of people with diabetes remain undiagnosed in mainland China compared with 53% in Hong Kong and Taiwan [8]. Other national surveys consisting of large migrant Chinese populations include those from Singapore [9] and Mauritius conducted in 1998 [10]. Both of these studies show 7–10% age- and sex-adjusted prevalence of diabetes, comparable to those reported in other Chinese populations living in affluent societies.

Using the latest figures from the InterAsia Study conducted in China in 2000, it is estimated that at least 40 million people have diabetes (fasting plasma glucose (FPG) ≥ 7 mmol l^{-1}) or impaired fasting glycemia (IFG) (FPG = 6–6.9 mmol l^{-1}). Amongst the 20 million Chinese people with diabetes based on FPG, only 30% were previously diagnosed (**Figure 15.2**). Compared with reports in the early 1980s, there have been major increases in disease prevalence with time. In agreement with WHO predictions [11], the major increase is observed in the young and middle-aged groups [12] (**Figure 15.3**). This has obvious socioeconomic implications associated with potential premature mortality and morbidity. Thus, despite differences in sampling methods and diagnostic criteria, the rising prevalence with time and effects of urbanization are clearly evident. In China, a 1% increase in adult prevalence will translate to approximately 1 million people with diabetes.

15.4 DIAGNOSIS OF HYPERGLYCEMIA IN CHINESE POPULATIONS

The rationale behind the use of a cutoff value of 2 h plasma glucose (PG) ≥ 11.1 mmol l^{-1} following the administration of a 75 g oral glucose tolerance test (OGTT) was originally based on the risk of microvascular complications. On the other hand, the use of FPG ≥ 7 mmol l^{-1} to define diabetes is more arbitrary [13]. During the last decade or so, the diagnostic criteria for diabetes have undergone several revisions, both by the WHO and the American Diabetes Association (ADA). Based on prospective data from many ethnic groups, IFG has now been redefined as an FPG between 5.5 and 6.9 mmol l^{-1} which is associated with increased risk of diabetes and CVDs [14, 15].

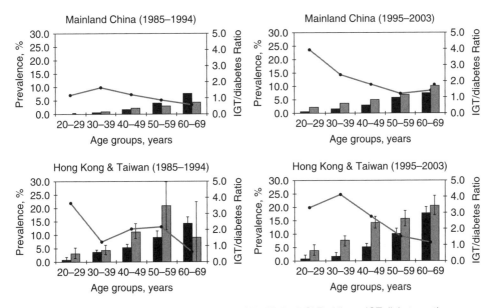

Red bar = diabetes with 95% CI Blue bar = IGT with 95% CI Red line = IGT:diabetes ratio

Figure 15.1 Consolidated prevalence rates of diabetes and impaired glucose tolerance (IGT) and IGT/diabetes ratios of the Chinese populations in mainland China, Hong Kong and Taiwan based on studies that applied an OGTT and WHO guidelines. (Wong, K.C. and Wang, Z. (2006) Prevalence of type 2 diabetes mellitus of Chinese populations in mainland China, Hong Kong, and Taiwan. *Diabetes Research and Clinical Practice*, 73 (2), 126–34.)

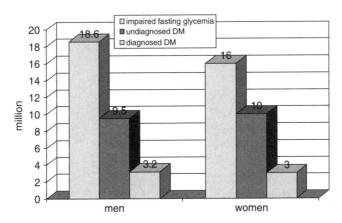

Figure 15.2 Prevalence of diagnosed and undiagnosed diabetes and impaired fasting glycemia in a recent national survey for diabetes and cardiovascular risk factors in Mainland China. An estimated 60.5 million people are expected to have or at risk of having diabetes. (Adapted from Gu, D. *et al.* (2003) *Diabetologia*, 46, 1190–8.)

In Hong Kong Chinese, a low sensitivity of FPG $\geq$ 7.8 mmol l^{-1} for the diagnosis of diabetes was reported in the early 1990s. Based on a quadratic model from 680 subjects, the predicted FPG corresponding to a 2 h PG $\geq$ 11.1 mmol l^{-1} was 5.7 mmol l^{-1}, whereas the predicted 2 h PG corresponding to an FPG $\geq$ 7.8 mmol l^{-1} was 15.2 mmol l^{-1}. Of those with a 2 h PG $\geq$ 11.1 mmol l^{-1}, 40% had an FPG $\geq$ 7.8 mmol l^{-1} and 50% had an FPG $\geq$ 7 mmol l^{-1} [16].

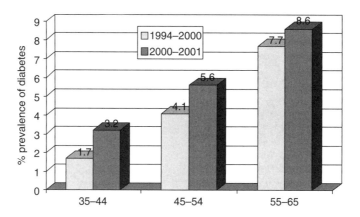

Figure 15.3 Diabetes prevalence in China has increased by 88%, 37% and 12% in adults aged 35–44, 45–54 and 55–64 respectively during the past decade. (Adapted from Gu, D. *et al.* (2003) *Diabetologia*, 46, 1190–8.)

In the Diabetes Epidemiology Collaborative Analysis of Diagnostic Criteria in Asia (DECODA), which examined data from 17 512 subjects aged 30–89 years without a previous history of diabetes, the prevalence of diabetes was 4.0% by the FPG criteria only (≥ 7 mmol l^{-1}) and 6.0% by the 2 h PG criteria only (≥ 11.1 mmol l^{-1}). The FPG value of 7.0 mmol l^{-1} gave a sensitivity for diabetes as defined by a 2 h PG ≥ 11.1 mmol l^{-1} of 46% and a specificity of 99%. The FPG associated with a 2 h PG ≥ 11.1 mmol l^{-1} with optimal sensitivity and specificity was 5.8 mmol l^{-1} (sensitivity 79%, specificity 85%) [17]. In a subsequent 5-year follow-up study involving Japanese and Asian Indian subjects, using a model containing FPG and 2 h PG, only 2 h PG in subjects with impaired glucose tolerance (IGT) or diabetes was predictive of all-cause or cardiovascular mortality with 1.3–3.3-fold increased risk compared with normal subjects [18]. In China, mild retinopathy has been reported in subjects with either newly diagnosed diabetes or IGT, suggesting either a long period of undiagnosed disease or a low glycemic threshold for developing microvascular complications [19].

In the Shanghai Diabetes Community-based Survey, the 3-year cumulative incidence of diabetes and impaired glucose regulation (IGR, mainly due to IGT) were 4.96% and 11.10%, in subjects without diabetes at baseline. Subjects with IGR (IGT and/or IFG) had 11.7 fold increased risk of diabetes compared to those with normal glucose tolerance (NGT). On further analysis, the respective relative

risk of diabetes in subjects with IFG, isolated IGT and combined IFG and IGT were 15.4, 9.2 and 27.6 (20). In Hong Kong, subjects with IFG or IGT developed diabetes at an annual rate of 4–10% depending on the presence of other risk factors [21, 22]. In the 1992 Singapore national survey, after an observational period of 10 years, subjects with IFG/IGT had 1.4-fold increased mortality and those with diabetes 2.5-fold increased mortality after adjustment for age, gender, ethnic group and educational level [23]. Taken together, the high IGT/diabetes ratio in various Chinese populations, ranging from 30 to 5, with the highest observed in the young age group [8] (see Figure 15.1), indicates that a large population of Chinese people is at risk of premature cardiovascular mortality and morbidity.

15.5 GESTATIONAL DIABETES MELLITUS

In a large-scale survey in China (1998 and 1999), 9471 women underwent initial screening (50 g glucose load) at 26–30 gestational weeks. Women with a serum glucose reading ≥ 7.8 mmol l^{-1} at 1 h were subjected to a 75 g hour OGTT. A total of 701 (79%) women took a subsequent OGTT. Of these, 174 women were confirmed to have gestational diabetes mellitus (GDM) (154 with IGT and 20 with diabetes). The prevalence of GDM was 2.3% (2.0% for IGT and 0.3% for diabetes), adjusting for serum glucose levels at the initial screening test. Independent predictors for GDM were maternal age, stature, prepregnancy body mass index (BMI), weight gain in pregnancy before screening, diabetes in first-degree relatives and habitual cigarette smoking during pregnancy. Women who smoked or had a short stature were more likely to develop GDM than their counterparts. PG levels at screening, maternal weight gain during pregnancy and gestational week at delivery were determinants of fetal birthweight [24, 25].

In Hong Kong, between 1990 and 1994, glycemic status was examined in 942 Chinese pregnant women with a median age of 27 years, using the 1998 WHO criteria. All subjects underwent a 75 g OGTT at 24–28 weeks of gestation. The prevalence of GDM was 14.2% according to the 1998 WHO criteria and 14.0% according to the 1985 WHO criteria. The similar prevalence was due to the fact that nearly all women with GDM had IGT, which was diagnosed on 2 h PG [26]. In a follow-up study of 800 women with a history of GDM/gestational IGT who underwent 75 g OGTT at 6 weeks postdelivery, the crude prevalence of IGT was 22% and that of diabetes was 13%. This was compared with 5% and 1% in age-matched control subjects. Women with a history of GDM also had a two- to eight-fold increased risk of obesity, hyperlipidemia, hypertension and dysglycemia compared with control subjects [27, 28].

15.6 CHILDHOOD OBESITY AND DIABETES

Despite the relatively low prevalence of classical type 1 diabetes (see later section), there is a growing 'epidemic' of young onset diabetes in China closely related to the rising prevalence of childhood obesity. On a global basis, the prevalence of childhood obesity has been estimated to be 10–15% in most affluent societies [29]. As early as 1970s, the rising prevalence of type 2 diabetes in Japanese children was reported and attributed to increased consumption of animal protein and fat together with reduced physical activity [30]. Recent studies in Hong Kong, Taiwan and Singapore have also reported high prevalence rates of obesity in Chinese children or adolescents, ranging from 10 to 50% depending on definitions, subject selection and study methods [31, 32]. In these young subjects, there is considerable overlap between the phenotypes of type 1 and type 2

diabetes, with obesity and autoimmunity both playing contributory roles in disease manifestation.

Recently, both Japan and Taiwan have embarked upon national screening programs (using urinalysis) for diabetes in all primary and secondary schools. In Japan, based on surveys conducted between 1974 and 2002, the overall annual incidence of type 2 diabetes in school children was 2.63 per 100 000 with a higher annual incidence in the period after 1981 compared with that before 1980 (2.76 per 100 000 versus 1.73 per 100 000, $p < 0.0001$). Secondary school adolescents tend to be affected more often than primary school children. Over 80% of affected children or adolescents were obese [33]. In Taiwan, based on a national survey in 1999, the prevalence of newly identified diabetes, based on an FPG $\geq$ 7 mmol l^{-1} after two positive urine tests for glucose, was 9.0 per 100 000 for boys and 15.3 per 100 000 for girls. Obesity, family history, hypertension and hypercholesterolemia were major risk factors [32, 34].

In Hong Kong, in a pilot study involving 271 primary school children, approximately 50% were obese or overweight. In these children, obesity or overweight was associated with clustering of cardiovascular risk factors, including insulin resistance. In addition, family history and formula feeding were risk factors for obesity [31]. In another study involving 30 Hong Kong school children aged 9–11 years, obesity was associated with increased carotid intima-media thickness (IMT) and endothelial dysfunction which improved after a sustained weight reduction and physical fitness program [35]. In a subsequent community-based study involving 14 secondary schools and 2000 adolescents aged 11–18 years, based on published definitions (three of five risk factors: fasting triglyceride $\geq$1.24 mmol l^{-1}; high-density lipoprotein cholesterol (HDL-C) $\leq$1.03 mmol l^{-1}; FPG $\geq$ 6.1 mmol l^{-1}; waist circumference $\geq$90th percentile value for age and sex from this sample population; blood pressure $\geq$90th percentile for age, sex and height based on data from the National Blood Pressure Education Program Working Group on High Blood Pressure in Children and Adolescents) [36], 2.4% of adolescents had metabolic syndrome (MetS). General obesity, a family history of diabetes and attendance at schools with average to low academic performances were independent risk factors. These findings suggest that both school and home environments are important determinants for obesity and MetS in children and adolescents [37].

In a study of 975 mainland Chinese children aged 6–13 years, 40% had maintained their relative positions of bodyweight after 6 years. Overweight children were 2.8 times as likely as all other children to become overweight adolescents, whereas underweight children were 3.6 times as likely to remain underweight as adolescents. Parental obesity and underweight, individuals' initial BMI, dietary fat intake, and family income predicted tracking and changes in BMI [38].

15.7 TYPE 1 DIABETES

In China, a two-sample capture–recapture method has been used to estimate case ascertainment of type 1 diabetes in 24 million young people. Between 1988 and 1996, 903 cases were registered in nine ethnic groups with an overall (ascertainment-corrected) incidence rate of 0.59 per 100 000 person-years (0.52 per 100 000 person-years for males and 0.66 per 100 000 person-years for females), ranging from 0.25 per 100 000 person-years to 3.06 per 100 000 person-years in different ethnic groups. Apart from a higher incidence in North China, there was also a significant increase in incidence with time between 1988 and 1996. Using age from 0 to 4 years as the referent, the relative risks for type 1 diabetes for ages from 5 to 9 years and from 10 to 14 years were 2.3 and 3.6 respectively [39].

Hong Kong has one of the highest incidence rates of type 1 diabetes within China. Based on a registry established in 1997 that ascertained all cases diagnosed under the age of 15 years, using medical records at all regional public hospitals and a survey of all registered practitioners in Hong Kong, 255 diabetes cases were identified, with 227 having type 1 diabetes mellitus (218 were Chinese), 18 had type 2 diabetes and 11 had secondary diabetes. The age-standardized incidence of type 1 diabetes was 1.4 per 100 000 person-years, with a higher incidence in females (1.7 per 100 000 person-years in females compared with 1.2 per 100 000 person-years in males) and the 10–14-year age-group [40]. Despite the overall low incidence of childhood type 1 diabetes in China compared with other countries, these data show considerable geographic and ethnic variability.

The etiology of type 1 diabetes remains unknown, but both genetic and environmental factors are believed to be important. The major histocompatibility complex (MHC) on chromosome 6p21 has been shown to contribute strongly to the familial clustering of type 1 diabetes with various combinations of DQ-DR haplotypes/genotypes/alleles associated with either increased or reduced risk of type 1 diabetes in different populations [41]. Studies conducted in Chinese from Hong Kong and Taiwan have reported DR3, DR9, DQA1*301, DQA1*0501, DQB1*0201 and DQB1*0303 [42–44] as risk alleles. In a study of young Chinese patients with diabetes (age of onset <35 years) with either type 1 ($n = 34$) or type 2 phenotypes ($n = 103$), the DRB1*03.DQA1*05.DQB1*02 haplotype was the major risk marker and DRB1*12.DQA1*06.DQB1*0301 was associated with a decreased risk of type 1 diabetes. Positivity for antibodies to glutamic acid decarboxylase (GAD), found in 26.5% persons with type 1 diabetes and 6.9% of persons with type 2 diabetes, was also associated with the DRB1*03 allele. Amongst the type 2 diabetes patients, those positive for both GAD antibodies and DRB1*03 appeared to have more aggressive disease, as indicated by earlier use of insulin therapy, whereas GAD-positive subjects carrying DRB1*12 appeared to be relatively protected against progression of the autoimmune process and to suffer limited β-cell loss [45].

In addition to the human leukocyte antigen (HLA) genes of the MHC, which encode molecules crucial to the immune system, another locus associated with type 1 diabetes lies within the 2q21–q33 region and has been attributed to a single nucleotide polymorphism (SNP) in the 3' untranslated region (UTR) of the cytotoxic T lymphocyte-associated protein 4 (*CTLA4*) gene. The latter encodes a costimulatory receptor involved in and conferring an inhibitory effect on T-cell activation [46]. At least two independent studies in China have reported 1.6–3.6-fold increased risk of type 1 diabetes in association with the *CTLA4* 49 G/G genotype or G allele [47, 48].

The ethnic differences in allele distributions and frequencies between Caucasians and non-Caucasians, including Chinese, are now well recognized [49, 50]. With the availability of public databases containing large amounts of information regarding genes and genetic variations such as the HAPMAP, together with high-throughput genotyping technology, more information regarding the genetic epidemiology of diabetes in different populations, including Chinese, is anticipated.

15.8 TYPE 2 DIABETES AND METABOLIC SYNDROME (METS)

The majority of people with diabetes have type 2 disease which is associated with multiple risk factors including high blood pressure, dyslipidemia (notably, high triglyceride, low HDL-C and small dense low-density lipoprotein cholesterol (LDL-C)), high blood glucose, increased inflammatory and prothombotic factors with central obesity as a major linking factor, frequently referred as MetS [51]. A recent WHO report, entitled 'Prevention of chronic diseases – a vital investment,' estimated that 1 billion people are overweight. Obesity is now considered as the main driving force for this epidemic of chronic diseases [1], with the majority of these people coming from developing countries, including China [52].

15.8.1 Definition of Obesity

Asian populations, including Chinese, have often been considered as 'nonobese.' However, several reports from Hong Kong in the early 1990s have highlighted the relatively low BMI of Chinese people with diabetes, averaging only 25 kg m^{-2}, compared with a BMI of approximately 23 kg m^{-2} in the general population. This compares with an average BMI of 27–30 kg m^{-2} in Caucasians with diabetes and 25 kg m^{-2} in Caucasians without diabetes [53, 54].

A large number of reports in the early 90's have reported the low threshold value of BMI or waist circumference for various cardiovascular risk factors in Chinese populations [55–57]. These findings have now been confirmed in the Obesity in Asia Collaboration, comprising 21 cross-sectional studies in the Asia-Pacific with information on more than 263,000 individuals, indicating that measures of central obesity, in particular, waist circumference (WC), are better discriminators of prevalent diabetes and hypertension in Asians and Caucasians, and are more strongly associated with prevalent diabetes (but not hypertension), compared

with BMI. For any given level of BMI, waist circumference or waist:hip ratio, the absolute risk of diabetes or hypertension tended to be higher among Asians compared with Caucasians, supporting the use of lower anthropometric cut-points to indicate overweight among Asians [58]. Similar recommendations have also been made by the WHO which recommends a lower threshold BMI value for action in high risk individuals such as Asian populations [59]. These recommendations are now further supported by long term prospective surveys showing that BMI and waist circumference are predictive of diabetes, cardiovascular and all cause mortality in Chinese populations [21, 60, 61].

In Shanghai, more than 600 Chinese men and women underwent magnetic resonance imaging to measure visceral fat area. Using receiver operator curve (ROC) analysis, a cutoff value for waist circumference at 90 cm gives 80% sensitivity and specificity in predicting a visceral fat area of 100 cm^2, a conventional definition for visceral obesity [62, 63]. Furthermore, in Hong Kong Chinese, mesenteric fat, which directly drains into the portal circulation, was found to explain most of the variance of cardiovascular risk factors compared with total visceral fat and preperitoneal and subcutaneous fat [64]. In this study, mesenteric fat thickness was also an independent predictor for fatty liver [65] and carotid IMT [66]. For every 1 mm increase in mesenteric fat thickness as measured by ultrasound scan, the odds ratio of MetS increased by 1.35-fold. Using ROC analysis, mesenteric fat thickness of 10 mm was found to be the optimal cutoff value to identify MetS with a sensitivity of 70% and specificity of 75% [67]. While the prognostic significance of visceral fat is now widely accepted [68], these findings suggest that the metabolic consequences of different depots of visceral fat need further investigations.

The IDF has recently proposed the use of ethnic specific cutoff values to define central obesity and MetS [69]. Using Singapore as an example, the prevalence of MetS has been reported to be 10.8%, 17.3% and 21.7% respectively in Chinese, Malay and Indian men if central obesity is defined as ≥102 cm in accordance with the National Cholesterol Education Program Adult Treatment Panel III (NCEP-ATP III) guideline. These figures increase to 18.1%, 24.7% and 32.4% respectively if the Asian definition of central obesity for men

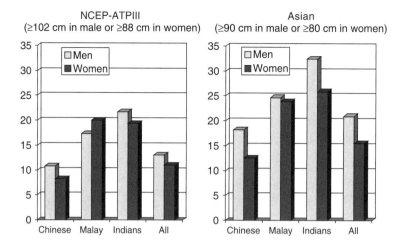

Figure 15.4 Prevalence of MetS in a multiethnic population in Singapore using the NCEP-ATP III criterion with US or Asian definitions of central obesity. (Adapted from Tan, C.E. *et al.* (2004) *Diabetes Care*, 27, 1182–6.)

($\geq$90 cm) is applied (**Figure 15.4**). Similarly, the prevalence of MetS using the NCEP-ATP III definition ($\geq$88 cm for women) were 8.3%, 20% and 19.3% respectively in Chinese, Malay and Indian women increasing to 12%, 23.8% and 15.5% respectively if the Asian definition is adopted ($\geq$80 cm in women) [70].

In China, if a BMI $\geq$ 30 kg m^{-2} is used to define obesity, then 80 million Chinese are obese and 13.7% (64 million) have MetS. If a BMI $\geq$ 25 kg m^{-2} is used, then 187 million Chinese are obese and 15.1% (71 million) have MetS [71]. These findings highlight the need to conduct epidemiological and interventional studies in specific ethnic groups.

15.8.2 Risk Factors for Type 2 Diabetes and MetS

The causes of diabetes and MetS are complex and involve genetic, environmental and lifestyle factors (**Figure 15.5**). Obesity, especially visceral obesity, is now considered to be the main cause for insulin resistance, defined as reduced insulin action at peripheral tissues, notably liver and muscle. Together with β-cell dysfunction, these two factors interact to give rise to diabetes. Positive energy balance due to excessive intake and inadequate expenditure, together with age- and stress-related hormonal changes lead to obesity. Adipocytes, especially visceral adipocytes, are metabolically active cells which can secrete an array of cytokines

and growth factors resulting in a proinflammatory and prothrombotic state, which contribute to insulin resistance and vascular dysfunction [51, 72].

Many risk factors for diabetes have now been reported [73, 74] and many of them have also been confirmed in Asians. Some of these risk factors include family history [54, 75], smoking, physical inactivity [28, 76–78], television watching (more than 2 h daily) [79], rapid acculturation, high caloric intake and consumption of fast foods [80].

There is now a trend to use self-assessment items to develop risk scores to select high-risk subjects [81] for screening for diabetes, IGT or MetS [82, 83]. While some of these Caucasian-derived risk scores have high precision value, they are often of low predictive value in Asian populations. In this regard, Asian relevant risk score using age, sex, waist circumference, body mass index, hypertension and family history of diabetes has been developed and validated to predict diabetes [84].

15.8.2.1 Socioeconomic Status

Both low socioeconomic status (SES) and low educational levels are independently associated with increased risk of diabetes and associated mortality and morbidity [85–87]. In China, low education is an independent risk factor for diabetes in subjects with high personal annual income [88]. In Hong Kong, Ko *et al.* [89] reported independent associations between low SES and low educational

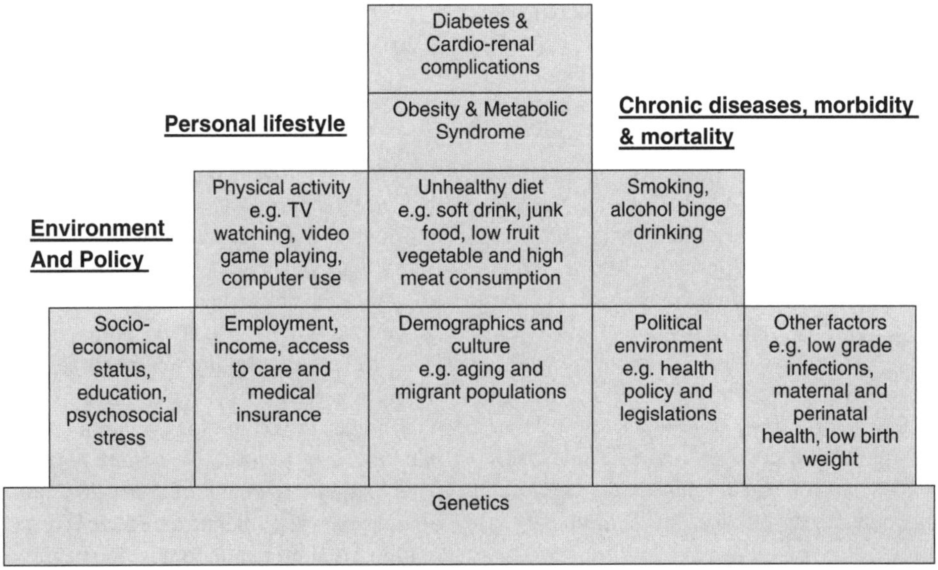

		Diabetes & Cardio-renal complications		
Personal lifestyle		Obesity & Metabolic Syndrome	**Chronic diseases, morbidity & mortality**	
Environment And Policy	Physical activity e.g. TV watching, video game playing, computer use	Unhealthy diet e.g. soft drink, junk food, low fruit vegetable and high meat consumption	Smoking, alcohol binge drinking	
Socio-economical status, education, psychosocial stress	Employment, income, access to care and medical insurance	Demographics and culture e.g. aging and migrant populations	Political environment e.g. health policy and legislations	Other factors e.g. low grade infections, maternal and perinatal health, low birth weight
Genetics				

Figure 15.5 Diabetes and MetS. A multidimensional challenge requiring multisectoral collaborations.

level as risk factors for diabetes. These findings suggest the interplay become national affluence and personal education in this epidemiological transition. While rich people in poor countries are at risk for diabetes, poor people in affluent countries are at increased risk. This finding may be of particular relevance in China given her rapid socioeconomic development but generally low educational level of her people.

15.8.2.2 Low Birthweight

In agreement with others [90], epidemiological data from China and Taiwan have confirmed that subjects with low birthweight (e.g. <2.5 kg) especially if followed by rapid catch up growth, have an increased risk of MetS [34, 91].

15.8.2.3 Gestational Diabetes

Based on a meta-analysis, a history of GDM is associated with a two- to three-fold increased risk of diabetes and may explain up to 10% of population attributable risks of diabetes [92]. Compared with Anglo-Celtic women in Australia, Chinese women have a sixfold increased risk of GDM (15% versus 3%) [93]. In Chinese women with GDM, novel risk factors for diabetes have been identified. Lao and co-workers [94–96] reported a

threefold increased risk of GDM in women with chronic hepatitis B virus (HBV) infection (see later section) and an 11-fold increased risk in subjects with α-thalassemia. Both of these conditions are associated with increased serum ferritin. Family members of diabetes subjects with α-thalassemia trait are more insulin resistant than relatives of diabetes subjects without thalassemia, even after adjustment of obesity [97]. In part due to their pro-oxidant capacity, abnormal iron metabolism has been implicated in the pathogenesis of diabetes as evidenced by increased risk of diabetes and liver dysfunction in subjects with hemachromatosis, including their relatives [98, 99].

15.8.2.4 Chronic Inflammation

Increased inflammatory markers such as high-sensitivity C reactive protein (hsCRP) and inter-leukin 6 are predictive of diabetes and CVDs in Caucasians [100, 101]. In Hong Kong men, hsCRP is an independent predictor of MetS [102]. In a prospective study, apart from 2 h PG and waist circumference [21], hsCRP also predicted the progression from IGT to diabetes in Hong Kong Chinese [103].

In 5757 Hong Kong Chinese patients with tuberculosis, 9.6% of patients had a known history of diabetes, with excess risk in men aged between

45 and 54 years [104]. In a group of Chinese type 2 diabetes patients, while the overall frequency of HBV infection was similar to that of the general population (10%), chronic HBV carriers had earlier onset of diabetes, worse glycemic control and were more likely to require insulin therapy than non-HBV carriers [105]. In Taiwan, based on a cohort of 359 Chinese subjects with chronic hepatitis C virus (HCV) infection, 34.6 % had glucose intolerance (27% diabetes, 7% IGT). Increased age, obesity, family history of diabetes and previous treatment with interferon were associated with glucose intolerance in these subjects [103, 106]. These findings may partly explain the association between low SES and risk of diabetes, as well as high rates of diabetes in developing countries despite low levels of obesity.

15.8.3   Phenotypic Heterogeneity of Diabetes

One of the earliest reports documenting patterns of diabetes in Chinese came from Hong Kong in the early 1990s. In a clinic-based population of 500 diabetes patients, classical type 1 diabetes (defined as acute ketotic presentation or requirement for continuous insulin therapy within 1 year of diagnosis) accounted for only 3% of the population. Even in subjects with age of onset less than 35 years, the proportion of type 1 diabetes was only 10% [53]. Since then, the rarity of classical type 1 diabetes in Chinese, using either clinical definition or autoimmune markers, or both, averaging only 10% even in young patients, has been confirmed in several surveys [53, 107–109].

Approximately 4–6% of Chinese type 2 diabetes patients, especially those with a lean phenotype, exhibit autoimmune markers suggesting a diagnosis of latent autoimmune diabetes in adults (LADA) [110]. As in Caucasians [111], Chinese patients with LADA show rapid decline in β-cell function, correlated with anti-GAD titers [112]. Additionally, some Chinese patients, often obese, present with severe hyperglycemia and mild to moderate ketosis but eventually revert to a clinical course more typical of type 2 disease. This form of diabetes was first reported in Afro-Americans [113], but has also been encountered, albeit infrequently, in Chinese patients [114, 115]. In young Chinese subjects with neither a type 1 phenotype nor autoimmune markers, over 50% have a positive family history. Many are obese and have features of MetS [110, 116–118].

Despite this low proportion of autoimmune type 1 diabetes, primary β-cell dysfunction remains an important feature in Asian type 2 diabetes patients [119, 120]. In a clinic-based cohort of Chinese type 2 diabetes patients, despite short duration of disease, over 40% had poor insulin reserve, as evidenced by a fasting C peptide <2 nmol l^{-1}, which correlated positively with BMI [121]. Some young type 2 diabetic patients present with advanced complications, such as nephropathy and retinopathy, suggesting long periods of undiagnosed disease [122, 123]. These findings corroborate reports from Japan, where the risk of nephropathy is considerably higher in young type 2 than in type 1 diabetes patients. In a prospective cohort of Japanese diabetes patients with age of onset less than 35 years old, 25 years after diagnosis, 25% of type 1 and 50% of type 2 diabetes patients develop nephropathy and renal impairment [124]. In a cross-sectional cohort of young type 2 diabetic patients in Hong Kong with less than 5 years of disease duration, more than 30% had increased albuminuria less [125] suggesting that many of these patients are at risk of developing cardiovascular and renal complications in the prime of life [126, 127].

15.8.3.1   Monogenic Diabetes

It is now increasingly recognized that type 2 diabetes is a heterogeneous condition composed of subtypes in which genetic susceptibility is strongly associated with environmental factors at one end of the spectrum and highly genetic forms at the other, especially in people with young onset of disease. Although some of them may have the typical forms of maturity-onset diabetes of the young (MODY) with an autosomal dominant inheritance and age of onset less than 25 years, less typical forms of disease have also been reported. A large number of genetic variants have now been identified from these families, many encoding for transcription factors (or their regulators) involved in the neogenesis and maturation of β cells, as well as in transcription and secretion of insulin [128]. These people with diabetes exhibit marked heterogeneity in their clinical course and treatment requirement. While mutations with glucokinase are typically associated with increased FPG, often from birth, the clinical course is usually mild and rarely leads to complications. On the other hand, mutations of the hepatic nuclear factor 1α (HNF-1α) are associated with more severe metabolic deterioration which, however, responds well to treatment with sulfonylurea [129]. Several case series have shown that 5–10% of young Chinese diabetes patients have glucokinase or HNF-1α mutations [116–118]. Some of these young people present with advanced complications due to late diagnosis, highlighting the importance of family screening in these subjects [122].

Other genetic factors that have been reported in Chinese patients include mitochondrial gene mutations, notably the *A3243G* mutation, found in 1–3% of type 1 or type 2 diabetes patients, often associated with maternal family history of diabetes, deafness and β-cell failure [130–132]. The importance of inter-ethnic differences is further reflected by the positive risk association of the 16189 variant of mitochondria in Asian [133] but not Caucasian population [134].

Another candidate for diabetes in Chinese subjects is amylin, a peptide cosecreted with insulin. Pancreatic amyloidosis in association with β-cell loss has been reported in both Caucasian and Chinese subjects, using autopsy samples [135–137]. Changes in the metabolic milieu or genetic variants encoding proteins involved in amylin metabolism may lead to structural changes to amylin leading to β-cell death [138]. In Chinese, Japanese and Pacific Islanders [139], genetic mutations of amylin, such as the *S20G* mutation, have been found in 2–3% of diabetes patients, especially with young-onset disease and a positive family history [140–142]

15.8.3.2 MetS

Owing to the multiple correlations amongst risk factors in MetS, factor analysis and structural equation modeling have been used to analyze their interrelationships. In Hong Kong Chinese, obesity, age and family history were found to be the major explanatory variables for the various components of MetS. Several factors loaded by blood pressure, lipid and glucose parameters identified by these analyses were more often linked by obesity than by insulin resistance variables [75, 143–146].

Based on a prospective cohort of 559 Chinese subjects recruited in Beijing, four factors in baseline data were identified (factor 1: fasting insulin levels, BMI and waist/hip ratio; factor 2: systolic and diastolic blood pressures; factor 3: 2 h postload PG, serum insulin and FPG; factor 4: total cholesterol and triglycerides). In nondiabetes subjects, factors

1 and 3 predicted new onset of diabetes; in diabetes subjects, however, factor 2 and glycemia were strongly associated with albuminuria. The authors concluded that insulin resistance alone did not underlie all features of MetS and that different physiological processes associated with various components of MetS contain unique information about diabetes risk [147].

In the Hong Kong Familial Diabetes Study involving 179 families and 913 first-degree relatives, ascertained mainly through a young proband with diabetes, 78% of families had at least one subject with early-onset diabetes. MetS was highly prevalent in probands (53%) and siblings (25%). Recurrence risk ratios in siblings were high for diabetes (4.3), hypertension (2.9) and central obesity (2.0). There were also high estimates of heritability ranging from 0.45 to 0.63 for all components of MetS, including homeostasis model assessment (HOMA)-β. Obesity indices showed the strongest phenotypic correlation with other traits, and were significantly influenced by genetic factors [148].

Using a genome-wide scan approach, groups from Hong Kong, Taiwan and China have reported linkage of diabetes and/or components of MetS to chromosomes 1, 9 and 20 [149–154] with the linkage signals in the chromosomal 1q region highly replicable in Pima Indians, Caucasians, Amish, Finnish and French populations. The recently discovered genetic variants near TCF7L2, SLC30A8, HHEX, CDKAL1, CDKN2A/B, IGF2BP2 and FTO using genome wide association studies have also been found to be significant in Asian including Chinese populations although there are major differences in allele frequencies and thus, population attributable risks between Asian and Caucasian populations [155].

15.8.3.3 Hormonal Dysregulation in MetS

Vague [156] was the researcher to report on the differential effects of android (central) and gynecoid (general) obesity on cardiovascular morbidity and mortality. Björntorp subsequently hypothesized that age-related changes in hormones, notably decreased growth hormone (GH) and testosterone, as well as stress-related increases in hormones such as hypercortisolemia, can lead to increased deposition of visceral fat and insulin resistance. The resultant hyperinsulinemia can then activate the sympathetic nervous system (SNS) to give rise to hypertension and to promote sodium and water retention and abnormal vascular cellular growth. Lipotoxicity and glucotoxicity further interact to worsen insulin resistance and β-cell dysfunction, thus giving rise to a series of vicious cycles [72, 157]. In support and in agreement with other reports, reduced GH, insulin-like growth factor (IGF-1) and testosterone, as well as hypercortisolemia and increased SNS activity, have been reported in Chinese subjects with type 2 diabetes and/or MetS [102, 158, 159].

Adiponectin is one of the few adipocytokines that confers protective effects against MetS and diabetes. Yang and Chuang [160] from Taiwan recently summarized the knowledge regarding the metabolism and genetic roles of adiponectin in MetS with particular reference to Chinese subjects. In agreement with other reports, adiponectin is protective against fatty liver, diabetes and atherosclerosis in Chinese subjects. Although risk associations of adiponectin genetic variants and components of MetS have been reported, interpretation is hampered by small sample size, variations in study design, differences in subject phenotypes and lack of replications.

15.9 DIABETIC COMPLICATIONS

In the InterHeart Study with more than 10 000 participants, subjects from China and Hong Kong had a lower mean BMI level than Caucasian populations. However, within each BMI category, increasing waist/hip ratio quintiles were associated with progressively increased risks of myocardial infarction. These data strongly support the prognostic significance of obesity, especially central obesity, in cardiovascular mortality and morbidity in both Caucasian and Asian populations [161].

In the Asia Pacific Cohort Collaboration involving 237 468 participants from 17 cohort studies in the Asia Pacific region (including China), which included 1661 stroke and 816 coronary heart disease (CHD) events, based on 1.2 million person-years of follow up, the authors identified continuous positive associations between FPG and CVD risks down to a concentration of 4.9 mmol l^{-1}. Overall, each 1 mmol l^{-1} lower FPG was associated with a 21% lower risk of total stroke and 23% lower risk of total CHD [162].

15.9.1 Pattern of Macrovascular Complications

In the WHO Multinational Study of Vascular Diseases in Diabetes (WHO-MSVDD), when compared with Caucasians, Chinese diabetes patients have a shorter duration of known diabetes, lower blood pressure, total blood cholesterol and BMI, lower rates of large-vessel disease (34% versus 18%; low rates of CHD and peripheral vascular disease (PVD) but high rates of stroke), but higher rates for retinopathy (47% versus 36%) and proteinuria (57% versus 25%) [163]. A collaborative study group in Asia has reported 30% of patients with stroke had diabetes as a major contributing factor. In these subjects, diabetes was an independent predictor for early death during the 12 months postevent period [164]. In asymptomatic Chinese type 2 diabetes patients, 20% had atherosclerosis involving the middle cerebral arteries (using transcranial ultrasound Doppler). This was associated with albuminuria, retinopathy, hypertension, dyslipidemia and PVD [165]. In agreement with the WHO-MSVDD study [163], recent reports also confirmed the low prevalence of CHD and PVD in Chinese type 2 diabetes patients, averaging 3–10% [166]. Despite these low rates, diabetes is a leading cause of acute myocardial infarction [167] and heart failure [168].

15.9.2 Pattern of Microvascular Complications

In the early 1990s, Chan and co-workers [169, 170] reported a 50% prevalence of micro- or macro-albuminuria in Hong Kong Chinese individuals attending a hospital-based diabetes clinic despite a mean disease duration of less than 5 years. These findings have been confirmed in a multicenter survey of 6000 hypertensive type 2 diabetes patients recruited from 11 Asian countries, 3000 of whom were Chinese. In this survey, 20% of patients had clinical proteinuria and 40% microalbuminuria, making Asians one of the populations with the highest rates of diabetic nephropathy [171]. Other workers report a 30–50% prevalence for other microvascular complications, such as erectile dysfunction and retinopathy, which correlate with glycemic and blood pressure control, disease duration and albuminuria and are predictive of cardio-renal complications and related mortality [172, 173].

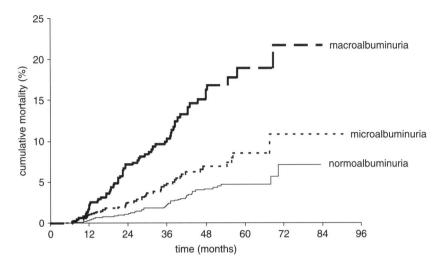

Figure 15.6 Cumulative mortality in 3773 Chinese type 2 diabetic patients after 3 years of follow up stratified by baseline albuminuric status. (Adapted from So, W.Y. *et al.* (2004) *Hypertension*, 44, 294–9.)

In approximately 50% of these patients, albuminuria coexisted with retinopathy, whereas albuminuria in the remaining subjects clustered with obesity, hypertension and dyslipidemia [75, 174]. Reports from Japan and China also indicate close associations between albuminuria and various components of MetS, including insulin resistance [174–177]. In addition, quintiles of white blood cell count within the normal range closely correlate with diabetic complications, independent of conventional risk factors and obesity [178]. In Hong Kong Chinese, increased albuminuria is highly predictive of death, cardiovascular and renal complications, with three- to five-fold increased risk compared with patients with normoalbuminuria [127, 179] (**Figure 15.6**).

15.9.3 Diabetic Kidney Disease

In the WHO-MSVDD, end-stage renal disease (ESRD) accounted for 10–15% of deaths in Hong Kong Chinese and in Japanese, in contrast to less than 5% of patients of European origin. Furthermore, the main cause of death due to CVDs was CHD in Caucasians, but was stroke in Chinese and Japanese patients [180]. The relative predilection of Asian patients to renal complications [180, 181] is now well established. In the Reduction of Endpoints in NIDDM with the Angiotensin II Antagonist Losartan (RENAAL) study [182],

which examined the renoprotective effect of an angiotensin receptor blocker (ARB; Losartan), in type 2 diabetes patients with nephropathy (albumin creatinine ratio ≥ 25 mg mmol^{-1}) and renal insufficiency (serum creatinine 110–260 μmol l^{-1}), receiving conventional antihypertensive drugs, 17% of subjects were enrolled from Asia (mainly from Japan and Hong Kong). The highest incidence of primary endpoint (death or ESRD defined as need for dialysis or doubling of baseline plasma creatinine) was observed in Asian patients treated with placebo with an annual rate approaching 15%. However, Asian subjects also benefited most from Losartan, which conferred a relative risk reduction for primary endpoint of 38%, compared with 28% for the cohort as a whole (**Figure 15.7**) [126].

The risk of CVD is increased in the presence of chronic kidney disease due to changes in the metabolic milieu, including anemia, increased calcium phosphate product with vascular calcification, oxidative stress and inflammation. In Chinese subjects, renal function is the major predictor of carotid IMT, a surrogate for atherosclerosis, which is predictive of cardiovascular events [183]. Close associations between glomerular filtration rate (GFR) and micro- and macro-vascular complications, independent of conventional risk factors and albuminuria, have been reported in Chinese type 2 diabetes patients [184]. Different grades of chronic

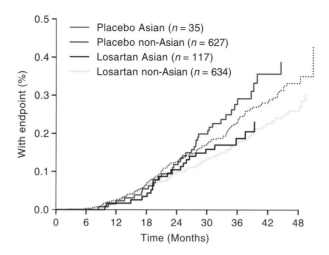

Figure 15.7 Effects of blockade of the renin angiotensin system using Losartan on incidence of ESRD in Asian and non-Asian type 2 diabetic patients with overt proteinuria and renal insufficiency in the RENAAL study. (Adapted from Brenner, B. *et al.* (2001) *New England Journal of Medicine*, 345, 861–9 and Chan, J.C.N. *et al.* (2004) *Diabetes Care* 27, 874–9.)

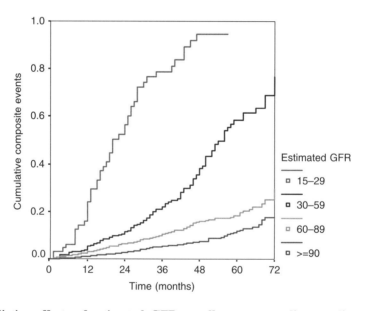

Figure 15.8 Predictive effects of estimated GFR on all-cause mortality, cardiovascular and renal endpoints in 4421 Chinese type 2 diabetes mellitus patients after 3.5 years of follow up. (Adapted from So, W.Y. *et al.* (2006) Diabetes Care 9:2046–2052.)

kidney disease (as classified by GFR) are also predictive of death, cardiovascular and renal endpoints in these patients [185] (**Figure 15.8**). Based on 4000 patients followed up for a mean duration of 3.5 years in Hong Kong, a risk equation has been developed which identifies blood hemoglobin, albuminuria and estimated

GFR (using the Modification of Diet in Renal Disease (MDRD) equation modified for Chinese population) as the main predictors for ESRD. The risk equation has sensitivity and specificity values approaching 90% with area under the ROC of 0.9. This risk equation, if externally validated, will be useful in identifying high-risk subjects [186].

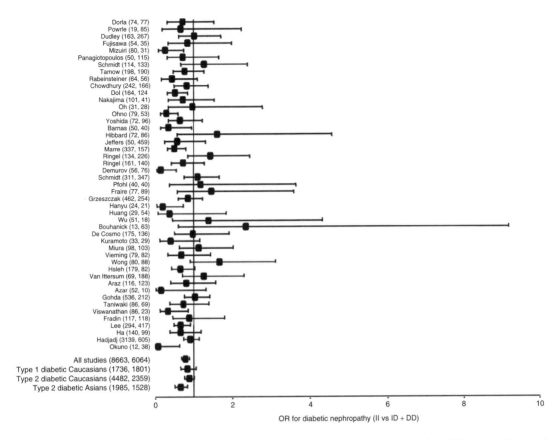

Figure 15.9 A meta-analysis showing the protective effects of ACE II genotype for diabetic nephropathy especially in Asian populations. (With kind permission from Springer Science & Business Media: Ng, D.P., Tai, B.C., Koh, D. et al. (2005) Angiotensin-I converting enzyme insertion/deletion polymorphism and its association with diabetic nephropathy: a meta-analysis of studies reported between 1994 and 2004 and comprising 14,727 subjects. *Diabetologia*, 48, 1008-16.)

The pathogenesis of diabetic nephropathy involves genetic, inflammatory, metabolic and hemobreakdynamic factors [187]. A large number of genetic variants encoding proteins in these pathways have been reported to be associated with diabetic nephropathy in Chinese subjects. Genetic variants that have been reported in large cohorts or replicated in separate Chinese populations include those encoding the aldose reductase [176, 188, 189], angiotensin converting enzyme (ACE) [190, 191], plasminogen activator inhibitor (PAI-1) [192], tumor necrosis factor (TNF-1α) [177], tumor growth factor (TGF-1β) [193] and various lipases and lipoproteins, notably apolipoprotein E, with possible gene–gene interactions [194–196]. Of particular note, the *ACE* insertion/deletion *II* genotype has now been shown to confer a

protective effect against diabetic nephropathy, especially amongst Asians, in a recent meta-analysis [197] (**Figures 15.9 and 15.10**).

Other factors include chronic inflammation, high prevalence of young-onset type 2 subjects with long disease duration (often undiagnosed or suboptimally treated), low relative risk for cardiovascular death, poor access to medical care and suboptimal control of risk factors. In a prospective cohort consisting of 2838 Chinese type 2 diabetes patients followed up for 3.5 years, chronic HBV infection was associated with a fourfold increased risk of ESRD independent of other all risk factors [105]. Similar findings have also been reported in Afro-Americans in whom chronic hepatitis C infection is associated with increased risk of ESRD [198, 199]. In Chinese type 2 diabetes patients with overt nephropathy

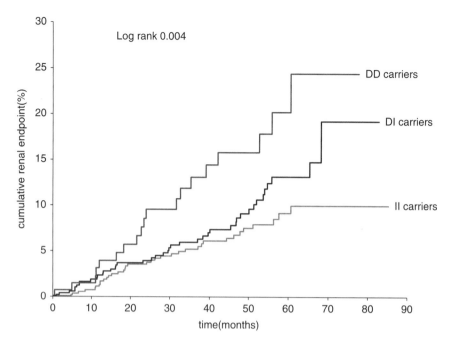

Figure 15.10 Independent predictive role of ACE DD/DI genotypes on renal endpoints in Chinese type 2 diabetic patients. (Adapted from Wang, Y. et al. (2004) Diabetes Care, 28, 348–54.)

and renal insufficiency, chronic HBV infection also predicts cardiovascular endpoints [200].

In Hong Kong, two clinic-based surveys in the early [179] and late 1990s [127] reported an annual mortality rate of 2–3% in known type 2 diabetes patients. In the earlier report [179], the majority of patients died from stroke and ESRD with equal contributions from both. In the more recent report by So et al. [127], 30% of diabetes patients died from cardiovascular causes (including stroke, CHD and heart failure), 15% died from ESRD and 30% from cancers.

Many Asian diabetes patients with ESRD do not have access to renal replacement therapy due to limited resources, old age and/or multiple comorbidities. In China, only 10% of patients on dialysis have diabetes [201], compared to more than 40% in Hong Kong Chinese patients [202].

15.10   FROM EPIDEMIOLOGY TO PREVENTION

Results of diabetes prevention programs [203, 204] suggest that improvement of lifestyle through education may alter the natural history of diabetes despite genetic predisposition. The lifestyle

modification program conducted by Pan et al. in China was a forerunner in this respect (**Figure 15.11**): 600 subjects with IGT were randomized (by clinic) to control, diet alone, diet plus exercise and exercise alone intervention groups. After 4 years, the risk of new onset of diabetes was significantly reduced by 30–50% in all three intervention groups compared with a control group. These beneficial results have now been confirmed in a 20-year follow up survey of the original cohort [205]. Since then, the beneficial effects of lifestyle modification have been independently confirmed in other populations (see additional reading list). Despite debates regarding cost effectiveness, there is a general consensus that opportunistic rather than population-based screening approaches should be adopted to identify risk subjects for intensive and structured prevention programs [206].

Pharmacological agents have also been shown in randomized clinical trials to reduce the risk of diabetes in high-risk subjects. In Chinese subjects, both metformin [207] and acarbose [208] have been shown to improve glucose tolerance in subjects with IGT and were generally well tolerated.

In Singapore, implementation of school-based programs, including features such as removal of

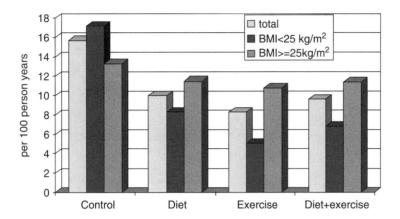

Figure 15.11 A 6-year lifestyle modification program in the Chinese Da Qing Diabetes Prevention Program showing 31–46% relative risk reduction for progression from impaired IGT to diabetes in both obese and nonobese Chinese subjects. The long term beneficial effects of this lifestyle modification program has recently been confirmed in a 20-year follow up study. (Adapted from Pan, X.R. *et al.* **(1997)** *Diabetes Care* **20, 537–44.)**

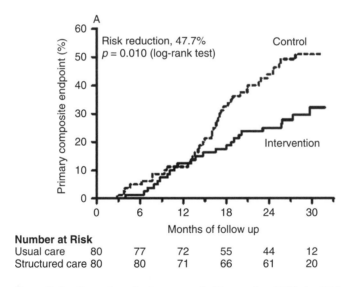

Number at Risk						
Usual care	80	77	72	55	44	12
Structured care	80	80	71	66	61	20

Figure 15.12 Prevention of death and end-stage renal disease by 50% in Chinese type 2 diabetic patients with overt nephropathy and renal insufficiency using structured care protocol delivered by a pharmacist-doctor team. (Reproduced from [215], Copyright © 2005, Elsevier.)

vending machines for beverages with high sugar content, compulsory physical education classes and provision of nutritionally balanced school meals, has been accompanied by an attenuated rising trend of obesity [209, 210].

A large number of randomized clinical trials confirm the beneficial effects of optimal control of blood pressure, blood glucose, LDL-C and appropriate use of RAS inhibitors and aspirin on cardiorenal complications. Each of these interventions is associated with 20–30% risk reduction. Multifaceted care targeting all risk factors has been shown to reduce risk of cardiovascular complications by 50% in Caucasians [211, 212]. Similar results have been reported in Chinese. Structured education and care programs using a

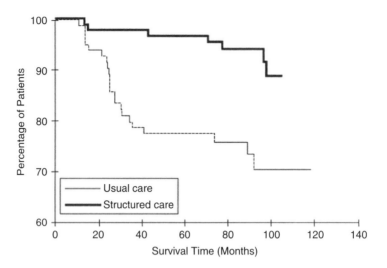

Figure 15.13 Prevention of death using structured care protocol delivered by a doctor-nurse team in Chinese hypertensive type 2 diabetic patients with no cardiovascular or renal complications at baseline. (Reproduced from [216], Copyright © 2003, Ascend Media.)

multidisciplinary approach can significantly improve metabolic control [213, 214] and clinical outcomes including death and ESRD [215–217]. Despite these encouraging findings, in the Diabcare-Asia 1998 study, which enrolled more than 20 000 young Asian type 1 and type 2 diabetes patients from 230 diabetes centers in 12 Asian countries, including China, the average HbA$_{1c}$ ranged from 8.5 to 9.9%. In 82% of the analysis population, the mean of centrally measured HbA$_{1c}$ was 8.6%. Of these subjects, 55% had values exceeding 8%, with China being one of the countries having a higher mean value than the overall mean [218].

15.11   CONCLUSION

In the past two decades, China has experienced a two- to three-fold increase in the prevalence of diabetes, with the highest rates observed in Chinese living in affluent societies such as Hong Kong, Singapore and Taiwan. The majority of these subjects remain undiagnosed. Even amongst the diagnosed, many (or even most) remain untreated or suboptimally treated. There are also high rates of gestational diabetes and childhood obesity in Chinese. Chinese develop diabetes at a lower level of obesity than Caucasians. Apart from genetic factors, diet and physical

inactivity, low birthweight, low-grade chronic infections, SES and education levels all have effects on diabetes and associated complications, giving rise to marked phenotypic and genotypic heterogeneity.

Compared with Caucasians, stroke and renal disease are more important causes of morbidity and mortality than CHD, and chronic kidney disease is a major determinant for cardiovascular events. Models of preventive programs for diabetes and associated complications have been developed in China. The main challenges lie in translating evidence to clinical practice to secure early diagnosis and optimal care.

References

1. World Health Organization (2006) Preventing Chronic Diseases: A Vital Investment. http://www .who.int/chp/chronic_disease_report/en/index .html (last accessed 1 June 2006).
2. Zimmet, P., Alberti, K.G. and Shaw, J. (2001) Global and societal implications of the diabetes epidemic. *Nature*, **414**, 782–787.
3. Yoon, K.H. Lee, J.H., Kim, J.W., *et al.* (2006) Epidemic obesity and type 2 diabetes in Asia. *Lancet*, **368**, 1681–1688.
4. Roglic, G., Unwin, N., Bennett, P. *et al.* (2005) The burden of mortality attributable to diabetes: realistic estimates for the year 2000. *Diabetes Care*, **28**, 2130–5.

5. International Diabetes Federation (2006) Facts and figures. Cost of diabetes, http://www.idf.org/home/ (last accessed on 1 June 2006).

6. Lin, T., Chou, P., Lai, M. *et al.* (2001) Direct cost-of-illness of patients with diabetes mellitus in Taiwan. *Diabetes Research and Clinical Practice*, **54** (Suppl 1), 43–6.

7. Chen, X., Tang, L. and Chen, H. (2003) Assessing the impact of complications on the costs of type 2 diabetes in urban China. *Chinese Journal of Diabetes*, **11**, 238–41.

8. Wong, K.C. and Wang, Z. (2006) Prevalence of type 2 diabetes mellitus of Chinese populations in mainland China, Hong Kong, and Taiwan. *Diabetes Research and Clinical Practice*, **73** (2), 126–34.

9. Cutter, J., Tan, B. and Chew, S. (2001) Levels of cardiovascular disease risk factors in Singapore following a national intervention programme. *Bulletin of the World Health Organization*, **79**, 908–15.

10. Soderberg, S., Zimmet, P., Tuomilehto, J. *et al.* (2005) Increasing prevalence of type 2 diabetes mellitus in all ethnic groups in Mauritius. *Diabetic Medicine: A Journal of the British Diabetic Association*, **22**, 61–8.

11. Wild, S., Roglic, G., Green, A. *et al.* (2004) Global prevalence of diabetes: estimates for the year 2000 and projections for 2030. *Diabetes Care*, **27**, 1047–53.

12. Gu, D., Reynolds, K., Duan, X., *et al.* (2003) Prevalence of diabetes and impaired fasting glucose in the Chinese adult population: International Collaborative Study of Cardiovascular Disease in Asia (InterASIA). *Diabetologia*, **46**, 1190–8.

13. Sayegh, H.A. and Jarrett, R.J. (1979) Oral glucose tolerance tests and the diagnosis of diabetes: results of a prospective study based on the Whitehall survey. *Lancet*, **II**, 432–3.

14. World Health Organization, Department of Noncommunicable Disease Surveillance (1999) *Definition, Diagnosis and Classification of Diabetes Mellitus and its Complications*. WHO, Geneva.

15. The Expert Committee on the Diagnosis and Classification of Diabetes Mellitus (2003) Follow-up report on the diagnosis of diabetes mellitus. *Diabetes Care*, **26**, 3160–7.

16. Cockram, C.S., Lau, J.T.F., Chan, A.Y.W. *et al.* (1992) Assessment of glucose tolerance test criteria for diagnosis of diabetes in Chinese subjects. *Diabetes Care*, **15**, 988–90.

17. Nakagami, T., Qiao, Q., Tuomilehto, J., *et al.* DECODA Study Group, Diabetes Epidemiology: Collaborative Analysis of Diagnostic Criteria in Asia; International Diabetes Epidemiology Group (2002) The fasting plasma glucose cut-point predicting a diabetic 2-h OGTT glucose level depends on the phenotype. *Diabetes Research and Clinical Practice*, **55**, 35–43.

18. Nakagami, T. (2004) Hyperglycaemia and mortality from all causes and from cardiovascular disease in five populations of Asian origin. *Diabetologia*, **47**, 385–94.

19. Hu, Y.H., Pan, X.R., Liu, P.A. *et al.* (1991) Coronary heart disease and diabetic retinopathy in newly diagnosed diabetes in Da Qing, China: the Da Qing IGT and Diabetes Study. *Acta Diabetologica*, **28**, 169–73.

20. Jia, W.P., Pang, C., Chen, L., *et al.* (2007) Epidemiological characteristics of diabetes mellitus and impaired glucose regulation in a Chinese adult population: the Shanghai Diabetes Studies, a cross-sectional 3-year follow-up study in Shanghai urban communities. *Diabetologia*, **50**, 286–292.

21. Cheung, B.M., Wat, N.M., Man, Y.B., *et al.* (2007) Development of diabetes in Chinese with the metabolic syndrome: a 6-year prospective study. *Diabetes Care*, **30**, 1430–1436.

22. Tso, A.W., Xu, A., Sham, P.C. *et al.* (2007) Serum adipocyte fatty acid binding protein as a new biomarker predicting the development of type 2 diabetes: a 10-year prospective study in a Chinese cohort. *Diabetes Care*, **30**, 2667–2672.

23. Ma, S., Cutter, J., Tan, C. *et al.* (2003) Associations of diabetes mellitus and ethnicity with mortality in a multiethnic Asian population: data from the 1992 Singapore National Health Survey. *American Journal of Epidemiology*, **158**, 543–52.

24. Yang, X., Zhang, H., Dong, L. *et al.* (2004) The effect of glucose levels on fetal birth weight: a study of Chinese gravidas in Tianjin, China. *The Journal of Diabetic Complications*, **18**, 37–41.

25. Yang, X., Hsu-Hage, B., Zhang, H. *et al.* (2003) Gestational diabetes mellitus in women of single gravidity in Tianjin City, China. *Diabetes Care*, **25**, 847–51.

26. Ko, G.T.C., Tam, W.H., Chan, J.C.N. and Rogers, M. (2002) Prevalence of gestational diabetes mellitus in Hong Kong based on the 1998 WHO criteria. *Diabetic Medicine: A Journal of the British Diabetic Association*, **19**, 180.

27. Ko, G.T.C., Chan, J.C.N., Tsang, L.W.W. *et al.* (1999) Glucose intolerance and other cardiovascular risk factors in Chinese women with a history of gestational diabetes mellitus. *Australian and New Zealand Journal of Obstetrics and Gynaecology*, **39**, 478–83.

28. Ko, G.T.C., Chan, J.C.N., Tsang, L.W.W. *et al.* (2000) Outcomes of screening for glucose intolerance in high risk Hong Kong Chinese. *Diabetes Care*, **23**, 1290–4.

29. Alberti, G., Zimmet, P., Shaw, J., *et al.* (2004) Type 2 diabetes in the young: the evolving epidemic: the International Diabetes Federation consensus workshop. *Diabetes Care*, **27**, 1798–811.

30. Kitagawa, T., Owada, M., Urakami, T. and Yamauchi, K. (1998) Increased incidence of non-insulin dependent diabetes mellitus among Japanese school children correlates with an increased intake of animal protein and fat. *Clinical Pediatrics*, **37**, 111–15.

31. Sung, R.Y., Tong, P.C.Y., Yu, C.W. *et al.* (2002) High prevalence of insulin resistance and metabolic syndrome in overweight/obese preadolescent Hong Kong Chinese children aged 9–12 years. *Diabetes Care*, **26**, 250–1.

32. Wei, J., Sung, F., Lin, C. *et al.* (2003) National surveillance for type 2 diabetes mellitus in Taiwanese children. *The Journal of the American Medical Association*, **290**, 1345–50.

33. Urakami, T., Kubota, S., Nitadori, Y. *et al.* (2005) Annual incidence and clinical characteristics of type 2 diabetes in children as detected by urine glucose screening in the Tokyo metropolitan area. *Diabetes Care*, **28**, 1876–81.

34. Wei, J., Sung, F., Li, C. *et al.* (2003) Low birth weight and high birth weight infants are both at an increased risk to have type 2 diabetes among schoolchildren in Taiwan. *Diabetes Care*, **26**, 343–8.

35. Woo, K.S., Chook, P., Yu, C.W. *et al.* (2004) Effects of diet and exercise on obesity-related vascular dysfunction in children. *Circulation*, **109**, 1981–6.

36. Cook, S., Weitzman, M., Auinger, P. *et al.* (2003) Prevalence of a metabolic syndrome phenotype in adolescents. *Archives of Pediatrics and Adolescent Medicine*, **157**, 821–7.

37. Ozaki, R. Qiao, Q., Wong, G.W. *et al.* (2007) Overweight, family history of diabetes and attending schools of lower academic grading are independent predictors for metabolic syndrome in Hong Kong Chinese adolescents. *Arch Dis Child*, **92**, 224–228.

38. Wang, Y., Ge, K. and Popkin, B. (2000) Tracking of body mass index from childhood to adolescence: a 6-years follow-up study in China. *The American Journal of Clinical Nutrition*, **72**, 1018–24.

39. Li, X., Li, T., Yang, Z. *et al.* (2000) A nine-year prospective study on the incidence of childhood type 1 diabetes mellitus in China. *Biomedical and Environmental Sciences*, **13**, 263–7.

40. Huen, K.F., Low, L.C., Wong, G.W. *et al.* (2000) Epidemiology of diabetes mellitus in children in Hong Kong: the Hong Kong childhood diabetes register. *Journal of Pediatrics Endocrinology and Metabolism*, **13**, 297–302.

41. Pociot, F. and McDermott, M. (2002) Genetics of type 1 diabetes. *Genes and Immunity*, **3**, 235–49.

42. Penny, M.A., Jenkins, D., Mijovic, C. *et al.* (1992) Susceptibility to IDDM in a Chinese population. Role of HLA class II alleles. *Diabetes*, **41**, 914–30.

43. Chuang, L., Jou, T., Hu, C. *et al.* (1994) HLA-DQB1 codon 57 and IDDM in Chinese living in Taiwan. *Diabetes Care*, **17**, 863–8.

44. Chuang, L., Jou, T., Wu, H. *et al.* (1995) HLA-DQA1 genotypes and its interaction with HLA-DQB1 in Chinese IDDM living in Taiwan. *Proceedings of the National Science Council, Republic of China. Part B, Life Sciences*, **19**, 73–9.

45. Kelly, M.A., Chan, J.C.N., Heward, J. *et al.* (2000) HLA typing and immunological characterization of young-onset diabetes mellitus in a Hong Kong Chinese population. *Diabetic Medicine: A Journal of the British Diabetic Association*, **18**, 22–8.

46. Ueda, H., Howson, J., Esposito, L. *et al.* (2003) Association of the T-cell regulatory gene *CTLA4* with susceptibility of autoimmune disesse. *Nature*, **423**, 506–11.

47. Lee, Y., Huang, F., Lo, F. *et al.* (2000) Association of *CTLA4* gene A–G polymorphism with type 1 diabetes in Chinese children. *Clinical Endocrinology*, **52**, 153–57.

48. Ma, Y., Tang, X., Chang, W. *et al.* (2002) *CTLA-4* gene A/G polymorphism associated with diabetes mellitus in Han Chinese. *Chinese Medical Journal*, **115**, 1248–50.

49. Altshuler, D., Brooks, L., Chakravarti, A., *et al.* (2005) A haplotype map of the human genome. *Nature*, **437**, 1299–320.

50. Ng, M.C.Y., Wang, Y., So, W.Y. *et al.* (2004) Ethnic differences in the linkage disequilibrium and distribution of single nucleotide polymorphisms in 35 candidate genes for cardiovascular diseases. *Genomics*, **83**, 559–65.

51. Eckel, R., Grundy, S. and Zimmet, P. (2005) The metabolic syndrome. *Lancet*, **365**, 1415–28.

52. Smyth, S. and Heron, A. (2006) Diabetes and obesity: the twin epidemics. *Nature Medicine*, **12**, 75–80.

53. Chan, J.C.N., Cheung, C.K., Swaminathan, R. *et al.* (1993) Obesity, albuminuria and hypertension among Hong Kong Chinese with non-insulin-dependent diabetes mellitus

(NIDDM). *Postgraduate Medical Journal*, **69**, 204–10.

54. Cockram, C.S., Woo, J., Lau, E. *et al.* (1993) The prevalence of diabetes mellitus and impaired glucose tolerance among Hong Kong Chinese adults of working age. *Diabetes Research and Clinical Practice*, **21**, 67–73.

55. Yajnik, C. and Yudkin, J. (2004) The Y–Y paradox. *Lancet*, **363**, 163.

56. He, M., Tan, K.C., Li, E.T. and Kung, A.W. (2001) Body fat determination by dual energy X-ray absorptiometry and its relation to body mass index and waist circumference in Hong Kong Chinese. *International Journal of Obesity and Related Metabolic Disorders*, **25**, 748–52.

57. Ko, G.T.C., Chan, J.C.N., Woo, J. and Cockram, C.S. (1999) Prediction of hypertension, diabetes, dyslipidaemia or albuminuria using simple anthropometric indexes in Hong Kong Chinese. *International Journal of Obesity*, **23**, 1136–42.

58. Huxley, R., James, W.P., Barzi, F. *et al.* (2008) Ethnic comparisons of the cross-sectional relationships between measures of body size with diabetes and hypertension. *Obes Rev*, **9** (Suppl 1), 53–61.

59. WHO Expert Consultation (2004) Appropriate body mass index for Asian populations and its implications for policy and intervention strategies. *Lancet*, **363**, 157–63.

60. Schooling, C.M., Lam, T.H., Li, Z.B. *et al.* (2006) Obesity, physical activity, and mortality in a prospective Chinese elderly cohort. *Archives of Internal Medicine*, **166**, 1498–1504.

61. Thomas, G.N., Schooling, C.M., McGhee, S.M. *et al.* (2007) Metabolic syndrome increases all-cause and vascular mortality: the Hong Kong Cardiovascular Risk Factor Study. *Clin Endocrinol (Oxf)*, **66**, 666–671.

62. Jia, W.P., Lu, J.X., Kiang, K.S. *et al.* (2003) Prediction of abdominal visceral obesity from body mass index, waist circumference and waist–hip ratio in Chinese adults: receiver operating characteristics curves analysis. *Biomedical and Environmental Sciences*, **2003**, 206–11.

63. Jia, W., Xiang, K., Chen, L. *et al.* (2002) Epidemiological study on obesity and its comorbidities in urban Chinese older than 20 years of age in Shanghai, China. *Obesity Reviews*, **3**, 157–65.

64. Liu, K., Chan, Y., Chan, W. *et al.* (2003) Sonographic measurement of mesenteric fat thickness and its association with cardiovascular risk factors: comparison with subcutaneous and preperitoneal fat thickness, magnetic resonance imaging and anthropometric indexes. *International Journal of Obesity*, **27**, 1267–73.

65. Liu, K., Chan, Y.L., Chan, J.C. *et al.* (2006) Mesenteric fat thickness as an independent determinant of fatty liver. *International Journal of Obesity*, **30**, 787–93.

66. Liu, K.H., Chan, Y.L., Chan, J.C.N. and Chan, W.B. (2005) Association of carotid intima-media thickness with mesenteric, preperitoneal and subcutaneous fat thickness. *Atherosclerosis*, **179**, 299–304.

67. Liu, K., Chan, Y., Chan, W. *et al.* (2006) Mesenteric fat thickness is an independent determinant of metabolic syndrome and defines subjects with increased carotid intima-media thickness. *Diabetes Care*, **29**, 379–84.

68. Despres, J.P., Lemieux, I., (2000) Abdominal obesity and metabolic syndrome. *Nature*, **444**, 881–887.

69. Alberti, K., Zimmet, P. and Shaw J. (2005) The metabolic syndrome – a new worldwide definition. *Lancet*, **366**, 1059–62.

70. Tan, C.E., Ma, S., Wai, D. *et al.* (2004) Can we apply the National Cholesterol Education Program Adult Treatment Panel Definition of the metabolic syndrome to Asians? *Diabetes Care*, **27**, 1182–6.

71. Gu, D., Reynolds, K., Wu X., *et al.* (2005) Prevalence of the metabolic syndrome and overweight among adults in China. *Lancet*, **365**, 1398–405.

72. Chan, J.C.N., Tong, P.C.Y. and Critchley, J.A.J.H. (2002) The insulin resistance syndrome – mechanism of clustering of cardiovascular risk. *Seminars in Vascular Medicine*, **2**, 45–57.

73. Alberti, K.G., Zimmet, P. and Shaw J. (2007) International Diabetes Federation: a consensus on Type 2 diabetes prevention. *Diabet Med*, **24**, 451–463.

74. Gillies, C.L., Abrams, K.R., Lambert P.C., *et al.* (2007) Pharmacological and lifestyle interventions to prevent or delay type 2 diabetes in people with impaired glucose tolerance: systematic review and meta-analysis. *Bmj*, **334**, 299

75. Chan, J.C.N., Cheung, J.C.K., Lau, E.M.C. *et al.* (1996) The metabolic syndrome in Hong Kong Chinese – the inter-relationships amongst its components analysed by structural equation modelling. *Diabetes Care*, **19**, 953–9.

76. Sawada, S., Lee, I., Muto, T. *et al.* (2003) Cardiorespiratory fitness and the incidence of type 2 diabetes: prospective study of Japanese men. *Diabetes Care*, **26**, 2918–22.

77. Nakanishi, N. Takatorige, T. and Suzuki K. (2005) Cigarette smoking and the risk of the metabolic syndrome in middle-aged Japanese male office workers. *Industrial Health*, **43**, 295–301.

78. Ko, G.T.C., Chan, J.C.N., Tsang, L.W. *et al.* (2000) Smoking and diabetes in Chinese men. *Postgraduate Medical Journal*, **77**, 240–3.

79. Hancox, R., Milne, B. and Poulton, R. (2004) Association between child and adolescent television viewing and adult health: a longitudinal birth cohort study. *Lancet*, **364**, 257–62.

80. Pereira, M., Kartashov, A., Ebbeling, C. *et al.* (2005) Fast-food habits, weight gain, and insulin resistance (the CARDIA study): 15-year prospective analysis. *Lancet*, **365**, 36–42.

81. Glumer, C., Carstensen, B., Sandbaek, A. *et al.* (2004) A Danish diabetes risk score for targeted screening: the Inter99 study. *Diabetes Care*, **27**, 727–33.

82. Meigs, J., Williams, K., Sullivan, L. *et al.* (2004) Using metabolic syndrome traits for efficient detection of impaired glucose tolerance. *Diabetes Care*, **27**, 1417–26.

83. Stern, M., Williams, K. and Haffner, S. (2002) Identification of persons at high risk for type 2 diabetes mellitus: do we need the oral glucose tolerance test? *Annals of Internal Medicine*, **136**, 575–81.

84. Aekplakorn, W., Bunnag, P., Woodward, M., *et al.* (2006) A risk score for predicting incident diabetes in the Thai population. *Diabetes Care*, **29**, 1872–1877.

85. Maty, S., Everson-Rose, S., Hann, M. *et al.* (2005) Education, income, occupation, and the 34-year incidence (1965–99) of type 2 diabetes in the Alameda County Study. *International Journal of Epidemiology*, **34**, 1274–81.

86. Connolly, V., Unwin, N., Sherriff, P. *et al.* (2000) Diabetes prevalence and socioeconomic status: a population based study showing increased prevalence of type 2 diabetes mellitus in deprived areas. *Journal of Epidemiology and Community Health*, **54**, 173–7.

87. Kumari, M., Head, J. and Marmot, M. (2004) Prospective study of social and other risk factors for incidence of type 2 diabetes in the Whitehall II Study. *Archives of Internal Medicine*, **164**, 1873–80.

88. Pan, X.R., Yang, W.Y., Li, G.W. and Liu, J. (1997) Prevalence of diabetes and its risk factors in China, 1994. National Diabetes Prevention and Control Cooperative Group. *Diabetes Care*, **20**, 1664–9.

89. Ko, G.T.C., Chan, J.C.N. and Cockram, C.S. (2001) A low socioeconomic class is associated with diabetes and metabolic syndrome in Hong Kong Chinese. *European Journal of Epidemiology*, **17**, 289–95.

90. Hales, C.N. and Barker, D.J.P. (1992) Type 2 (non-insulin-dependent) diabetes mellitus: the thrifty phenotype hypothesis. *Diabetologia*, **35**, 595–601.

91. Mi, J., Law, C., Zhang, K.L. *et al.* (2000) Effects of infant birthweight and maternal body mass index in pregnancy on components of the insulin resistance syndrome in China. *Annals of Internal Medicine*, **132**, 253–60.

92. Cheung, N. and Byth, K. (2003) Population health significance of gestational diabetes. *Diabetes Care*, **26**, 2005–9.

93. Yue, D., Molyneaux, L., Ross, G. *et al.* (1996) Why does ethnicity affect prevalence of gestational diabetes? The underwater volcano theory. *Diabetic Medicine: A Journal of the British Diabetic Association*, **13**, 748–52.

94. Lao, T.T., Tse, K.Y., Chan, L.Y. *et al.* (2003) HBsAg carrier status and the association between gestational diabetes with increased serum ferritin concentration in Chinese women. *Diabetes Care*, **26**, 3011–16.

95. Lao, T.T. and Ho, L.F. (2001) Alpha-thalassaemia trait and gestational diabetes mellitus in Hong Kong. *Diabetologia*, **44**, 966–71.

96. Lao, T.T., Chan, P.L. and Tam, K.F. (2001) Gestational diabetes mellitus in the last trimester – a feature of maternal iron excess? *Diabetic Medicine: A Journal of the British Diabetic Association*, **18**, 218–23.

97. Tong, P.C.Y., Ng, M.C.Y., Ho, C.S. *et al.* (2001) Thalassemia minor is associated with insulin resistance in high-risk subjects for diabetes. *Diabetes*, **50** (Suppl 2), A103.

98. Fernandez-Real, J-M., Ricart-Engel, W., Arroyo, E. *et al.* (1998) Serum ferritin as a component of the insulin resistance syndrome. *Diabetes Care*, **21**, 62–68.

99. Ferrannini, E. (2000) Insulin resistance, iron, and the liver. *Lancet*, **355**, 2181–2.

100. Pradhan, A.D., Manson, J.E., Rifai, N. *et al.* (2001) C-reactive protein, interleukin 6 and risk of developing type 2 diabetes mellitus. *The Journal of the American Medical Association*, **286**, 327–34.

101. Mendall, M.A. (1998) Inflammatory responses and coronary heart disease: the dirty chicken hypothesis of cardiovascular risk factors. *British Medical Journal*, **316**, 953–4.

102. Tong, P.C.Y., Ho, C.S., Yeung, V.T.F. *et al.* (2005) Low testosterone and insulin-like growth factor-I but high C-reactive protein are independent predictors for metabolic syndrome in Chinese middle-aged men with a family history of type 2 diabetes. *The Journal of Clinical Endocrinology and Metabolism*, **90**, 6418–23.

103. Tan, K.C., Wat, N.M., Tam, S.C. *et al.* (2003) C-reactive protein predicts the deterioration of glycemia in Chinese subjects with impaired glucose tolerance. *Diabetes Care*, **26**, 2323–8.

104. Tam, C.M., Leung, C.C., Noertjojo, K. *et al.* (2003) Tuberculosis in Hong Kong – patient characteristics and treatment outcome. *Hong Kong Medical Journal*, **9**, 83–90.

105. Cheng, A.Y.S., Kong, A.P.S., Wong, V.W.S. *et al.* Chronic hepatitis B viral infection independently predicts renal outcome in type 2 diabetic patients. (2006) *Diabetologia*, **49** (8), 1777–84.

106. Chen, L., Hwang, S., Tsai, S. *et al.* (2000) Glucose intolerance in Chinese patients with chronic hepatitis C. *World Journal of Gastroenterology*, **9**, 505–8.

107. Ko, G.T.C., Chan, J.C.N., Yeung, V.T.F. *et al.* (1998) Antibodies to glutamic acid decarboxylase in young Chinese diabetic patients. *Annals of Clinical Biochemistry*, **35**, 761–7.

108. Thai, A.C., Ng, W.Y., Loke, K.Y. *et al.* (1997) Anti-GAD antibodies in Chinese patients with youth and adult-onset IDDM and NIDDM. *Diabetologia*, **40**, 1425–30.

109. Pan, C.Y., So, W.Y., Khalid, B.A. *et al.* (2004) Metabolic, immunological and clinical characteristics in newly diagnosed Asian diabetes patients aged 12–40 years. *Diabetic Medicine: A Journal of the British Diabetic Association*, **21**, 1007–13.

110. Ng, M.C.Y., Lee, S.C., Ko, G.T.C. *et al.* (2001) Familial early onset type 2 diabetes in Chinese: the more significant roles of obesity and genetics than autoimmunity. *Diabetes Care*, **24**, 667–71.

111. Turner, R.C., Stratton, I., Horton, V. *et al.* (1997) UKPDS 25: autoantibodies to islet-cell cytoplasm and glutamic acid decarboxylase for prediction of insulin requirement in type 2 diabetes. UK Prospective Diabetes Study Group. *Lancet*, **350**, 1288–93.

112. Yang, L., Zhou, Z.G., Huang, G. *et al.* (2005) Six-year follow-up of pancreatic beta cell function in adults with latent autoimmune diabetes. *World Journal of Gastroenterology*, **11**, 2900–5.

113. Banerji, M.A., Chaiken, R.L., Huey, H. *et al.* (1994) GAD antibody negative NIDDM in adult Black subjects with diabetic ketoacidosis and increased frequency of human leukocyte antigen DR3 and DR4. Flatbush Diabetes. *Diabetes*, **43**, 741–5.

114. Tan, K.C.B., Mackay, I.R., Zimmet, P.Z. *et al.* (2000) Metabolic and immunologic features of Chinese patients with atypical diabetes mellitus. *Diabetes Care*, **23**, 335–8.

115. Li, J.K.Y., Chan, J.C.N., Zimmet, P.Z. *et al.* (2000) Young Chinese adults with new onset of diabetic ketoacidosis – clinical course, autoimmune status and progression of pancreatic beta cell function. *Diabetic Medicine: A Journal of the British Diabetic Association*, **17**, 295–8.

116. Chan, J.C.N. and Ng, M.C.Y. (2003) Lessons learned from young onset diabetes in China. *Current Diabetes Reports*, **3**, 101–7.

117. Xu, J.Y., Dan, Q.H., Chan, V. *et al.* (2005) Genetic and clinical characteristics of maturity-onset diabetes of the young in Chinese patients. *European Journal of Human Genetics*, **13**, 422–7.

118. Xu, J.Y., Chan, V., Zhang, W.Y. *et al.* (2002) Mutations in the hepatocyte nuclear factor-1alpha gene in Chinese MODY families: prevalence and functional analysis. *Diabetologia*, **45**, 744–6.

119. Yoon, K., Ko, S., Cho, J. *et al.* (2003) Selective beta-cell loss and alpha-cell expansion in patients with type 2 diabetes mellitus in Korea. *The Journal of Clinical Endocrinology and Metabolism*, **88**, 2300–8.

120. Boyko, E., Leonetti, D., RW, B. and Fujimoto, W. (1997) Fasting insulin level underestimates risk of non-insulin-dependent diabetes mellitus due to confounding by insulin secretion. *American Journal of Epidemiology*, **145**, 18–23.

121. Chan, W.B., Tong, P.C.Y., Chow, C.C. *et al.* (2004) The associations of body mass index, C peptide and metabolic status in Chinese type 2 diabetic patients. *Diabetic Medicine: A Journal of the British Diabetic Association*, **21**, 349–53.

122. Ng, M.C.Y., Li, J.K.Y., So, W.Y. *et al.* (2000) Nature or nurture – an insightful illustration from a Chinese family with hepatocyte nuclear factor 1-alpha diabetes (MODY3). *Diabetologia*, **43**, 816–18.

123. Chan, J.C.N., Hawkin, B.R. and Cockram, C.S. (1990) A Chinese family with non-insulin-dependent diabetes of early onset. *Diabetic Medicine: A Journal of the British Diabetic Association*, **7**, 211–14.

124. Yokoyama, H., Okudaira, M., Otani, T. *et al.* (1998) High incidence of diabetic nephropathy in early onset Japanese NIDDM patients. Risk analysis. *Diabetes Care*, **21**, 1080–5.

125. Ko, G.T.C., Chan, J.C.N., Lau, M.S.W. and Cockram, C.S. (2000) Diabetic microangiopathic complications in young Chinese diabetic patients – a clinic-based cross-sectional study. *Journal of Diabetes and its Complications*, **13**, 300–6.

126. Chan, J.C.N., Wat, N.M.S., So, W.Y. *et al.* (2004) RAAS blockade and renal disease in type 2 diabetic patients: an Asian perspective from the RENAAL Study. *Diabetes Care*, **27**, 874–9.

127. So, W.Y., Chan, N., Tong, P.C.Y. *et al.* (2004) Effect of RAAS inhibition on survival and renal

outcomes in 3737 Chinese type 2 diabetic patients. *Hypertension*, **44**, 294–9.

128. Fajans, S.S., Bell, G.I. and Polonsky, K.S. (2001) Molecular mechanisms and clinical pathophysiology of maturity onset diabetes of the young. *The New England Journal of Medicine*, **345**, 971–80.

129. Hattersley, A. and Pearson, E. (2006) Minireview: Pharmacogenetics and beyond: the interaction of therapeutic response, β-cell physiology and genetics in diabetes. *Endocrinology*, **147** (6), 2657–63.

130. Ng, M.C.Y., Yeung, V.T.F., Chow, C.C. *et al.* (2000) Mitochondrial DNA *A3243G* mutation in patients with early or late onset type 2 diabetes mellitus in Hong Kong Chinese. *The Journal of Endocrinology*, **52**, 557–64.

131. Ji, L., Hou, X. and Han, X. (2001) Prevalence and clinical characteristics of mitochondrial tRNA leu(UUR) mt 3243 A→G and *ND-1* gene mt 3316 G→A mutations in Chinese patients with type 2 diabetes. *Diabetes Research and Clinical Practice*, **114**, 1205–7.

132. Xiang, K., Wang, Y., Wu, S. *et al.* (1997) Mitochondrial tRNA(Leu(UUR)) gene mutation diabetes mellitus in Chinese. *Chinese Medical Journal*, **110**, 372–8.

133. Park, K.S., Chan, J.C., Chuang, L.M. *et al.* (2008) A mitochondrial DNA variant at position 16189 is associated with type 2 diabetes mellitus in Asians. *Diabetologia*, **51**, 602–608.

134. Chinnery, P.F., Elliott, H.R., Patel, S. *et al.* (2005) Role of the mitochondrial DNA 16184–16193 poly-C tract in type 2 diabetes. *Lancet*, **366**, 1650–1.

135. Zhao, H.L., Lai, F.M.M., Tong, P.C.Y. *et al.* (2003) Prevalence and clinicopathological characteristics of islet amyloid in Chinese patients with type 2 diabetes. *Diabetes*, **52**, 2759–66.

136. Clark, A. and Nilsson, M.R. (2004) Islet amyloid: a complication of islet dysfunction or an aetiological factor in type 2 diabetes? *Diabetologia*, **47**, 157–69.

137. Clark, A., Wells, C.A., Buley, I.D. *et al.* (1988) Islet amyloid, increased A-cells, reduced B-cells and exocrine fibrosis: quantitative changes in the pancreas in type 2 diabetes. *Diabetes Research (Edinburgh, Lothian)*, **9**, 151–9.

138. Hayden, M.R., Tyagi, S.C., Kerklo, M.M. and Nicolls, M.R. (2005) Type 2 diabetes mellitus as a conformational disease. *Journal of Pancreas*, **6**, 287–302.

139. Poa, N., Cooper, G. and Edgar, P. (2003) Amylin gene promoter mutations predispose to type 2 diabetes in New Zealand Maori. *Diabetologia*, **46**, 574–8.

140. Lee, S.C., Hashim, Y., Li, J.K.Y. *et al.* (2001) The islet amyloid polypeptide (amylin) gene *S20G* mutation in Chinese subjects: evidence for associations with type 2 diabetes and cholesterol levels. *The Journal of Endocrinology*, **54**, 541–6.

141. Seino S. (2001) *S20G* mutation of the amylin gene is associated with type II diabetes in Japanese. Study Group of Comprehensive Analysis of Genetic Factors in Diabetes Mellitus. *Diabetologia*, **44**, 906–9.

142. Ma, Z., Westermark, G.T., Sakagashira, S. *et al.* (2001) Enhanced in vitro production of amyloid-like fibrils from mutant (*S20G*) islet amyloid polypeptide. *Amyloid*, **8**, 242–9.

143. Anderson, P.J., Critchley, J.A.J.H., Chan, J.C.N. *et al.* (2001) Factor analysis of the metabolic syndrome: obesity versus insulin resistance as the central abnormality. *International Journal of Obesity*, **25**, 1782–8.

144. Chan, J.C.N., Cheung, J.C.K., Stehouwer, C.D.A. *et al.* (2002) The central roles of obesity-associated dyslipidaemia, endothelial activation and cytokines in the metabolic syndrome – an analysis by structural equation modelling. *International Journal of Obesity*, **26**, 994–1008.

145. Pladevall, M., Singal, B., Williams, L. *et al.* (2006) A single factor underlies the metabolic syndrome: a confirmatory factor analysis. *Diabetes Care*, **29**, 113–22.

146. Ang, L., Ma, S., Cutter, J. *et al.* (2005) The metabolic syndrome in Chinese, Malays and Asian Indians. Factor analysis of data from the 1998 Singapore National Health Survey. *Diabetes Research and Clinical Practice*, **67**, 53–62.

147. Wang, J., Qiao, Q., Miettinen, M. *et al.* (2004) The metabolic syndrome defined by factor analysis and incident type 2 diabetes in a Chinese population with high postprandial glucose. *Diabetes Care*, **27**, 2429–37.

148. Li, J.K.Y., Ng, M.C.Y., So, W.Y. *et al.* (2006) Phenotypic and genetic clustering of diabetes and metabolic syndrome in Chinese families with type 2 diabetes mellitus. *Diabetes/Metabolism Research and Reviews*, **22**, 46–52.

149. Ng, M.C., So, W.Y., Cox, N.J. *et al.* (2004) Genome wide scan for metabolic syndrome and related quantitative traits in Hong Kong Chinese and confirmation of a susceptibility locus on chromosome 1q21–25. *Diabetes*, **53**, 2676–83.

150. Xiang, K., Wang, Y., Zheng, T. *et al.* (2004) Genome-wide search for type 2 diabetes/impaired glucose homeostasis susceptibility genes in the Chinese: significant linkage to chromosome

6q21–q23 and chromosome 1q21–q24. *Diabetes*, **53**, 228–34.

151. Zhao, J., Xiong, M., Huang, W. *et al.* (2005) An autosomal genomic scan for loci linked to type 2 diabetes in northern Han Chinese. *Journal of Molecular Medicine*, **83**, 209–15.

152. Ng, M.C.Y., So, W.Y., Cox, N.J. *et al.* (2004) Genome wide scan for type 2 diabetes loci in Hong Kong Chinese and confirmation of a susceptibility locus on chromosome 1q21–q25. *Diabetes*, **53**, 1609–13.

153. Chiu, Y., Chuang, L., Hsiao, C. *et al.* (2005) An autosomal genome-wide scan for loci linked to prediabetic phenotypes in nondiabetic Chinese subjects from the Stanford Asia-Pacific Program of Hypertension and Insulin Resistance Family Study. *Diabetes*, **54**, 1200–6.

154. Luo, T., Zhao, Y., Li, G. *et al.* (2001) A genome-wide search for type II diabetes susceptibility genes in Chinese Hans. *Diabetologia*, **44**, 501–6.

155. Ng, M.C., Park, K.S., Oh, B. *et al.* (2008) Implication of Genetic Variants near TCF7L2, SLC30A8, HHEX, CDKAL1, CDKN2A/B, IGF2BP2 and FTO in Type 2 Diabetes and Obesity in 6719 Asians. *Diabetes*.

156. Vague J. (1991) *Regulation of the Fat Mass. Obesities*, John Libbey & Co. Ltd./Edition Solal, Marseille, France, pp. 25–34.

157. Björntorp, P. (1991) Metabolic implications of body fat distribution. *Diabetes Care*, **14**, 1132–43.

158. Lee, Z.S.K., Critchley, J.A.J.H., Tomlinson, B. *et al.* (2001) Urinary epinephrine and norepinephrine with obesity, insulin and the metabolic syndrome in Hong Kong Chinese. *Metabolism: Clinical and Experimental*, **50**, 135–43.

159. Lee, Z.S.K., Chan, J.C.N., Yeung, V.T.F. *et al.* (1999) Plasma insulin, growth hormone, cortisol and central obesity among young Chinese type 2 diabetic patients. *Diabetes Care*, **22**, 1450–7.

160. Yang, W. and Chuang, L. (2006) Human genetics of adiponectin in the metabolic syndrome. *Journal of Molecular Medicine*, **84**, 112–21.

161. Yusuf, S., Hawken, S., Ounpuu, S. *et al.* (2005) Obesity and the risk of myocardial infarction in 27,000 participants from 52 countries: a case-control study. *Lancet*, **366**, 1640–9.

162. Lawes, C., Parag, V., Bennett, D., *et al.* (2004) Blood glucose and risk of cardiovascular disease in the Asia Pacific region. *Diabetes Care*, **27**, 2836–42.

163. Chi, Z., Lee, E., Lu, M. *et al.* (2001) Vascular disease prevalence in diabetic patients in China: standardised comparison with the 14 centres in the WHO Multinational Study of Vascular Disease in Diabetes. *Diabetologia*, **44** (Suppl 2), S82–6.

164. Wong, K.S. (1999) Risk factors for early death in acute ischemic stroke and intracerebral hemorrhage. A prospective hospital-based study in Asia. *Stroke; A Journal of Cerebral Circulation*, **30**, 2326–30.

165. Thomas, G.N., Lin, J.W., Lam, W.W. *et al.* (2003) Middle cerebral artery stenosis in type II diabetic Chinese patients is associated with conventional risk factors but not with polymorphisms of the rennin–angiotensin system genes. *Cerebrovascular Diseases (Basel, Switzerland)*, **16**, 217–23.

166. Thomas, G.N., Critchley, J.A.J.H., Tomlinson, B. *et al.* (2003) Peripheral vascular disease in type 2 diabetic Chinese patients: associations with metabolic indices, concomitant vascular disease and genetic factors. *Diabetic Medicine: A Journal of the British Diabetic Association*, **20**, 988–95.

167. Hu, D.Y., Pan, C.Y., Yu, J.M. *et al.* (2006) The relationship between coronary artery disease and abnormal glucose regulation in China: the China Heart Survey. *European Heart Journal*, **27**, 2573–2579.

168. Sanderson, J.E., Chan, S.K., Chan, W.W. *et al.* (1995) The aetiology of heart failure in the Chinese population of Hong Kong – a prospective study of 730 consecutive patients. *International Journal of Cardiology*, **51**, 29–35.

169. Chan, J.C.N. and Cockram, C.S. (1997) Diabetes mellitus in Chinese and its implications on health care. *Diabetes Care*, **20**, 1785–90.

170. Chan, J.C.N., Ng, M.C.Y., Critchley, J.A.J.H. *et al.* (2001) Diabetes mellitus – a special medical challenge from a Chinese perspective. *Diabetes Research and Clinical Practice*, **54**, S19–27.

171. Wu, A.Y., Kong, N.C., de Leon, F.A. *et al.* (2005) An alarmingly high prevalence of diabetic nephropathy in Asian type 2 diabetic patients: the MicroAlbuminuria Prevalence (MAP) Study. *Diabetologia*, **48**, 1674–5.

172. Tong, P.C., Kong, A.P., So, W.Y. *et al.* (2007) Interactive effect of retinopathy and macroalbuminuria on all-cause mortality, cardiovascular and renal end points in Chinese patients with Type 2 diabetes mellitus. *Diabet Med*, **24**, 741–746.

173. Ma, R.C., So, W.Y., Yang, X. *et al.* (2008) Erectile dysfunction predicts coronary heart disease in type 2 diabetes. *J Am Coll Cardiol*, **51**, 2045–2050.

174. Chan, J.C.N., Tomlinson, B., Nicholls, M.G. *et al.* (1996) Albuminuria, insulin resistance and dyslipidaemia in Chinese patients with non-insulin-dependent diabetes (NIDDM).

Diabetic Medicine: A Journal of the British Diabetic Association, **13**, 150–5.

175. Tanaka, H., Shiohira, Y., Uezu, Y. *et al.* (2006) Metabolic syndrome and chronic kidney disease in Okinawa, Japan. *Kidney International*, **69**, 369–74.

176. Wang, Y., Ng, M.C.Y., Lee, S.C. *et al.* (2003) Phenotypic heterogeneity associations of two aldose reductase gene polymorphisms with nephropathy and retinopathy in type 2 diabetes. *Diabetes Care*, **26**, 2410–15.

177. Wang, Y., Ng, M.C.Y., So, W.Y. *et al.* (2005) Tumor necrosis factor alpha G-308A polymorphism increased the risk of nephropathy in obese Chinese type 2 diabetic patients. *Nephrology, Dialysis, Transplantation*, **20**, 2733–8.

178. Tong, P.C.Y., Lee, K.F., So, W.Y. *et al.* (2004) Association of white blood cell counts with macrovascular and microvascular complications in Chinese patients with type 2 diabetes. *Diabetes Care*, **27**, 216–22.

179. Chan, J.C.N., Cheung, C.K., Cheung, M.Y.F. *et al.* (1995) Abnormal albuminuria as a predictor of mortality and renal impairment in Chinese patients with NIDDM. *Diabetes Care*, **18**, 1013–14.

180. Morrish, N.J., Wang, S., Stevens, L.K. *et al.* (2001) Mortality and causes of death in the WHO Multinational Survey of Vascular Diseases in Diabetes. *Diabetologia*, **44**, S14–21.

181. Karter, A., Ferrara, A., Liu, J. *et al.* (2002) Ethnic disparities in diabetic complications in an insured population. *The Journal of the American Medical Association*, **287**, 2519–27.

182. Brenner, B.M., Cooper, M.E., De Zeeuw, D., *et al.* (2001) Effects of Losartan on renal and cardiovascular outcomes in patients with type 2 diabetes and nephropathy. *The New England Journal of Medicine*, **345**, 861–9.

183. Chan, W.B., Chan, N.N., Lai, C.W.K. *et al.* (2006) Vascular defect beyond the endothelium in type 2 diabetic patients with overt nephropathy and moderate renal insufficiency. *Kidney International*, **70** (4), 711–6.

184. Kong, A.P., So, W.Y., Szeto, C.C. *et al.* (2006) Assessment of glomerular filtration rate in addition to albuminuria is important in managing type II diabetes. *Kidney International*, **69**, 383–7.

185. So, W.Y., Kong, A.P., Ma, R.C., *et al.* (2006) Glomerular filtration rate, cardiorenal end points, and all-cause mortality in type 2 diabetic patients. *Diabetes Care*, **29**, 2046–2052.

186. Yang, X.L., So, W.Y., Kong, A.P.S., *et al.* (2006) End-stage renal disease risk equations for Hong Kong Chinese type 2 diabetic patients – the Hong

Kong Diabetes Registry. *Diabetologia*, **49** (10), 2299–308.

187. Cooper, M. (1998) Pathogenesis, prevention and treatment of diabetic nephropathy. *Lancet*, **352**, 213–19.

188. Zhao, H.L., Tong, P.C., Lai, F.M. *et al.* (2005) Association of glomerulopathy with the 5′-end polymorphism of the aldose reductase gene and renal insufficiency in type 2 diabetic patients. *Diabetes*, **53**, 2984–91.

189. Liu, Y., Wat, N., Chung, S. *et al.* (2002) Diabetic nephropathy is associated with the 5′-end dinucleotide repeat polymorphism of the aldose reductase gene in Chinese subjects with type 2 diabetes. *Diabetic Medicine: A Journal of the British Diabetic Association*, **19**, 113–18.

190. Wang, Y., Ng, M.C.Y., So, W.Y. *et al.* (2004) Prognostic effect of insertion/deletion polymorphism of the *ACE* gene on renal and cardiovascular clinical outcomes in Chinese patients with type 2 diabetes. *Diabetes Care*, **28**, 348–54.

191. Lee, Y. and Tsai, J. (2002) *ACE* gene insertion/deletion polymorphism associated with 1998 World Health Organization definition of metabolic syndrome in Chinese type 2 diabetic patients. *Diabetes Care*, **25**, 1002–8.

192. Wong, T.Y.H., Poon, P., Szeto, C.C. *et al.* (2000) Association of plasminogen activator inhibitor-1 4G/4G genotype and type 2 diabetic nephropathy in Chinese patients. *Kidney International*, **57**, 632–8.

193. Wong, T.Y., Poon, P., Chow, K.M. *et al.* (2003) Association of transforming growth factor-beta (TGF-beta) T869C (Leu 10Pro) gene polymorphisms with type 2 diabetic nephropathy in Chinese. *Kidney International*, **63**, 1831–5.

194. Baum, L., Ng, M.C.Y., So, W.Y. *et al.* (2005) The hepatic lipase (HL) 514C T polymorphism and its interactions with ApoC3 482C T and ApoE exon 4 polymorphisms on risk of nephropathy in Chinese type 2 diabetic patients. *Diabetes Care*, **28**, 1704–9.

195. Ng, M.C.Y., Baum, L., So, W.Y. *et al.* (2006) Association of lipoprotein lipase S447X, apolipoprotein E exon 4, and ApoC3 455T→C polymorphisms on the susceptibility of diabetic nephropathy. *Clinical Genetics*, **70** (1), 20–8.

196. Liu, L., Xiang, K., Zheng, T. *et al.* (2003) Co-inheritance of specific genotypes of *HSPG* and *ApoE* gene increases risk of type 2 diabetic nephropathy. *Molecular and Cellular Biochemistry*, **254**, 353–8.

197. Ng, D.P., Tai, B.C., Koh, D. *et al.* (2005) Angiotensin-I converting enzyme insertion/ deletion polymorphism and its association with

diabetic nephropathy: a meta-analysis of studies reported between 1994 and 2004 and comprising 14,727 subjects. *Diabetologia*, **48**, 1008–16.

198. Crook, E., Penumalee, S., Gavini, B. and Filippova, K. (2005) Hepatitis C is a predictor of poorer renal survival in diabetic patients. *Diabetes Care*, **28**, 2187–91.

199. Soma, J., Saito, T. and Taguma, Y. *et al.* (2000) High prevalence and adverse effect of hepatitis C virus infection in type II diabetic-related nephropathy. *Journal of the American Society of Nephrology*, **11**, 690–9.

200. Lo, M.K.W., Lee, K.F., Chan, N. *et al.* (2004) Effects of gender, *Helicobacter pylori* (HP) and hepatitis B virus serology status on cardiovascular and renal complications in Chinese type 2 diabetic patients with overt nephropathy. *Diabetes, Obesity and Metabolism*, **6**, 223–30.

201. Hou, F. (2006) Cardiovascular risk in Chinese patients with chronic kidney diseases: where do we stand? *Chinese Medical Journal*, **118**, 883–6.

202. Lui, S.F., Ho, Y.W., Chau, K.F. *et al.* (1999) Hong Kong Renal Registry 1995–1999. *Hong Kong Journal of Nephrology*, **1**, 53–60.

203. Knowler, W.C., Barrett-Connor, E., Fowler, S.E. *et al.* (2002) Reduction in the incidence of type 2 diabetes with lifestyle intervention or metformin. *The New England Journal of Medicine*, **346**, 393–403.

204. Lindstrom, J., Ilanne-Parikka, P., Peltonen, M. *et al.* (2006) Sustained reduction in the incidence of type 2 diabetes by lifestyle intervention: follow-up of the Finnish Diabetes Prevention Study. *Lancet*, **368**, 1673–1679.

205. Li, G., Zhang, P., Wang, J. *et al.* (2008) The long-term effect of lifestyle interventions to prevent diabetes in the China Da Qing Diabetes Prevention Study: a 20-year follow-up study. *Lancet*, **371**, 1783–1789.

206. Engelgau, M. (2005) Trying to predict the future for people with diabetes: a tough but important task. *Annals of Internal Medicine*, **143**, 301–2.

207. Li, C., Pan, C., Lu, J. *et al.* (1999) Effect of metformin on patients with impaired glucose tolerance. *Diabetic Medicine: A Journal of the British Diabetic Association*, **16**, 477–81.

208. Yang, W., Lin, L., Qi, J. *et al.* (2001) The preventive effect of acarbose and metformin on the progression to diabetes mellitus in the IGT population: a 3-year multicentre prospective study. *Chinese Journal of Endocrinology and Metabolism*, **17**, 131–136.

209. Toh, C., Cutter, J. and Chew, S. (2002) School based intervention has reduced obesity in Singapore. *British Medical Journal*, **324**, 427.

210. Sahota, P., Rudolf, M., Dixey, R. *et al.* (2001) Evaluation of implementation and effect of primary school based intervention to reduce risk factors for obesity. *British Medical Journal*, **323**, 1027–29.

211. Gaede, P., Lund-Andersen, H., Parving, H.H. *et al.* (2008) Effect of a multifactorial intervention on mortality in type 2 diabetes. *N Engl J Med*, **358**, 580–591.

212. Gaede, P., Vedel, P., Larsen, N. *et al.* (2003) Multifactorial intervention and cardiovascular disease in patients with type 2 diabetes. *The New England Journal of Medicine*, **348**, 383–93.

213. Ko, G.T.C., Li, J.K., Kan, E.C. and Lo, M.K. (2004) Effects of a structured health education program by a diabetes educator nurse on cardiovascular risk factors in Chinese type 2 diabetic patients: a 1-year prospective randomised study. *Diabetic Medicine: A Journal of the British Diabetic Association*, **21**, 1274–9.

214. Wong, F.K., Mok, M.P., Chan, T. and Tsang, M.W. (2005) Nurse follow-up of patients with diabetes: randomized controlled trial. *Journal of Advanced Nursing*, **50**, 391–402.

215. Leung, W.Y.S., So, W.Y., Tong, P.C.Y. *et al.* (2005) Effects of structured care by a pharmacist–diabetes specialist team in patients with type 2 diabetic nephropathy *The American Journal of Medicine*, **118**, 1414.e21–7.

216. So, W.Y., Tong, P.C.Y., Ko, G.T. *et al.* (2003) The effects of protocol driven care versus usual outpatient clinic care on survival rates in type 2 diabetic patients. *The American Journal of Managed Care*, **9**, 606–15.

217. Wu, J.Y.F., Leung, W.Y.S., Chang, S. *et al.* (2006) Effectiveness of telephone counselling by a pharmacist in reducing mortality in patients receiving polypharmacy: randomised controlled trial *British Medical Journal*, **333** (7567), 522–5.

218. Chuang, L., Tsai, S., Huang, B. and Tai T. (2002) The status of diabetes control in Asia – a cross-sectional survey of 24 317 patients with diabetes mellitus in 1998. *Diabetic Medicine: A Journal of the British Diabetic Association*, **19**, 978–85.

Further Reading

Bhatt, D., Steg, P., Ohman, E., *et al.* (2006) International prevalence, recognition, and treatment of cardiovascular risk factors in outpatients with atherothrombosis.

The Journal of the American Medical Association, **11**, 180–9.

King, H., Keuky, L., Seng, S. *et al.* (2005) Diabetes and associated disorders in Cambodia: two epidemiological surveys. *Lancet*, **366**, 1633–9.

Kosaka, K., Noda, M. and Kuzuya, T. (2005) Prevention of type 2 diabetes by lifestyle intervention: a Japanese trial in IGT males. *Diabetes Research and Clinical Practice*, **67**, 152–62.

Lo, C. (2004) *The Misunderstood China. Uncovering the Truth Behind the Bamboo Curtain*, Pearson/Prentice Hall, Singapore.

Ramachandran, A., Snehalatha, C., Mary, S., *et al.* (2006) The Indian Diabetes Prevention Programme shows that lifestyle modification and metformin prevent type 2 diabetes in Asian Indian subjects with impaired glucose tolerance (IDPP-1). *Diabetologia*, **49**, 289–97.

16

Epidemiology of Diabetes in South East Asia

Ambady Ramachandran and Chamukuttan Snehalatha

India Diabetes Research foundation & Dr. A. Ramachandran's Diabetes Hospitals,
Chennai, India

16.1 DIABETES: BURDEN, GLOBAL PREVALENCE AND PROJECTIONS

Chronic diseases pose a primary challenge for the health care system in this century [1] and account for 46% of the global burden of disease and 59% of the 57 million deaths annually [2]. Diabetes is emerging as the most common noncommunicable disease of the globe, and there are 194 million diabetic subjects today. The impact of this worldwide explosion of type 2 diabetes mellitus (which accounts for approximately 85–95% of all cases of diabetes) will remain centered in the developing countries. Of the 194 million, 100 million live in the developing world – a majority in the Indian subcontinent and China [3]. India already faces a grave problem with the largest number of subjects with diabetes (approximately 33 million in 2003) that is expected to escalate further, with the number increasing to 57 million in the year 2025 [3, 4] and over 80 million by the year 2030 [5]. The rise in the incidence of type 2 diabetes is a result of environmental and lifestyle changes.

16.2 SCENARIO IN SOUTH EAST ASIA

The World Health Organization (WHO)–South East Asia (SEA) region comprises 11 countries: Bangladesh, Bhutan, Democratic People's Republic of Korea, India, Indonesia, Maldives, Myanmar, Nepal, Sri Lanka, Thailand and Timor-Leste. Most of these countries have witnessed considerable improvement in socioeconomic conditions in recent years [6]. They are also experiencing rapid urbanization, resulting in drastic changes in lifestyle with attendant health problems. Although several infectious and parasitic diseases have been controlled to a great extent, the noncommunicable diseases are becoming increasingly common, causing a double burden on many of the countries in this region. Although significant economic improvement has occurred in countries like India, the large population is a hurdle in effectively reducing the problem of poverty and malnutrition.

According to the world population prospects it would reach 6.1 million by mid 2000. Six countries of the world account for almost 50% of the annual increase, of which three are from the region: India, China and Pakistan contribute 21%, 12% and 5% respectively [6].

In the year 2000, the population in the SEA region was 1.53 billion. It is expected to increase by 1.75 billion by the year 2010. It is also projected that, by 2050, India's population will exceed that of China's. The density of population in the SEA region is projected by the fact that although only 5% of the global land mass is covered by the region, but 25% of the world population lives there.

In the developed countries, further urbanization is likely to be limited and the future incidence of type 2 diabetes will be primarily due to aging of the population rather than to increase in size or lifestyle changes seen, including eating habits to societal levels. The majority of the Indian population lives in rural areas and the rural population is also

The Epidemiology of Diabetes Mellitus, second edition Edited by Jean-Marie Ekoé, Marian Rewers, Rhys Williams and Paul Zimmet
© 2008 John Wiley & Sons, Ltd

Table 16.1a Prevalence of type 2 diabetes in South East Asia: Indian subcontinent.

	Year (Ref.)	Prevalence (%)	
		Urban	Rural
India	1972 [7]	2.3	
	1979 [8]	3.0	1.3
	1988 [9]	5.0	
	1992 [10]	8.2	2.4
	1997 [10]	11.6	
	2000 [10]	12.1	
	2006 [11]	14.3	
	2008 [12]	18.6	9.2
Pakistan	1995 [13]	10.8	6.5
Bangladesh	1997 [14]	4.5	
	2000 [15]		3.8
Sri Lanka	1994 [16]		5.0 (semiurban)
	1995 [17]	8.1	

Table 16.1b Prevalence of type 2 diabetes in South East Asia: other countries.

		Year (Ref.)	Prevalence (%)	
			Urban	Rural
Singapore				
	Chinese	1984 [18]	4.0	
		1992	8.0	
	Malaysia	1984	7.6	
		1992	9.3	
	Migrant Indians	1984	8.9	
		1992	12.8	
Philippines		1992 [19]	8.4–12.0	3.8–9.7
Malaysia		1982 [20]	2.1	
		1986	6.3	
		1996	8.3	
		1999 [21]	10.5	
Thailand		1971 [22]	2.5	
		1986	6.0	6.0
		1989		
		1997	13.9	
Vietnam		2001 [23]	3.8	
Cambodia		2005 [24]	11.0	5.0
			(semiurban)	

undergoing a transition in their lifestyle. All these changes have benefited the population in terms of a better living standard, but the darker side of the advancements seems to be an increase in the incidence of lifestyle-related diseases, especially type 2 diabetes. Chronic diseases have replaced acute diseases as the major cause of mortality and morbidity. The life span of people has increased, but with a reduced quality of life. In the last two decades, epidemiological studies in several SEA countries, including India, have revealed a high prevalence of type 2 diabetes among the urban population in the homelands [7–25] (**Table 16.1a** and **b**).

16.3 RISING PREVALENCE OF DIABETES IN THE INDIAN SUBCONTINENT

The epidemic of diabetes in India needs to be viewed within the larger demographic and socioeconomic context. India is the second most populous country and has diverse groups of people with reference to caste and religion, habitat, socioeconomic status, education level, lifestyles, food habits and so on. The population of India has roughly tripled since the country's independence in 1947, although the population growth has declined from 2.3% in 1975–1990 to 2.0% in 1990–2001.

Life expectancy has doubled from 32 years in 1941–1951 to 64 years in 2002, while the death rate has declined from 41/1000 to 25/1000 and the birth rate from 25/1000 to 9/1000. The infant mortality rate has declined from 148/1000 live births in 1951 to 129/1000 in 1975 to 69/1000 in 2002 ('Population – a human and social development,' http://planningcommission.nic.in/data/dt_pophsd.pdf). India has also witnessed impressive macroeconomic and industrial development [25, 26]. The gross domestic product (GDP) of India was a meager US$54 billion in 1950. By 1975, the country's GDP had grown to a 325 billion purchasing power parity (PPP) dollars. India's GDP grew at 4.9% per annum during 1990–2001, 1.97 trillion in 1995 and to 2.91 trillion in 2001, making India the world's fourth largest economy. In addition,

Table 16.2 Studies showing a rising trend in the prevalence of type 2 diabetes in India.[a]

Year	Author	Place	Area	Prevalence (%) Urban	Rural
1971	Tripathy et al.	Cuttack	Central	1.2	
1972	Ahuja et al.	New Delhi	North	2.3	
1979	Gupta et al.	Multicentre		3.0	1.3
1984	Murthy et al.	Tenali	South	4.7	
1986	Patel	Bhadran	West	3.8	
1988	Ramachandran et al.	Kudremukh	South	5.0	
1989	Kodali et al.	Gangavathi	South		2.2
1989	Rao et al.	Eluru	South		1.6
1991	Ahuja et al.	New Delhi	North	6.7	
1992	Ramachandran et al.	Madras	South	8.2	2.4
1997	Ramachandran et al.	Madras	South	11.6	
2000	Ramankutty et al.	Kerala	South	12.4	2.5
2001	Ramachandran et al.	National Urban (DESI)		12.1	
2001	Misra et al.	New Delhi	North	10.3	
2002	Mohan et al.	Chennai	South	12.1	
2004[b]	Sadikot et al.	National		5.6	2.7
2006	Mohan et al.	Chennai	South	14.3	
2008	Ramachandran et al.	Chennai [11, 12, 27]	South	18.6	9.2

[a]Ramachandran et al. 2004 (Ref. [12, 27]).
[b]Different sample selection criteria.

the average per capita income rose from US$530 in 1975 to US$2820 in 2001, and the proportion of people below the poverty line fell from 55% in 1974 to 41% in 1992 and to 26% in 2001 [25, 26].

There have been several studies from various parts of India revealing a rising trend in the prevalence of type 2 diabetes in the urban population [11, 12, 27] (**Table 16.2**). A multicentric epidemiological study carried out by the Indian Council of Medical Research (ICMR) in the early 1970s reported the prevalence of diabetes to be 2.3% in urban areas and 1.5% in rural areas [7]. The WHO criteria were not available then.

A series of studies from Chennai showed that the percentage of adult urban subjects affected had increased from 5.2% in 1984 to 8.2% in 1989, to 11.6% in 1995, 13.9% in 2000 and 18.6% in 2006 [10, 12] (**Figure 16.1**). A National Urban Diabetes Survey in 2000 showed that the prevalence of diabetes in urban India was 12.1% in subjects aged ≥20 years [28]. The prevalence in all the cities was more than 9% (varied from 9.3 to 16.6%). This

study revealed that the prevalence of diabetes in southern parts was higher than in the eastern and northern parts of India (Chennai: 13.5%; Bangalore: 12.4%; Hyderabad: 16.6%; Kolkata: 11.7%; New Delhi: 11.6%; Mumbai: 9.3%) [28]. The Prevalence of Diabetes in India Study (PODIS) survey [29] reported a low prevalence rate when compared with other previous studies (5.6%), but the sampling criteria and population size were different. However, the final estimated prevalence of diabetes with reference to actual numbers is similar (33 million) to that derived from earlier studies. The urban population is exposed to a more detrimental lifestyle that is characterized by high fat, refined diet, sedentary habits, lack of physical exercise, obesity, smoking and stressful behavior, etc., contributing to the high prevalence of diabetes in the urban areas.

A fourfold urban–rural difference in the rates of prevalence of diabetes was evident in the last decade. In the rural population of South India in the year 1990, and the prevalence rate was reported to be 2.4% [10]. The population was representative

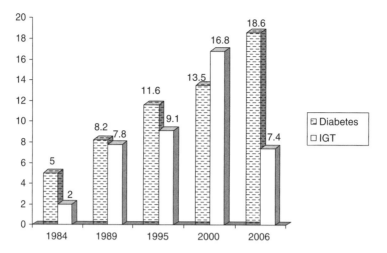

Figure 16.1 The increasing prevalence of diabetes mellitus (DM) and impaired glucose tolerance (IGT) in urban India [10, 12].

of people with low income, poor socioeconomic background, illiterate and most of them were hard-working laborers. The study also reported a 3:1 ratio of newly detected to known diabetes, an implication of poor socioeconomic condition and health care. Another study in the semiurban parts reported a prevalence rate of 5.9%, midway between the urban (11.6%) and the rural (2.4%) [31]. The sample population resembled the rural population in some habits but had access to certain urban facilities.

A study done in rural southern India after 14 years (2003) was an indicator of the lifestyle transition occurring in the rural population and it showed

a striking increase in the rate of prevalence of diabetes (6.4%) [32]. The contributing factors were chiefly the improved socioeconomic conditions, which encompassed an increase in family income, educational status, availability of motorized transport and a shift in occupational structure. As a consequence of the lifestyle transition there was also an increase in the prevalence of diabetes in the rural population (from 2.2% to 6.4%) [32] (**Figure 16.2**).

Studies among the migrant Asian Indian populations had shown the effect of migration to a more affluent environment among a population

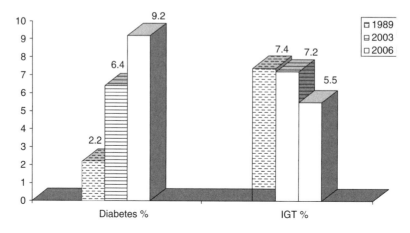

Figure 16.2 The temporal changes in prevalence of diabetes and impaired glucose tolerance (IGT) in rural southern India [12].

ethnically predisposed to develop diabetes. In several countries, prevalence of diabetes in Asian Indians was high compared with the host population and other migrant ethnic groups [33, 34]. Irrespective of the differences in anthropometry, dietary and socioeconomic factors and migratory patterns, the migrant Indians showed a higher prevalence of type 2 diabetes than Europeans [34]. Change in environmental factors is believed to unmask the increased ethnic propensity for diabetes [35]. Unmasking of ethnic propensity was highlighted in another epidemiological study from Mauritius [36]. It is a multiethnic population, with 68% of Asian Indian origin and the remainder comprising of Chinese, African and Creole population. The prevalence of type 2 diabetes was found to be 18% in Indian migrants, 17% in Creoles and 11% in Chinese. The rate of prevalence of type 2 diabetes in the migrant Indian population of Mauritius was similar to many of the urban rates of prevalence of diabetes on the mainland. In contrast, the prevalence of diabetes was high among the Chinese migrants, who have low rates of diabetes in mainland China. A similar situation was also evident in the Chinese migrants in Singapore [18].

16.4 IMPAIRED GLUCOSE TOLERANCE AND IMPAIRED FASTING GLUCOSE

A high prevalence of impaired glucose tolerance (IGT) has been reported in several recent epidemiological studies in developing nations such as India [12], Pakistan [13], Bangladesh [14], South Korea [37] and Africa [38]. Even when a marked urban–rural difference was seen in the prevalence of diabetes, the prevalence of IGT was similar in many Asian populations [10, 13, 14]. This probably indicates a genetic basis for type 2 diabetes, as IGT is a prediabetic condition in most of the ethnic groups.

Prevalence of impaired fasting glucose (IFG) is also high in Indians and in many other Asian populations [15, 39]. IGT and IFG show several metabolic aberrations which are risk factors for diabetes and cardiovascular disease (CVD). They include insulin resistance, presence of hypertension and obesity. Clustering of the risk factors was also common in these conditions [40].

IGT and IFG are the forerunners of diabetes. These stages are not only indicators of future diabetes, but also an index of impending rise in CVDs [41]. The prevalence of IGT in urban and rural populations had also increased steadily, suggesting the possibility for further rise in diabetes due to this large pool of susceptible subjects. IGT occurs at a young age in Indians in the age group <40 years [29]. The risk associations with anthropometric variables such as body mass index (BMI) and with family history of diabetes were also different. The prevalence of IGT increased with age, whereas IFG did not. Prevalence of IFG and IGT were similar in urban Indians (8.7% and 8.1% respectively) [39]. A study from Jaipur, in the western part of India, reported a prevalence of IFG of 5.3% in males and 5.2% in females [42]. The Hoorn Study in the Netherlands [43] and the Botnia Study in Finland [44] showed similar prevalences in IFG and IGT.

It is also interesting to note that in most of the studies reported the prevalence of IGT was similar in both urban (8.1%) and rural (7.8%) areas, despite the wide urban–rural difference in the prevalence of diabetes (2.4% in rural areas and 13.9% in urban areas) [12]. PODIS, on the other hand, reported a difference in the prevalence rates in the IGT between the urban and rural populations. The present estimate of approximately 33 million adults in India having diabetes may be an underestimation due to the rapid rate of urbanization occurring in many parts of the country [30]. Reports from Kerala in southern India [45] and other regions in India [46] have also highlighted the increasing trend in the prevalence of diabetes and IGT. It is a matter of concern that not only is the number of diabetic subjects increasing, but it also seems to be affecting the younger population in the most productive years of their life. Social, economic and psychological impacts of these escalating health hazards could be a major national health problem.

The risk variables associated with diabetes are similar in most parts of the world, but their expression and intensity vary widely between races and between geographical regions. The role of genetic environmental interaction is well known. Indians have the high genetic risk for diabetes and they seem to be susceptible to multiple environmental factors, which are independently associated with diabetes. Many of the environmental risk factors are modifiable.

16.5 GENETIC FACTORS

Racial predisposition is evident from the studies in immigrant Indians [33-36,47]. Asian Indian migrants living in different countries have high rates of glucose intolerance compared with inhabitants of other racial origin. Evidence for a genetic component comes from the increased concordance of diabetes in monozygotic twins, a high prevalence in the offspring of diabetic parents and a high prevalence in certain ethnic groups [48]. Type 2 diabetes is a polygenic disorder with many candidate genes identified in different populations, but none has been shown to be involved in the development of the disorder. The genetic risk factors for type 2 diabetes are complex and still elusive. However, the genetic predisposition is obvious from the heritable nature of the disease.

16.6 ACQUIRED RISK FACTORS

16.6.1 Age

An analysis by the International Diabetes Epidemiology Group comparing the profile of type 2 diabetes in European and Asian populations showed that Indians had the strongest age-associated risk for diabetes among all the groups [49]. Asian Indians develop diabetes at a much younger age than the Western population [12, 49, 50] (**Figure 16.3**). In developed Western countries, diabetes generally occurs in individuals aged ≤65 years. In developing countries, onset of diabetes occurs at a younger age [49] (45–65 years). The National Urban Diabetes Study (NUDS) showed that more than 50% of diabetic cases developed the disorder before the age of 50 years [12]. The association between age and diabetes was higher in the Indian and the Maltese populations than in all other populations studied, after correcting for other confounding variables such as BMI (Europeans, Chinese and Japanese) [49]. In each age group, the fasting and 2 h plasma glucose during an oral glucose tolerance test (OGTT) were significantly higher for Indians than for Chinese and Japanese populations. The age- and sex-specific prevalence and the peak prevalence of diabetes were higher in the Indian and Singapore cohorts than in the Chinese and Japanese cohorts [49]. Reports form Pakistan also showed age-related diabetes prevalence data similar to that in India. The peak age was in the age group of 55–64 years [13].

An early occurrence of diabetes in the population has a severe economic impact, as severe morbidity and early mortality occur in the most productive years of life. The diabetic subjects live long enough to develop the debilitating vascular complications of diabetes.

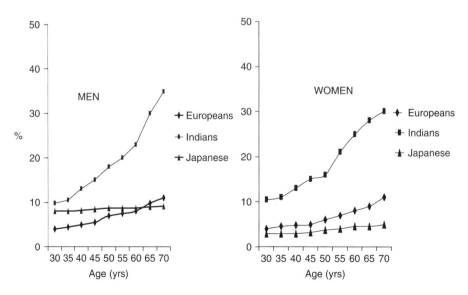

Figure 16.3 Age-specific prevalence of diabetes in Asian Indians, Europeans and Japanese. (With kind permission from Springer Science & Business Media: Nakagami, T., Qiao, Q., Carstensen, B. et al. (2003) Age, body mass index and type 2 diabetes - associations modified by ethnicity. *Diabetologia*, 46, 1063-70.)

16.6.2 Family History of Diabetes

The prevalence of diabetes increases with increasing family history of diabetes. Strong familial aggregation of the disease has been noted in Indians and in other Asian populations. In India, nearly 75% of type 2 diabetic patients have a first-degree family history of diabetes. The risk of the offspring developing diabetes with a parental history increases above 50% and it is around 40% if the proband has a diabetic sibling.

Familial aggregation of diabetes with a high prevalence among first-degree relatives and vertical transmission through more than two generations is commonly seen in Asian Indians [48].

16.7 ENVIRONMENTAL RISK FACTORS

16.7.1 Obesity and Central Adiposity

Obesity is a strong risk factor for type 2 diabetes, and its effects are compounded by several heterogeneous factors. Asian Indians have a leaner BMI than many other races, but BMI is strongly associated with glucose intolerance as in other populations. This suggests that increase in body weight, although within the ideal levels of BMI, confers high risk in this population. Even within a normal range of body weight, weight gain could increase the risk of diabetes, especially in the presence of a familial predisposition. The healthy BMI for an Asian Indian is shown to be $>23 \, kg \, m^{-2}$, as suggested by studies in Indian migrants in the United States [51] and by our study [52]. Adverse changes in insulin sensitivity and in blood glucose level result from small increments in body weight. An excess of body fat, especially concentrated within the abdomen, has a range of potential harmful effects. This includes increased risk for diabetes, blood pressure, dyslipidemia, insulin resistance, coronary artery disease and some forms of cancer. For diabetes, obesity (and specifically abdominal obesity) is a major risk factor. Indians have a phenotype characterized by lean BMI, upper body adiposity and high body-fat percentage, which probably explains their high insulin resistance (**Table 16.3**). The risk of metabolic disease increases progressively above $22 \, kg \, m^{-2}$ in Asian Indians. A WHO expert group has considered a BMI of $\geq 23 \, kg \, m^{-2}$ as the cutoff for normal in Asian population [53].

Table 16.3 Comparison of body fat and BMI in Indians and in the White population.[a]

	BMI $(kg \, m^{-2})$	Fat (%)
Men		
Asian Indian	21.4 ± 3.7	21.3 ± 7.6
	22.0^{b}	22.7^{b}
	24.5 ± 2.5	33 ± 7.00
White	25.2 ± 3.1	21.2 ± 7.8
Women		
Asian Indian	23.3 ± 5.5	35.4 ± 5.0
	22.7^{b}	37.4^{b}
White	23.3 ± 3.7	30.3 ± 8.6

[a]Reproduced from [28]. Copyright © 2004, The Association of Physicians of India.
[b]Median values.

Similarly, the waist circumference, an index of upper body adiposity, is also lower in the Asian population. The WHO and the Adult Treatment Panel III (ATP III) criteria recommend a cutoff limit for waist circumference of 102 cm in men and 88 cm in women [54]. However, the recent studies have shown that the cutoff for normal waist circumference is significantly lower for the Asian population. The risk of diabetes becomes significant above a waist circumference of 85 cm for men and 80 cm for women in the Indian population [52]. Recognizing these variations in Asian populations, the recent International Diabetes Federation criteria for cutoff values for waist circumference in Asian Indians have been defined as 90 cm for men and 85 cm for women [55].

16.7.2 Physical Inactivity and Sedentary Occupation

The role of physical activity in maintaining normal metabolic functions is well recognized. Physical inactivity as an independent factor in triggering the epidemic of type 2 diabetes. The impact of physical inactivity is manifested markedly in populations who have been accustomed to habitual heavy physical activity. Migration from rural areas to urban slums in metropolitan cities leads to obesity, glucose intolerance and dyslipidemia [56, 57]. The risk of developing diabetes was more in subjects who followed a sedentary lifestyle [32, 58] (**Figure 16.4**). In Fiji, among Melanesian and Indian men, the prevalence of diabetes was more

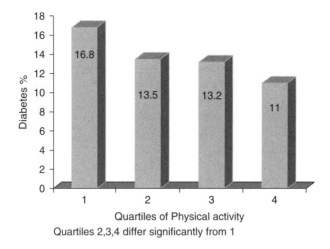

Figure 16.4 The influence of physical activity on prevalence of diabetes [12].

than twofold higher in subjects with sedentary or light activity than in those performing moderate or heavy exercise [59].

16.7.3   Urbanization

The developing countries are undergoing rapid urbanization and migration of population to urban areas. In the next 30 years a major redistribution of the population will occur, and by the year 2030 60% of the world's population could be living in urban areas. According to the WHO estimates, in the last five decades a two- to five-fold increase in urban population has occurred in most of the SEA countries. In India, the percentage of the urban population was 25.5% in 1990, 28.4%, in 2000 and it is expected to increase to 45.8% in 2030 [6]. A transition from a traditional to modern life has produced several health hazards in many populations, including the Asian Indians. Urbanization is associated with increasing obesity, decreasing physical activity and other risk factors associated with development of diabetes (**Figure 16.5**).

The impact of urbanization on the prevalence of diabetes was evident from two studies conducted in Chennai, India. In the first study, the prevalence of diabetes in a semiurban area was found to be 5.9% in comparison with a prevalence of 2.4% in the rural population and 11.6% in the urban population [10, 31]. These people led a more sedentary lifestyle than the rural population. The social and economic changes occurring in rural India have produced

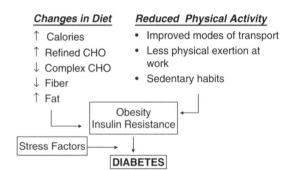

Figure 16.5 The changes occurring in lifestyle factors due to urbanization [32].

significant changes in te occupational, dietary and activity levels. Also, increasing numbers of people seek jobs involving less manual labor and migrate to urban areas. Better transport facilities are available and physical activity levels are significantly reduced (**Table 16.4**). Increased calorie consumption with more of fat and refined carbohydrates has also become common.

The changing demography of diabetes is evident from studies in Singapore and Malaysia [18, 19]. A phenomenal increase in diabetes has occurred in Singapore: it rose from 2% in 1975 to 4.7% in 1984, to 8.6% in 1992 and to 9% in 1998 in the age-group 18–69 years. Malays (14.3%) and Indians (men 16.7%, women 16.7%) had the highest prevalence. In addition, another 15% had IGT. A sedentary lifestyle and an increasing rate of obesity were

Table 16.4 Improvements in living conditions in the villages in the last 14 years.[a]

Factor	Past	Present	Chi square[b]
Regular use of motorized transport	86.6	93.4	31.6
Electricity	50.6	95.1	605.8
Water supply near residence	68.6	96.3	319.6
Medical facility	87.5	96.6	68.1
Watching television regularly	23.8	78.6	732.4
Three regular meals	57.2	70.1	42.8
Regular access to city	54	74	102.5
Monthly income (Rs)[c]	254 ± 100	1413 ± 1023	—

[a]Values are percentages unless otherwise stated. Ramachandran *et al.* 2004 (Ref. [32]).
[b]$p < 0.001$.
[c]Means $\pm$ SD (income corrected for rate of inflation), $p < 0.0001$.

strongly associated with an increasing prevalence of glucose intolerance.

16.7.4 Gestational Diabetes

Gestational diabetes mellitus (GDM) is a strong indicator of future diabetes. It is major health hazard in women, as it adversely affects both maternal and fetal outcomes of the pregnancy unless a tight glycemic control is maintained. It was reported that 34% of Danish women with previous diet-treated GDM had abnormal glucose tolerance 11–12 years after pregnancy, compared with 5% in a control group [61]. Prospective studies on GDM are not available in the Indian population. A study by Seshiah *et al.* [62] reported a prevalence of 17.7% of GDM in the urban population.

16.7.5 Stress Factors

The impact of stress, both physical and mental, is very strong on diabetogenesis, especially in those with a strong genetic background. A clinic-based prospective study from our center had clearly shown the effect of stress on diabetes [63].

16.7.6 Insulin Resistance and Metabolic Syndrome

Clustering of the risk factors common for diabetes and CVD has been demonstrated in populations, especially in those with a high prevalence of type 2 diabetes, including Asian Indians [64–67]. The presence of combinations of each risk factor with one or more of the other factors occurs more frequently than expected by chance in several populations, including the Asian Indians, indicating the presence of metabolic syndrome.

The consensus on the definition of the syndrome by the ATP III [54] and the WHO [68] has provided the opportunity to assess and compare the prevalence of metabolic syndrome in various populations. Metabolic syndrome is highly prevalent among Asian Indians in their homeland or in migrant Indians [65, 66, 69].

Diabetes mellitus itself increases the risk of CVD by two- to four-fold. The vicious cycle involving insulin resistance, glucose intolerance and cardiovascular risk seems to exist in a large proportion of Asian Indians, especially in urban areas [65–67].

Abdominal adiposity is a strong indicator of insulin resistance. A modified criteria for abdominal obesity is more appropriate for Asian Indians who have a lean BMI than the Western populations [65, 67]. Ramachandran's modification of the ATP III criteria for waist circumference to >90 cm for men and >85 cm for women (derived using mean plus one standard deviation for nondiabetic, nonobese healthy people) was appropriate for Asian Indian adults to denote abdominal obesity [65]. Using these cutoff values for waist circumference and the cutoff values mentioned in ATP III criteria for other parameters, we found that 41.1% of the adult population of Chennai, India, had metabolic syndrome. Metabolic syndrome was present in 27.9% of subjects with fasting plasma glucose

(FPG) $<110\,\mathrm{mg\ dl^{-1}}$ and its prevalence increased to $>70\%$ with higher FPG values. It was more common in women than in men and also in older people.

Another study by Mohan *et al.* also confirmed the high prevalence of metabolic syndrome in the same population [70]. In a study of the socially deprived urban slum dwellers in New Delhi, Misra *et al.* also observed a high prevalence of obesity, dyslipidemia, diabetes (10.3%) and increased body fat in the population [56].

A familial predisposition to metabolic syndrome exists. Abdominal obesity and general obesity have a high familial inheritance in the southern Asian Indian population, as in the case of type 2 diabetes [71].

16.8 DIABETES RISK SCORE

Screening for diabetes is impractical in India, which has a very large population. Screening of the high-risk group has been advocated as a feasible strategy to identify early diabetes. If the high-risk population can be identified using a risk score from a simple questionnaire and anthropometric measurements and no laboratory investigations, then this would be practical and also cost effective. Indians have several peculiarities in the risk factors for diabetes; therefore, the risk score that has been developed in the white population would not apply to Indians. We have developed a simple risk score using the risk variables including age, BMI, waist circumference, physical activity levels and presence of family history of diabetes. This was specific for the Indian population and this simple score can be used in any clinical setting without any special investigations (**Table 16.5**). It is found to be highly specific for the population and is sensitive in picking up the high-risk group [60].

16.9 PREVENTION OF DIABETES

The etiological factors for diabetes include genetic and environmental influences, both of which are equally strong. An interaction of these factors leads to the final expression of the disease. While the genetic component cannot be corrected, many of the environmental factors are modifiable. Obesity, diet and physical activity are the modifiable factors. The interaction of diet and exercise influences the body fat pattern, which has a significant

Table 16.5 Indian diabetes risk score.[a,b]

Variable	Risk score
Age (years)	
30–44	10
45–59	18
>59	19
Family history of diabetes mellitus	7
BMI ($\geq 25\,\mathrm{kg\ m^{-2}}$)	7
Waist (men: >85 cm; women: >80 cm)	5
Sedentary physical activity	4
Maximum score	42

[a] A receiver operating characteristic procedure showed a cutoff score of ≥ 21 having sensitivity and specificity close to 60%.
[b] Ramachandran *et al.* 2005 (Ref. [60]).

role in determining insulin sensitivity. Traditional lifestyles characterized by a diet including less saturated fat and complex carbohydrates and by greater physical activity may protect against the development of cardiovascular risk factors and diabetes, even in the presence of a potential genetic predisposition.

A few prospective studies in white populations and also in Chinese had shown the beneficial effects of lifestyle modification in reducing the risk of diabetes [72–74]. Subjects with IGT or with history of GDM have been studied in the prevention programs.

Primary prevention of diabetes is urgently needed in India as it is facing an enormous burden from the large number of subjects with diabetes. In order to answer several unanswered questions on the feasibility of prevention of diabetes in the Indian population, a 3-year prospective study in subjects with IGT was conducted in Chennai. It was a randomized control study in which 531 subjects with persistent IGT were included.

The four arms of the study were

1. control group with no intervention;
2. advised with lifestyle modification (LSM);
3. treated with 500 mg of metformin (MET);
4. LSM + MET.

The median follow-up period was 30 months and the 3-year cumulative incidences of diabetes were

Table 16.6 Comparison of the outcome in the intervention groups at 3 years.[a]

	Group 1 control	Group 2 LSM	Group 3 MET	Group 4 LSM + MET
Number	133	120	128	121
Cumulative incidence of diabetes third year (%)	55.0	39.3	40.5	39.5
95% CI (%)	46.0–63.5	30.4–48.5	32.0–49.7	30.9–48.9
Absolute risk reduction (%)	—	15.7	14.5	15.5
Relative risk reduction (%)	—	28.5	26.4	28.2
95% CI (%)		20.5–37.3	19.1–35.1	20.3–37.0
P value versus control group (Cox's regression equation)	—	0.018	0.029	0.022
Number needed to treat for 3 years to prevent diabetes in one case	—	6.4	6.9	6.5

[a]Ramachandran *et al.* 2006 (Ref. [75]).

55%, 39.3%, 40.5% and 39.5% in groups one to four respectively.

The relative risk reduction in LSM (28.5%), MET (26.4%) and LSM + MET (28.2%) compared with the control group was very similar (**Table 16.6**). The study showed that progression from IGT to diabetes was high in Indians. Both LSM and MET were equally effective and there was no added benefit from combining them. The study thus showed that primary prevention of diabetes was possible in a comparatively lean, but highly insulin-resistant Indian population by moderate change in physical activity and diet modifications [75] (**Table 16.6**). Screening for glucose intolerance for preventive measures at an early age is a requisite in Indians, as they develop hyperglycemia at a younger age.

16.10 CHRONIC COMPLICATIONS OF DIABETES

The burden of diabetes involves health care delivery to a large number of diabetic subjects and also the treatment of vascular complications. There is a lack of population-based data on the prevalence of micro- and macro-vascular complications from different parts of the developing world. It is being reported that retinopathy is prevalent in approximately 30% of type 2 diabetes and its prevalence is significantly high in the Asian and Pacific Island nations [38]. High rates of CVD

are reported from India [76, 77] and other Asian countries and also in the migrant Indian populations [78]. No discernable pattern relating to geographical distribution was apparent for nephropathy or amputations. Although it is reported that the prevalence of peripheral vascular disease (PVD) is lower in the Indian population, the number of people suffering from foot complications is quiet high on account of its large population [79].

Long-standing diabetes mellitus is associated with an increased prevalence of microvascular and macrovascular diseases. Data from Chennai show that the prevalence of complications of type 2 diabetes are as follows: retinopathy 23.7%, nephropathy 5.5%, peripheral neuropathy 27.5%, coronary heart disease (CHD) 11.4%, PVD 4.0% and stroke 0.9%. Prevalence of hypertension is also high (38.0%) [76] (**Table 16.7**). Similar rates of prevalence of diabetic complications have been reported by other workers also. Prevalence of retinopathy is high among the Indian type 2 diabetic subjects. A study by Rema *et al.* in South India showed a prevalence of 34.1% of retinopathy [80]. The prevalence of nephropathy in India was less (8.9% in Vellore [81], 5.5% in Chennai [76]) when compared with the prevalence of 22.3% in Asian Indians in the United Kingdom in the study by Samanta *et al.* in 1991 [79]. Diabetic nephropathy is one of the leading causes of chronic renal failure in India. A strong familial clustering of diabetic nephropathy in Indian type 2 diabetic patients was

Table 16.7 Vascular complications in type 2 diabetes.[a, b]

	Prevalence (%)
Microvascular complications	
Retinopathy	23.7
BDR[c]	20
PDR[c]	3.7
Nephropathy	5.5
Peri-neuropathy	27.5
Macrovascular complications	
Coronary heart disease	11.4
Peripheral vascular disease	4.0
Cerebrovascular accidents	0.9
Hypertension	38.0

[a] Random sample of $n = 3010$, male:female $=$ 1892:1118; mean age 52 ± 9.7 years.
[b] Ramachandran *et al.* 1999 (Ref. [76]).
[c] BDR: background diabetic retinopathy; PDR: proliferative diabetic retinopathy.

noted [82]. The study showed that proteinuria was present in 50% and microalbuminuria in 26.7% of the siblings of probands with diabetic nephropathy. In contrast, the prevalence of proteinuria and microalbuminuria among siblings of probands with normoalbuminuria was nil and 3.3% respectively [82].

Recent studies in India show that the prevalence of CHD in Indians may be as high as in the immigrant Indians [66]. The prevalence of CHD indicated by major Q wave changes was found to be 3.9%; this is similar to the prevalence in Asian Indians in the United Kingdom (4.0%), as shown by McKeigue *et al.* [83]. Another 10.3% had other abnormal electrocardiogram changes. A similar prevalence of major Q wave changes was shown by studies in northern India by Chadha *et al.* [84] (3.2%) and Gupta *et al.* (2.8%) [85]. A study showed that, in Asian Indian subjects admitted with acute coronary syndrome, abnormal glucose tolerance was present in nearly 84% of the subjects [86].

Prevalence of PVD in Asian Indians is comparatively low compared with the white population (9.3%). Low prevalences of PVD were demonstrated in Indian patients by Premalatha *et al.* [87] (overall 3.2%, 6.3% in diabetes) and also in our study (4.0%) [76].

Diabetic foot infections are a major problem and a common cause for hospital admission of diabetic patients in India [79]. Although the prevalence of PVD is low, neuropathy is very common and is an associated risk factor for foot infections, which often tend to recur.

16.11 TYPE 2 DIABETES IN CHILDREN

Recent studies on migrants in the United Kingdom and the United States [88], studies in India [89] and among Japanese [90] show a rising trend in type 2 diabetes in children and adolescents. The association of obesity with metabolic diseases like diabetes and CVD is well recognized. Childhood obesity leads to overweight in adulthood. Reports of increasing obesity among children are abundant from the developed countries. Similar trends have been seen in children in urban India. This is probably an indicator of the impending danger of an increased prevalence of metabolic diseases in the next generation also.

In a study in urban southern India, the prevalence of overweight was 17.8% among boys and 15.8% among girls aged 14–19 years [91]. There was a strong association of overweight with lack of physical activity and higher socioeconomic group.

A high prevalence of maturity-onset diabetes in the young has been reported in southern India [92]. There are also reports of type 2 diabetes in Indian children. The emerging epidemic of diabetes and obesity can be reduced only with implementation of strategies to educate the public regarding preventive measures for the above risk variables, which should start in the preteen ages.

16.12 COSTS OF TREATING DIABETES

The WHO estimates that 2.5–15% of annual health budgets are spent on diabetes-related illness. If the predictions of diabetes prevalence are realized, then the health care expenditure being spent in 2025 will go even higher, with high-prevalence countries spending nearly 40% of their budget [93]. The costs involved in the care and management of diabetes are quite considerable, for both the individual and the health care system. The nature of the disorder is such that it not only involves a direct cost that is borne by the affected individual, their family and the health care authorities, but also indirect and intangible costs which hold a substantial proportion of health costs. An estimate of the direct costs of diabetes was made as early as 1997 by the American Diabetes Association (ADA), and was estimated at US$44 billion per year [94]. In India, the annual cost of diabetes care (direct cost) was at US$310 per patient in a secondary care facility for type 1 diabetes; it was US$100 per patient for type 2 diabetes in the same set up. The cost was at US$343 per patient annually for those with foot and other complications [95–97]. Patients in the low socioeconomic group spent nearly one-quarter of their annual income on diabetes care, whereas in the high income group the expenditure was 3.5% of their total income [97]. Direct costs to individuals and their families include medical care, drugs and other supplies, in addition to other personal costs such as increased payments for health and insurances. Direct costs to the health care sector include hospital services, physician services, laboratory tests and the daily management of diabetes. Hospital inpatient costs for the treatment of complications are the largest single contributor to direct health care costs. The medical costs incurred by a person with diabetes are two to five times higher than those who are without diabetes.

The indirect costs are the result of lost production as a consequence of time off from work, inability to work because of disability, premature retirement and even premature mortality because of complications. Indirect costs may be even greater than direct costs of diabetes, which ADA estimated were US$54 billion [98]. Intangible costs are those that reduces the quality of life after the onset of the disease, ranging from pain, anxiety, stress to the influence in the personal relationship and leisure time activities.

India needs to implement preventive measures to reduce the burden of diabetes, as it poses a medical challenge which is not matched by the budget allocations for diabetes care in India. It is estimated that the annual cost of diabetes care is approximately Rs 90 200 million. The average expenditure per patient per year would be a minimum of Rs 4500. There is an urgent need to implement preventive measures to reduce the cost of the disease, which involves direct and indirect costs to the patient and to society.

ACKNOWLEDGMENTS

We thank Dr A. Yamuna and Dr S. Sivasankari for help in the preparation of the manuscript. We also thank Ms A. Bobby for secretarial assistance.

References

1. Beaglehole, R., Irwin, A. and Prentice, T. *et al.* (2004) *World Health Report: Changing History*, WHO, Geneva.
2. WHO (2005) Global Strategy on Diet, Physical Activity and Health: Facts Related to Chronic Diseases, WHO, Geneva.
3. Wild, S., Roglic, G., Green, A. *et al.* (2004) Global prevalence of diabetes: estimates for the year 2000 and projections for 2030. *Diabetes Care*, **27**, 1047–53.
4. Fall, C.H. (2001) Non-industrialized countries and affluence. *British Medical Bulletin*, **60**, 33–50.
5. Bjork, S., Kapur, A., King, H. *et al.* (2003) Global policy aspects of diabetes in India. *Health Policy*, **66**, 61–72.
6. WHO South East Asia Region (2002) *Health Situation in the South East Asian Region 1998–2000*, World Health Organization, Regional Office for South East Asia, New Delhi, India.
7. Ahuja, M.M.S. (1979) Epidemiological studies on diabetes mellitus in India, in *Epidemiology of Diabetes in Developing Countries* (ed M.M.S. Ahuja), Interprint, New Delhi, pp. 29–38.
8. Gupta, O.P., Joshi, M.H. and Dave, S.K. (1978) Prevalence of diabetes in India. *Advances in Metabolic Disorders*, **9**, 147–65.
9. Ramachandran, A., Jali, M.V., Mohan, V. *et al.* (1988) High prevalence of diabetes in an urban population in South India. *British Medical Journal*, **297**, 587–90.
10. Ramachandran, A., Snehalatha, C., Dharmaraj, D. and Viswanathan, M. (1992) Prevalence of glucose intolerance in Asian Indians: urban-rural difference and significance of upper body adiposity. *Diabetes Care*, **15**, 1348–55.
11. Ramachandran, A., Snehalatha, C., Latha, E. *et al.* (1997) Rising prevalence of NIDDM in urban population in India. *Diabetologia*, **40**, 232–37.
12. Ramachandran, A., Snehalatha, C., Kapur, A. *et al.* (2001) High prevalence of diabetes and impaired glucose tolerance in India: National Urban Diabetes Survey. *Diabetologia*, **44**, 1094–101.
13. Shera, A.S., Rafique, G., Khawaja, I.A. *et al.* (1999) Pakistan National Diabetes Survey. Prevalence of glucose intolerance and associated factors in Baluchistan Province. *Diabetes Research and Clinical Practice*, **44**, 49–58.

14. Abu Sayeed, M., Zafirul Hussain, M., Banu, A. *et al*. (1997) Prevalence of diabetes in a suburban population of Bangladesh. *Diabetes Research and Clinical Practice*, **34**, 149–55.

15. Abu Sayeed, M., Mahtab, H., Khanam, P.A. *et al*. (2003) Diabetes and impaired fasting glycemia in a rural population of Bangladesh. *Diabetes Care*, **26**, 1034–9.

16. Fernando, D.J.S., Siribaddana, S. and de Silva, D. (1994) Impaired glucose tolerance and diabetes mellitus in a suburban Sri Lankan community. *Postgraduate Medical Journal*, **70**, 347–9.

17. Samrage, S.M. (1995) Some epidemiological aspects of non insulin dependent diabetes mellitus in a defined population in the Kalutara District of Sri Lanka. Thesis submitted for the Degree of Doctor of Medicine, University of Colombo.

18. Lee, W.R.W. (2000) The changing demography of diabetes mellitus in Singapore. *Diabetes Research and Clinical Practice*, **50**, 35–9.

19. Khalid, B.A.K., Rani, U., Ng, M.L. *et al*. (1990) Prevalence of diabetes, hypertension and renal disease amongst railway workers in Malaysia. *The Medical Journal of Malaysia*, **45**, 8–13.

20. Institute of Public Health (1985, 1996) *National Health and Morbidity Survey 1 & 2*, Institute of Public Health, Ministry of Health, Malaysia.

21. Mafauzy, M., Mokhtar, N., Mohamad, W.B. and Musalmah, M. (1999) Diabetes mellitus and associated cardiovascular risk factors in north-east Malaysia. *Asia-Pacific Journal of Public Health*, **11**, 16–19.

22. Tandhanand, S. and Vannasaeng, S. (1986) Diabetes mellitus in Thailand, in *World Book of Diabetes in Practice*, Vol. **2** (ed L.P. Krall), Elsevier Science, Amsterdam, pp. 252–7.

23. Puavilai, G., Kheesukapan, P., Chanprasertyotin, S. *et al*. (2001) Random capillary plasma glucose measurement in the screening of diabetes mellitus in high-risk subjects in Thailand. *Diabetes Research and Clinical Practice*, **51**, 125–31.

24. Duc Son, L.E.N.T., Kusama, K., Hung, N.T.K. *et al*. (2004) Prevalence and risk factors for diabetes in Ho Chi Minh City, Vietnam. *Diabetic Medicine*, **21**, 371–6.

25. Singh, D.L. and Bhattarai, M.D. (2003) High prevalence of diabetes and impaired fasting glycaemia in urban Nepal (Letter). *Diabetic Medicine*, **20**, 170–1.

26. The World Bank. (2003) eWorld Development Indicators. The World Bank, Washington, DC. http://www.worldbank.org/data/wdi (last accessed April 2008).

27. Committee on Vision 2020 for India (2002) Report of the Committee on India Vision 2020, Planning Commission, Government of India, New Delhi. http://www.planningcommission.nic.in/plans/plan-rel/pl_vsn2020.pdf (last accessed April 2008).

28. Ramachandran, A. (2005) Epidemiology of diabetes in India – three decades of research. *Journal of the Association of Physicians of India*, **53**, 35–8.

29. Ramachandran, A., Snehalatha, C. and Vijay, V. (2002) Temporal changes in prevalence of type 2 diabetes and impaired glucose tolerance in urban southern India. *Diabetes Research and Clinical Practice*, **58**, 55–60.

30. Sadikot, S.M., Nigam, A., Das, A. *et al*. (2004) The burden of diabetes and impaired glucose tolerance in India using the WHO 1999 criteria: Prevalence of Diabetes in India Study (PODIS). *Diabetes Research and Clinical Practice*, **66**, 301–7.

31. Ramachandran, A., Snehalatha, C., Latha, E. *et al*. (1999) Impacts of urbanisation on the life style and on the prevalence of diabetes in native Asian Indian population. *Diabetes Research and Clinical Practice*, **44**, 207–13.

32. Ramachandran, A., Snehalatha, C., Baskar, A.D.S. *et al*. (2004) Temporal changes in prevalence of diabetes and impaired glucose tolerance associated with lifestyle transition occurring in the rural population in India. *Diabetologia*, **47**, 860–5.

33. De Courten, M., Benett, P.H., Tuomilehto, J. *et al*. (1997) Epidemiology of NIDDM in non-Europids, in *International Textbook of Diabetes Mellitus*, 2nd edn (eds K.G.M.M. Alberti, P. Zimmet, R.A. DeFronzo), John Wiley & Sons, Ltd, Chichester, pp. 143–70.

34. Simmons, D., Williams, D.R.P. and Powell, M.J. (1989) Prevalence of diabetes in a predominantly Asian community: preliminary findings of the Coventry Diabetes Study. *British Medical Journal*, **298**, 18–21.

35. Zimmet, P., Taylor, R. and Ram, P. (1983) Prevalence of diabetes and impaired glucose tolerance in the biracial Melanesian and Indian population of Fiji. A rural urban comparison. *American Journal of Epidemiology*, **118**, 673–88.

36. Soderberg, S., Zimmet, P. and Tuomilehto, J. *et al*. (2005) Increasing prevalence of type 2 diabetes mellitus in all ethnic groups in Mauritius. *Diabetic Medicine*, **22**, 61–8.

37. Park, Y., Lee, H., Koh Chang, S. *et al*. (1995) Prevalence of diabetes and IGT in Yonchon County, South Korea. *Diabetes Care*, **18**, 545–8.

38. International Diabetes Federation (2003) *Diabetes Atlas, Executive Summary*, 2nd edn, International Diabetes Federation, Brussels.

39. Ramachandran, A., Snehalatha, C., Satyavani, K. *et al*. (2003) Impaired fasting glucose and impaired

glucose tolerance in urban population in India. *Diabetic Medicine*, **20**, 220–4.

40. Snehalatha, C., Ramachandran, A., Satyavani, K. *et al.* (2003) Clustering of cardiovascular risk factors in impaired fasting glucose and impaired glucose tolerance. *International Journal of Diabetes in Developing Countries*, **23**, 58–60.

41. Donahue, R.P. and Orchard, T.J. (1992) Diabetes mellitus and macrovascular complications: an epidemiological perspective. *Diabetes Care*, **15**, 1141–55.

42. Gupta, A., Gupta, R., Sarma, M. *et al.* (2003) Prevalence of diabetes, impaired fasting glucose and insulin resistance syndrome in an urban Indian population. *Diabetes Research and Clinical Practice*, **61**, 69–76.

43. De Vegt, F., Nijpels, G., Dekker, J.M. *et al.* (1998) The 1997 American Diabetes Association criteria versus the 1985 World Health Organisation criteria for the diagnosis of abnormal glucose tolerance. Poor agreement in the Hoorn study. *Diabetes Care*, **21**, 1686–90.

44. Tripathy, D.C.M., Almgren, P., Isomaa, B. *et al.* (2000) Insulin secretion and insulin sensitivity in relation to glucose tolerance: lessons from the Botnia Study. *Diabetes*, **49**, 975–80.

45. Kutty, V.R., Soman, C.R., Joseph, A. *et al.* (2000) Type 2 diabetes in southern Kerala. Variation in prevalence among geographic divisions within a region. *The National Medical Journal of India*, **13**, 287–92.

46. Zargar, A.H., Khan, A.K., Masoodi, S.R. *et al.* (2000) Prevalence of type 2 diabetes mellitus and impaired glucose tolerance in the Kashmir Valley of the Indian subcontinent. *Diabetes Research and Clinical Practice*, **47**, 135–46.

47. Zimmet, P.Z. (1999) Diabetes epidemiology as a tool to trigger diabetes research and care. *Diabetologia*, **42**, 499–518.

48. Viswanathan, M., McCarthy, M.I., Snehalatha, C. *et al.* (1996) Familial aggregation of type 2 (non-insulin-dependent) diabetes mellitus in South India: absence of excess maternal transmission. *Diabetic Medicine*, **13**, 232–7.

49. Nakagami, T., Qiao, Q., Carstensen, B. *et al.* (2003) Age, body mass index and type 2 diabetes – associations modified by ethnicity. *Diabetologia*, **46**, 1063–70.

50. Harris, M.I., Flegal, K.M., Cowie, C.C. *et al.* Prevalence of diabetes, impaired fasting glucose and impaired glucose tolerance in US adults. The Third Nation Health and Nutrition Examination Survey, 1988–1994. *Diabetes Care*, **21** (4), 518–24.

51. Banerji, M.A., Faridi, N., Atluri, R. *et al.* (1999) Body composition, visceral fat, leptin and insulin resistance in Asian Indian men. *The Journal of Clinical Endocrinology and Metabolism*, **84**, 137–44.

52. Snehalatha, C., Vijay, V. and Ramachandran, A. (2003) Cut off values for normal anthropometric variables in Asian Indian adults. *Diabetes Care*, **26**, 1380–4.

53. World Health Organisation, International Association for the Study of Obesity, International Obesity TaskForce (2000) *The Asia Pacific Perspective on Redefining Obesity and its Treatment*, Health Communications, Sydney.

54. Expert Panel on Detection, Evaluation and Treatment of High Blood Cholesterol in Adults (2001) Executive Summary of the Third Report of the National Cholesterol Education Program (NCEP) of high blood cholesterol in adults (Adult Treatment Panel III). *Journal of the American Medical Association*, **285**, 2486–97.

55. Zimmet, P., Alberti, G. and Jonathan, S. (2005) A new IDF worldwide definition of the metabolic syndrome. *Diabetes Voice*, **50**, 31–3.

56. Misra, A., Pandey, R.M., Ramadevi, J. *et al.* (2001) High prevalence of diabetes, obesity and dyslipidaemia in urban slum population in northern India. *International Journal of Obesity*, **25**, 1–8.

57. Misra, A., Chaudhary, D., Vikram, N.K. *et al.* (2002) Insulin resistance and clustering of atherogenic risk factors in women belonging to low socio-economic strata in urban slums of North India. *Diabetes Research and Clinical Practice*, **56**, 73–5.

58. Mohan, V., Shanthirani, C.S. and Deepa, R. (2003) Glucose intolerance (diabetes and IGT) in a selected south Indian population with special reference to family history, obesity and life style factors – the Chennai urban population study (CUPS 14). *The Journal of the Association of Physicians of India*, **51**, 771–7.

59. Taylor, R., Ram, P., Zimmet, P. *et al.* (1984) Physical activity and prevalence of diabetes in Melanesian and Indian men in Fiji. *Diabetologia*, **27**, 578–82.

60. Ramachandran, A., Snehalatha, C., Vijay, V. *et al.* (2005) Derivation and validation of diabetes risk score for urban Asian Indians. *Diabetes Research and Clinical Practice*, **70**, 63–70.

61. Lauenborg, J., Hansen, T., Jensen, D.M. *et al.* (2004) Increasing incidence of diabetes after gestational diabetes – a long term follow-up in a Danish population. *Diabetes Care*, **27**, 1194–9.

62. Seshiah, S., Balaji, V. and Madhuri, S.B. (2004) Gestational diabetes mellitus in India. *The Journal of the Association of Physicians of India*, **52**, 707–11.

63. Ramachandran, A., Snehalatha, C., Shobana, R. *et al.* (1999) Influence of life style factors in development of diabetes in Indians – scope for primary prevention. *The Journal of the Association of Physicians of India*, **47**, 764–6.

64. Zimmet, P.Z., Collins, V.R., Dowse, G.K. *et al.* (1994) Is hyperinsulinaemia a central characteristic of a chronic cardiovascular risk factor clustering syndrome? Mixed findings in Asian Indian, Creole, and Chinese Mauritians. *Diabetic Medicine*, **11**, 388–96.

65. Ramachandran, A., Snehalatha, C., Satyavani, K. *et al.* (2003) Metabolic syndrome in urban Asian Indian adults – a population study using modified ATP III criteria. *Diabetes Research and Clinical Practice*, **60**, 199–204.

66. Ramachandran, A., Snehalatha, C., Latha, E. *et al.* (1998) Clustering of cardiovascular risk factors in urban Asian Indians. *Diabetes Care*, **21**, 967–71.

67. Shashank Joshi, R. (2003) Metabolic syndrome – emerging clusters of the Indian phenotype. *The Journal of the Association of Physicians of India*, **51**, 445–6.

68. World Health Organization (1999) *Definition, Diagnosis and Classification of Diabetes Mellitus and its Complications. Part 1: Diagnosis and Classification of Diabetes Mellitus, Department of Non communicable Disease Surveillance*, WHO, Geneva.

69. Misra, A. and Vikram, N.K. (2002) Insulin resistance syndrome (metabolic syndrome) and Asian Indians. *Current Science*, **83**, 1483–96.

70. Mohan, V., Shanthirani, S., Deepa, R. *et al.* (2001) Intra-urban differences in the prevalence of the metabolic syndrome in southern India – the Chennai Urban Population Study. *Diabetic Medicine*, **18**, 280–7.

71. Davey, G., Ramachandran, A., Snehalatha, C. *et al.* (2000) Familial aggregation of central adiposity among southern Indians. *International Journal of Obesity*, **24**, 1523–7.

72. Knowler, W.C., Barrett-Connor, E., Fowler, S.E. *et al.* (2002) Reduction in the incidence of type 2 diabetes with lifestyle intervention or metformin. *The New England Journal of Medicine*, **346**, 393–403.

73. Tuomilehto, J., Lindstrom, J., Eriksson, J.G. *et al.* (2001) Prevention of type 2 diabetes mellitus by changes in lifestyle among subjects with impaired glucose tolerance. *The New England Journal of Medicine*, **344**, 1343–50.

74. Pan, X.R., Li, G.W., Hu, Y.H. *et al.* (1997) Effects of diet and exercise in preventing NIDDM in people with impaired glucose tolerance: the Da Qing IGT and Diabetes Study. *Diabetes Care*, **20**, 537–44.

75. Ramachandran, A., Snehalatha, C., Mary, S. *et al.* (2006) The Indian Diabetes Prevention Programme shows that lifestyle modification and metformin prevent type 2 diabetes in Asian Indian subjects with impaired glucose tolerance (IDPP 1). *Diabetologia*, **49**, 289–97.

76. Ramachandran, A., Snehalatha, C., Satyavani, K. *et al.* (1999) Prevalence of vascular complications and their risk factors in type 2 diabetes. *The Journal of the Association of Physicians of India*, **47**, 1152–6.

77. Mohan, V., Vijaya Prabha, R. and Rema, M. (1996) Vascular complications in long term south Indian NIDDM of over 25 years duration. *Diabetes Research and Clinical Practice*, **31**, 133–40.

78. Samanta, A., Burden, A.C. and Jagger, C. (1991) A comparison of the clinical features and vascular complications of diabetes between migrant Asian and Caucasian in Leicester, U.K. *Diabetes Research and Clinical Practice*, **14**, 205–14.

79. Vijay, V. (1999) Prevention of diabetic foot complications (review). *Endocrine Update*, **1**.

80. Rema, R., Ponnaiya, M. and Mohan, V. (1996) Prevalence of retinopathy in non insulin dependent diabetes mellitus at a diabetes centre in southern India. *Diabetes Research and Clinical Practice*, **34**, 29–36.

81. John, L., Sundar Rao, P.S.S. and Kanagasabapathy, A.S. (1991) Prevalence of diabetic nephropathy in non-insulin dependent diabetics. *The Indian Journal of Medical Research*, **94**, 24–9.

82. Vijay, V., Snehalatha, C., Shina, K. *et al.* (1999) Familial aggregation of diabetic kidney disease in type 2 diabetes in South India. *Diabetes Research and Clinical Practice*, **43**, 167–71.

83. McKeigue, P.M., Shah, B. and Marmot, M.G. (1991) Relation of central obesity and insulin resistance with high diabetes prevalence and cardiovascular risk in South Indians. *The Lancet*, **337**, 382–6.

84. Chadha, S.L., Radhakrishnan, S., Ramachandran, K. *et al.* (1990) Epidemiological study of coronary heart disease in urban population in Delhi. *The Indian Journal of Medical Research*, **92**, 424–30.

85. Gupta, R., Prakash, H., Majumdar, S. *et al.* (1995) Prevalence of coronary heart disease and coronary risk factors in an urban population of Rajasthan. *Indian Heart Journal*, **47**, 331–8.

86. Ramachandran, A., Snehalatha, C., Sathyamurthy, I. *et al.* (2005) High incidence of glucose intolerance in Asian Indian subjects with acute coronary syndrome. *Diabetes Care*, **28**, 2492–6.

87. Premalatha, G., Shanthirani, S., Deepa, R. *et al.* (2000) Prevalence and risk factors of peripheral vascular disease in a selected South Indian population. *Diabetes Care*, **23**, 1295–300.

88. American Diabetes Association (2000) Type 2 diabetes in children and adolescents. *Pediatrics*, **105**, 671–80.

89. Ramachandran, A., Snehalatha, C., Satyavani, K. *et al.* (2003) Type 2 diabetes in Asian-Indian urban children. *Diabetes Care*, **26**, 1022–5.

90. Kitagawa, T., Owada, M., Urakami, T. *et al.* (1998) Increased incidence of non-insulin dependent diabetes mellitus among Japanese school children correlates with an increased intake of animal protein and fat. *Clinical Pediatrics*, **37**, 111–16.

91. Ramachandran, A., Vinitha, R., Thayyil, Megha *et al.* (2002) Prevalence of overweight in urban Indian adolescent school children. *Diabetes Research and Clinical Practice*, **57**, 185–90.

92. Mohan, V., Ramachandran, A., Snehalatha, C. *et al.* (1985) High prevalence of maturity onset diabetes of the young (MODY) among Indians. *Diabetes Care*, **8**, 371–4.

93. Williams, R. (2003) The economic impact of diabetes, in *Diabetes Atlas*, 2nd edn (eds B. Allgot, P. Gan, H. King *et al.*), International Diabetes Federation, Brussels, pp. 175–92.

94. American Diabetes Association (1998) Economic consequences of diabetes mellitus in the US in 1997. *Diabetes Care*, **21**, 296–309.

95. Shobana, R., Rama Rao, P., Lavanya, A. *et al.* (2000) Expenditure on health care incurred by diabetic subjects in a developing country – a study from southern India. *Diabetes Research and Clinical Practice*, **48**, 37–42.

96. Shobana, R., Rama Rao, P., Lavanya, A. *et al.* (2001) Foot care economics – cost burden to diabetic patients with foot complications: a study from southern India. *Journal of the Association of Physicians of India*, **49**, 530–3.

97. Shobana, R., Rama Rao, P., Lavanya, A. *et al.* (2002) Costs incurred by families having type 1 diabetes in a developing country – a study from southern India. *Diabetes Research and Clinical Practice*, **55**, 45–8.

98. Williams, R. (2002) Diabetes: its indirect costs: the cost of lost production. *Diabetes Voice*, **47**, 41–5.

17

The Epidemiology of Diabetes in Pacific Island Populations

Stephen Colagiuri,[1] Taniela Palu,[2] Satupaitea Viali,[3] Zafiml Hussain[1] and Ruth Colagiuri[4]

[1]Department of Endocrinology, Diabetes and Metabolism, Prince of Wales Hospital, Randwick, Australia
[2]Diabetes Centre, Vaiola Hospital, Nulu'alofa, Tonga
[3]Oceania Medical School, Apia, Samoa
[4]Diabetes Unit, Australian Health Policy Unit, Sydney University, Sydney, New South Wales, Australia

17.1 INTRODUCTION

Diabetes is an increasing global health problem. It is the fourth or fifth leading cause of death in most developed countries and is epidemic in many developing and newly westernized nations. Complications from diabetes, such as coronary artery and peripheral vascular disease, stroke, diabetic neuropathy, amputations, renal failure and blindness are resulting in increasing disability, reduced life expectancy and enormous health costs for virtually every society.

Diabetes and other noncommunicable diseases are a major threat to the populations of the Pacific Islands. Some of the earliest data on the emerging worldwide epidemic of diabetes came from studies in the Pacific Island of Nauru [1]. The disturbing increase in diabetes prevalence not only impacts on individuals, but is also a major threat to health systems throughout the Pacific which are struggling to cope with the system and financial challenges posed by noncommunicable diseases.

17.2 GEOGRAPHY

The Pacific Ocean has an estimated 20 000–30 000 islands, which are often collectively called Oceania (which includes Australia and New Zealand). The Pacific Island populations represent a diverse group of peoples which are divided into three geoethnic groups: Polynesia, Micronesia and Melanesia (see **Figure 17.1**). The term 'Polynesia' was first coined by Charles de Brosses in 1756 [2] and originally applied to all the islands of the Pacific. In 1831, Jules Dumont d'Urville proposed a restriction on the use of this term and also introduced the terms *Micronesia* and *Melanesia* [3]. This division into three distinct Pacific subregions remains in widespread use today and reflects the different racial and ethnic groups whose origins can be traced to Southeast Asia, Europeans, Americans, Chinese and Indians (found mostly in Fiji) and various migrations to the region over several thousand years.

Polynesia means many islands and includes Samoa, American Samoa, Tonga, Niue, Tuvalu, Tokelau, the Cook Islands, French Polynesia, Wallis and Futuna Islands, the Hawaiian Islands, the Midway Islands and Easter Island. Polynesians are the most homogeneous in culture, language and physical appearance, being of tall stature and generally lighter skinned than Micronesians or Melanesians. Micronesia means small islands and includes the Marianas, Guam, Wake Island,

The Epidemiology of Diabetes Mellitus, second edition   Edited by Jean-Marie Ekoé, Marian Rewers, Rhys Williams and Paul Zimmet

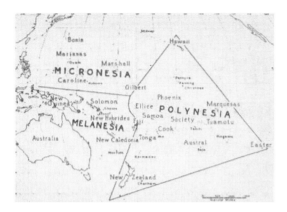

Figure 17.1 Pacific Island groups.

Palau, the Marshall Islands, Kiribati, Nauru, and the Federated States of Micronesia. Melanesia means Black islands and includes New Guinea, New Caledonia, Vanuatu, Fiji and the Solomon Islands. Although there are several distinct types of native peoples in Melanesia, virtually all are dark skinned and have tightly curled hair.

17.3 EPIDEMIOLOGICAL TRANSITION

Like the rest of the developing world, Pacific Island populations have been undergoing a major change from a traditional to a Western lifestyle. Although the great diversity of the Pacific Islands makes it difficult to generalize, the traditional lifestyle has common features throughout the region. Pacific Islanders depended on subsistence farming and, especially on the coasts, on fishing. Traditional diets included various kinds of marine life, and plants such as taro, cassava, yams, breadfruit, bananas, coconuts and other fruits.

The past 50 years has seen dramatic changes to this traditional lifestyle. Diets have been transformed with the general abundance of available food, the introduction of processed foods and sweetened beverages, and the establishment of supermarkets and take-away food outlets. Motor vehicles and public transport and sedentary leisure time activities, such as television watching and computers, have resulted in a marked decrease in levels of physical activity. Other harmful health activities, such as smoking, have also been embraced by many throughout the region. Unfortunately, many of these changes have been promoted and encouraged by

governments as a means of raising revenue. These changes have led to a change in disease pattern and burden of disease from communicable disease and high infant mortality to noncommunicable diseases, of which diabetes is a leading contributor.

All theories explaining the increase in diabetes in this region revolve around lifestyle changes exposing a genetic predisposition. Neel [4] was the first to propose that the genes which supported a hunter–gatherer lifestyle became deleterious in times of food abundance and that insulin resistance subsequently emerged as the underlying reason for this genetic protection. While changes in diet, increasing weight and decreased physical activity are all important factors, the specific mechanism by which the environment has unmasked the genetic predisposition remains unclear. Possibilities include the effect of poor fetal and infant nutrition [5] and changes in quantity and quality of dietary carbohydrate [6].

17.4 GENERAL

Diabetes prevalence has been studied in many Pacific Islands over the past decades, and, like other parts of the world, diabetes prevalence varies widely, but common to all has been the increase in diabetes. Direct comparison between studies is often difficult because of the use of different methods and diagnostic criteria for diagnosing diabetes. The effects of these changes can be substantial. Shaw *et al.* [7] compared diabetes prevalence diagnosed by the current World Health Organization (WHO) [8] and American Diabetes Association (ADA) [9] criteria and reported that in some populations the prevalence of diabetes increased by up to 30% while others showed a fall of up to 19%. While these differences are important, they cannot alone account for the differences in prevalence rates, as many comparative studies have been made within and between countries using the same diagnostic criteria.

Another limitation of the data is that in many countries the data are 20 years old and there is a lack of recent studies. Therefore, the true current status of diabetes in many of the Pacific Island countries is not known and estimates of the present magnitude of the problem can only be based on extrapolations from data from other similar countries and general trends throughout the Pacific. More up-to-date information will become available through the WHO STEPwise approach to Surveillance (STEPS) surveillance survey which is initially being carried out in Fiji, Samoa, the Federated States of Micronesia and Rarotonga in the Cook Islands [10].

The major form of diabetes in this region is type 2 diabetes and most reports have focused on this. There are no published data on gestational diabetes or childhood type 2 diabetes, which is known to be an emerging global problem.

17.5 PREVALENCE OF DIABETES

Table 17.1 shows the prevalence of diabetes and impaired glycemic regulation by ethnographic region and by country. Data are presented as age-standardized rates, either from the publication or calculated from data contained in the publication. In some instances only crude prevalence rates are presented where the publication did not contain sufficient data to calculate age-standardized rates. This limits direct comparisons in some instances. Another limiting consideration is differences in diagnostic criteria between surveys.

17.5.1 Polynesia

Overall rates of diabetes vary throughout Polynesia, but recent surveys show generally high prevalence rates of 15–20%.

17.5.1.1 Samoa (Formerly Western Samoa)

In 1978, Zimmet *et al.* [27] performed a prevalence study in rural and urban communities of Samoa. A repeat survey was carried out in 1991 [13] in the same geographical locations. Using 1985 WHO diagnostic criteria [28], between the 1978 and 1991 survey, the age-standardized prevalence of diabetes in urban Apia increased from 8.1% (95% confidence interval (CI) 5.2−11.0) to 9.5% (95% CI 6.8−12.1) in men and from 8.2% (95% CI 5.8−10.7) to 13.4% (95% CI 10.8−16.0) in women. In the two rural locations, prevalence increased significantly from 0.1% (95% CI 0.0−2.0) to 5.3% (95% CI 2.9−7.6) in men, whereas it was similar in women (5.4% (95% CI 1.5−9.3) versus 5.6% (95% CI 2.8−8.5)) in Poutasi and from 2.3% (95% CI 0.4−4.3) to 7.0% (95% CI 4.2−9.8) in men and 4.4% (95% CI 1.6−7.1) to 7.5% (95% CI 4.8−10.2) in women in Tuasivi.

A STEPS survey [10] was conducted in 2002 of 2728 people aged 20–64 sampled from six urban villages in Apia and five rural villages in each of the islands of Upolu and Savaii. An oral glucose tolerance test (OGTT) was not performed and diabetes was diagnosed by measuring fasting capillary glucose using an Advantage meter. Diabetes was defined by history of known diabetes, and also by the 1999 WHO diagnostic criteria using a fasting capillary blood glucose level of ≥ 6.1 mmol l^{-1} to diagnose diabetes [8]. Using these criteria, the age-standardized prevalence of diabetes was 22.5% (Viali, S., personal communication, 2005).

Comparisons of age-standardized prevalence of diabetes diagnosed by fasting glucose alone for people aged 25–64 years shows an increase from 5.8% (95% CI 4.5–7.0) in 1978 to 10.4% (95% CI 9.1–11.7) in 1991 and to 22.5% (95% CI 21.0–24.0) in 2002. This increase has occurred across all ages, as shown in **Figure 17.2**.

The early Samoan studies showed a clear urban–rural difference in prevalence of diabetes. Although a difference is still apparent in the latest survey, this is less marked than the original survey in 1978, which probably reflects a decreasing difference in lifestyles between urban and rural areas (**Table 17.2**).

In addition to diabetes, impaired glucose tolerance (IGT) and impaired fasting glycemia (IFG) are also common. In the 1991 survey, age-standardized prevalence of IGT in rural Poutasi was 7.4% (95% CI 4.0–10.9) in men and 8.0% (95% CI 4.7–11.4) in women and was similar in urban Apia: 5.7% (95% CI 3.6–7.9) in men and 9.7% (95% CI 7.0–12.5) in women. Prevalence of IFG in the 2002 survey was 38.6% (95% CI 33.1–44.2).

17.5.1.2 Tonga

The most recent published data on diabetes prevalence in the Pacific comes from Tonga. Conducted in 1998–2000, the survey included 1024 people aged ≥ 15 years from Tongatapu, Ha'apai and Vav'u. The age-standardized prevalence of diabetes in people aged 20 years and over was 10.6% (95% CI 8.9–12.3), 9.2% (95% CI 6.7–11.6) in men and 12.0% (95% CI 9.5–14.5) in women, of which approximately 80% was undiagnosed [15]. A repeat survey in 2004 of 1007 people from the same locations showed an increase in prevalence over a 5-year period to 12.0% (95% CI 9.1–14.9) (Colagiuri, S., personal communication, 2006).

Table 17.1 Prevalence of diabetes and impaired glycemic regulation in Pacific Islands.

Country	Reference	Year of study	Test method and criteria	Sample size	Age (years)	BMI (mean ± SD)	Total diabetes prevalence (%)[a] (95% CI)	Ratio known:new diabetes	IGT (%)[a]	IFG (%)[a]
Polynesia Cook Islands Rarotonga	King *et al.* [11]	1980	OGTT (1985 WHO and National Diabetes Data Group 1979)	1102	≥20	M: 28.4 W: 30.0	M: 5.3 W: 8.3	No data	M: 9.8 W: 10.8	No data
Manihiki Atoll	Weinstein *et al.* [12]	1980	OGTT (1985 WHO)	133	≥20	M: 28.3 ± 8.3 W: 30.5 ± 8.3	*Crude prevalence* M + F: 9.1 M: 8.0 W: 10.3	No data	*Crude prevalence* M + F: 18.0 M: 8.0 W: 31.0	No data
Niue	King *et al.* [11]	1980	OGTT (1985 WHO and National Diabetes Data Group 1979)	1128	≥20	M: 26.0 W: 27.8	M: 5.6 W: 8.6	No data	M: 6.9 W: 6.8	No data
Samoa	Collins *et al.* [13]	First survey: 1978 Second survey: 1991	OGTT (1985 WHO)	*1978* 1206 *1991* 1772	≥25	*1978* M: 27.5, W: 29.8 *1991* M: 30.4, W: 32.9	*1978 rural* Poutasi: M: 0.1 (0.0–2.0) W: 5.4 (1.5–9.3) *1991 rural* Poutasi: M: 5.3 (2.9–7.6) W: 5.6 (2.8–8.5) *1978 urban* Apia: M: 8.1 (5.2–11.0) W: 8.2 (5.8–10.7) *1991 urban* Apia: M: 9.5 (6.8–12.1) W: 13.4 (10.8–16.0)	*1978* 1.0:3.4 *1991* 1.0:1.7	*1978 rural* Poutasi: M: 7.9 (2.5–13.3) W: 4.6 (1.5–7.7) *1991 rural* Poutasi: M: 7.4 (4.0–10.9) W: 8.0 (4.7–11.4) *1978 urban* Apia: M: 6.8 (4.0–9.7) W: 9.5 (6.3–12.6) *1991 urban* Apia: M: 5.7 (3.6–7.9) W: 9.7 (7.0–12.5)	No data

Country	Reference	Year	Criteria	n	Age	BMI		Ratio		
Samoa	Viali S et al. personal communication	2002	WHO 1998 fasting capillary glucose only	2728	20–64	31.8 ± 6.4	M: 17.2 (15.4–19.0) W: 22.2 (17.3–27.1)	1.0:2.5	No data	38.6 (33.1–44.2)
Tonga	Finau et al. [14]	1973	OGTT fasting glucose: ≥6.7 mmol l⁻¹ 2 h glucose: ≥8.9 mmol l⁻¹	791	20–69	Estimated BMI Urban Nuku'alofa: M: 28.3, W: 29.5 Rural Foa Island: M: 25.6, W: 27.1	Urban Nuku'alofa: M: 5.5, W: 9.7 Rural Foa Island: M: 4.7, W: 10.1	1.0:6.7	No data	No data
	Colagiuri et al. [15]	1998–2000	WHO 1998	1024	≥15	M + F: 32.3 ± 6.1 M: 30.2 ± 5.4 F: 33.8 ± 6.2	≥20 years M + F: 10.6 (8.9–12.3) M: 9.2 (6.7–11.6) W: 12.0 (9.5–14.5)	1.0:4.9	M + F: 5.8 (4.5–7.1) M: 4.8 (3.3–6.4) W: 6.4 (4.5–8.3)	No data
	Colagiuri S et al. personal communication	2004	WHO 1998	1007	≥15	Combined: 33.0 ± 6.5 M: 30.9 ± 5.7 W: 34.6 ± 6.6	≥20 years M + F: 13.1 (11.1–15.1) M: 12.0 (9.1–14.9) W: 14.2 (11.3–17.0)	1.0:3.9	M + F: 7.1 (5.5–8.7) M: 5.0 (2.9–7.0) W: 8.9 (6.4–11.3)	M + F: 13.4 (10.5–16.2) M: 11.8 (8.1–15.5) W: 15.3 (11.0–19.6)
Wallis Islands	Taylor et al. [16]	1980	OGTT (1980 WHO and National Diabetes Data Group 1979)	579	≥20	M: 27.0 ± 4.5 W: 29.0 ± 5.1	3.2 (1.6–4.8)	1:2.8	7.3 (4.8–9.9)	No data
Wallis Island and New Caledonia	Taylor et al. [17]	1980	OGTT (1980 WHO and National Diabetes Data Group 1979)	WI: 579 NC: 564	WI: ≥20 NC: M: 25–64 F: 20–64	WI: 28.0 NC: 31.3	WI (≥20 years): 3.1 (1.5–4.6) NC (25–64 years): 12.1 (8.9–15.4)	WI: 1:3.8 NC: M: 1:4.3 F: no data	WI: M: 4.0 ± 1.7 W: 9.3 ± 2.3 NC: M: 9.9 ± 2.1 W: 8.5 ± 1.6	No data

(continued overleaf)

Table 17.1 (*continued*)

Country	Reference	Year of study	Test method and criteria	Sample size	Age (years)	BMI (mean ± SD)	Total diabetes prevalence (%)[a] (95% CI)	Ratio known:new diabetes	IGT (%)[a]	IFG (%)[a]
Micronesia										
Federated States of Micronesia	Shmulewitz et al. [18]	1994	OGTT (WHO 1999)	2167	20–85	31.0 ± 5.7	*Crude prevalence*: 12	No data	No data	No data
Kiribati	King et al. [19]	1981	OGTT (1980 WHO)	2938	≥20	M + F: 26.8 M: 26.8 W: 26.8 Urban: 28.0 Rural: 24.7	Urban: M: 9.1, W: 8.7 Rural: M: 3.0, W: 3.3	No data	Urban: M:16.1, W:17.9 Rural: M:10.6, W:13.7	No data
Nauru	Zimmet et al. [1]	1975	≥8.9 mmol l^{-1} 2 h after OGTT	221	≥15	*Mean ± SD weight (kg)* M: 85.0 ± 1.6 W: 79.5 ± 1.8	≥20 years: 46.0 (38.3–53.7)	1.0:2.3	No data	No data
	Zimmet et al. [20]	1976	≥8.9 mmol l^{-1} 2 h after OGTT	417	≥10	*New diabetes*: M: 33.2 ± 4.7 W: 36.1 ± 6.6 *Known diabetes*: M: 30.3 ± 4.7 W: 35.0 ± 9.2 *No diabetes*: M: 31.1 ± 6.3 W: 34.7 ± 7.1	≥20 years: 48.2 (42.3–54.2)	1:2	No data	No data

Dowse et al. [21]	1987	OGTT (1985 WHO)	1975–1976: 421 1982: 1406 1987: 1201	≥20	IGT subjects: 1975–76: 33.5 1982: 35.8 1987: 37.5 No diabetes: 1975–1976: 32.8 1982: 33.3 1987: 34.2	1975–1976 survey: M + F: 27.9 (23.8–32.0) M: 30.1 (24.0–36.1) W: 25.9 (20.4–31.3) 1982 survey: M + F: 24.7 (22.7–26.6) M: 24.7 (21.9–27.5) W: 24.6 (21.8–27.3) 1987 survey: M + F: 24.0 (22.1–25.9) M: 23.8 (20.9–26.7) W: 24.1 (21.5–26.6)	No data	1975–1976 survey: M + F: 21.1 (17.0–25.3) M: 17.2 (11.6–22.7) W: 24.9 (18.9–30.9) 1982 survey: M + F: 17.4 (15.4–19.3) M: 17.5 (14.6–20.4) W: 17.2 (14.5–19.8) 1987 survey: M + F: 8.7 (7.1–10.3) M: 7.6 (5.6–9.7) W: 9.5 (7.2–11.8)	No data
Melanesia Fiji									
Zimmet et al. [22]	1980	OGTT (1980 WHO and National Diabetes Data Group 1979)	2638 Indian: M: 595 W: 703 Melane-sian: M: 640 W: 700	≥20	Indian urban: M: 22.8 ± 3.9, W: 23.9 ± 5.9 Indian rural: M: 21.5 ± 3.8, W: 23.5 ± 5.8 Melanesians urban: M: 25.8 ± 3.8, W: 27.9 ± 5.8	Indian urban: M: 12.9, W: 11.0 Indian rural: M: 12.1, W: 11.3 Melanesians urban: M: 3.5, W: 7.1	No data	Indian urban: M: 8.3, W: 11.8 Indian rural: M: 10.2, W: 9.6 Melanesians urban: M: 7.3, W: 13.2	No data

(continued overleaf)

Table 17.1 (continued)

Country	Reference	Year of study	Test method and criteria	Sample size	Age (years)	BMI (mean ± SD)	Total diabetes prevalence (%)[a] (95% CI)	Ratio known:new diabetes	IGT (%)[a]	IFG (%)[a]
						Melanesians rural: M: 25.5 ± 3.7, W: 26.3 ± 4.7	*Melanesians rural:* M: 1.1, W: 1.2		*Melanesians rural:* M: 5.7, W: 8.5	
New Caledonia	Zimmet et al. [23]	1979	OGTT (1980 WHO and National Diabetes Data Group 1979)	1108	≥20		*Crude prevalence:*	1:6.2	*Crude prevalence:*	No data
		Melanesians and part-Polynesians (Melanesian–Polynesians)				Touho (Melanesians): M: 24.1 ± 3.1 W: 24.5 ± 4.3	Touho (Melanesians): M: 2.2, W: 0.2		Touho (Melanesians): M: 6.7, W: 4.9	
						Ouvea (Melanesians): M: 24.6 ± 15.0 W: 26.4 ± 5.6	Ouvea (Melanesians): M: 0.0, W: 3.9		Ouvea (Melanesians): M: 3.5, W: 6.2	
						Ouvea (part-Polynesians): M: 24.0 ± 3.2 W: 26.8 ± 2.0	Ouvea (part-Polynesians): M: 6.7, W: 7.2		Ouvea (part-Polynesians): M: 4.9, W: 10.1%	
Solomon Islands	Eason et al. [24]	1985	OGTT (1980 WHO)	1504	≥18	*Obesity prevalence:* M: BMI ≥ 27 kg m^{-2} W: BMI ≥ 25 kg m^{-2}		No clear indication about known and new diabetes		No data

Country	Reference	Year	Diagnostic criteria	n	Study population	Age (years)	Prevalence of obesity (%) / mean BMI	Crude prevalence	Crude prevalence
								No data	No data
				Munda: 873	Munda: urban Melanesian		Munda: M: 12%, W: 37%	Munda (urban Melan): M: 0.0, W: 1.4	Munda: M: 0.2, W: 0.7
				Paradise: 330	Paradise: rural Melanesian		Paradise: M: 10%, W: 45%	Paradise (rural Melan): M: 0.0, W: 1.5	Paradise: M: 0.0, W: 0.0
				Solstar: 301	Solstar: rural Micronesian		Solstar: M: 41%, W: 71%	Solstar (rural Micro): M: 4.3, W: 7.9	Solstar: M: 2.2, W: 4.5
Papua New Guinea	King *et al.* [25]	1983	OGTT (1985 WHO)	799		≥20	Masilakaiufa: M: 23.3, W: 21.6	*Crude prevalence:* Masilakaiufa: 0.0 (M: 0.0, W: 0.0)	*Crude prevalence:* Masilakaiufa: 1.9 (M: 1.7, W: 2.2)
							Napapar: M: 23.6, W: 22.9	Napapar: 0.7 (M: 1.6, W: 0.0)	Napapar: 0.0 (M: 0.0, W: 0.0)
							Matupit: M: 23.3, W: 24.2	Matupit: 4.0 (M: 4.8, W: 3.4)	Matupit: 0.7 (M: 0.8, W: 0.7)
								No data	No data
Vanuatu	Taylor [26]	1985	OGTT (1980 WHO and National Diabetes Data Group 1979)	1378		≥20	Rural: M: 22.6, W: 22.9	Rural: M: 1.0, W: 0.9	Rural: M: 2.6, W: 2.1
							Semirural: M: 24.1, W: 25.4	Semirural: M: 2.1, W: 1.1	Semirural: M: 1.8, W: 2.6
							Urban: M: 25.9, W: 27.9	Urban: M: 2.1, W: 12.1	Urban: M: 2.1, W: 3.2

Age-standardized for study population to local population distribution, unless stated.

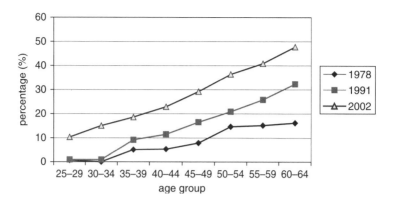

Figure 17.2 Comparison of prevalence of diabetes diagnosed by fasting glucose in the Samoan 1978, 1991 and 2002 surveys across various age groups.

The first Tongan population based diabetes prevalence survey was conducted in 1973 on the islands of Tongatapu and Foa [14]. A total of 791 people aged 20–69 years participated in the survey. The interpretation of the OGTT used a fasting plasma glucose ≥ 6.7 mmol l^{-1} or a 2 h result ≥ 8.9 mmol l^{-1} to diagnose diabetes. The age-adjusted prevalence for total diabetes was 7.5%, 5% in males and 9.8% in females. Using the current WHO diagnostic criteria, the previous study would have tended to overestimate the prevalence of diabetes. Despite this, comparison of the prevalence rates for diabetes between the two published surveys indicates at least a doubling in prevalence over the past 25 years.

17.5.1.3   Cook Islands

In 1980, King *et al.* [11] conducted a population-based study in Rarotonga in the Cook Islands, a location which has been considerably influenced by sociocultural modernization and tourism. The age-standardized prevalence of diabetes in men was

Table 17.2 Comparison of diabetes diagnosed by fasting plasma glucose in urban and rural areas of samoa for people aged 25-64 years.

	Upolu (%)		Rural Savaii (%)
	Urban	Rural	
1978	9.9	2.3	5.6
1991	17.9	9.2	10.7
2002	28.6	22.9	19.1

5.3% and in women 8.3%, and the age-standardized prevalence of IGT in men was 9.8% and in women 10.8%.

Another 1980 survey of 133 adults from the Manihiki Atoll in the Cook Island group, revealed a prevalence of diabetes of 9.1% (males 8.0%, females 10.3%) and IGT (males 8.0%, females 31.0%) [12].

17.5.1.4   Niue

King *et al.* [11] also studied people in Niue in 1980 and reported an age-standardized prevalence of diabetes of 5.6% in men and 6% in women, and the age-standardized prevalence of IGT in men was 6.9% and in women 6.8%.

17.5.1.5   Wallis Islands

An interesting study of Wallis Islanders demonstrated the effects of a change in lifestyle over a relatively short period of time. Taylor *et al.* [17] compared diabetes prevalence in Wallis Islanders living a traditional lifestyle in the Wallis Islands and first-generation Wallis Islanders who had migrated to Noumea in New Caledonia. The Wallis Islanders who were still resident on the Wallis Islands had a crude prevalence of diabetes of 2.6% and 6.6% for IGT, but rates were considerably higher for those who were living in Noumea, being 12% for diabetes and 9.1% for IGT.

17.5.2   Micronesia

There is considerable variation in the rates of diabetes throughout Micronesia. Diabetes in the small island of Nauru has topped the Pacific-region prevalence charts since the earliest surveys. In contrast, other locations have shown more modest rates.

17.5.2.1 Nauru

The most studied Island in the Pacific region has been Nauru, with reports beginning with the 1975–1976 survey [1]. The most recent survey, done in 1994 [18], shows an overall diabetes prevalence in people aged 25 years and older of 32.3% and a prevalence in people aged 45 years and older of over 50%. Nauru has been exposed to westernization since the turn of the twentieth century with the discovery of rich phosphate reserves, income from which has given Nauruans significant wealth and resulted in a rapid change from their traditional lifestyle, especially for diet to an almost total reliance on imported foods and drinks.

The trends in prevalence of type 2 diabetes and IGT have been examined in the surveys performed in 1975–1976, 1982 and 1987 using the 1985 WHO diagnostic criteria [13]. The age-standardized prevalence of diabetes has remained relatively constant: 27.9% (men 30.1%, women 25.9%) in 1975–1976, 24.7% (men 24.7%, women 24.6%) in 1982 and 24.0% (men 23.8%, women 24.1%) in 1987. However, the prevalence of IGT had decreased significantly from 21.1% in 1975–1976 to 8.7% in 1987.

Balkau et al. [29] examined the incidence of diabetes (defined by 1980 WHO criteria [30]) in 266 Nauruans classified as not having diabetes in 1975–1976. Retesting of these subjects in 1982 showed an annual incidence of 1.6% for type 2 diabetes. The factor most consistently associated with incident diabetes was baseline 2 h plasma glucose.

17.5.2.2 Kiribati

A population-based diabetes prevalence survey of 2938 individuals in Kiribati was conducted in 1981 and analyzed using 1980 WHO diagnostic criteria. In men, the age-standardized prevalence of diabetes in the urban areas was 9.1% and in the rural areas 3.0%, while in women the age-standardized prevalence of diabetes in the urban areas was 8.7% and in the rural areas 3.3%. The overall age-standardized prevalence of IGT in the rural

areas was 10.6% in men and 13.7% in women. In the urban areas, the age-standardized prevalence of IGT in men was 16.1% and in women 17.9%.

17.5.2.3 Federated States of Micronesia

Shmulewitz et al. [18] recently surveyed 2167 people aged >20 years in the island of Kosrae in the Federated States of Micronesia. Diabetes was found in 12% based on the 1999 WHO criteria. Obesity (defined as a (body mass index) BMI $\geq$ 35 kg m^{-2}) was found in 24%, hypertension in 17% and dyslipidemia in 20% of the population.

17.5.3 Melanesia

Some of the lowest rates of diabetes have been reported in this region of the Pacific; however, most studies are dated and recent data are limited.

17.5.3.1 Papua New Guinea

A diabetes survey was conducted in the highlands of Papua New Guinea in 1983 [19]. A total of 308 people from two traditional villages in the Eastern Highlands Province were studied and diabetes was diagnosed using the 1980 WHO criteria. No case of type 2 diabetes was detected. The prevalence of IGT was 2%.

17.5.3.2 Vanuatu

In 1985, Taylor et al. [26] reported low rates of diabetes in various communities in Vanuatu. In men, the age-standardized prevalence of diabetes in the urban areas was 2.1%, in the semirural areas 2.1% and in the rural areas 1.0%. In women, the age-standardized prevalence of diabetes in the urban areas was 12.1%, in the semirural areas 1.1% and in the rural areas 0.9%.

17.5.3.3 Solomon Islands

Eason et al. [24] examined diabetes in a 1985 study in the Solomon Islands. Among 1504 people aged 18 years and over, age-standardized prevalence of diabetes was low in urban and rural Melanesians (none in males and 1.5% in females), whereas rates were considerably higher in rural Micronesians (4.3% in males and 7.9% in females). The authors suggested that this study showed that rates of diabetes are inherently low in Melanesians.

17.5.3.4   Fiji

In 1980, Zimmet *et al.* [22] examined rural–urban and ethnic differences in diabetes and IGT in the biracial population of Fiji (Melanesian and Indian). The age-standardized prevalence of diabetes in rural Melanesian males was one-third that of urban males (1.1% versus 3.5%). In females, there was a sixfold rural–urban difference (1.2% versus 7.1%). By contrast, rural and urban Indians had similar rates (12.1% versus 12.9% for males; 11.3% versus 11.0% for females). No statistically significant differences existed in age-standardized IGT prevalence between rural and urban groups or between Melanesians and Indians.

17.5.3.5   New Caledonia

The 1979 survey in New Caledonia showed low rates in this Melanesian population, with an overall crude prevalence of 3.9%.

17.6   RATES OF UNDIAGNOSED DIABETES

Asymptomatic hyperglycemia is a significant public health problem, and people with undiagnosed diabetes have high rates of coronary heart disease and increased risk of cardiovascular disease [31]. Lowe *et al.* [32] reported 22-year follow-up data that asymptomatic hyperglycemia confers increased risk of mortality in middle aged men.

Unfortunately, a substantial proportion of the diabetic population in Pacific countries is undiagnosed (**Table 17.1**). Ratios of diagnosed to undiagnosed of 1:4 (i.e. 80% undiagnosed) are common. This compares with rates of 1:1 in developed countries [33]. The low proportion of diagnosed diabetes is likely to contribute to the high rates of complications and the frequent presentation with diabetes-related problems, especially foot sepsis.

The low ratio of diagnosed to undiagnosed diabetes in Pacific countries probably reflects differences in health care and health promotion compared with the more developed countries, which are more likely to offer routine health care checks and conduct campaigns aimed at identifying people with undiagnosed diabetes. Although undiagnosed cases of diabetes are probably a function of less testing, the possibly that hyperglycemia is accompanied by fewer symptoms in Pacific Islanders cannot be excluded. In addition, there is a prevailing attitude of seeking medical advice only for advanced problems.

17.7   DIAGNOSING UNDIAGNOSED DIABETES

The majority of people with undiagnosed diabetes in Pacific Island surveys have elevations in both fasting and 2 h plasma glucose. Consequently, diabetes can be diagnosed on the basis of a fasting plasma glucose alone. For example, in the Tonga study, 90% could be detected by fasting glucose alone [15]. Similarly, in the 1978 and 1991 Samoa surveys, 84% and 97% respectively of people with new diabetes could be diagnosed on the basis of the fasting plasma glucose with only an additional 16% and 3% respectively being diagnosed on the basis of an elevated 2 h plasma glucose following an OGTT [13].

The implication of this observation is that programs for the detection of undiagnosed diabetes in the Pacific can be based on measurement of fasting glucose alone in the knowledge that this will detect the majority. The risk factors which are associated with having undiagnosed diabetes are similar to those found in the rest of the world.

17.8   SCREENING FOR UNDIAGNOSED DIABETES

A number of screening programs have been developed for detecting individuals with undiagnosed diabetes. Most programs include a two-step procedure involving an assessment of risk factors to identify high-risk individuals, using either an aggregated risk factor score or a predictive model, and then testing these high-risk individuals biochemically [34].

The Tonga 1998–2000 [15] survey was used to explore risk factor assessment for undiagnosed diabetes. A predictive model which included age, waist circumference, blood pressure and family history of diabetes performed well with an receiver operating characteristic curve area of 0.81 (95% CI 0.75–0.87) and a sensitivity of 76.3% and a specificity of 75.7% at the optimal cut-point. A risk score also performed well, with an aggregate score of ≥27 having a sensitivity of 78.0% and a specificity of 73.1% for detecting undiagnosed diabetes. Therefore, either method could be used to detect undiagnosed type 2 diabetes. However, a risk score calculation is easier to perform in the primary care setting and may be the preferred method for detecting high-risk individuals, who should then have plasma glucose testing.

17.9 DIABETES COMPLICATIONS

Complications are common in people with diabetes in the Pacific. The first survey was performed by King *et al.* [35], who reported a prevalence of retinopathy of 24% in diabetic people in Nauru. The prevalence of albuminuria was also high in Nauruans: 26% and 30% of men and women respectively had microalbuminuria and 13% of both sexes had macroalbuminuria. Of the subjects with macroalbuminuria, 66% had diabetes. The prevalence increased with worsening glucose tolerance: 26% of subjects with normal glucose tolerance had either micro- or macro-albuminuria, increasing to 43% of subjects with IGT, 63% of newly diagnosed diabetic subjects and 75% of previously diagnosed diabetic subjects [36].

The 1991 population-based study in Samoa examined the prevalence of diabetic retinopathy and nephropathy [37]. Proliferative diabetic retinopathy was found in 4.5% of known diabetic subjects. The prevalence of an elevated urinary albumin was 15.0% in subjects with IGT, 26.0% in newly diagnosed diabetes subjects and 23.4% in known diabetes subjects. Duration of diabetes and level of glycemia were the most important associated factors.

Brooks *et al.* [38] compared rates of diabetes complications in Fiji and an Australian diabetes center. Although the prevalence of diabetic retinopathy increased linearly with duration of diabetes, it was higher in Fiji for the same duration of diabetes. Of people with retinopathy in Fiji, more than half had moderate to severe nonproliferative diabetic retinopathy or proliferative diabetic retinopathy, which is significantly higher than the Australian cohort.

In 1995, 195 people with type 2 diabetes attending the Vaiola Hospital Diabetes Clinic in Tonga were assessed for metabolic status and presence of diabetic complications and compared with an age, sex and duration of diabetes matched Australian sample attending the Diabetes Centre at the Prince of Wales Hospital, Sydney (**Table 17.3**). The Tongans had considerably worse diabetes control and at least twice the rate of blindness, retinopathy and signs of early kidney disease, and six times the rate of amputation.

Hospitalization is frequent among people with diabetes in the Pacific. For example, there are approximately 1500 admissions a year to the main medical ward in the National Hospital in Apia, Samoa, of which 25% have diabetes. Diabetes sepsis accounts for about 40% of diabetes admission, of whom one-third required an amputation, amounting to 52 people who had an amputation in 2002 (Viali, S., personal communication, 2006).

17.10 OBESITY

Obesity is a well-documented risk factor for diabetes. However, Pacific Islanders are a heterogeneous group and vary considerably in body habitus. Polynesians are generally of large build, whereas Melanesians are traditionally smaller people. There is currently no agreed cut-point for defining obesity which is specific for Pacific Islanders with a large body habitus. Applying the widely used WHO BMI classification for adults to the Tongan population means that 0.1% would be classified as underweight, 10.8% as normal weight, 28.8% as overweight and 60.4% as obese (BMI $\geq$ 30.0 kg m^{-2}). Data examining optimal BMI cut-points for identifying cardiovascular risk factors in Tongan people suggest a BMI of 30 kg m^{-2} in men and 32 kg m^{-2} in women.

Table 17.3 Comparison of complications after matching for age, gender and duration of diabetes in Tongans and an Australian cohort.

	Tongan	Australian
HbA$_{1c}$ (%)	9.8	8.1
Blind[a] (%)	7.2	1.4
Retinopathy (%)	41.6	21.3
Neuropathy	30.2	16.4
Foot ulcer (%)	4.4	1.1
Amputation	7.8	0
Microalbuminuria (%)	62.5	33.9

Visual acuity <6/60 in at least one eye.

While an appropriate ideal weight for Pacific Island countries and people of different ethnocultural background has not been determined, weight in the region continues to increase. For example, in the 1973 Tongan survey Finau *et al.* [14] reported a mean weight of 83.4 kg in men and 76.3 kg in women. In the 1998–2000 survey [15], mean weight had increased to 93.2 kg in men and 93.0 kg in women, representing a substantial gain in weight over this 25-year period.

17.11 CONCLUSION

The health status of Pacific Island populations in terms of life expectancy and general morbidity has improved significantly in recent years, and infectious diseases are largely under control and infant mortality rates are low. However, these health gains are being increasingly threatened by the alarming increase in noncommunicable diseases, especially diabetes. Diabetes is a major and growing public health problem in the Pacific that is impacting on individual and population health. Rates continue to increase at an alarming rate and show no signs of abating. Prevention public health strategies are urgently needed to address this epidemic.

References

1. Zimmet, P., Taft, P., Guinea, A. *et al.* (1977) The high prevalence of diabetes mellitus on a central Pacific Island. *Diabetologia*, **13**, 111–15.
2. De Brosses, M. (1756) *Histoire des Navigations aux Terres Australes, Contenant ce que l'on sait des Moeurs et des Productions des Contrées Découvertes Jusqu'à ce Jour*, Durand, Paris (English translation by J. Callender, Edinburgh, 1766–8).
3. Wikipedia (2006) http://en.wikipedia.org/wiki/Jules_Dumont_d%27Urville (accessed July 2008).
4. Neel, J.V. (1962) Diabetes mellitus: a thrifty genotype rendered detrimental by progress. *American Journal of Human Genetics*, **14**, 353–62.
5. Hales, C.N. and Barker, D.J.P. (1992) Type 2 (non-insulin-dependent) diabetes mellitus: the thrifty phenotype hypothesis. *Diabetologia*, **35**, 595–601.
6. Brand Miller, J. and Colagiuri, S. (1994) The carnivore connection: dietary carbohydrate in the evolution of NIDDM. *Diabetologia*, **37**, 1280–6.
7. Shaw, J.E., Courten, M.D., Boyko, E.J. and Zimmet, P.Z. (1999) Impact of new diagnostic criteria for diabetes on different populations. *Diabetes Care*, **22**, 762–6.
8. World Health Organization (1999) *Definition, Diagnosis and Classification of Diabetes Mellitus and its Complications: Report of a WHO Consultation. Part 1: Diagnosis and Classification of Diabetes Mellitus*, World Health Organization, Geneva.
9. The Expert Committee on the Diagnosis and Classification of Diabetes Mellitus (2003) Follow-up report on the diagnosis of diabetes mellitus. *Diabetes Care*, **26**, 3167
10. Bonita, R., de Courten, M., Dwyer, T. *et al.* (2001) *Surveillance of Risk Factors for Noncommunicable Diseases: The WHO STEPwise Approach*, World Health Organization, Geneva, www.who.int/entity/ncd_surveillance/media/en/269.pdf (accessed March 2006).
11. {King}, H., Taylor, R., Koteka, G. *et al.* (1986) Glucose tolerance in Polynesia. Population-based surveys in Rarotonga and Niue. *The Medical Journal of Australia*, **145**, 505–10.
12. Weinstein, S., Sedlak-Weinstein, E., Taylor, R. and Zimmet, P. (1981) The high prevalence of impaired glucose tolerance and diabetes mellitus in an isolated Polynesian population, Manihiki, Cook Islands. *The New Zealand Medical Journal*, **94**, 411–13.
13. Collins, V.R., Dowse, G.K., Toelupe, P.M. *et al.* (1994) Increasing prevalence of NIDDM in the pacific island population of Western Samoa over a 13-year period. *Diabetes Care*, **17**, 288–96.
14. Finau, S.A., Stanhope, J.M., Prior, I.A.M. and Joseph, J.G. (1983) The Tonga cardiovascular and metabolic study: design, demographic aspects and medical findings. *Community Health Studies*, **vii**, 67–77.
15. Colagiuri, S., Colagiuri, R., Na'ati, S. *et al.* (2002) The prevalence of diabetes in the kingdom of Tonga. *Diabetes Care*, **25**, 1378–83.
16. Taylor, R.J., Bennett, P.H., LeGonidec, G. *et al.* (1983) The prevalence of diabetes mellitus in a traditional-living Polynesian population: the Wallis Island Survey. *Diabetes Care*, **6**, 334–40.
17. Taylor, R., Bennett, P., Uili, R. *et al.* (1985) Diabetes in Wallis Polynesians: a comparison of residents of Wallis Island and first generation migrants to Noumea, New Caledonia. *Diabetes Research and Clinical Practice*, **1**, 169–78.
18. Shmulewitz, D., Auerbach, S.B., Lehner, T. *et al.* (2001) Epidemiology and factor analysis of obesity, type II diabetes, hypertension, and dyslipidemia (Syndrome X) on the Island of Kosrae, Federated States of Micronesia. *Human Heredity*, **51**, 8–19.
19. King, H., Heywood, P., Zimmet, P. *et al.* (1984) Glucose tolerance in a highland population in

Papua New Guinea. *Diabetes Research*, **1** (1), 45–51.

20. Zimmet, P., Arblaster, M. and Thoma, K. (1978) The effect of westernization on native populations. Studies on a Micronesian community with a high diabetes prevalence. *Australian and New Zealand Journal of Medicine*, **8**, 141–6.

21. Dowse, G., Zimmet, P., Finch, C. and Collins, V. (1991) Decline in incidence of epidemic glucose intolerance in Nauruans: implications for the thrifty genotype. *American Journal of Epidemiology*, **133**, 1093–104.

22. Zimmet, P., Taylor, R., Ram, P. *et al.* (1983) Prevalence of diabetes and impaired glucose tolerance in the biracial (Melanesian and Indian) population of Fiji: a rural–urban comparison. *American Journal of Epidemiology*, **118**, 673–88.

23. Zimmet, P., Canteloube, D., Genelle, B. *et al.* (1982) The prevalence of diabetes mellitus and impaired glucose tolerance in Melanesians and part-Polynesians in rural New Caledonia and Ouvea (Loyalty Island). *Diabetologia*, **23**, 393–8.

24. Eason, R.J., Pada, J., Wallace, R. *et al.* (1987) Changing patterns of hypertension, diabetes, obesity and diet among Melanesians and Micronesians in the Solomon Islands. *The Medical Journal of Australia*, **146**, 465–73.

25. King, H., Finch, C., Collins, A. *et al.* (1989) Glucose tolerance in Papua New Guinea: ethnic differences, association with environmental and behavioural factors and the possible emergence of glucose intolerance in a highland community. *The Medical Journal of Australia*, **151**, 204–10.

26. Taylor, R., Jalaludin, B., Levy, S. *et al.* (1991) Prevalence of diabetes, hypertension and obesity at different levels of urbanisation in Vanuatu. *The Medical Journal of Australia*, **155**, 86–90.

27. Zimmet, P., Faaiuso, S., Ainuu, J. *et al.* (1981) The prevalence of diabetes in the rural and urban Polynesian population of Western Samoa. *Diabetes*, **30**, 45–51.

28. World Health Organization (1985) Diabetes Mellitus: Report of a WHO Study Group. Tech. Rep. Ser., No. 727, World Health Organization, Geneva.

29. Balkau, B., King, H., Zimmet, P. and Raper, L.R. (1985) Factors associated with the development of diabetes in the micronesian population of Nauru. *American Journal of Epidemiology*, **122**, 594–605.

30. World Health Organization Expert Committee on Diabetes Mellitus (1980) Diabetes Mellitus. 2nd report. Tech. Rep. Ser. No. 646, World Health Organization, Geneva.

31. Eastman, R.C., Cowie, C.C. and Harris, M.I. (1997) Undiagnosed diabetes or impaired glucose tolerance and cardiovascular risk. *Diabetes Care*, **20**, 127–28.

32. Lowe, L.P., Liu, K., Greenland, P. *et al.* (1997) Diabetes, asymptomatic hyperglycemia, and 22-year mortality in black and white men. The Chicago Heart Association Detection Project in Industry Study. *Diabetes Care*, **20**, 163–9.

33. Dunstan, D.W., Zimmet, P.Z., Welborn, T.A. *et al.* (2002) The rising prevalence of diabetes and impaired glucose tolerance: the Australian Diabetes, Obesity and Lifestyle Study. *Diabetes Care*, **25**, 829–34.

34. Roglic, G., Williams, R. and Colagiuri, S. (2004) Screening for diabetes – the World Health Organisation perspective, in *Prevention of Type 2 Diabetes* (ed M. Ganz), John Wiley & Sons, Ltd, England.

35. King, H., Zimmet, P., Taylor, R. *et al.* (1983) Characteristics associated with diabetic retinopathy in Nauruans. *The Tohoku Journal of Experimental Medicine*, **141** (Suppl), 343–53.

36. Collins, V.R., Dowse, G.K., Finch, C.F. *et al.* (1989) Prevalence and risk factors for micro- and macroalbuminuria in diabetes subjects and entire population of Nauru. *Diabetes*, **38**, 1602–10.

37. Collins, V.R., Dowse, G.K., Plehwe, W.E. *et al.* (1995) High prevalence of diabetic retinopathy and nephropathy in Polynesians of Western Samoa. *Diabetes Care*, **18**, 1140–9.

38. Brooks, B., Chong, R., Ho, I. *et al.* (1999) Diabetic retinopathy and nephropathy in Fiji: comparison with data from an Australian diabetes centre. *Australian and New Zealand Journal of Ophthalmology*, **27**, 9–13.

Further Reading

WHO (2006) Global InfoBase Online. www.who.int/ncd_urveillance/infobase Unpublished data from International Diabetes Institute (accessed 25 May 2006).

18

Epidemiology of Type 2 Diabetes in North America

Linda S. Geiss,[1] Jing Wang,[1] Edward W. Gregg[2] and Michael M. Engelgau[3]

[1]Division of Diabetes Translation, Centers for Disease Control and Prevention,
Atlanta, GA, USA

[2]Department of Epidemiology, Graduate School of Public Health,
University of Pittsburgh, Pittsburgh, PA, USA

[3]Division of Diabetes Translation, National Center for Chronic Disease Prevention and
Health Promotion, Centers for Disease Control and Prevention, Atlanta, GA, USA

18.1 INTRODUCTION

Diabetes is a common, serious and costly health problem in North America. It is likely to become even more common as the North American population ages, as the minority populations most at risk for diabetes grow in number, as diabetes incidence continues to increase and as survival improves among persons with diabetes. This report on the epidemiology of type 2 diabetes in North America describes the prevalence and incidence of diabetes, its risk factors and the consequences of diabetes, including mortality and the complications of diabetes and their trends. Although many definitions of North America include Mexico, this review is limited to the United States and Canada. Data on Mexico are provided in Chapter 12. Further, most of the epidemiologic sources of data on diabetes are unable to distinguish between types of diabetes. Because the vast majority of people with diabetes in North America have type 2 diabetes, the data presented within this report reflect the burden experience of people with type 2 diabetes.

18.2 NORTH AMERICAN SOURCES OF DATA TO MONITOR DIABETES

Both the United States and Canada have national diabetes surveillance systems (NDSSs) to monitor and track the burden of diabetes [1, 2]. Although other types of data sources are incorporated into these systems, the US system relies primarily on national health survey data and the fledging Canadian system relies primarily on health care administrative data from participating provinces and territories. In addition to national survey and administrative data, population-based research has monitored special populations with diabetes and provided valuable insight into the morbidity and mortality associated with diabetes.

18.2.1 National Health Survey Data

Nationally representative health interview surveys within the United States and Canada are conducted either face to face or by telephone. Conducted continuously since 1957, the National Health Interview Survey of the Centers for Disease Control and Prevention (CDC) is the oldest household interview survey in North America. Other health surveys used to monitor diabetes in the United States include CDC's state-based Behavioral Risk Factor Surveillance System and CDC's National Health and Nutrition Examination Survey (NHANES). The latter survey includes an examination component that contains blood and biochemical measurements that, when combined with interview data, allow the estimation of

The Epidemiology of Diabetes Mellitus, second edition   Edited by Jean-Marie Ekoé, Marian Rewers, Rhys Williams and Paul Zimmet

undiagnosed diabetes and thus the determination of the prevalence of all persons with diabetes (i.e. both diagnosed and undiagnosed diabetes). Health surveys within Canada include Statistics Canada's National Population Health Survey and the Canadian Community Health Survey. Recently, the Joint Canada–United States Health Survey—a one-time, random telephone survey conducted between November 2002 and March 2003 using the same methodology in both the United States and Canada—was conducted by CDC and Statistics Canada to facilitate international comparisons.

18.2.2   Health Care Administrative Data

The most recent report from the Canadian NDSS used 1999–2000 data from the health insurance programs of eight provinces and three territories, accounting for over 95% of the Canadian population [2]. In addition, some provinces, including Manitoba [3] and Ontario [4], have published their own reports. In the United States, such health care administrative data typically exist only for special populations whose health care is provided for or paid by a governmental agency, such as the Medicare, Medicaid, Veterans Administration and the Indian Health Service (IHS) populations. Typically, hospitalization and physician claims or encounter data are used to identify cases of diabetes in health care administrative data.

18.2.3   Population-based Research

Cross-sectional and longitudinal population-based studies conducted in selected North American communities and populations have contributed to our understanding of the prevalence and incidence of diabetes. Cohort studies, which follow people over time, are particularly useful for studying the natural history of disease, including investigating the incidence of diabetes and its risk factors, as well as the morbidity and mortality among people with diabetes.

18.2.4   Data Limitations

Survey data and administrative data can identify only those people with diagnosed disease and, therefore, do not account for people with undiagnosed diabetes. However, both survey data and administrative data are moderately sensitive and highly specific in identifying people with diagnosed diabetes [5, 6]. The use of telephones to conduct health surveys may introduce bias

because households without telephones are not included. Although the presence of household telephones is generally high in North America, the lack of a household telephone is more common in lower socioeconomic population groups that are disproportionately burdened by diabetes. In addition, administrative data have limited information on patient demographic characteristics, socioeconomic status, health behaviors and risk factors. Although population-based studies may overcome several of the limitations of survey and administrative data, data from population-based studies reflect small geographic areas or special population subgroups that may not represent the experience of the US and Canada populations. Further, such studies also tend to differ in methodology, time period studied, definitions used and length of follow-up, making summary statements difficult.

18.3   CURRENT AND FUTURE PREVALENCE OF DIABETES

18.3.1   Current and Projected Numbers of People with Diabetes

In 1958, 1.6 million Americans reported that they had been diagnosed with diabetes [7] (**Figure 18.1**). By 2005 (nearly 50 years later) that number had grown over eightfold to 14.6 million Americans [8]. This number is expected to increase to 39.0 million by 2050 [9]. Furthermore, the actual and potential burden of diabetes in the United States is underestimated by these statistics on diagnosed diabetes, because nearly a third of diabetes is undiagnosed [10]. When the additional 6.2 million persons who were unaware that they had the disease are added to the number of those with diagnosed disease, an estimated 20.8 million Americans had diabetes in 2005 [8].

In 1999–2000, there were 1.2 million adult Canadians with diagnosed diabetes [11]. This number is projected to increase to 2.4 million people by 2016 [12]. If the ratio of undiagnosed to total diabetes among Canadians was similar to that of Americans, about 2 million adult Canadians had diabetes in 1999–2000.

18.3.2   Prevalence and Trends

The prevalence of diagnosed diabetes among Americans of all ages increased from 0.9% in 1958 [7] to 5.1% in 2004 [1] (**Figure 18.1**), and is expected to increase to 9.7% in 2050 [9]. It

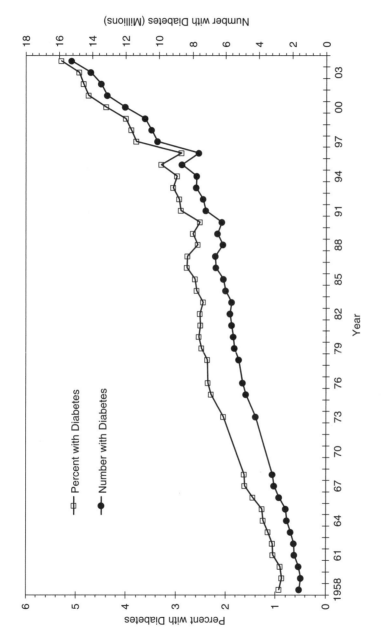

Figure 18.1 Number of people with diagnosed diabetes and prevalence of diagnosed diabetes in the United States, 1958–2004.

is predicted that 33% of American children born in the year 2000 will be diagnosed with diabetes during their lifetime [13]. However, these statistics do not include data on undiagnosed diabetes. When these data are incorporated into 2005 prevalence estimates, an estimated 7.0% of the total US population, 9.6% of the population aged 20 years or older, and 20.9% of the population aged 60 years or older had diabetes [8]. Mirroring increasing trends in diagnosed diabetes, the total prevalence of diabetes (diagnosed and undiagnosed) also increased over five consecutive NHANES between 1960 and 2000 [14] and was higher in the 1999–2002 NHANES than in the 1988–1994 NHANES [10]. In the past quarter of a century, the growth in diagnosed diabetes in the United States is apparent in all age groups, in both sexes and in all racial/ethnic groups for which data are available [1], and the prevalence of diabetes has increased sharply since 1990 (**Figure 18.1**). Increases in the prevalence of diagnosed diabetes also occurred across the adult populations of all the states that form the United States (**Figure 18.2**). These increases mirrored increasing rates of obesity in the states.

Provincial health care data from the Canadian NDSS and from Manitoba and Ontario also indicate increasing trends in diabetes prevalence. From 1989 to 1998, the prevalence of diagnosed diabetes in Manitoba adults increased among both First Nation women (from 18.2 to 24.9%) and First Nation men (from 10.4 to 17.0%) and in non-First Nation men (from 4.2 to 6.0%) and women (from 3.7 to 5.4%) [3]. From 1995 to 2005, the prevalence of diagnosed diabetes in Ontario adults increased 82%, from 4.9% to 8.9% [4]. Aggregated provincial administrative data show that prevalence among Canadian adults increased, from 4.3% in 1997–1998 to 5.1% in 1999–2000 [2]. Furthermore, national survey data from 1994–1995 to 2000–2001 show a 32% increase (from 3.4% to 4.5%) in the prevalence of diagnosed diabetes among Canadian adults [15]. In these data, prevalence increased across all age groups, but the increases were significant only among those less than 65 years of age. These data also show that the prevalence of diagnosed diabetes increased among both men and women, with prevalence among men increasing at a greater rate, such that their prevalence rate became significantly greater than that of women

by the end of the time period. A similar trend is seen in US surveillance data, which indicate that the age-adjusted prevalence of men and women began to diverge in the late 1990s, with rates for men rising above rates for women [1]. However, this sex-based difference in the United States is due to differences in rates among the majority White population. In contrast to rates among Whites, the prevalence of diagnosed diabetes among racial and ethnic minorities is greater among women than men [1, 3, 10, 16]. These differences by race may be due to different patterns of overweight and obesity by sex and race.

A one-time, random telephone survey conducted in 2003 in both the United States and Canada facilitates cross-national comparison of diagnosed diabetes prevalence. One study using these survey data found that the prevalence of diagnosed diabetes among US adults (6.7%) was more than 40% higher than that in Canadian adults (4.7%) [17]. This study also found that obesity and sedentary lifestyle (known risk factors for diabetes) were more common among US adults. However, the different racial and ethnic makeup of the non-Caucasian populations of each country (e.g. Blacks and Hispanics are more prevalent in the US population) complicates the comparison of prevalence between the two countries.

18.3.3 Undiagnosed Diabetes

Among American adults, the prevalence of undiagnosed diabetes (as measured by no self-reported history of diabetes and a fasting glucose value of $\geq 126\,\mathrm{mg}\,\mathrm{dl}^{-1}$) was 2.8% in 1999–2002 [10]; this was not significantly different from the prevalence of undiagnosed diabetes in 1988–1994 (2.7%). Consistent with these findings, three consecutive NHANES from 1976 to 2000 suggest that there has been no decrease in the prevalence of undiagnosed diabetes [14]. However, this trend varied by body mass index (BMI). Among those most obese (BMI ≥ 35), there was a large decrease in the prevalence of undiagnosed diabetes, accompanied by a large increase in diagnosed diabetes, suggesting detection of diabetes may have improved in this group.

Like diagnosed diabetes, undiagnosed diabetes in adult Americans increases with age [10, 18]. Unlike diagnosed diabetes, the age–sex-standardized prevalence of undiagnosed diabetes among American adults does not vary by race. Also,

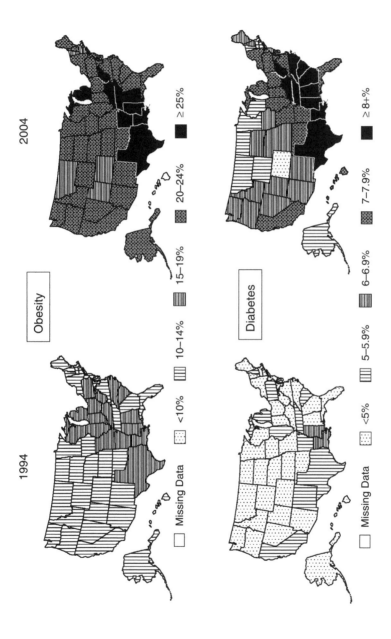

Figure 18.2 Prevalence of obesity and diagnosed diabetes per 100 adult population, United States, 1994 and 2004.

gender differences in prevalence exist only among non-Hispanic Whites and not among non-Hispanic Blacks or Mexican Americans [10].

18.3.4 Vulnerable Groups

In North America, elderly minority groups and those with lower socioeconomic status are disproportionately burdened by diabetes. In the general population, glucose tolerance worsens with age [19, 20]. Generally (although sometimes dropping in the oldest age group, probably due to selective mortality), the prevalence of diabetes increases sharply with age in all sex and race groups [1, 4, 10, 15]. In 1999–2002, the prevalence of diagnosed and undiagnosed diabetes was 21.6% among Americans aged 65 years and older, compared with only 2.3% among those aged 20–39 years [10]. Race/ethnicity is a risk factor for diabetes incidence [1, 3, 16, 21–26] and the prevalence of diabetes generally is at least twice as common in racial and ethnic minority populations [1, 3, 7, 10, 16, 27, 28]. Furthermore, diabetes develops at younger ages in minority populations, leaving individuals in those populations even more vulnerable to develop diabetes complications at younger ages. Although there is significant variability across populations and tribes, American Indians and Alaska Natives in the United States and the First Nations communities in Canada are disproportionately affected by diabetes, with rates two to five times greater than the rate among Caucasians [3, 8, 16, 27]. Most other minority populations within the United States, including Hispanic/Latino American, non-Hispanic Blacks and Asian Americans and Pacific Islanders, also have a higher prevalence of diabetes than do their Caucasian counterparts [1, 8, 10]. In 1999–2002, the age- and sex-standardized prevalence of diagnosed and undiagnosed diabetes for non-Hispanic Black (11.0%) and Mexican American (10.4%) adults was at least twice that of non-Hispanic White adult Americans (5.2%) [10]. The prevalence of diabetes among the elderly of these minority groups was particularly high, exceeding 30%. Higher rates of diabetes among minority populations may reflect greater genetic susceptibility, higher levels of risk factors for diabetes, or a combination of these and other factors. The associations of age and race/ethnicity with diabetes have important implications in light of demographic trends in North America: As the Canadian and the US populations age and as their minority populations grow, the incidence and prevalence of diabetes are likely to increase.

When measured by either income or educational level, lower socioeconomic status is associated with an elevated risk of diabetes [4, 15, 23, 29–31]. Those with lower socioeconomic status may possess higher levels of risk factors for diabetes and other chronic diseases [21, 31], may have less access to care and higher levels of stress, and may have low levels of health literacy that may affect self- and medical care [32].

18.3.5 Prediabetes and Total Hyperglycemia

People with prediabetes have impaired fasting glucose (IFG), defined as fasting glucose of $100–125\,\text{mg dl}^{-1}$, impaired glucose tolerance (IGT), defined as glucose of $140–199\,\text{mg dl}^{-1}$ after a 2 h oral glucose tolerance test, or both IFG and IGT. In a cross-sectional sample of US adults aged 40–74 years, who were tested during the period 1988–1994, 33.8% had IFG, 15.4% had IGT and 40.1% had prediabetes (IGT or IFG or both) [8]. When these percentages were applied to the US population in 2000, an estimated 35 million adults aged 40–74 years had IFG, 16 million had IGT and 41 million had prediabetes. Estimates for 2002 based on more recent NHANES data (1999–2002) indicate that 54 million US adults aged 20 years or older have IFG [10].

Although more recent nationally representative data are not available on IGT, the 1999–2002 prevalence of IFG in the US population aged 20 years and older was 26.0% [10]. This is not significantly greater than the prevalence of 24.7% in 1988–1994. In both time periods, the prevalence of IFG increased with age and in 1999–2002 IFG prevalence reached a high of 39.1% among people aged 65 years and older. IFG is also higher among men than among women, and higher among non-Hispanic Whites and Mexican Americans than among non-Hispanic Blacks.

When prevalence estimates for diagnosed and undiagnosed diabetes and IFG are combined, 35.3% of the US adult population in 1999–2002 had abnormal glucose levels [10]. As with the prevalence of IFG, there was no significant increase in the percentage of those with abnormal glucose levels between the periods 1988–1994 and 1999–2002 in the US adult population.

18.4 INCIDENCE OF DIABETES

18.4.1 Magnitude and Trend

Prospective population-based incidence studies that perform serial diagnostic tests for diabetes are rare and have been conducted on populations that are not nationally representative; for example, Pima Indians [28] and participants in the San Antonio Heart Study [22]. Most incidence studies in the United States and Canada, particularly those that are nationally representative, use cross-sectional survey data, medical records, registries or health care administrative data to identify newly diagnosed cases of diabetes and are unable to detect new cases of disease that have not been diagnosed.

In the United States, the incidence of diagnosed diabetes increased during the 1960s but changed little between 1968 and 1992 [7]. However, from 1997 to 2003, the incidence of diagnosed diabetes in the US population aged 18–79 years increased 41%, from 4.9 per 1000 to 6.9 per 1000 [23]. During this period, incidence increased in most sociodemographic subgroups in the United States. Medicare administrative data indicate that incidence is also increasing among the aged [25]. Between 1994 and 2001, incidence increased 37% in this high-risk population. Similarly, among Canadian adults followed over a 6-year period from 1994–1995 to 2000–2001, incidence increased from 4.0 per 1000 person years to 6.7 per 1000 person years and, as in the United States, incidence increased in most sociodemographic subgroups [15]. Canadian administrative data from Manitoba indicate that incidence also increased between 1989 and 1998 for First Nation men and non-First Nation men and women [3]. Also, Ontario administrative health data from 1997 through 2003 indicated a 31% increase in age- and sex-adjusted incidence. The amount of increase varied by age, with those aged 20–49 years experiencing a 44% increase compared with a 19% increase among those aged 50 years or older [4].

Population-based studies in the United States conducted in earlier periods and using different methodologies also indicate that incidence is increasing [22, 28, 33–35]. For example, between the periods 1970–1974 and 1990–1994, age-adjusted incidence in Rochester, Minnesota, residents aged 30 years or older rose 67% for men and 42% for women [33]. Also, incidence

increased rapidly (almost tripling) from 1987 to 1996 among Mexican Americans and non-Hispanic Whites aged 25–64 years participating in the San Antonio Heart Study [22].

In 2005, an estimated 1.5 million Americans were newly diagnosed with diabetes [8]. Each year, the annual number of newly diagnosed cases of diabetes exceeds the number of deaths among adults with diabetes [3, 25] adding to the increasing prevalence of diabetes. This imbalance between the number of deaths among people with diabetes and the number of people entering the prevalent pool is likely to continue to grow (see Section 18.6).

18.4.2 Modifiable Risk Factors

The increasing trends in diabetes incidence and prevalence coincide with increasing trends in BMI in both the United States and Canada [36–44]. Various measures of adiposity are associated with the incidence of diabetes. Diabetes incidence increases sharply with BMI, and obesity is a major factor in the development of diabetes [15, 24, 35, 45–50]. Incidence is also higher among people who are overweight [15, 23, 48], and weight gain is associated with incidence, regardless of BMI [51–54]. Also, regardless of BMI, abdominal fat and waist circumference are also associated with diabetes incidence [53, 55, 56].

Physical inactivity, independent of the effects of obesity, further elevates the risk of diabetes [48, 50, 57]. In addition, a number of other lifestyle factors are associated with incidence, including smoking [48, 58, 59], no or excessive alcohol consumption [59–61] and various aspects of diet [48, 62–65].

18.5 DIABETES COMPLICATIONS

Most of the human and economic costs of diabetes are due to its devastating but largely preventable complications, including kidney failure, amputation and heart disease and stroke.

18.5.1 Preventing Complications

Over the last few decades, numerous public health agencies and other private and public organizations within the United States and Canada sought to prevent and control these disabling consequences of diabetes by increasing the use of preventive care practices and reducing risk factors for complications among people with diabetes. The efficacy of preventive care practices (e.g. timely eye and foot care, adult vaccinations) and risk-factor reduction (e.g. glycemia, blood pressure, and lipid control) in preventing complications is summarized elsewhere [66]. In the United States, national representative survey data and administrative data from the Centers for Medicare and Medicaid Services (CMS), the Department of Veterans Affairs (VA) and the IHS all indicate that rates of many preventive care practices increased [67–71].

Favorable changes have also occurred among risk factors for complications. In the US adult population with diabetes, the prevalence of high total cholesterol, high blood pressure and smoking declined over the three decades between 1971 and 2000 [72]. Between the periods 1950–1966 and 1977–1995, Framingham Heart study participants with diabetes who were 45–64 years at enrollment also experienced declines in systolic blood pressure and total cholesterol [73]. Recently, other favorable changes in risk factors have also been reported in the United States by the IHS and VA [67, 70, 71].

Along with favorable changes in preventive care practices and risk factors, there are encouraging trends in the rates of some complications (see the sections on the various types of complications below). Some complication rates are no longer increasing and others are decreasing. In general, however, even when complication rates decrease, the number of events continues to increase as the number of people with diabetes continues to grow. Furthermore, despite encouraging trends, preventive care practices remain suboptimal, the level of risk factors for complications remains high and rates of diabetes complications remain high [13, 67, 69].

18.5.2 Cardiovascular Disease

Cardiovascular disease is the leading cause of death among people with diabetes [74]. Diabetes is associated with a two- to four-fold increased risk of heart disease and stroke incidence and death. This excess risk may be due to higher levels of cardiovascular risk factors, such as high blood pressure and lipid disorders [75]. Furthermore, the presence of one or more of the risk factors may have a greater impact on clinical outcomes in people with diabetes than in those without diabetes [75]. Recent evidence, however, suggests

that cardiovascular risk factors among Americans with diabetes improved over the last 30 years [72]. Recent evidence also indicates a reduction in the rate of cardiovascular events, such as hospitalization and death in the North American population with diabetes [1, 68, 73, 76].

18.5.3 Eye, Kidney and Lower-extremity Disease

Diabetes is the leading cause of kidney failure, lower-extremity amputation and blindness of working-age adults [75, 77–79]. About 25% of all Americans with diabetes have considerable visual impairment, a rate approximately twice that of persons without diabetes [69]. Between 1988 and 1994, the prevalence and severity of diabetic retinopathy among Americans 40 years of age and older with type 2 diabetes was greater in non-Hispanic Blacks and Mexican Americans than in non-Hispanic Whites [18].

In Ontario, from 1995 to 2000, the proportion of new dialysis patients who had diabetes grew from 38% to 51% [80]. However, this increase was not due to a greater need for dialysis among people with diabetes, but was due to the growth of the total number of people with diabetes during this period. In 2003, about 53% of new cases of end-stage renal disease (ESRD) in the United States were caused by diabetes [81]. Encouragingly, after many years of increase, the overall incidence of ESRD among Americans with diabetes is now declining [1, 78] (**Figure 18.3**). However, trends vary by sex and by race/ethnicity. From 1997 to 2002, ESRD incidence decreased among persons <65 years of age, women and Whites, and it stopped increasing among persons aged 65–74 years, men and Blacks [78]. ESRD incidence also declined among American Indian and Alaska Natives in the southwest of the United States, a group having disproportionately high rates of ESRD [82].

Rates of lower-extremity amputation among Americans with diabetes are decreasing in the United States (**Figure 18.3**) [1, 67, 68]. However, disparities still exist, with Blacks having higher rates than Whites and men having higher rates than women [1, 68]. From 1995 to 1999, amputation rates in Ontario also declined [83]. As in the United States, rates in Ontario increased with age, were higher among men than women, and higher among First Nation people [16, 83]. Amputation rates were

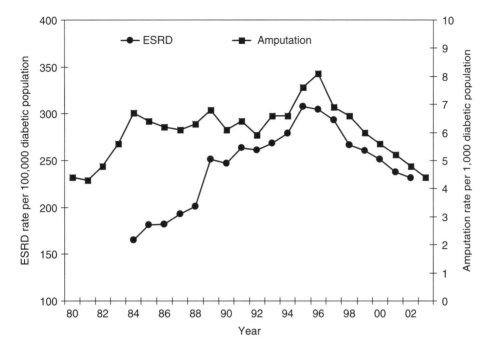

Figure 18.3 Age-adjusted incidence of ESRD treatment and rate of hospital discharge for nontraumatic lower-extremity amputation in the US population with diabetes, 1980–2003.

also inversely related to socioeconomic status, and lack of access to regular care was an important predictor of amputation.

18.5.4 Acute Complications

Hypoglycemia, diabetic ketoacidosis and hypersomolar coma are acute complications of diabetes that can lead to death if untreated. However, there are encouraging trends in the rates of these acute complications. Between 1994 and 1999, hospitalization and emergency department treatments of hyper- and hypo-glycemic emergencies decreased in Ontario [84]. People living in rural areas and aboriginal communities were about twice as likely to experience an acute complication as were those living elsewhere. In the United States, hospitalizations and deaths rates due to diabetic ketoacidosis and hypersomolar coma declined from 1985 to 2002 [1, 85]; and in the elderly Medicare population, rates of emergency department admissions for metabolic crisis and ketoacidosis declined from 1992 to 2001 [68]. Generally, in the United States, incidence and death rates due to acute complications are higher among Blacks than among Whites [1, 68, 85].

18.6 MORTALITY

According to death certificate data, diabetes is the sixth leading cause of death in the United States and Canada [86]. However, typical death certificate data substantially underestimate the impact of diabetes on the mortality of persons with the disease [74, 87]. Age-adjusted mortality among adults with diabetes is about twice that of people who do not have diabetes. Among middle-aged people with diabetes, life expectancy is reduced by 5–10 years [74]. Reduction in life expectancy is greater for women than for men and for those with complications. Reduction in life expectancy also decreases with increasing age at diagnosis.

The leading cause of death in persons with diabetes is heart disease. The risk of heart disease and ischemic heart disease is two to four times higher for persons with diabetes than for those without diabetes [74]. This excess risk cannot be fully explained by higher levels of risk factors in people with diabetes and is greater among women and those using insulin.

Few studies have examined temporal trends in mortality among persons with diabetes. In a nationally representative cohort study of US adults aged 35–74 years, no significant changes occurred between 1971 and 1993 in all-cause mortality, heart disease and ischemic heart disease mortality among people with diabetes, while a substantial decline occurred in people without diabetes [88]. However, other studies, some occurring in more recent time periods, have found decreasing death rates among people with diabetes. For example, a 14% decline in death rates was observed in Rochester, Minnesota, residents with diabetes from 1970 to 1994 [89]. However, this decline was less than the 21% decline among persons without diabetes. From 1994 to 2001, death rates in the elderly Medicare population with diabetes decreased from 92.1 per 1000 to 87.2 per 1000, while there was no decrease among those without diabetes [25]. Also, from 1997 to 2002, mortality rates among adults with diabetes living in North Dakota declined about 35%, from 74.1 per 1000 to 47.5 per 1000 persons with diabetes [90]. Over an 8-year period, from 1992 to 2000, adults with diabetes in Ontario experienced declines in all-cause mortality as well as in mortality due to acute myocardial infarction and stroke [76]. In general, the magnitudes of these reductions in mortality were similar to those without diabetes. More recent data from Ontario indicate that declines in all-cause mortality among adults with diabetes continue, with age- and sex-adjusted death rates falling by 25% between 1995 and 2005 [4].

Over the last few decades, the health of the North American population has improved, as evidenced by declining mortality rates, reductions in cardiovascular risk factors and declines in cardiovascular disease death rates [91–93]. Altogether, declines in mortality, reductions in cardiovascular risk factors and declines in cardiovascular events and other complications seen among people with diabetes also suggest improvements in the health of the population with diabetes.

18.7 SUMMARY

In the North American population with diabetes, encouraging trends are now being seen in rates of preventive care, levels of risk factors, rates of some complications and in survival. However, despite improvements, diabetes care remains suboptimal, risk factors for complications are too prevalent, rates of complications and death are too high and

disadvantaged populations are disproportionately affected. Furthermore, even if complication and mortality rates decrease further, the absolute numbers of people adversely affected may continue to increase as the population with diabetes continues to increase.

Diabetes, already a major public health problem in North America, is likely to become even more common as the North American population ages, as race and ethnic populations at disproportionate risk for diabetes grow in number, as diabetes incidence continues to increase, and as survival improves among persons with diabetes. Since the 1990s, the prevalence and incidence of diabetes have increased at an alarming rate. Overweight and obesity have reached epidemic proportions in North America and the increasing adiposity is probably the most important single factor in the increasing incidence of diabetes. Recent clinical trials have shown that moderate weight loss and exercise can prevent or delay type 2 diabetes among adults at high risk of diabetes. With such compelling evidence, the prevention of diabetes presents a major challenge and opportunity to stem the diabetes burden in North America.

References

1. Centers for Disease Control and Prevention (2006) National Diabetes Surveillance System. Available at: http://www.cdc.gov/diabetes/statistics/index.htm (accessed 4 May 2006).
2. Health Canada (2002) *Diabetes in Canada*, 2nd edn, Health Protection Branch, Health Canada, Ottawa, ON, available at: http://www.phac-aspc.gc.ca/publicat/dic-dac2/english/01cover_e.html (accessed 4 May 2006).
3. Green, C., Blanchard, J.F., Young, T.K. and Griffith, J. (2003) The epidemiology of diabetes in the Manitoba-registered First Nation population: current patterns and comparative trends. *Diabetes Care*, **26**, 1993–8.
4. Lipscombe, L.L. and Hux, J.E. (2007) Trends in diabetes prevalence, incidence, and mortality in Ontario, Canada 1995–2005: a population-based study. *Lancet*, **369**, 750–6.
5. Hux, J.E., Ivis, F., Flintoft, V. and Bica, A. (2002) Diabetes in Ontario: determination of prevalence and incidence using a validated administrative data algorithm. *Diabetes Care*, **25**, 512–16.
6. Saydah, S.H., Geiss, L.S., Tierney, E. *et al.* (2004) Review of the performance of methods to identify diabetes cases among vital statistics, administrative,

and survey data. *Annals of Epidemiology*, **14**, 507–16.

7. Kenny, S.J., Aubert, R.E. and Geiss, L. (1995) Prevalence and incidence of non-insulin-dependent diabetes, in *Diabetes in America* (eds M. Harris, C. Cowie, M. Stern *et al.*), National Institutes of Health, Bethesda, MD, pp. 47–67.

8. Centers for Disease Control and Prevention (2005) National Diabetes Fact Sheet: General Information and National Estimates on Diabetes in the United States, 2005, US Department of Health and Human Services, Centers for Disease Control and Prevention, Atlanta, GA, available at: http://www.cdc.gov/diabetes/pubs/factsheet05.htm (accessed 4 May 2006).

9. Honeycutt, A.A., Boyle, J.P., Broglio, K.R. *et al.* (2003) A dynamic Markov model for forecasting diabetes prevalence in the United States through 2050. *Health Care Management Science*, **6**, 155–64.

10. Cowie, C.C., Rust, K.F., Byrd-Holt, D.D. *et al.* (2006) Prevalence of diabetes and impaired fasting glucose in adults in the U.S. population, National Health and Nutrition Examination Survey 1999–2002. *Diabetes Care*, **29**, 1263–8.

11. Health Canada (2006) Diabetes Facts and Figures, available at: http://www.phac-aspc.gc.ca/ccdpc-cpcmc/ndss-snsd/english/facts_figures_e.html (accessed 4 May 2006).

12. Ohinmaa, A., Jacobs, P., Simpson, S. and Johnson, J.A. (2004) The projection of prevalence and cost of diabetes in Canada: 2000 to 2016. *Canadian Journal of Diabetes*, **28**, 116–23.

13. Narayan, K.M., Boyle, J.P., Thompson, T.J. *et al.* (2003) Lifetime risk for diabetes mellitus in the United States. *The Journal of the American Medical Association*, **290**, 1884–90.

14. Gregg, E.W., Cadwell, B.L., Cheng, Y.J. *et al.* (2004) Trends in the prevalence and ratio of diagnosed to undiagnosed diabetes according to obesity levels in the U.S. *Diabetes Care*, **27**, 2806–12.

15. Millar, W.J. and Young, T.K. (2003) Tracking diabetes: prevalence, incidence and risk factors. *Health Reports*, **14**, 35–47.

16. Shah, B.R., Anand, S., Zinman, B. and Duong-Hua, M. (2003) Diabetes and first nations people, in *Diabetes in Ontario: An ICES Practice Atlas* (eds J.E. Hux, G.L. Booth, P.M. Slaughter and A. Laupacis), Institute for Clinical Evaluative Sciences, Toronto, pp. 13.231–248.

17. Lasser, K.E., Himmelstein, D.U. and Woolhandler, S. (2006) Access to care, health status, and health disparities in the United States and Canada: results of a cross-national population-based survey. *American Journal of Public Health*, **96** (7), 1300–7.

18. Harris, M.I., Flegal, K.M., Cowie, C.C. *et al.* (1998) Prevalence of diabetes, impaired fasting glucose, and impaired glucose tolerance in U.S. adults. The Third National Health and Nutrition Examination Survey, 1988–1994. *Diabetes Care*, **21**, 518–24.

19. Cowie, C.C. and Harris, M.I. (1995) Physical and metabolic characteristics of persons with diabetes, in *Diabetes in America* (eds M. Harris, C. Cowie, M. Stern *et al.*), National Institutes of Health, Bethesda, MD, pp. 117–64.

20. Shimokata, H., Muller, D.C., Fleg, J.L. *et al.* (1991) Age as independent determinant of glucose tolerance. *Diabetes*, **40**, 44–51.

21. Brancati, F.L., Kao, W.H., Folsom, A.R. *et al.* (2000) Incident type 2 diabetes mellitus in African American and white adults: the Atherosclerosis Risk in Communities Study. *The Journal of the American Medical Association*, **283**, 2253–9.

22. Burke, J.P., Williams, K., Gaskill, S.P. *et al.* (1999) Rapid rise in the incidence of type 2 diabetes from 1987 to 1996: results from the San Antonio Heart Study. *Archives of Internal Medicine*, **159**, 1450–6.

23. Geiss, L.S., Pan, L., Cadwell, B. *et al.* (2006) Changes in incidence of diabetes in U.S. Adults, 1997–2003. *American Journal of Preventive Medicine*, **30**, 371–7.

24. Lee, E.T., Welty, T.K., Cowan, L.D. *et al.* (2002) Incidence of diabetes in American Indians of three geographic areas: the Strong Heart Study. *Diabetes Care*, **25**, 49–54.

25. McBean, A.M., Li, S., Gilbertson, D.T. and Collins, A.J. (2004) Differences in diabetes prevalence, incidence, and mortality among the elderly of four racial/ethnic groups: Whites, Blacks, Hispanics, and Asians. *Diabetes Care*, **27**, 2317–24.

26. Resnick, H.E., Valsania, P., Halter, J.B. and Lin, X. (1998) Differential effects of BMI on diabetes risk among black and white Americans. *Diabetes Care*, **21**, 1828–35.

27. Burrows, N.R., Geiss, L.S., Engelgau, M.M. and Acton, K.J. (2000) Prevalence of diabetes among Native Americans and Alaska Natives, 1990–1997: an increasing burden. *Diabetes Care*, **23**, 1786–90.

28. Knowler, W.C., Pettitt, D.J., Saad, M.F. and Bennett, P.H. (1990) Diabetes mellitus in the Pima Indians: incidence, risk factors and pathogenesis. *Diabetes/Metabolism Reviews*, **6**, 1–27.

29. Choi, B.C. and Shi, F. (2001) Risk factors for diabetes mellitus by age and sex: results of the National Population Health Survey. *Diabetologia*, **44**, 1221–31.

30. Robbins, J.M., Vaccarino, V., Zhang, H. and Kasl, S.V. (2001) Socioeconomic status and type 2 diabetes in African American and non-Hispanic white women and men: evidence from the Third

National Health and Nutrition Examination Survey. *American Journal of Public Health*, **91**, 76–83.

31. Robbins, J.M., Vaccarino, V., Zhang, H. and Kasl, S.V. (2005) Socioeconomic status and diagnosed diabetes incidence. *Diabetes Research and Clinical Practice*, **68**, 230–6.

32. Berkman, N.D., DeWalt, D.A., Pignone, M.P. *et al.* (2004) Literacy and Health Outcomes, Evidence Report/Technology Assessment Report No. 87, Agency for Healthcare Research and Quality, Rockville, MD, available at: http://www.ncbi.nlm.nih.gov/books/bv.fcgi?rid=hstat1a.chapter.32213 (accessed 4 May 2006).

33. Burke, J.P., O'Brien, P., Ransom, J. *et al.* (2002) Impact of case ascertainment on recent trends in diabetes incidence in Rochester, Minnesota. *American Journal of Epidemiology*, **155**, 859–65.

34. Leibson, C.L., O'Brien, P.C., Atkinson, E. *et al.* (1997) Relative contributions of incidence and survival to increasing prevalence of adult-onset diabetes mellitus: a population-based study. *American Journal of Epidemiology*, **146**, 12–22.

35. Lipton, R.B., Liao, Y., Cao, G. *et al.* (1993) Determinants of incident non-insulin-dependent diabetes mellitus among blacks and whites in a national sample. The NHANES I Epidemiologic Follow-up Study. *American Journal of Epidemiology*, **138**, 826–39.

36. Belanger-Ducharme, F. and Tremblay, A. (2005) Prevalence of obesity in Canada. *Obesity Reviews*, **6**, 183–6.

37. Flegal, K.M., Carroll, M.D., Kuczmarski, R.J. and Johnson, C.L. (1998) Overweight and obesity in the United States: prevalence and trends, 1960–1994. *International Journal of Obesity and Related Metabolic Disorders*, **22**, 39–47.

38. Katzmarzyk, P.T. (2002) The Canadian obesity epidemic: an historical perspective. *Obesity Research*, **10**, 666–74.

39. Katzmarzyk, P.T. and Ardern, C.I. (2004) Overweight and obesity mortality trends in Canada, 1985–2000. *Canadian Journal of Public Health*, **95**, 16–20.

40. Mokdad, A.H., Ford, E.S., Bowman, B.A. *et al.* (2000) Diabetes trends in the U.S.: 1990–1998. *Diabetes Care*, **23**, 1278–83.

41. Mokdad, A.H., Bowman, B.A., Ford, E.S. *et al.* (2001) The continuing epidemics of obesity and diabetes in the United States. *The Journal of the American Medical Association*, **286**, 1195–200.

42. Ogden, C.L., Fryar, C.D., Carroll, M.D. and Flegal, K.M. (2004) Mean body weight, height, and body mass index, United States 1960–2002. Advance Data from Vital and Health Statistics, no. 347,

National Center for Health Statistics, Hyattsville, MD.

43. Ogden, C.L., Carroll, M.D., Curtin, L.R. *et al.* (2006) Prevalence of overweight and obesity in the United States, 1999–2004. *The Journal of the American Medical Association*, **295**, 1549–55.

44. Tremblay, M.S., Katzmarzyk, P.T. and Willms, J.D. (2002) Temporal trends in overweight and obesity in Canada, 1981–1996. *International Journal of Obesity and Related Metabolic Disorders*, **26**, 538–43.

45. Edelstein, S.L., Knowler, W.C., Bain, R.P. *et al.* (1997) Predictors of progression from impaired glucose tolerance to NIDDM: an analysis of six prospective studies. *Diabetes*, **46**, 701–10.

46. Gurwitz, J.H., Field, T.S., Glynn, R.J. *et al.* (1994) Risk factors for non-insulin-dependent diabetes mellitus requiring treatment in the elderly. *Journal of the American Geriatrics Society*, **42**, 1235–40.

47. Hara, H., Egusa, G. and Yamakido, M. (1996) Incidence of non-insulin-dependent diabetes mellitus and its risk factors in Japanese-Americans living in Hawaii and Los Angeles. *Diabetic Medicine*, **13**, S133–42.

48. Hu, F.B., Manson, J.E., Stampfer, M.J. *et al.* (2001) Diet, lifestyle, and the risk of type 2 diabetes mellitus in women. *The New England Journal of Medicine*, **345**, 790–7.

49. Stevens, J., Couper, D., Pankow, J. *et al.* (2001) Sensitivity and specificity of anthropometrics for the prediction of diabetes in a biracial cohort. *Obesity Research*, **9**, 696–705.

50. Weinstein, A.R., Sesso, H.D., Lee, I.M. *et al.* (2004) Relationship of physical activity vs body mass index with type 2 diabetes in women. *The Journal of the American Medical Association*, **292**, 1188–94.

51. Colditz, G.A., Willett, W.C., Rotnitzky, A. and Manson, J.E. (1995) Weight gain as a risk factor for clinical diabetes mellitus in women. *Annals of Internal Medicine*, **122**, 481–6.

52. Ford, E.S., Williamson, D.F. and Liu, S. (1997) Weight change and diabetes incidence: findings from a national cohort of US adults. *American Journal of Epidemiology*, **146**, 214–22.

53. Koh-Banerjee, P., Wang, Y., Hu, F.B. *et al.* (2004) Changes in body weight and body fat distribution as risk factors for clinical diabetes in US men. *American Journal of Epidemiology*, **159**, 1150–9.

54. Oguma, Y., Sesso, H.D., Paffenbarger, R.S. Jr and Lee, I.M. (2005) Weight change and risk of developing type 2 diabetes. *Obesity Research*, **13**, 945–51.

55. Cassano, P.A., Rosner, B., Vokonas, P.S. and Weiss, S.T. (1992) Obesity and body fat distribution in relation to the incidence of non-insulin-dependent

diabetes mellitus. A prospective cohort study of men in the normative aging study. *American Journal of Epidemiology*, **136**, 1474–86.

56. Wei, M., Gaskill, S.P., Haffner, S.M. and Stern, M.P. (1997) Waist circumference as the best predictor of noninsulin dependent diabetes mellitus (NIDDM) compared to body mass index, waist/hip ratio and other anthropometric measurements in Mexican Americans—a 7-year prospective study. *Obesity Research*, **5**, 16–23.

57. Kriska, A.M., Saremi, A., Hanson, R.L. *et al.* (2003) Physical activity, obesity, and the incidence of type 2 diabetes in a high-risk population. *American Journal of Epidemiology*, **158**, 669–75.

58. Manson, J.E., Ajani, U.A., Liu, S. *et al.* (2000) A prospective study of cigarette smoking and the incidence of diabetes mellitus among US male physicians. *The American Journal of Medicine*, **109**, 538–42.

59. Rimm, E.B., Chan, J., Stampfer, M.J. *et al.* (1995) Prospective study of cigarette smoking, alcohol use, and the risk of diabetes in men. *British Medical Journal*, **310**, 555–9.

60. Wei, M., Gibbons, L.W., Mitchell, T.L. *et al.* (2000) Alcohol intake and incidence of type 2 diabetes in men. *Diabetes Care*, **23**, 18–22.

61. Koppes, L.L., Dekker, J.M., Hendriks, H.F. *et al.* (2005) Moderate alcohol consumption lowers the risk of type 2 diabetes: a meta-analysis of prospective observational studies. *Diabetes Care*, **28**, 719–25.

62. Hu, F.B., van Dam, R.M. and Liu, S. (2001) Diet and risk of type II diabetes: the role of types of fat and carbohydrate. *Diabetologia*, **44**, 805–17.

63. Liu, S., Manson, J.E., Stampfer, M.J. *et al.* (2000) A prospective study of whole-grain intake and risk of type 2 diabetes mellitus in US women. *American Journal of Public Health*, **90**, 1409–15.

64. Salmeron, J., Ascherio, A., Rimm, E.B. *et al.* (1997) Dietary fiber, glycemic load, and risk of NIDDM in men. *Diabetes Care*, **20**, 545–50.

65. Schulze, M.B., Liu, S., Rimm, E.B. *et al.* (2004) Glycemic index, glycemic load, and dietary fiber intake and incidence of type 2 diabetes in younger and middle-aged women. *The American Journal of Clinical Nutrition*, **80**, 348–56.

66. Narayan, K.M., Gregg, E.W., Engelgau, M.M. *et al.* (2000) Translation research for chronic disease: the case of diabetes. *Diabetes Care*, **23**, 1794–8.

67. Geiss, L., Engelgau, M., Pogach, L. *et al.* (2005) A national progress report on diabetes: successes and challenges. *Diabetes Technology and Therapeutics*, **7**, 198–203.

68. Kuo, S., Fleming, B.B., Gittings, N.S. *et al.* (2005) Trends in care practices and outcomes among

medicare beneficiaries with diabetes. *American Journal of Preventive Medicine*, **29**, 396–403.

69. Saaddine, J.B., Cadwell, B., Gregg, E.W. *et al.* (2006) Improvements in diabetes processes of care and intermediate outcomes: United States, 1988–2002. *Annals of Internal Medicine*, **144**, 465–74.

70. Sawin, C.T., Walder, D.J., Bross, D.S. and Pogach, L.M. (2004) Diabetes process and outcome measures in the Department of Veterans Affairs. *Diabetes Care*, **27** (Suppl 2), B90–4.

71. Wilson, C., Gilliland, S., Cullen, T. *et al.* (2005) Diabetes outcomes in the Indian health system during the era of the special diabetes program for Indians and the Government Performance and Results Act. *American Journal of Public Health*, **95**, 1518–22.

72. Imperatore, G., Cadwell, B.L., Geiss, L. *et al.* (2004) Thirty-year trends in cardiovascular risk factor levels among US adults with diabetes: National Health and Nutrition Examination Surveys, 1971–2000. *American Journal of Epidemiology*, **160**, 531–9.

73. Fox, C.S., Coady, S., Sorlie, P.D. *et al.* (2004) Trends in cardiovascular complications of diabetes. *The Journal of the American Medical Association*, **292**, 2495–9.

74. Geiss, L.S., Herman, W.H. and Smith, P.J. (1995) Mortality in non-insulin-dependent diabetes, in *Diabetes in America* (eds M. Harris, C. Cowie, M. Stern *et al.*), National Institutes of Health, Bethesda, MD, pp. 233–57.

75. Stamler, J., Vaccaro, O., Neaton, J.D. and Wentworth, D. (1993) Diabetes, other risk factors, and 12-yr cardiovascular mortality for men screened in the Multiple Risk Factor Intervention Trial. *Diabetes Care*, **16**, 434–44.

76. Booth, G.L., Kapral, M.K., Fung, K. and Tu, J.V. (2006) Recent trends in cardiovascular complications among men and women with and without diabetes. *Diabetes Care*, **29**, 32–7.

77. Centers for Disease Control and Prevention (2003) Hospital discharge rates for nontraumatic lower extremity amputation by diabetes status—United States, 1997. *Morbidity and Mortality Weekly Report*, **50**, 954–8.

78. Centers for Disease Control and Prevention (2005) Incidence of end-stage renal disease among persons with diabetes - United States, 1990–2002. *Morbidity and Mortality Weekly Report*, **54**, 1097–100.

79. Klein, R. and Klein, B.E.K. (1995) Vision disorders in diabetes, in *Diabetes in America* (eds M. Harris, C. Cowie, M. Stern *et al.*), National Institutes of Health, Bethesda, MD, pp. 293–338.

80. Oliver, M.J., Charmaine, E.L., Shi, J. and Rothwell, D. (2003) Dialysis therapy for persons with diabetes, in *Diabetes in Ontario: An ICES Practice Atlas*, (eds J.E. Hux, G.L. Booth, P.M. Slaughter and A. Laupacis), Institute for Clinical Evaluative Sciences, Toronto, pp. 8.165–80.

81. US Renal Data System (2005) USRDS 2005 Annual Data Report: Atlas of End-Stage Renal Disease in the United States, National Institutes of Health, National Institute of Diabetes and Digestive and Kidney Diseases, Bethesda, MD. Available at: http://www.usrds.org/adr.htm (accessed 10 May 2006).

82. Burrows, N.R., Narva, A.S., Geiss, L.S. *et al.* (2005) End-stage renal disease due to diabetes among southwestern American Indians, 1990–2001. *Diabetes Care*, **28**, 1041–4.

83. Hux, J.E., Jacka, R., Fung, K. and Rothwell, D. (2003) Diabetes and peripheral vascular disease, in *Diabetes in Ontario: An ICES Practice Atlas* (eds J.E. Hux, G.L. Booth, P.M. Slaughter and A. Laupacis), Institute for Clinical Evaluative Sciences, Toronto, pp. 6.129–50.

84. Booth, G.L., Hux, J.E., Fang, J. and Chan, B.T. (2005) Time trends and geographic disparities in acute complications of diabetes in Ontario, Canada. *Diabetes Care*, **28**, 1045–50.

85. Wang, J., Williams, D.E., Narayan, K.M. and Geiss, L.S. (2006) Declining death rates from hyperglycemic crisis among adults with diabetes, United States, 1985–2002. *Diabetes Care*, **29**, 2018–22.

86. Anderson, R.N. and Smith, B.L. (2005) Deaths: leading causes for 2002. National Vital Statistics Reports, vol 53, no 17, National Center for Health Statistics, Hyattsville, MD.

87. Tierney, E.F., Geiss, L.S., Engelgau, M.M. *et al.* (2001) Population-based estimates of mortality associated with diabetes: use of a death certificate check box in North Dakota. *American Journal of Public Health*, **91**, 84–92.

88. Gu, K., Cowie, C.C. and Harris, M.I. (1999) Diabetes and decline in heart disease mortality in US adults. *The Journal of the American Medical Association*, **281**, 1291–7.

89. Thomas, R.J., Palumbo, P.J., Melton, L.J. III *et al.* (2003) Trends in the mortality burden associated with diabetes mellitus: a population-based study in Rochester, Minn, 1970–1994. *Archives of Internal Medicine*, **163**, 445–51.

90. Tierney, E.F., Cadwell, B.L., Engelgau, M.M. *et al.* (2004) Declining mortality rate among people with diabetes in North Dakota, 1997–2002. *Diabetes Care*, **27**, 2723–5.

91. Arias, E. (2004) United States life tables, 2002. National Vital Statistics Reports, vol 53, no 6, National Center for Health Statistics, Hyattsville, MD.

92. Gregg, E.W., Cheng, Y.J., Cadwell, B.L. *et al.* (2005) Secular trends in cardiovascular disease risk factors according to body mass index in US adults. *The Journal of the American Medical Association*, **293**, 1868–74.

93. Kochanek, K.D., Murphy, S.L., Anderson, R.N. and Scott, C. (2004) Deaths: final data for 2002. National Vital Statistics Reports, vol 53, no 5, National Center for Health Statistics, Hyattsville, MD.

19

Non-Caucasian North American Populations: Native Americans

Meda E. Pavkov,[1] K. M. Venkat Narayan,[2] Robert G. Nelson,[1]
Robert L. Hanson[1] and William C. Knowler[1]

[1]National Institute of Diabetes and Digestive and Kidney Diseases, Phoenix, AZ, USA
[2]National Center for Chronic Disease Prevention and Health Promotion, Centers for
Disease Control and Prevention, Atlanta, GA, USA

19.1 NATIVE AMERICANS

Indigenous peoples lived in every region of North America for thousands of years before Europeans arrived. In this chapter, the term *Native American* will be used to refer to the descendents of these indigenous peoples. The Native American founder populations migrated from Asia into America through the Bering Strait sometime during the Pleistocene [1]. The number of these migrations and the size of the ancestral populations, however, remain a topic of debate.

The terms *American Indians* (AIs) and *Alaska Natives* (ANs) refer to members of the more than 560 federally recognized tribes in the United States and Alaska. The AN population includes Eskimos, Aleuts and Indians (Athabascan, Tsimpsian, Haida and Tlingit). A common term for the indigenous peoples of what is now Canada is *Aboriginal peoples*. Canada recognizes three distinct Aboriginal groups: North American Indian, Métis and Inuit. Of these Aboriginal peoples who are not Inuit or Métis, *First Nations* is the most common term of self-identification. The official term for First Nations people is *Indian* [2]. The principal Mexican indigenous group at the time of the Spanish conquest was the Nahuas, better known as the *Aztecs*. The descendants of these early people belong to as many as 22 distinct pueblos and tribes. Estimates for the numbers of unmixed indigenous peoples in Mexico vary from 10 to 30% of the population [3].

While one of the smallest minorities in the United States, AI/ANs are a very diverse group, representing a variety of cultures and traditions. Their members often live on reservations and in rural communities, mostly in the western United States and in Alaska. In addition to their tribal affiliations, AI/ANs are often distinguished by language and/or cultural groups, some of which extend across the United States, Canada and Mexico [4]. Approximately 3.2 million people in the United States identify themselves as AI/AN [5]. According to the 2001 Census, over 1.3 million Canadians reported at least some Aboriginal origin [6]. In general, Native Americans face widespread economic and educational disadvantage [7].

19.2 DIABETES IN NATIVE AMERICANS

Diabetes was either rare or unrecognized among Native Americans until the middle part of the twentieth century [8–10]. Since then diabetes has become one of the most common serious diseases in many Native American tribes [11]. Diabetes occurring in Native Americans is almost exclusively type 2 diabetes [11]. The Pima Indians of Arizona, who have participated in a longitudinal study of diabetes, obesity and diabetes complications since 1965 [12], have among the highest recorded prevalence and incidence of type 2 diabetes in

The Epidemiology of Diabetes Mellitus, second edition Edited by Jean-Marie Ekoé, Marian Rewers, Rhys Williams and Paul Zimmet
© 2008 John Wiley & Sons, Ltd

the world [13, 14]. Insulin resistance and impaired insulin secretion are the major early abnormalities in the pathogenesis of diabetes [15, 16]. Although the reasons for the high prevalence and incidence of diabetes in this population are not known with certainty, genetic factors and the increasing prevalence of obesity associated with rapid changes in lifestyle may be responsible. The prevalence of diabetes in the Pima Indians living in a remote area of the Sierra Madre Mountains in Mexico is low [17], despite a low estimated genetic distance between these people and the Pima Indians of Arizona [18], supporting the notion that, despite genetic predisposition, a traditional lifestyle may protect against the development of obesity and diabetes. High rates of diabetes have also been observed in other Native American tribes [11, 19, 20] and in diverse societies worldwide that have recently adopted Western culture [21–23].

19.3 MAGNITUDE OF THE PROBLEM OF TYPE 2 DIABETES IN NATIVE AMERICANS

19.3.1 Prevalence

Prevalence is the proportion of individuals in a population who have the disease at a specific point in time. Estimates of diabetes prevalence are influenced by the method of ascertainment and by the definition of diabetes. A large number of studies have reported the prevalence of clinically diagnosed diabetes among Native Americans in the United States [24–27]. The prevalence of diagnosed diabetes varies across tribes and is generally higher than in the US population as a whole [24–27]. In 2003, the estimated prevalence of diabetes was 15.1% among the AI/AN population ≥20 years old who were receiving care from Indian Health Service (IHS) medical facilities [28], increasing by 31% since 1994 [29]. AI/ANs are 2.2 times as likely to have diabetes as non-Hispanic Whites. Age-adjusted prevalence in AI/ANs is lowest among ANs (8.1%) and highest among AIs in the southwestern United States (26.7%). However, the rates of diagnosed diabetes among ANs may also be increasing [30]. The reported age-standardized prevalence of diagnosed diabetes among ANs ranges from 0.2% among Chukchi and Eskimo of Chukota [31], to 1.8% among Eskimo-Inuit and Athapaskan Indians of Alaska and to 4.9% among

Aleuts in Alaska [32]. Between 1990 and 2001, the largest increase was noted among Eskimos (110%) and Aleuts (81%) [32]. Age–sex-adjusted prevalence varies from 3.2% in rural Alaska to 4.8% in the Alaska Gulf Coast region [33]. In the Canadian Aboriginal Peoples Survey of 2001, the overall prevalence of self-reported diabetes in Aboriginal people was 6.0%, and varied from 2.3% in Inuit (Eskimo), to 5.9% in Métis and to 8.3% in Indians [34]. By contrast, diabetes is rare among indigenous communities of Mexico. The highest reported prevalence of type 2 diabetes was 4.4% in 91 Otomi Indians aged 15–77 years old [35]. Among 193 Tepehuano, Huichol and Mexicanero tribe members from Durango, Mexico, aged 30–64 years old without known racial admixture and minimal Western influence on lifestyle, no prevalent cases of diabetes were found between 1991 and 1997 [36].

Studies based on clinically diagnosed cases rather than systematic testing underestimate the prevalence of diabetes because a large proportion of type 2 diabetes may remain undiagnosed [37]. Prevalence studies of diabetes in Native Americans based on systematic testing in the community are available for only a few tribes [38–41], and are summarized in **Table 19.1**. Among the studies reported in **Table 19.1**, the longitudinal study in Pima Indians [38] uses the 1985 World Health Organization (WHO) criteria [42] for diabetes diagnosis, and the date of diagnosis and age of onset are determined at biennial research examinations or from review of clinical records if diabetes was diagnosed in the course of routine medical care. The Navajo Health and Nutrition Survey [39] estimated diabetes prevalence based on oral glucose tolerance testing and the 1980 WHO criteria in subjects 20 years and older [43]. Lee *et al.* [40] estimated the prevalence of diabetes based on fasting plasma glucose and oral glucose tolerance test results. The other study [41] tested glucose tolerance only in people meeting certain criteria on other tests.

In a population-based study among Algonquin communities in Quebec, the age–sex-standardized prevalence of type 2 diabetes, diagnosed by serum glucose level 2 h after a 75 g oral glucose tolerance test, among people ≥15 years old was 19.1% in Lac Simon and 9.0% in River Desert [44]. In the same two communities, the prevalence among 30–64-year-olds was 48.6% in women and 23.9% in

Table 19.1 Prevalence of diabetes from population-based studies in Native Americans.

Author	Study population	Prevalence (%)[a]		
		M	F	T
Knowler et al.[b]	Pima Indians aged $\geq$5 years, Gila River Indian Community in Arizona	26	30	29
Will et al. [39]	Navajo Health and Nutrition Survey	17	23	23
Lee et al. [40]	Men and women aged 45–74 years:			
	Pima/Maricopa/Papago, Arizona Apache	65	72	70
	Caddo, Comanche, Delaware, Fort Sill Apache, Kiowa, Wichita, Oklahoma Oglala, Sioux	38	42	40
	Cheyenne River Sioux, Devils Lake Sioux, North and South Dakota	33	46	40
Rith-Najarian et al. [41]	Men and women of all ages, Red Lake Chippewa Indians	13	16	15

[a]Prevalence rates are standardized to US general population for the relevant ages.
[b]Updated from Ref. [38].

men [45]. Mexican Americans in the United States who derive to a large extent from Native Americans with admixture from Caucasians also have high rates of diabetes, and their prevalence ranges from 3.8% among 20–44-year-olds to 23.9% among 45–74-year-olds [46]. Overall, the prevalence of diabetes in Native Americans is higher than the rate of 7.3% in the US general population [29].

Much of the information about the impact of diabetes in AI/AN communities comes from ongoing studies with the Pima Indians who live in a geographically defined area in Arizona, United States. Compared with the predominantly White population of Rochester, Minnesota, the age–sex-adjusted prevalence of diabetes was 12.7 times as high in the Pima Indians [13].

19.3.2 Incidence

Incidence rates quantify the number of new cases of a disease that develop in a population of individuals at risk during a specified time interval. High incidence of diabetes has been reported in a number of Native American tribes in the United States [40], and Canada [47]. In the Pima Indians, the incidence of diagnosed diabetes was 19 times that in the predominantly White population of Rochester, Minnesota [13], and was one of the highest reported

in the world. The increasing prevalence of obesity and increasing prevalence of diabetes in pregnant women observed over the last decades have shifted the onset of diabetes to younger ages [48].

19.4 DETERMINANTS OF TYPE 2 DIABETES

19.4.1 Genetic Factors

Genetic factors may be important determinants of type 2 diabetes in Native Americans. The prevalence of type 2 diabetes is higher in individuals of full Native American heritage than in those with genetic admixture [40, 49–51], possibly because full-heritage Native Americans have a greater dose of diabetes susceptibility genes than admixed individuals. Familial aggregation of diabetes occurs in several AI/AN populations [40, 52, 53]. For example, among Pimas, a parent who developed diabetes at a younger age is more likely to transmit diabetes to an offspring than is a parent with an older age of onset (**Figure 19.1**) [38]. Thus, individuals who develop diabetes at younger ages may have a greater burden of diabetes susceptibility genes than those who develop the disease later in life. Similarly, the prevalence of type 2 diabetes is higher in relatives of leaner diabetic Pimas than

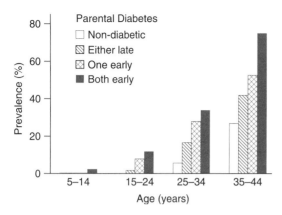

Figure 19.1 Prevalence of diabetes by age of onset of diabetes in parents. Diabetes was defined as of the last examination in the parents. Parents whose onset of diabetes was before age 45 were classified as 'early.' (Updated from data in Ref. [38].)

in relatives of heavier individuals with the disease [54], suggesting that the genetic factors which result in type 2 diabetes are at least partially separate from those that cause obesity.

While familial aggregation of disease suggests the potential importance of genetic factors, segregation analysis can determine whether this aggregation is consistent with a particular mode of inheritance. Among Seminoles, analyses of 1 h postload glucose concentrations were consistent with the hypothesis that a single genetic locus has a major effect on these levels, but the degree of dominance at this putative locus could not be determined [55]. Among Pimas, segregation analyses were consistent with a major effect of a single locus influencing age of onset of disease [56]. On the basis of these analyses, it is tempting to speculate that familial aggregation of type 2 diabetes among Native Americans may be explained in large part by the action of a single genetic locus or a few loci.

More precise knowledge of the genetics of type 2 diabetes would be obtained if a particular genetic marker was linked to or associated with the disease. In linkage studies, cosegregation of the disease with alleles at one or more genetic markers is assessed within families, while the co-occurrence of specific alleles with the disease in the population is analyzed in association studies. Linkage studies can identify susceptibility loci (the chromosomal

location of putative susceptibility genes, typically in a fairly broad region) and association studies may identify particular susceptibility variants, but until very recently have not been feasible on a genome-wide basis.

Most such molecular studies of type 2 diabetes in Native Americans have been conducted in two populations, the Pimas of Arizona (United States) and the Oji-Cree of Ontario (Canada). Genome-wide linkage studies in the Pimas have identified potential susceptibility loci for young-onset diabetes on chromosomes 1q and 7q and a diabetes–obesity locus on chromosome 11q [57], while linkage studies in the Oji-Cree have identified potential diabetes susceptibility loci on chromosomes 6q and 16 [58]. The chromosome 1q region is also linked to type 2 diabetes in several Caucasian and Asian populations [59]. To date, particular variants in these regions that confer susceptibility to diabetes have not been conclusively identified.

A proline–alanine substitution at the 12th codon in the peroxisome proliferator activated receptor-γ (*PPARγ*) gene has shown a consistent association with type 2 diabetes in many populations, although the strength of association is modest (odds ratio is 1.25 for homozygotes at the proline allele compared with carriers of the alanine allele) [60]. This polymorphism is not significantly associated with diabetes in either the Pimas or the Oji-Cree; the direction of association in the Pimas is similar to that observed in other populations (odds ratio 1.36), while in the Oji-Cree it is in the opposite direction (odds ratio 0.75) [61, 62]. Variants in the *calpain-10* gene, which have been proposed to confer susceptibility to type 2 diabetes in some populations, show little evidence for such association in either Pimas or Oji-Cree [63, 64].

Modest, but statistically significant, evidence for association has been identified in the Pimas between diabetes and alleles at several candidate genes, including insulin receptor substrate-1 (*IRS1*) on chromosome 2q, *HLA-A2* on chromosome 6p and protein phosphatase 1 regulatory subunit 3A (*PPP1R3A*) on chromosome 7q [65–68]. In the Oji-Cree, a mutation in codon 319 of hepatocyte nuclear factor 1-α (*HNF-1α*), a gene on chromosome 12q in which other mutations can cause maturity-onset diabetes of youth, is strongly associated with diabetes [69, 70]. This mutation causes a glycine to serine substitution in the protein and

33% of those with diabetes are carriers of the serine allele, compared with only 17% of non-diabetic individuals, a difference that is highly statistically significant ($p = 0.0002$; odds ratio 2.43). The mutation appears to be rare in Pimas [71] and in Caucasian populations, but its role in other Native American populations has not been examined to our knowledge. It is often difficult to determine the functional relevance of particular polymorphisms, but transfection of the serine allele into HeLa cells results in decreased *HNF-1α* transcriptional activity and this suggests that the polymorphism may have functional consequences [72]. At present, however, the significance of these findings and those of other genetic studies, with respect to the etiologic mechanisms of type 2 diabetes in Native Americans, remains unclear. Future research into the genetics of type 2 diabetes will hopefully lead to a better understanding of the pathogenesis of the disease.

19.4.2   Perinatal Factors

As mentioned above, diabetes is a familial disease, occurring more frequently in those with a diabetic father or mother. However, the diabetic intrauterine environment presents a risk for the early development of diabetes in Pima Indians which is in addition to the genetic predisposition [73]. Before the age of 10 years, type 2 diabetes is almost entirely limited to children whose mothers had diabetes during the pregnancy, and half of the offspring of diabetic pregnancies have already developed diabetes by the time they reach childbearing age. This effect results in a vicious cycle of diabetes begetting diabetes [74]. Higher rates of diabetes are found among adults who were at the extremes of birthweight [75–77]. Rates of diabetes among those with birthweights below 2.5 kg or above 4.5 kg are nearly twice as high as among those with intermediate weights.

Breastfeeding for a period of at least 2 months is associated with a 50% reduction in rates of diabetes [78]. The reasons for this finding have not been fully explored, but may relate to a nutritional intake more suited to an infant's growing needs, either because of differences in breast- and bottle-feeding per se or because mothers who choose to breastfeed continue to feed their children differently than those who do not.

19.5   POTENTIALLY MODIFIABLE RISK FACTORS

A number of factors, which are potentially modifiable, including obesity, dietary composition and physical inactivity, are thought to contribute to the progression from genetic susceptibility to type 2 diabetes [79–81].

19.5.1   Obesity

Obesity is a powerful and well-established risk factor for the development of type 2 diabetes [52]. As shown in **Figure 19.2** the age–sex-adjusted incidence of diabetes in Pima Indians increases with body mass index (BMI), a measure of obesity.

Throughout its range, BMI is a strong predictor of type 2 diabetes risk in Pima Indians and is not significantly improved by combining it with other measures of general adiposity or body fat distribution [82]. Furthermore, the incidence of diabetes increases with the duration of obesity (BMI ≥ 30 kg m^{-2}). Compared with Pima Indians with less than 5 years of obesity, those with 5–10 years of obesity have 1.4 times the incidence of type 2 diabetes, and those with at least 10 years of obesity have 2.4 times the incidence [83]. Persons who gain weight most rapidly are most likely to develop diabetes, whereas those who lose weight are at the lowest risk [84].

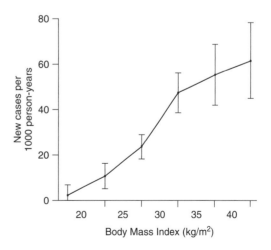

Figure 19.2 Age–sex-adjusted incidence of diabetes in adult Pima Indians by body mass index (BMI), with 95% confidence intervals. (Updated from Ref. [38].)

Table 19.2 Percentage of AI/AN with obesity, by sex and region, Behavioral Risk Factor Surveillance System 1997–2000.[a]

	Men (%)	Women (%)	Both sexes (%)
Total non-AI/AN	18.9	18.4	18.7
Total AI/AN	23.9	23.8	23.9
Alaska	26.9	31.1	29.0
East	22.9	25.2	23.9
Northern Plains	22.8	25.7	24.2
Pacific Coast	23.4	20.2	21.6
Southwest	26.2	24.6	26.4

[a]$BMI \geq 30\,kg\,m^{-2}$. Weighted and standardized to the 2000 US projected population.

The prevalence of obesity among AI/ANs is higher than in the US general population in both males and females and at all ages (**Table 19.2**) [85]. The overall prevalence of obesity (BMI $\geq$ $31.1\,kg\,m^{-2}$ for men, $\geq 32.3\,kg\,m^{-2}$ for women) among AI/ANs was 13.7% for men and 16.5% for women, higher than the US rates of 9.1% and 8.2% respectively [85]. Among the Navajo, overweight was uncommon 40 years ago [86]. By 1979, DeStefano et al. [87] found that a quarter of Navajo men and half of Navajo women were overweight. A recent survey indicates that the prevalence of overweight remains high among Navajo adults [88]. Data from the Pimas are consistent with this finding. Moreover, Pima children have become heavier, on average, during the last century, and continue to do so [89].

19.5.2 Diet

Diet has been linked to the development of diabetes for over 2500 years [90], but the precise role of dietary factors, which is reviewed elsewhere [91], remains ambiguous. Few data are available in Native Americans linking dietary factors with the development of type 2 diabetes, except for one study in the Pima Indians which found that a high caloric diet may predict diabetes [92]. The traditional Pima diet, derived from local agricultural produce, is believed to have been high in fiber and low in fat [38], but the Pima diet changed during the last century and is now nutritionally similar to the diet in the rest of the United States [93]. Pimas who identified their diet as being traditional had a lower incidence of diabetes than those who reported eating a

Western diet; among those same individuals, no specific dietary components, as identified by dietary questionnaires, predicted development of diabetes [94].

Similar secular changes in the diet of other Native American populations have also occurred; in particular, the fat content of Native American diets appears to have increased dramatically from 17% of total calories in the pre-European contact diet to 38% in the current diet [95].

19.5.3 Physical Activity

The adoption and maintenance of a physically active lifestyle can play a significant role in preventing type 2 diabetes. Increased physical activity may have a protective effect on the development of type 2 diabetes [80]. When the age-adjusted diabetes incidence rates were examined by levels of activity stratified by tertile of BMI, the incidence rate of diabetes remained lower in more active men and women than in less active men and women from all BMI groups, with the exception of the middle BMI tertile in men ($p < 0.05$ in women only, **Figure 19.3**). Among 37–57-year-old subjects, those with the highest levels of physical activity also had the lowest prevalence of diabetes [96]. Similarly, Zuni Indians without diabetes were more likely to have exercised frequently than those with diabetes [97].

The evidence that BMI is positively predictive of diabetes incidence is strong and consistent between observational studies, but the evidence for dietary composition or physical activity as predictors of diabetes is weaker. Yet a number of randomized clinical trials have tested whether intervention

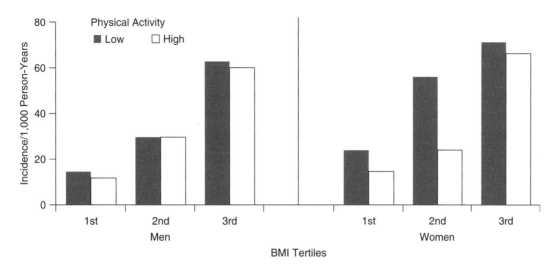

Figure 19.3 Diabetes incidence rates per 1000 person-years by total physical activity and body mass index (BMI; adjusted for age), Gila River Indian Community, 1987–2000. Dark bar, low activity; light bar, high activity. (From data in Ref. [96].)

on these risk factors will reduce the incidence of diabetes. One such clinical trial, the Diabetes Prevention Program, included Native Americans [98]. In this trial in individuals at high risk of developing diabetes, the incidence was reduced by 58% in persons assigned to an intensive weight loss intervention with the goals of reducing weight, reducing total calories and calories from fat and increasing moderate physical activity. The benefits of the interventions were uniform across race/ethnic group, including AIs.

19.6 COMPLICATION OF TYPE 2 DIABETES

The frequency of several important vascular and nonvascular complications of type 2 diabetes in Native Americans is examined, with particular emphasis on those that exert a significant influence on mortality.

19.6.1 Cardiovascular Disease

Recent IHS data indicate that the incidence of cardiovascular disease (CVD) has increased among AI/ANs, CVD being now the leading cause of death among AI/ANs [99]. Tribal variations in death rates due to CVD, however, are striking, just as they are for the prevalence of CVD. Southwestern tribes, such as the Navajo and Pima/Maricopa/Papago

Indians, have low mortality rates from CVD, nearly all of which is found in those with diabetes [100, 101], whereas the Northern Plains Indians have rates as high or higher than the general population of the United States, and a much greater proportion of cardiovascular deaths are found in those without diabetes, particularly among men [101].

The Strong Heart Study [102] examined the prevalence of myocardial infarction and coronary heart disease (CHD) in 4549 subjects from 13 AI tribes in Arizona, Oklahoma and North and South Dakota. The prevalence of CHD in these subjects is shown in **Figure 19.4** according to sex, diabetes and center [103]. Although the prevalence of diabetes was highest among AIs in Arizona, CHD prevalence was lower than among AIs in other centers. The lower prevalence of CHD among Indians in Arizona may be related, in part, to their low cigarette smoking and to their low concentrations of total and low-density lipoprotein cholesterol compared with other tribal groups [103]. Between 1965 and 1998, the rate of death from CHD remained stable in nondiabetic Pima Indians but increased among those with diabetes [104]. This finding suggests that, in the absence of diabetes, the underlying susceptibility to CHD in this population has not changed. Conversely, the emergence of CHD as a leading underlying cause of death in diabetic Pima Indians can be attributed largely to the availability

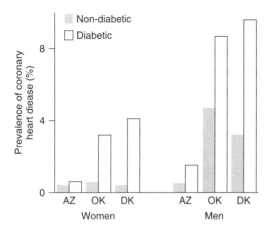

Figure 19.4 Prevalence of coronary heart disease by sex, study center and presence of diabetes in the Strong Heart Study, 1989–1992. Data from [103]. Criteria for coronary heart disease included definite myocardial infarction, evidence in the medical record of coronary angioplasty or bypass surgery, thrombolytic therapy, a positive angiogram or angina pectoris by Rose questionnaire when accompanied by Minnesota Code 4.1 or 5.1 or a verified history of myocardial infarction.

of renal replacement therapy and the resulting shift from death due to diabetic nephropathy (DN) to other underlying causes of death [105]. Since DN and CHD share many of the same risk factors [100, 106], substantial reductions in deaths from DN probably made a rise in CHD death rates inevitable. This finding suggests that a change in clinical practice, rather than a worsening of cardiovascular risk per se [105], is responsible for the current epidemic of CHD among diabetic patients in this population.

Compared with other US populations, incidence rates for stroke are similar in AI women and lower in men, and the incidence of CHD in AI men and women is almost twofold higher than the US population (**Figure 19.5**) [107–109]. However, diabetes had a strong independent effect on this outcome after adjustment for other risk factors.

Among ANs, the overall incidence of confirmed myocardial infarction is 8.1 cases per 1000 person-years [110], with men having a higher incidence than women. Eskimos have the lowest rate (6.2 cases per 1000 person-years) and Aleuts the

highest (10.2 cases per 1000 person-years). By contrast, the incidence of stroke is highest among Eskimos (17.6 cases per 1000 person-years) and lowest among Alaska Indians (11.5 cases per 1000 person-years), and women have a higher incidence of stroke than men. Moreover, diabetic AN women were found to have higher rates of myocardial infarction and stroke than diabetic White women in the Nurses Health Study Cohort [111].

19.6.2 Lower-extremity Amputations

More than 50 000 amputations each year are performed on diabetic patients in the United States [112], and the amputation rate among diabetic patients is about 15 times that in nondiabetic patients [113]. Longitudinal studies of amputation rates in Pima Indians and in Indians from Oklahoma indicate substantially higher incidence rates of lower-extremity amputations in these AI/AN populations than in the general US population [114, 115]. ANs on the other hand, have a lower age–sex-adjusted amputation rate than other AIs with diabetes [116], which is attributable in part to a shorter duration of diabetes and effective foot-care programs [117].

19.6.3 Microvascular Complications

Nearly all of the excess mortality associated with either type of diabetes is found in persons with proteinuria [106, 118, 119]. **Figure 19.6** shows the age–sex-adjusted death rate among Pima Indians according to the presence or absence of diabetes and proteinuria. The death rate in diabetic subjects without proteinuria was no greater than in nondiabetic subjects, but the rate in those with clinical proteinuria was nearly four times as high. The excess deaths in diabetic subjects with proteinuria are due principally to cardiovascular or renal disease [106, 119, 120], leading to the inference that proteinuria reflects widespread vascular damage in both small and large vessels [121]. The frequency with which proteinuria leads to life-threatening CVD or to kidney failure in persons with diabetes depends on the frequency of other risk factors for these diseases. For example, persons in whom type 2 diabetes develops later in life may have a higher risk of death from CVD than persons in whom diabetes develops at a younger age, because of greater exposure to risk factors for CVD that precede the onset of diabetes [122].

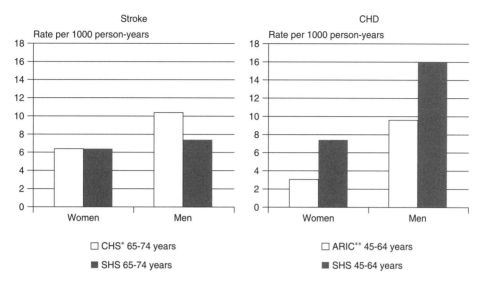

Figure 19.5 Stroke and CHD incidence (fatal and nonfatal) in AIs compared with other US population data from the CHS [108] and ARIC [109] studies. SHS, Strong Heart Study. *3.3-year average follow-up; **5.2-year average follow-up. CHD includes fatal and nonfatal events plus revascularization.

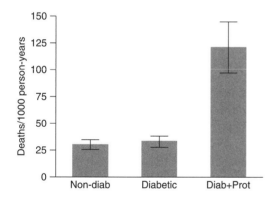

Figure 19.6 Age–sex-adjusted death rates and 95% confidence intervals in 1426 Pima Indians ≥45 years of age. Rates are shown for nondiabetic subjects without proteinuria (Non-diab), diabetic subjects without proteinuria (Diabetic), and diabetic subjects with proteinuria (Diab+Prot). Proteinuria was defined by a protein-to-creatinine ratio ≥1.0 g g⁻¹. (Reference [106].)

Persons who develop type 2 diabetes before 20 years of age are at considerable risk for nephropathy [123] and eventual renal failure as young adults, particularly if their risk of CVD is low [100].

Although a rise in urinary albumin excretion characteristically occurs after the onset of type 2 diabetes, it may also precede the onset of diabetes. The prevalence of elevated urinary albumin excretion (albumin-to-creatinine ratio ≥30 mg g⁻¹) is twice as high in Pima Indians with impaired glucose tolerance as in those with normal glucose tolerance (**Figure 19.7**) [124]. This finding suggests that even small elevations of the plasma glucose concentration may have an impact on vascular function.

With the onset of type 2 diabetes, the prevalence of elevated urinary albumin excretion is even higher, and both the magnitude and frequency of the elevation are related to the duration of diabetes. Among Pima Indians with diabetes of up to 5 years' duration, the prevalence is 29%, and in those with diabetes ≥20 years it is 86% (**Figure 19.7**). Microalbuminuria (albumin-to-creatinine ratio 30–300 mg g⁻¹) accounts for 82% of the prevalent cases among Pima Indians with <5 years of diabetes, but for only 22% in those with diabetes ≥20 years. Hence, the majority of Pima Indians with diabetes of long duration are at increased risk of premature death from vascular disease. A high prevalence of elevated urinary albumin excretion has also been reported in persons with diabetes from other AI/AN tribes [125, 126].

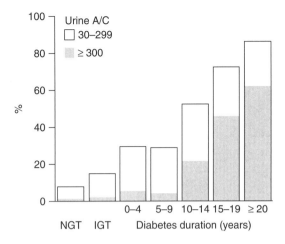

Figure 19.7 Prevalence of elevated urinary albumin-to-creatinine ratios in 2728 Pima Indians ≥15 years of age with normal glucose tolerance (NGT), impaired glucose tolerance (IGT), and in diabetic subjects by duration of type 2 diabetes. (Adapted from data in Ref. [124].)

19.6.4 Kidney Disease

Among the Pima Indians, half of those with type 2 diabetes develop nephropathy within 20 years of the diagnosis of diabetes [128], and the presence of proteinuria is usually associated with an irreversible deterioration of renal function that often leads to end-stage renal disease (ESRD). The incidence of proteinuria increased over the past 36 years in diabetic Pima Indians, due principally to a higher proportion of people with long duration of diabetes [129]. On the other hand, the incidence of diabetic ESRD, defined as dialysis or death due to DN, increased until 1990 and then began to decline [130]. The decline coincides with the introduction and widespread use within this community of medicines that block the renin-angiotensin system and increased use of other medicines for blood pressure and glycemic control [131].

The prevalence of ESRD is 3.5 times as great in AI/ANs as in White Americans [132], but varies widely by tribe [133–137]. Among the Zuni Indians, the age–sex-adjusted prevalence of ESRD is 18.5-fold higher than among White Americans and 5.3-fold higher than among other AIs [138]. In contrast to the Pima Indians, in whom 93% of ESRD is attributable to diabetes [135], ESRD in the Zuni

Indians is attributable to high rates of nondiabetic and diabetic kidney disease [138, 139]. Among southwestern AIs residing in Arizona, Colorado, Nevada, New Mexico and Utah, the incidence rate of diabetic ESRD declined between 1993 and 2001. The age-specific incidence of diabetic ESRD decreased in all age groups. The increasing use of RAS inhibitors among diabetic AIs and a reduction in risk factors for diabetes-related ESRD were proposed as factors contributing to the decline in ESRD incidence in this population [140].

In Pima Indians, DN was the leading cause of death in those with diabetes, accounting for 23% of the deaths from natural causes during the years from 1975 to 1984 [141]. Recently, however, ischemic heart disease has emerged as the leading cause of death due largely to the availability of renal replacement therapy and to changes in the pattern of death among those with DN [105]. In recent years, Pimas have also survived longer after the onset of ESRD, giving them a greater opportunity for developing fatal CVD [142, 143].

19.6.5 Retinopathy

Retinopathy is a frequent complication of diabetes in all populations, and Native Americans are no exception [144]. The frequency of vision-threatening proliferative diabetic retinopathy, however, is much higher in AI/AN than in Whites with type 2 diabetes [145–147]. The prevalence of more severe grades of retinopathy is higher in people with longer durations of diabetes [148]. The risk of retinopathy differed by age at diagnosis: rates were lower in those in whom diabetes was diagnosed in youth [123]. In fact, retinopathy did not occur in any subject before 20 years of age, whereas nephropathy was present even in subjects aged 10–15 years. Among Pima Indians, mild non-proliferative diabetic retinopathy (NPDR) is more likely to improve than worsen at a subsequent examination. However, more severe NPDR is unlikely to regress. Duration of diabetes, hyperglycemia, pharmacological treatment for diabetes, and macroalbuminuria appear to be the major factors associated with the development of any level of retinopathy, as diagnosed by either retinal photographs or fundoscopy. Once retinopathy has been established, hyperglycemia and macroalbuminuria remain risk factors for its progression [149].

19.6.6 Nonvascular Complications

Diabetic persons are generally considered more susceptible to bacterial and fungal infections than are nondiabetic persons [150]. In accordance with this observation, diabetic Sioux Indians were four times as likely to have tuberculosis as those without diabetes [151], and southwestern Indians with diabetes were more likely to have disseminated coccidioidomycosis than those without [152]. In Pima Indians, infection is the only major cause of death other than ischemic heart disease and DN that is related to the duration of diabetes (**Figure 19.8**) [127]. Nevertheless, the death rate from infections in diabetic Pima Indians was not significantly greater than in those without diabetes in 1975–1984 [127].

19.6.7 Periodontal Disease

Periodontal disease, a chronic inflammatory disease of the periodontal tissues, is a complication of diabetes that is frequently overlooked. It is exceedingly common even in persons without diabetes, but prospective studies in Pima Indians indicate the age–sex-adjusted incidence is nearly three times as high in subjects with diabetes as in those without [153], and 75% of diabetic Pima Indians are edentulous after 20 years of diabetes. Although the rates of periodontal disease in other AI/AN populations are not known, they are likely to be high given the high rates of type 2 diabetes. The inflammatory

nature of periodontal disease may hinder metabolic control [154] and may inhibit proper dietary intake [155, 156]. Periodontal disease is associated with increased mortality from cardiovascular and kidney disease in diabetic Pima Indians [157].

19.7 CONCLUSION

In summary, diabetes affects Native Americans disproportionately compared with other racial/ethnic populations and is almost exclusively type 2 diabetes. Genetic factors and the increasing prevalence of obesity associated with the transition from a traditional to a modern lifestyle may be responsible for the increasing prevalence of diabetes among Native Americans. Moreover, the increase in obesity among youth and the increasing prevalence of diabetes in pregnant women over recent decades has shifted the onset of type 2 diabetes to younger ages. Earlier onset of diabetes presents an additional public health concern, as these patients will have costly and disabling diabetes-related complications during their most productive years.

The principal contributors to mortality in type 2 diabetes are renal and CVD. The frequency with which each of these complications occurs may depend on factors such as age, duration of diabetes and underlying genetic susceptibility. Proteinuria is the marker of diabetic kidney disease and strong predictor of CVD. Nearly all the excess mortality in diabetes befalls those with gross proteinuria. AI/ANs, have higher rates of type 2 diabetes than many other populations and often develop diabetes at a young age. Consequently, they have higher frequencies of these life-threatening complications. Moreover, they also have higher frequencies of other complications that may not lead to premature death, but which substantially reduce their quality of life.

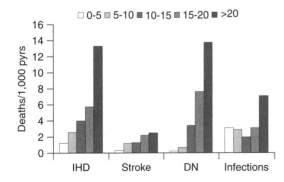

Figure 19.8 Age–sex-adjusted cause-specific death rates in diabetic Pima Indians aged ≥35 years for ischemic heart disease ($n = 147$), stroke ($n = 42$), diabetic nephropathy ($n = 124$) and infections ($n = 102$), according to duration of diabetes. (Updated Ref. [127].)

ACKNOWLEDGMENTS

We are grateful to the members of the Gila River Indian Community for their enormous contribution toward the understanding of diabetes in Native Americans through their participation in a longitudinal study since 1965. This review was supported, in part, by the Intramural Research Program of the National Institute of Diabetes and Digestive and Kidney Diseases.

References

1. Cavalli-Sforza, L.L., Piazza, A. and Menozzi, P. (1994) *History and Geography of Human Genes*, Princeton University Press, Princeton, NJ.

2. Indian Act(R.S., c. I-5) (1985) http://laws.justice .gc.ca/en/ShowFullDoc/cs/I-5///en (last access April 2008).

3. History of Mexico, available at http://en.wikipedia .org/wiki/Mexico (last access April 2008).

4. Ghodes, D. (1995) Diabetes in North American Indians and Alaska Natives, in *Diabetes in America* (ed N. Harris), NIH Publication No. 95-1468, US Department of Health and Human Services, Washington, DC, pp. 683–701.

5. Indian Health Service (2006) Fact Sheet http:// www.ihs.gov/PublicInfo/PublicAffairs/Welcome_ Info/ThisFacts.asp (accessed 16 February 2006).

6. Statistics Canada (2006) Definitions, http:// www12.statcan.ca/english/census01/Products/ Analytic/companion/abor/definitions (accessed 16 February 2006).

7. US Bureau of Census (1992) Minority Economic Profiles, 24 July, Tables CPH-L-92, 93 and 95, and unpublished data.

8. West, K.M. (1974) Diabetes in American Indians and other native populations of the New World. *Diabetes*, **23**, 841–55.

9. Sievers, M.L. and Fisher, J.R. (1981) Diseases of North American Indians, in *Biocultural Aspects of Disease* (ed H.R. Rothschild), Academic Press, New York, pp. 191–252.

10. Joslin, E.P. (1940) The universality of diabetes. *Journal of the American Medical Association*, **115**, 2033–8.

11. Sievers, M.L. and Fisher, J.R. (1985) Diabetes in North American Indians, in *Diabetes in America*, (eds M.I. Harris and R.F. Hamman), NIH Publication No 85-1468, US Department of Health and Human Services, Washington, DC, pp. xi 1–20.

12. Bennett, P.H., Burch, T.A. and Miller, M. (1971) Diabetes mellitus in American (Pima) Indians. *Lancet*, **ii**, 125–8.

13. Knowler, W.C., Bennett, P.H., Hamman, R.F. and Miller, M. (1978) Diabetes incidence and prevalence in Pima Indians: a 19-fold greater incidence than in Rochester, Minn. *American Journal of Epidemiology*, **108**, 497–504.

14. King, H. and Rewers, M. (1991) Diabetes in adults is now a Third World problem. *Bulletin World Health Organization*, **69** (6), 643–8.

15. Saad, M.F., Knowler, W.C., Pettitt, D.J. *et al.* (1989) Sequential changes in serum insulin concentration during development of non-insulin-dependent diabetes. *Lancet*, **i**, 1356–9.

16. Lillioja, S., Mott, D.M., Spraul, M. *et al.* (1993) Insulin resistance and insulin secretory dysfunction as precursors of non-insulin-dependent diabetes mellitus. *The New England Journal of Medicine*, **329**, 1988–92.

17. Ravussin, E., Valencia, M.E., Esparza, J. *et al.* (1994) Effects of a traditional lifestyle on obesity in Pima Indians. *Diabetes Care*, **17**, 1067–74.

18. Tishkoff, S.A. and Kidd, K.K. (2004) Implications of biogeography of human populations for 'race' and medicine. *Nature Genetics*, **36**, 1–7.

19. Gohdes, D.M. (1983) Diabetes in American Indians: a growing problem. *Diabetes Care*, **6**, 609–13.

20. Young, T.K. and Shah, C. (1987) Extent and magnitude of the problem, in *Diabetes in the Canadian Native Population: Bicultural Perspectives* (ed K.T. Young), Canadian Diabetes Association, Toronto, pp. 11–25.

21. Cameron, W.I., Moffit, P. and Williams, D.R.R. (1986) Diabetes mellitus in the Australian Aborigines of Bourke, New South Wales. *Diabetes Research and Clinical Practice*, **2**, 307–14.

22. Prior, I.A.M. and Tasman-Jones, C. (1981) New Zealand Maori and Pacific Polynesians, in *Western Diseases: Their Emergence and Prevention* (eds H.C. Trowell and D.D. Bunkitt), Edward Arnold, London, pp. 227–67.

23. Zimmet, P., Dowse, G., Finch, S. *et al.* (1990) The epidemiology and natural history of NIDDM: lessons from the South Pacific. *Diabetes/Metabolism Reviews*, **6**, 91–124.

24. Carter, J., Horowitz, R., Wilson, R. *et al.* (1989) Tribal differences in diabetes: prevalence among American Indians in New Mexico. *Public Health Reports*, **104**, 665–9.

25. Freeman, W.L., Hosey, G.M.H., Diehr, P. and Gohdes, D. (1989) Diabetes in American Indians of Washington, Oregon, and Idaho. *Diabetes Care*, **12**, 282–8.

26. Acton, K., Rogers, B., Campbell, G. *et al.* (1993) Prevalence of diagnosed diabetes and selected related conditions of six reservations in Montana and Wyoming. *Diabetes Care*, **16** (Suppl 1), 263–5.

27. Valway, S., Freeman, W. and Kaufman, S. (1993) Prevalence of diagnosed diabetes among American Indians and Alaska Natives, 1987. *Diabetes Care*, **16** (Suppl 1), 271–6.

28. Centers for Disease Control and Prevention (2005) National Diabetes Fact Sheet: General Information and National Estimates on Diabetes in the United States, 2005, US Department

of Health and Human Services, Centers for Disease Control and Prevention, Atlanta, GA, http://www.diabetes.org/uedocuments/National DiabetesFactSheetRev.pdf.

29. Acton, K.J., Burrows, N.R., Geiss, L.S. and Thompson, T. (2003) Diabetes prevalence among American Indians and Alaska Natives and the overall population – United States, 1994–2002. *Morbidity and Mortality Weekly Report*, **52**, 702–4.

30. Schraer, C.D., Bulkow, L.R., Murphy, N.J. and Lanier, A.P. (1993) Diabetes prevalence, incidence and complications among Alaska Natives, 1987. *Diabetes Care*, **16** (Suppl 1), 257–9.

31. Young, T.K., Schraer, C.D., Shubnikoff, E.V. *et al.* (1992) Prevalence of diagnosed diabetes in circumpolar indigenous populations. *International Journal of Epidemiology*, **21**, 730–5.

32. Hall, L.D., Sberna, J. and Utermohle, C.J. (2001) Diabetes in Alaska, 1991–2000. Results from the Behavioral Risk Factor Surveillance System, State of Alaska Epidemiology Bulletin Recommendations and Reports, Vol. 5, No. 4, Department of Health and Human Services, Division of Public Health.

33. Hall, L.D., Stillwater, B., Stolz, G. and Utermohle, C.J. (2005) The Prevalence of Diabetes Among Adult Alaskans, 2002–2004, State of Alaska Epidemiology Bulletin Recommendations and Reports, Vol. 9, No. 3, Department of Health and Human Services, Division of Public Health.

34. O'Donnell, V. and Tait, H. (2003) *Aboriginal Peoples Survey 2001 – Initial Findings: Well-being of the Non-reserve Aboriginal Population*, Catalogue no. 89-589-XIE, Statistics Canada, Ottawa. Available at http://www.statcan.ca/english/freepub/89-589-XIE/89-589-XIE2003001.pdf (last access April 2008).

35. Alvarado-Osuna, C., Milian-Suazo, F. and Vallez-Sanchez, V. (2001) Prevalence of diabetes mellitus and hyperlipemias in Otomi Indians. *Salud Publica de Mexico*, **43**, 459–63.

36. Guerrero-Romero, F., Rodriguez-Moran, M. and Sandoval-Herrera, F. (1997) Low prevalence of non-insulin-dependent diabetes mellitus in indigenous communities of Durango, Mexico. *Archives of Medical Research*, **28**, 137–40.

37. Harris, M.I., Hadden, W.C., Knowler, W.C. and Bennett, P.H. (1987) Prevalence of diabetes and impaired glucose tolerance and plasma glucose levels in US populations aged 20–74 yr. *Diabetes*, **36**, 523–34.

38. Knowler, W.C., Pettitt, D.J., Saad, M.F. and Bennett, P.H. (1990) Diabetes mellitus in the Pima

Indians: incidence, risk factors and pathogenesis. *Diabetes/Metabolism Reviews*, **6**, 1–27.

39. Will, J.C., Strauss, K.F., Mendlein, J.M. *et al.* (1997) Diabetes mellitus among Navajo Indians: findings from the Navajo Health and Nutrition Survey. *The Journal of Nutrition*, **127** (Suppl 10), 2106S–13S.

40. Lee, E.T., Howard, B.V., Savage, P.J. *et al.* (1995) Diabetes mellitus and impaired glucose tolerance in three American Indian populations aged 45–74 years: the Strong Heart Study. *Diabetes Care*, **18**, 599–609.

41. Rith-Najarian, S.J., Valway, S.E. and Gohdes, D.M. (1993) Diabetes in a northern Minnesota Chippewa tribe. *Diabetes Care*, **16** (Suppl 1), 266–70.

42. World Health Organization (1985) Diabetes Mellitus: Report of a WHO Study Group. WHO Tech. Rep. Ser. 727, WHO, Geneva.

43. World Health Organization (1980) WHO Expert Committee on Diabetes Mellitus. 2nd report, WHO Tech. Rep. Ser. 646, WHO, Geneva.

44. Delisle, H.F. and Ekoé, J. (1993) Prevalence of non-insulin-dependent diabetes mellitus and impaired glucose tolerance in two Algonquin communities in Quebec. *Canadian Medical Association Journal*, **148**, 41–7.

45. Delisle, H.F., Rivard, M. and Ekoé, J. (1995) Prevalence estimates of diabetes and other cardiovascular risk factors in two largest Algonquin communities of Quebec. *Diabetes Care*, **18**, 1255–9.

46. Flegal, K.M., Ezzati, T.M., Harris, M.I. *et al.* (1991) Prevalence of diabetes in Mexican Americans, Cubans, and Puerto Ricans for the Hispanic Health and Nutrition Examination Survey, 1982–1984. *Diabetes Care*, **14** (Suppl 3), 628–38.

47. Young, T.K. and Harris, S.B. (1994) Risk of clinical diabetes in a northern Native Canadian cohort. *Arctic Medical Research*, **53**, 64–70.

48. Dabelea, D., Hanson, R.L., Bennett, P.H. *et al.* (1998) Increasing prevalence of type II diabetes in American Indian children. *Diabetologia*, **41**, 904–10.

49. Drevets, C.C. (1965) Diabetes mellitus in Choctaw Indians. *Journal of the Oklahoma State Medical Association*, **58**, 322–9.

50. Brousseau, J.D., Eelkema, R.C., Crawford, A.C. and Abe, T.A. (1979) Diabetes among three affiliated tribes: correlation with degree of Indian inheritance. *American Journal of Public Health*, **69**, 1277–8.

51. Knowler, W.C., Williams, R.C., Pettitt, D.J. and Steinberg, A.C. (1988) Gm3; 5, 13, 14 and type 2 diabetes mellitus: an association in American

Indians with genetic admixture. *American Journal of Human Genetics*, **43**, 520–6.

52. Knowler, W.C., Pettitt, D.J., Savage, P.J. and Bennett, P.H. (1981) Diabetes incidence in Pima Indians: contributions of obesity and parental diabetes. *American Journal of Epidemiology*, **113**, 144–56.

53. Lee, E.T., Anderson, P.S., Bryan, J. *et al.* (1985) Diabetes, parental diabetes, and obesity in Oklahoma Indians. *Diabetes Care*, **8**, 107–113.

54. Hanson, R.L., Pettitt, D.J., Bennett, P.H. *et al.* (1995) Familial relationships between obesity and NIDDM. *Diabetes*, **44**, 418–22.

55. Elston, R.C., Namboodiri, K.K., Nino, H.V. and Pollitzer, W.S. (1974) Studies on blood and urine glucose in Seminole Indians: indications for segregation of a major gene. *American Journal of Human Genetics*, **26**, 13–34.

56. Hanson, R.L., Elston, R.C., Pettitt, D.J. *et al.* (1995) Segregation analysis of non-insulin-dependent diabetes mellitus in Pima Indians: evidence for a major-gene effect. *American Journal of Human Genetics*, **57**, 160–70.

57. Hanson, R.L., Ehm, M.G., Pettitt, D.G. *et al.* (1998) An autosomal genomic scan for loci linked to type II diabetes mellitus and body-mass index in Pima Indians. *American Journal of Human Genetics*, **63**, 1130–8.

58. Hegele, R.A., Sun, E., Harris, S.B. *et al.* (1999) Genome-wide scanning for type 2 diabetes susceptibility genes in Canadian Oji-Cree using 190 microsatellite markers. *Journal of Human Genetics*, **44**, 10–14.

59. McCarthy, M.I. (2003) Growing evidence for diabetes susceptibility genes from genome scan data. *Current Diabetes Reports*, **3**, 159–67.

60. Altshuler, D., Hirschorn, J.N., Klannemark, M. *et al.* (2000) The common PPARγ Pro12Ala polymorphism is associated with decreased risk of type 2 diabetes. *Nature Genetics*, **26**, 76–80.

61. Muller, Y.L., Bogardus, C., Beamer, B.A. *et al.* (2003) A functional variant in the peroxisome proliferator-activated receptor γ2 promoter is associated with predictors of obesity and type 2 diabetes. *Diabetes*, **52**, 1864–71.

62. Hegele, R.A., Cae, H., Harris, S.B. *et al.* (2000) Peroxisome proliferator-activated receptor-γ2 P12A and type 2 diabetes in Canadian Oji-Cree. *The Journal of Clinical Endocrinology and Metabolism*, **85**, 2014–19.

63. Baier, L.J., Permana, P.A., Yang, X. *et al.* (2000) A *calpain-10* gene polymorphism is associated with reduced muscle mRNA levels and insulin resistance. *The Journal of Clinical Investigation*, **106**, R69–R73.

64. Hegele, R.A., Harris, S.B., Zinman, B. *et al.* (2001) Absence of association of type 2 diabetes with *CAPN10* and *PC-1* polymorphisms in Oji-Cree. *Diabetes Care*, **24**, 1498–9.

65. Baier, L.J. and Hanson, R.L. (2004) Genetic studies of the etiology of type 2 diabetes in Pima Indians: hunting for pieces to a complicated puzzle. *Diabetes*, **53**, 1181–6.

66. Kovacs, P., Hanson, R., Lee, Y.-H. *et al.* (2003) The role of insulin receptor substrate-1 gene (*IRS1*) in type 2 diabetes mellitus in Pima Indians. *Diabetes*, **52**, 3005–9.

67. Williams, R.C., Knowler, W.C., Butler, W.J. *et al.* (1981) *HLA-A2* and type 2 diabetes mellitus in Pima Indians: an association of allele frequency with age. *Diabetologia*, **21**, 460–3.

68. Xia, J., Scherer, S.W., Cohen, P.T. *et al.* (1998) A common variant in *PPP1R3* associated with insulin resistance and type 2 diabetes. *Diabetes*, **47**, 1519–24.

69. Hegele, R.A., Cao, H., Harris, S.B. *et al.* (1999) The hepatic nuclear factor 1-a *G319S* is associated with early-onset type 2 diabetes in Canadian Oji-Cree. *The Journal of Clinical Endocrinology and Metabolism*, **84**, 1077–82.

70. Hegele, R.A., Zinman, B., Hanley, A.J.G. *et al.* (2003) Genes, environment and Oji-Cree type 2 diabetes. *Clinical Biochemistry*, **36**, 163–70.

71. Baier, L.J., Permana, P.A., Traurig, M. *et al.* (2000) Mutations in the genes for nuclear factor (HNF)-1α, −4α, −1β and −3β; the dimerization cofactor of HNF-1 and insulin promoter factor 1 are not common causes of early-onset type 2 diabetes in Pima Indians. *Diabetes Care*, **23**, 302–4.

72. Triggs-Raine, B.L., Kirkpatrick, R.D., Kelly, S.L. *et al.* (2002) HNF-1α *G319S*, a transactivation-deficient mutant, is associated with altered dynamics of diabetes onset in an Oji-Cree community. *Proceedings of the National Academy of Sciences of the United States of America*, **99**, 4614–19.

73. Pettitt, D.J., Aleck, K.A., Baird, H.R. *et al.* (1988) Congenital susceptibility to NIDDM: role of intrauterine environment. *Diabetes*, **37**, 622–8.

74. Pettitt, D.J. and Bennett, P.H. (1995) Long-term outcome of infants of diabetic mothers, in *Diabetes Mellitus in Pregnancy: Principles and Practice*, 2nd edn (eds E.A. Reece and D. Coustan), Churchill Livingstone, New York, pp. 379–88.

75. McCance, D.R., Pettitt, D.J., Hanson, R.L. *et al.* (1994) Birth weight and non-insulin-dependent diabetes: thrifty phenotype, or surviving small baby genotype? *British Medical Journal*, **308**, 942–5.

76. Young, T.K., Martens, P.J., Taback, S.P. *et al.* (2002) Type 2 diabetes mellitus in children: prenatal and early infancy risk factors among native Canadians. *Archives of Pediatrics and Adolescent Medicine*, **156**, 651–5.

77. Lindsay, R.S., Walker, J.D., Halsall, I. *et al.* (2003) Insulin and insulin propeptides at birth in offspring of diabetic mothers. *The Journal of Clinical Endocrinology and Metabolism*, **88**, 1664–71.

78. Pettitt, D.J., Forman, M.R., Hanson, R.L. *et al.* (1997) Breastfeeding and incidence of non-insulin-dependent diabetes mellitus in Pima Indians. *Lancet*, **350**, 166–8.

79. Saad, M.F., Knowler, W.C., Pettitt, D.J. *et al.* (1988) The natural history of impaired glucose tolerance in the Pima Indians. *The New England Journal of Medicine*, **319**, 1500–6.

80. Tuomilehto, J., Knowler, W.C. and Zimmet, P. (1992) Primary prevention of non-insulin-dependent diabetes mellitus. *Diabetes Metabolism Reviews*, **8**, 339–53.

81. Knowler, W.C., Narayan, K.M.V., Hanson, R.L. *et al.* (1995) Preventing non-insulin-dependent diabetes mellitus. *Diabetes*, **44**, 483–8.

82. Tulloch-Reid, M.K., Williams, D.E., Looker, H.C. *et al.* (2003) Do measures of body fat distribution provide information on the risk of type 2 diabetes in addition to measures of general obesity? Comparison of anthropometric predictors of type 2 diabetes in Pima Indians. *Diabetes Care*, **26**, 2556–61.

83. Everhart, J.E., Pettitt, D.J., Bennett, P.H. and Knowler, W.C. (1992) Duration of obesity increases the incidence of NIDDM. *Diabetes*, **41**, 235–40.

84. Hanson, R.L., Narayan, K.M.V., Pettitt, D.J. *et al.* (1995) Rate of weight gain, weight fluctuation and incidence of NIDDM. *Diabetes*, **44**, 261–6.

85. Center for Disease Control (2003) Surveillance for health behaviors of American Indians and Alaska Natives: findings from the Behavioral Risk Factor Surveillance System, 1997–2000. *Morbidity and Mortality Weekly Report CDC Surveillance Summaries*, **52** (SS07), 1–13.

86. Sandstead, H.R., McGanity, W.J., Smith, H.H. *et al.* (1956) A study of the dietary background and nutriture of the Navajo Indian. III. Physical findings. *The Journal of Nutrition*, **60**, 35–62.

87. DeStefano, F., Coulehan, J.L. and Wiant, M.K. (1979) Blood pressure survey in the Navajo Indian reservation. *American Journal of Epidemiology*, **109**, 335–45.

88. White, L.L., Ballew, C., Gilbert, T.J. *et al.* (1997) Weight, body image, and weight control practices of Navajo Indians: findings from the Navajo Health and Nutrition Survey. *The Journal of Nutrition*, **127**, 2094S–8S.

89. Knowler, W.C., Pettitt, D.J., Saad, M.F. *et al.* (1991) Obesity in the Pima Indians: its magnitude and relationship with diabetes. *The American Journal of Clinical Nutrition*, **53**, 1543S–51S.

90. Shree Gulabkunverba Ayurvedic Society (transl) (1949) *Charaka Samhita (600 BC)*, Ayurvedic Society, Jamnagar, India.

91. Knowler, W.C., McCance, D.R., Nagi, D.K. and Pettitt, D.J. (1993) Epidemiologic studies of the causes of non-insulin-dependent diabetes mellitus, in *Causes of Diabetes* (ed R.D.G. Leslie), John Wiley & Sons, Ltd, Chichester, pp. 187–218.

92. Bennett, P.H., Knowler, W.C., Baird, H.R. *et al.* (1984) Diet and development of non-insulin-dependent diabetes mellitus: an epidemiological perspective, in *Diet, Diabetes and Atherosclerosis* (eds G. Pozza, P. Micossi, A.L. Catapano and R. Paoletti), Raven Press, New York, pp. 109–19.

93. Smith, C.J., Nelson, R.G., Hardy, S.A. *et al.* (1996) Survey of the diet of Pima Indians using quantitative food frequency assessment and 24-hour recall. *Journal of the American Dietetic Association*, **96**, 778–84.

94. Williams, D.E., Knowler, W.C., Smith, C.J. *et al.* (2001) The effect of Indian or Anglo dietary preference on the incidence of diabetes in Pima Indians. *Diabetes Care*, **24**, 811–16.

95. Jackson, M.Y. (1994) Diet, culture, and diabetes, in *Diabetes as a Disease of Civilization: The Impact of Culture Change on Indigenous Peoples* (eds J.R. Joe and R.S. Young), Mouton de Gruyter, New York, pp. 381–406.

96. Kriska, A.M., Saremi, A., Hanson, R.L. *et al.* (2003) Physical activity, obesity, and the incidence of type 2 diabetes in a high-risk population. *American Journal of Epidemiology*, **158**, 669–75.

97. Benjamin, E., Mayfield, J. and Gohdes, D. (1993) Exercise and incidence of NIDDM among Zuni Indians. *Diabetes*, **42** (Suppl 1), 203A.

98. Knowler, W.C., Barrett-Connor, E., Fowler, S.E. *et al.* (2002) Reduction in the incidence of type 2 diabetes with lifestyle intervention or metformin. *The New England Journal of Medicine*, **346**, 393–403.

99. Galloway, J.M. (2005) Cardiovascular health among American Indians and Alaska Natives. Successes, challenges and potentials. *American Journal of Preventive Medicine*, **29** (S1), 11–17.

100. Nelson, R.G., Sievers, M.L., Knowler, W.C. *et al.* (1990) Low incidence of fatal coronary heart disease in Pima Indians despite high prevalence of

non-insulin-dependent diabetes. *Circulation*, **81**, 987–95.

101. Welty, T.K. and Coulehan, J.L. (1993) Cardiovascular disease among American Indians and Alaska Natives. *Diabetes Care*, **16** (Suppl 1), 277–83.

102. Lee, E.T., Welty, T.K., Fabsitz, R. *et al.* (1990) The Strong Heart Study. A study of cardiovascular disease in American Indians: design and methods. *American Journal of Epidemiology*, **132**, 1141–55.

103. Howard, B.V., Lee, E.T., Cowan, L.D. *et al.* (1995) Coronary heart disease prevalence and its relation to risk factors in American Indians. The Strong Heart Study. *American Journal of Epidemiology*, **142**, 254–68.

104. Hoehner, C.M., Williams, D.E., Sievers, M.L. *et al.* (2006) Trends in heart disease death rates in diabetic and nondiabetic Pima Indians. *Journal of Diabetes and Its Complications*, **20**, 8–13.

105. Pavkov, M.E., Sievers, M.L., Knowler, W.C. *et al.* (2004) An explanation for the increase in heart disease mortality rates in diabetic Pima Indians. *Diabetes Care*, **27**, 1132–6.

106. Nelson, R.G., Pettitt, D.J., Carraher, M.J. *et al.* (1988) Effect of proteinuria on mortality in NIDDM. *Diabetes*, **37**, 1499–504.

107. Howard, B.V., Lee, E.T., Cowan, L.D. *et al.* (1999) Rising tide of cardiovascular disease in American Indians: the Strong Heart Study. *Circulation*, **99**, 2389–95.

108. Manolio, T.A., Kronmal, R.A., Burke, G.L. *et al.* (1996) Short-term predictors of incident stroke in older adults: The Cardiovascular Health Study. *Stroke*, **27**, 1479–86.

109. Chambless, L.E., Heiss, G., Folsom, A.R. *et al.* (1997) Association of coronary heart disease incidence with carotid arterial wall thickness and major risk factors: The Atherosclerosis Risk in Communities (ARIC) Study, 1987 to 1993. *American Journal of Epidemiology*, **146**, 483–94.

110. Naylor, J.L., Schraer, C.D., Mayer, A.M. *et al.* (2003) Diabetes among Alaska Natives: a review. *International Journal of Circumpolar Health*, **62**, 363–87.

111. Manson, J.E., Colditz, G.A., Stampfer, M.J. *et al.* (1991) A prospective study of maturity-onset diabetes mellitus and risk of coronary heart disease and stroke in women. *Archives of Internal Medicine*, **151**, 1141–7.

112. Graves, E.J. (1992) National Hospital Discharge Survey: annual summary, 1990. Vital and Health Statistics, Series 13: Data From the National Health Survey, No. 112, National Center for Health Statistics, Hyattsville, MD.

113. Most, R.S. and Sinnock, P. (1983) The epidemiology of lower extremity amputations in diabetic individuals. *Diabetes Care*, **6**, 87–91.

114. Nelson, R.G., Gohdes, D.M., Everhart, J.E. *et al.* (1988) Lower extremity amputations in NIDDM: 12-yr follow-up study in Pima Indians. *Diabetes Care*, **11**, 8–16.

115. Lee, J.S., Lu, M., Lee, V.S. *et al.* (1993) Lower-extremity amputation: incidence, risk factors, and mortality in the Oklahoma Indian Diabetes Study. *Diabetes*, **42**, 876–82.

116. Schraer, C.D., Mayer, A.M., Vogt, A.M. *et al.* (2001) The Alaska Native diabetes program. *International Journal of Circumpolar Health*, **60**, 487–94.

117. Schraer, C.D., Adler, A.I., Mayer, A.M. *et al.* (1997) Diabetes complications and mortality among Alaska Natives: eight years of observation. *Diabetes Care*, **20**, 314–21.

118. Andersen, A.R., Christiansen, J.S., Andersen, J.K. *et al.* (1983) Diabetic nephropathy in type 1 (insulin dependent) diabetes: an epidemiological study. *Diabetologia*, **25**, 496–501.

119. Borch-Johnsen, K., Andersen, P.K. and Deckert, T. (1985) The effect of proteinuria on relative mortality in type 1 (insulin-dependent) diabetes mellitus. *Diabetologia*, **28**, 590–6.

120. Jensen, T., Borch-Johnsen, K., Kofoed-Enevoldsen, A. and Deckert, T. (1987) Coronary heart disease in young type 1 (insulin-dependent) diabetic patients with and without diabetic nephropathy: incidence and risk factors. *Diabetologia*, **30**, 144–8.

121. Deckert, T., Feldt-Rasmussen, B., Borch-Johnsen, K. *et al.* (1989) Albuminuria reflects widespread vascular damage. The Steno hypothesis. *Diabetologia*, **32**, 219–26.

122. Jarrett, R.J. and Shipley, M.J. (1988) Type 2 (non-insulin-dependent) diabetes mellitus and cardiovascular disease – putative association via common antecedents; further evidence from the Whitehall Study. *Diabetologia*, **31**, 737–40.

123. Krakoff, J., Lindsay, R.S., Looker, H.C. *et al.* (2003) Incidence of retinopathy and nephropathy in youth-onset compared with adult-onset type 2 diabetes. *Diabetes Care*, **26**, 76–81.

124. Nelson, R.G., Kunzelman, C.L., Pettitt, D.J. *et al.* (1989) Albuminuria in type 2 (non-insulin-dependent) diabetes mellitus and impaired glucose tolerance in Pima Indians. *Diabetologia*, **32**, 870–6.

125. Hanley, A.J.G., Harris, S.B., Mamakeesick, M. *et al.* (2005) Complications of type 2 diabetes among Aboriginal Canadians: prevalence and associated risk factors. *Diabetes Care*, **28**, 2054–7.

126. Robbins, D.C., Knowler, W.C., Lee, E.T. *et al.* (1996) Regional differences in albuminuria among American Indians: an epidemic of renal disease. *Kidney International*, **49**, 557–63.

127. Sievers, M.L., Nelson, R.G., Knowler, W.C. and Bennett, P.H. (1992) Impact of NIDDM on mortality and causes of death in Pima Indians. *Diabetes Care*, **15**, 1541–9.

128. Kunzelman, C.L., Knowler, W.C., Pettitt, D.J. and Bennett, P.H. (1989) Incidence of proteinuria in type 2 diabetes mellitus in the Pima Indians. *Kidney International*, **35**, 681–7.

129. Pavkov, M.E., Knowler, W.C., Bennett, P.H. and Nelson, R.G. (2004) Increasing incidence of proteinuria in Pima Indians with type 2 diabetes. *Diabetologia*, **47** (Suppl 1), I–VIII, A63.

130. Pavkov, M.E., Knowler, W.C., Krakoff, J. and Nelson, R.G. (2004) Trends in renal replacement therapy among Pima Indians with type 2 diabetes. *Journal of the American Society of Nephrology*, **15**, 393A.

131. Looker, H.C., Krakoff, J., Nelson, R.G. *et al.* (2005) Trends in treatment for diabetes and blood pressure: 1989–2003. *Diabetes*, **54** (Suppl 1), A611.

132. Narva, A.S. (2002) Kidney disease in Native Americans. *Journal of the National Medical Association*, **94**, 738–42.

133. Megill, D.M., Hoy, W.E. and Woodruff, S.D. (1988) Rates and causes of end-stage renal disease in Navajo Indians, 1971–1985. *The Western Journal of Medicine*, **149**, 178–82.

134. Hoy, W.E., Megill, D.M. and Hughson, M.D. (1987) Epidemic renal disease of unknown etiology in the Zuni Indians. *American Journal of Kidney Diseases*, **9**, 485–96.

135. Nelson, R.G., Newman, J.M., Knowler, W.C. *et al.* (1988) Incidence of end-stage renal disease in type 2 (non-insulin-dependent) diabetes mellitus in Pima Indians. *Diabetologia*, **31**, 730–6.

136. Narva, A.S. (1985) End stage renal disease. *The IHS Primary Care Provider*, **10**, 82–5.

137. US Renal Data System (2004) USRDS 2004 Annual Data Report: Atlas of End-Stage Renal Disease in the United States, National Institutes of Health, National Institute of Diabetes and Digestive and Kidney Diseases, Bethesda, MD.

138. Shah, V.O., Scavini, M., Stidley, C.A. *et al.* (2003) Epidemic of diabetic and non-diabetic renal disease among the Zuni Indians: The Zuni Kidney Project. *Journal of the American Society of Nephrology*, **14**, 1320–9.

139. Shah, V.O., Scavini, M., Stidley, C.A. *et al.* (2005) Kidney disease among the Zuni Indians:

The Zuni Kidney Project. *Kidney International – Supplement*, **68** (97), S126–31.

140. Burrows, N.R., Narva, A.S., Geiss, L. *et al.* (2005) End-stage renal disease due to diabetes among southwestern American Indians, 1990–2001. *Diabetes Care*, **28**, 1041–4.

141. Kleinman, J.C., Donahue, R.P., Harris, M.I. *et al.* (1988) Mortality among diabetics in a national sample. *American Journal of Epidemiology*, **128**, 389–401.

142. Nelson, R.G., Hanson, R.L., Pettitt, D.J. *et al.* (1996) Survival during replacement therapy for diabetic end-stage renal disease in Pima Indians. *Diabetes Care*, **19**, 1333–7.

143. Pavkov, M.E., Bennett, P.H., Sievers, M.L. *et al.* (2005) Predominant effect of kidney disease on mortality in Pima Indians with or without type 2 diabetes. *Kidney International*, **68**, 1267–74.

144. Gohdes, D. (1995) Diabetes in North American Indians and Alaska Natives, in *Diabetes in America*, 2nd edn (eds M.I. Harris, C.C. Cowie, M.P. Stern *et al.*), NIH Publication No. 95/1468, Vol. **5**, National Diabetes Data Group, US Department of Health and Human Services, Bethesda, MD, pp. 683–702.

145. Nelson, R.G., Wolfe, J.A., Horton, M.B. *et al.* (1989) Proliferative retinopathy in NIDDM: incidence and risk factors in Pima Indians. *Diabetes*, **38**, 435–40.

146. Lee, E.T., Lee, V.S., Kingsley, R.M. *et al.* (1992) Diabetic retinopathy in Oklahoma Indians with NIDDM. *Diabetes Care*, **15**, 1620–7.

147. Lee, E.T., Lee, V.S., Lu, M. and Russell, D. (1992) Development of proliferative retinopathy in NIDDM. A follow-up study of American Indians in Oklahoma. *Diabetes*, **41**, 359–67.

148. Looker, H.C., Krakoff, J., Knowler, W.C. *et al.* (2003) Longitudinal studies of incidence and progression of diabetic retinopathy assessed by retinal photography in Pima Indians. *Diabetes Care*, **26**, 320–6.

149. Liu, Q.Z., Pettitt, D.J., Hanson, R.L. *et al.* (1993) Glycated haemoglobin, plasma glucose and diabetic retinopathy: cross-sectional and prospective analyses. *Diabetologia*, **36**, 428–32.

150. Tofte, R.W. and Sabath, L.D. (1982) Infection in patients with, diabetes mellitus or obesity, in *Diabetes Mellitus and Obesity* (eds S. Bleicher and B. Bradoff), Williams and Wilkins, Baltimore, MD, pp. 577–83.

151. Mori, M.A., Leonard, G. and Welty, T.K. (1992) The benefits of isoniazid chemoprophylaxis and risk factors for tuberculosis among Oglala Sioux Indians. *Archives of Internal Medicine*, **152**, 547–50.

152. Sievers, M.L. (1977) Prognostic factors in disseminated coccidioidomycosis among southwestern American Indians, in *Coccidioidomycosis: Current Clinical and Diagnostic Status* (ed L. Ajello), Symposium Specialists, Miami, FL, pp. 63–78.

153. Nelson, R.G., Shlossman, M., Budding, L.M. *et al.* (1990) Periodontal disease and NIDDM in Pima Indians. *Diabetes Care*, **13**, 836–40.

154. Taylor, G.W., Burt, B.A., Becker, M.P. *et al.* (1996) Severe peridontitis and risk for poor glycemic control in subjects with non-insulin-dependent diabetes mellitus. *Journal of Periodontology*, **67**, 1085–93.

155. Gottsegan, R. (1983) Dental and oral aspects of diabetes mellitus, in *Diabetes Mellitus: Theory and Practice* (eds M. Ellenberg and H. Rifkin), Medical Examination Publishing, New York, pp. 895–906.

156. Williams, R.C. Jr and Mahan, C.J. (1960) Periodontal disease and diabetes in young adults. *Journal of the American Medical Association*, **172**, 776–8.

157. Saremi, A., Nelson, R.G., Tulloch-Reid, M. *et al.* (2005) Periodontal disease and mortality in type 2 diabetes. *Diabetes Care*, **28**, 27–32.

20

Epidemiology of Type 2 Diabetes in Hispanic North Americans

Judith Baxter and Richard F. Hamman

Colorado School of Public Health, University of Colorado Denver, Aurora, CO, USA

20.1 INTRODUCTION

Over the last 25 years, national surveys and large population-based studies of diabetes and heart disease have contributed significantly to our understanding of the epidemiology of these diseases in the US population. These include, but are not limited to, the Pima Studies, the San Luis Valley Diabetes Study, the San Antonio Heart Study, the Rancho Bernardo Studies, the Honolulu Heart Study, Insulin Resistance and Atherosclerosis Studies and ARIC. Specifically, these studies have established that type 2 diabetes is a significant health problem occurring at substantially higher rates in minority populations. The morbidity and mortality associated with type 2 diabetes is a major health concern for Native American, African-American and Hispanic populations. Increasing prevalence of diabetes leads to increases in rates of diabetes complications, mortality and health care costs, together with poorer quality of life. Minority populations carry a disproportionate share of this burden, resulting from both the excess prevalence in these populations and those forces which contribute to the many health disparities (discrimination, lack of access to health care, differential care based on group status, etc.). Examining the epidemiology of type 2 diabetes in these populations provides an understanding of the nuances of disease etiology and offers opportunity for assessing and developing prevention and treatment strategies applicable across groups, as well as ones tailored to the unique risk factors profiles and cultural circumstances of minority groups.

This chapter reviews the epidemiology of type 2 diabetes in the US Hispanic population, while other chapters focus on Native American, African American and Asian American populations. The specific objectives of this chapter are to: (i) provide a brief demographic profile of the US Hispanic population, examining its size, composition and distribution; (ii) examine recent prevalence and incidence data in type 2 diabetes in the Hispanic compared with non-Hispanic White US population; (iii) describe the mortality burden associated with diabetes; and (iv) examine differential risk factor patterns. Where possible we attempt to examine the demographic, morbidity and mortality patterns over time to assess changing trends and assess the directions for future investigation that the data reviewed here suggest.

20.2 HISPANIC POPULATION PROFILE

Hispanic Americans are a diverse and fast-growing segment of the US population. The US Census Bureau has consistently identified and described this ethnic group since the 1970 Census, when the Spanish/Hispanic origin question was included on the sample enumeration questionnaire. With the 1980 full enumeration questionnaire, all persons were asked if they were of Spanish or Hispanic origin or

The Epidemiology of Diabetes Mellitus, second edition   Edited by Jean-Marie Ekoé, Marian Rewers, Rhys Williams and Paul Zimmet
© 2008 John Wiley & Sons, Ltd

descent, with positive subgroup categories permitting persons to self-identify as Mexican, Mexican American and Chicano; Puerto Rican, Cuban and other Spanish/Hispanic. Although language and origins from Latin America or Spain are elements shared by Hispanic Americans, there is significant diversity that is only hinted at in the subgroup identifications used by the Census Bureau. Persistent differences in historical, cultural, social and socioeconomic circumstances exist. In combining all Hispanic subgroups together in order to identify epidemiological trends clearly, much of the ability to understand and explain these observations is lost.

We will first attempt to describe some of the underlying diversity of this population in terms of its size, composition and distribution and the historical and cultural circumstances that are important to consider when examining type 2 diabetes trends. Unfortunately, much of the available epidemiologic data is not produced for Hispanic subpopulations at

this level of detail, so some degree of homogenization is required.

20.3   SIZE AND DISTRIBUTION OF HISPANIC POPULATION— REGIONAL TRENDS

In 1990, the Hispanic population comprised 9.0% of the US population. By the year 2000 it had increased to 12.5% of the total population [1, 2]. Current estimates for 2004 place the total Hispanic population at 41 322 070, or approximately 14.3% of the US population [3].

The demographic profile of the Hispanic population in 2000 shown in **Table 20.1** includes self-identified subgroup diversity, regional distribution and selected social and economic characteristics. Persons self-identifying as Mexican American and other Hispanic comprise 7.3% and 3.6% of the total US population respectively. Among the total Hispanic population, these two groups make

Table 20.1 Selected characteristics of Hispanic persons and subgroups in the United States: 2000.

	Total	Mexican	Puerto Rican	Cuban	Other
Hispanic population	35 305 818	20 640 711	3 406 178	1 241 685	10 017 244
Fraction of total 2000 US population, 281 421 906 (%)	12.50	7.30	1.20	0.40	3.60
Fraction of total 2000 regional populations					
Northeast (%)	9.8	0.90	3.90	0.30	4.7
Midwest (%)	4.9	3.40	0.50	0.10	0.9
South (%)	11.60	6.50	0.80	0.90	3.3
West (%)	24.30	18.00	0.40	0.20	5.7
Fraction of total Hispanic population[a] (%)	100	58.50	9.60	3.50	28.40
Population change 1990–2000 (%) [1, 2]	57.9	52.9	24.9	18.9	96.9
Median age years	25.9 (35.4)	24.2	27.3	40.7	24.7[a]
Fraction living below poverty level 2001 (%) [4]	21.4	22.8	26.1	16.5	17.7[a]
Fraction of population with at least a high school education 2002 (%) [4]	57.00	50.6	66.8	70.8	74.0[a]

[a]Other Hispanic, excluding Central and South Americans.

up nearly 90% of all Hispanic persons. A majority of persons identifying as 'other Hispanic' do not provide further specification; others in this subgroup include Spaniards and those from the Dominican Republic and Central and South America. Many of this unspecified 'other Hispanic' group include those in the US Southwest that trace ancestry to the early Spanish explorers that came from Mexico. National origin or descent is a major but not sole determinant of subgroup identification and carries with it distinct and varied historical, social and cultural attributes, including attitudes, beliefs and values about food, physical activity and social roles. These may well play a role in the diversity of prevalence and incidence estimates of type 2 diabetes seen in the Hispanic population overall and certainly deserve attention when designing interventions and treatment strategies.

The Hispanic population and particular subgroups have grown rapidly. Overall, the population increased 57.9% between 1990 and 2000, with the greatest increase occurring in the western United States. In contrast, the total US population increased by 13.2% in the same period. The two largest subgroups, Mexican Americans and other Hispanics, had a remarkable population increase between 1990 and 2000, 52.9% and 96.9% respectively. Puerto Rican and Cuban subgroups also increased, but not as much [5].

The regional distribution of the Hispanic subgroups and the population change between 1990 and 2004 are detailed in **Table 20.1** and **Figures 20.1 and 20.2** [1–3]. As of the 2000 census, 36% of all US Hispanics live in the west and south; in 1990 these two regions held only 27%. In 2000, 77% of US Hispanics lived in seven states, with California and Texas having the greatest number and percentage of population [5]. **Figure 20.1** shows the Hispanic population by county in the year 2000 and underscores these facets of the population distribution. As seen in **Figure 20.2**, for three time-periods spanning 14 years, the Hispanic population is increasing in all regions. However, as a proportion of the total population, the percentage change is greatest in the Midwestern and Southern (includes Texas) regions of the United States.

20.4 AGE AND SOCIOECONOMIC CHARACTERISTICS

The median age of the Hispanic population is nearly 10 years younger than that of the total US population (25.9 years versus 35.4 years). This reflects the younger age structure of the Hispanic population due in large part to higher birth rates, lower percentage of population over the age of 65 years, and immigration patterns of younger persons. In 2000, the median age of Mexican American and other Hispanics was 25 years, Puerto Ricans were slightly older at 27 years and Cuban Americans had a substantially older median age of 41 years. This substantially older age of the Cuban subgroup reflects the sporadic and limited nature of the immigration patterns of the last 40 years.

Educational attainment also varies among Hispanic populations (**Table 20.1**). Overall, 57% of Hispanic persons over the age of 25 years had at

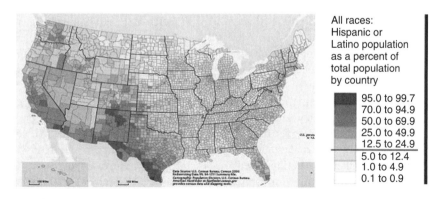

All races: Hispanic or Latino population as a percent of total population by country

95.0 to 99.7
70.0 to 94.9
50.0 to 69.9
25.0 to 49.9
12.5 to 24.9
5.0 to 12.4
1.0 to 4.9
0.1 to 0.9

Figure 20.1 Hispanics as a percentage of total US population by county, 2000. (Data source: US Census Bureau, Census 2000 Redistricting Data (PL 94-171) Summary File. Cartography: Population Division, US Census Bureau).

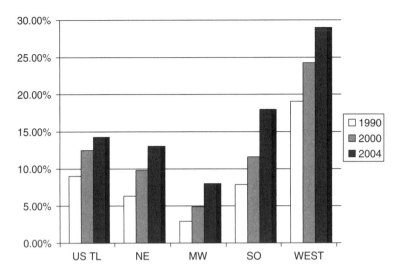

Figure 20.2 Percentage of total US population reporting Hispanic origin by region: 1990, 2000, 2004 [1, 2, 6].

least a high school education. This proportion was markedly different from the non-Hispanic White (NHW) population where 89% had attained this level of education. In 2002, Mexican Americans had the lowest percentage of those 25 years and older having graduated from high school (51%) compared with other Hispanic subgroups, which ranged from 67 to 74%. Similar patterns exist for other socioeconomic indicators, including poverty level measures for 2001. Three times the number of all Hispanic persons lived below the poverty line compared with NHW persons (21% versus 8%). Among Hispanic subgroups the range in the percentage living below the poverty line was 16–26%, with Cubans and other Hispanics with the fewest persons living in poverty and Mexican Americans and Puerto Rican groups with the highest percentages.

As a cautionary note, when using and interpreting population-based data, issues associated with population enumeration and ascertainment of endpoints need to be considered when examining morbidity and mortality rates within this ethnic group and between population subgroups. Segments of the Hispanic population are likely to be underenumerated in the census or in other population-based surveys that provide the denominators for rates. Such underenumeration can occur differentially across regions of the United States and across the different subgroups. An undercounted denominator with a numerator that is more complete will result in

apparently higher rates or greater disparity between minorities and the majority population. Conversely, if the ascertainment of an endpoint is incomplete for segments of the population and the population denominator is accurate or has been corrected, then there may be an under estimation of the true rates and possibly an even greater disparity when compared with other population groups that are not as subject to these biases. Unfortunately, there is no simple way to determine the possible direction of such biases in much of the available data.

20.5 PREVALENCE OF DIABETES

Prevalence measures the number of existing cases of diabetes at a point in time in a defined population. Thus, it includes only current survivors with diabetes. Changes in prevalence over time are influenced by the age structure of the population (with older average age resulting in higher diabetes prevalence), the amount of screening and detection of diabetes by health care providers, the correctness of reporting by individuals (if self-report is the outcome) and by improving trends in survivorship (notably for cardiovascular disease (CVD) and diabetes itself [7]). Studies in Europe have suggested that the increased prevalence of diabetes can be almost fully explained by stable risk (incidence) and changing survivorship and age of the population [8], though incidence rate increases have been reported in several US populations (see below), making it likely that, in addition to the factors noted above, rising prevalence also reflects higher risk in later time periods.

Table 20.2 summarizes recent studies of diabetes prevalence among Hispanics in the United States. Older studies have been reviewed previously [9]. The prevalence of diabetes by self-report in 2004 using data from the US National Health Interview Survey (NHIS) accessible through the Diabetes Surveillance System of the Centers for Disease Control and Prevention (CDC) is shown in **Table 20.2** for Hispanics and non-Hispanic Whites

[10]. Overall, Hispanics have 1.5–1.7 times higher reported diabetes prevalence than NHWs for each age group over the age of 45 years, with a prevalence of approximately 15% at ages 45–64 years and 25–30% in the 65–74-year age group. Prevalence is somewhat lower over the age of 75 years (20–25%), which may be the result of either increased mortality at older ages or a 'cohort effect,' where older persons have a lower risk of developing diabetes at the oldest ages since they belonged to cohorts which at younger ages (and decades ago) were less exposed to risk factors such as obesity. Hispanic males have higher prevalence than Hispanic females

Table 20.2 Summary of recent studies of Hispanic prevalence of diabetes (per 100).

Study, year, author, method	Race/ethnicity (gender)	Age group (years)			
CDC NHIS, 2004 [10], self-report		**0–44**	**45–64**	**65–74**	**>75**
	Hispanic (M)	1.1	14.4	30.1	19.4
	NHW (M)	1.0	9.6	20.4	16.7
	Hispanic (F)	1.3	13.5	23.0	24.0
	NHW (F)	1.3	7.8	13.9	13.8
BRFSS, 1998–2002 [12], self-report		**18–44**	**45–54**	**55–64**	**> 65**
California	Hispanics (M + F)	3.2	11.7	24.6	25.6
Florida			6.1	12.8	20.6
Illinois		2.0	15.9	19.8	25.8
New York/New Jersey		2.4	10.5	15.9	17.7
Texas		2.8	13.0	20.8	25.4
NHANES, 1999–2002 [13], fasting plasma glucose		**20–39**	**40–59**	**60 +**	
	Mexican-American (M)	0.2	11.0	25.6	
	NHW (M)	1.6	5.5	14.5	
	Mexican-American (F)	2.6	12.0	24.5	
	NHW (F)	0.8	3.7	12.3	
Medicare, 2001 [14], medical claims data					**>67**[a]
	Hispanic (M + F)				33.4
	NHW (M + F)				18.4
HEPESE, 1999 [15], self-report		**65–74**	**75–84**	**> 85**	
	Hispanic (M + F)	24.6	18.4	12.0	

[a] Age and sex adjusted.

except at the youngest and oldest ages, a pattern shared with NHWs. Since most diabetes in any population is type 2, these prevalence results primarily reflect excess type 2 diabetes among Hispanics. The absence of important differences in prevalence at ages < 45 years is due in part to similar or lower prevalence of diabetes in Hispanic youth compared with NHWs [11].

The Hispanic Health and Nutritional Examination Survey (HANES) from 1982 to 1984 was the first to document prevalence of diabetes in Hispanic subpopulations carefully [16]. Among men and women 45–74 years of age, the prevalence of both diagnosed and undiagnosed diabetes was high for both Mexican Americans (23.9%) and Puerto Ricans in New York City (26.1%) compared with Cubans in south Florida (15.8%) or NHWs in 1976–1980 (12%). The total prevalence of diabetes was not significantly different for Mexican Americans and Puerto Ricans but was significantly lower for Cubans. Since this study included both diagnosed and oral glucose tolerance test (OGTT)-detected diabetes, the prevalence is higher than that reported in interviews, but the pattern of lower prevalence rate among Cuban Americans seen here is consistent with the Florida Behavioral Risk Factor Surveillance System (BRFSS) data shown in **Table 20.2**.

Prevalence of type 2 diabetes can also be assessed using fasting glucose levels and American Diabetes Association criteria [17] to identify both diagnosed and previously undiagnosed diabetes. The most recent analysis of representative US population data using fasting glucose criteria as well as previously diagnosed diabetes comes from the 1999–2002 National Health and Nutrition Examination Survey (NHANES) [13]. In this report, prevalence was similar to that from NHIS [10] (**Table 20.2**). In both reports, males had higher rates than females, and Hispanics had excess diabetes in all age groups compared with NHWs. However, once results were standardized for age, there was no difference in the previously undiagnosed (screen detected) diabetes rates between Hispanics and NHWs [13].

Impaired fasting glucose (IFG; fasting glucose level 5.6–7.0 mmol l^{-1}) is a high-risk state that may precede the development of diabetes. In the NHANES, the age-adjusted prevalence of IFG in Hispanics age > 20 years was 32%, compared with 26% in NHWs ($p = 0.008$) [13]. Thus, not only is

diagnosed diabetes more prevalent in Hispanic persons, but so is IFG, together resulting in an adjusted prevalence of glucose intolerance (both diabetes and IFG) among Hispanics of 45% compared with 34% in NHWs (prevalence ratio 1.33).

Results from most US population survey data do not include large numbers of elderly subjects. Recent reports using Medicare data [14] suggest that elderly Hispanics (aged > 67 years) who have Medicare benefits had a prevalence 1.8 times higher than Whites in the same record system (**Table 20.2**). Black *et al.* [15] presented prevalence of self-reported diabetes among community-dwelling elderly Hispanics aged 65 years and over from Texas, California, New Mexico, Arizona and Colorado in a survey representing over 500 000 Mexican Americans in this region. Prevalence was somewhat lower in this community-dwelling sample than that reported from the Medicare survey (which included institutionalized persons) [14]. Prevalence was lower at older ages and was also lower among immigrants (19.9%) than among US-born Hispanics (23.8%).

From these recent results, it appears that US Hispanics have 1.5–2-fold higher diabetes prevalence across the age span than do US NHWs, with higher prevalence in males than females in most studies.

20.6 INCIDENCE OF DIABETES

Incidence rates measure the risk of newly developing diabetes in a defined period of time (usually per year) in a defined population. There are very few recent reports of incidence among Hispanic populations by age and sex. Older data from the San Luis Valley Diabetes Study [18] have shown that Hispanics have higher incidence of clinically diagnosed type 2 diabetes at each age, and that the peak age of onset is about 10 years earlier (**Figure 20.3**).

The San Antonio Heart Study also reported the 8-year incidence of diabetes using an OGTT and the 1979 World Health Organization (WHO) criteria [19], a method which is more sensitive in detecting diabetes than self-report or clinical diagnosis alone. The results are compared in **Figure 20.3** after calculating the average annual incidence rates per 1000 person-years for both studies. Though the age groups are somewhat different, it shows a similar pattern of two- to three-fold excess in age-specific incidence of type 2 diabetes in Hispanic compared

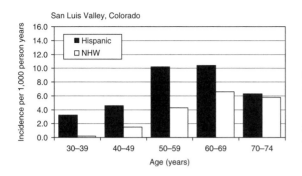
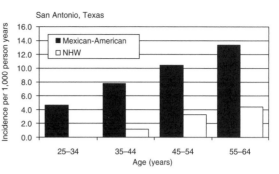

Figure 20.3 Incidence of diabetes (per 1000 per year) by age and race/ethnic group. Left: San Luis Valley, Colorado [18]; right: San Antonio, Texas [19].

with NHW persons. Burke *et al.* [20] have also shown that the incidence of type 2 diabetes is approximately two times higher in San Antonio low-income Mexican Americans than in similar residents of Mexico City, which was not explained by body mass index (BMI) differences.

The Nurses Health Study has recently reported diabetes incidence rates based on 20-year follow-up by race/ethnic group [21]. Hispanic nurses without diabetes at baseline ($n = 613$) had higher age-adjusted risk of developing self-reported diabetes than for NHW nurses (risk ratio RR = 1.76, 95% confidence interval (CI) 1.32–2.34). Adjustment for BMI increased the excess (RR = 1.86) and further adjustment for smoking, diet and physical activity reduced it only slightly (multivariate RR = 1.73, 1.30–2.31). Thus, Hispanic nurses had higher diabetes incidence which was not accounted for by differing patterns of obesity, diet or physical activity.

20.7 LIFETIME RISK

Narayan *et al.* [22] used a Markov model incorporating prevalence, incidence and mortality rates to estimate the cumulative lifetime risk of developing diabetes in the United States among a hypothetical cohort of births in the year 2000. Combining all race/ethnic groups, men had a 33% lifetime risk and women had a 39% risk (**Figure 20.4**). Hispanics had the highest estimated risk of any group (men, 45%; women, 53%). These lifetime risk estimates show the opposite gender pattern to prevalence/incidence data, likely due to higher mortality in males. Nearly one-half of Hispanics born in the year 2000 can

be expected to develop diabetes in the absence of major preventive interventions.

20.8 TRENDS IN DIABETES PREVALENCE AND INCIDENCE

Using data from the US NHIS conducted annually on the civilian noninstitutionalized household population, long-term trends in prevalence and incidence of diabetes have been established [10]. As shown in **Figure 20.5**, over the period from 1990 to 2004, the annual age-adjusted prevalence of self-reported diabetes increased among US NHWs from 2.7% to 4.3% in females and from 2.6% to 5.1% in males. Methods changed slightly in 1997; so, using the most comparable data, the percentage increase for 1997–2004 was 37.8% among NHW males and 19.4% among females. Obviously, the longer term increase has been even greater. For Hispanic persons, 1997 was the first year with adequate sample size to determine stable prevalence estimates. The prevalence has increased from 6.3% in 1997 to 6.8% in 2004 among females, and from 6.2% to 7.0% among males, a percentage increase of 12.9% to 7.9% respectively. Most of the increase has occurred among persons aged 45 years and older. Since these data are age adjusted to the 2000 US census standard population, differences in age make-up of the population over time do not influence these trends. Trends in prevalence appear similar for Hispanic and NHW populations in the United States.

In a recent publication of the combined results from several US Health and Nutritional Examination surveys (NHANES, Hispanic HANES) dating from 1960 to 2000, Gregg *et al.* [23] reported a

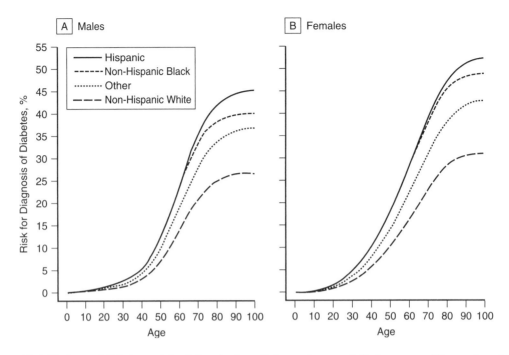

Figure 20.4 Estimated lifetime risk of developing diabetes by race/ethnic group. (Reproduced from [22], Copyright © 2003, the American Medical Association.)

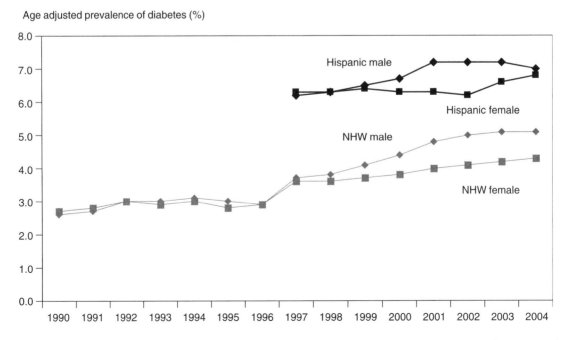

Figure 20.5 Average annual prevalence (%) of self-reported diabetes by year (3-year moving average), race/ethnicity and sex. United States National Health Interview Survey [10].

55% increase in total diabetes prevalence (both diagnosed and previously undiagnosed), due at least in part to an overall increase in obesity. However, when stratifying by BMI category, no important increases in diabetes prevalence were seen. Increasing trends in *diagnosed* diabetes occurred in all groups, suggesting that increased testing for diabetes was occurring, and especially in more obese groups. In a related analysis, the authors found that the proportion of diagnosed diabetes had risen dramatically, from 41% of total cases diagnosed in 1976–1980 to 83% in 1999–2000 [24]. These results are important when considering trends in self-reported diabetes since, as the population becomes more obese, simultaneous increases in detection appear to be happening among more obese persons, augmenting an apparent trend when self-reported outcomes are used. Other factors relevant to increases in prevalence include greater survivorship to older age groups from competing causes (leading to increased chances to be diagnosed with diabetes), reduction in CVD risk among persons with diabetes [25], lowering of the diagnostic glucose criteria for diabetes, as well as increased health care surveillance for diabetes, independent of real changes in incidence. There are no specific data for Hispanics presented

in these publications due to only recent addition of Hispanic populations large enough for analysis, though it seems likely that such trends would affect the Hispanic population as well, though perhaps to a lesser degree due to lower health care access [26].

Using NHIS self-reported data restricted to those persons diagnosed within the calendar year of the survey allows incidence rates to be estimated (**Figure 20.6**). From 1997 through 2004, the age-adjusted incidence of diagnosed diabetes increased 43% in Whites (from 4.6 per 1000 to 6.6 per 1000) and increased 34% in Hispanics (from 7.4 per 1000 to 9.9 per 1000) [10]. This effect was primarily seen in those older than age 45 years. Geiss *et al.* [27] showed that incidence was 1.9 per 1000 among normal weight persons and significantly higher (17.8 per 1000) among those with a BMI $\geq$ 30 kg m^{-2} in the period 2001–2003. Since these results are based on self-report, the potential influence of obesity may be partly due to more diabetes screening among obese persons [24], as noted for prevalence.

McBean *et al.* [14] also explored trends in older persons using Medicare Fee for Service beneficiaries data from 1994 to 2001. Among Hispanic persons older than 67 years there was

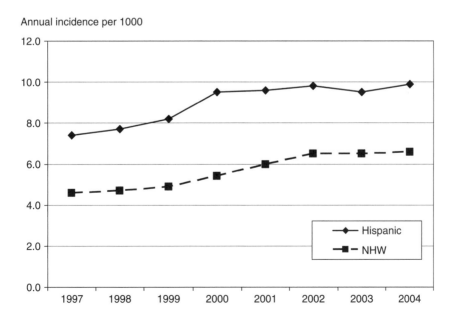

Figure 20.6 Trends in average annual incidence rates (per 1000) for Hispanic and NHW persons in the United States, 1997–2004 [10].

a significant 55% increase in incidence of diabetes among those without diabetes at baseline, consistent with data among younger age groups. Among NHWs, the increase was 37%. This dataset avoids self-reporting biases and has reasonable sensitivity and specificity for a diagnosis of diabetes.

A comparison of 7- to 8-year incidence trends for type 2 diabetes among both Hispanics and NHWs in San Antonio, Texas, is shown in **Figure 20.7** [28]. Nondiabetic subjects were enrolled over different years during the study and each person was followed for 7 to 8 years and retested using an OGTT for the development of diabetes. The rates shown in **Figure 20.7** have been annualized for comparison with other reports. Overall, incidence rates were 1.6 times higher among Hispanics than NHWs and the average increase was ∼ 10% per year and of similar magnitude in both racial/ethnic groups. Excluding subjects with impaired glucose tolerance (IGT) did not eliminate the secular trend, suggesting that it was not due simply to higher proportions of subjects with IGT at later examinations. Given the repeated testing design of the same cohort over 8 years, these results strongly suggest that Hispanic (and NHW) incidence is increasing rapidly over a surprisingly short time interval. It also indicates that higher incidence rates have been occurring among Hispanic populations throughout the 1980s, and the rise is not restricted to the mid–late 1990s.

There has also been a statistically significant increasing trend in BMI in both San Antonio and Mexico City Hispanics [29] between the 1980s and the 1990s. In Mexico City, it appears that the increasing BMI trend lines are similar to obesity prevalence that occurred in San Antonio perhaps 20 years earlier. Focusing only on the proportion of participants with BMI $\geq$ 30 kg m^{-2} (obese subjects), there was an increase in obesity of 2.7% per year in San Antonio (from 35% to 50% over a decade) compared with 1.5% per year in Mexico City (from 30% to 35% obese). The increasing trends in incidence rates reported from San Antonio [28] were adjusted for changes in obesity, as well as age, sex and type of neighborhood. Overall, obesity changes accounted for 28% of the increased risk of diabetes seen in San Antonio. There did not appear to be a decrease in the average age at onset among Hispanics in San Antonio [29], consistent with that seen in other US populations over a similar time period [27].

20.9 FUTURE PROJECTIONS

Using 1998 prevalence, incidence, mortality and population projections, Boyle *et al.* [30] at the CDC estimated the future growth of diabetes in the United States to the year 2050. In 2000, they estimated that the number of persons in the United States with

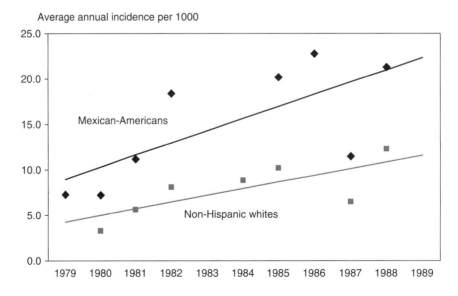

Figure 20.7 Average annual incidence of type 2 diabetes by oral glucose tolerance testing among persons in San Antonio, Texas, followed for 7–8 years [28].

diabetes was ~11 million and would increase to over ~29 million persons, an increase in prevalence from 3.99% (2000) to 7.21% (2050). Since 1998, incidence rates have increased and the relative risk of dying among persons with diabetes has decreased, so Narayan *et al.* recently updated these projections [31]. They now estimate that the 2005 prevalence (5.62%) will increase to 12.00% by 2050 with an estimated 48.28 million persons having diabetes. Hispanics are expected to increase from a prevalence of 5.47% (2005) to 12.39% (2050), a 127% increase. These projections are likely to be conservative, especially for Hispanics, since diabetes incidence is modeled to be constant from 2004 forward, whereas it is actually increasing, and since projections of the future number of Hispanics are likely to be low. Thus, the future burden of diabetes will be enormous in the United States, and especially among Hispanics.

The available data indicate that incidence rates are increasing in Hispanic (and other groups) in the United States. This results in increased prevalence, which is also increased due to decreases in mortality risk and increased screening in an aging population. Together, these forces are driving population prevalence substantially higher, a trend that is likely to continue well into this century. It is less clear what the cause(s) of the increased incidence are likely to be. While trends of increased obesity are clearly underway [28, 32–35], studies that have explored Hispanic to NHW differences in risk have usually found that they are incompletely explained by obesity and other lifestyle differences [21]. In addition, the temporal trends in incidence which were modeled in San Antonio Hispanics suggested that only approximately 28% of the increase might be explained by changes in obesity [28]. It is likely that this is a minimal estimate, since it did not account for age at onset of obesity or for duration of obesity, both factors known to be independently associated with diabetes risk in addition to current BMI [36, 37].

20.10 DIABETES MORTALITY TRENDS

Disease-specific mortality rates and trends impact observed prevalence and are another indicator of the burden of a disease in a population. Specific causes of death are reported in two ways: as 'any mention'

of a disease on death certificates (contributory and/or underlying) or as the 'underlying cause.' The first provides a picture of the general contribution a disease has to the overall mortality burden, whereas the latter provides a more specific assessment of the prevailing cause. Though most formal national vital statistics data generally use the underlying cause of death, comparing diabetes mortality rates based on the 'any mention' versus the underlying cause can be informative. Since diabetes is a major risk factor for CVD and other diabetes complications, its impact on mortality is broader than the underlying rates would suggest. A recent assessment from the Translating Research into Action for Diabetes (TRIAD) study [38] examines the reporting of diabetes as a cause of death among persons with known diabetes and describes trends over time. This recent assessment found any mention of diabetes in 39% of deaths and mentioned as the underlying cause in 10%, suggesting that this pattern of underreporting of diabetes continues to be a persistent problem [39, 40].

Figure 20.8 shows the percent of all deaths by age group for each ethnic group. Deaths attributed to diabetes as the underlying cause of death account for about 7% of all Hispanic deaths compared to 2.5% of NHW deaths. This excess in deaths due to diabetes for Hispanics is consistent across all age groups. The percentage of all deaths due to diabetes rises from early middle age and peaks as a percentage of all deaths in the 55–64 years range for both ethnicities. Over the age of 65 years there are other competing causes of death. Diabetes ranks

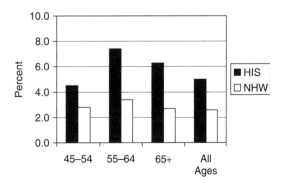

Figure 20.8 Percentage of all deaths due to diabetes as an underlying cause by ethnicity for selected age groups. HIS, Hispanic: black bars; NHW: white bars.

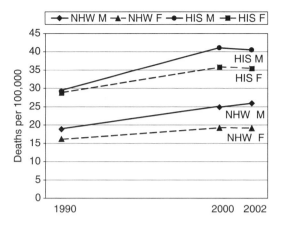

Figure 20.9 US age-adjusted death rates with diabetes as underlying cause of death by gender and ethnicity 1990, 2000, 2002. HIS: Hispanic.

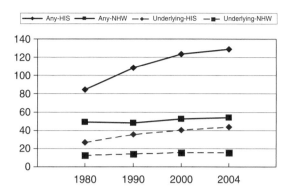

Figure 20.10 Colorado age-adjusted death rates with any and underlying cause of death mention of diabetes per 100 000 by ethnicity for 1980, 1990, 2000 and 2004. 'Any': any mention of diabetes; 'underlying': diabetes as underlying cause of death; HIS: Hispanic.

as the fifth and as the seventh leading cause in Hispanic and NHW deaths respectively [41].

Ethnic- and gender-specific trends in diabetes mortality as an underlying cause from three time points (1990, 2000, 2002) are shown in **Figure 20.9**, directly standardized to the 2000 population (Colorado Vital Statistics, Health Statistics Section, Colorado Department of Public Health & Environment, unpublished analysis). Hispanic men and women have consistently had substantially higher death rates in each year analyzed. Although the pattern of increasing death rates due to diabetes from 1990 to 2000 is reflected in both ethnic groups, the slope of the increase is much steeper for Hispanic men and women. The rates were 25% and 19% higher for NHW men and women respectively compared with 41% and 36% respectively for Hispanic men and women. In the short time between 2000 and 2002 there were few rate changes.

Figure 20.10 shows data for both 'any mention' and 'underlying cause' of death in Colorado for the period 1980–2004. Rates for 'any mention' of diabetes show the same pattern but with much higher mortality rates than rates of diabetes as 'underlying cause' (**Figure 20.10**). Death rates based on 'any mention' of diabetes are 3–3.5 times higher than the rates based on 'underlying cause' of death for both ethnic groups across all time periods. This underscores the significance of diabetes morbidity as a contributing factor to the overall mortality experience.

Patterns in Hispanic subgroup mortality are rarely described in the literature [42, 43] and difficult to compare due to different time-periods examined and characteristics of the populations studied (e.g. foreign born versus all Hispanics). Smith and Barnett [43], in comparing diabetes-related (underlying and contributing) mortality for Mexican Americans, Puerto Ricans and Cubans over the age of 35 using National Vital Statistics Data for 1996–1997, found a graded and substantial difference across subgroups. Mexican Americans had the highest rates (251 per 100 000), Puerto Ricans at 204 per 100 000 and Cubans having rates considerably lower at 101 per 100 000 (all adjusted to the 2000 US population). In all subgroups, diabetes-related death rates were higher for men than for women. Socioeconomic differences of lower educational attainment, lower income and higher percentages of persons living in poverty all mirror the subgroup differences observed [43].

Over 20 years ago, Markides and Coreil [44] made an observation concerning the *Hispanic epidemiological paradox* where, despite a more disadvantage socioeconomic position, Hispanic health outcomes, most notably mortality, were similar to or better than other non-Hispanic populations with socioeconomic advantages. In contrast to all-cause- and selected-cause-specific mortality patterns comparing Hispanics with non-Hispanic populations that have led to this observation, diabetes-related mortality patterns clearly do not fit the paradox. There remains a major health disparity for diabetes-related mortality for the Hispanic population. Hispanics have age-adjusted death rates due to diabetes 1.5–2 times those for NHW persons. This disparity has worsened, as NHW death rates due to diabetes have been relatively stable over 20–25 years and Hispanic death rates have steadily increased. Whether this is due to changes in classification of cause of death differentially by ethnic group over time or to real changes that mirror trends in prevalence and incidence rates is unanswered at present.

20.11   RISK FACTORS

Risk factors for type 2 diabetes among Hispanic Americans have been reasonably well studied. Metabolic risk factors for type 2 diabetes have been explored recently among Whites in the Framingham offspring cohort in Massachusetts and compared with NHWs and Mexican Americans in San Antonio, Texas [45]. **Figure 20.11** compares the age-adjusted percentage of each population with selected metabolic risk factors for males and females separately.

Among males, Mexican Americans have elevated levels of most risk factors compared with NHWs in San Antonio, though for several risk factors they are similar to males in Framingham. Among females, most metabolic risk factors are higher in Mexican Americans than females of both comparison groups,

except for hypertension and elevated fasting plasma glucose.

Trends in obesity and physical activity in the United States have recently been published [46]. **Figure 20.12** shows the prevalence of overweight and obesity over time among Hispanics compared with NHWs from the late 1970s through 2004. In each time period, Hispanics have a greater prevalence of overweight and obesity (BMI $\geq$ 25) with an increasing prevalence over time. Among adults classified as obese (BMI $\geq$ 30), Hispanic females have the highest prevalence, with Hispanic males being more similar to NHW persons, mirroring the results from San Antonio shown in **Figure 20.11** above. Since obesity is the major risk factor for type 2 diabetes, these trends are consistent both with the rising prevalence and incidence of type 2 regardless of race/ethnicity, and also with Hispanic excess risk.

The pattern of excess obesity in Hispanics is established early in life (**Figure 20.13**). Results from the National Health and Nutrition Examination Survey (1999–2000) showed that, over the age of 6 years, Hispanic youth were more obese than their NHW counterparts [47].

Figure 20.14 shows recent results from the NHIS for persons reporting no physical activity, another major risk factor for type 2 diabetes [46]. Almost 55% of Hispanic persons in the United States report being physically inactive, a prevalence significantly higher than among NHWs, among whom about 45% reported being inactive. Persons who live in poverty

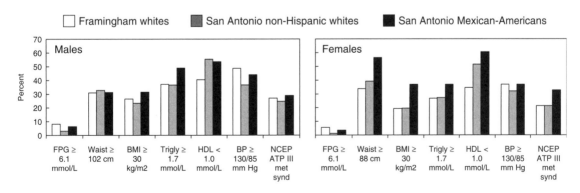

Figure 20.11 Age-adjusted percentage of population with risk factor levels above cut-point, by sex. White bars: Framingham offspring cohort; gray bars: NHWs in San Antonio, Texas; black bars: Mexican Americans in San Antonio, Texas. FPG: fasting plasma glucose; waist: waist circumference; BMI: body mass index; Trigly: triglyceride level; HDL: high-density lipoprotein cholesterol level; BP: blood pressure; NCEP ATP III: National Cholesterol Education Program Adult Treatment Panel III.

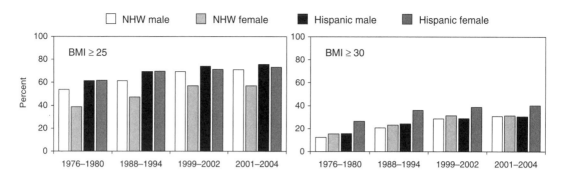

Figure 20.12 Percentage of US population with BMI ≥ 25 (left panel) or BMI ≥ 30 (right panel) by sex, time period and race/ethnic group; age adjusted to the 2000 US population [46].

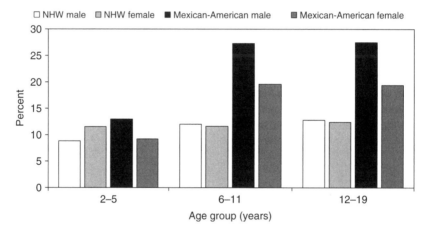

Figure 20.13 Percentage of youth with BMI ≥ 95th percentile for age, by sex and race/ethnic group. United States, 1999–2000 [47].

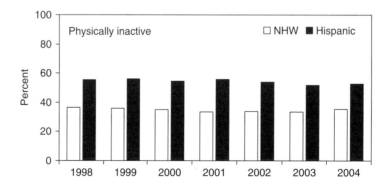

Figure 20.14 Percentage of US population who report no physical activity by race/ethnic group by year; age adjusted to the 2000 US population [46].

report less regular physical activity than those who do not live in poverty, and this is magnified among poor Hispanic populations, who report less physical activity than NHW persons in the same social strata.

As shown above, the Hispanic population has a higher prevalence of several major behavioral and metabolic risk factors for type 2 diabetes. However, studies that have directly examined the impact of measured risk factors on diabetes incidence have found that they act similarly in both Hispanic and NHW persons [9, 48, 49]. Obesity, central adiposity, lack of physical activity, higher intake of dietary fats, smoking and prenatal factors such as gestational diabetes in the mother confer similar levels of increased risk. Glucose intolerance, especially IGT, confers higher risk of diabetes in multiple populations, including among Hispanics in both Colorado and Texas [50]. Among persons with IGT who were randomized to either the intensive lifestyle or metformin interventions of the Diabetes Prevention Program (DPP), the reduction in diabetes incidence was similar in all race/ethnic groups, including persons of Hispanic ethnicity [51], again suggesting that the combination of risk factors present in persons with IGT act similarly in all race/ethnic groups.

Metabolic factors, including higher levels of insulin resistance and lower insulin secretion, have also been shown to predict diabetes independent of obesity and they appear to confer similar levels of increased risk in both Hispanic and NHW populations [52, 53].

As examples from recent data, the age–sex-adjusted prevalence was higher in both Hispanics and NHWs with lower levels of education, greater obesity and lack of participation in vigorous physical activity, but it did not vary by presence of health insurance in the six-state BRFSS data (**Figure 20.15**) [12]. No attempt was made in these results to determine if the Hispanic excess was explained by these factors.

Risk factors, including several markers of obesity and fat patterning, though acting similarly in both Hispanic and NHW populations, did not explain the 1.9-fold excess prevalence of type 2 diabetes in Hispanics in rural Colorado [54]. In San Antonio, Texas, the excess obesity and weight change seen in Hispanics compared with NHWs was also found not to explain the excess incidence [52]. In the most comprehensive evaluation of multiple risk factors to explain Hispanic excess diabetes, Shai *et al.* [21] explored the 20-year incidence of type 2 diabetes among Hispanic compared with NHW nurses in the Nurses Health Study. As noted above, after adjustment for BMI at baseline as well as for smoking, dietary intake (including fiber, trans fats, total calories) and physical activity, Hispanic nurses had 73% higher diabetes incidence over 20 years (95% CI: 30–231%).

There is relatively little documentation in large studies about the variability of risk factor patterns in meaningful subgroups of the Hispanic population. Evidence that social and cultural factors may play a role in obesity provides evidence that there may be important differences within this ethnic group. Sundquist and Winkleby [55, 56], in analyses of the third wave of the National Health and Nutrition Examination Survey (1988–1994), have examined

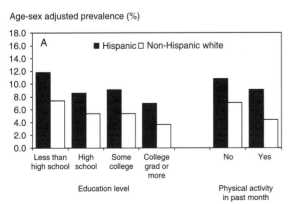
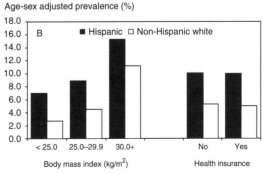

Figure 20.15 Age–sex-adjusted prevalence of self-reported diabetes by race/ethnic group and by selected risk factors. Black bars: Hispanic persons; white bars: NHWs.

country of birth, language and other risk factors in relation to obesity and risks of CVD. Adjusted for known covariates, Mexican-American men and women born in Mexico were least obese and had lower cardiovascular risk, whereas US-born English-speaking persons were intermediate on both outcomes, and US-born Spanish-speaking men and women had the highest levels obesity and were at highest risk for CVD. Although limited in number, such reports suggest that there is heterogeneity in diabetes and cardiovascular risk that may be important within the Hispanic population. Particular dimensions of variability, such as country of birth, language spoken and acculturation status, may also be critical variables in designing interventions for both prevention and treatment.

20.12　GENETIC ADMIXTURE

It appears that risk factors such as obesity, insulin resistance and secretion, physical activity and dietary patterns do not explain the excess Hispanic type 2 diabetes risk. This suggests that genetic factors, and/or gene-environment interaction is likely operating to increase the risk among Hispanics in the United States, especially those in the southwest, were Native American admixture is common. Genetic factors in the etiology of type 2 diabetes are reviewed in detail in Chapter 8 and will not be repeated here. However, the unique genetic data that bear on the excess risk among Hispanic populations suggests that the degree of individual American Indian admixture is associated with elevated risk of type 2 diabetes in southern Colorado Hispanics [57], as was first noted in San Antonio using older polymorphic protein markers [58].

Overall, Hispanics in the San Luis Valley of Colorado were estimated to be 65% European, 34% Native American and less than 1% African. The odds ratio for type 2 diabetes and admixture using a panel of 21 admixture informative markers was 8.1 (95% CI: 1.3–59) [57], which was reduced to 5.5 (0.8–41) when income was added to the model. Interestingly, addition of BMI to the age–sex–admixture-adjusted model had no impact, implying that obesity does not account for the admixture effect. These results suggest some degree of gene–environment interaction with income as a marker for socioeconomic and cultural influences. They also support the idea that

introduction of American Indian genes (probably occurring well over seven to eight generations ago [57]) has led to the higher risk of type 2 diabetes in southwestern Hispanics.

20.13　POSSIBILITIES FOR PREVENTION

Several recent randomized clinical trials have now shown that type 2 diabetes may be delayed for 3 to 7 years [59] and perhaps prevented altogether in a proportion of high-risk persons [60]. In the DPP conducted in the United States from 1992 to 2001, minority populations, including Hispanic persons from several different states, were recruited to participate [61]. Slightly over 1000 persons were randomized to each of the interventions: intensive lifestyle or metformin compared with blinded placebo. The largest reduction in risk occurred in the lifestyle group (58% lower risk over 2.8 years of follow-up) compared with placebo. The metformin group had a 33% lower risk. As shown in **Figure 20.16**, the risk reduction for both intervention groups was not different between persons of Hispanic origin and Caucasians (or for other race/ethnic groups) [51]. While the DPP randomized persons of several Hispanic origins, including in south Florida (Cuban Americans), New York (Puerto Rican Hispanics) and the US Southwest (Mexican Americans), no analysis of differences in these Hispanic subgroups has been reported, probably due to relatively small sample size.

One other randomized controlled prevention trial was conducted among Latina women in California. The TRoglitazone In the Prevention Of Diabetes (TRIPOD) trial was a single-center 5-year study to determine whether troglitazone prevented or delayed the onset of type 2 diabetes in high-risk Latina women with a history of gestational diabetes mellitus (GDM) [62, 63]. Two hundred and sixty-six women with confirmed GDM were randomized to placebo or 400 mg of troglitazone per day and 235 had at least one follow-up visit. The primary endpoint was the development of OGTT diabetes. After a median of 30 months of follow-up, the incidence rate in the placebo group was 12.3 per 100 person-years and was 5.4 per 100 person-years in the troglitazone group (hazard ratio 0.45, 95% CI

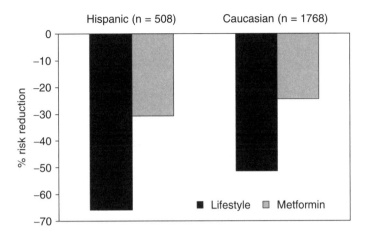

Figure 20.16 Percentage reduction in risk of developing diabetes over 2.8 years by intervention and race/ethnicity. Diabetes Prevention Program 1992–2002 [51].

$= 0.25\text{--}0.83, p = 0.001$). Troglitazone was discontinued in the study on removal from the market in 2000. Subgroup analysis showed that the majority of the effect was in women who improved their insulin sensitivity and reduced β-cell workload. In the subgroup considered nonresponders to treatment (lowest tertile of insulin sensitivity S_i change), diabetes developed at 9.8% per year, whereas in the responders (upper two tertiles) it was 3.0% per year.

These are the only randomized prevention trials that have included Hispanic persons. They both indicate that diabetes prevention using either lifestyle modification or medication is effective in Hispanics as in other population groups. This argues for a common biologic mechanism leading to reduced risk across multiple race/ethnic groups. However, they provide no data on the best individual and/or community-based prevention strategies to maximize risk reduction in the heterogeneous Hispanic communities throughout the United States, since these subgroups have different cultural, dietary and physical activity patterns that must be accounted for in planning such interventions.

20.14 PREVENTIVE PRACTICES FOR COMPLICATIONS

There are a number of evidence-based preventive care strategies that can reduce the risk of subsequent complications among persons with diabetes [64].

These include, among others, an annual dilated eye examination, home self-monitoring for blood glucose levels, hemoglobin ^{A1c} tests at least twice a year and an annual foot examination. During interviews conducted by most state health departments as a part of the BRFSS, persons with diabetes are asked about these preventive care practices [10]. **Figure 20.17** summarizes these findings among Hispanic persons in 42 states in 2004 and compares them with NHWs in the same states, adjusted for age. For each preventive practice, Hispanics report a somewhat lower frequency of receiving the care or testing their glucose at home. The frequency of these care practices has increased in both Hispanics and NHWs since 1994, when data were first reported; differences between Hispanics and NHWs have narrowed since then. The largest change has been in home glucose-monitoring, which rose 187% among Hispanics from 1994 to 2004, from 18% to 50%; among NHWs it increased 62%, from 37% to 61%. In both Hispanics and NHWs, there remain 30–50% of persons with diabetes who do not report using these preventive practices, suggesting that future complications will not be decreased to an optimal level. In addition, these process measures do not reflect the actual test outcomes. That is, having two ^{A1c} tests a year (process) does not imply good glucose control (outcome). Thus, while there are relatively small differences as of 2004 in the process of preventive practices, little is known about the outcomes of such care for Hispanics. In

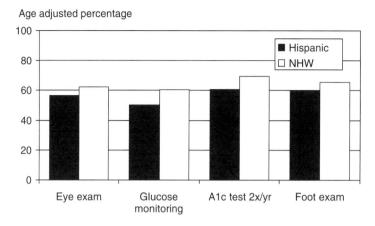

Age adjusted percentage

Figure 20.17 Age-adjusted proportion of persons with diabetes reporting preventive care practices in 2004 Behavioral Risk Factor Surveillance System, 42 states, by race/ethnic group. Black bars: Hispanic persons; white bars: NHW persons. Eye exam is dilated annual fundus examination; glucose monitoring is at home; A_{1c} is hemoglobin A_{1c} test at least twice a year; foot examination is annual. [10].

general, the more that process indicators are met, the better is the patient satisfaction and self-rated quality of diabetes care, but not levels of $A1_c$ or blood pressure [65].

There are a limited number of outcome studies of these practices among US Hispanics. As seen in other studies [66], Haffner *et al.* [67] found that Mexican Americans in San Antonio had similar prevalence of hypertension to NHWs; however, Mexican Americans had worse levels of hypertension control after adjustment for age, sex, obesity, fat distribution and education [67].

Kirk *et al.* [68] recently reviewed the available literature on ethnic disparities in outcomes of care. Levels of glycemic control as measured by Hb^{A1c} were higher in Hispanics than in NHWs in all eight studies reporting these levels, and a greater proportion of Hispanic persons had glycemia levels above a specified cut-point (e.g. $HbA_{1c} > 8\%$) in an additional six out of eight studies identified. Less consistency was seen for elevated blood pressure, though a trend was suggested for higher blood pressure and/or poorer control in Hispanic subjects than in NHW controls. Low-density lipoprotein cholesterol levels were consistently slightly lower among Hispanics than among NHWs in most studies reviewed. These limited data suggest that Hispanic persons have worse glycemic and blood pressure control, both major risk factors for microvascular complications in the future.

20.15 DIRECTIONS FOR FUTURE RESEARCH

As this chapter has described, the US Hispanic population is a young, socioeconomically disadvantaged, rapidly growing diverse ethnic group. Within this group, diverse national origins, immigration patterns and social and cultural traditions are represented which may impact health. This population has higher prevalence and incidence of type 2 diabetes than NHW populations. Hispanic type 2 prevalence is expected to increase 127% by 2050 and these projections are likely to be conservative, given the growth and age structure of this population. Although risk factors seem to be operating similarly in Hispanics and NHWs, the Hispanic population is characterized as having a higher prevalence of many of the risk factors for type 2 diabetes. This population is further characterized as having an earlier peak age of onset and increased risks of complications, especially microvascular complications. Diabetes-related mortality is also in excess and increasing for Hispanics. Thus, the future burden of diabetes in the US Hispanic population will be enormous.

Twenty years of examining the natural history of diabetes in population-based studies have not yet been able to fully explain the excess of diabetes in Hispanics. Future research needs to identify the combination of factors responsible for the increasing trends in diabetes risk with a focus on those modifiable at the population level. While obesity is clearly a major factor, early life factors such as obesity and diabetes during pregnancy, and early breast feeding habits, need to be considered. These studies should also include current genetic markers for diabetes so that potential gene–environment interactions can be explored to determine how much of the elevated risk in Hispanics is due to genes, to environment and to the interaction of these factors. In addition to the risk factors associated with obesity, physical activity and metabolic syndrome, further elaboration of the impact of social and cultural (particularly socioeconomic) factors on risk within and across populations is needed.

Although the number of studies examining meaningful subgroups of the Hispanic population are limited in depth and number, what do exist give clear indications that there is heterogeneity in risk diabetes and major complications *within* the Hispanic population. Particular dimensions of variability, such as country of birth, language spoken and acculturation status, may be critical variables in understanding risk, as well as for designing interventions for both prevention and treatment. Comprehensive multiethnic studies are required over longer time periods to address modifiable factors that can reduce future complications risk. Many of the intervening variables between the process and outcomes of care are influenced by personal and cultural values, socioeconomic status and acculturation. Whether the risk of complications can be reduced in Hispanic persons to the same degree as in persons of other race/ethnic groups is presently unknown and should be studied.

References

1. US Census Bureau (2006) Census 1990, Summary File 1, Matrices P3, P4, PCT4, PCT4, PCT8 and PCT11.
2. US Census Bureau (2006) Census 2000, Summary File 1, Matrices P3, P4, PCT4, PCT4, PCT8 and PCT11.
3. US Census Bureau (2005) Population Division. Annual Estimates of the Population by Race Alone and Hispanic or Latino Origin for the United States and States, July 1, 2004 (Table 4). (SC-EST2004-04).
4. Ramirez, R.R. and de la Cruz, G.P. (2003) The Hispanic Population in the United States: March 2002, Current Population Reports, P20-545, US Department of Commerce, Economics and Statistics Division, US Census Bureau, Washington, DC.
5. Guzman, B. (2001) The Hispanic Population: Census 2000 Brief, C2KBR/01-3, US Department of Commerce, Economics and Statistics Division, US Census Bureau, Washington, DC.
6. US Census Bureau (2007) Current Population Survey Annual Social and Economic Supplement, 2004 Tables 19.2, 18.2.
7. Gu, K., Cowie, C.C. and Harris, M.I. (1999) Diabetes and decline in heart disease mortality in US adults. *Journal of American Medical Association*, **281**, 1291–7.
8. Green, A., Stovring, H., Andersen, M. and Beck-Nielsen, H. (2005) The epidemic of type 2 diabetes is a statistical artefact. *Diabetologia*, **48**, 1456–8.
9. Stern, M.P., Mitchell, B.D. (1995) Diabetes in Hispanic Americans, in *Diabetes in America*, 2nd edn, NIH, Bethesda, pp. 631–59.
10. Centers for Disease Control and Prevention (2006) Diabetes Surveillance System, http://www.cdc.gov/diabetes/statistics/index.htm (accessed October 2006).
11. The SEARCH for Diabetes in Youth Study Group (2006) The burden of diabetes among U.S. youth: prevalence estimates from the SEARCH for diabetes in youth study. *Pediatrics*, **118**, 1510–18.
12. Burrows, N.R., Valdez, R., Geiss, L.S. and Engelgau, M. (2004) Prevalence of diabetes among Hispanics – selected areas, 1998–2002. *Morbidity and Mortality Weekly Report*, **53**, 941–4.
13. Cowie, C.C., Rust, K.F., Byrd-Holt, D.D. *et al.* (2006) Prevalence of diabetes and impaired fasting glucose in adults in the U.S. population: National Health and Nutrition Examination Survey 1999–2002. *Diabetes Care*, **29**, 1263–8.
14. McBean, A.M., Li, S., Gilbertson, D.T. and Collins, A.J. (2004) Differences in diabetes prevalence, incidence, and mortality among the elderly of four racial/ethnic groups: Whites, Blacks, Hispanics, and Asians. *Diabetes Care*, **27**, 2317–24.
15. Black, S.A., Ray, L.A. and Markides, K.S. (1999) The prevalence and health burden of self-reported diabetes in older Mexican Americans: findings from the Hispanic established populations for epidemiologic studies of the elderly. *American Journal of Public Health*, **89**, 546–52.
16. Flegal, K.M., Ezzati, T.M., Harris, M.I. *et al.* (1991) Prevalence of diabetes in Mexican Americans, Cubans, and Puerto Ricans from the Hispanic Health and Nutrition Examination Survey, 1982–1984. *Diabetes Care*, **14**, 628–38.

17. American Diabetes Association (1997) Report of the Expert Committee on the Diagnosis and Classification of Diabetes Mellitus. *Diabetes Care*, **20**, 1183–97.

18. Baxter, J., Hamman, R.F., Lopez, T.K. *et al.* (1993) Excess incidence of known non-insulin-dependent diabetes mellitus (NIDDM) in Hispanics compared with non-Hispanic whites in the San Luis Valley, Colorado. *Ethnicity and Disease*, **3**, 11–21.

19. Haffner, S.M., Hazuda, H.P., Mitchell, B.D. *et al.* (1991) Increased incidence of type II diabetes mellitus in Mexican-Americans. *Diabetes Care*, **14**, 102–8.

20. Burke, J.P., Williams, K., Haffner, S.M. *et al.* (2001) Elevated incidence of type 2 diabetes in San Antonio, Texas, compared with that of Mexico City, Mexico. *Diabetes Care*, **24**, 1573–8.

21. Shai, I., Jiang, R., Manson, J.E. *et al.* (2006) Ethnicity, obesity, and risk of type 2 diabetes in women: a 20-year follow-up study. *Diabetes Care*, **29**, 1585–90.

22. Narayan, K.M., Boyle, J.P., Thompson, T.J. *et al.* (2003) Lifetime risk for diabetes mellitus in the United States. *Journal of American Medical Association*, **290**, 1884–90.

23. Gregg, E.W., Cheng, Y.J., Cadwell, B.L. *et al.* (2005) Secular trends in cardiovascular disease risk factors according to body mass index in US adults. *Journal of American Medical Association*, **293**, 1868–74.

24. Gregg, E.W., Cadwell, B.L., Cheng, Y.J. *et al.* (2004) Trends in the prevalence and ratio of diagnosed to undiagnosed diabetes according to obesity levels in the U.S. *Diabetes Care*, **27**, 2806–12.

25. Imperatore, G., Cadwell, B.L., Geiss, L. *et al.* (2004) Thirty-year trends in cardiovascular risk factor levels among US adults with diabetes: National Health and Nutrition Examination Surveys, 1971–2000. *American Journal of Epidemiology*, **160**, 531–9.

26. Gary, T.L., Narayan, K.M., Gregg, E.W. *et al.* (2003) Racial/ethnic differences in the healthcare experience (coverage, utilization, and satisfaction) of US adults with diabetes. *Ethnicity and Disease*, **13**, 47–54.

27. Geiss, L.S., Pan, L., Cadwell, B. *et al.* (2006) Changes in incidence of diabetes in U.S. adults, 1997–2003. *American Journal of Preventive Medicine*, **30**, 371–7.

28. Burke, J.P., Williams, K., Gaskill, S.P. *et al.* (1999) Rapid rise in the incidence of type 2 diabetes from 1987 to 1996: results from the San Antonio Heart Study. *Archives of Internal Medicine*, **159**, 1450–56.

29. Williams, K., Stern, M.P. and Gonzalez-Villalpando, C. (2004) Secular trends in obesity in Mexico City and in San Antonio. *Nutrition Reviews*, **62**, S158–62.

30. Boyle, J.P., Honeycutt, A.A., Narayan, K.M. *et al.* (2001) Projection of diabetes burden through 2050: impact of changing demography and disease prevalence in the U.S. *Diabetes Care*, **24**, 1936–40.

31. Narayan, K.M.V., Boyle, J.P., Geiss, L.S. *et al.* (2006) Impact of recent increase in incidence on future diabetes burden: U.S., 2005–2050. *Diabetes Care*, **29**, 2114–16.

32. Ford, E.S., Mokdad, A.H., Giles, W.H. *et al.* (2005) Geographic variation in the prevalence of obesity, diabetes, and obesity-related behaviors. *Obesity Research*, **13**, 118–22.

33. Ford, E.S., Mokdad, A.H. and Ajani, U.A. (2004) Trends in risk factors for cardiovascular disease among children and adolescents in the United States. *Pediatrics*, **114**, 1534–44.

34. Mokdad, A.H., Ford, E.S., Bowman, B.A. *et al.* (2003) Prevalence of obesity, diabetes, and obesity-related health risk factors, 2001. *Journal of the American Medical Association*, **289**, 76–9.

35. Mokdad, A.H., Bowman, B.A., Ford, E.S. *et al.* (2001) The continuing epidemics of obesity and diabetes in the United States. *Journal of the American Medical Association*, **286**, 1195–200.

36. Lindsay, R.S., Cook, V., Hanson, R.L. *et al.* (2002) Early excess weight gain of children in the Pima Indian population. *Pediatrics*, **109**, E33.

37. Black, E., Holst, C., Astrup, A. *et al.* (2005) Long-term influences of body-weight changes, independent of the attained weight, on risk of impaired glucose tolerance and type 2 diabetes. *Diabetes*, **22**, 1199–205.

38. McEwen, L.N., Kim, C., Haan, M. *et al.* (2006) Diabetes reporting as a cause of death: results from the Translating Research into Action for Diabetes (TRIAD) study. *Diabetes Care*, **29**, 247–53.

39. Bild, D.E. and Stevenson, J.M. (1992) Frequency of recording of diabetes on US death certificates: analysis of the 1986 National Mortality Followback Survey. *Journal of Clinical Epidemiology*, **45** (3), 275–81.

40. Ochi, J.W., Melton, L.J., Palumbo, P.J. and Chu, C.P. (1985) A population-based study of diabetes mortality. *Diabetes Care*, **8**, 224–9.

41. National Center for Health Statistics, National Vital Statistics System (2006) WISQARS Leading Causes of Death Report (2000–2003), Office of Statistics and Programming National Center for Injury Prevention and Control, Centers for Disease Control and Prevention.

42. Rosenwaike, I. (1987) Mortality differentials among persons born in Cuba, Mexico, and Puerto Rico residing in the United States, 1979–1981. *American Journal of Public Health*, **77** (5), 603–6.

43. Smith, C.A.S. and Barnett, E. (2005) Diabetes-related mortality among Mexican Americans, Puerto Ricans, and Cuban Americans in the United States. *Pan American Journal of Public Health*, **18** (6), 381–7.

44. Markides, K.S. and Coreil, J. (1986) The health of Hispanics in the southwestern United States: an epidemiologic paradox. *Public Health Reports*, **101**, 253–65.

45. Meigs, J.B., Wilson, P.W., Nathan, D.M. *et al.* (2003) Prevalence and characteristics of the metabolic syndrome in the San Antonio Heart and Framingham Offspring studies. *Diabetes*, **52**, 2160–7.

46. National Center for Health Statistics (2006) *Health, United States, 2006 With Chartbook on Trends in the Health of Americans*, DHHS Pub. No. 2006-1232, U.S. Department of Health and Human Services, Centers for Disease Control and Prevention, National Center for Health Statistics, Hyattsville, MD.

47. Ogden, C.L., Flegal, K.M., Carroll, M.D. and Johnson, C.L. (2002) Prevalence and trends in overweight among US children and adolescents, 1999–2000. *Journal of the American Medical Association*, **288**, 1728–32.

48. Dabelea, D. and Hamman, R.F. (2003) The epidemiology of type 2 diabetes mellitus, in *Diabetes: A Fundamental and Clinical Text*, 2nd edn (eds D. LeRoith, S.I. Taylor and J.M. Olefsky), Lippincott-Raven, Philadelphia, PA.

49. Monterrosa, A.E., Haffner, S.M., Stern, M.P. and Hazuda, H.P. (1995) Sex difference in lifestyle factors predictive of diabetes in Mexican-Americans. *Diabetes Care*, **18** (4), 448–56.

50. Edelstein, S.L., Knowler, W.C., Bain, R.P. *et al.* (1997) Predictors of progression from impaired glucose tolerance to non-insulin-dependent diabetes mellitus: an analysis of six prospective studies. *Diabetologia*, **46**, 701–10.

51. The Diabetes Prevention Program Research Group (2002) Reduction in the incidence of type 2 diabetes with lifestyle intervention or metformin. *New England Journal of Medicine*, **346**, 393–403.

52. Haffner, S.M., Miettinen, H. and Stern, M.P. (1997) Are risk factors for conversion to NIDDM similar in high and low risk populations? *Diabetologia*, **40**, 62–6.

53. Baxter, J., Hamman, R.F., Hoag, S. *et al.* (1993) Hyperinsulinemia does not explain the ethnic difference in incidence of glucose intolerance between Hispanics (H) and non-Hispanic whites (NHW). The San Luis Valley Diabetes Study (Abstract). *Diabetes*, **42** (Supp 1), 30A.

54. Marshall, J.A., Hamman, R.F., Baxter, J. *et al.* (1993) Ethnic differences in risk factors associated with the prevalence of non-insulin-dependent diabetes mellitus: The San Luis Valley Diabetes Study. *American Journal of Epidemiology*, **137**, 706–18.

55. Sundquist, J. and Winkleby, M.A. (1999) Cardiovascular risk factors in Mexican American adults: a transcultural analysis of NHANES III, 1988-1994. *American Journal of Public Health*, **89**, 723–30.

56. Sundquist, J. and Winkleby, M.A. (2000) Country of birth, acculturation status and abdominal obesity in a national sample of Mexican-American women and men. *International Journal of Epidemiology*, **29**, 470–77.

57. Parra, E.J., Hoggart, C.J., Bonilla, C. *et al.* (2004) Relation of type 2 diabetes to individual admixture and candidate gene polymorphisms in the Hispanic-American population of San Luis Valley, Colorado. *Journal of Medical Genetics*, **41**, e116.

58. Chakraborty, R., Ferrell, R.E., Stern, M.P. *et al.* (1986) Relationship of prevalence of non-insulin-dependent diabetes mellitus to Amerindian admixture in the Mexican Americans of San Antonio, Texas. *Genetic Epidemiology*, **3**, 435–54.

59. Hamman, R.F. and Dabelea, D. (2007) Prevention of type 2 and gestational diabetes, in *The Evidence Base for Diabetes Care*, 2nd edn (eds W.H. Herman, A.L. Kinmonth, N. Wareham and R.L. Williams), John Wiley & Sons, Ltd, London.

60. Herman, W.H., Hoerger, T.J., Brandle, M. *et al.* (2005) The cost-effectiveness of lifestyle modification or metformin in preventing type 2 diabetes in adults with impaired glucose tolerance. *Annals of Internal Medicine*, **142**, 323–32.

61. Fujimoto, W.Y. (2000) Background and recruitment data for the U.S. diabetes prevention program. *Diabetes Care*, **23** (Suppl 2), B11–13.

62. Azen, S.P., Peters, R.K., Berkowitz, K. *et al.* (1998) TRIPOD (TRoglitazone In the Prevention Of Diabetes): a randomized, placebo-controlled trial of troglitazone in women with prior gestational diabetes mellitus. *Controlled Clinical Trials*, **19**, 217–31.

63. Buchanan, T.A., Xiang, A.H., Peters, R.K. *et al.* (2002) Preservation of pancreatic beta-cell function and prevention of type 2 diabetes by pharmacological treatment of insulin resistance in high-risk Hispanic women. *Diabetes*, **51**, 2796–803.

64. Williams, R.L., Tuomilehto, J. and Herman, W.H. (2002) *The Evidence Base for Diabetes Care*, John Wiley & Sons, Ltd, London.

65. Ackermann, R.T., Thompson, T.J., Selby, J.V. *et al.* (2006) Is the number of documented diabetes process-of-care indicators associated with cardiometabolic risk factor levels, patient satisfaction, or self-rated quality of diabetes care? The Translating Research Into Action for Diabetes (TRIAD) study. *Diabetes Care*, **29**, 2108–13.

66. Shetterly, S.M., Rewers, M., Hamman, R.F. and Marshall, J.M. (1994) Patterns and predictors of hypertension incidence among Hispanics and non-Hispanic Whites: the San Luis Valley Diabetes Study. *Journal of Hypertension*, **12**, 1095–102.

67. Haffner, S.M., Morales, P.A., Hazuda, H.P. and Stern, M.P. (1993) Level of control of hypertension in Mexican Americans and non-Hispanic Whites. *Hypertension*, **21**, 83–8.

68. Kirk, J.K., Bell, R.A., Bertoni, A.G. *et al.* (2005) Ethnic disparities: control of glycemia, blood pressure, and LDL cholesterol among US adults with type 2 diabetes. *Annals of Pharmacotherapy*, **39**, 1489–501.

21

Non-Caucasian North American Populations: African Americans

Mary A. Banerji and Harold Lebovitz

SUNY Health Science Center, New York, NY, USA

21.1 INTRODUCTION

Present-day African Americans originated in West Africa and came to the New World during the eighteenth-century slave trade. Their present heterogeneous West African, Native American and European genetic background may be the basis for their 1.5–2-fold greater prevalence of diabetes than whites. The majority of diabetes in adults is type 2 diabetes. Some of the predisposing factors for diabetes in blacks are similar to whites (age, sex, family history), some are different (generalized obesity, impaired glucose tolerance) and for some there are no reliable data (regional obesity, diet, physical activity). The excess prevalence of diabetes in African Americans is unexplained by the known risk factors and may be related to their specific genetic and environmental interactions.

A unique pathophysiological aspect of type 2 diabetes in African Americans is the presence of insulin-resistant and insulin-sensitive variants. In contrast, insulin resistance predominates in many other populations, such as whites and Hispanics. The insulin-sensitive variant, compared with the insulin-resistant variant, has a lower cardiovascular disease risk. This may explain the paradox among blacks, who, despite a high prevalence of diabetes and hypertension, have lower rates of coronary artery disease. The insulin-sensitive variant, characterized by insulin deficiency, may comprise up to 30% of diabetes in some African-American groups. Insulin resistance appears to be more importantly linked with the amount of visceral adipose tissue

in both African-American men and women with diabetes and not with subcutaneous adipose tissue. Serum triglycerides levels are also linked to visceral adipose tissue volume and liver fat content. Thus, the actual frequency of the insulin-sensitive and insulin-resistant subtypes may be related to the degree of visceral adiposity in the particular population, which is likely to be both environmentally and genetically determined.

There are unusual clinical variants of type 2 diabetes among African Americans: among those presenting with severe symptomatic hyperglycemia there is a component of pancreatic β-cell recovery resulting in long-term remissions (>3 years) off antidiabetic therapy without marked weight loss. In addition, adults not infrequently present with diabetic ketoacidosis (DKA) yet have type 2 diabetes: they are glutamic acid decarboxylase and islet cell antibody negative, insulin resistant, with relatively decreased insulin levels. They are obese, have family histories of diabetes and a clinical course typical of type 2 diabetes, requiring diet, oral agents or insulin for control of hyperglycemia.

In contrast to adults, in whom type 2 diabetes is more common than in whites, among children type 1 diabetes is much less frequent than in whites but more frequent than in native Africans, in whom it is uncommon. This is thought to be due to a genetic admixture with European diabetes susceptibility genes. Among children and adolescents there is a distinct maturity-onset diabetes of youth (MODY): acute hyperglycemic presentation, with and without diabetic ketoacidosis, variable obesity, positive

The Epidemiology of Diabetes Mellitus, second edition   Edited by Jean-Marie Ekoé, Marian Rewers, Rhys Williams and Paul Zimmet
© 2008 John Wiley & Sons, Ltd

family history of diabetes, absence of autoimmune markers and absence of an absolute requirement for insulin treatment.

The microvascular complications of diabetes, particularly retinopathy, nephropathy and amputations, affect African Americans disproportionately while the rates of macrovascular disease are lower.

21.2 PREVALENCE

Prevalence data for African Americans with type 2 diabetes comes from the National Health Interview Survey (NHIS), an annual population-based interview of physician-diagnosed illnesses [1] and the second National Health and Nutrition Examination Survey (NHANES II), 1976–1980, which screened for diabetes mellitus using the 2 h oral glucose tolerance test [2, 3]. NHANES II data should be interpreted with some caution because of the small numbers of African Americans who completed the oral glucose tolerance test compared with whites ($n = 351$ versus 3348). These epidemiologic data did not distinguish African Americans by their complex genetic background including European, West African and Native American Indian [4, 5].

The age-adjusted prevalence of physician-diagnosed diabetes is comparable in African Americans and whites below the age of 45, twofold greater over age 45 years and 16% in African Americans over age 75 years (**Figure 21.1**). These represent large numbers of subjects with diagnosed diabetes (**Table 21.1**). The prevalence of diabetes in adults has increased fourfold from 1963 to 1990 (**Figure 21.2**) with African-American women having the highest rates and largest increases [6].

NHANES II, using oral glucose tolerance testing, found nearly half of both African-American (and

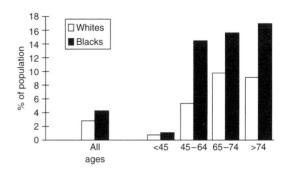

Figure 21.1 Percentage of diagnosed diabetes among US blacks and whites, 1994, NHIS. (National Center for Health Statistics [1].)

white) individuals with diabetes in the United States are undiagnosed, suggesting a large burden of potential diabetic complications [2, 7]. **Figure 21.3** shows total rates of diabetes (diagnosed and undiagnosed) by race, sex and age [7]. African-American women have higher rates at all ages except in the oldest age group of 65–74 years. **Figure 21.4** shows the separate rates of previously and newly diagnosed diabetes and impaired glucose tolerance by age in African Americans and whites [2]. The overall age-standardized prevalence of diagnosed and undiagnosed diabetes in African Americans is 1.5 times that of whites.

NHANES III (1988–1994) and NHANES 1999–2002 also shed light on prevalence. NHANES 1999–2002 screened for diabetes using fasting plasma glucose levels, not an oral glucose tolerance test. The overall population age- and sex-standardized prevalence rates of diagnosed and undiagnosed diabetes reported were 5.2% for whites 10.4% for Mexican Americans and 11.0% for

Table 21.1 Number of persons (in 1000s) with diagnosed diabetes, US 1992– 94 (NHIS).

Age (years)	1992 Black	1992 White	1993 Black	1993 White	1994 Black	1994 White	1992–1994 Average Black	1992–1994 Average White
<45	216	1033	304	1151	260	1086	260	1090
45–64	408	2238	578	2413	740	2314	575	2322
65–74	367	1710	292	1576	242	1572	300	1619
≥75	155	1106	141	1161	164	1053	153	1107
Total	1146	6087	1315	6331	1406	6025	1288	6138

Sources: National Center for Health Statistics [1, 203, 204].

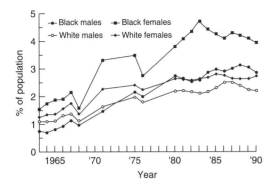

Figure 21.2 Time trends in the percentage of black and white men and women with diagnosed diabetes, US, 1963–90 (NHIS). (National Center for Health Statistics [202].)

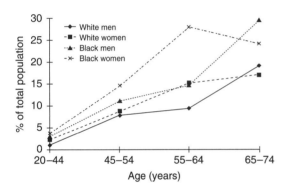

Figure 21.3 Percentage of the population with diagnosed and undiagnosed diabetes (WHO criteria), by age, sex and race, 1976–80 (NHANES II). (Reproduced from [7] by permission.)

non-Hispanic blacks. Significant changes in prevalence rates were found only in non-Hispanic blacks, with a 30% overall increase from 8.4% to 11.0% while there were no significant increase in whites and Mexican Americans [8].

21.3   INCIDENCE

The incidence of diabetes in African Americans has been estimated from NHANES I (1971–1975) follow-up data until 1987 [9]. Among 11 097 participants (9532 white and 1566 black) who were between the ages of 20 and 70 years at baseline, 880 incident cases developed. Since blood glucose was not originally measured, it is possible that some

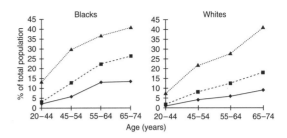

Figure 21.4 Percentage of the population with glucose intolerance—WHO criteria (diagnosed diabetes [solid line], undiagnosed diabetes [dashed line] impaired glucose tolerance [dotted line]) by race and age. (Reproduced from [2] by permission.)

of the cases which developed represent previously undiagnosed diabetes. The age-adjusted incidence of diabetes over the duration of the study was 15.0% in African-American women and 10.9% in men (comparable data in whites was 7% for both sexes).

21.4   RISK FACTORS FOR TYPE 2 DIABETES

Information on risk factors is derived from cross-sectional studies, since there are no good longitudinal data.

21.4.1   Age, Sex and Family History of Diabetes

Both age and sex are risk factors for diabetes, with African-American women having a greater risk than men and both sexes having a greater risk with increasing age; see **Figure 21.3** [1–3, 9].

Family history of diabetes was determined in NHANES II: among previously and newly diagnosed African-American diabetic subjects, age 20–54 years, 25% had a parent with diabetes and ~50% had a sibling with diabetes. In contrast, in individuals without diabetes, 19% had a parent with diabetes and 8% had a sibling with diabetes. The age-standardized prevalence of diabetes increased with numbers of diabetic first-degree relatives (**Table 21.2**). African-American individuals with 0, 1 and ≥2 relatives with diabetes had prevalence rates of diabetes of 7.8%, 11.8% and 23.3% respectively; the corresponding rates for whites

Table 21.2 Family history of diabetes as a risk factor for diabetes.

	Relative rates of diabetes* by number of family members with diabetes	
	1 vs 0	≥2 vs 0
Black	1.5	3.0
White	1.8	3.6

*Ratios of age standardized rates of diagnosed and undiagnosed diabetes, age 20–74.
Source: Reproduced by permission from Harris MI. Epidemiological correlates of Type 2 diabetes in Hispanics, whites and blacks in the US population. *Diabetes Care* (1991); **14** (suppl 3): 639–648.

were 4.6%, 8.4% and 16.3% [10]. This supports a possible dose effect for inherited diabetes risk factors [11].

21.4.2 Candidate Genes and Diet

There are few data on African Americans on the relationship of these factors to diabetes. While candidate genes do not explain the common forms of diabetes [12–15], the Z †4allele of the glucokinase gene was found to have an age-, sex- and body mass index (BMI)-adjusted odds ratio of 2.9 with onset of diabetes 10 years earlier in subjects of African ancestry [16, 17]. Mutations in *PAX4* have been identified in individuals with diabetic ketoacidosis of West African origin. PAX4 is a transcription factor which is responsible for the differentiation of β-cell progenitor cells into differentiated insulin-producing beta cells. These data must be replicated in order to assess their validity in light of a significant background population heterogeneity in *PAX4* in persons of West African origin [18]. NHANES II dietary data showed similar nutrient distributions among African American and white diabetics [7].

21.4.3 Physical Inactivity

Although higher levels of habitual physical activity are associated with lower prevalence of diabetes in various population studies [19–27], cross-sectional data showed increased work activity and decreased diabetes (previously and newly diagnosed) in Mexican Americans but not in African Americans or

whites [11]. African Americans report numerous barriers to exercise, including environmental (unsafe walking areas) and disease related (peripheral neuropathy and degenerative joint disease) [28].

21.4.4 Socioeconomic Status

In NHANES II, the rate of diabetes in African Americans declined with increasing income from poverty to middle income without a further decline in the upper income level [7, 11, 27]. Less than elementary school education was associated with a higher rate of diabetes compared with education beyond this. After adjusting for obesity and age, however, income and education were not strong risks for diabetes in African Americans. Data from NHANES 1999–2002 show similar trends.

21.4.5 Impaired Glucose Tolerance (IGT)

Often considered a prediabetic state [29], impaired glucose tolerance (IGT) constitutes nearly two-thirds of the total glucose intolerance in the United States population (IGT, diagnosed and undiagnosed diabetes) [30]. In contrast to diabetes, age-specific prevalence rates are similar in African Americans and whites. In whites and African-American males, IGT increases with age, but IGT declines after age 55 years in African-American females. Among African-American women age 65–74 years, the lower rate of IGT is not due to greater conversion to diabetes, since the total glucose intolerance is lower [2] and may reflect increased mortality in this group.

21.4.6 Obesity

Table 21.3 shows diabetic subjects are more obese than nondiabetic subjects; African-American women are more obese than white women regardless of glucose tolerance status [26]. The percentage of African American (58.8%) and white (45.2%) women with type 2 diabetes who are obese (BMI > 30 kg m^{-2}) is greater than African-American or white men (24.4% and 20.5% respectively) and highest among African-American women [29].

The increased prevalence of type 2 diabetes among African Americans is unlikely to be due simply to increased obesity. After adjusting for co-variates, obesity was associated with a higher risk of diabetes among African Americans relative to whites [31]: at ideal body weight, the risk of

Table 21.3 Mean body mass index (BMI) in persons age 20–74 years, NHANES II, (1976–80), based on diabetes status.

	Black		White	
	Men	Women	Men	Women
Previously DX diabetes	29.4	31.0	26.9	28.2
Newly Dx diabetes	*	31.4	26.7	31.3
Impaired glucose tolerance	27.5	29.7	27.4	27.4
Non-diabetic	25.3	26.0	25.2	24.2

Source: Cowie CC, Harris M et al. *Diabetes in America*, 2nd edn. National Institute of Health, 1995: appendix 7.9, p. 141, reproduced by permission.

diabetes was similar in African Americans and whites, but rose to 1.7 times at 150% of ideal bodyweight. This may be because BMI is not the ideal measure for metabolically important risk factor(s) for diabetes; measures of central or visceral adipose tissue may be better markers of increased risk. In other groups, longitudinal studies show the progression of normal to IGT is associated with an increase in insulin but without an increase in bodyweight in 30% of cases; these cases had an increase in central obesity [32, 33].

21.4.7 Regional Obesity

Although central obesity is associated with numerous adverse health outcomes [34–36], its role in African Americans is uncertain due to inadequate longitudinal studies. Whether the adverse effects of central obesity are mediated through insulin resistance or whether it is simply a marker for other defects is unknown. Beginning in childhood, nondiabetic African Americans have greater central obesity than whites [37–39]. Among whites, diabetes is more frequent with increased central obesity [35, 36]. Longitudinal NHANES I follow-up data suggest that higher central obesity predicts diabetes in both African Americans and whites [7]. However, cross-sectional NHANES II data show the frequency of diabetes is independent of central obesity (subscapular: triceps skinfold thickness) in blacks but

not whites [29]. Similarly, glucose-intolerant and normoglycemic Afro-Caribbean men had similar measures of central obesity (waist/hip ratio (WHR), waist/thigh ratio, sagittal abdominal diameter), whereas glucose-intolerant European men had greater central obesity than their normoglycemic counterparts [40]; Afro-Caribbean men had lower waist girths and Afro-Caribbean women had higher waist girths than their respective European counterparts [40–42]. These inconsistencies suggest that central obesity, as measured anthropometrically, may not be an optimum interracial yardstick for metabolically important fat depots: Conway *et al.* [43] and others [44, 45] report that the WHR (anthropometry) measures 23% less visceral adipose tissue as determined by magnetic resonance imaging in African-American women compared with white women. Thus, the diabetes risk of regional obesity must be assessed with direct techniques.

A unifying hypothesis may be that, among African Americans, insulin deficiency is as important a risk factor for diabetes as central obesity with its attendant insulin resistance [43–45]. Longitudinal studies are needed to delineate the relative roles of insulin deficiency and general versus regional obesity as risk factors for diabetes.

21.4.8 Insulin Resistance

Using cross-sectional data, an increase in underlying insulin resistance in African Americans has been proposed to explain their increased prevalence of diabetes [46, 47]. Insulin resistance is typically inferred from elevated fasting plasma insulin levels or from insulin responses to oral or intravenous glucose. The frequently sampled intravenous glucose tolerance test (FSIVGTT) [48, 49] and the euglycemic insulin clamp ('gold standard') are used less often to determine insulin resistance [50].

The case for increased insulin resistance among African Americans compared with whites is difficult to make with certainty from the cross-sectional data available. Variable fasting plasma insulin levels have been reported in African Americans compared with whites (higher in six studies [51–55] including children [56], the same in eight studies [42, 57–63] and lower in one study of newly diagnosed diabetics [64]). There is no consistent relationship between the fasting plasma insulin and the insulin responses to oral or intravenous glucose.

All five studies which measured insulin responses showed higher insulin responses in African Americans than in whites, but only one reported higher fasting plasma insulin; the rest were similar to whites. Additionally, higher insulin responses to stimuli may represent decreased hepatic extraction [42, 61] or differences in proinsulin/insulin ratios [65]; also, fasting plasma insulin is not a good measure of insulin resistance [66]. Thus, based on plasma insulin as a surrogate for insulin resistance, it is not clear whether African Americans are more insulin resistant than whites.

Using the FSIVGTT-S1, Osei and co-workers [46, 61] reported that nondiabetic African Americans without significant differences in BMI were more insulin resistant than whites. Similarly, the Insulin Resistance Atherosclerosis Study (IRAS) epidemiology study [55] found that nondiabetic African Americans compared with whites were more insulin resistant after multivariate adjustment for the increased obesity, smoking and sedentary behavior in African Americans. Osei and Cottrell [46] report that, among African Americans, nondiabetic first-degree relatives of type 2 diabetic subjects were as insulin resistant as nondiabetic controls and had similar insulin and glucose responses to oral glucose despite a greater BMI ($28 \, \text{kg m}^{-2}$ versus $24 \, \text{kg m}^{-2}$). In contrast, among whites, the first-degree relatives had a greater BMI and were more insulin resistant than controls. Comparing the African-American and white relatives, despite a 52% greater insulin resistance in blacks, their insulin levels in response to oral glucose were paradoxically similar. Osei and Cottrell's data suggest: (i) relative to their insulin resistance, African Americans are relatively insulin deficient; (ii) in the range of 24–$28 \, \text{kg m}^{-2}$, the BMI may not equally measure physiologically equivalent obesity in whites as in African Americans.

In contrast, two studies in nondiabetic African-American subjects used the euglycemic insulin clamp and reported no differences in insulin action compared with whites: one studied overweight African-American and white men with similar body mass indices ($30.8 \, \text{kg m}^{-2}$ versus $32.9 \, \text{kg m}^{-2}$) and percentage body fat levels (25% versus 30%) [63] and the other [67] studied lean, young nonhypertensive African-American men (BMI $23.8 \, \text{kg m}^{-2}$) in whom insulin action was similar to published data in control subjects [68, 69].

Thus, whether underlying insulin resistance, independent of obesity, is a risk factor for the excess prevalence of diabetes in African Americans is complex and unknown at present.

21.5 IS THERE A METABOLIC INSULIN RESISTANCE SYNDROME IN AFRICAN AMERICANS?

Insulin resistance, glucose intolerance, hyperinsulinemia, central obesity, dyslipidemia, hypertension and macrovascular disease are components of metabolic insulin resistance syndrome [70]. If the syndrome exists in a population and the components are causally related, then targeting the primary defect might eliminate the cascade of abnormalities. Selective reporting of the components makes assessment difficult in African Americans; the association of hyperinsulinemia and hypertension is weakest (**Table 21.4**). A perennial and controversial issue is whether disease risks associated with metabolic syndrome are more than what would be expected from its individual components alone.

21.5.1 Hyperinsulinemia

Increased plasma insulin levels were associated with higher triglyceride, glucose and low-density lipoprotein (LDL)-cholesterol levels in both African-American and white nondiabetic subjects; this association was strongest for lean subjects and less so for obese subjects [54, 71]. Among young African-American subjects, after adjusting for percentage body fat, WHR was associated with various cardiovascular risk factors (triglyceride, high-density lipoprotein (HDL)-cholesterol, LDL-cholesterol (women only), apolipoprotein A-1 and B, uric acid, systolic blood pressure (BP)); fasting plasma insulin only partly explained these associations [43, 59], suggesting that hyperinsulinemia may be a marker and not the basis for metabolic syndrome. Reports show that African Americans have more favorable lipid profiles than whites, including lower triglycerides and higher HDL-cholesterol levels despite similar or higher fasting plasma insulin levels, central obesity and glucose intolerance [51, 52, 58, 72, 73]. However, within the African-American population, plasma insulin is related to central obesity, glucose and plasma triglycerides [51, 52, 58]; **Table 21.4.** For

Table 21.4 Association of plasma insulin or insulin resistance to the components of the metabolic syndrome X in black subjects.

	Plasma insulin	Insulin resistance	Blood pressure	Glucose intolerance	Trig	HDL-chol	Central obesity SSST/waist/WHR	Comments
Fontbonne								Associations found in groups based on high and low plasma insulin level
Telecom [51]	X		Yes	Yes	Yes	Yes		
Freedman [57]	X				Yes	Yes		Children and adolescents–selected by extremes of plasma VLDL and LDL cholestrol levels
Jiang								
Bogalusa [75]	X		No					Ref. [54]: X-sectional data, association with central fat not seen in thin or sexually immature children; Ref. [73]: 6-year longitudinal data
McKeigue [41]	X		Yes	Yes	Yes		Yes	Association reported for mean only
Nabulsi [54]	X		No	Yes	Yes		Yes	Associations stronger for lean versus obese subjects
Folsom								
ARIC [209]	X						Yes	
Folsom [53]	X				Yes	Yes	Yes	Association of % body fat and CV risk factors not explained entirely by plasma insulin levels
Manolio						Yes	Yes	
CARDIA [59]	X							
Karter		X					Yes	
IRAS [62]								
Chaturved [52]	X			Yes	Yes			
Cruikshank [42]	X		No					Association found in whites but not blacks
Falkner [67]	X	X	Yes					Young lean hypertensive and normotensive men
Saad [63]	X	X	No					Young modestly obese US men
Osei [76]	X				No	No	Yes	1st-degree non-diabetic relatives of Type 2 diabetic subjects
Gaillard [77]	X		No	Yes	Yes*	No		1st-degree relatives of Type 2 diabetes US blacks n = 200 *association only in highest insulin quintile
Chaiken [78]		X	No		Yes	Yes*		Diabetic subjects *men only
Banerji [87, 89]		X			Yes		Yes	Diabetic subjects; Central obesity = total visceral fat measured by computed tomography

Trig = serum trigylceride levels HDL–chol = serum HDL–cholesterol levels SSST = subscapular or skinfold thickness WHR = waist to hip ratio the association of hyperinsulinemia and hypertension, some show a relationship [51, 58, 67], but the majority do not [42, 54, 6374–77]. A key regulator of plasma triglyceride levels is lipoprotein lipase, and some investigators have reported that the activity of this enzyme may not be related to insulin resistance (S1 derived from the FSIVGG) in African Americans as has been reported in Caucasians [71].

21.5.2 Insulin Resistance

Several reports show an inverse relationship between clamp-derived insulin resistance and triglycerides in African-American diabetic subjects [74, 78]. Chaiken [78] found no relationship with insulin resistance and hypertension in diabetic African-American subjects; Saad *et al.* [63] found similar results in nondiabetic African American but not white men. Karter reported an association of insulin resistance (SI derived from FSIVGTT) and waist circumference among African Americans which was weaker than in Hispanics and whites [62].

Metabolic syndrome was initially described using research measures of insulin resistance. When other associated features of elevated plasma insulin levels, elevated triglycerides, hypertension and central obesity were appreciated as well as their link with increased mortality, various organizations developed standardized *clinical* criteria to define the metabolic syndrome. In 1998, the World Health Organization (WHO) published a first definition followed by a modification, and in 2001 the US-based National Cholesterol Education Program (NCEP) Adult Treatment Panel III came out [79]. In response to a proliferation of definitions, the International Diabetes Federation (IDF) finally proposed a single definition. It should be remembered that these are all based upon expert consensus only and are described below.

1. The NCEP criteria required three of five of the following: (i) waist circumference >102 cm for men and >88 cm for women; (ii) plasma triglyceride >150 mg dl^{-1}; (iii) plasma HDL-cholesterol of <40 mg dl^{-1} in men and >50 mg dl^{-1} in women; (iv) BP > 130/85; (v) fasting plasma glucose >110 mg dl^{-1} (6.1 mmol l^{-1}).

2. The WHO criteria were (i) hyperinsulinemia, (ii) fasting plasma glucose >110 mg dl^{-1}, 2 h post prandal glucose >140 mg dl^{-1} or

a diagnosis of diabetes or use of diabetes medications, *plus* two of the following: (i) abdominal obesity (WHR > xx or BMI > 30 kg m^{-2}); (ii) dyslipidemia (plasma triglyceride >150 mg dl^{-1} and/or HDL-cholesterol <35 mg dl^{-1} in men and 37 mg dl^{-1} in women); (iii) BP > 140/90.

3. The IDF criteria: central adiposity defined ethnically, *plus* two of the following four factors: (i) high fasting plasma triglycerides (>150 mg dl^{-1}); (ii) low HDL-cholesterol (<40 mg dl^{-1} for men and <50 mg dl^{-1} for women); (iii) high systolic BP (≥130 mmHg) or high diastolic BP (≥85 mmHg); (iv) high fasting blood glucose (≥100 mg dl^{-1}) or a diagnosis of diabetes.

The frequency of metabolic syndrome in African Americans, Mexican Americans and whites among participants in the National Health and Nutrition Survey 1999–2002 are presented in **Figure 21.5** [79]. Overall, African-American men have the lowest rates compared with Mexican American or white men. A meta-analysis reports that metabolic syndrome using the NCEP or WHO criteria explains 6–7% of all-cause mortality, 12–17% of cardiovascular disease and 30–52% of diabetes [80].

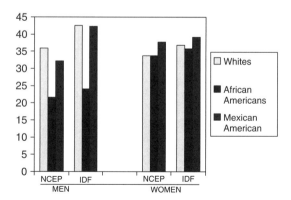

Figure 21.5 Comparison of frequencies of the metabolic syndrome in different racial groups from NHANES 1992–2002 using the NCEP or the IDF criteria. African American Men have the lowest rates of metabolic syndrome using wither criteria. Reproduced from [84].

21.6 PATHOGENESIS OF TYPE 2 DIABETES IN AFRICAN AMERICANS

Insulin-sensitive and -resistant variants in type 2 diabetes in African-Americans is a heterogeneous disorder with insulin-sensitive and insulin-resistant variants identified using the euglycemic insulin clamp method [81]. In contrast, most studies [4, 8, 68, 82], with few exceptions [83–85], report type 2 diabetes to be a disorder of insulin resistance. The two variants are notably different in terms of cardiovascular risk factors and body composition [74, 86, 87]. The insulin-sensitive variant has low lipid levels, whereas the insulin-resistant variant has higher lipid levels.

The relationship of insulin action to obesity was studied: most obese African-American type 2 diabetes subjects (BMI > 30 kg m^{-2}) were insulin resistant, but below this level they were equally likely to be insulin resistant as insulin sensitive [88]. Further, body composition studies using 23 scan computed tomographic techniques showed among modestly obese to lean diabetics (BMI 26.3 kg m^{-2} men and 27.7 kg m^{-2} women) that insulin-sensitive subjects had significantly lower visceral or intra-abdominal adipose tissue volume than the insulin-resistant variants [87]. In contrast,

there were no differences in subcutaneous adipose tissue volume. Comparing men and women with type 2 diabetes, total visceral adipose tissue volume was not different, whereas total or subcutaneous adipose tissue was twofold greater in women [87]. Insulin-mediated glucose disposal, derived using euglycemic clamp studies, was inversely related to visceral adipose tissue in both men and women, whereas there was no such relationship with subcutaneous adipose tissue (**Figure 21.6**). Increased visceral adipose tissue was related to increased liver fat (measured by computed tomography density) [89]. Liver fat content may alter the dynamics of hepatic insulin clearance [90]; thus, insulin resistance and hyperinsulinemia may both be the result of increased visceral adipose tissue and hepatic fat. Whether insulin sensitivity or visceral adipose tissue is genetically or environmentally determined is not known; however, differences in HLA-DQ subtyping in the resistant and sensitive variants [91] suggest a genetic component.

Insulin-sensitive subjects have low plasma LDL-cholesterol and triglyceride levels compared with insulin-resistant subjects, suggesting markedly different cardiovascular disease outcomes [74, 86]. Serum triglyceride is inversely related to

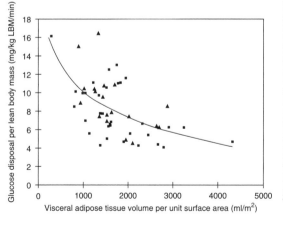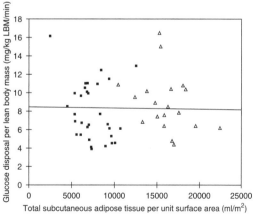

Figure 21.6 Relationship of insuline-mediated gluscose disposal (mg. kg lean body mass (LBM)$^{-1}$.min^{-1}) during a 1 mU.kg^{-1}.min^{-1} euglycemic insulin clamp with adipose tissue distribution in black men (filled squares) and women (open triangles) with Type 2 diabetes. Panel A: Glucose disposal and total visceral adipose tissue volume (ml/m^2 body surface area, BSA); equation for line shown is $y = -4.15 \ln(x) + 38.86$. Correlation coefficient $= -0.58, p = 0.0001$. Panel B: Glucose disposal and toal subcutaneous adipose tissue volume (ml/m^2 body surface area, BSA), correlation coefficient $= -0.27, p =$ not significant. (Reproduced from [87] by permission.)

insulin mediated glucose disposal levels, visceral fat and liver fat [89]. The presence of insulin-resistant and insulin-sensitive diabetic subtypes with differing cardiovascular risk factors is consistent with the lower serum triglyceride levels and higher HDL-cholesterol levels found among African Americans and Afro-Caribbeans compared with whites [51, 54, 58, 72] and their lower rates of cardiovascular disease [6, 42].

Several studies estimate the frequency of insulin-sensitive compared with insulin-resistant subtypes. Chaiken *et al.* [78] report that 30% (or 27 of 90) unselected African-American clinic-based type 2 diabetes subjects with a BMI $< 30 \, \text{kg m}^{-2}$ were insulin sensitive (euglycemic insulin clamp technique). Ginsberg and Rayfield [92] showed that, following treatment of hyperglycemia, some African-American type 2 diabetes subjects were normally insulin sensitive. In contrast, a small subset of the IRAS population-based study showed that only 11% of African-American type 2 diabetes subjects with a BMI $< 30 \, \text{kg m}^{-2}$ ($n = 60$) were insulin sensitive, using the FSIVGTT-S1 [47].

Whether differences in frequency of insulin sensitivity among studies of African Americans with type 2 diabetes are due to differences in amounts of visceral adipose tissue, inherent population differences or technique is not known. Insulin action measured by the FSIVGTT-S1 may not be equivalent to the euglycemic insulin clamp technique in diabetic subjects [48]. Therefore, based on the evidence, one can conclude that above a BMI of $30 \, \text{kg m}^{-2}$ African Americans with diabetes are likely to be insulin resistant, and up to 30% are likely to be insulin sensitive below this.

21.6.1 Pancreatic β-Cell Failure

Since diabetes in African Americans is metabolically heterogeneous [6, 64, 69, 72, 73, 81, 85], this suggests that a larger proportion of diabetes may be accounted for by poorer β-cell reserve occurring in the absence of marked insulin resistance. This concept is supported by: (i) UK Prospective Diabetes Study data showing Afro-Caribbeans had lower insulin secretion and were more insulin sensitive than European caucasians based on the homeostatic model assessment method [64]; (ii) physiological data showing markedly insulin-deficient (insulin-sensitive) versus relatively insulin-deficient (insulin-resistant) subtypes

in African Americans [81], as well as South African black data showing marked insulin deficiency with type 2 diabetes [93]; and (iii) epidemiological data showing that more African-American adults with diabetes use insulin than whites [88]. Insulin deficiency as a primary etiology for diabetes has also been reported in non-African-American populations (lean white US male veterans, Swedish and Japanese subjects [83–85]).

Further evidence that blacks compared with whites and Mexican Americans have altered insulin clearance and impaired β-cell function comes from data showing that black men and women had lower C-peptide levels than Mexican Americans did and had lower molar ratios of insulin to C-peptide [94].

Longitudinal data in several populations show that the development of diabetes is associated with a marked decrease in β-cell function and insulin secretion despite the presence of coexisting insulin resistance [94]. In contrast, individuals with normal glucose tolerance, followed over time, generally increase their body weight and become more insulin resistant but compensate by *increasing* insulin secretion. The observations are consistent with data in insulin-sensitive and insulin-resistant diabetic African Americans with near-normal glycemia who relapse into marked hyperglycemia; this transition is associated in both subtypes with a marked fall in insulin secretion [88].

21.7 CLINICAL VARIANTS OF DIABETES IN AFRICAN AMERICANS

21.7.1 Remission in Diabetes

African-American subjects with type 2 diabetes who present with severe hyperglycemia may develop long-lasting remissions [95, 96]. At the time of presentation, these individuals require hospitalization for severe symptomatic hyperglycemia (mean glucose $600 \, \text{mg dl}^{-1}$, 33.3 mm) and following a period of treatment, with antidiabetic pharmacologic agents they are able to discontinue these agents and remain in near normoglycemic remission with normal HbAlC levels. They are able to maintain this for years on their own version of a 'diet' including occasional ice cream, cake and barbecue [95, 97–102].

The development of remission is not associated with: (i) marked weight loss; (ii) reversal of stressful illness; or (iii) a 'transient honeymoon', or variant of immunologically mediated type 1 diabetes as evidenced by absent islet cell and glutamic acid decarboxylase antibodies [95].

The clinical characteristics of 72 individuals who developed remission were mean age 48 years and BMI 27.6 kg m^{-2} (range 21–35 kg m^{-2}); two-thirds were men. All had newly diagnosed type 2 diabetes and remission developed within 12 months. Most patients participated in intensive glycemic monitoring and regulation. Although the hemoglobin AlC was within normal range and mean fasting plasma glucoses were 110 mg dl^{-1} (6.1 mmol l^{-1}), oral glucose tolerance testing showed that 36/72 (50%) had a diabetic glucose tolerance test (2 h plasma glucose of 239 mg dl^{-1} or 13.3 mmol l^{-1}), 24/72 (33%) had IGT and 12/72 (25%) had normal glucose tolerance. Nearly all the individuals with normal glucose tolerance were insulin sensitive, whereas only half of those who were diabetic or had IGT were insulin sensitive, using the euglycemic insulin clamp technique.

Long-term follow-up of 8 years showed that remission off all medications was maintained for a median of 39 months, or 3.3 years (**Figure 21.7**) [96]. A small subset, not included in the analysis, has been in remission for 10–15 years. Additionally, once in remission, the usual medical or surgical 'stresses' did not perturb glucose homeostasis and precipitate a relapse to hyperglycemia. Mauvais-Jarvis *et al.* [103] also report durations of remissions of 40 months; these patients were either on a diet or low does of oral antidiabetes agents.

To determine the frequency of remission, all newly diagnosed type 2 diabetes subjects hospitalized with symptomatic hyperglycemia over 300 mg dl^{-1} (16.7 mmol l^{-1}) were treated intensively after discharge with multiple doses of insulin, diet and diabetes education. The hypothesis was that intensive glycemic regulation would reverse any element of glucose toxicity and potentially allow for the recovery of pancreatic β-cell secretory capacity essential for the remission. Of the first 26 patients followed for 120 days, 40% developed a remission [104]. Comparing those who did and did not develop a remission, presenting plasma glucoses, BMI, change in weight with treatment and HbAlC levels achieved with treatment were similar. This series has been extended to over 100 patients with similar results. In other racial groups, using continuous insulin infusions, remission rates were up to 90% in the first few months after therapy [105, 106]. Some studies have described remissions in patients of West African origin who present with ketoacidosis [107–113]. Morrison *et al.* [113] has reported 'phasic diabetes' in Afro-Caribbeans who present with severe symptomatic hyperglycemia and then do not return for treatment for prolonged periods and are asymptomatic despite hyperglycemia.

21.7.2 Recovery of β-Cell Function

Longitudinal studies show the transition from normal to IGT and type 2 diabetes in the context of insulin resistance is associated with progressive loss of β-cell function and decreased insulin secretion [114]. Worsening glycemia is associated

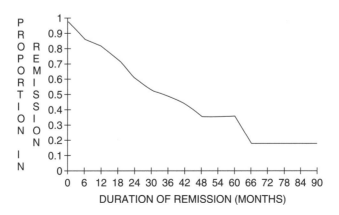

Figure 21.7 Proportion of black individuals remaining in remission over time:survival curve. (Reproduced from [96], Figure 1, by permission.)

with declining β-cell function [115]. If worsening glycemia is due to declining β-cell function, then improved glycemia as seen during remission may be due to improved β-cell function. The data in African Americans support this concept. The mechanism for remission must in some way be based on the recovery of β-cell function, since those who developed a remission had a greater recovery of insulin secretion [104]. On the basis of a previous series, individuals who are in remission are as likely to be insulin resistant as insulin sensitive; therefore, this would not distinguish remitters from nonremitters. Remission has also been described in other populations besides those of African origin, including Turks, Koreans, Chinese and Canadians [105, 106]. In addition to human studies, recovery of β-cell function is associated with normalization of the blood glucose concentration in a rat model as well as in cell culture systems [116–118].

21.7.3   Preservation of β-Cell Function

Intensive glycemic control at the onset of the diagnosis of diabetes is associated with the recovery of β-cell function and the question arises as to whether this improvement can be extended. This would allow for a prolonged period of normoglycemia. Data show that remission can be prolonged with low doses of pharmacologic agents. In a small double-blind placebo-controlled study, treatment with glipizide (1.25–2.5 mg day^{-1}) for 3.5 years significantly prolonged the duration of remission compared with placebo [119]. Umpierrez et al. [112] report that initial insulin treatment of African-American subjects presenting with severe hyperglycemia results in a partial recovery of insulin secretory capacity with good glycemic control being maintained with low doses of sulfonylurea.

Thus, near normoglycemic remissions, with normal HbAlC levels, occur in a predictable percentage of newly diagnosed African-American type 2 diabetes subjects who are intensively treated at the outset; this phenomenon is unassociated with weight loss, reversal of medical illness or 'stress', islet cell antibodies and does not appear to occur in longstanding diabetes. The duration of remission is significant and can be prolonged with low doses of sulfonylureas. The mechanism is related to the recovery of pancreatic β-cell function. Low-dose sulfonylureas preserve β-cell

function. One concludes that this phenomenon is likely to be an inherent feature of β cells and hence a novel treatment target for newly identified diabetes.

21.7.4   DKA in African-American Adults with Type 2 Diabetes

This entity was named *Flatbush diabetes* after the neighborhood in Brooklyn where it was first described. Subsequent authors have termed this *ketosis-prone diabetes mellitus* (KPDM).

Adult African Americans may present with DKA as their initial manifestation of diabetes, often without any precipitating events. A series of 21 cases (80% were newly diagnosed) showed that, following treatment, these individuals had a clinical course of type 2 diabetes [120]. Their mean presenting plasma glucose was 693 mg dl^{-1} (38.5 mm), pH 7.18, age 45 years and BMI 28.7 kg m^{-2}. Metabolic studies performed several months after the episode found all were insulin resistant, with significant residual C-peptide levels (but less than normal controls) in response to oral glucose stimulation. Because of the clinical course, metabolic studies and the absence of glutamic acid decarboxylase antibodies, these subjects are considered to be type 2 diabetes. Interestingly, these subjects had an increase in either HLA-DR3 or -DR4. This finding was confirmed by Mauvais-Jarvis et al. [103] but not others. Morrison et al. [113] has reported DKA Afro-Caribbean patients (Jamaicans) who are ultimately not insulin dependent.

Umpierrez and co-workers [121, 122] also reported African Americans presenting with DKA, all of whom were eventually considered to be type 2 diabetes: none had islet cell antibodies and 25/35 obese patients with DKA and 16/22 hyperglycemic patients without DKA were able to discontinue insulin treatment during follow-up. Initially, insulin response to carbohydrate stimulus was minimal; however, after 3 months, there was significant improvement, albeit not to normal. Among 56 consecutive admissions of African-American patients who presented to hospital with DKA, 25% were newly presenting and 75% were previously diagnosed. Among the latter, 67% had stopped their insulin, 14% had an infection, 5% had other illnesses and 14% had no identifiable cause [123]. Others have also described diabetic ketoacidosis in adults, among patients of African origin [107–111] and also among Japanese, Chinese, Native American, Hispanic and Caucasian populations. Among African-American patients who present with DKA, leanness and a prior history of DKA suggest that the patient is likely to be markedly insulin deficient even after initial treatment and have islet-cell-related autoantibodies or glutamic acid decarboxylase antibodies, implying an autoimmune etiology.

21.7.5 Atypical Diabetes of Childhood

Not all diabetes in childhood represents autoimmune type 1 diabetes and a distinct minority has an atypical version. Winter *et al.* [124] described African-American youths who presented with severe hyperglycemia and varying degrees of obesity, with and without ketoacidosis, who subsequently did not have an obligate requirement for insulin. There was no evidence of autoimmune markers, nor of an increase in frequency of HLA DR3 and HLA DR4. They represented ~9% of their clinic population. In a community incidence study, Lipton and Fivecoate [125] found that 7% of African-American boys and 16% of African-American girls were obese and many had positive family histories of diabetes suggesting atypical diabetes. Another clinic-based study notes that 50% of African-American children and adolescents with type 2 diabetes had presented with diabetic ketoacidosis and were obese. Type 2 diabetes was diagnosed by virtue of the lack of insulin dependence for short-term survival and lack of autoimmune markers. They did not identify an autosomal dominant mode of inheritance [126].

Umpaichitra *et al.* [127] described obese, mostly African-American children with type 2 diabetes with decreased but measurable C peptide and increased glucagon responses to a mixed meal challenge. Thus, relative hypoinsulinemia and hyperglucagonemia represent pancreatic β- and α-cell dysfunctions in children with type 2 diabetes. The severity of both β- and α-cell dysfunctions appears to be determined by the duration of diabetes. A recent study reported that these types of patient did not have hyperglucagonemia [128].

21.7.6 Insulin-Dependent Diabetes Mellitus in African-American Children

Among African-American children, type 1 diabetes is much less common than among whites [129]. The incidence of type 1 diabetes among African-American children <15 years of age varies geographically from 12.0 per 100 000 per year to 3.3 per 100 000 per year [130–132]. In contrast, among whites, the incidence ranges from 13.8 per 100 000 per year to 16.9 per 100 000 per year. As with other groups, diabetes is diagnosed less often in the summer. There may be a higher prevalence among girls than boys [125, 131–135]. The frequency of childhood diabetes in African Americans, whose slave ancestors originated in western Africa, is intermediate between western African children (in whom it is rare) and American whites [136, 137]. Therefore, it has been hypothesized that type 1 diabetes occurs in African Americans primarily as a result of an influx of Caucasian-derived diabetes susceptibility genes [138–140]. The regional differences in frequency of type 1 diabetes in US blacks may reflect differences in genetic admixture with Caucasians or different genetic–environmental interactions.

Type 1 diabetes is an autoimmune disorder. Polymorphism among certain class II immunoregulatory amino acid residues is strongly associated with type 1 diabetes. In humans, the class II genes are found in the major histocompatibility complex in the HLA-D region of the short arm of chromosome 6. Specific alterations in amino acid sequences affect peptide-binding and antigen-presenting capacities of the major histocompatibility complex [141]. There is an increased frequency of HLA DR3 and HLA DR4 in type 1 diabetes populations, the highest frequency being associated with heterozygous HLA DR3/HLA DR4 genotypes [142]. While the frequency of HLA DR3 and HLA DR4 is lower in the African-American population [121] compared with whites, their frequencies are increased in African American, Afro-Caribbean (black) and white type 1 diabetes populations [142–144]. HLA DR7 and HLA DR9 are also positively associated with type 1 diabetes in blacks but not in whites [145]. Among blacks, the HLA-DR and HLA-DQ relationships are different from whites: the HLA DQA1 allele, DQA1*0301 and the HLA DQB1 alleles, DQB1*0201 and DQB1*0302 are positively associated with type 1 diabetes [146].

The presence of aspartic acid at the 57th position of the HLA-DQ β-chain confers resistance to type 1 diabetes, while a nonaspartic acid residue is strongly associated with susceptibility in many populations, including African Americans [140, 147, 148]. Interestingly, there was no difference in the frequency of this marker among African Americans and whites with type 1 diabetes.

21.8 COMPLICATIONS OF DIABETES

21.8.1 Retinopathy

African Americans with diabetes have more retinopathy than whites [149]: up to 40% more severe retinopathy (self-reported, NHIS, 1977) [7] and 30–300% more blindness in diabetic African-American men and women respectively compared with their white counterparts [150–152]. This may be related to a greater frequency or to risk factors and to inadequate health care delivery: a report of 51 adult African-American diabetic subjects who received an initial ophthalmologic examination showed the median time to be 11.5 years after diagnosis and 37.5% had severe retinopathy [153].

Although African Americans do have more retinopathy than whites, the data do not suggest that they are inherently more susceptible to retinopathy than whites. NHANES III data, using fundal photography in diagnosed diabetics, showed that while any retinopathy was 46% higher in African Americans than whites (prevalence 18.2% versus 26.5%, $p = 0.07$), there was no difference after adjusting for risk factors for retinopathy, including BP and severity of diabetes (duration of diabetes, hemoglobin A1C level, treatment with insulin and oral agents) [151]. The prevalence of proliferative retinopathy was similar in the two groups (0.9% and 1.8% for African Americans and whites respectively). Similarly, there was no difference in nonproliferative retinopathy (direct ophthalmoscopy) in Afro-Caribbean Jamaicans compared with whites with type 2 diabetes after correcting for glycemia and other risk factors [133].

Among 70 consecutive newly diagnosed type 2 diabetic African-American subjects who presented with symptoms of hyperglycemia, 15% had background retinopathy when examined within 0–9 months of diagnosis (seven field fundal photographs) [154], which is similar to that in another study of urban blacks [155]. These data are comparable to other populations [156].

21.8.2 Nephropathy End-Stage Renal Disease (ESRD) Prevalence and incidence

Among both African Americans and whites with end-stage renal disease (ESRD), diabetes accounts for 30% of ESRD [157, 158]. Data from the Michigan Kidney Registry, from 1974 to 1983 (470 African American and 861 white diabetics with ESRD), shows an annual age-adjusted rate of 127.8 per 100 000 African-American diabetics and 50.2 per 100 000 white diabetics, with an African American: white incidence ratio of 2.55 [159]. **Figure 21.8** shows that that the incidence in African Americans is bimodal with peaks at ages 20 and 60 years [2] while whites have a single peak at age 30 years. Thus, the excess incidence of diabetic ESRD is attributable to type 2 diabetes and not to type 1 diabetes (African American: white incidence ratio 4.31 (95% confidence interval (CI) 3.6–5.52) and 1.03 (95% CI 0.73–1.36) respectively). Stephens reported similar data [160]. Most African Americans with diabetic ESRD had type 2 diabetes (77%) and most whites had type 1 diabetes (58%) [138]. Pugh et al. [161] confirm these data in African Americans with ESRD (84% type 2 diabetes, 13% type 1 diabetes) but differ in whites (59% type 2 diabetes, 39% type 1 diabetes). Recent data from the United States Renal Data Systems (USRDS) suggests that the incidence rates of ESRD are declining overall and have not risen among blacks [162–165]. The reason for these promising findings is not known, but may include improved diabetes, BP or lipid management

The risk of diabetic ESRD depends on type of diabetes and race [159, 162–165]. The estimated 10-year risk of diabetic ESRD, for African Americans and whites combined, is 5.2% for type 1 diabetes and 0.50% for type 2 diabetes (African Americans have an eightfold higher and whites have a 20-fold higher risk). The 10-year risk of diabetic ESRD is four times greater in African Americans than in whites with type 2 diabetes (1.06% versus 0.27%) and 1.62 times greater with type 1 diabetes (8.7% versus 5.38%).

Analysis of the NHANES and USRDS data showed that although the prevalence of chronic renal insufficiency (glomerular filtration rates (GFR) rates between 15 and 59 ml min^{-1} per 1.73 m^2) was not different in whites and blacks, the incidence of progression to new cases of ESRD was significantly greater (5% in blacks and only 1% in whites).

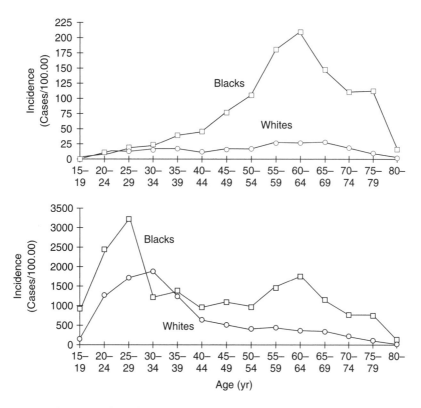

Figure 21.8 Age-specific rates of the incidence of diabetic end-stage renal disease among blacks and whites in Michigan, 1974–1983 Panel A shows the incidence per 100 000 general population and panel B the incidence per 100 000 diabetic patients. (Reproduced from [159], Figure 1, page 1076, by permission.)

These findings were only modestly affected by adjustments in gender, age and diabetes. Therefore, the increased incidence of ESRD in blacks was due to a greater likelihood of *progression* from chronic renal insufficiency, not to an increased population prevalence of chronic renal insufficiency [162–165] (**Figures 21.9** and **21.10**). The increased prevalence of diabetes appears to play a significant role in the increased numbers of individuals treated for ESRD accounting for 27% of the excess cases [162–165].

Overall, the 5-year *survival with diabetes and ESRD* is 24–30% compared with 48% with nondiabetic ESRD [157]. Paradoxically, despite a higher prevalence of hypertension and incidence of diabetic ESRD, African Americans have *better survival on dialysis treatment* than whites [166–168]. Data from the Michigan kidney registry in patients with age of onset of ESRD ≤65 years during the years 1974–1983 and followed through 1988 (284 African American and 311 white patients)

showed the median survival time was 27 months for Africans with type 2 diabetes and 16 months for whites (45% longer in African Americans than in whites). In contrast, transplantation was associated with equal and lower death rate than dialysis for both races without significant differences by type of diabetes [169]. This advantage in survival persists after adjusting for various comorbidities known to affect survival, including type of diabetes. Data from this study showed that, at the time of ESRD, African Americans had a significantly higher prevalence of left ventricular hypertrophy and higher BP but, interestingly, lower frequency of congestive heart failure (CHF) (58.5 versus 71.5, $p < 0.05$), lower frequency of myocardial infarction (MI) (23.5% versus 33.1%, $p < 0.10$) and a longer duration between first MI and ESRD (56.3 months versus 34.9 months, $p < 0.10$).

The reason for the higher rates of ESRD in African Americans is not known. Variations in

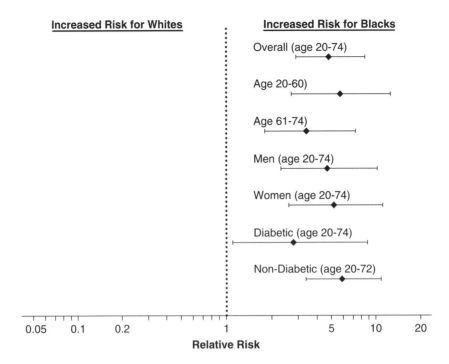

Figure 21.9 Black *versus* white relative risks for progression from chronic renal insufficiency (CRI) to ESRD cases, overall and by subgroup. Reproduced from [207].

BP, glycemic control, socioeconomic status and access to health care are reported as not accounting for the observed fourfold increase in African Americans versus whites with type 2 diabetes [170]. For example, after controlling for the increased prevalence of type 2 diabetes, glucose, BP, male sex and CHF, the likelihood of a serum creatinine >2 mg dl^{-1} was 91% higher in African Americans than in whites [171].

Inherited or genetic factors may account for the higher rates of ESRD. Freedman *et al.* [172] report a familial predisposition for ESRD among African Americans with type 2 diabetes with an eightfold greater increase in ESRD in individuals with a close relative with ESRD independent of glycemic control (after adjusting for smoking, hypertension and cholesterol levels). The susceptibility to ESRD is independent of the presence of type 2 diabetes in African Americans and is similar to data from Pima Indians and whites with type 1 diabetes [173, 174]. HLA associations may mark African-American type 2 diabetes patients with hypertension at risk for nephropathy compared with those without hypertension [175].

21.8.3 Early Diabetic Nephropathy

Since ESRD takes years to develop and itself causes hypertension, it is difficult to determine the relative roles of antecedent versus subsequently developing hypertension, glycemic control, duration of diabetes, microalbuminuria and hyperfiltration in the pathogenesis of diabetic nephropathy [176–178]. In cross-sectional and longitudinal studies, Chaiken *et al.* [177] report the natural history of early nephropathy in terms of duration of diagnosed diabetes and hypertension in 194 African-American type 2 diabetes subjects. Overt nephropathy (albumin excretion rates (AERs) >300 mg/24 h) was correlated with: (i) duration of diabetes; (ii) decrease in GFRs (measured with ^{125}I-iothalamate infusion) and increase in serum creatinine, and all these patients were hypertensive. Incipient nephropathy (AER 30–300 mg/24 h) was correlated with duration of diabetes and 80% of this group were hypertensive. Analysis in terms of the duration of diabetes and the presence or absence of hypertension showed that subjects who remained normotensive had normal renal function regardless of duration of diabetes (normal GFR and serum

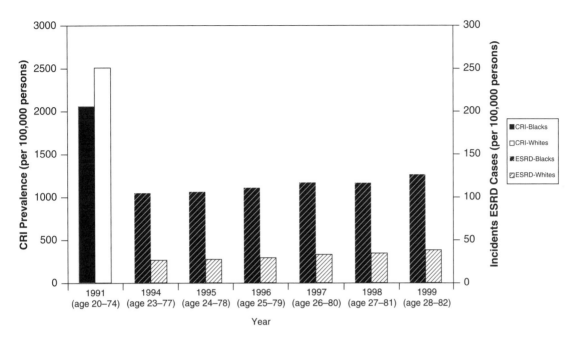

Figure 21.10 US prevalence of chronic renal insufficiency (CRI) in 1991 and incident cases of ESRD. CRI defined as proportion of people with CRI in 1991 from the Third National Health and Nutrition Examination Surveys projected to the overall population in 1991. Incident cases od ESRD defined as new cases form the United States Renal Data Systems in a particular year for a birth cohort divided by overall population in 1991. Reproduced from [207].

creatinine). In hypertensive subjects with type 2 diabetes, Chaiken *et al.* [177] found: (i) a decrease in GFR with duration of diabetes of greater than 1 year; (ii) with type 2 diabetes >10 years, 36% had impaired renal function (GFR < 80 ml m^{-2} and/or serum creatinine >1.4 mg dl^{-1}); 75% of these subjects have microalbuminuria or proteinuria. Within the group with longstanding diabetes, subjects who developed their hypertension after the diagnosis of diabetes were more likely to have nephropathy than those who developed hypertension prior to or at the time of diagnosis of diabetes (17/20 (85%) versus 7/13 (54%) respectively, $p < 0.05$), suggesting that nephropathy resulted in hypertension.

Within the first year of diagnosis of type 2 diabetes in African Americans, Chaiken *et al.* [177] showed an absence of microalbuminuria in subjects (mean age 47 years) with or without hypertension. In contrast, Goldschmid *et al.* [176] reported 30% to have microalbuminuria (mean age 52 years). The reason for this difference is unknown, but may be due to the older age or delay in presentation of diabetes in Goldschmid *et al.*'s patients. Similarly

to Chaiken *et al.*, they found that the risk factors for nephropathy were duration of diabetes and hypertension; multivariate analysis showed HbAlC did not predict nephropathy. Dasmahaptra *et al.* [178] reported that 50 out of 116 African-American clinic-based patients had increased AER, but did not report data for new-onset patients. AER correlated with age of onset, hypertension and BMI, but not with duration of diabetes, age, HbA1C or lipids. African Americans without diabetes had a twofold increase in micro- or macro-albumimuria than whites did after adjusting for confounders in the NHANES III epidemiological study [179].

Thus, early diabetic nephropathy, characterized by microalbuminuria, is associated with duration of diabetes and hypertension. The role of glycemia is not clear. It is not known whether urinary microalbumin excretion rates are associated with cardiovascular risk as in some groups [180, 181].

Early glomerular hyperfiltration has been variably associated with subsequent nephropathy in type 1 diabetes [182–185] but not in type 2 diabetes [186–189]. Chaiken *et al.* report hyper-filtration in 36% (15/42) of newly diagnosed (<1 year) African-American type 2 diabetic subjects in good glycemic control (GFRs ≥ 140 ml min^{-1} m^{-2} measured using a constant infusion of ^{125}I-iothalamate) [190–192]. Hyperfiltration occurred mostly in younger patients and up to age 62 years and persisted up to 10 years after the diagnosis of diabetes in 14–20% of subjects. It did not predict deterioration of renal function [192].

21.8.4   Amputations and Peripheral Vascular Disease

Based on hospital discharge records, amputations are higher for African Americans with diabetes than for whites [193]. Statewide data from California (1991) estimated that age-adjusted amputation rates were 95.3 per 100 000 versus 55.0 per 100 000 for African American and white diabetics respectively [194]. A major problem with such statistics is lack of long-term data integrating glycemic control, comorbid conditions and socioeconomic factors, including access to health care and delay in diagnosis. African Americans appear to have more lower extremity arterial disease than whites when measured using the ratio of the ankle systolic BP to the brachial systolic BP [195].

Based on these and other data, it is likely that neuropathy is greater in African Americans with diabetes, but few data are available.

21.8.5   Cardiovascular Disease

African Americans with diabetes have more macrovascular disease than those without diabetes [196, 197]. However, among patients with diabetes, African Americans have less atherosclerotic cardiovascular disease than whites. The frequency of angina and MI was 2.3–3.0 times greater in newly diagnosed and 50–20% higher in previously diagnosed whites compared with African-American diabetic subjects in NHANES II [7]. This is of interest because newly diagnosed African-Americans smoked more than whites (42% versus 28.7%) and smoking is a major cardiovascular risk factor [7]. Not only are African Americans with type 2 diabetes at lower risk for clinical coronary artery disease than whites with type 2 diabetes, in families enriched for type 2 diabetes, African-American men had

lower levels of coronary and carotid artery calcified plaque than white men despite increased conventional risk factors and increased carotid intimal medial thickness. Similarly, Afro-Caribbean blacks in England had half the hospitalizations for heart attacks (6% versus 13%) than whites, despite the greater rate (31% versus 14%) of diabetes [7, 9].

The lower rate of MI and angina in African Americans than in whites with type 2 diabetes is consistent with their lower serum triglycerides and higher HDL-cholesterol levels (adjusted for BMI) [10]. African-American men and women with diabetes versus those without had significantly lower total LDL-cholesterol and triglycerides and higher HDL-cholesterol (NHANES II) [72] **(Figure 21.11)**. In contrast, LDL-cholesterol was slightly higher in white diabetics than in nondiabetics [70]. These epidemiologic data showing lower rates of macrovascular disease and favorable lipids are consistent with the heterogeneous pathophysiology of type 2 diabetes in African Americans: up to 30% of African-American diabetics are insulin sensitive with lower triglyceride and LDL-cholesterol levels [69, 74]. Also, nondiabetic African Americans, compared with whites, have higher HDL-cholesterol levels and lower triglyceride levels [198–201].

Hypertension is a major risk factor for both macrovascular and microvascular disease, and African Americans with and without diabetes have higher BP than whites do [7]. The frequency of hypertension in the general population increases with age; however, among African Americans and whites with diabetes, the frequency of hypertension decreases after the age of 55 years. This may be related to increased mortality of diabetic subjects with hypertension. The majority of nondiabetic African Americans and whites do not have hypertension (60% and 70% respectively). The majority of diabetics do have hypertension: 63–80% among African Americans and 40–60% among whites.

Microalbuminuria is a risk factor for early nephropathy and cardiovascular mortality. Treatment with angiotensin-converting enzyme inhibitors improves both microalbuminuria and clinical outcomes. Among African-American patients with diabetes, persistent microalbuminuria despite ACE-I treatment appears to be associated with impaired vascular reactivity and may be a

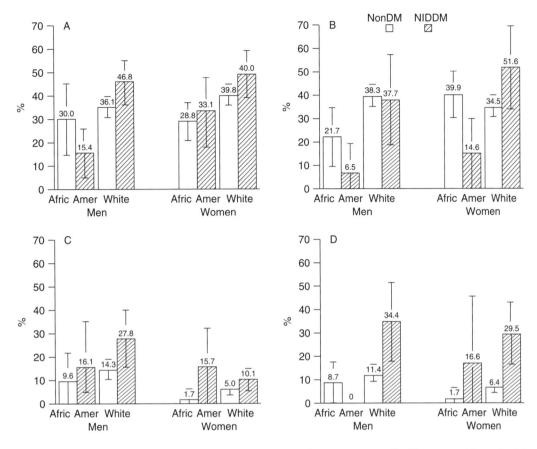

Figure 21.11 Frequency of dyslipidemia in black and white adults, age 40–69 years with and without Type 2 diabetes, US 1976–80. NHANES II. Panel A: total cholestral > 240 mg/dl, (B) LDL-cholestrol > 160 mg/dl, (C) HDL-cholestrol < 35 mg/dl, (D) fasting triglyceride < 250 mg/dl. (Reproduced from [72] by permission.)

marker for poor cardiovascular outcomes in this population [8].

21.8.6 Mortality of Diabetes

Twenty-two-year mortality data from the NHANES I study showed that the age-adjusted mortality rate for non-Hispanic blacks with type 2 diabetes was 23% higher than for non-Hispanic whites [202]. The mortality for African-American women and men with diabetes was significantly higher than for those without diabetes (40% and 50% respectively) [202, 203]. Diabetes was listed as an underlying cause of death in only 7.7% of diabetic men and 13.4% of diabetic women. This confirms that mortality data among African Americans (and others) with diabetes suffers from severe underreporting: the data are derived from hospital death certificates,

which list proximal cause but not underlying illness [1]. Mortality rates for African Americans and whites are similar at age <15 years for type 1 diabetes (0.1 per 100 000 population) [204–207].

References

1. Adams, P.F. and Marano, M.A. (1995) *Current Estimates from the National Health Interview Survey, 1994.* Vital and Health Statistics, Series 10, No. 193, National Center for Health Statistics, Hyattsville, MD.
2. Harris, M.I., Hadden, W.C., Knowler, W.C. and Bennett, P.H. (1987) Prevalence of diabetes and impaired glucose tolerance and plasma glucose levels in the US population age 20–74 yrs. *Diabetes Care*, **36**, 523–34.
3. Hadden, W.C. and Harris, M.I. (1987) *Prevalence of Diagnosed Diabetes, Undiagnosed Diabetes,*

and Impaired Glucose Tolerance in Adults 20–74 Years of Age, United States, 1976–80. Vital and Health Statistics Series, Series 11, No. 237, National Center for Health Statistics, Hyattsville, MD.

4. Reed, E.T. (1969) Caucasian genes in American Negroes. *Science*, **165**, 762–8.

5. Engerman, S.L. and Genovese, E.D. (1975) *Race and Slavery in the Western Hemisphere*, Princeton University Press, Princeton, NJ, pp. 107–28.

6. Kenny, S.J., Aubert, R.E. and Geiss, L.S. (1995) Prevalence and incidence of non-insulin dependent diabetes, in *Diabetes in America*, 2nd edn (eds M.I. Harris, C.C. Cowie, M.P. Stern *et al.*), NIH Publication No. 95-1468, National Institute of Health, National Institute of Diabetes and Digestive Diseases, Bethesda, MD, pp. 47–67.

7. Harris, M.I. (1990) Non-insulin dependent diabetes mellitus in black and white Americans. *Diabetes/Metabolism Reviews*, **6**, 71–90.

8. Cowie, C.C., Englegau, M.M., Rust, K.F. *et al.* (2006) Prevalence of diabetes and impaired fasting glucose in adults in the U.S. population. National Health and Nutrition Examination Survey 1999–2002. *Diabetes Care*, **29**, 1263–8.

9. Lipton, R.B., Liao, Y., Cao, G. *et al.* (1993) Determinants of non-insulin dependent diabetes mellitus among blacks and whites in a national sample. The NHANES I epidemiologic follow-up study. *American Journal of Epidemiology*, **138**, 826–39.

10. Cowie, C.C. and Harris, M. (1995) Physical and metabolic characteristics of persons with diabetes, in *Diabetes in America*, 2nd edn (eds M.I. Harris, C.C. Cowie, M.P. Stern *et al.*), NIH Publication No. 95-1468, National Institute of Health, National Institute of Diabetes and Digestive Diseases, Bethesda, MD.

11. Harris, M. (1991) Epidemiologic correlates of NIDDM in Hispanics, whites and blacks in the US population. *Diabetes Care*, **14** (Suppl 30), 639–48.

12. Cox, N.J., Epstein, P.A. and Spielman, R.S. (1989) Linkage studies on NIDDM and insulin and insulin-receptor genes. *Diabetes*, **38**, 653–8.

13. Murakami, K., Wilk, J., Nishida, K. *et al.* (1990) *Hep-G2* glucose transporter gene polymorphism in Caucasian, black and Hispanic and Japanese patients with NIDDM. *Diabetes Research and Clinical Practice*, **9**, 115–21.

14. Matsutani, A., Koraanyi, L., Cox, N. and Permutt, M.A. (1990) Polymorphisms of *GLUT2* and *GLUT4* genes: use in evaluation of genetic susceptibility to NIDDM in blacks. *Diabetes*, **39**, 1534–42.

15. Velho, G., Froguel, P., Clement, K. *et al.* (1992) Primary pancreatic beta cell secretory defect caused by mutations in glucokinase gene in kindreds of maturity onset diabetes of the young. *Lancet*, **340**, 444–8.

16. Chiu, K.C., Province, M.A. and Permutt, M.A. (1992) Gluco-kinase gene is genetic marker for NIDDM in American blacks. *Diabetes*, **41**, 843–9.

17. Chiu, K.C., Province, M.A., Dowse, G.K. *et al.* (1992) A genetic marker at the glucokinase gene locus for type 2 (non-insulin dependent) diabetes mellitus in Mauritian Creoles. *Diabetologia*, **35**, 632–8.

18. Mauvais-Jarvis, F., Smith, S.B., Le May, C. *et al.* (2004) *PAX4* gene variations predispose to ketosis-prone diabetes. *Human Molecular Genetics*, **13**, 3151–9.

19. Stern, M.P., Gonzales, C., Mitchell, B.D. *et al.* (1992) Genetic and environ- mental determinants of type II diabetes in Mexico City and San Antonio. *Diabetes*, **41**, 484–92.

20. Zimmet, P., Faaiuso, S., Ainuu, J. *et al.* (1981) The prevalence of diabetes in the rural and urban Polynesian population of Western Samoa. *Diabetes*, **30**, 45–51.

21. Zimmet, P., Seluka, A., Collins, J. *et al.* (1977) Diabetes mellitus in an urbanized isolated Polynesian population. The Funafuti study. *Diabetes*, **26**, 1101–8.

22. Wicking, J., Ringrose, H., Whitehouse, S. and Zimmet, P. (1981) Nutrient intake in a partly westernized isolated Polynesian population. The Funafuti study. *Diabetes Care*, **4**, 92–5.

23. Chen, M.K. and Lowenstein, F.W. (1986) Epidemiological factors related to self-reported diabetes among adults. *American Journal of Preventive Medicine*, **2**, 14–19.

24. Manson, J.E., Rimm, E.B., Stampfer, M.J. *et al.* (1991) Physical activity and incidence of non-insulin-dependent diabetes mellitus in women. *Lancet*, **338**, 774–8.

25. Manson, J.E., Nathan, D., Krowleski, A.S. *et al.* (1992) A prospective study of exercise and incidence of diabetes among US male physicians. *Journal of the American Medical Association*, **268**, 63–7.

26. Helmrich, S.P., Ragland, D.R., Leung, R.W. and Paffenbarger, R.S. Jr (1991) Physical activity and reduced occurrence of non-insulin dependent diabetes mellitus. *The New England Journal of Medicine*, **325**, 147–52.

27. Pan, X-R., Li, G-W., Hu, Y-H. *et al.* (1997) Effects of diet and exercise in preventing NIDDM in people with impaired glucose tolerance. The Da

Qing IGT and Diabetes Study. *Diabetes Care*, **20**, 537–44.

28. Duttin, G.R., Bodenlos, J.S., Johnson, J. *et al.* (2005) Barriers to physical activity among predominantly low-income African American patients with type 2 diabetes. *Diabetes Care*, **28**, 1209–10.

29. Cowie, C.C. and Harris, M. (1995) Physical and metabolic characteristics of persons with diabetes, in *Diabetes in America*, 2nd edn (eds M.I. Harris, C.C. Cowie, M.P. Stern *et al.*), NIH Publication No. 95-1468, National Institute of Health, National Institute of Diabetes and Digestive Diseases, Bethesda, MD, p. 143.

30. Cowie, C.C. and Harris, M. (1995) Physical and metabolic characteristics of persons with diabetes, in *Diabetes in America*, 2nd edn (eds M.I. Harris, C.C. Cowie, M.P. Stern *et al.*), NIH Publication No. 95-1468, National Institute of Health, National Institute of Diabetes and Digestive Diseases, Bethesda, MD, p. 141.

31. Cowie, C., Harris, M.I., Silverman, R.E. *et al.* (1993) Effect of multiple risk factors on differences between blacks and whites in the prevalence of non-insulin dependent diabetes mellitus in the United States. *American Journal of Epidemiology*, **137**, 719–32.

32. Lillioja, S., Mott, D.M., Spraul, M. *et al.* (1993) Insulin resistance and insulin secretory dysfunction as precursors of non-insulin dependent diabetes mellitus. *The New England Journal of Medicine*, **329**, 1988–92.

33. Bergstrom, R.W., Newell-Morris, L.L., Leonetti, D.L. *et al.* (1990) Association of elevated fasting C-peptide level and increased intra-abdominal fat distribution with development of NIDDM in Japanese-American men. *Diabetes*, **39**, 104–111.

34. Fujimoto, W.Y., Newell-Morris, L.L., Grote, M. *et al.* (1991) Visceral fat obesity and morbidity: NIDDM and atherogenic risk in Japanese American men and women. *International Journal of Obesity*, **15**, 41–4.

35. Larsson, B., Svardsudd, K., Welin, L. *et al.* (1984) Abdominal adipose tissue distribution, obesity and risk of cardiovascular disease and death: 13 year follow-up of participant in the study of men born in 1913. *British Medical Journal*, **288**, 1401–4.

36. Lapidus, L., Bengtsson, C., Larsson, B. *et al.* (1984) Distribution of adipose tissue and risk of cardiovascular disease and death: a 12 year follow-up in the population study of women in Gothenburg, Sweden. *British Medical Journal*, **289**, 1257–61.

37. Mueller., W.H. (ed) (1988) Ethnic differences in fat distribution in childhood, in *Fat Distribution During Growth and Later Health Outcomes*, Alan R. Liss, New York. pp. 127–45.

38. Stevens, J., Keil, J.E., Rust, P.F. *et al.* (1992) Body mass index and body girths as predictors of mortality in black and white women. *Archives of Internal Medicine*, **152**, 1257–62.

39. Kumanyika, S. (1987) Obesity in black women. *Epidemiologic Reviews*, **9**, 31–50.

40. Chaturvedi, N., McKeigue, P.M. and Marmot, M.G. (1994) Relationship of glucose intolerance to coronary risk in Afro-Caribbeans compared with Europeans. *Diabetologia*, **37**, 765–72.

41. McKeigue, P.M., Shah, B. and Marmot, M.G. (1991) Relation of central obesity and insulin resistance with high diabetes prevalence and cardiovascular risk in South Asians. *Lancet*, **337**, 382–6.

42. Cruikshank, J.K., Cooper, J., Burnett, M. *et al.* (1991) Ethnic differences in fasting plasma C-peptide in relation to glucose tolerance and blood pressure. *Lancet*, **338**, 842–7.

43. Conway, J.M., Yanovski, S.Z., Avila, N.A. and Hubbard, V.S. (1995) Visceral adipose tissue differences in black and white women. *The American Journal of Clinical Nutrition*, **61**, 765–71.

44. Duncan, B.B., Chambless, L.E., Schmidt, M.I. *et al.* (1995) Correlates of body fat distribution. Variation across categories of race, sex, and body mass in the atherosclerosis risk in communities study. The Atherosclerosis Risk in Communities (ARIC) Study Investigators. *Annals of Epidemiology*, **5**, 192–200.

45. Wang, J., Thornton, J.C., Burastero, S. *et al.* (1996) Comparisons for body mass index and body fat among Puerto Ricans, blacks, whites and Asians living in the New York City area. *Obesity Research*, **4**, 377–84.

46. Osei, K. and Cottrell, D.A. (1994) Minimal model analysis of insulin sensitivity and glucose-dependent glucose disposal in black and white Americans: a study of persons at risk for type 2 diabetes. *European Journal of Clinical Investigation*, **24**, 843–50.

47. Haffner, S.M., Howard, G., Mayer, E. *et al.* (1997) Insulin sensitivity and insulin response in African Americans, non-Hispanic whites and Hispanics with NIDDM: the insulin resistance atherosclerosis study. *Diabetes*, **46**, 63–9.

48. Saad, M.F., Anderson, R.L., Laws, A. *et al.* (1994) A comparison between the minimal model and the glucose clamp in the assessment of insulin sensitivity across the spectrum of glucose tolerance. Insulin Resistance Atherosclerosis Study. *Diabetes*, **439**, 1114–21.

49. Bergman, R.N., Finegood, D.T. and Ader, M. (1985) Assessment of insulin sensitivity in vivo. *Endocrine Reviews*, **6**, 45–86.

50. DeFronzo, R.A., Tobin, J.D. and Andres, R. (1979) Glucose clamp technique: a method for quantifying insulin secretion and resistance. *The American Journal of Physiology*, **2376**, E214–23.

51. Fontbonne, A., Papoz, L., Eschwege, E. *et al.* (1992) Features of the insulin-resistance syndrome in men from French Caribbean islands. The Telecom Study. *Diabetes*, **41**, 1385–9.

52. Chaturvedi, N., McKeigue, P.M. and Marmot, M.G. (1994) Relationship of glucose intolerance to coronary risk in Afro-Caribbeans compared to Europeans. *Diabetologia*, **37**, 765–72.

53. Folsom, A.R., Burke, G., Ballew, C. *et al.* (1989) Relation of body fatness and its distribution to cardiovascular risk factors in young blacks and whites. The role of insulin. *American Journal of Epidemiology*, **130**, 911–24.

54. Nabulsi, A.A., Folsom, A.R., Heiss, G. *et al.* (1995) Fasting hyperinsulinemia and cardiovascular disease risk factors in non-diabetic adults: stronger associations in lean versus obese subjects. *Metabolism*, **44**, 914–22.

55. Haffner, S.M., D'Agostino, R., Saad, M.F. *et al.* (1996) Increased insulin resistance and insulin secretion in non-diabetic African-Americans and Hispanics compared with non-Hispanic whites: the Insulin Resistance Atherosclerosis Study. *Diabetes*, **45**, 742–8.

56. Svec, F., Nastasi, K., Hilton, C. *et al.* (1992) Black–white contrasts in insulin levels during pubertal development. The Bogalusa Heart Study. *Diabetes*, **41**, 313–17.

57. Freedman, D.S., Srinivasan, S.R., Burke, G.L. *et al.* (1987) Pattern of body fat distribution to hyperinsulinemia in children and adolescents: the Bogalusa Heart Study. *The American Journal of Clinical Nutrition*, **46**, 403–10.

58. McKeigue, P.M., Shah, B. and Marmot, M.G. (1991) Relation of central obesity and insulin resistance with high diabetes. *Lancet*, **337**, 382–6.

59. Manolio, T.A., Savage, P.J., Burke, G.L. *et al.* (1991) Correlates of fasting insulin levels in young adults: the CARDIA study. *Journal of Clinical Epidemiology*, **44**, 571–8.

60. Osei, K., Cottrell, D.A. and Harris, B. (1992) Differences in basal and poststimulation glucose homeostasis in non-diabetic first degree relatives of black and white patients with type 2 diabetes mellitus. *The Journal of Clinical Endocrinology and Metabolism*, **75**, 82–6.

61. Osei, K. and Schuster, D.P. (1994) Ethnic differences in secretion, sensitivity and hepatic extraction of insulin in black and white Americans. *Diabetic Medicine*, **11**, 755–62.

62. Karter, A.J., Mayer-Davis, E.J., Selby, J.V. *et al.* (1996) Insulin sensitivity and abdominal obesity in African-American, Hispanic, and non-Hispanic white men and women. The Insulin Resistance and Atherosclerosis Study. *Diabetes*, **45**, 1547–55.

63. Saad, M.F., Lillioja, S., Nyomba, B.L. *et al.* (1991) Racial differences in the relationship between blood pressure and insulin resistance. *The New England Journal of Medicine*, **324**, 733–9.

64. UK Prospective Diabetes Study Group (1994) UKPDS study XII: differences between Asian, Afro-Caribbean and white Caucasian type 2 diabetic patients at diagnosis of diabetes. *Diabetic Medicine*, **11**, 670–7.

65. Clark, P.M., Levy, J.C. and Cox, L. (1992) Immuno-radiometric assay of insulin, intact proinsulin and 32–33 split pro-insulin and radioimmunoassay of insulin in diet treated type 2 (non-insulin dependent) diabetic subjects. *Diabetologia*, **35**, 469–74.

66. Boyko, E.J., Leonetti, D.L., Bergstrom, R.W. and Fujimoto, W.Y. (1997) Fasting insulin underestimates risk of non-insulin-dependent diabetes mellitus due to confounding by insulin secretion. *American Journal of Epidemiology*, **145**, 18–23.

67. Falkner, B., Hulman, S., Tannenbaum, J. and Kusher, H. (1990) Insulin resistance and blood pressure in young black men. *Hypertension*, **16**, 706–11.

68. DeFronzo, R.A., Simonson, D. and Ferrannini, E. (1982) Hepatic and peripheral insulin resistance: a common feature of type II (non-insulin dependent diabetes mellitus. *Diabetologia*, **23**, 313–19.

69. Chaiken, R.L., Banerji, M.A., Pasmantier, R.M., (1991) Patterns of glucose and lipid abnormalities in black NIDDM subjects. *Diabetes Care*, **14**, 1036–42.

70. Reaven, G.M. (1988) The role of insulin resistance in human disease. *Diabetes*, **37**, 1595–607.

71. Sumner, A.E., Vega, G.L., Genovese, D.J. (2005) Normal triglyceride levels despite insulin resistance in African Americans: role of lipoprotein lipase. *Metabolism*, **54**, 902–9.

72. Cowie, C.C., Howard, B.V. and Harris, M.I. (1994) Serum lipoproteins in African Americans and whites with non-insulin dependent diabetes in the US population. *Circulation*, **90**, 1185–93.

73. Summerson, J.H., Konen, J.C. and Dignan, M.B. (1992) Racial differences in lipid and lipoprotein levels in diabetes. *Metabolism*, **41**, 851–5.

74. Banerji, M.A. and Lebovitz, H.E. (1991) Coronary heart disease risk factor profiles in black patients with non- insulin dependent diabetes. *The American Journal of Medicine*, **91**, 51–8.

75. Jiang, X., Srinivasan, S.R., Bao, W. and Berenson, G.S. (1993) Association of fasting insulin with longitudinal changes in blood pressure in children and adolescents. The Bogalusa Heart Study. *American Journal of Hypertension*, **6**, 564–9.

76. Osei, K., Cottrell, D.A. and Bassetti, B. (1991) Relationship of obesity to serum insulin and lipoproteins in relatives of black patients with non-insulin-dependent diabetes mellitus (NIDDM). *International Journal of Obesity*, **15**, 441–51.

77. Gaillard, T.R., Schuster, D.P., Basad, B.M. (1997) The impact of socio-economic status on cardiovascular risk factors in African Americans at high risk for type II diabetes. Implications for syndrome X. *Diabetes Care*, **20**, 745–52.

78. Chaiken, R.L., Banerji, M.A., Huey, H. and Lebovitz, H.E. (1993) Do blacks with NIDDM have an insulin-resistance syndrome? *Diabetes*, **42**, 444–9.

79. Ford, E.S. (2005) Prevalence of the metabolic syndrome defined by the International Diabetes Federation among adults in the US. *Diabetes Care*, **28**, 2745–9.

80. Ford, E.S. (2005) Risks of all cause mortality cardiovascular disease associated with the metabolic syndrome. *Diabetes Care*, **28**, 1769–78.

81. Banerji, M.A. and Lebovitz, H.E. (1989) Insulin sensitive and insulin resistant variants in NIDDM. *Diabetes*, **38**, 784–801.

82. Swislocki, A.L.M., Donner, C.C. and Fraze, E. (1987) Can insulin resistance exist as a primary defect in non-insulin dependent diabetes mellitus? *Journal of Endocrinology and Metabolism*, **64**, 778–82.

83. Arner, P., Pollare, T. and Lithell, H. (1991) Different aetiologies of type 2 (non-insulin dependent) diabetes mellitus in obese and non-obese subjects. *Diabetologia*, **34**, 483–7.

84. Kelley, D.E., Mokan, M. and Mandarino, L.J. (1993) Metabolic pathways of glucose in skeletal muscle of lean NIDDM patients. *Diabetes Care*, **16**, 1158–66.

85. Taniguchi, A., Nakai, Y. and Fukushima, M., (1992) Pathogenic factors responsible for glucose intolerance in patients with NIDDM. *Diabetes*, **41**, 1540–6.

86. Banerji, M.A., Chaiken, R.L. and Gorden, D. (1995) Does intra-abdominal adipose tissue in black men determine whether NIDDM is insulin resistant or insulin-sensitive? *Diabetes*, **44**, 141–6.

87. Banerji, M.A., Lebowitz, J. and Chaiken, R.L. (1997) The relationship of visceral adipose tissue and glucose disposal is independent of sex in black NIDDM subjects. *The American Journal of Physiology: Endocrinology and Metabolism*, **273**, E425–32.

88. Banerji, M.A. and Lebovitz, H.E. (1992) Insulin action in black Americans with non-insulin dependent diabetes mellitus. *Diabetes Care*, **15**, 1295–302.

89. Banerji, M.A., Buckley, C. and Chaiken, R.L. (1995) The relationship of liver fat, triglycerides and visceral adipose tissue in insulin-resistant and insulin-sensitive black men with NIDDM. *International Journal of Obesity*, **19**, 846–50.

90. Bjorntorp, P. (1990) 'Portal' adipose tissue as a generator of risk factors for cardiovascular disease and diabetes. *Arteriosclerosis*, **10**, 493–6.

91. Banerji, M.A., Norin, A.J., Chaiken, R.L. and Lebovitz, H.E. (1993) HLA-DQ associations distinguish insulin-resistant and insulin-sensitive variants of NIDDM in black Americans. *Diabetes Care*, **16**, 429–33.

92. Ginsberg, H. and Rayfield, E.J. (1981) Effect of insulin therapy on insulin resistance in type II diabetic subjects: evidence for heterogeneity. *Diabetes*, **30**, 739–45.

93. Joffe, B., Panz, V.R. and Wing, J.R. (1992) Pathogenesis of non-insulin-dependent diabetes mellitus in the black population of southern Africa. *Lancet*, **340**, 460–2.

94. Harris, M.I., Cowie, C.C., and Gu, K. (2002) Higher fasting insulin but lower fasting C-peptide in Africans in the US population. *Diabetes/Metabolism Research and Reviews*, **18**, 149–55.

95. Banerji, M.A. and Lebovitz, H.E. (1990) Remission in non-insulin dependent diabetes mellitus: clinical characteristics of remission and relapse in black patients. *Medicine*, **69**, 176–85.

96. Banerji, M.A., Chaiken, R.L. and Lebovitz, H.E. (1996) Long term remission in NIDDM in blacks. *Diabetes*, **45**, 337–41.

97. Rendell, M., Zarriello, J. and Drew, H.M. (1981) Recovery from decompensated non-insulin dependent diabetes mellitus: studies of C-peptide secretion. *Diabetes Care*, **4**, 354–9.

98. Cheng, T.O., Jahraus, R.C. and Traut, E.F. (1953) Extreme hyperglycemia and severe ketosis with spontaneous remission of diabetes mellitus. *Journal of the American Medical Association*, **152**, 1531–3.

99. Crump, W.J. (1978) The honeymoon period in non-insulin-dependent diabetes mellitus. *The Journal of Family Practice*, **25**, 78–80.

100. Peck, F.B. Jr, Kirtley, W.R., Peck, F.B. Sr (1958) Complete remission of severe diabetes. *Diabetes*, **7**, 93–7.

101. Genuth, S.M. (1970) Clinical remission in diabetes mellitus. Studies of insulin secretion. *Diabetes*, **19**, 116–21.

102. Pirart, J. and Lauvaux, J.P. (1971) Remission in diabetes, in *Handbook of Diabetes Mellitus*, Vol. II (ed E. Pieffer), J.F. Lehmann Verlag, Munchen, pp. 443–502.

103. Mauvais-Jarvis, F., Sobngwi, E. and Porcher, R. (2004) Ketosis-prone type 2 diabetes in patients of sub-Saharan African origin: clinical pathophysiology and natural history of beta-cell dysfunction and insulin resistance. *Diabetes*, **53**, 645–53.

104. McFarlane, S., Chaiken, R.L. and Hirsch, S., (2001) Near-normoglycaemic remission in African-Americans with type 2 diabetes mellitus is associated with recovery of beta cell function. *Diabetic Medicine*, **18**, 10–16.

105. Ilkova, H., Glaser, B. and Tunckale, A. (1997) Induction of long term glycemic control in newly diagnosed diabetic patients by transient intensive insulin treatment. *Diabetes Care*, **20**, 1353–6.

106. Li, Y., Xu, W. and Liao, Z. (2004) Induction of long term glycemic control in newly diagnosed diabetic patients is associated with improvement in beta cell function. *Diabetes Care*, **27**, 2597–602.

107. Sobngwi, E., Vexiau, P., Levy, V. *et al.* (2002) Metabolic and immunogenetic prediction of long-term insulin remission in African patients with atypical diabetes. *Diabetic Medicine*, **19**, 832–5.

108. Sobngwi, E., Mauvais-Jarvis, F. and Vexiau, P. (2002) Diabetes in Africans. Part 2: ketosis-prone atypical diabetes mellitus. *Diabetes and Metabolism*, **28**, 5–12.

109. Maldonado, M., Hampe, C.S. and Gaur, L.G. (2003). Ketosis-prone diabetes: dissection of a heterogeneous syndrome using an immunogenetic and β-cell functional classification, prospective analysis, and clinical outcomes. *The Journal of Clinical Endocrinology and Metabolism*, **88**, 5090–8.

110. Balasubramanyam, A., Zern, J.W., Hyman, D.J. and Pavlik, V. (1999) New profiles of diabetic ketoacidosis: type 1 vs. type 2 diabetes and the effect of ethnicity. *Archives of Internal Medicine*, **159**, 2317–22.

111. Piñero-Piloña, A. and Raskin, P. (2001) Idiopathic type 1 diabetes. *Journal of Diabetes and its Complications*, **15**, 328–35.

112. Umpierrez, G.E., Clark, W.S. and Steen, M.T. (1997) Sulfonylurea treatment prevents recurrence

113. Morrison, E.Y., Ragoobirsingh, D., Thompson, H. *et al.* (1995) Phasic insulin dependent diabetes mellitus: manifestations and cellular mechanisms. *The Journal of Clinical Endocrinology and Metabolism*, **80**, 1996–2001.

114. Weyer, C., Bogardus, C., Mott, D.M. and Pratley, R.E. (1999) The natural history of insulin secretory function and insulin resistance in the pathogenesis of type 2 diabetes mellitus. *The Journal of Clinical Investigation*, **104**, 787–94.

115. U.K. Prospective Diabetes Study Group (1995) U.K. Prospective Diabetes Study 16. Overview of 6 years' therapy of type II diabetes: a progressive disease. *Diabetes*, **44**, 1249–58.

116. Kaisser, N., Nesher, R. and Donath, M.Y. (2005) *Psammomys obesus*, a model for environment–gene interactions in type 2 diabetes. *Diabetes*, **54** (Suppl 2), S137–44.

117. Kaiser, N., Yuli, M. and Üçkaya, G. (2005) Dynamic changes in beta cell mass and pancreatic insulin during the evolution of nutrition dependent diabetes in *Psammomys obesus*: impact of glycemic control. *Diabetes*, **54**, 138–45.

118. Guz, Y., Torres, A. and Teitelman, G. (2002) Detrimental effect of protracted hyperglycemia on beta cell neogenesis in a mouse murine model of diabetes. *Diabetologia*, **45**, 1689–96.

119. Banerji, M.A., Chaiken, R.L. and Lebovitz, H.E. (1995) Prolongation of near normoglycemic remission in NIDDM with sulfonylureas treatment. *Diabetes*, **44**, 44–7.

120. Banerji, M.A., Chaiken, R.L. and Huey, H. (1994) GAD antibody negative NIDDM in black subjects with DKA and increased frequency of HLA DR3 and DR4. *Diabetes*, **43**, 741–5.

121. Umpierrez, G.E., Casals, M.M.C. and Gebhart, S.S.P. (1995) Diabetic ketoacidosis in obese African Americans. *Diabetes*, **44**, 790–5.

122. Umpierrez, G.E., Woo, W. and Hagopian, W.A. (1999) Immunogenetic analysis suggests different pathogenesis for obese and lean African-Americans with diabetic ketoacidosis. *Diabetes Care*, **22**, 1517–23.

123. Musey, V.C., Lee, J.K. and Crawford, R. (1995) Diabetes in Urban African Americans: I. Cessation of insulin therapy is the major precipitating cause of diabetic ketoacidosis. *Diabetes Care*, **18**, 483–9.

124. Winter, W.E., Maclaren, N.K. and Riley, W.J. (1987) Maturity onset diabetes of youth in black. Americans. *The New England Journal of Medicine*, **316**, 285–91.

of hyperglycemia in obese African-American patients with a history of hyperglycemic crises. *Diabetes Care*, **20**, 479–83.

125. Lipton, R.B. and Fivecoate, J.A. (1995) High risk of IDDM in African American and Hispanic children in Chicago, 1985–1990. *Diabetes Care*, **18**, 476–82.

126. Pinhas-Hamiel, O., Dolan, L.M. and Zeitler, P.S. (1997) Diabetic ketoacidosis among obese African-American adolescents with NIDDM. *Diabetes Care*, **20**, 484–6.

127. Umpaichitra, V., Bastian, W. and Taha, D. (2001) C-peptide and glucagon profiles in minority children with type 2 diabetes mellitus. *The Journal of Clinical Endocrinology and Metabolism*, **86**, 1605–9.

128. Elder, D.A., Prigeon, R.L., Wadwa, R.P. and Dolan, L.M. (2006) D'Alessio beta cell function, insulin snesititvity and glucose tolerance in obese, diabetic and non diabetic adolescents and young adults. *The Journal of Clinical Endocrinology and Metabolism*, **91**, 185–91.

129. Tull, E.S. and Roseman, J.M. (1995) Diabetes in African Americans, in *Diabetes in America*, 2nd edn (eds M.I. Harris, C.C. Cowie, M.P. Stern *et al.*), NIH Publication No. 95-1468, National Institute of Health, National Institute of Diabetes and Digestive Diseases, Bethesda, MD, p. 622.

130. Tull, E.S., Makame, M.H., DERI Group (1992) Evaluation of type I diabetes in black African heritage populations: no time for further neglect. *Diabetic Medicine*, **9**, 513–21.

131. LaPorte, R.E., Tajima, N., Dorman, J.S. *et al.* (1986) Differences between blacks and whites in the epidemiology of insulin-dependent diabetes mellitus in Allegheny County, Pennsylvania. *American Journal of Epidemiology*, **123**, 592–603.

132. Wagenkrecht, L.E., Roseman, J.M. and Alexander, W.J. (1989) Epidemiology of IDDM in black and white children in Jefferson County, Alabama, 1979–1985. *Diabetes*, **38**, 629–33.

133. Lorenzie, M., Cogliero, E. and Schmidt, N.J. (1985) Racial differences in incidence of juvenile-onset type 1 diabetes: epidemiologic studies in southern California. *Diabetologia*, **28**, 734–8.

134. Lipman, T.H. (1993) The epidemiology of type 1 diabetes in children 0–14 years of age in Philadelphia. *Diabetes Care*, **16**, 922–8.

135. Tull, E.S., Roseman, J.M. and Christian, C.L.E. (1991) Epidemiology of childhood insulin-dependent diabetes mellitus in the US Virgin Islands from 1979–1988: evidence of an epidemic in the early 1980's and variation by degree of racial admixture. *Diabetes Care*, **14**, 558–64.

136. MacDonald, M.J., Famuyiwa, O.O. and Nwabuelo, I.A. (1986) HLA-DR associations in black type 1 diabetes in Nigeria: further support for models of inheritance. *Diabetes*, **35**, 583–89.

137. MacDonald, M.J. (1988) Speculation on the evolution of insulin-dependent diabetes genes. *Metabolism*, **37**, 1182–4.

138. Reitnauer, P.J., Go, R.C.P. and Acton, R.T. (1982) Evidence of genetic admixture as a determinant in the occurrence of insulin-dependent diabetes mellitus. *Diabetes*, **31**, 532–7.

139. Chakraborty, R., Mohammed, K.I., Nwankwo, M. and Ferrell, R.E. (1992) Caucasian genes in African Americans. *American Journal of Human Genetics*, **50**, 145–55.

140. Todd, J.A., Mijovic, C.H. and Fletcher, J.A. (1989) Identification of susceptibility loci for insulin dependent diabetes by transracial gene mapping. *Nature*, **338**, 587–9.

141. Garrett, T.P., Saper, M.A. and Bjorkman, P.J. (1989) Specific pockets for the side chains of peptide antigens in HLA-Aw68. *Nature*, **342**, 692–6.

142. Dunston, G.M., Henry, L.Q., Christian, J.Q. and Callender, C.O. (1989) HLA DR3, DQ heterogeneity in American blacks is associated with susceptibility and resistance to insulin-dependent diabetes mellitus. *Transplantation Proceedings*, **21**, 653–5.

143. Wang, C., Rivas, M.L. and Burghen, G.A. (1989) C4 and Bf phenotypes in black and Caucasian patients with childhood onset insulin-dependent diabetes mellitus. *Journal of Clinical and Laboratory Immunology*, **30**, 183–90.

144. Rodey, G.E., White, N. and Frazer, T.O. (1979) HLA-DR specificities among black Americans with juvenile-onset diabetes. *The New England Journal of Medicine*, **301**, 810–12.

145. Fletcher, J., Mijovic, C. and Odugbesan, O. (1988) Trans-racial studies implicate HLA-DQ as a component of genetic susceptibility to type 1 (insulin-dependent) diabetes. *Diabetologia*, **31**, 864–70.

146. Mijovic, C.H., Jenkins, D. and Jacobs, K.H. (1991) HLA-DQA1 and -DQB1 alleles associated with genetic susceptibility to IDDM in a black population. *Diabetes*, **40**, 748–53.

147. Dorman, J.S., LaPorte, R.E., Stone, R.A. and Trucco, M. (1990) Worldwide differences in the incidence of type 1 diabetes are associated with the amino acid variation at position 57 of the HLA-Dq beta chain. *Proceedings of the National Academy of Sciences of the United States of America*, **87**, 7370–4.

148. Todd, J.A., Bell, J.I. and McDevitt, H.O. (1987) HLA-DQ beta gene contributes to susceptibility and resistance to insulin-dependent diabetes mellitus. *Nature*, **329**, 599–604.

149. Rabb, M.F., Gagliano, D.A. and Sweeney, N.E. (1990) Diabetic retinopathy in blacks. *Diabetes Care*, **13**, 1202–26.

150. Kahn, H.A. and Hiller, R. (1974) Blindness caused by diabetic retinopathy. *American Journal of Ophthalmology*, **78**, 58–67.

151. Harris, I., Klein, R. and Cowie, C.C. (1998) Is the risk of diabetic retinopathy greater in non-Hispanic blacks and Mexican-Americans than in non-Hispanic whites with type 2 diabetes: a US population study. *Diabetes Care*, **21**, 1230–5.

152. Cruikshank, J.K. and Alleyne, S.A. (1987) Black West Indian and matched white diabetics in Britain compared with diabetes in Jamaica: body mass, blood pressure and vascular disease. *Diabetes Care*, **10**, 170–9.

153. Appiah, A.P., Ganthier, R. Jr and Watkins, N. (1991) Delayed diagnosis of diabetic retinopathy in black and Hispanic patients with diabetes mellitus. *Annals of Ophthalmology*, **23**, 156–8.

154. Banerji, M.A., Berman, D., Chaiken, R.L. and Lebovitz, H.E. Frequency of retinopathy in newly diagnosed diabetes (unpublished data).

155. El-Kebbi, I.M., Ziemer, D.C., Gallina, D.L. and Phillips, L.S. (1998) Diabetes in urban African-Americans. Utility of fasting or random glucose in identifying poor glycemic control. *Diabetes Care*, **21**, 501–5.

156. Davis, T.M., Stratton, I.M., Fox, C.J. *et al.* (1997) UK Prospective Diabetes Study 22. Effect of age at diagnosis on tissue damage during the first 6 years of NIDDM. *Diabetes Care*, **20**, 1435–41.

157. Held, P.J. and Pork, F.K. (1991) Webb RL USRDS 1991. *American Journal of Kidney Diseases*, **19** (Suppl 2), 1.

158. US Renal Data System (1994) US Renal Data System 1994 Annual Report, National Institute of Health, National Institute of Diabetes and Digestive Diseases, Division of Kidney, Urologic and Hematologic Diseases, Bethesda, MD.

159. Cowie, C.C., Pork, F.K. and Wolfe, R.A. (1989) Disparities in the incidence of end-stage renal disease; according to race and type of diabetes. *The New England Journal of Medicine*, **321**, 1074–9.

160. Stephens, G.W., Gillaspy, J.A. and Clyne, D. (1990) Racial differences in the incidence of end-stage renal disease in type I and II diabetes mellitus. *American Journal of Kidney Diseases*, **15**, 562–7.

161. Pugh, J.A., Medina, R.A., Cornell, J.C. and Basu, S. (1995) NIDDM is the major cause of diabetic end-stage renal disease. More evidence from a triethnic community. *Diabetes*, **44**, 1375–80.

162. Burrows, N.R., Wang, L.S. and Geiss, M.A. (2005) Incidence of end stage renal disease among persons with diabetes – Unites States 1990–2002. *Morbidity and Mortality Weekly Report*, **54** (43), 1097–100.

163. Nelson, C.B., Port, F.K., Wolfe, R.A. and Guire, K.E. (1992) Comparison of continuous ambulatory peritoneal dialysis and hemodialysis patients' survival with evaluation of trends during the 1980s. *Journal of the American Society of Nephrology*, **3**, 1147–55.

164. Wolfe, R.A., Port, F.K., Hawthorne, V.M. and Guire, K.E. (1990) A comparison of survival among dialytic therapies of choice: in-center hemodialysis versus continuous ambulatory peritoneal dialysis at home. *American Journal of Kidney Diseases*, **25**, 433–40.

165. US Renal Data System (1990) USRDS Annual Data Report, National Institute of Health, National Institute of Diabetes and Digestive Diseases, Bethesda, MD,.

166. Cowie, C.C., Pork, F.K., Rust, K.F. and Harris, M.I. (1994) Differences in survival between black and white patients with diabetic end-stage renal disease. *Diabetes Care*, **17**, 681–7.

167. Brancati, F.L., Whittle, J.C. and Whelton, P.K. (1992) The excess incidence of diabetic end-stage renal disease among blacks. *Journal of the American Medical Association*, **268**, 3079–84.

168. Tierney, W.M., McDonald, C.J. and Lutt, F.C. (1989) Renal disease in hypertensive adults: effect of race and type II diabetes. *American Journal of Kidney Diseases*, **13**, 485–93.

169. Freedman, B.I., Tuttle, A.B. and Spray, B.J. (1995) Familial predisposition to nephropathy in African-Americans with non-insulin dependent diabetes mellitus. *American Journal of Kidney Diseases*, **25**, 710–13.

170. Seaquist, E.R., Goeta, F.C., Rich, S. and Barbosa, J. (1989) Familial clustering of diabetic kidney disease: evidence for genetic susceptibility to diabetic nephropathy. *The New England Journal of Medicine*, **320**, 1161–5.

171. Petit, D.J., Saad, M.F. and Bennett, P.H. (1990) Familial predisposition to renal disease in two generations of Pima Indians with type II (non-insulin dependent) diabetes mellitus. *Diabetologia*, **33**, 428–43.

172. Acton, R.T., Bell, D.S.H. and Roseman, J. (1993) Association of HLA phenotypes with hypertension in African Americans and Caucasoid Americans with type II diabetes, a population at risk for

renal disease. *Transplantation Proceedings*, **25**, 2400–3.

173. Goldschmid, M.G., Domin, W.S. and Ziemer, D.C. (1995) Diabetes in urban African Americans. *Diabetes Care*, **18**, 955–61.

174. Chaiken, R.C., Palmissano, J., Norton, M.E. *et al.* (1995) Interaction of hypertension and diabetes on renal function in black NIDDM subjects. *Kidney International*, **47**, 1697–702.

175. Dasmahaptra, A., Bale, A., Raghuwanshi, A.P. *et al.* (1997) Incipient and overt diabetic nephropathy in African Americans with NIDDM. *Diabetes Care*, **17**, 297–304.

176. Bryson, C.L., Ross, H.J., Boyko, E.J. and Young, B.A. (2006) Racial and ethnic variations in albuminuria in the US Third National Health and Nutrition Examination Survey (NHANES III) population: association with diabetes and level of CKD. *American Journal of Kidney Diseases*, **48**, 720–6.

177. Haffner, S.M., Stern, M.P. and Gruber, K.K. (1990) Microalbuminuria potential marker for increased cardiovascular risk factors in non-diabetic subjects. *Arteriosclerosis*, **10**, 727–31.

178. Yudkin, J.S., Forrest, R.D. and Jackson, C.A. (1988) Microalbuminuria as a predictor of vascular disease in non-diabetic subjects. *Lancet*, **ii**, 530–3.

179. Mogenson, C. (1971) Glomerular hyperfiltration rate and renal plasma flow in short term and long term juvenile diabetes mellitus. *Scandinavian Journal of Clinical and Laboratory Investigation*, **28**, 91–100.

180. Mogenson, C.E. and Christiansen, C.K. (1984) Predicting diabetic nephropathy in insulin-dependent patients. *The New England Journal of Medicine*, **311**, 89–93.

181. Jones, S.L., Wiseman, M.J. and Viberti, G.C. (1991) Glomerular hyperfiltration as a risk factor for diabetic nephropathy: five year report of a prospective study. *Diabetologia*, **34**, 59–60.

182. Lervang, H.H., Jensen, S., Brochner-Mortensen, J. and Ditzel, J. (1988) Early glomerular hyperfiltration and the development of late nephropathy in type 1(insulin-dependent) diabetes mellitus. *Diabetologia*, **31**, 723–9.

183. Herman, W.H. and Teutsch, S.M. (1985) Kidney diseases associated with diabetes, in *Diabetes in America*, vol. XIV (eds M.I. Harris, C.C. Cowie, M.P. Stern *et al.*), NIH Publication No. 85-1468, US Government Printing Office, Washington, DC, pp. 1–31.

184. Damsgaard, E.M. and Mogenson, C.E. (1986) Microalbuminuria in elderly, hyperglycemic patients and controls. *Diabetic Medicine*, **3**, 430–5.

185. Silveiro, S.P., Friedman, R. and Jobim de Azevedo, M. (1996) Five year prospective study of glomerular filtration rate and albumin excretion rate in normofiltering and hyperfiltering normo-albuminuria NIDDM patients. *Diabetes Care*, **19**, 171–4.

186. Vedel, P., Obel, J. and Nielsen, F.S. (1996) Glomerular hyperfiltration in microalbuminuria NIDDM patients. *Diabetologia*, **39**, 1584–9.

187. Lebovitz, H.E. and Palmisano, J. (1990) Cross-sectional analysis of renal function in black Americans with NIDDM. *Diabetes Care*, **13** (Suppl 4), 1186–90.

188. Palmissano, J. and Lebovitz, H.E. (1989) Renal function in black Americans with type II diabetes. *Journal of Diabetes and its Complications*, **3**, 40–4.

189. Chaiken, R.L., Eckert-Norton, M. and Bard, M. (1998) Hyperfiltration in African American patients with type 2 diabetes mellitus: cross-sectional and longitudinal data. *Diabetes Care*, **21**, 2129–34.

190. Center for Disease Control and Prevention (1993) *Diabetes Surveillance, 1993*, US Department of Health and Human Services, Atlanta, GA, pp. 87–93.

191. Reiber, G., Boyko, E.J. and Smith, D.G. (1995) Lower extremity foot ulcers and amputations in diabetes, in *Diabetes in America*, NIH Publication No 95-1468, 2nd edn (eds M.I. Harris, C.C. Cowie, M.P., Stern *et al.*), National Diabetes Data Group, Bethesda, MD, p. 416.

192. Zheng, Z.J., Rosomond, W.D., Chambless, L.E. *et al.* (2005) Lower extremity arterial disease assessed by ankle–brachial index in a middle aged population of African Americans and whites: the Atherosclerosis Risk in Communities (ARIC) study. *American Journal of Physical Medicine*, **29**, 42–9.

193. Robertson, W.B. and Strong, J.P. (1968) Atherosclerosis in persons with hypertension and diabetes mellitus. *Laboratory Investigation*, **18**, 538–51.

194. Shafer, S.Q., Bruun, B. and Richter, R.W. (1990) Brain infarction risk factors in black New York City stroke patients. *Journal of Chronic Diseases*, **27**, 127–33.

195. Otten, M.W. Jr, Tentsch, S.M., Williamson, D.F. and Marks, J.S. (1990) The effect of known risk factors in the excess mortality of black adults in the United States. *Journal of the American Medical Association*, **263**, 845–85.

196. Keil, J.E., Sutherland, S.E. and Knapp, R.G. (1993) Mortality rates and risk factors for coronary disease in black as compared to white men and

women. *The New England Journal of Medicine*, **329**, 73–8.

197. Gillum, R.F. and Grant, C.T. (1982) Coronary heart disease in black populations. II. Risk factors. *American Heart Journal*, **4**, 852–64.

198. Kannel, W.B. and McGee, D.L. (1979) Diabetes and cardio-vascular disease: the Framingham Study. *Journal of the American Medical Association*, **24**, 2035–8.

199. Gu, K., Cowie, C.C. and Harris, M.I. (1998) Mortality in adults with and without diabetes in a national cohort of the US population, 1971–93. *Diabetes Care*, **21**, 1138–45.

200. Lowe, L.P., Liu, K. and Greenland, P. (1997) Diabetes, asymptomatic hyper-glycemia and 22-years mortality in black and white men. The Chicago Heart Association Detection Project in Industry Study. *Diabetes Care*, **20**, 163–9.

201. Tull, E.S. and Roseman, J.M. (1995) Diabetes in African Americans, in *Diabetes in America*, 2nd edn (eds M.I. Harris, C.C. Cowie, M.P., Stern *et al.*), NIH Publication No. 95-1468, National Institute of Health, National Institute of Diabetes and Digestive Diseases, Bethesda, MD, p. 625.

202. National Center for Health Statistics (1963–1990) Current estimates from the National Health Interview Survey. Vital and Health Statistics, National Center for Health Statistics, Hyattsville, MD

203. National Center for Health Statistics (1994) Current estimates from the National Health Interview Survey, 1992. Vital and Health Statistics, Series 10, No. 189, National Center for Health Statistics, Hyattsville, MD.

204. National Center for Health Statistics (1994) Current estimates from the National Health Interview Survey, 1993. Vital and Health Statistics, Series 10, No. 190, National Center for Health Statistics, Hyattsville, MD.

205. Platz, P., Jakobsen, B.K., Morling, N. *et al.* (1981) HLA-D and DR antigens in the genetic analysis of insulin-dependent diabetes mellitus. *Diabetologia*, **21**, 108–15.

206. McAlpine, D.D., Liu, J. and Li, S. (2004) Differences between blacks and whites in the incidence of end-stage renal disease and associated risk factors. *Advances in Renal Replacement Therapy*, **11**, 5–13.

207. Hsu, C.Y., Lin, F., Vittinghoff, E. and Shlipak, M.G. (2003) Racial differences in the progression from chronic renal insufficiency to end-stage renal disease in the United States. *Journal of the American Society of Nephrology*, **14**, 2902–7.

208. Muntner, P., Coresh, J., Powe, N.R. and Klag, M.J. (2003) The contribution of increased diabetes prevalence and improved myocardial infarction and stroke survival to the increase in treated end-stage renal disease. *Journal of the American Society of Nephrology*, **14**, 1568–77.

209. Folsom, A.R., Eckfeldt, J.H., Weitzman, S. *et al.* (1994) Relation of carotid artery wall thickness to diabetes mellitus, fasting glucose and insulin, body size and physical activity. *Stroke*, **25**, 66–73.

Further Reading

Chaiken, R.L., Khawaja, R. and Bard, M. (1997) Utility of untimed urinary albumin measurements in assessing albuminuria in black NIDDM subjects. *Diabetes Care*, **20**, 709–13.

Kolterman, O.G., Gray, G.S. and Griffin, J. (1970) Receptor and post-receptor defects contribute to the insulin resistance in non-insulin dependent diabetes mellitus. *The Journal of Clinical Investigation*, **49**, 2151–60.

Reitnauer, P.J., Roseman, J.M. and Barger, B.O. (1981) HLA associations in a sample of the American black population. *Tissue Antigens*, **1**, 286–93.

22

Epidemiology of Diabetes in Asian North Americans

Marguerite J. McNeely and Wilfred Y. Fujimoto

University of Washington, Department of Medicine, Seattle WA, USA

22.1 INTRODUCTION

Asians began immigrating to North America more than a century ago. Following an initial wave of immigration from China and Japan in the 1800s, immigration of non-Europeans was severely restricted until the mid 1960s [1]. Since then, immigration of people from Asia to North America has steadily increased [2]. Today, Asian North Americans represent a very diverse population of at least 24 different ethnicities. Some Asian families, particularly those originally from China and Japan, have resided in North America for several generations, whereas many others are more recent immigrants.

The vast majority of published information about the epidemiology of diabetes in Asian North Americans comes from the United States, although Asians are also a significant ethnic minority group in Canada. In the United States, over 85% of Asian Americans trace their ancestry to China, The Philippines, India, Vietnam, Korea or Japan [2] **(Figure 22.1)**. About a third of Asian Americans are US born, about a third are foreign-born naturalized citizens and about a third are foreign-born residents [2]. On average, Asian Americans are younger, more likely to be married and more likely to have a college degree than other Americans. The median annual family income for Asians is above the US median income, but the poverty rate for Asian Americans is similar to the national average [2]. About 80% of Asian Americans speak a language other than English at home, and 60% report that they speak English 'very well' [2]. Over half of Asian Americans live in the states of California, New York and Hawaii [3]. About 14% of Asian Americans report their race as mixed, most commonly Asian and Caucasian [3]. Even though Asian Americans comprise about 4.2% of the US population [3], little national health data is available on this ethnic group [4]. Compared with other ethnic minorities in the United States, relatively few studies of diabetes risk and diabetic complications have been conducted in Asian Americans [5].

22.2 PREVALENCE OF TYPE 1 DIABETES IN ASIAN NORTH AMERICANS

There is very little information about the prevalence of type 1 diabetes in Asian North Americans. Lorenzi et al. [6] retrospectively reviewed medical charts of children aged 0–19 years who were diagnosed with type 1 diabetes in San Diego, California, and found a statistically significantly lower than expected number of cases in Asian Americans than in Caucasians.

22.3 PREVALENCE OF TYPE 2 DIABETES IN ASIAN NORTH AMERICANS

The US Medicare program, a national program that provides health care insurance for the vast majority of elderly Americans, is one of the few sources of national health information that is linked to Asian ethnicity. Medicare data on adults aged 67 years and

The Epidemiology of Diabetes Mellitus, second edition   Edited by Jean-Marie Ekoé, Marian Rewers, Rhys Williams and Paul Zimmet
© 2008 John Wiley & Sons, Ltd

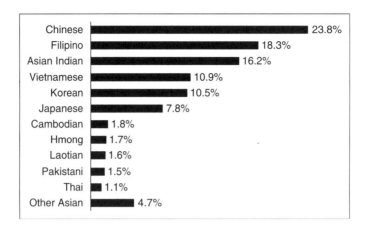

Figure 22.1 Ethnic distribution of Asian Americans. Other Asian group includes: Bangladeshi, Bhutanese, Burmese, Indo Chinese, Indonesian, Iwo Jiman, Malaysian, Maldivian, Nepalese, Okinawan, Singaporean, Sri Lankan, Taiwanese and unspecified Asian [3]. (US Census Bureau, Census 2000, special tabulations [2].)

older showed the age- and sex-adjusted prevalence of diagnosed diabetes was 24.3% in Asians and 18.4% in Caucasians. Furthermore, between 1993 and 2001, the prevalence of diagnosed diabetes in elderly Asian Americans increased by 68% compared with an increase of 36% for the overall Medicare population [7]. Another important source of national health information that includes data on Asian Americans is the Behavioral Risk Factor Surveillance System. Based on data from this national health telephone survey conducted in 2001, the prevalence of type 2 diabetes was about 60% higher in Asians than in Caucasians, after accounting for the lower body mass index (BMI) in Asians [8].

Several regional studies have also shown a high prevalence of type 2 diabetes in Asian North Americans (**Table 22.1**). In Hawaii, residents with Chinese, Filipino, Korean and Japanese ancestry each had a higher prevalence of diabetes than was observed in Caucasian residents [9]. The prevalence of diabetes in Asian Indians residing in Atlanta, Georgia was 22.5% for men and 13.6% for women, which was higher than in Caucasians [10]. In the Japanese American Community Diabetes Study in Seattle, Washington, the prevalence of type 2 diabetes in second-generation Japanese Americans aged 45–74 years was 16% for women and 20% for men [11, 12], compared with 13% of US Caucasians aged 40–74 years [13] using the 1985 World Health Organization (WHO) criteria [14]. In the Honolulu

Heart Program, 17% of elderly Japanese-American men reported a diagnosis of diabetes, and 23% of those without known diabetes met criteria based on an oral glucose tolerance test [15], compared with 13% for diagnosed diabetes in elderly US Caucasians [13]. In the Filipino Women's Health Study of women aged 50–69 years living in southern California, the prevalence of diabetes was 36% in Filipino women and 9% in Caucasian women [16]. Furthermore, the odds of prevalent type 2 diabetes were over six times higher in Filipino women than in Caucasians after adjusting for age, truncal fat, smoking, alcohol, exercise, estrogen use, hypertension and lipids. South Asian and Southeast Asian Canadian children were found to be at increased risk for type 2 diabetes mellitus compared with Caucasian Canadian children in Toronto, Ontario, although prevalence data were not reported [17]. Of all known children with type 2 diabetes in Toronto, 48% were South Asian or Southeast Asian and 14% were Caucasian, which was strikingly disproportionate to their percentage of the Toronto general population (17.4% South Asian or Southeast Asian and 68% Caucasian). In summary, the available evidence indicates that Asian North Americans have a prevalence of type 2 diabetes that is approximately 1.3–4 times higher than Caucasians.

Comparisons of diabetes prevalence among Asian subgroups in North America are sparse. Two studies reported a higher prevalence of diabetes in

Table 22.1 Prevalence of type 2 diabetes in Asian and Caucasian Americans.

Study	Asian-American study population	Diabetes ascertainment	Prevalence in Asian Americans	Prevalence in Caucasians	Crude prevalence ratio	Adjusted prevalence ratio
Medicare [7]	Asian Americans (national sample)	Diagnostic code database	24.3% Men and women ≥67 years old	18.4% Men and women ≥67 years old	—	1.3 age, sex
BRFSS [8]	Asian Americans (national sample)	Self-reported diagnosis	5% Men and women ≥30 years old	6.9% Men and women ≥30 years old	0.7	1.0 age, sex 1.6 age, sex, BMI
Sloan [9]	Chinese in Hawaii	Glucose screening with physician confirmation	1.8% Men and women ≥15 years old	1.1% Men and women ≥15 years old	1.6	2.1 age
Sloan [9]	Filipinos in Hawaii	Glucose screening with physician confirmation	3.5% Men and women ≥15 years old	1.1% Men and women ≥15 years old	3.2	3.1 age
Sloan [9]	Koreans in Hawaii	Glucose screening with physician confirmation	1.9% Men and women ≥15 years old	1.1% Men and women ≥15 years old	1.7	2.9 age
Sloan [9]	Japanese in Hawaii	Glucose screening with physician confirmation	1.9% Men and women ≥15 years old	1.1% Men and women ≥15 years old	1.7	2.9 age

(continued overleaf)

Table 22.1 (*continued*)

Reference	Population	Criteria	Prevalence	Prevalence	Ratio	Notes
Venkataraman et al. [10]	Asian Indians in Atlanta, GA	Self-reported diagnosis	18.1% Men and women ≥20 years old	4.8%[a] Men and women ≥20 years old	3.8	—
JACDS [11]	Japanese in Seattle, WA	Diabetes treatment or 1985 WHO criteria	16% Women 45–74 years old	13.4%[a] Men and women 40–74 years old	1.2	—
JACDS [12]	Japanese in Seattle, WA	Diabetes treatment or 1985 WHO criteria	20% Men 45–74 years old	13.4%[a] Men and women 40–74 years old	1.5	—
HHP [15]	Japanese in Hawaii	Self-reported diagnosis	17% Men >70 years old	13.2%[a] Men ≥75 years old	1.3	—
Araneta et al. [16]	Filipinos in San Diego, CA	Self-reported diagnosis or 1999 WHO criteria	36% Women 50–69 years old	9% Women 50–69 years old	4.0	6.1 age, truncal fat, comorbidities.

[a]Diabetes prevalence in Caucasians is from the Third National Health and Nutrition Examination Survey [13]; prevalence for ≥20 years old is standardized for age and sex to US population. BRFSS, behavioral risk factor surveillance system; HHP, Honolulu Heart Program; JACDS: Japanese American Community Diabetes Study.

Filipinos than in other Asian-American subgroups [9, 18]. One of these studies also found that multiple-race Asians also had a high prevalence of diabetes compared with other Asian subgroups [18].

22.4 INCIDENCE OF TYPE 2 DIABETES IN ASIAN NORTH AMERICANS

According to 2001 Medicare data, the annual incidence of newly diagnosed diabetes in Asian Americans aged 67 years and older was 49.4 per 1000, which was 48% higher that the annual incidence observed for Caucasians [7]. Two studies have reported diabetes incidence using a 2 h oral glucose tolerance test in Japanese Americans. In a cohort of 1144 Japanese Americans aged 40–60 years living in Los Angeles and Hawaii, the cumulative 6-year incidence of diabetes was 10.8% [19]. This is very similar to the approximately 5-year incidence of 11% and 10-year incidence of 18% observed in a similar aged cohort of second-generation and third-generation Japanese Americans from Seattle, Washington [20].

22.5 RISK FACTORS FOR TYPE 2 DIABETES IN ASIAN NORTH AMERICANS

22.5.1 Age, Sex and Family History

As observed in other populations, the risk of type 2 diabetes increases with age in Asian Americans [10, 21].

Sex is not clearly associated with diabetes prevalence in the US population overall [13], although Medicare data indicate the prevalence of diagnosed diabetes is about 2–9% higher in elderly American men than in women [7]. Hara *et al.* [19] reported the incidence of diabetes was 1.25 times higher in Japanese-American men than women from Los Angeles and Hawaii. However, in Japanese Americans from Seattle, there was no significant difference in the incidence of diabetes by sex [21].

The available information about family history as a risk factor for diabetes in Asian Americans is somewhat inconsistent. Nakanishi *et al.* [22]. reported that a family history of diabetes was associated with an increased risk of incident diabetes in Japanese-American women but not in men. In

the Honolulu Heart Program, parental history of diabetes was associated with a twofold increase in diabetes incidence among Japanese-American men under age 55 years, but not in older men, after adjustment for covariates including age, BMI, triglycerides, glucose, hypertension, physical activity and blood pressure [23]. In Japanese Americans from Seattle, a family history of diabetes in a parent or sibling was associated with a 2.3-fold increase in the 5-year incidence of diabetes in subjects aged 55 years and older, after adjustment for age, sex, BMI and smoking. However, family history was not associated with diabetes incidence in younger Japanese Americans [21].

22.5.2 Diet and Physical Activity

In the early 1980s, the prevalence of diabetes was four times higher in Japanese Americans than in native Japanese, leading to the hypothesis that westernized lifestyle involves changes in diet and physical activity that increase the risk of diabetes [24]. Japanese Americans living in Los Angeles and Hawaii eat a more westernized diet (higher fat and higher simple carbohydrates) and have a higher prevalence of diabetes than native Japanese [25]. In Japanese Americans from Seattle, a diet higher in animal protein and animal fat was associated with a significantly higher prevalence of diabetes [26]. In the Honolulu Heart Program, a more traditional Asian diet (higher in carbohydrates, lower in fat and animal protein), was associated with a 30% lower prevalence of type 2 diabetes mellitus among Japanese-American men, after adjustment for age, BMI and physical activity [27]. However, in this same study, the 6-year incidence of diabetes was not associated with Western diet [23]. While less is known about diet, acculturation and diabetes risk in other Asian-American subgroups, Jonnalagadda and Diwan [28] reported that a higher degree of American identity was associated with higher fat intake in Asian Indian Americans. Overall, these results support the hypothesis that the typical Western diet is higher in fat and animal protein than a traditional Asian diet, and that adoption of a Western diet is associated with increased risk of type 2 diabetes in Asian North Americans [24].

There are few studies on physical activity and diabetes risk in Asian North Americans, but the available evidence indicates that a more sedentary lifestyle is a risk factor for diabetes.

In the Honolulu Heart Program, higher amounts of physical activity were associated with a lower incidence of diabetes in Japanese-American men [29]. For Japanese Americans living in Seattle, less physical activity was associated with higher diabetes prevalence [30].

22.5.3 Social Factors

Research on social risk factors for diabetes in Asian North Americans has focused on acculturation and time since immigration. In a study of recent Japanese immigrants residing in Westchester County, New York, the age-adjusted prevalence of diagnosed diabetes was 4.6% for Japanese adults, which was significantly lower than the 6.8% prevalence observed for other residents of this county [31]. The prevalence was also much lower than in second-generation Japanese Americans from Seattle, where the prevalence was 16% for woman and 20% for men [11, 12]. In the Honolulu Heart Program, more years spent living in Japan was associated with lower diabetes prevalence in Japanese-American men [27]. Overall, these results suggest that recent Asian immigrants may be at lower risk for diabetes than Asians who have resided in North America for longer periods of time. These results also support the hypothesis that longer exposure to a westernized lifestyle is associated with increased risk of diabetes [24].

There is little information regarding the effect of socioeconomic status on diabetes risk in Asian North Americans. In second-generation Japanese Americans, any college education was associated with decreased prevalence of diabetes, a finding that was not readily explained by differences in physical activity, income, occupation, age or BMI [32].

22.5.4 Obesity

Increased BMI is a strong risk factor for diabetes prevalence in Asian Americans, with odds ratios similar to those observed in other Americans [33]. In Japanese Americans, the association between diabetes incidence and overweight status (BMI $\geq 25\,kg\ m^{-2}$) was particularly strong for those under age 55 years compared with older subjects [21]. Chinese Americans and Japanese Americans have a lower BMI than other Asian Americans, whereas being born in the United States is a risk factor for overweight status in all Asian-American

subgroups [18]. Unlike all other ethnic minority groups in the United States, Asians have a lower average BMI than Caucasians, and relatively few are obese (BMI $\geq 30\,kg\ m^{-2}$) [8]. Initially, this may seem incongruous with the higher prevalence of diabetes in Asian Americans. However, BMI is affected by skeletal proportions, bone mass and muscle mass in addition to fat mass. For a given level of BMI, Asian Americans have more body fat measured by dual-photon absorptiometry than Caucasians do [34]. It is likely that the association between BMI and body fat varies among subgroups of Asian North Americans, since these associations reportedly differ by Malay, Chinese and Indian ancestry in residents of Indonesia, Singapore and Hong Kong [35].

22.5.5 Central Obesity

Central obesity refers to disproportionately higher fat deposition in the torso than in the extremities. Central obesity is frequently measured as waist circumference. Central obesity is increasingly recognized as a form of obesity that is even more strongly associated with type 2 diabetes than BMI [36]. However, waist circumference cut-offs currently used to define central obesity in the general US population ($\geq 108\,cm$ in men and $\geq 88\,cm$ in women) [37] are insensitive for determining diabetes risk in second- and third-generation Japanese Americans because few Japanese Americans have a waist circumference this large [21]. The proportion of body fat located within the abdominal cavity, referred to as *intra-abdominal fat* or *visceral fat*, is thought to be an especially important fat depot with regard to diabetes risk [38]. It is widely believed that waist circumference is more strongly associated with diabetes risk than BMI because it is a surrogate marker for visceral fat. However, in Filipino women, the correlation between waist circumference and visceral fat area was lower than in Caucasian women [39]. Despite having similar average waist circumference and BMI, Filipino women had larger amounts of visceral fat and a higher prevalence of diabetes than Caucasian women. Park *et al.* [40] also found that Asian-American women had more visceral fat than Caucasian women, after adjusting for age and total amount of body fat. These studies support the opinion that thresholds for waist circumference used to define central obesity in Caucasians may be inappropriately high for Asians [41]. Visceral adiposity will be discussed in more detail later in this chapter.

22.5.6 Genetic Risk Factors

Neel [42] hypothesized that during times of plentiful food, optimal energy storage conferred a survival advantage when there was insufficient food and proposed that diabetes was a consequence of this 'thrifty genotype.' The thrifty genotype hypothesis has been advanced as a reason for the epidemic of type 2 diabetes currently occurring among populations throughout the world, including Asians. Thus, as populations in which this disease was previously uncommon gained easier access to food and exercised less, the prevalence of diabetes increased.

The strong genetic basis for type 2 diabetes is supported by the very high concordance among identical twins. Therefore, although the thrifty genotype hypothesis is interesting, there is a need to identify the specific genetic causes of type 2 diabetes. The genes that are of greatest interest are those that may influence the pathophysiology associated with type 2 diabetes, namely β-cell dysfunction, insulin resistance and obesity. Although the data about specific genes associated with diabetes in Asian Americans are very sparse and virtually all are from Japanese Americans, there are several reports that are of interest. Whether these findings are applicable to other Asian-American groups remain to be determined.

Glucokinase (GCK) plays an important role in regulation of insulin secretion [43]. Because several mutations of the GCK gene have been identified in cases of maturity-onset diabetes of the young (MODY), this was examined in Japanese Americans who had a history of type 2 diabetes in one or more first-degree relatives [44]. Six variants of the GCK gene were identified in 21 subjects, but none was significantly associated with either impaired glucose tolerance (IGT) or diabetes, although a nonsignificant increase in the G $\rightarrow$ A substitution at nucleotide-30 in the β-cell-specific promoter was observed in subjects with abnormal glucose tolerance. To examine more closely whether this substitution in the β-cell-specific promoter was related to β-cell function, Stone et al. [45] subsequently reported that by using the insulinogenic index during the first 30 min of the 75 g oral glucose tolerance test divided by fasting insulin (Δinsulin-30/Δglucose-30/fasting insulin) as an estimate of β-cell function, this GCK promoter variant was indeed associated with reduced β-cell function in 125 unrelated, middle-aged, nondiabetic Japanese-American men [45].

The β_3-adrenergic receptor is thought to be involved in thermogenesis and lipolysis in humans and a high frequency of the Trp64Arg variant of its gene has been found in Pima Indians who have among the highest prevalence of type 2 diabetes in the world [46]. Pima Indians who were homozygous for this mutation had earlier onset of diabetes and slightly lower metabolic rate. Among Finns, an association of the Trp64Arg variant was found with increased hip-to-waist ratio, hyperinsulinemia and insulin resistance [47]. Based upon these earlier findings, the Trp64Arg variant has been looked for in Japanese Americans. Kawamura et al. [48] reported that, among Japanese-American men with IGT in Hawaii, this variant was associated with higher fasting and 2 h insulin levels and homeostasis model assessment of insulin resistance (HOMA-IR). This association was not seen, however, among men with either normal glucose tolerance or diabetes. On the other hand, Stone et al. [49] found that this variant was associated with abnormal glucose tolerance but not with fasting insulin or body fat distribution.

The peroxisome proliferator-activated receptor-γ (PPARγ) is a transcription factor that plays a pivotal role in adipocyte differentiation and expression of adipocyte-specific genes [50]. Of the two isoforms, PPARγ1 and PPARγ2, the expression in human adipocytes of only the latter is influenced by obesity and nutritional factors [51]. Hence, a number of studies have looked at the relationship of the PPARγ2 gene to obesity, insulin resistance and type 2 diabetes. A Pro12Ala substitution in PPARγ2 was found to be associated with lower BMI and improved insulin sensitivity in nondiabetic Finns [52]. In the same study, the Pro/Pro genotype was significantly associated with type 2 diabetes in 300 Japanese-American men and women, with a trend for individuals who carried the Ala allele in each of the three glucose tolerance groups (normal, IGT and diabetes) to have lower fasting insulin and BMI. These findings in Japanese Americans were consistent with results from two studies among native Japanese. One of these showed the Ala allele to be associated with lower fasting insulin and HOMA-IR [53] and the other showed reduced risk for diabetes [54]. Nemoto *et al.* [55] later reported from a comparison of 105 native Japanese and 145 Japanese Americans that the Pro allele was significantly associated with diabetes in Japanese Americans but not in native Japanese. These authors also showed that diabetic Japanese Americans with the Pro/Pro genotype had significantly higher BMI and fasting insulin than diabetic native Japanese with the same genotype and suggested that the interaction of genotype with a Western lifestyle might be important in the development of type 2 diabetes. In another study carried out in a native Asian population, BMI was not associated with the Pro12Ala genotype in Korea [56].

22.6 PATHOGENESIS OF TYPE 2 DIABETES IN ASIAN NORTH AMERICANS

It is now commonly accepted that both insulin resistance and impaired pancreatic islet β-cell function occur in the pathogenesis of type 2 diabetes. Whether insulin resistance, β-cell dysfunction or both are the primary abnormality, and whether one abnormality precedes the other, has been debated, however. Furthermore, although obesity has been implicated in the pathogenesis of insulin resistance, there is much evidence that a central pattern of body fat distribution may be even more important than overall adiposity. Particularly important may be visceral adiposity. The role of body fat and its distribution, insulin resistance and β-cell dysfunction in the pathogenesis of type 2 diabetes in Asian Americans will be reviewed in this section. Most of these reports have come from studies in Japanese Americans.

22.6.1 Body Fat and Body Fat Distribution

It is quite clear that being overweight or obesity increases the risk of type 2 diabetes. Moreover, increased body fat is associated with insulin resistance, which is found in the majority of cases of type 2 diabetes. These relationships between body weight and type 2 diabetes and insulin resistance are also present in Asian Americans. However, it has also become clear that this association between body weight and diabetes and insulin resistance

may occur in Asian Americans at a BMI that is still within the normal range ($<25\,\mathrm{kg\,m^{-2}}$).

As described above, BMI does not take into account the pattern of distribution of adipose tissue. It is now clear that the preferential accumulation of body fat centrally is associated with diabetes and insulin resistance. Moreover, the central pattern characterized by increased visceral fat is especially important, as was first shown by computed tomography in Japanese-American men 20 years ago by Shuman *et al.* [57], who reported that increased fat in this but no other adipose depot was associated with type 2 diabetes. A subsequent prospective study over 2.5 years in the same population showed visceral fat to be a risk factor for incident type 2 diabetes, an association that remained after adjusting for BMI or total fat, although disappearing after taking into consideration glycemia [58]. A later prospective study, this time including both men and women who had a mean BMI $< 25\,\mathrm{kg\,m^{-2}}$ and carried out over an approximately 10-year follow-up interval, showed visceral adiposity to precede the development of diabetes, independent of fasting insulin, insulin secretion, glycemia, total and regional adiposity and family history of diabetes [59]. Furthermore, an association between visceral adiposity and risk of IGT was also shown over approximately 10 years of follow-up in Japanese-American men and women who were generally not overweight at a mean BMI $< 24\,\mathrm{kg\,m^{-2}}$, and this was independent of fasting insulin, insulin secretion and other adipose depots [60].

22.6.2 Insulin Resistance

An elevated fasting C-peptide level was shown by Bergstrom *et al.* [58] to precede the development of type 2 diabetes in Japanese-American men who were followed for 2.5 years, and this association remained after adjustment for fasting glucose. Fasting C-peptide was interpreted to be elevated as a compensatory response to an underlying insulin-resistant state and, hence, was used as a surrogate marker for insulin resistance. Moreover, fasting C-peptide was significantly correlated with intra-abdominal fat, a finding that suggested insulin resistance and visceral adiposity were antecedent events in the development of type 2 diabetes. A subsequent analysis of additional information obtained in nondiabetic Japanese Americans followed for 5 and 10 years showed, however, that higher fasting insulin, C-peptide and leptin at baseline predicted visceral fat accumulation in both men and women and this relationship was independent of baseline visceral fat or change in subcutaneous fat over time [61]. Although these findings do not agree with the notion that increased visceral fat precedes the development of insulin resistance, a possible explanation is that the baseline data may not be representative of the actual baseline; that is, at the time that the 'baseline' measurements were made, the study participants were already on the path to body fat accumulation, insulin resistance and eventually, diabetes. An earlier report in Japanese Americans showed that increased baseline leptin levels were associated with increased risk of developing diabetes in men but not in women, and this was independent of baseline fat, glycemia, fasting insulin, insulin resistance and age [62]. The reasons for this sex difference and the mechanism whereby leptin is associated with diabetes risk were not elucidated by this study.

Chiu *et al.* [63] reported intriguing differences in insulin sensitivity from a comparison of β-cell function and insulin sensitivity assessed using the hyperglycemic clamp technique in glucose-tolerant Asian Americans, African Americans, Mexican Americans and Caucasians. A significant difference in insulin sensitivity was found among these groups, with Caucasians being the most sensitive. Pairwise comparisons showed no differences among the other groups. On the other hand, β-cell function appropriately compensated for the differences in insulin sensitivity, thereby preserving normal glucose tolerance. Further analysis showed that ethnicity was an independent determinant of insulin sensitivity. Finally, waist-to-hip ratio was significantly different among the groups, with Asian Americans having the lowest ratio. However, they were more insulin resistant than Caucasians.

22.6.3 β-cell Dysfunction

Studies of persons with type 2 diabetes, as well as those at high risk of progressing to type 2 diabetes, have shown that β-cell dysfunction is not only evident in those who already are diabetic, but also in those at risk who still have fasting glucose levels well within the normal range [64]. It is now well known that insulin secretion is affected by a large number of factors, one of which is insulin sensitivity. The importance of insulin sensitivity

as a determinant of the amount of insulin that is secreted has been eloquently demonstrated by Kahn *et al.* [65]. Thus, in order to maintain normal glucose homeostasis in the presence of insulin resistance, the β-cell must compensate by secreting more insulin. By understanding this relationship, the role of insulin resistance as a determinant of hyperglycemia becomes clearer. Hyperglycemia develops with insulin resistance in those individuals who have an impairment of insulin secretion.

First-degree relatives of persons with type 2 diabetes are themselves at increased risk for this disease. The American Diabetes Association's (ADA's) genetics of non-insulin-dependent diabetes mellitus study recruited African-American, Asian-American, Caucasian and Hispanic-American families that had at least two first-degree relatives with type 2 diabetes. In a comparison of the effect of ethnicity upon insulin sensitivity and β-cell function among those family members who had no history of diabetes in themselves, Jensen *et al.* [66] found significant differences in both insulin resistance, estimated from HOMA-IR, and insulin secretion, measured as the insulinogenic index between Asian Americans and the other ethnic groups. Although in all ethnic groups the insulin resistance increased and insulin secretion decreased as glucose tolerance worsened, Asian Americans were less insulin resistant and had the lowest insulinogenic index. These findings regarding insulin resistance and insulin secretion are different from those reported by Chiu *et al.* [63] discussed earlier. However, when the insulinogenic index was adjusted for insulin resistance by dividing by HOMA-IR, there was no longer any significant difference from the other ethnic groups. Hence, Asian Americans are not different from other ethnicities in terms of the effects of insulin resistance and β-cell dysfunction in determining abnormal glucose tolerance.

There are several reports from Japanese Americans that have examined the temporal relationship between β-cell dysfunction, insulin resistance, visceral adiposity and type 2 diabetes. Chen *et al.* [67] reported that, in initially nondiabetic Japanese-American men, accumulation of visceral fat preceded the development of type 2 diabetes and that impaired insulin secretion preceded the development of visceral adiposity. In addition to low insulin secretion, Boyko *et al.* [68] reported that high fasting insulin and C-peptide at baseline preceded visceral fat accumulation measured at 5 years in nondiabetic Japanese-American men. However, as was pointed out for the study by Tong *et al.* [61], a possible explanation is that the baseline data may not have represented the true baseline for insulin resistance, since at the time of those baseline measurements they may already have been on the path to body fat accumulation, insulin resistance and, eventually, diabetes. Finally, because abnormal elevation of plasma proinsulin in relationship to plasma insulin has been reported in type 2 diabetes, this was examined in nondiabetic Japanese-American men and was found to be increased at baseline in those who subsequently developed diabetes [69]. The risk of developing diabetes with elevated proinsulin remained after adjustment for fasting insulin, indicating that proinsulin was not merely a marker for fasting insulin. Thus, inefficient processing of proinsulin to insulin may be another marker of the β-cell dysfunction associated with type 2 diabetes in Asian Americans.

22.7 DIAGNOSIS OF DIABETES IN ASIAN NORTH AMERICANS

The ADA and the WHO both currently define diabetes as a fasting plasma glucose $\geq 7.0 \, \text{mmol} \, l^{-1}$ or a 2 h postload glucose $\geq 11.1 \, \text{mmol} \, l^{-1}$; however, the ADA criteria emphasize the use of fasting glucose in clinical practice [70, 71]. In a cohort of Japanese Americans from Seattle followed for 10 years, 99% of those with incident diabetes met criteria based on 2 h glucose, but only 28% of these subjects also met criteria based on fasting glucose (Fujimoto WY, unpublished results). In a separate cohort of Japanese Americans from Hawaii and Los Angeles, only 40% diagnosed by 2 h glucose also met fasting glucose criteria [72]. These results in Japanese Americans are consistent with studies performed in Asian countries, where the majority of residents with diabetes met criteria based on 2 h glucose but not fasting glucose [73]. However, in European populations, only about 31% with diabetes met criteria based on 2 h glucose but not fasting glucose [74]. Anand *et al.* [75] examined ethnic differences in the prevalence of abnormal 2 h glucose and fasting glucose in a Canadian population. Canadians of Chinese or Asian Indian ancestry were more likely to have

elevated 2 h glucose without elevation in fasting glucose compared with Caucasians. Taken together, these results indicate that reliance on fasting glucose to diagnose diabetes is likely to result in a greater proportion of missed diabetes diagnoses in Asian North Americans compared with Caucasians.

22.8 COMPLICATIONS OF DIABETES IN ASIAN NORTH AMERICANS

22.8.1 Retinopathy

The only information about the risk of retinopathy in Asian North Americans comes from the Behavioral Risk Factor Surveillance System telephone survey of US residents. In this study, the prevalence of self-reported retinopathy in diabetic Asian Americans was similar that to reported by other diabetic Americans [76].

22.8.2 Nephropathy

In the United States, Asian Americans have a higher incidence of end-stage renal disease (ESRD) due to diabetes [77]. Among 429 918 US veterans with diabetes, diabetic ESRD prevalence was 80% higher in Asian Americans than in Caucasians, after adjusting for age, sex, comorbidity, frequency of medical visits, geographic region and other covariates [78]. However, in this same study there was no significant difference between Asian Americans and Caucasians in the prevalence of early diabetic nephropathy. In a population of 62 432 diabetic patients enrolled in the Kaiser Permanente Medical Care Program in Northern California, the incidence of diabetic ESRD was 85% higher in Asian Americans compared with Caucasians [79]. Despite having a higher incidence and prevalence of diabetic ESRD, Asian Americans have longer survival after initiation of treatment than Caucasians do [77]. The reasons for this increased survival are unknown. Renal transplantation is commonly used to treat ESRD in the United States, but the odds of finding a suitably matched donor can be affected by ethnicity, due to variation in the frequency of specific human leukocyte antigen antigens in minority populations relative to the majority population. In a study of subjects with type 1 diabetes, Asian Americans with ESRD were as likely to get a kidney transplant as Caucasians were, but were less likely to get simultaneous pancreatic–kidney transplant [80]. These findings may not apply to the pattern of renal transplantation in Asian Americans with type 2 diabetes, which is far more common than type 1 diabetes.

22.8.3 Foot Ulcers, Amputations and Peripheral Vascular Disease

The prevalence of a self-reported history of diabetic foot ulcers is about the same in Asian Americans as in Caucasians, but is lower than in Hispanics, Native Americans and Pacific Islanders [76]. Among US veterans with diabetes, Asian Americans had a 69% lower incidence of lower extremity amputation than Caucasians did, after adjusting for age, geographic region and other comorbidities [81]. In diabetic patients followed in the Kaiser Permanente Medical Care Program, the incidence of lower extremity amputation was also about 60% lower in Asian Americans than in Caucasians [79]. There are no data specifically on peripheral vascular disease in Asian North Americans.

22.8.4 Cardiovascular Disease

In US veterans with diabetes, the prevalence of cardiovascular disease was about 33% lower in Asian Americans than in Caucasians, after adjustment for covariates such as age, sex, comorbidity, geographic region and number of visits [78]. In the Kaiser study, diabetic Asian Americans had a 32% lower incidence of myocardial infarction and a 24% lower incidence of stroke [79] than Caucasians did. The decreased risk of stroke may reflect a lower risk of stroke in the Asian-American population overall rather than a decreased risk of stroke specifically related to diabetes. The incidence of stroke was 40% lower in a general population of elderly Japanese-American men from Hawaii than in Caucasian men from Framingham, Massachusetts [82].

22.8.5 Mortality

Young et al. [78] monitored the 18-month incidence of mortality in a cohort of 429 918 US veterans with diabetes, and found no significant differences between Asian Americans and Caucasians. In a large Medicare study of elderly Americans, the relative risk (RR) of mortality from diabetes during 4-year follow-up was also about the same in Asian Americans (RR 1.95) as in Caucasians (RR 1.86) [83].

22.9 CONCLUSIONS

Asian North Americans are a heterogeneous, understudied minority population with ties to more than 20 different Asian countries. The prevalence of type 2 diabetes is approximately 1.3–4 times higher in Asians than in the majority Caucasian population, despite having lower than average BMI. The reasons for this increased risk of diabetes are not fully understood, but possible contributing factors include a higher proportion of body fat for a given level of BMI and a greater propensity for visceral fat deposition, both of which contribute to insulin resistance. Asian North Americans are more likely to have a missed diagnosis of diabetes than Caucasians if fasting glucose is used instead of an oral glucose tolerance test. In Asian Americans with diabetes, the prevalence of diabetic ESRD is about 80% higher, the prevalence of lower extremity amputation is about 60–69% lower and the risk of cardiovascular disease is about 24–33% lower than in diabetic Caucasians. However, the incidence of mortality from diabetes is about the same in Asian Americans as in Caucasians.

References

1. Carlson, A.W. (1985) One century of foreign immigration to the United States: 1880–1979. *The International Migration*, **23**, 309–34.
2. Reeves, T.J. and Bennett, C.E. (2004) We the People: Asians in the United States. Census 2000 Special Report CENSR-17, US Census Bureau. Available at http://www.census.gov/population/www/cen2000/briefs.html#sr (accessed 22 February 2006).
3. Barnes, J.S., Bennett, C.E. (2002) The Asian Population: 2000 (C2KBR/01-16), US Census Bureau, Population Division. Available at http://www.census.gov/population/www/cen2000/briefs.html (accessed 22 February 2006).
4. Ghosh, C. (2003) Healthy People 2010 and Asian Americans/Pacific Islanders: defining a baseline of information. *American Journal of Public Health*, **93**, 2093–8.
5. Carter, J.S., Pugh, J.A. and Monterrosa, A. (1996) Non-insulin-dependent diabetes mellitus in minorities in the United States. *Annals of Internal Medicine*, **125**, 221–32.
6. Lorenzi, M., Cagliero, E. and Schmidt, N.J. (1985) Racial differences in incidence of juvenile-onset type 1 diabetes: epidemiologic studies in southern California. *Diabetologia*, **28**, 734–8.

7. McBean, A.M., Li, S., Gilbertson, D.T. and Collins, A.J. (2004) Differences in diabetes prevalence, incidence, and mortality among the elderly of four racial/ethnic groups: Whites, Blacks, Hispanics, and Asians. *Diabetes Care*, **27**, 2317–24.

8. McNeely, M.J. and Boyko, E.J. (2004) Type 2 diabetes prevalence in Asian Americans: results of a national health survey. *Diabetes Care*, **27**, 66–9.

9. Sloan, N.R. (1963) Ethnic distribution of diabetes mellitus in Hawaii. *The Journal of the American Medical Association*, **183**, 419–24.

10. Venkataraman, R., Nanda, N.C., Baweja, G. *et al.* (2004) Prevalence of diabetes mellitus and related conditions in Asian Indians living in the United States. *The American Journal of Cardiology*, **94**, 977–80.

11. Fujimoto, W.Y., Leonetti, D.L., Kinyoun, J.L. *et al.* (1987) Prevalence of diabetes mellitus and impaired glucose tolerance among second-generation Japanese-American men. *Diabetes*, **36**, 721–9.

12. Fujimoto, W.Y., Leonetti, D.L., Bergstrom, R.W. *et al.* (1991) Glucose intolerance and diabetic complications among Japanese-American women. *Diabetes Research and Clinical Practice*, **13**, 119–29.

13. Harris, M.I., Flegal, K.M., Cowie, C.C. *et al.* (1998) Prevalence of diabetes, impaired fasting glucose, and impaired glucose tolerance in U.S. adults. The Third National Health and Nutrition Examination Survey, 1988–1994. *Diabetes Care*, **21**, 518–24.

14. World Health Organization (1985) Diabetes Mellitus: Report of a WHO Study Group. Tech. Rep. Ser., No. 727, World Health Organization, Geneva.

15. Rodriguez, B.L., Curb, J.D., Burchfiel, C.M. *et al.* (1996) Impaired glucose tolerance, diabetes, and cardiovascular disease risk factor profiles in the elderly. The Honolulu Heart Program. *Diabetes Care*, **19**, 587–90.

16. Araneta, M.R., Wingard, D.L. and Barrett-Connor, E. (2002) Type 2 diabetes and metabolic syndrome in Filipina-American women: a high-risk nonobese population. *Diabetes Care*, **25**, 494–9.

17. Zdravkovic, V., Daneman, D. and Hamilton, J. (2004) Presentation and course of type 2 diabetes in youth in a large multi-ethnic city. *Diabetic Medicine*, **21**, 1144–8.

18. Gomez, S.L., Kelsey, J.L., Glaser, S.L. *et al.* (2004) Immigration and acculturation in relation to health and health-related risk factors among specific Asian subgroups in a health maintenance organization. *American Journal of Public Health*, **94**, 1977–84.

19. Hara, H., Egusa, G. and Yamakido, M. (1996) Incidence of non-insulin-dependent diabetes mellitus and its risk factors in Japanese-Americans living in Hawaii and Los Angeles. *Diabetic Medicine*, **13**, S133–42.

20. McNeely, M.J., Boyko, E.J., Leonetti, D.L. *et al.* (2003) Comparison of a clinical model, the oral glucose tolerance test, and fasting glucose for prediction of type 2 diabetes risk in Japanese Americans. *Diabetes Care*, **26**, 758–63.

21. McNeely, M.J., Boyko, E.J., Shofer, J.B. *et al.* (2001) Standard definitions of overweight and central adiposity for determining diabetes risk in Japanese Americans. *The American Journal of Clinical Nutrition*, **74**, 101–7.

22. Nakanishi, S., Yamane, K., Kamei, N. *et al.* (2003) Relationship between development of diabetes and family history by gender in Japanese-Americans. *Diabetes Research and Clinical Practice*, **61**, 109–15.

23. Burchfiel, C.M., Curb, J.D., Rodriguez, B.L. *et al.* (1995) Incidence and predictors of diabetes in Japanese-American men. The Honolulu Heart Program. *Annals of Epidemiology*, **5**, 33–43.

24. Fujimoto, W.Y., Bergstrom, R.W., Boyko, E.J. *et al.* (2000) Type 2 diabetes and the metabolic syndrome in Japanese Americans. *Diabetes Research and Clinical Practice*, **50** (Suppl 2), S73–6.

25. Nakanishi, S., Okubo, M., Yoneda, M. *et al.* (2004) A comparison between Japanese-Americans living in Hawaii and Los Angeles and native Japanese: the impact of lifestyle westernization on diabetes mellitus. *Biomedicine and Pharmacotherapy*, **58**, 571–7.

26. Tsunehara, C.H., Leonetti, D.L. and Fujimoto, W.Y. (1990) Diet of second-generation Japanese-American men with and without non-insulin-dependent diabetes. *The American Journal of Clinical Nutrition*, **52**, 731–8.

27. Huang, B., Rodriguez, B.L., Burchfiel, C.M. *et al.* (1996) Acculturation and prevalence of diabetes among Japanese-American men in Hawaii. *American Journal of Epidemiology*, **144**, 674–81.

28. Jonnalagadda, S.S. and Diwan, S. (2005) Health behaviors, chronic disease prevalence and self-rated health of older Asian Indian immigrants in the U.S. *Journal of Immigrant Health*, **7**, 75–83.

29. Burchfiel, C.M., Sharp, D.S., Curb, J.D. *et al.* (1995) Physical activity and incidence of diabetes: the Honolulu Heart Program. *American Journal of Epidemiology*, **141**, 360–8.

30. Fujimoto, W.Y., Bergstrom, R.W., Boyko, E.J. *et al.* (1994) Diabetes and diabetes risk factors in second- and third-generation Japanese Americans in Seattle, Washington. *Diabetes Research and Clinical Practice*, **24** (Suppl 1), S43–52.

31. Hosler, A.S. and Melnik, T.A. (2003) Prevalence of diagnosed diabetes and related risk factors:

Japanese adults in Westchester County, New York. *American Journal of Public Health*, **93**, 1279–81.

32. Leonetti, D.L., Tsunehara, C.H., Wahl, P.W. and Fujimoto, W.Y. (1992) Educational attainment and the risk of non-insulin-dependent diabetes or coronary heart disease in Japanese-American men. *Ethnicity and Disease*, **2**, 326–36.

33. McNeely, M.J. and Boyko, E.J. (2004) Type 2 diabetes prevalence in Asian subjects: response to Sone *et al*. *Diabetes Care*, **27**, 1252.

34. Wang, J., Thornton, J.C., Burastero, S. *et al.* (1996) Comparisons for body mass index and body fat percent among Puerto Ricans, blacks, whites and Asians living in the New York City area. *Obesity Research*, **4**, 377–84.

35. Deurenberg, P., Deurenberg-Yap, M. and Guricci, S. (2002) Asians are different from Caucasians and from each other in their body mass index/body fat per cent relationship. *Obesity Reviews*, **3**, 141–6.

36. Janssen, I., Katzmarzyk, P.T. and Ross, R. (2002) Body mass index, waist circumference, and health risk: evidence in support of current National Institutes of Health guidelines. *Archives of Internal Medicine*, **162**, 2074–9.

37. Expert Panel on the Identification Evaluation and Treatment of Overweight and Obesity in Adults (1998) Executive summary of the clinical guidelines on the identification, evaluation, and treatment of overweight and obesity in adults. *Archives of Internal Medicine*, **158**, 1855–67.

38. Fujimoto, W.Y. (1996) Overview of non-insulin-dependent diabetes mellitus (NIDDM) in different population groups. *Diabetic Medicine*, **13**, S7–10.

39. Araneta, M.R. and Barrett-Connor, E. (2005) Ethnic differences in visceral adipose tissue and type 2 diabetes: Filipino, African-American, and white women. *Obesity Research*, **13**, 1458–65.

40. Park, Y.W., Allison, D.B., Heymsfield, S.B. and Gallagher, D. (2001) Larger amounts of visceral adipose tissue in Asian Americans. *Obesity Research*, **9**, 381–7.

41. Steering Committee of the Western Pacific Region of the World Health Organization the International Association for the Study of Obesity and the International Obesity Task Force (2000) *The Asia-Pacific Perspective: Redefining Obesity and its Treatment*, Health Communications Australia Pty Limited, Melbourne, Australia.

42. Neel, J.V. (1962) Diabetes mellitus: a "thrifty" genotype rendered detrimental by "progress"? *American Journal of Human Genetics*, **14**, 353–62.

43. Matschinsky, F., Liang, Y., Kesavan, P. *et al.* (1993) Glucokinase as pancreatic beta cell glucose sensor and diabetes gene. *The Journal of Clinical Investigation*, **92**, 2092–8.

44. Stone, L.M., Kahn, S.E., Deeb, S.S. *et al.* (1994) Glucokinase gene variations in Japanese-Americans with a family history of NIDDM. *Diabetes Care*, **17**, 1480–3.

45. Stone, L.M., Kahn, S.E., Fujimoto, W.Y. *et al.* (1996) A variation at position −30 of the beta-cell glucokinase gene promoter is associated with reduced beta-cell function in middle-aged Japanese-American men. *Diabetes*, **45**, 422–8.

46. Walston, J., Silver, K., Bogardus, C. *et al.* (1995) Time of onset of non-insulin-dependent diabetes mellitus and genetic variation in the beta 3-adrenergic-receptor gene. *The New England Journal of Medicine*, **333**, 343–7.

47. Widen, E., Lehto, M., Kanninen, T. *et al.* (1995) Association of a polymorphism in the beta 3-adrenergic-receptor gene with features of the insulin resistance syndrome in Finns. *The New England Journal of Medicine*, **333**, 348–51.

48. Kawamura, T., Egusa, G., Okubo, M. *et al.* (1999) Association of beta3-adrenergic receptor gene polymorphism with insulin resistance in Japanese-American men. *Metabolism*, **48**, 1367–70.

49. Stone, L.M., Kahn, S.E., Fujimoto, W.Y. *et al.* (1996) Association of the Trp64Arg β3-adrenergic receptor substitution with abnormal glucose tolerance but not body fat distribution or fasting insulin levels in Japanese Americans. *Diabetes*, **45** (Suppl 2), 293A.

50. Spiegelman, B.M. (1998) PPAR-gamma: adipogenic regulator and thiazolidinedione receptor. *Diabetes*, **47**, 507–14.

51. Vidal-Puig, A.J., Considine, R.V., Jimenez-Linan, M. *et al.* (1997) Peroxisome proliferator-activated receptor gene expression in human tissues. Effects of obesity, weight loss, and regulation by insulin and glucocorticoids. *Journal of Clinical Investigation*, **99**, 2416–22.

52. Deeb, S.S., Fajas, L., Nemoto, M. *et al.* (1998) A Pro12Ala substitution in PPARgamma2 associated with decreased receptor activity, lower body mass index and improved insulin sensitivity. *Nature Genetics*, **20**, 284–7.

53. Hara, K., Okada, T., Tobe, K. *et al.* (2000) The Pro12Ala polymorphism in PPAR gamma2 may confer resistance to type 2 diabetes. *Biochemical and Biophysical Research Communications*, **271**, 212–16.

54. Mori, H., Ikegami, H., Kawaguchi, Y. *et al.* (2001) The Pro[12] → Ala substitution in PPAR-gamma is associated with resistance to development of diabetes in the general population: possible involvement in

impairment of insulin secretion in individuals with type 2 diabetes. *Diabetes*, **50**, 891–4.

55. Nemoto, M., Sasaki, T., Deeb, S.S. *et al.* (2002) Differential effect of PPARgamma2 variants in the development of type 2 diabetes between native Japanese and Japanese Americans. *Diabetes Research and Clinical Practice*, **57**, 131–37.

56. Oh, E.Y., Min, K.M., Chung, J.H. *et al.* (2000) Significance of Pro12Ala mutation in peroxisome proliferator-activated receptor-gamma2 in Korean diabetic and obese subjects. *The Journal of Clinical Endocrinology and Metabolism*, **85**, 1801–4.

57. Shuman, W.P., Morris, L.L., Leonetti, D.L. *et al.* (1986) Abnormal body fat distribution detected by computed tomography in diabetic men. *Investigative Radiology*, **21**, 483–7.

58. Bergstrom, R.W., Newell-Morris, L.L., Leonetti, D.L. *et al.* (1990) Association of elevated fasting C-peptide level and increased intra-abdominal fat distribution with development of NIDDM in Japanese-American men. *Diabetes*, **39**, 104–11.

59. Boyko, E.J., Fujimoto, W.Y., Leonetti, D.L. and Newell-Morris, L. (2000) Visceral adiposity and risk of type 2 diabetes: a prospective study among Japanese Americans. *Diabetes Care*, **23**, 465–71.

60. Hayashi, T., Boyko, E.J., Leonetti, D.L. *et al.* (2003) Visceral adiposity and the risk of impaired glucose tolerance: a prospective study among Japanese Americans. *Diabetes Care*, **26**, 650–5.

61. Tong, J., Fujimoto, W.Y., Kahn, S.E. *et al.* (2005) Insulin, C-peptide, and leptin concentrations predict increased visceral adiposity at 5- and 10-year follow-ups in nondiabetic Japanese Americans. *Diabetes*, **54**, 985–90.

62. McNeely, M.J., Boyko, E.J., Weigle, D.S. *et al.* (1999) Association between baseline plasma leptin levels and subsequent development of diabetes in Japanese Americans. *Diabetes Care*, **22**, 65–70.

63. Chiu, K.C., Cohan, P., Lee, N.P. and Chuang, L.M. (2000) Insulin sensitivity differs among ethnic groups with a compensatory response in beta-cell function. *Diabetes Care*, **23**, 1353–8.

64. Kahn, S.E., Porte, D. Jr (1996) Pathophysiology of type II diabetes mellitus, in *Diabetes Mellitus* (eds D. Porte Jr and R.S. Sherwin), Elsevier Science, New York, pp. 487–512.

65. Kahn, S.E., Prigeon, R.L., McCulloch, D.K. *et al.* (1993) Quantification of the relationship between insulin sensitivity and beta-cell function in human subjects. Evidence for a hyperbolic function. *Diabetes*, **42**, 1663–72.

66. Jensen, C.C., Cnop, M., Hull, R.L. *et al.* (2002) Beta-cell function is a major contributor to oral glucose tolerance in high-risk relatives of four ethnic groups in the U.S. *Diabetes*, **51**, 2170–8.

67. Chen, K.W., Boyko, E.J., Bergstrom, R.W. *et al.* (1995) Earlier appearance of impaired insulin secretion than of visceral adiposity in the pathogenesis of NIDDM. 5-year follow-up of initially nondiabetic Japanese-American men. *Diabetes Care*, **18**, 747–53.

68. Boyko, E.J., Leonetti, D.L., Bergstrom, R.W. *et al.* (1996) Low insulin secretion and high fasting insulin and C-peptide levels predict increased visceral adiposity. 5-year follow-up among initially nondiabetic Japanese-American men. *Diabetes*, **45**, 1010–15.

69. Kahn, S.E., Leonetti, D.L., Prigeon, R.L. *et al.* (1995) Proinsulin as a marker for the development of NIDDM in Japanese-American men. *Diabetes*, **44**, 173–9.

70. Alberti, K.G. and Zimmet, P.Z. (1998) Definition, diagnosis and classification of diabetes mellitus and its complications. Part 1: diagnosis and classification of diabetes mellitus provisional report of a WHO consultation. *Diabetic Medicine*, **15**, 539–53.

71. Expert Committee on the Diagnosis and Classification of Diabetes Mellitus (1997) Report of the Expert Committee on the Diagnosis and Classification of Diabetes Mellitus. *Diabetes Care*, **20**, 1183–97.

72. Okubo, M., Watanabe, H., Fujikawa, R. *et al.* (1999) Reduced prevalence of diabetes according to 1997 American Diabetes Association criteria. *Diabetologia*, **42**, 1168–70.

73. Qiao, Q., Nakagami, T., Tuomilehto, J. *et al.* (2000) Comparison of the fasting and the 2-h glucose criteria for diabetes in different Asian cohorts. *Diabetologia*, **43**, 1470–5.

74. The DECODE-Study Group on behalf of the European Diabetes Epidemiology Study Group (1999) Is fasting glucose sufficient to define diabetes? Epidemiological data from 20 European studies. *Diabetologia*, **42**, 647–54.

75. Anand, S.S., Razak, F., Vuksan, V. *et al.* (2003) Diagnostic strategies to detect glucose intolerance in a multiethnic population. *Diabetes Care*, **26**, 290–6.

76. McNeely, M.J. and Boyko, E.J. (2005) Diabetes-related comorbidities in Asian Americans: results of a national health survey. *Journal of Diabetes and its Complications*, **19**, 101–6.

77. Cowie, C.C. (1993) Diabetic renal disease: racial and ethnic differences from an epidemiologic perspective. *Transplantation Proceedings*, **25**, 2426–30.

78. Young, B.A., Maynard, C. and Boyko, E.J. (2003) Racial differences in diabetic nephropathy, cardiovascular disease, and mortality in a

national population of veterans. *Diabetes Care*, **26**, 2392–9.

79. Karter, A.J., Ferrara, A., Liu, J.Y. *et al.* (2002) Ethnic disparities in diabetic complications in an insured population. *The Journal of the American Medical Association*, **287**, 2519–27.

80. Isaacs, R.B., Lobo, P.I., Nock, S.L. *et al.* (2000) Racial disparities in access to simultaneous pancreas–kidney transplantation in the United States. *American Journal of Kidney Diseases*, **36**, 526–33.

81. Young, B.A., Maynard, C., Reiber, G. and Boyko, E.J. (2003) Effects of ethnicity and nephropathy on lower-extremity amputation risk among diabetic veterans. *Diabetes Care*, **26**, 495–501.

82. Rodriguez, B.L., D'Agostino, R., Abbott, R.D. *et al.* (2002) Risk of hospitalized stroke in men enrolled in the Honolulu Heart Program and the Framingham Study: a comparison of incidence and risk factor effects. *Stroke*, **33**, 230–6.

83. Bertoni, A.G., Kirk, J.K., Goff, D.C. and Wagenknecht, L.E. Jr (2004) Excess mortality related to diabetes mellitus in elderly Medicare beneficiaries. *Annals of Epidemiology*, **14**, 362–7.

23

Epidemiology of Type 2 Diabetes in Children and Adolescents

Jonathan E. Shaw[1] and Dana M. Dabelea[2]

[1]Baker IDI Heart & Diabetes Institute, Caulfield, Victoria, Australia
[2]University of Colorado School of Medicine, Denver, CO, USA

23.1 INTRODUCTION

Type 2 diabetes has traditionally been viewed as a disorder of adults, most commonly seen in those who are middle-aged and elderly. Indeed, onset of diabetes after the age of 30 or 40 years has frequently been used as both a clinical and research tool to distinguish type 2 diabetes from type 1 diabetes. However, as the prevalence of type 2 diabetes has risen in recent decades, type 2 diabetes has appeared in younger adults, and is now occurring in adolescents and youth. The information on the patterns and epidemiology of type 2 diabetes in youth is currently patchy, primarily due to the relative rarity of the disorder, the infrequency of formal registries to capture information on all cases and the small number of appropriate, population-based studies available. Nevertheless, it is now clear that type 2 diabetes is an emerging problem among the youth of many societies around the world, particularly among those ethnic groups known to have high prevalences of type 2 diabetes in adults, although it has also been reported in low-prevalence European populations. Furthermore, increasing data are emerging to indicate that, for both microvascular and macrovascular diabetic complications, type 2 diabetes carries a risk for youth that is at least equal to, and may exceed, that seen in type 1 diabetes.

This chapter will present data on the patterns and epidemiology of type 2 diabetes in youth from studies around the world, drawing not only on the small number of population-based studies in which formal screening for undiagnosed cases has been included, but also on the rather larger number of clinic and registry-based studies.

23.2 PREVALENCE AND INCIDENCE

23.2.1 Population-based Studies

It is generally accepted that population-based studies, in which all individuals within a geographical target area undergo blood glucose testing, represent the ideal method of determining the prevalence of diabetes. The advantage of the method is that it captures all of the asymptomatic and undiagnosed cases, which may represent over 50% of the total number of cases within a given population. However, there are very few such studies of type 2 diabetes in children and adolescents available. Even in those that have been conducted, the use of the oral glucose tolerance test (OGTT) (the gold standard for diabetes diagnosis) is uncommon, and the studies often lack the key data required to differentiate type 2 diabetes from type 1 diabetes precisely.

In the United States, the National Health and Nutrition Examination Survey (NHANES) III provided prevalence data on a national sample of 2867 12–19-year-olds, collected between 1988 and 1994 [1]. Thirteen adolescents were found to have diabetes, of whom four were considered to have type 2 diabetes, and all four were either non-Hispanic Black or Mexican American. A further 22 adolescents had $HbA_{1c} > 6\%$, but did not

The Epidemiology of Diabetes Mellitus, second edition   Edited by Jean-Marie Ekoé, Marian Rewers, Rhys Williams and Paul Zimmet
© 2008 John Wiley & Sons, Ltd

meet the formal criteria for diabetes. The paper does not provide a prevalence of type 2 diabetes (though it does for total diabetes), but this can be calculated to be 0.13%. The differentiation between type 1 and type 2 diabetes was based only on the use of insulin, which is unfortunate, as a high proportion of youth with type 2 diabetes are, in fact, treated with insulin, and so it is uncertain to what extent adolescents with type 2 diabetes in this study were misclassified as having type 1 diabetes. Data from NHANES 1999–2002 provide a much more recent update for the US population [2]. The prevalence of diabetes (types 1 and 2) was 0.5%, among over 4000 adolescents completing self-report information. Again, no prevalence was provided for type 2 diabetes, but 8 out of 18 of these diabetes cases were classified as being type 2 diabetes (on the basis of not using insulin), with a further two cases being on both insulin and tablets, and hence probably having type 2 diabetes. Unfortunately, although fasting glucose was measured on over 1400 adolescents, and the prevalence of impaired fasting glucose (IFG) was found to be 11%, using a cut-off for IFG of 5.6 mmol l^{-1}, and 1.5%, using a cut-off of 6.1 mmol l^{-1} (unchanged from the NHANES III data from a decade earlier), no data were provided on undiagnosed diabetes. Data from a single US school district [3] showed a diabetes prevalence of 0.4%. A study surveying Mexican American fourth graders found an overall type 2 diabetes prevalence of 0.3%, and a prevalence of 0.14% of each of impaired glucose tolerance (IGT) and IFG [4]. A study of eighth graders from four schools in the southern United States, selected because of the high proportion of children from high-risk ethnic groups (56% Hispanic, mean age 13.6 years), reported that 6.2% had IFG (fasting plasma glucose (FPG) ≥ 6.1 mmol l^{-1}), 2.3% had IGT and 0.4% had undiagnosed diabetes (FPG ≥ 7.0 mmol l^{-1}) [5]. Accurate surveillance of the Pima Indian population over the last 40 years has shown rising rates of glucose intolerance over time, as well as a female preponderance [6]. From 1967–1976 to 1987–1996 the prevalence of type 2 diabetes in youth increased from 2.4% in males and 2.7% in females to 3.8% in males and 5.3% in females, the highest rates reported in children to date. A study of American Indian (AI) and Alaskan Native adolescents reported that the prevalence of type 2

diabetes increased by 68% from 1990 to 1998 among those aged 15–19 years (0.32–0.54%) [7].

SEARCH for Diabetes in Youth is a large, six-site, collaborative study of physician-diagnosed diabetes in youth aged <20 years in the United States. SEARCH was initiated in 2000 to address gaps in knowledge about the epidemiology of diabetes in US youth, particularly with respect to race/ethnicity and diabetes type. The study began conducting population-based ascertainment of cases of diabetes in youth less than 20 years of age in 2001, and continues to ascertain incident cases from 2002 onwards. SEARCH identified 6379 youth with diabetes (prevalent in 2001), in a population of approximately 3.5 million youth [8]. Among the 1349 cases in children aged 0 to 9 years, a total of 11 cases had type 2 diabetes (0.01 per 1000 general population). In this age group, type 1 was the most prevalent type of diabetes. Among youth aged 10–19 years the highest prevalence of type 2 diabetes was observed among AI youth (1.74 per 1000). African American (AA) youth exhibited the second highest prevalence of type 2 diabetes (1.05 per 1000), followed by Asian/Pacific Islander (API) (0.54 per 1000), Hispanic (0.48 per 1000) and non-Hispanic White (NHW) youth (0.19 per 1000). In this age group type 2 diabetes accounted for about 6% of diabetes diagnosed among NHW adolescents. In all other racial/ethnic groups type 2 diabetes accounted for a sizeable proportion of diabetes types, ranging from 22% in Hispanic youth, 33% in AA youth, 40% in API youth, to 76% in AI youth.

Undoubtedly, the largest surveillance of type 2 diabetes in youth has been undertaken in Japan and Taiwan, where screening programs for renal disease, involving urine dipsticking of millions of schoolchildren, have been harnessed to screen for diabetes by follow-up of those with glycosuria. Once again, significant methodological limitations apply with this design, as glycosuria is a relatively insensitive screening tool for diabetes, picking up only those with more severe hyperglycemia. In the most recent report from the Japanese study, involving almost 9 million children screened between 1974 and 2002 [9], the overall annual incidence of type 2 diabetes was 2.63 per 100 000. The annual incidence after 1981 was significantly higher than that before 1980 (1.73 versus 2.76 per 100 000, $p < 0.0001$). However, there was no statistical change in the incidence of type 2 diabetes from 1981 to 2002. Not surprisingly, the annual incidence was significantly higher for junior high school students compared with primary school students (6.43 per 100 000 versus 0.78 per 100 000, $p < 0.0001$). Over 80% of those with diabetes were obese, and almost 60% had a positive family history of diabetes in first- or second-degree relatives.

A screening program in which fasting blood glucose was measured in those with persistent glycosuria, carried out in 3 million students (aged 6–18 years) in Taiwan [10], found the prevalence of undiagnosed diabetes to be 9.0 per 100 000 and 15.3 per 100 000 for boys and girls respectively. The prevalence of undiagnosed diabetes was 62% higher in girls than in boys, after adjustment for other factors, and the cases were most commonly identified between the ages of 12 and 14 years. A 3-year follow-up of the clinical outcomes of these cases showed that 54% had type 2 diabetes, 10% had type 1 diabetes, 9% had secondary diabetes, 20% were nondiabetic and 8% had no definite diagnosis. The cases identified as having type 2 diabetes had higher mean body mass index (BMI), cholesterol and blood pressure than those with a normal fasting glucose, suggesting that cardiovascular risk was starting to rise in those with diabetes even at this young age.

Another very large study recently reported data on over 70 000 17-year-old Israeli military conscripts [11]. Type 2 diabetes (diagnostic fasting, 2 h or random blood glucose, but not treated with insulin) was found in 0.036% of males and 0.01% of females. A study of Turkish adolescents, in which 1647 adolescents had an FPG, identified 1.96% with IFG, but no cases of type 2 diabetes [12]. Data from a Saudi Arabian study [13] showed that, in the under 14-year-old age-group, type 2 diabetes was present in 0.12% and IGT in a further 0.25%. In those aged 14–29 years, the prevalence of type 2 diabetes was 0.79% and IGT was 0.21%. Considering the variations in age groups in the studies reported here, the Saudi data point to a relatively high prevalence and, as such, are consistent with data in adults showing that the prevalence of diabetes in the Middle East is probably higher than among any other populations, apart from Pacific Islanders and indigenous peoples from North America and Australasia [14].

23.2.2 Clinic-based and Register Studies

A large number of studies have published data collected from diabetes clinics and from diabetes registers. These have focused on providing estimates of the ratio of type 1 to type 2 diabetes, as well as descriptions of the phenotype of type 2 diabetes, and some have attempted to estimate the prevalence or incidence of type 2 diabetes, on the assumption that the cases in the clinic represent all of those from within a definable population. While the strength of such studies is that the assignment of diabetes type is usually done by pediatricians (though not always in a uniform manner) and, therefore, are likely to be more accurate than can be achieved in population-based studies, it is often unclear how representative any particular clinic population is of other clinic populations. Furthermore, publication bias almost certainly exists, in which clinics finding high rates of type 2 diabetes are likely to analyze and publish their data, while those with low rates of type 2 diabetes are less likely to do so. Regional and national registries should solve most of these problems. However, those set up for childhood type 1 diabetes do not always cope well with type 2 diabetes. They do not always capture the appropriate information to differentiate between the diabetes types, and they often depend on well-organized links between a small number of pediatricians, although adolescents with type 2 diabetes may be managed in primary care or by adult physicians. Changes in incidence rates over time also need to be interpreted cautiously. At least two factors that are unrelated to actual changes in the incidence of type 2 diabetes may contribute to apparent secular rises in the incidence of type 2 diabetes. First, assignment of diabetes type has varied over time, and while several years ago almost all youth presenting with diabetes would be assumed to have type 1 diabetes, this is increasingly recognized to be incorrect, and the need for insulin, as well as even the presence of diabetic ketoacidosis, is now no longer taken to be diagnostic of type 1 diabetes. Second, there is likely to be an element of increasing awareness and surveillance that leads to better identification of undiagnosed type 2 diabetes. Thus, cases that might have remained undiagnosed until adulthood 15 years ago may now be being diagnosed in adolescence. The effect of these factors on secular changes in the numbers of people being referred to diabetes clinics, and diagnosed with type 2 diabetes, cannot usually be determined, but is likely to be a contributing factor to the reported rises in incidence.

Several studies in the United States have reported increases in the incidence of type 2 diabetes. Using data from the medical records of 735 AA and Latino children with insulin-treated diabetes in Chicago [15] the incidence of type 2 diabetes was shown to rise by 9% per year from 1985 to 1994, with the incidence being higher in African Americans than Latinos (15.2 versus 10.7 per 100 000 per year). Presentation was typically around puberty, and 62% of those with type 2 diabetes were girls (compared with 50% of those with type 1). Among 1027 consecutive diabetic patients attending a diabetic clinic in Cincinnati [16], a 10-fold increase in type 2 diabetes incidence rates, from 0.7 per 100 000 per year in 1982 to 7.2 per 100 000 per year in 1994, was observed. Onset was typically around puberty again for type 2 diabetes, and the female:male ratio was 1.7:1. Amongst 569 children and adolescents presenting to a Florida clinic with diabetes between 1994 and 1998 [17], the proportion with type 2 diabetes rose from 9.4% of new cases to 20% of new cases over the 5-year period. Within the group as a whole, being Hispanic, Black or female significantly increased the likelihood of having type 2 diabetes. Similarly, a study in Thailand [18] reported a rise from 5 to 17% from 1997 to 1999 in the proportion with type 2 diabetes referred to a diabetic clinic in that country. A study from a clinic in Hungary from 1989 to 2001 also reported rising incidence rates over time, with 57% of all their cases of type 2 diabetes within the 13-year period and 77% of all cases of IGT being diagnosed in the last 6 years of the 13-year study [19].

A detailed study from the only pediatric diabetic clinic serving an Australian population of approximately 2 million has documented a rise in the incidence of type 2 diabetes amongst children aged 0–17 years [20]. Between 1990 and 2002, average annual rises of the incidence of type 2 diabetes of 23% in the indigenous population and 31% in the nonindigenous population were observed. By the end of the study period, the estimated annual incidences were approximately 16 per 100 000 per year in the indigenous population and 1 per 100 000 per year in the nonindigenous population, which compares with an incidence of just over 20 per 100 000 per year for type 1 diabetes in children nationally. Among the 43 children identified during the study period with type 2 diabetes, the peak age at diagnosis was 13–14 years old, and 65% were girls. In an analysis of 14–20-year-olds attending an adolescent diabetes clinic in New Zealand, the prevalence of type 2 diabetes within the clinic population rose from 1.8% in 1996 to 11.0% in 2002 [21]. While only 12.5% of new cases of diabetes were classified as type 2 diabetes in 1997–1999, this figure rose to 35.7% for 2000–2001. Amongst the 18 patients with type 2 diabetes attending the clinic in 2002, all were either Maori or Pacific Islanders; and in contrast to most other studies, only 50% were female, perhaps reflecting the fact that most of the patients in this study developed diabetes after puberty (mean age of onset 15 years), while most other studies report populations with a slightly younger diabetes onset, much closer to puberty. Indeed, Taiwanese data reveal that the female bias decreases with increasing age, and within the 16–18-year-old group the incidence of diabetes was equal for males and females [10].

While there seems to be much evidence of increasing incidence and prevalence of type 2 diabetes among youth in the United States and in other populations, it is possible that this is predominantly a feature of high-risk ethnic groups. A series of studies from Europe indicate that type 2 diabetes remains a rarity in these populations. Well-designed studies from Germany, Austria, France and the United Kingdom [22–24] all show type 2 diabetes accounting for only 1–2% of all cases of diabetes. A survey in which 177 British pediatric diabetes centers reported information on all children (aged 0–16 years) with diabetes found that less than 1% of all cases were due to type 2 diabetes, and the risks of type 2 diabetes were higher in South Asians and in girls [25]. A single center in France [23] reported that only 2% of 382 children (aged 1–16 years) with diabetes had type 2 diabetes. Using a national register in Austria, Rami et al. [26] showed that of all newly diagnosed cases of diabetes under the age of 15 in the 3 years from 1999 to 2001, 1.5% of cases were due to type 2 diabetes, giving an incidence of 0.25 per 100 000 per year.

Several possible explanations exist for the much lower numbers of type 2 diabetes reported in these European studies, compared with many other studies. First, this may accurately reflect the differences between populations, and may arise from the relatively small numbers of people from high-risk ethnic groups in these European populations. Second, there may be a greater degree of underdiagnosis of type 2 diabetes in parts of Europe than in other parts of the world, though such a difference is not an obvious feature of adult-onset type 2 diabetes. Third, it is noteworthy that most of these European studies draw data from national or regional registers or from a large, national collection of diabetes centers. By comparison, the reports from single centers may be biased to the small number that by chance or because of their particular population have seen rapid rises in their numbers with type 2 diabetes. However, even the population-based data from the United States [2] showed a prevalence of diagnosed type 2 diabetes among 12–19-year-olds that was approximately 1000-fold higher than the estimates based on the British data [25] on 0–16-year-olds (0.2% versus 0.0002%). It seems unlikely that such a huge difference exists or that this can be due to ethnic differences, as even the prevalence in British South Asian children was only 0.001% [25], but the full explanation for these discrepancies remains uncertain.

23.3 PROFILE OF CHILDREN AND ADOLESCENTS WITH TYPE 2 DIABETES

Most of the studies published to date on type 2 diabetes in youth have focused on estimates of its prevalence and its risk factors. However, information on its management, presentation and natural history, particularly in reference to the development of complications, is also essential in the understanding of the epidemiology of this disease. In one of the most comprehensive studies published so far on the description of children with type 2 diabetes, data from 331 patients aged up to 18 years old, attending 56 centers in Australia and nine Southeast and East Asian countries, were collated [27]. There was a 20% excess of females and the mean age of onset of diabetes was 12 years. There was somewhat surprisingly good glycemic control, with a median HbA_{1c} of 7.0%, and an association between more frequent home blood glucose monitoring and a lower HbA_{1c}, though that may have been confounded

by an association with better care facilities in the wealthier countries. Overall, 25% were managed without pharmacological glucose-lowering therapy, 49% were on oral agents, and 26% were on insulin alone (11%) or in combination with oral agents (15%), with excellent glycemic control being achieved (median HbA_{1c} 6.0%) in those on diet alone. Hypertension was detected in 24% and microalbuminuria in 8%, with retinopathy and neuropathy being present in only 0.6% and 1.2% respectively. The study was biased toward regular clinic attenders (77% of the study population reported four or more clinic visits in the previous 12 months), who might have been expected to have a worse profile than those attending less frequently if frequency of attendance is based on need for care. However, if frequency of attendance is related to access and economics, then frequent attenders are likely to be healthier than infrequent attenders.

A study of 1501 children (aged ≥ 18 years) with diabetes (including 68 with type 2 diabetes) from a single center in Australia examined the prevalence of complications in type 1 and type 2 diabetes [28]. Comparing type 1 with type 2 diabetes, glycemic control was worse (HbA_{1c} 8.5% versus 7.3%) and diabetes duration was longer (6.8 years versus 1.3 years) in type 1 diabetes, but ages were similar. Retinopathy was more common in type 1 diabetes (20% versus 0%), while microalbuminuria was more common in type 2 diabetes (28% versus 6%). Hypertension was also more common in type 2 diabetes (36% versus 16%), but there were no differences in the occurrence of neuropathy. Interestingly, while hypertension and age were independently associated with microalbuminuria in those with type 1 diabetes, the only predictor of microalbuminuria in type 2 diabetes was HbA_{1c}, though the small numbers of individuals with type 2 diabetes limits the power of multivariate analyses. Perhaps one of the most concerning and important study findings was that 18% of those with type 2 diabetes had developmental and psychosocial problems.

A Japanese study examined the incidence of nephropathy in 620 patients with type 1 diabetes and 958 with type 2 diabetes diagnosed at under 30 years of age [29]. After 30 years of diabetes, 44% of those with type 2 and 20.2% of those with type 1 had developed nephropathy. Whereas the incidence of nephropathy declined over the study period among those with type 1 diabetes, it did not change in type 2 diabetes. Krakoff *et al.* [30] investigated whether or not age at diabetes onset was related to the risk of developing retinopathy and nephropathy amongst Pima Indians, by following up those diagnosed with type 2 diabetes at under 20 years of age (youth), 20–39 years (young adults) and 40–59 years of age (older adults). At less than 5 years' duration of type 2 diabetes, nephropathy was present in all age groups (incidence: 13 per 1000 person-years for youth, 8 per 1000 person-years for young adults and 7 per 1000 person-years for older adults). However, retinopathy only appeared among those with youth-onset diabetes after 5–10 years' duration (incidence: 10 per 1000 person-years for youth, 29 per 1000 person-years fot young adults and 35 per 1000 person-years for older adults).

A study of 51 New Zealand Maori with diabetes onset before the age of 30 years, and including 18 with type 1 diabetes and 28 with type 2 diabetes [31], reported that microalbuminuria or nephropathy was present in 62% of type 2 patients, but only 18% of the type 1 group, despite having similar mean duration of diabetes and HbA$_{1c}$. It should be noted, however, that the mean age was nine years older for type 2 diabetes, and that it was unclear whether or not all of the nephropathy was diabetic. Those with type 2 diabetes also had higher prevalences of retinopathy and hypertension.

Among 2868 SEARCH participants, at least two cardiovascular disease (CVD) risk factors were present in 92% of youth with type 2 diabetes and 14% of those with type 1 diabetes ($p < 0.0001$). In multivariate analyses, age, race/ethnicity (minority versus NHW) and diabetes type (type 2 versus type 1) were independently associated with having at least two CVD risk factors [32]. Similarly, SEARCH found that 7% of youth with type 1 diabetes had hypertension (blood pressure >95th percentile for age and height by sex, or medication) versus 29% of those with type 2 diabetes [32]. A spot urine sample was obtained from 2755 SEARCH youth with diabetes. In logistic regression, adjusted for age, gender, race/ethnicity, diabetes duration, hemoglobin A1c and systolic blood pressure, youth with type 2 diabetes were 2.5 (95% confidence interval (CI) 1.5–4.0) times as likely to have an elevated urinary albumin:creatinine ratio (≥ 30 μg mg^{-1}) as those with type 1 diabetes, independent of demographics (sex, race/ethnicity), hyperglycemia (HbA$_{1c}$,

diabetes duration) and insulin-resistance-related factors (lipids, blood pressure, BMI) [33].

Perhaps the most concerning report of complications in type 2 diabetes comes from First Nation (indigenous) Canadians. Patients who developed type 2 diabetes as children were then resurveyed as young adults, aged between 18 and 33 years. Of the 51 subjects, 9% had died, 6% were on dialysis, one had a toe amputation and one was blind [34].

A number of studies have reported on the prevalence of type 2 diabetes and IGT amongst obese youth. As long ago as 1965 there was evidence of abnormal glucose tolerance in obese children, with an IGT prevalence of 23% reported in 66 children attending an obesity clinic [35]. More recently, another study from the United States examined a group of 167 children and adolescents attending an obesity clinic [36]. IGT was present in 25% of the 4–10-year-olds and 21% of the 11–18-year-olds. An additional 4% had type 2 diabetes. However, other studies have reported much lower rates of diabetes in obese youth. In a study of 121 overweight (mean BMI 27 kg m^{-2}) and 104 normal children in the United States (aged 6–11 years), IGT was present in 4.1% of the overweight group and in none of the normals [37]. Among almost 500 German children with obesity, 7.5% had IGT and 1.2% had type 2 diabetes [38], although these are almost certainly underestimates, as OGTTs were only done in the 20% who had an elevated fasting glucose or other diabetes risk factor. Among 710 obese Italian children, 4.5% had IGT and only one had diabetes [39]. The reason for the large difference in prevalence between these studies of obese children is somewhat unclear, but probably relates to differences in severity of obesity and in ethnic composition. Clearly, the ability to extrapolate from one clinic population to another may be limited, and this must be considered when interpreting some of the data above on the prevalence and incidence of type 2 diabetes in clinic-based populations.

23.4 FACTORS IN THE DEVELOPMENT OF TYPE 2 DIABETES

The etiology of type 2 diabetes in children and adolescents has only come under scrutiny in the last few years; consequently, the literature is not as robust as for adults. However, data so far available suggest,

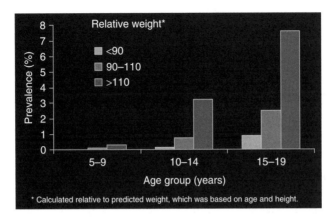

Figure 23.1 Prevalence of diabetes among Pima Indians according to age and relative weight. (Reproduced from Dabelea, D., Hanson, R.L., Bennett, P.H. et al. (1998) Increasing prevalence of type II diabetes in American Indian children. *Diabetologia*, **41 (8), 904–10, with kind permission from Springer Science and Business Media.)**

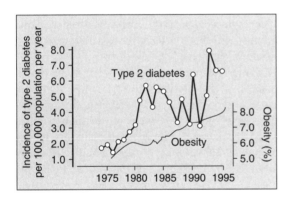

Figure 23.2 Incidence of type 2 diabetes and prevalence of obesity in Japanese children, 1976–1995. (Reproduced from [44], Copyright © 1998, Sage Publications Ltd.)

as would be expected, that many of the risk factors that have been identified for adult type 2 diabetes also apply to children and adolescents. Some of the more important factors are discussed below.

23.4.1 Ethnicity

Ethnicity is widely recognized as an important risk factor in the development of type 2 diabetes in adults. The data so far available would suggest that, if anything, the influence of ethnicity is even stronger for youth-onset than for adult-onset type 2 diabetes. Indeed, in a number of studies, the only cases of type 2 diabetes in

children and adolescents have been among those of non-European backgrounds. Higher prevalences have been seen in Asians, Hispanics, indigenous peoples (USA, Canada, Australia) and AAs, with some of the highest rates in the world being observed amongst Pima Indians [7, 40]. For instance, from the period 1967–1976 to 1987–1996 the prevalence of type 2 diabetes in Pimas increased four- to six-fold, reaching a prevalence of 22.3 per 1000 for 10–14-year-olds and 50.9 per 1000 for 15–19-year-olds by 1992–1996 [41].

23.4.2 Obesity, Diet and Activity

On a global basis, the rise in type 2 diabetes rates seems to mirror the growth in urbanization and economic development. Closely associated with this is the increase in overweight and obesity. Indeed, as has been described many times in studies of adults, there is a strong relationship, in children and adolescents, between obesity and the prevalence of type 2 diabetes (**Figure 23.1**).

Obesity has been linked to changing patterns in diet and physical activity levels [42, 43]. Allied to this are studies from Japan which have demonstrated a parallel rise in type 2 diabetes incidence in children and levels of obesity from 1975 to 1995 [44] (see **Figure 23.2**). Of note is that over this time period there have also been significant increases in fat and animal protein intake among Japanese youth, now mirroring the kind of westernized diets consumed by Japanese-Americans [45].

Dietary changes are not only confined to the home environment. A survey of Californian public schools found that 85% sold fast food, which in turn accounted for 70% of all food sales [46]. Of concern is that almost 70% of school districts allowed advertising on campus, with 24% allowing advertising in exchange for cash or equipment.

The prevalence of obesity among Japanese children increased from 5% to 8% from 1976 to 1992 and is similar to data reported from the United States [47]. In the United States, the National Longitudinal Survey of Youth, which is a prospective cohort study conducted from 1986 to 1998, showed that over this time period the overweight prevalence increased annually by 3.2% in NHWs, 5.8% in AAs and 4.3% in Hispanics. Thus, by 1998, 21.5% of AAs, 21.8% of Hispanics and 12.3% of NHWs were overweight [48].

A more recent study of nearly 5000 children in the United States has shown that, during 1999–2000, 15% of 6–19-year-olds were overweight, compared with 11% in 1994–1998. The biggest rises were recorded in AA and Mexican American adolescents [49]. This study also showed that the prevalence of being overweight (BMI $\geq$ 25 kg m^{-2}) reached a staggering 65% in US adults. Increasing obesity is also a problem in Australia, with a recent study examining children aged 7–15 years reporting that the prevalence of obesity has increased two- to four-fold from 1985 to 1997 [50].

The problem of obesity also extends to developing nations, particularly in the more affluent urban areas. In India, a recent study found that the age-adjusted prevalence of being overweight among 13–18-year-olds was around 18%. Prevalence rates increased with age and decreasing physical activity and with higher socioeconomic status [51]. Other factors also thought to be important amongst Indian Asians are low birthweight (LBW) and insulin resistance (IR) [52].

Obesity is also being increasingly observed in indigenous populations, such as the Objiwa-Cree community in Canada, where a study found that 48–51% of children aged 4–19 years have a weight >90th percentile [53]. Changes in traditional lifestyles among indigenous communities, such as a reduction in hunting and gathering, as well as the adoption of a more sedentary life with

a westernized diet, are thought to contribute to rising obesity levels [54]. Currently, some 85% of children with type 2 diabetes are either overweight or obese at diagnosis [55].

Inactivity is one of the major contributors to being overweight. In the developed world, use of computers and increasing time spent in front of the television are some of the factors impacting on activity [43, 49].

A recent longitudinal study showed a marked decline in physical activity in adolescent girls, with 56% of Black and 31% of White girls aged 16–17 years having no habitual leisure-time physical activity [56]. Pregnancy, cigarette smoking, higher BMI and lower parental education at baseline were all associated with a subsequent decline in physical activity. Another study highlighting racial differences in physical activity levels found that White students in the United States have generally higher physical activity levels than other ethnic groups, with boys usually more active than girls, whatever the race [57].

A lifestyle predisposing to obesity and type 2 diabetes seems to characterize families with adolescents who have type 2 diabetes. Specifically, they have shown that members of such families tend to be overweight, inactive and have a tendency to high fat intake and even binge eating [58]. Overall in the United States, only 50% of young people aged 12–21 years are regularly involved in physical activity, with some 25% admitting to no physical activity at all. Even in schools there is a decline in physical education, with participation rates down from 41.6% in 1991 to 24.5% in 1995 [59].

A recent detailed study on 1732 9- and 15-year-olds related a composite metabolic score (including IR, lipids, blood pressure, obesity and fitness) to physical activity assessed objectively by accelerometry [60]. The risk of having an elevated metabolic score only began to fall when more than 60 min per day of moderate activity was accumulated, suggesting that the current targets of 30 min per day may be inadequate.

23.4.3 Insulin Resistance

The onset of type 2 diabetes is frequently reported around puberty and is thought to coincide with a physiological rise in IR associated with puberty, where insulin sensitivity may be reduced by as much as 30% [61]. Healthy young adolescents compensate for the peripubertal rise in IR by increasing insulin secretion as they have normal pancreatic β-cell function. This is not the case with adolescents with type 2 diabetes, where both insulin action and eventually β-cell function are impaired [55].

There appear to be ethnic differences in IR, with AA children being more hyperinsulinemic and insulin resistant than Europids [62]. Similarly, the Bogalusa Heart Study has shown that, compared with Europids, AAs, especially girls, had higher insulin levels and insulin:glucose ratios [63].

Further, a recent study, using the hyperinsulinemic–euglycemic clamp, has further characterized hyperinsulinemia in AA children by demonstrating that, compared with Europids, AAs have a combination of both lower insulin clearance and higher insulin secretion [64]. Using a frequently sampled intravenous glucose tolerance test, both AA and Hispanic children demonstrated greater IR than Europid children [65]. Further analysis showed no ethnic differences in the first-phase insulin secretion. However, second-phase secretion was significantly higher among Hispanics than among AAs, due to lower hepatic insulin clearance among AAs.

IR may be lowered by simple means, such as increasing activity levels. This has been demonstrated in obese children and more recently in nondiabetic, normal-weight children [66], where the more active children had lower fasting insulin and greater insulin sensitivity.

23.4.4   Acanthosis Nigricans

Acanthosis nigricans (AN) is thought to be a physical marker of IR and is reported to occur in up to 60–90% of young people with type 2 diabetes [40]. This seems to be especially true for AAs and some Native Americans, but so far not demonstrated in other populations, such as in Japan [45]. However, despite its ubiquitous occurrence in some populations with type 2 diabetes, it should not exclusively be used as a reliable marker of hyperinsulinemia and IR.

In one study, only 35% of obese children with hyperinsulinemia had AN, whether AA or White [67]. Similarly a recent survey of obese Hispanic children (BMI $\geq$ 95th percentile) found that there was no association between AN and markers of IR. In contrast, AN was positively associated with BMI, but negatively with birthweight [68].

23.4.5   Polycystic Ovary Syndrome

Polycystic ovary syndrome is associated with menstrual irregularities, hyperandrogenism and IR [69]. It is also said to affect up to 5–10% of females in their reproductive years [70] and is thought to predispose to glucose intolerance, with studies showing up to 30–40% being affected by IGT and up to 7–10% with type 2 diabetes [69, 71, 72]. It may explain the female preponderance in type 2 diabetes rates amongst adolescents [61, 69].

23.4.6   Family History

Many studies show a strong family history among affected youth, with 45–80% having at least one parent with diabetes and 74–100% having a first- or second-degree relative with type 2 diabetes [55, 73]. Children with diabetes are also more likely to have a family history of CVD, with one study showing that up to 28% have a positive family history of CVD [74].

The Bogalusa Heart Study [75] has shown that children of individuals with type 2 diabetes were more likely to be obese and have higher blood pressures, fasting insulin, glucose and triglycerides. In a study among Pima Indians, it was shown that the cumulative incidence of type 2 diabetes was highest in offspring if both parents had diabetes [76].

23.4.7   Intrauterine Environment

The intrauterine environment has been increasingly recognized as being an important contributor to disease both in childhood and in adult life. Both LBW (<2500 g), and high birthweight are associated with the development of type 2 diabetes in later life [77, 78], including among children as young as age 10 years [79], and both genetic and environmental factors are likely to be involved in mediating this relationship. The hypothesis linking LBW to diabetes has been termed the thrifty phenotype, and suggests that the fetal response to intrauterine malnutrition leads to IR and impaired β-cell development, as well as LBW, with the metabolic abnormalities increasing the risk of diabetes later in life. Studies of monozygotic and dizygotic twins have shown that the lower birthweight twin has a greater risk of diabetes in adulthood, suggesting the importance of environmental and intrauterine factors [80, 81]. Birthweight may also be influenced by genetic

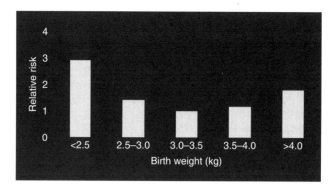

Figure 23.3 Risk of developing youth-onset type 2 diabetes according to birthweight [83]. (Copyright © 2003 American Diabetes Association, from *Diabetes Care*®,Vol.26, 2003; 343-348, reprinted with permission from The American Diabetes Association.)

factors, with a recent study suggesting that paternal type 2 diabetes may play a role [82]. Children born to a father with type 2 diabetes weighed an average of 186 g less than children from nondiabetic parents. This was not affected by birth order, father's height or social class. No significant differences were seen in birthweight of offspring between diabetic and nondiabetic mothers.

A recent nationwide survey from Taiwan has shown a U-shaped curve for birthweight and risk of type 2 diabetes in childhood (**Figure 23.3**), in which the risk was increased in those with either high birthweight (≥4000 g) (odds ratio (OR) 1.78, 95% CI 1.04–3.06) or LBW (<2500 g), (OR 2.91, 95% CI 1.25–6.76) [83]. This held true after taking into account age, sex and family history of type 2 diabetes. The likelihood is that the two extremes of birthweight represent two separate types of risk for diabetes: the thrifty phenotype for LBW, and the genetic and, possibly, environmental risk associated with high birthweight and maternal diabetes during pregnancy.

A study from India found that IR in children was inversely related to birthweight [84]. Children with LBW were also more likely to develop later hypertension and dyslipidemia. In comparison with White Caucasian babies, Indian babies are lighter, have more subcutaneous fat [85] and higher cord insulin and leptin levels [86]. The propensity to fat deposition seems to extend to Indian children born in the United Kingdom, who appear to have a greater tendency to central adiposity than their White Caucasian counterparts [87]. A study examining 152 South African children aged 7 years old

found an inverse correlation between birthweight and insulin secretion following an OGTT [88]. In addition, children with LBW but high weights at 7 years had higher insulin concentrations and indices of obesity than those with LBW who remained at a low weight by 7 years of age. There was also a positive correlation between weight velocity and IR as measured by the homeostasis model assessment.

LBW followed by catch-up growth in childhood appears to carry a particularly high risk of subsequent diabetes, as shown in both animal experimental [77, 89] and human observational studies [90–92]. A recent prospective, population-based survey from India found that subjects with IGT or type 2 diabetes as adults tended to have LBWs but accelerated increases in BMI from 2–12 years of age [93].

Recent data have shown that exposure to maternal diabetes *in utero* is a significant risk factor for obesity, IGT and type 2 diabetes in youth, independent of any effect that is transmitted genetically.

In a prospective study, Silverman *et al.* [94] followed a cohort of offspring of diabetic mothers and found that, although neonatal macrosomia disappears after the first year of life, by the age of 8 years almost half of the offspring have a weight greater than the 90th percentile. A direct correlation was found between amniotic fluid insulin concentration at weeks 32–34 of pregnancy and obesity at ages 6 and 8 years, suggesting a possible mechanism of this excessive growth [95]. Investigators also measured glucose and insulin concentrations fasting and 2 h after oral glucose, yearly from the age of 1.5 years. On their most recent evaluation (age 12.3 years), offspring of diabetic mothers had a significantly higher prevalence of IGT than an age- and sex-matched control group (19.3% versus 2.5%), and two offspring had developed type 2 diabetes.

There is evidence that the excess obesity and type 2 diabetes in offspring of diabetic mothers is not solely due to genetic factors. Within Pima Indian families with nondiabetic offspring, BMI was significantly higher ($+2.6 \, \text{kg m}^{-2}$) in the 62 siblings born after their mothers were diagnosed with type 2 diabetes (exposed to the diabetic intrauterine environment) than in the 121 siblings born before [96]. Similarly, within the same Pima Indian family, siblings born after mother's diagnosis of diabetes have over a threefold higher risk of developing diabetes at an early age than siblings born before the diagnosis of diabetes in the mother (OR 3.0, $p < 0.01$). Since these differences were not seen in the families of diabetic fathers, it is unlikely that these findings are due to cohort or birth order effects. Among Pima Indian youth of Arizona, exposure to maternal diabetes in pregnancy and obesity accounted for most of the dramatic increase in type 2 diabetes prevalence over the last 30 years [6]. Obesity itself is a long-term consequence of such exposure in this population. However, the actual extent to which exposure to maternal diabetes *in utero* and obesity account for the development of type 2 diabetes in other populations is unknown.

23.5 CONCLUSIONS

The emerging evidence of the presence of type 2 diabetes in children and adolescents, while still imprecise, is entirely consistent with the increasing prevalence of type 2 diabetes in adults, the falling age of onset of type 2 diabetes in adults and the rapidly increasing prevalence of obesity in both adults and children. In addition to describing the prevalence of type 2 diabetes in children and adolescents accurately, several challenges lie ahead. These include improving the ability to distinguish type 2 from type 1 diabetes in adolescents and identifying interventions that will succeed in making the necessary lifestyle changes in obese adolescents with type 2 diabetes. The evidence of the high risk of complications in this group, particularly in relation to microalbuminuria and

CVD risk factors, makes the need to develop such interventions very urgent.

References

1. Fagot-Campagna, A., Saaddine, J.B., Flegal, K.M. and Beckles, G.L. (2001) Diabetes, impaired fasting glucose, and elevated HbA1c in U.S. adolescents: the Third National Health and Nutrition Examination Survey. *Diabetes Care*, **24** (5), 834–7.

2. Duncan, G.E. (2006) Prevalence of diabetes and impaired fasting glucose levels among US adolescents: National Health and Nutrition Examination Survey, 1999–2002. *Archives of Pediatrics and Adolescent Medicine*, **160** (5), 523–8.

3. Dolan, L.M., Bean, J., D'Alessio, D. *et al.* (2005) Frequency of abnormal carbohydrate metabolism and diabetes in a population-based screening of adolescents. *The Journal of Pediatrics*, **146** (6), 751–8.

4. Hale, D.E., Danney, M.M., Caballero, M. *et al.* (2002) Prevalence of type 2 diabetes mellitus in urban, Mexican American 4th graders. *Diabetes*, **51** (Suppl 2), A25.

5. Baranowski, T., Cooper, D.M., Harrell, J. *et al.* (2006) Presence of diabetes risk factors in a large U.S. eighth-grade cohort. *Diabetes Care*, **29** (2), 212–17.

6. Dabelea, D., Hanson, R.L., Bennett, P.H. *et al.* (1998) Increasing prevalence of type II diabetes in American Indian children. *Diabetologia*, **41** (8), 904–10.

7. Acton, K.J., Burrows, N.R., Moore, K. *et al.* (2002) Trends in diabetes prevalence among American Indian and Alaska Native children, adolescents, and young adults. *American Journal of Public Health*, **92** (9), 1485–90.

8. The SEARCH for Diabetes in Youth Study Group (2006) The burden of diabetes mellitus among US youth: prevalence estimates from the SEARCH for Diabetes in Youth Study. *Pediatrics*, **118** (4), 1510–18.

9. Urakami, T., Kubota, S., Nitadori, Y. *et al.* (2005) Annual incidence and clinical characteristics of type 2 diabetes in children as detected by urine glucose screening in the Tokyo metropolitan area. *Diabetes Care*, **28** (8), 1876–81.

10. Wei, J.N., Sung, F.C., Lin, C.C. *et al.* (2003) National surveillance for type 2 diabetes mellitus in Taiwanese children. *The Journal of the American Medical Association*, **290** (10), 1345–50.

11. Bar Dayan, Y., Elishkevits, K., Grotto, I. *et al.* (2005) The prevalence of obesity and associated

morbidity among 17-year-old Israeli conscripts. *Public Health*, **119** (5), 385–9.

12. Uckun-Kitapci, A., Tezic, T., Firat, S. *et al.* (2004) Obesity and type 2 diabetes mellitus: a population-based study of adolescents. *Journal of Pediatric Endocrinology and Metabolism*, **17** (12), 1633–40.

13. El-Hazmi, M.A. and Warsy, A.S. (2000) Prevalence of overweight and obesity in diabetic and non-diabetic Saudis. *Eastern Mediterranean Health Journal*, **6** (2–3), 276–82.

14. Sicree, R., Shaw, J.E. and Zimmet, P. (2003) The global burden of diabetes, in *Diabetes Atlas*, 2nd edn (ed D. Gan), International Diabetes Federation,Brussels, pp. 15–71.

15. Lipton, R., Keenan, H., Onyemere, K.U. and Freels, S. (2002) Incidence and onset features of diabetes in African-American and Latino children in Chicago, 1985–1994. *Diabetes/Metabolism Research and Reviews*, **18** (2), 135–42.

16. Pinhas-Hamiel, O., Dolan, L.M., Daniels, S.R. *et al.* (1996) Increased incidence of non-insulin-dependent diabetes mellitus among adolescents. *The Journal of Pediatrics*, **128** (5 Pt 1), 608–15.

17. Macaluso, C.J., Bauer, U.E., Deeb, L.C. *et al.* (2002) Type 2 diabetes mellitus among Florida children and adolescents, 1994 through 1998. *Public Health Reports*, **117** (4), 373–9.

18. Likitmaskul, S., Kiattisathavee, P., Chaichanwatanakul, K. *et al.* (2003) Increasing prevalence of type 2 diabetes mellitus in Thai children and adolescents associated with increasing prevalence of obesity. *Journal of Pediatric Endocrinology and Metabolism*, **16** (1), 71–7.

19. Korner, A.M. (2002) Rising tide of type 2 diabetes mellitus and impaired glucose tolerance among Hungarian children and adolescents. *Diabetologica Hungarica*, **10** (Suppl 2), 22–7.

20. McMahon, S.K., Haynes, A., Ratnam, N. *et al.* (2004) Increase in type 2 diabetes in children and adolescents in Western Australia. *The Medical Journal of Australia*, **180** (9), 459–61.

21. Hotu, S., Carter, B., Watson, P.D. *et al.* (2004) Increasing prevalence of type 2 diabetes in adolescents. *Journal of Paediatrics and Child Health*, **40** (4), 201–4.

22. Schober, E., Holl, R.W., Grabert, M. *et al.* (2005) Diabetes mellitus type 2 in childhood and adolescence in Germany and parts of Austria. *European Journal of Pediatrics*, **164** (11), 705–7.

23. Ortega-Rodriguez, E., Levy-Marchal, C., Tubiana, N. *et al.* (2001) Emergence of type 2 diabetes in an hospital based cohort of children with diabetes mellitus. *Diabetes and Metabolism*, **27** (5 Pt 1), 574–8.

24. Feltbower, R.G., McKinney, P.A., Campbell, F.M. *et al.* (2003) Type 2 and other forms of diabetes in 0–30 year olds: a hospital based study in Leeds, UK. *Archives of Disease in Childhood*, **88** (8), 676–9.

25. Ehtisham, S., Hattersley, A.T., Dunger, D.B. and Barrett, T.G. (2004) First UK survey of paediatric type 2 diabetes and MODY. *Archives of Disease in Childhood*, **89** (6), 526–9.

26. Rami, B., Schober, E., Nachbauer, E. and Waldhor, T. (2003) Type 2 diabetes mellitus is rare but not absent in children under 15 years of age in Austria. *European Journal of Pediatrics*, **162** (12), 850–2.

27. Eppens, M.C., Craig, M.E., Jones, T.W. *et al.* (2006) Type 2 diabetes in youth from the Western Pacific region: glycaemic control, diabetes care and complications. *Current Medical Research and Opinion*, **22** (5), 1013–20.

28. Eppens, M.C., Craig, M.E., Cusumano, J. *et al.* (2006) Prevalence of diabetes complications in adolescents with type 2 compared with type 1 diabetes. *Diabetes Care*, **29** (6), 1300–6.

29. Yokoyama, H., Okudaira, M., Otani, T. *et al.* (2000) Higher incidence of diabetic nephropathy in type 2 than in type 1 diabetes in early-onset diabetes in Japan. *Kidney International*, **58** (1), 302–11.

30. Krakoff, J., Lindsay, R.S., Looker, H.C. *et al.* (2003) Incidence of retinopathy and nephropathy in youth-onset compared with adult-onset type 2 diabetes. *Diabetes Care*, **26** (1), 76–81.

31. McGrath, N.M., Parker, G.N. and Dawson, P. (1999) Early presentation of type 2 diabetes mellitus in young New Zealand Maori. *Diabetes Research and Clinical Practice*, **43** (3), 205–9.

32. Rodriguez, B.L., Fujimoto, W.Y., Mayer-Davis, E.J. *et al.* (2006) Prevalence of cardiovascular disease risk factors in U.S. children and adolescents with diabetes: The SEARCH for Diabetes in Youth Study. *Diabetes Care*, **29** (8), 1891–6.

33. Dabelea, D., Maahs, D.M., Snively, B.M. *et al.* (2005) High prevalence of elevated albumin excretion in youth with type 2 diabetes: The SEARCH for Diabetes in Youth Study. *Diabetologia*, **48** (Suppl 1), A53–4.

34. Dean, H.F.B. (2002) Natural history of type 2 diabetes diagnosed in childhood: long term follow-up in young adult years. *Diabetes*, **51** (Suppl 2), A24.

35. Paulsen, E.P., Richenderfer, L. and Ginsberg-Fellner, F. (1968) Plasma glucose, free fatty acids, and immunoreactive insulin in sixty-six obese children. Studies in reference to a family history of diabetes mellitus. *Diabetes*, **17** (5), 261–9.

36. Sinha, R., Fisch, G., Teague, B. *et al.* (2002) Prevalence of impaired glucose tolerance among

children and adolescents with marked obesity. *The New England Journal of Medicine*, **346** (11), 802–10.

37. Uwaifo, G.I., Elberg, J. and Yanovski, J.A. (2002) Impaired glucose tolerance in obese children and adolescents. *The New England Journal of Medicine*, **347** (4), 290–2.

38. Wiegand, S., Maikowski, U., Blankenstein, O. *et al.* (2004) Type 2 diabetes and impaired glucose tolerance in European children and adolescents with obesity—a problem that is no longer restricted to minority groups. *European Journal of Endocrinology*, **151** (2), 199–206.

39. Invitti, C., Guzzaloni, G., Gilardini, L. *et al.* (2003) Prevalence and concomitants of glucose intolerance in European obese children and adolescents. *Diabetes Care*, **26** (1), 118–24.

40. Scott, C.R., Smith, J.M., Cradock, M.M. and Pihoker, C. (1997) Characteristics of youth-onset noninsulin-dependent diabetes mellitus and insulin-dependent diabetes mellitus at diagnosis. *Pediatrics*, **100** (1), 84–91.

41. Fagot-Campagna, A., Pettitt, D.J., Engelgau, M.M. *et al.* (2000) Type 2 diabetes among North American children and adolescents: an epidemiologic review and a public health perspective. *The Journal of Pediatrics*, **136** (5), 664–72.

42. Pinhas-Hamiel, O. and Zeitler, P. (2000) ''Who is the wise man?—the one who foresees consequences:'' childhood obesity, new associated comorbidity and prevention. *Preventive Medicine*, **31** (6), 702–5.

43. Ebbeling, C.B., Pawlak, D.B. and Ludwig, D.S. (2002) Childhood obesity: public-health crisis, common sense cure. *Lancet*, **360** (9331), 473–82.

44. Kitagawa, T., Owada, M., Urakami, T. and Yamauchi, K. (1998) Increased incidence of non-insulin dependent diabetes mellitus among Japanese school children correlates with an increased intake of animal protein and fat. *Clinical Pediatrics*, **37** (2), 111–15.

45. Tajima, N. (2002) Type 2 diabetes in children and adolescents in Japan. *International Diabetes Monitor*, **14** (4), 1–5.

46. Craypo, L., Purcell, A., Samuels, S.E. *et al.* (2002) Fast food sales on high school campuses: results from the 2000 California high school fast food survey. *The Journal of School Health*, **72** (2), 78–82.

47. Kitagawa, T., Owada, M., Urakami, T. and Tajima, N. (1994) Epidemiology of type 1 (insulin-dependent) and type 2 (non-insulin-dependent) diabetes mellitus in Japanese children. *Diabetes Research and Clinical Practice*, **24** (Suppl), S7–13.

48. Strauss, R.S. and Pollack, H.A. (2001) Epidemic increase in childhood overweight, 1986–1998. *The Journal of the American Medical Association*, **286** (22), 2845–8.

49. Ogden, C.L., Flegal, K.M., Carroll, M.D. and Johnson, C.L. (2002) Prevalence and trends in overweight among US children and adolescents, 1999–2000. *The Journal of the American Medical Association*, **288** (14), 1728–32.

50. Booth, M.L., Chey, T., Wake, M. *et al.* (2003) Change in the prevalence of overweight and obesity among young Australians, 1969–1997. *The American Journal of Clinical Nutrition*, **77** (1), 29–36.

51. Ramachandran, A., Snehalatha, C., Vinitha, R. *et al.* (2002) Prevalence of overweight in urban Indian adolescent school children. *Diabetes Research and Clinical Practice*, **57** (3), 185–90.

52. Narayan, K.M. (2001) Type 2 diabetes in children: a problem lurking for India? *Indian Pediatrics*, **38** (7), 701–4.

53. Dean, H. (1998) Diagnostic criteria for non-insulin dependent diabetes in youth (NIDDM-Y). *Clinical Pediatrics*, **37** (2), 67–71.

54. Young, T.K., Dean, H.J., Flett, B. and Wood-Steiman, P. (2000) Childhood obesity in a population at high risk for type 2 diabetes. *The Journal of Pediatrics*, **136** (3), 365–9.

55. American Diabetes Association (2000) Type 2 diabetes in children and adolescents. *Diabetes Care*, **23** (3), 381–9.

56. Kimm, S.Y., Glynn, N.W., Kriska, A.M. *et al.* (2002) Decline in physical activity in black girls and white girls during adolescence. *The New England journal of medicine*, **347** (10), 709–15.

57. Troiano, R.P. (2002) Physical inactivity among young people. *The New England Journal of Medicine*, **347** (10), 706–7.

58. Pinhas-Hamiel, O., Standiford, D., Hamiel, D. *et al.* (1999) The type 2 family: a setting for development and treatment of adolescent type 2 diabetes mellitus. *Archives of Pediatrics and Adolescent Medicine*, **153** (10), 1063–7.

59. Nesmith, J.D. (2001) Type 2 diabetes mellitus in children and adolescents. *Pediatrics in Review*, **22** (5), 147–52.

60. Andersen, L.B., Harro, M., Sardinha, L.B. *et al.* (2006) Physical activity and clustered cardiovascular risk in children: a cross-sectional study (The European Youth Heart Study). *Lancet*, **368** (9532), 299–304.

61. Dabelea, D., Pettitt, D.J., Jones, K.L. and Arslanian, S.A. (1999) Type 2 diabetes mellitus in minority children and adolescents. An emerging

problem. *Endocrinology and Metabolism Clinics of North America*, **28** (4), 709–29.

62. Gutin, B., Islam, S., Manos, T. *et al.* (1994) Relation of percentage of body fat and maximal aerobic capacity to risk factors for atherosclerosis and diabetes in black and white seven- to eleven-year-old children. *The Journal of Pediatrics*, **125** (6 Pt 1), 847–52.

63. Svec, F., Nastasi, K., Hilton, C. *et al.* (1992) Black–white contrasts in insulin levels during pubertal development. The Bogalusa Heart Study. *Diabetes*, **41** (3), 313–17.

64. Arslanian, S.A., Saad, R., Lewy, V. *et al.* (2002) Hyperinsulinemia in African American children: decreased insulin clearance and increased insulin secretion and its relationship to insulin sensitivity. *Diabetes*, **51** (10), 3014–19.

65. Goran, M.I., Bergman, R.N., Cruz, M.L. and Watanabe, R. (2002) Insulin resistance and associated compensatory responses in African American and Hispanic children. *Diabetes Care*, **25** (12), 2184–90.

66. Schmitz, K.H., Jacobs, D.R. Jr, Hong, C.P. *et al.* (2002) Association of physical activity with insulin sensitivity in children. *International Journal of Obesity and Related Metabolic Disorders*, **26** (10), 1310–16.

67. Nguyen, T.T., Keil, M.F., Russell, D.L. *et al.* (2001) Relation of acanthosis nigricans to hyperinsulinemia and insulin sensitivity in overweight African American and white children. *The Journal of Pediatrics*, **138** (4), 474–80.

68. Hirschler, V., Aranda, C., Oneto, A. *et al.* (2002) Is acanthosis nigricans a marker of insulin resistance in obese children? *Diabetes Care*, **25** (12), 2353.

69. Lewy, V.D., Danadian, K., Witchel, S.F. and Arslanian, S. (2001) Early metabolic abnormalities in adolescent girls with polycystic ovarian syndrome. *The Journal of Pediatrics*, **138** (1), 38–44.

70. Palmert, M.R., Gordon, C.M., Kartashov, A.I. *et al.* (2002) Screening for abnormal glucose tolerance in adolescents with polycystic ovary syndrome. *The Journal of Clinical Endocrinology and Metabolism*, **87** (3), 1017–23.

71. Ehrmann, D.A., Barnes, R.B., Rosenfield, R.L. *et al.* (1999) Prevalence of impaired glucose tolerance and diabetes in women with polycystic ovary syndrome. *Diabetes Care*, **22** (1), 141–6.

72. Dowling, H.J. and Pi-Sunyer, F.X. (1993) Race-dependent health risks of upper body obesity. *Diabetes*, **42** (4), 537–43.

73. Sinha, A.K., O'Rourke, S., O Leonard, D., Yarker. J. (2000) Early onset type 2 diabetes (T2DM) in the indigenous communities of far north Queensland (FNQ). In *Australian Diabetes Society Annual Scientific Meeting, Cairns, Australia*, p. 90.

74. Glowinska, B., Urban, M. and Koput, A. (2002) Cardiovascular risk factors in children with obesity, hypertension and diabetes: lipoprotein(a) levels and body mass index correlate with family history of cardiovascular disease. *European Journal of Pediatrics*, **161** (10), 511–18.

75. Berenson, G.S., Radhakrishnamurthy, B., Bao, W. and Srinivasan, S.R. (1995) Does adult-onset diabetes mellitus begin in childhood? The Bogalusa Heart Study. *The American Journal of the Medical Sciences*, **310** (Suppl 1), S77–82.

76. McCance, D.R., Pettitt, D.J., Hanson, R.L. *et al.* (1994) Glucose, insulin concentrations and obesity in childhood and adolescence as predictors of NIDDM. *Diabetologia*, **37** (6), 617–23.

77. Ozanne, S.E. and Hales, C.N. (2002) Early programming of glucose–insulin metabolism. *Trends in Endocrinology and Metabolism*, **13** (9), 368–73.

78. Phillips, D.I. (1998) Birth weight and the future development of diabetes. A review of the evidence. *Diabetes Care*, **21** (Suppl 2), B150–5.

79. Dabelea, D., Pettitt, D.J., Hanson, R.L. *et al.* (1999) Birth weight, type 2 diabetes, and insulin resistance in Pima Indian children and young adults. *Diabetes Care*, **22** (6), 944–50.

80. Poulsen, P., Vaag, A.A., Kyvik, K.O. *et al.* (1997) Low birth weight is associated with NIDDM in discordant monozygotic and dizygotic twin pairs. *Diabetologia*, **40** (4), 439–46.

81. Bo, S., Cavallo-Perin, P., Scaglione, L. *et al.* (2000) Low birthweight and metabolic abnormalities in twins with increased susceptibility to type 2 diabetes mellitus. *Diabetic Medicine: A Journal of the British Diabetic Association*, **17** (5), 365–70.

82. Hypponen, E., Smith, G.D. and Power, C. (2003) Parental diabetes and birth weight of offspring: intergenerational cohort study. *British Medical Journal*, **326** (7379), 19–20.

83. Wei, J.N., Sung, F.C., Li, C.Y. *et al.* (2003) Low birth weight and high birth weight infants are both at an increased risk to have type 2 diabetes among school children in Taiwan. *Diabetes Care*, **26** (2), 343–8.

84. Yajnik, C.S. (2001) The insulin resistance epidemic in India: fetal origins, later lifestyle, or both? *Nutrition Reviews*, **59** (1 Pt 1), 1–9.

85. Yajnik, C.S., Fall, C.H., Coyaji, K.J. *et al.* (2003) Neonatal anthropometry: the thin–fat Indian baby. The Pune Maternal Nutrition Study. *International Journal of Obesity and Related Metabolic Disorders*, **27** (2), 173–80.

86. Yajnik, C.S., Lubree, H.G., Rege, S.S. *et al.* (2002) Adiposity and hyperinsulinemia in Indians

are present at birth. *The Journal of Clinical Endocrinology and Metabolism*, **87** (12), 5575–80.

87. Peters, J. and Ulijaszek, S.J. (1992) Population and sex differences in arm circumference and skinfold thicknesses among Indo-Pakistani children living in the East Midlands of Britain. *Annals of Human Biology*, **19** (1), 17–22.

88. Crowther, N.J., Cameron, N., Trusler, J. and Gray, I.P. (1998) Association between poor glucose tolerance and rapid post natal weight gain in seven-year-old children. *Diabetologia*, **41** (10), 1163–7.

89. Wolf, G. (2003) Adult type 2 diabetes induced by intrauterine growth retardation. *Nutrition Reviews*, **61** (5 Pt 1), 176–9.

90. Yajnik, C.S. (2003) Nutrition, growth, and body size in relation to insulin resistance and type 2 diabetes. *Current Diabetes Reports*, **3** (2), 108–14.

91. Hales, C.N. and Barker, D.J. (2001) The thrifty phenotype hypothesis. *British Medical Bulletin*, **60**, 5–20.

92. Yajnik, C. (2000) Interactions of perturbations in intrauterine growth and growth during childhood on the risk of adult-onset disease. *The Proceedings of the Nutrition Society*, **59** (2), 257–65.

93. Bhargava, S.K., Sachdev, H.S., Fall, C.H. *et al.* (2004) Relation of serial changes in childhood body-mass index to impaired glucose tolerance in young adulthood. *The New England Journal of Medicine*, **350** (9), 865–75.

94. Silverman, B.L., Metzger, B.E., Cho, N.H. and Loeb, C.A. (1995) Impaired glucose tolerance in adolescent offspring of diabetic mothers. Relationship to fetal hyperinsulinism. *Diabetes Care*, **18** (5), 611–17.

95. Metzger, B.E., Silverman, B.L., Freinkel, N. *et al.* (1990) Amniotic fluid insulin concentration as a predictor of obesity. *Archives of Disease in Childhood*, **65** (10), 1050–2.

96. Dabelea, D., Hanson, R.L., Lindsay, R.S. *et al.* (2000) Intrauterine exposure to diabetes conveys risks for type 2 diabetes and obesity: a study of discordant sibships. *Diabetes*, **49** (12), 2208–11.

24

Global Epidemiology of Type 1 Diabetes

Lars C. Stene[1], Jaakko Tuomilehto[2] and Marian Rewers[3]

[1]Division of Epidemiology, Norwegian Institute of Public Health, Oslo, Norway

[2] Department of Epidemiology and Health Promotion, National Public Health Institute, Helsinki, Finland

[3] Barbara Davis Center For Childhood Diabetes, University of Colorado School of Medicine, Aurora, Colorado, USA

24.1 INTRODUCTION

Type 1 diabetes is a result of immune-mediated destruction of the pancreatic β-cells, and patients need exogenous insulin for maintenance of normal blood glucose concentrations and survival. In most populations, type 1 diabetes constitutes about 5–15% of the total patients with diabetes mellitus, although classification can be difficult in older age groups. Compared with many other complex diseases, type 1 diabetes is relatively easy to diagnose; and at least in childhood, the time of the clinical onset of the disease can be defined. Thus, information on incidence rates from standardized population-based registries for childhood-onset type 1 diabetes is available from many regions of the world. The causes of type 1 diabetes are essentially unclear, but several genetic factors are known to be involved, and environmental factors thus far unknown are also thought to contribute to the disease development. This chapter describes the occurrence of type 1 diabetes around the world, with a view to identifying clues that can aid us in identifying potentially etiological environmental factors.

24.2 NATURAL HISTORY AND ISLET AUTOANTIBODIES

At diagnosis of type 1 diabetes, immune cells of various types are found in the pancreatic islets, and newly diagnosed individuals have a varying degree of β-cell destruction [1, 2].

Clinical disease can appear at any age [3], but the disease process seems to have been less progressive in patients diagnosed at older ages [1, 4]. Clinical characteristics do not seem to vary too much depending on family history, human leukocyte antigen (HLA) susceptibility genes or age at onset within the childhood range [4–7]. In young adults or older persons, however, the clinical picture and classification becomes increasingly difficult to distinguish from type 2 diabetes.

The subclinical prediabetic period, during which pancreatic β-cells are destroyed, can vary from months to years, during which serological markers may be detected in the blood [8]. These are not thought to be pathogenic, but merely markers of the disease process. Particularly predictive of type 1 diabetes are autoantibodies to insulin, to the enzyme glutamate decarboxylase (GAD) and to the protein tyrosine phosphatase-like protein IA-2/ICA512 [8, 9]. It seems that insulin autoantibodies tend to appear first in young children, whereas antibodies to IA-2 often are the last to appear before clinical disease [10]. Other islet autoantibodies have also been described, such as the newly discovered autoantibodies to a zinc transporter exclusively expressed in the pancreatic β-cells [11], but the predictive value of these other islet autoantibodies remains to be thoroughly validated.

Islet autoantibodies are present in most childhood cases of type 1 diabetes and in a large proportion of adult patients [11, 12], and they might be

The Epidemiology of Diabetes Mellitus, second edition Edited by Jean-Marie Ekoé, Marian Rewers, Rhys Williams and Paul Zimmet
© 2008 John Wiley & Sons, Ltd

identified in the cord blood of a small proportion of newborns and in healthy children [13–15]. Not all autoantibodies are associated with the disease, and the origin of them in cord blood is often obscure [15]. The ability of islet autoantibodies to predict type 1 diabetes is critically dependent on several factors related to the population (age, sex, ethnicity, genetic susceptibility) and various assay-related issues [10, 11, 16, 17].

An early review indicated a correlation between the prevalence of islet cell antibodies islet cell antibody (ICAs) in school children and the incidence of type 1 diabetes in certain countries [13], but methods were not standardized. With stricter criteria to define islet autoimmunity, there was little difference in prevalence between English and Lithuanian school children, despite a large difference in background incidence of type 1 diabetes [14]. A study from Finland found regional differences in incidence of islet autoimmunity, and the difference persisted after adjusting for high-risk HLA genotype [18]. Using standardized methodology, there was no significant between-country difference for prevalence of high-titre ICA in first-degree relatives of persons with type 1 diabetes from countries with different background incidence of type 1 diabetes [19].

The modest between-country difference in prevalence of islet autoimmunity despite large differences in incidence of type 1 diabetes (see below) has been interpreted as evidence that there are no important environmental triggers of islet autoimmunity [20]. It is argued that differences in diabetes rates between populations are due to differences in factors influencing the rate of progression from islet autoimmunity to clinical type 1 diabetes. An analysis of this concept is complex. Data from Finland show both some regional difference in incidence of islet autoimmunity and seasonal variation in the appearance of islet autoantibodies, but this can only indirectly be considered as evidence for a potential role of environmental triggers on islet autoimmunity [18, 21, 22].

24.3 INCIDENCE OF TYPE 1 DIABETES IN DIFFERENT COUNTRIES

The efforts of the Diabetes Epidemiology Research International (DERI) Group [23], the World Health Organization (WHO) DIAbetes MONDiale (DIAMOND) [24] and EUROpe and DIABetes (EURODIAB) [25, 26] in standardizing registration principles of childhood-onset type 1 diabetes have made unique contributions to the type 1 diabetes epidemiology. Reporting is population based and based on notification by the diagnosing physician, age at onset at the date of first insulin injection and residence in a defined region at time of diagnosis. Most type 1 diabetes registries have been prospective and used one primary and one secondary source, and estimation of ascertainment has been done under the assumption that the two sources are independent [27, 28]. If sources are not completely independent, then the degree of ascertainment can be overestimated. However, dependencies and effects of covariates can be modeled when three or more sources are available [28], but this has rarely been applied to type 1 diabetes.

24.3.1 Childhood-onset Type 1 Diabetes by Country

Incidence rates of childhood-onset type 1 diabetes vary enormously around the world, from less than 1 per 100 000 to more than 40 per 100 000 person-years found in Finland. The highest incidence rates are found in the Italian island Sardinia, the other Nordic countries (except Iceland) and Kuwait [25, 29–31]. Although data from many parts of the world are scarce, particularly from Africa, the lowest incidences seem to be found in Asian countries, such as China, Japan and Pakistan, and in South American countries, such as Paraguay and Venezuela. European countries are well represented with registries, and there is an approximately 10-fold difference between the highest and lowest incidence countries in Europe [25, 26], with the apparently lowest rate of 3.6 per 100 000 in Macedonia during 1989–1994 [25]. Centres from central and southern Europe have intermediate incidence rates around 10 per 100 000, whereas most of the former Eastern Europe had low rates below 10 per 100 000 (**Figure 24.1**).

Standardized incidence data and time trends from nationwide registries with data during the 1990s are presented in **Table 24.1**. **Table 24.2** includes incidence data from the 1990s from centers in countries with less than nationwide coverage. The United States is represented with Allegheny County in Pennsylvania, Chicago, and Jefferson County

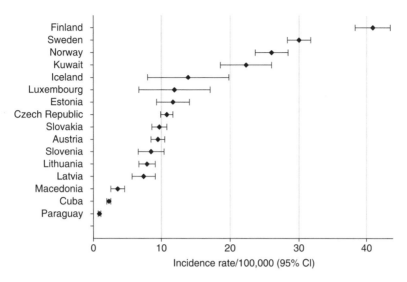

Figure 24.1 Incidence rate (per 100 000 person-years) of type 1 diabetes below age 15 years from selected nationwide registries during 1989–1999, based on [26, 31–34]. Incidences standardized to virtual population with equal proportion of individuals among males and females in the age-groups 0–4, 5–9 and 10–14 years. Standardized incidences for the Czech Republic and from Norway for the years 1990–1999 were kindly provided by personal communication with Dr Ondrej Cinek and Dr Geir Joner respectively. Horizontal bars represent 95% confidence intervals (CI) for the incidence rate.

in Alabama with incidences during the 1990s in the range of 11–18 per 100 000, depending on ethnic group. Alberta and Calgary in Canada had slightly higher rates around 23 per 100 000 [31], but a separate study from the Avalon Peninsula, Newfoundland, Canada, has found a higher incidence of 35.9 per 100 000 [35]. In South America, centers in Venezuela, Paraguay and Colombia have rates of less than 1 per 100 000, Chile (Santiago) has around 4 per 100 000, whereas Argentina and Brazil have an average of around 8 per 100 000. Many centers in Central America and the West Indies generally have low rates, except the US Virgin Islands and Puerto Rico where the rates are over 10 per 100 000. Oceania is represented only with New Zealand and parts of Australia, which have moderately high rates, although Maoris of New Zealand have much lower rates than non-Maoris [36]. In Asia, China is represented with data from 23 centers during the early 1990s, showing varying incidence rates from 0.1 per 100 000 to 4.5 per 100 000, with a mean of 0.8 per 100 000, Japan has a slightly higher average rate of 1.7 per 100 000 among three centers, whereas Kuwait stands out with a high incidence of 22 per 100 000. Only five countries from Africa are

included in the DIAMOND study, namely Algeria, Libya, Mauritius, Sudan and Tunisia. Earlier data also exist from Khartoum, Sudan, with an incidence of 6.4 per 100 000 [29]. Incidence rates reported from Africa range from low to intermediate, but the Bantus of sub-Saharan mainland Africa have barely been studied. Data from the 1980s exist only from Dar es Salaam, Tanzania, indicating a very low incidence of 0.8 per 100 000 [29], but in the Tanzanian population a considerable admixture with non-Bantu ethnic groups exists. Thus, there is a real need for incidence data from most African countries [37]. Problems with poverty, high infant death rates, deaths at onset without diagnosis of type 1 diabetes and lack of insulin, of course, make this task difficult.

24.3.2 Regional Variation within Countries

Regional variation in incidence of type 1 diabetes within countries has been documented in many studies [31, 32, 48–54]. For instance, the incidence among children in Norway tended to be relatively low in the northernmost county during the 1970s and 1990s [32, 48] and relatively high in the southernmost county during the 1990s [32]. Additional regional variation within Norway has also been

Table 24.1 Incidence rate and time trends for childhood-onset type 1 diabetes (<15 years at diagnosis) from countries with nationwide registries from 1989–1999, by ascending incidence.[a]

Country	Study period	Incidence rate per 10^5 person-years (95% CI)	Relative increase per year (95% CI)[b]	Ref.[c]
Finland[d]	1990–1999	40.9 (39.6, 42.2)	4.2% (3.1, 5.3)	[31]
Sweden[d]	1990–1999	30.0 (29.1, 30.8)	3.6% (2.6, 4.7)	[31]
Norway[d]	1990–1999	26.0 (24.8, 27.2)	0.04% ($p > 0.8$)	[32, 33]
Kuwait[d]	1992–1999	22.3 (20.5, 24.2)	7.0% (3.0, 11.1)	[31]
Denmark	1996–2000	19.5 (18.5, 19.5)	1.2% (0.7, 1.8)	[38]
Netherlands	1996–1999	18.6 (17.7, 19.4)	—	[39]
Iceland[d]	1989–1998	13.9 (11.2, 17.1)	−1% (−5, 4)[e]	[25, 26]
Luxembourg[d]	1989–1998	11.9 (9.5, 14.7)	4% (−12, 22)[e]	[25, 26]
Estonia[d]	1990–1999	11.7 (10.6, 13.0)	3.7% (0.1, 7.5)	[31]
Czech Republic[d]	1990–1999	10.8 (10.4,11.3)	6.6% ($p < 0.01$)	[34]
Slovakia[d]	1990–1999	9.7 (9.2, 10.3)	6.3% (4.3, 8.5)	[31]
Austria[d]	1989–1998	9.5 (9.0, 10.0)	5.8% (0.3, 11.7)[e]	[25, 26]
Slovenia[d]	1990–1998	8.5 (7.6, 9.5)	−2.9% (−13, 8.5)[e]	[25, 26]
Lithuania[d]	1990–1999	7.9 (7.3, 8.5)	2.5% (−0.2, 5.3)	[31]
Switzerland	1991–1994	7.9 (7.1, 8.7)	—	[25]
Latvia[d]	1990–1999	7.4 (6.6, 8.3)	3.1% (−0.6, 6.8)	[31]
Israel	1990–1993	6.0 (5.4, 6.7)	7.6% (−2.0, 18)	[25]
Dominica	1990–1993	5.7 (2.4, 12.6)	−46%	[31]
Macedonia[d]	1989–1998	3.6 (3.1, 4.1)	1% (−10, 14)[e]	[25, 26]
Jordan	1992–1996	3.2	—	[40]
Cuba[d]	1990–1999	2.3 (2.2, 2.5)	−11% (−13.4, −8.2)	[31]
Barbados	1990–1993	2.0 (0.6, 4.1)	−2.2% (−27.8, 32.3)	[31]
Mauritius	1990–1994	1.3 (0.8, 2.0)	—	[31]
Paraguay[d]	1990–1999	0.9 (0.8, 1.0)	−0.5% (−5.7, 4.9)	[31]

[a]The degree of ascertainment was generally estimated to be over 90% in most cases with a few exceptions, and in some countries ascertainment was not estimated (e.g. Finland, Estonia, Sweden, Barbados and Switzerland). Standardized incidences for the Czech Republic and from Norway for the years 1990–1999 were kindly provided from Dr Ondrej Cinek and Dr Geir Joner respectively.

[b]Based on log-linear (Poisson) modeling. A negative percentage increase indicates decrease. A 95% confidence interval (CI) for the percentage increase including zero indicates no significant increase at the 5% level.

[c]Some of the data are from EURODIAB [25], but age-standardized rates from 1990 onwards are presented by the DIAMOND Project [31] to make periods slightly more comparable. Data from DIAMOND [31] and EURODIAB [25] standardized to populations with equal proportion of boys and girls in age groups 0–4, 5–9 and 10–14. Few populations differ markedly from this distribution, and nonstandardized rates from the other studies, therefore, are likely to differ little from the standardized rates.

[d]Incidence rate shown in Figure 24.1. The remaining countries had incidence data from five calendar years or less.

[e]Trend estimate based on shorter time span, 1989–1994, based on [25].

Table 24.2 Incidence rate of childhood-onset type 1 diabetes during the 1990s from countries and regions from countries without nationwide registries, alphabetically by region.

Country/area[a]	Study period	Incidence rate per 10^5 person-years (95% CI)	Relative increase per year (95% CI)	Ref.
Africa			**3.0%**[b]	[31]
Algeria/Oran	1990–1999	8.6 (7.6, 9.8)	11.6% (5.5, 18.0)	[31]
Libya/Benghazi	1991–1999	9.0 (8.0, 10.2)	−0.9% (−5.6, 4.0)	[31]
Mauritius	1990–1994	1.3 (0.8, 2.0)	−2.2% (−28, 32)	[31]
Sudan/Gezira	1990	5.0 (3.8, 6.5)	—	[31]
Tunisia (4 centres)	1990–1999	7.4	0.7% (−3.5, 5.2)	[31]
Asia			**4.0%**[b]	[31]
China (22 centres)	1990–1994	0.84	−0.1% (−5.7, 5.8)	[31]
Japan	1990–1993	1.7	−3.5% (−16, 11)	[31]
South Korea/Seoul	1990–1991	1.1 (0.9, 1.5)	—	[31]
Pakistan/Karachi	1990–1999	0.5 (0.4, 0.6)	−5.6% (−11, 0.3)	[31]
Iran/Fars province	1991–1996	3.7 (3.3, 4.1)	—	[41]
Russia, Novosibirsk	1990–1999	6.9 (6.3, 7.6)	6.6% (3.0, 10)	[31]
Europe			**3.2%**[b]	[31]
Belgium/Antwerp	1989–1998	11.8 (10.1, 13.6)	10% (−1, 23)[c]	[26]
Bulgaria (2 centres)	1990–1999	9.4	5.1% (2.8, 7.5)	[31]
Croatia/Zagreb	1989–1998	6.6 (5.5, 7.8)	3% (−9, 17)[b]	[26]
France (4 centres)	1990–1994	8.5 (7.9, 9,1)	4.8% (−0.5, 10)	[31]
Germany/Düsseldorf	1998–1998	13.2 (12.1, 14.4)	—	[26]
Germany/Baden-Württemberg	1990–1999	12.6 (12.1, 13.2)	2.6% (1.0, 4.1)	[31]
Germany/estim. nationwide	1993–1995	14.2 (12.9, 15.5)	—	[42]
Greece (2 centres)	1989–1999	8.1	0.9% (−2.0, 3.8)	[26, 31, 43]
Hungary (18 centres)	1990–1994	9.1 (8.5, 9.8)	6.1% (0.7, 12)	[31]
Italy (7 centres)	1990–1999	10.5	0.9% (−0.9, 2.7)	[31, 44]
Italy/Sardinia	1990–1998	37.8 (35.5, 40.3)	1.4% (−1.1, 3.9)	[31]
Netherlands (5 centres)	1990–1994	13.0 (11.7, 14.4)	3.4 (−4.0, 11)	[31]
Poland (5 centres)	1989–1999	6.5	7.5% (4.6, 11)	[26, 31, 45]
Portugal (3 centres)	1989–1999	14.1	2.0% (−4.1, 8.4)[c]	[26, 31]
Madeira Island	1990–1999	6.9 (5.0, 9.4)		[31]
Romania/Bucharest	1989–1998	5.0 (4.1, 5.8)	2.4% (−10, 17)[c]	[26]
Spain (2 centres)	1990–1999	12.4 (11.7, 13.1)	−1.9% (−3.7, 0.0)	[31, 46]
UK/Scotland	1990–1999	26.4 (25.4, 27.4)	—[d]	[31]
UK/Northern Ireland	1989–1998	19.7 (17.8, 21.4)	—[d]	[26]
UK (4 centres)	1998–1999	17.0	—[d]	[26, 31]
North America			**5.3%**[b]	[31]
Canada (3 centres)	1990–1999	22.8	5.1% (1.9, 8.5)	[31]
USA/Allegheny county, PA	1990–1994	17.8 (15.5, 20.3)	—[d]	[31]
USA/Chicago, IL, African-Am	1990–1999	17.3 (15.8, 18.9)	—[d]	[31]

(*continued*)

Table 24.2 *(continued)*

Country/area[a]	Study period	Incidence rate per 10^5 person-years (95% CI)	Relative increase per year (95% CI)	Ref.
USA/Chicago, IL, Hispanic	1990–1999	11.4 (10.0, 12.9)	—[d]	[31]
USA/Chicago, IL, others	1995–1999	18.3 (15.7, 22.2)	—[d]	[31]
USA/Jefferson County, AL	1990–1995	14.1 (12.2, 18.2)	—[d]	[31]
South America			**5.3%**[b]	[31]
Argentina [4]	1990–1999	7.5	0.4% (−8.8, 11)	[31]
Brazil [2]	1990–1999	7.5	−16% (−49, 37)	[31]
Chile/Santiago	1990–1999	3.7 (3.4, 4.0)	7.5% (4.3, 11)	[31]
Colombia/Cali	1995–1999	0.5 (0.3, 0.7)	29% (−6.4, 79)	[31]
Colombia/Santafe de Bogota	1990	3.8 (2.9, 4.9)	—	[31]
Peru/Lima	1990–1994	0.5 (0.4, 0.7)	12.1% (−7.5, 36)	[31]
Uruguay/Montevideo	1992	8.3 (5.4, 11.8)	—	[31]
Venezuela/Caracas	1990–1994	—	−6.8% (−25, 15)	[31]
Central America/West Indies			**−3.6% (−5.0, 2.2)**[b]	[31]
Mexico/Veracruz	1990–1993	1.5 (0.7, 2.9)	—	[31]
Puerto Rico (US)	1990–1999	16.8 (16.0, 17.6)	−1.0% (−2.7, 0.7)	[31]
Virgin Islands (US)	1990–1996	12.8 (8.1, 18.8)	7.1% (−13, 32)	[31]
Oceania			**3.2% (−0.4, 6.9)**[b]	[31]
Australia/New South Wales	1990–1993	14.5 (13.5, 15.6)	4.1% (−2.5, 6.9)	[31, 47]
New Zealand [2]	1990–1999	18.0	2.8% (−1.4, 7.2)	[31]

[a]The degree of ascertainment was generally estimated to >90%, with some exceptions, such as variable from 51 to 100 in Chicago, 37–85 in Sardinia and in some centers it was not estimated. Percentage change is based on the DIAMOND Project [31] unless stated otherwise. Simple mean of all centers is shown (population size represented by the center was ignored): Argentina: Avellaneda 1990–1996, Cordoba 1991–1992, Corrientes 1992–1999, Tierra del Fuego 1993–1996; Bulgaria: Varna, West-Bulgaria; Brazil: Sao Paulo 1990–1992, Passo Fundo 1996–1999; Canada: Alberta 1990–1996, Calgary 1990–1999 and Prince Edward Island 1990–1993; Greece: Attica 1990–1999 based on [31], 'five northern regions' 1989–1998 based on [26]. Italy: seven centers, except Sardinia: Lazio, Lombardia 1990–1995, Marche, Pavia, eastern Sicily 1990–1994, Turin based on [31], Liguria 1989–1998 based on [44]; Japan: Chiba, Hokkaido, Okinawa; New Zealand: Auckland 1990–1996, Canterbury; Poland: Krakow 1990–1999 and Wielkopolska 1990 based on [31], Upper Silesia region 1989–1998 based on [45], Gliwice 1989–1998 and 'three cities' 1989–1998 based on [26]; Portugal: data from Coimbra and Madeira Island based on [31], data from Algarve and Portalegre based on [26]; Spain: Catalonia based on [31], Caceres (1988–1999, retrospective) based on [46]; Tunisia: Beja, Kairoan, Gafsa Monastir; UK: Leicester, Leeds, Oxford 1989–1998, based on [26], Plymouth 1990–1999, based on [31].

[b]The combined estimate includes also countries in Table 24.1. The change was significant in all regions except where confidence interval is indicated.

[c]Trend based on shorter period 1990–1994 [31].

[d]The combined percentage change for the United Kingdom based on the DIAMOND Project [31] was 3.1% (1.8, 4.3); The combined change in the United States was 5.5% (3.0, 8.0).

found at the municipality level [55]. A north–south gradient was found among 0–34-year-olds in Norway's neighbor country Sweden [51], with additional between-municipality difference in parts of Sweden [56]. Also, in the United Kingdom, large-scale [52] and small-scale regional variation has been described [57]. In Finland, high-risk areas were found in the wide belt crossing the central part of the country [53]. In Sardinia, the highest rate was in the southern part of the island and the lowest in the northwestern part [54]. Regional patterns have changed to some extent over time within at least some countries, such as Norway [32, 48] and Finland [53].

In some countries, there have been higher incidences in urban areas than in rural areas [41, 49, 58]. Other studies have found lower incidences in urban centers [59]. In Finland, the incidence was highest in the rural heartland areas, whereas the increase in incidence was strongest in urban areas; and the level of urbanization seems to explain only a part of the regional variation [60]. Still other studies have not found significant rural–urban differences. Interpretation depends on many local factors and the definition of urban. Population density is often used for defining urban areas, and higher incidence rates of type 1 diabetes were found in small areas in Northern Ireland [61] and Yorkshire, UK [62], with low population density, while other studies have not found a significant association with population density. Thus, the role of urbanization on the risk of type 1 diabetes remains unclear.

24.3.3 Incidence of Type 1 Diabetes by Sex

The majority of populations studied show less than 10–15% difference in incidence rate among males and females: high-incidence countries tend to have a male preponderance, whereas the opposite is true in low-incidence countries [63]. In addition, a male preponderance seems to be more pronounced with increasing age, particularly after puberty [63–65]. Also, in children aged 4 years or under, the incidence tends to be higher in males than in females. The peak incidence tends to be reached at a somewhat younger age in females than in males, and this did not change much during a period of decreasing age at onset in Sweden [66]. There is no satisfactory explanation for the sex differences in incidence, but hormonal and hypothetical environmental exposures have been

discussed. Some studies have found sex-specific associations of putative environmental factors with type 1 diabetes, but these are usually difficult to interpret [67–70].

24.3.4 Incidence of Type 1 Diabetes by Age

From birth, the incidence rate increases to peak around puberty in many populations [48, 57, 66, 71–73]. From age 15 years, the incidence tends to decrease and stabilize up to age 20–30 years, as seen, for example, in Norway during 1978–1982 (**Figure 24.2**).

Despite variation in absolute incidence rates, patterns similar to **Figure 24.2** have also been seen in many other countries [58, 66, 74]. Although most populations display a steady increase in incidence up to ages 10–15 years, recent data from Finland indicate that the age pattern has gradually changed, with the onset age has become younger. Thus, the incidence in the 0–4-year-olds which is nearly as high as that in 10–14-year-olds, but Finland is currently an exception in this regard [31]. Nevertheless, a similar tendency that the onset age is becoming younger has been observed in many other populations. A recent study collected standardized incidence data for the age group 15–29 years from eight European centers during 1996–1997 [65]. The relative differences in incidence between countries seem to be smaller in the higher age group. For instance, the overall incidence rate among 15–29-year-olds was not higher in Sardinia than in other centers such as in Spain, the United Kingdom and Belgium, which have much lower incidences among children [65]. Data from age groups above 35 years are particularly scarce. Population-based registries in Sweden, Antwerp (Belgium) and Lithuania have included cases of type 1 diabetes to age 34 or 39 years [58, 66, 75]. In Turin, Italy, the incidence and clinical characteristics have recently been described in 30–49-year-olds [76]. The only published population-based incidence studies covering the incidence of type 1 diabetes over the whole age span is one from Rochester, Minnesota, 1945–69 [77] and from Denmark during 1973–1977 [3]. The latter study indicated, in addition to smaller peaks at younger ages, a peak in incidence in the eighth decade of life and that the cumulative probability of developing type 1 diabetes before age 80 is in the range of 1–1.5%.

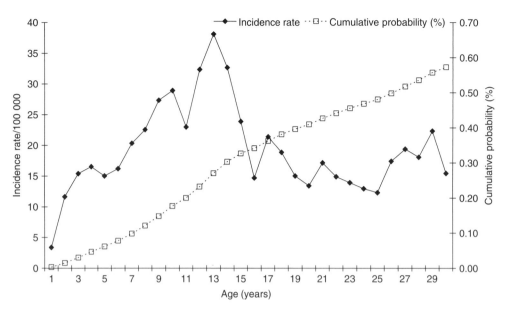

Figure 24.2 Incidence rate (per 100 00 per year) and cumulative probability (percentage of the birth cohort) of developing disease from birth until the age of 30 years in Norway during 1978–1982, based on data from [48, 73] and personal communication (G. Joner).

24.3.5   Seasonal Variation in Onset of Type 1 Diabetes

Gamble [71] reviewed early data and described a consistent peak in the autumn and winter and a low incidence in the spring or summer, which was consistent in many countries both in the northern and southern hemispheres. Although there is some variation in exact peaks and nadirs between countries, age groups, sexes and periods, this general pattern has later been seen in several studies with adequate sample sizes [36, 47, 72, 78–80]. A pooled analysis of more than 20 000 incident cases of childhood-onset type 1 diabetes from 21 European countries during 1989–1998 found that the typical seasonal pattern described above was strongest among the 10–14-year-olds, and only weak (but statistically significant) among the 0–4-year-olds [26]. Analysis of a large data set from Finland revealed some seasonal variation in incidence with somewhat lower incidence around June compared with the rest of the year, with no increase in incidence during winter [271]. Interpretation of seasonal variation must be done in light of the long and variable preclinical phase in type 1 diabetes. A trigger with seasonal variation, such as a viral infection, may well exist but remain undetected if the latency period is highly variable between

individuals. Furthermore, such seasonally varying etiological factors may theoretically have different effects in different age groups, and there may be different epidemic patterns of different viruses or virus serotypes that cancel out any seasonal pattern in the onset of disease. The seasonal pattern, therefore, probably reflects the effect of precipitating viral infections, but triggering effects cannot be completely ruled out. Much of the seasonal variation observed is due to random variation in the relatively small number of cases diagnosed each month in a particular population, since type 1 diabetes is a rare event among childhood populations.

24.3.6   Time Trends

An increasing incidence of childhood-onset type 1 diabetes has been noted in most countries [25, 30, 31, 48, 81–84]. Early studies from Norway indicated incidence rates below 10 per 100 000 among children from the end of the 1920s to the 1960s [85–87], compared with 28 per 100 000 during 1999–2003 [33], although methods were not strictly comparable. In Finland, the incidence has more than doubled since the mid 1960s [83]. Kuwait has experienced an extremely rapid increase, from around 4 per 100 000 during 1980–1981 to about 20 per 100 000 during 1992–1997 [79]. Several other populations have experienced a more than 50% increase in incidence of childhood-onset type 1 diabetes over a 20–30-year period [47, 49, 88–90]. Some year-to-year variation in incidence may be due to chance, but significant epidemic-like patterns have been described in many populations, often superimposed on a steady increase over time [49, 57, 83, 90, 91]. The most recent DIAMOND data showed an increase in incidence rate of 2.8% per year during 1990–1999 as the average for all included centers, roughly similar on every continent. In Central America and the West Indies the overall incidence fell on average by 3.6% per year [31], but changes in the degree of case ascertainment might be the reason for this decrease; in addition, given the small number of cases in these populations, this may also reflect random variation. In contrast to data from Europe showing that low-incidence countries tended to experience the highest relative increase during the early 1990s [25], the most recent trends also indicate a very high relative increase over time in high-incidence countries [31]. For instance, in Finland, where the incidence has been always the highest, the increase is still continuing. The latest data from Finland has shown that the incidence in children is no longer increasing linearly, but since the mid 1990s faster than before and now approaching 60/100,000 [92].

A greater relative increase in incidence among younger children than among the older children, leading to a younger average age at onset among 0–14-year-old children, has been reported in many but not all centers in Europe [25]. Measured on the absolute scale, the difference over time may be more similar in different age groups [34]. More recent data support the earlier findings from Europe and demonstrate a similar pattern in Australia and New Zealand; but in Asia and North America, the relative increase over time is not steeper in the 0–4-year age-group than among 5–14-year-olds [31]. The less steep increase over time among older individuals has also been seen in European studies covering wider age ranges. In France, there was increasing incidence during 1988–1997 in age groups 0–14 years, but stable incidence among the 15–19-year-olds [93]. In West Yorkshire during 1991–1999 the incidence increased with similar relative magnitude among 0–4, 5–9 and 10–14-year-olds, whereas the incidence rates were

stable among 15–29-year-olds [94]. The Swedish and Belgian data for type 1 diabetes have shown an increasing incidence among children, whereas the incidence among young adults has tended to decrease during the same calendar periods [58, 66, 75]. This latter observation is in line with a model where a certain pool of genetically susceptible individuals contract the disease at younger ages, which would lead to an 'early harvest' effect [20, 66]. However, it should be noted that the small amount of available data is not entirely consistent with the 'spring harvest hypothesis,' as the incidence has increased more among adult males than among male children in Lithuania (whereas the pattern among females is consistent with a possible 'early harvest effect') [58] and the incidence rate has increased in age groups over 15 years in the Turin province in Italy [95]. The 'early harvest' model dictates that an increasing incidence over time among the younger is accompanied, or followed, by a decreasing incidence in the older, and the magnitude of changes should cancel each other out to give a stable cumulative incidence at 'older' age. This pattern was clearly seen among Swedish men, but not as clearly among women [66]. In the Swedish study, the average age of onset decreased over time, but there was little change in the peak age at onset [66]. Furthermore, a detailed analysis of the Finish incidence data for children during 1965–1996 showed that, although the mean age at onset have changed over calendar time, the average age at onset had not changed significantly when analyzed by birth cohort [96]. Although early data from the 1946, 1958 and 1970 birth cohorts from England [97] were cited as evidence for an early harvest effect, it should be noted that the cumulative incidence at 23 years of age was much higher in the 1946 birth cohort than in the 1958 birth cohort, and the methods of case detection were not standardized in these studies. The latest analysis of the Finnish data showed that the absolute increase in incidence took place at the same rate in all ages in the childhood range [92], and there was also an increasing incidence in the population aged 15–39 years [98]. It thus seems that the ''spring harvest'' hypothesis needs to be re-considered. However, we cannot with the currently available data evaluate whether there has been a change in incidence of type 1 diabetes in age-groups above 40–50 years.

24.3.7   Birth Cohort or Period Effects?

If the incidence rate increases steadily (linearly or log-linearly) over time, then the increase may be attributable to a steadily increasing exposure to one or more risk factors or steadily decreased exposure to protective factors, as opposed to nonlinear or epidemic-like patterns in incidence rates, which may point toward factors changing in a similar manner over time. Nonlinear birth cohort effects, for instance, would be consistent with an 'epidemic-like' exposure operating prenatally, such as infections or other exposures *in utero*. However, effects of a prenatal exposure would depend on whether the latency period is uniform or variable; the latter would lead to increases within a certain birth cohort at any age, while the former would lead to an increased incidence in specific age groups and in specific birth cohorts only. Specific exposures may operate at different ages postnatally; and, given the multifactorial etiology of type 1 diabetes, specific patterns in time trends may be difficult to attribute to specific etiological factors. The linear dependence between age, period and cohort makes linear or log-linear increases over time (often called *drift*) impossible to attribute to either birth cohort or period on a statistical basis alone [99–101]. Constraints must be employed, and it is recommended to estimate deviations from a linear drift term [101]. It is potentially instructive to examine whether time trends appear to be attributable primarily to period effects or birth cohort effects, although the two are not mutually exclusive.

Increasing rates of childhood-onset type 1 diabetes in Poland during 1970–1985, Sweden during 1978–1987, Finland during 1965–1984 and Yorkshire during 1978–1990 were attributed to calendar period effects, rather than to birth cohort effects [57, 91, 102, 103]. A later analysis of Swedish children during 1978–1997 [104] indicated a further increase over periods, a steeper increase in the youngest children and no clear trend in cumulative incidence over birth cohorts. The recent Finnish nationwide data on the incidence of type 1 diabetes in both children [92] and young adults [98] strongly suggest that the period effect plays a stronger role than the birth cohort effect does. Modeling the incidence in Denmark during 1970–1976, 1980–1984 and 1996–2000 indicated a more prominent cohort effect [38]. Long-term data from army conscripts in Sardinia, the Netherlands and Switzerland have

shown nonlinear increases in incidence by birth cohorts [105–107]. In an age–period–cohort analysis of incidence in the age groups below 15 years during 1973–1982 and 1989–2003 in Norway, overall cohort effects were not significant, but there was a significant nonlinear calendar period effect with increasing incidence over time. However, when taking geographic location into account in a combined age–period–cohort–area model, some specific areas were found to exhibit significant cohort effects [55]. Other studies have also attempted to study cohort and period effects, with no clear distinction between the two, in some instances probably because of either small data sets or no formal modeling [66, 94, 95].

24.4   FAMILIAL AGGREGATION AND RELATION TO OTHER DISEASES

24.4.1   Familial Aggregation of Type 1 Diabetes

Familial aggregation of type 1 diabetes is well established, and the highest risk is seen in monozygotic twin siblings of persons with type 1 diabetes [108–110]. The absolute risk in first-degree relatives (other than monozygotic twins) of persons with type 1 diabetes seems to be about 4–7%, approximately 10–15 times the risk in the corresponding general populations [111–114]. Although part of this could theoretically be due to shared environmental factors, the majority of the familial aggregation is likely to be due to genetic factors. In Europe, 4–15% of newly diagnosed cases had a parent or sibling with type 1 diabetes, with higher proportions in high-incidence countries [115]; overall, 3.6% of cases had a sibling, 1.8% a mother and 3–4% a father with type 1 diabetes. A roughly twofold higher risk in children of fathers with type 1 diabetes compared with children of mothers with type 1 diabetes has been observed [115–118]. In a large cohort study in Finland where the parents rather than the children were probands, the cumulative risk by age 20 years was 7.8% in children of Finnish fathers with type 1 diabetes, compared with 5.3% among mothers with diabetes, which is an approximately 10-fold increased risk over the general population overall [118]. Many factors may influence studies of familial patterns of disease, both design and analysis issues and biological factors [119], so results must be interpreted with caution.

Models involving genetic imprinting, preferential transmission of risk alleles and selective embryonic or fetal loss have been considered, but no satisfactory explanation of the paternal versus maternal diabetes effect has been given.

24.4.2 Aggregation of Other Diseases

Aggregation of type 2 diabetes among relatives of patients with type 1 diabetes has been suggested in some studies, but other studies have suggested that many of the familial cases may have been misclassified and were really type 1 [120]. Aggregation of other autoimmune diseases in the families of patients with type 1 diabetes have been seen, often different diseases in different individuals within the families [121–123]. In light of the so-called Th1/Th2 paradigm, recent studies have found some evidence for an inverse association between type 1 diabetes and Th2-biased atopic disorders in individuals [124–127]. A correlation between the occurrence of type 1 diabetes and atopic disorders over different populations is tentatively explained by similar genetic or nongenetic risk factors, whereas the disease process of either disease reduces the risk in individuals of developing the other disease [128].

24.5 EPIDEMIOLOGIC EVIDENCE FOR ENVIRONMENTAL RISK FACTORS

24.5.1 General Epidemiological Evidence

For the fundamental aim of preventing type 1 diabetes, we need to identify modifiable environmental factors. If several factors contribute to the disease risk, then it is important to understand that factors contributing to the individual risk do not necessarily explain the variation in population incidence between regions or the increasing incidence over time within populations. Much of the data presented above supports a role of environmental factors in the etiology of type 1 diabetes. Available evidence from twin studies [108–110] and migration studies [129] provides evidence for involvement of both genetic and nongenetic factors. There is evidence that some of the between-country difference in incidence may be explained by different frequencies of the high-risk HLA genotype in different countries [130], but there are also examples of large

differences in incidence between populations that have related ethnic backgrounds, such as Iceland versus Norway [131] and Finland versus neighboring countries Estonia [132] and the Karelian Republic of Russia [133], although there may be genetic differences between these populations. In Finland, one HLA haplotype that confers a very high risk of type 1 diabetes and that has not been found in any other population explains probably about 10% of the cases of the cases of type 1 diabetes and, thus, specifically contributes to the high incidence in this population [272]. Data from Sardinia show that the children born to Sardinian parents who had moved to mainland Italy had an identical incidence to children living in Sardinia [273]. The observation that the proportion of newly diagnosed children with type 1 diabetes who carry the high-risk HLA genotype (DR4–DQ8/DR3–DQ2) seems to have decreased over time in several populations suggests that environmental factors may have contributed to the development of type 1 diabetes in more children with moderate-risk HLA genotypes [274].

It has been argued that environmental factors may operate *in utero* and early in life, but it is difficult to envisage that such exposure can explain all type 1 diabetes. Some evidence for epidemic-like patterns in incidence might suggest that some factors may have a relatively short induction time and operate also after 5 years of age [33, 57, 80, 90, 134, 135]. There is some evidence for a modest space–time clustering at birth or at diagnosis, often only in some subgroups of sex, region and age or using only a specific set of critical values for space- and time-clustered pairs [72, 136–139]. Helgason and Jonasson [67] observed that males with type 1 diabetes tended to be born in October, and attributed this to nitrosamines in smoked mutton eaten around Christmas. Many studies have since investigated the distribution of birth month in cases of type 1 diabetes, but the pattern does not seem to be consistent between countries, and many studies have not found any significant variation [140]. Also, a number of ecologic studies have found a correlation between incidence of childhood-onset type 1 diabetes and a variety of nongenetic factors, but such studies are prone to serious bias [141, 142]. Many consider infectious agents the most plausible candidates for initiators of autoimmunity, and perhaps also for progression of the disease process [22]. Nevertheless, despite extensive research, such agents have not been detected and, therefore, this theory remains speculative. Many other factors have also been implicated, including nutritional factors and perinatal factors, and these are reviewed below.

24.5.2 Microbial Factors

Infectious etiological agents in type 1 diabetes have been suspected for many decades, with many studies and different approaches [22, 143, 144]. More recently, it has also been suggested that some infections may reduce the risk of type 1 diabetes [144–146]. Agents studied in humans include enteroviruses, rubella, mumps virus, cytomegalovirus, endogenous retroviruses and Epstein–Barr virus. Various symptoms of infectious disease and general indicators of microbial exposure, such as day-care attendance [147], have also been studied. Both maternal infections during pregnancy and postnatal exposure have been studied. The utility of different methods of measuring exposure to microbial factors depend on the specific hypothesis to be tested and the study design. Several detailed reviews of potential molecular mechanisms linking viral infections and type 1 diabetes have been published; see [144, 148–150] for instance. Etiological roles of viral infections may, in general, be mediated thorough direct cytolytic effects or various forms of host-response-mediated pathologic effects, such as bystander activation of autoreactive T-cells and molecular mimicry.

24.5.2.1 Congenital Rubella Infection

Although rubella is now eradicated in many populations with high incidence of type 1 diabetes, congenital rubella infection has been associated with a high risk of diabetes: approximately 10–20% in some studies [151, 152], but lower risks have also been reported [153–155]. Rubella virus has been recovered from the pancreas of infected children [156, 157], but rubella infection in the neonatal period or later in childhood does not seem to be associated with type 1 diabetes [158], and islet autoimmunity after rubella vaccination is rare, transient and low titre [159]. Patients with congenital rubella syndrome and type 1 diabetes seem to have a similar distribution of HLA risk alleles to other patients with type 1 diabetes [160, 161]. However, studies of congenital rubella

syndrome and diabetes often include an apparently heterogeneous group of adults with impaired glucose tolerance, diabetes not treated with insulin and insulin-treated diabetes, sometimes with limited information on clinical characteristics [151, 152, 162–164]. None of 25 Finnish and 12 Polish adolescents with congenital rubella infections had markers of islet autoimmunity, and only one had type 1 diabetes [154]. In summary, congenital rubella infections are associated with increased risk of diabetes, but it seems reasonable to question whether all the patients identified in previous studies really had 'common' type 1 diabetes.

24.5.2.2 Enteroviruses

Human enteroviruses comprise many serotypes, and infections are common but mostly asymptomatic [165]. The earliest seroepidemiological case–control studies of type 1 diabetes reported a higher frequency of positivity for Coxsackievirus antibodies in cases than in controls [71], and a famous study reported that a Coxsackie B4 virus isolated from the pancreas of a child produced diabetes by adoptive transfer to mice [166]. In another study of pancreata from 250 children with fatal infections, viral cytopathology of the islets of Langerhans was found in four of seven cases of Coxsackievirus B infection [157], while no evidence of enterovirus RNA by in situ hybridization was detected in a study of 29 pancreata from patients who had died of recent-onset type 1 diabetes [167]. A recent analysis of pancreatic tissue from 6 type 1 diabetic and 26 control organ donors using immunohistochemistry, electron microscopy, whole-genome ex vivo nucleotide sequencing, and cell culture demonstrated beta-cell specific Coxsackie B4 enterovirus in specimens from 3 of the 6 patients, with no indication of infection in controls [168]. There was evidence for functional impairment of infected beta-cells, but a predominantly nondestructive islet inflammation, mediated by natural killer cells was indicated. This is an intriguing observation, but raises the question whether these infected cases really had common type 1 diabetes. Many seroepidemiological case–control studies have corroborated the initial findings, but studies have also found an inverse or no association [169].

Increased risk of childhood-onset type 1 diabetes was associated with antibodies against enteroviruses in frozen serum from Finnish mothers taken at the end of the first trimester [170] and in serum from Swedish mothers at delivery [171]. A later Swedish study using enterovirus RNA or IgM antibodies in serum from early pregnancy supported the earlier findings [172], but a later, larger Finnish study using a battery of enterovirus antibodies or serum enterovirus RNA from the first trimester was unable to confirm findings from the earlier study [173]. No significant results were found in other smaller studies from Finland using cord blood [174] and from Germany using enterovirus antibodies in serum taken at delivery [175]. A larger Swedish study of blood spots from newborn (2–3-day-old) children found a significant relation between RNA in blood spots and risk of type 1 diabetes during childhood, although only a small proportion of the newborn samples was positive for enterovirus RNA [176].

Using both serum enterovirus antibodies and enterovirus RNA as indications of infection, prospective studies from Finland have found enterovirus to be associated with increased risk of islet autoimmunity and type 1 diabetes [170, 177, 178], but use of different methods of data analysis makes interpretation of some of the Finnish studies somewhat difficult. A report from the Diabetes Prediction and Prevention Study (DIPP), which included 41 cases, seemed to support an increased risk of islet autoimmunity associated with enterovirus infections, particularly in the 6-month interval before seroconversion for islet autoantibodies [178]. A similar association was also found among 19 cases of islet autoimmunity and 84 controls from the Trial to Reduce IDDM in the Genetically at Risk (TRIGR) dietary intervention study [174]. In the Diabetes Autoimmunity Study in the Young (DAISY) Study, no association was found between enterovirus RNA in serum or in rectal swabs, and islet autoimmunity in a nested case–control study with 26 cases of islet autoimmunity [179]. No association was found between a panel of Coxsackievirus serotype-specific antibodies during childhood and development of islet autoimmunity in children of diabetic mothers or fathers in the German BabyDiab study [175]. Additional details and potential mechanisms of viral pathogenesis in type 1 diabetes with particular focus on enteroviruses are found in recent reviews [22, 149, 180].

24.5.2.3 Other Specific Virus Infections

Among other viruses associated with human type 1 diabetes, mumps was among the first to be described, but most of the evidence is circumstantial or conflicting [158, 167, 171, 181]. Human cytomegalovirus has been associated with type 1 diabetes in some studies [157, 182], but not in others [158, 183, 184], although the potential latency of this common virus and specific mechanisms involved [185] may require more specific investigations. Human endogenous retroviruses encoding a superantigen have been implicated in one study [186, 187], but others does not support a specific role in type 1 diabetes [188, 189]. Epstein–Barr virus has been implicated in a couple of studies, but others did not support this [170]. Serological evidence for rotavirus infections was found to correlate with positivity for islet autoantibodies in a prospective study including transiently autoantibody positive children at risk of type 1 diabetes [190], but no association was found in a Finnish study [191] using different analytic methods and assay.

24.5.2.4 Infectious Symptoms and the 'Hygiene Hypothesis'

The so-called 'hygiene hypothesis' proposes that the decline in nonspecific infectious and microbial exposure in many populations over the past few decades has caused the concomitant increase in incidence of type 1 diabetes [145, 146]. Some infections and microbial agents reduce the incidence of autoimmune diabetes in experimental animals [150]. Epidemiological studies have investigated nonspecific infections [192–194] or markers of microbial exposure, such as day-care attendance [147, 195], but the results have been quite inconsistent. Many earlier studies reported an increased risk with an increasing number (or markers) of infections, but more recent studies have reported reduced risk of type 1 diabetes associated with early infections, including studies based on medical records rather than recall [192–194]. Two cohort studies of islet autoimmunity did not find any association with neonatal or early childhood infectious diseases or symptoms of infections [69, 196]. In the DAISY cohort study of islet autoimmunity, we found significantly lower risk associated with maternal symptoms of infections during pregnancy [69]. A few case–control studies of general symptoms of maternal infections during pregnancy and risk of type 1 diabetes in children have not found any significant association [193, 197], but these were prone to recall or selection bias. A recent meta-analysis concluded that there is some evidence for a lower risk of type 1 diabetes among children who attended day-care centers early in life, although the amount of heterogeneity between studies makes it difficult to draw strong conclusions [147]. No association with day-care attendance before 2 years of age was found in the DAISY cohort study of autoimmunity [69].

24.5.2.5 The 'Polio Model'

The potential analogy of so-called 'polio model' with type 1 diabetes was pointed out a long time ago [71], and based on an observation from Finland that the occurrence of enterovirus infections seems to have decreased among infants and pregnant women; the authors proposed that this may explain part of the increasing incidence of type 1 diabetes via decreasing protection from maternal enterovirus antibodies [198]. These findings were replicated in studies that included additional countries [199, 200], but they remain only indirect tests of the hypothesis that maternal antibodies may protect against type 1 diabetes. Indirect evidence not supporting the polio model includes the prediction that the age at onset of type 1 diabetes should have increased over time, which is contrary to what is observed, and the apparent lack of association between socioeconomic status and type 1 diabetes (see below).

24.5.2.6 Vaccinations

Vaccinations provide a further aspect of the possible relation between viral infections and type 1 diabetes. A workshop on vaccines and risk of type 1 diabetes held in the late 1990s concluded that there was no evidence supporting an increasing risk of type 1 diabetes associated with common vaccines [201]. This conclusion has been enforced by more recent data and reviews [202–205]. Also, the available data clearly indicate that none of the currently available vaccinations introduced has reduced the risk of type 1 diabetes.

24.5.3 Dietary Factors

Studies published in the early 1980s stimulated the research about the role of diet in the etiology of type 1 diabetes [206–208].

24.5.3.1 Duration of Breast-feeding and Age at Introduction of Cow's Milk

The possible protective role of breast-feeding and detrimental role of early introduction of cow's milk in the development of type 1 diabetes have been hotly debated [209]. Several possible plausible mechanisms have been proposed to explain the epidemiological observations, including 'molecular mimicry,' a detrimental effect of bovine insulin in cow's milk, covered in detail in several reviews (see [208] and references therein). The fact that the majority of women breast-feed their children for several months in Western countries, including Scandinavian countries, does not support a major effect of breast-feeding in explaining the secular trends or differences between countries. A few prospective studies using islet autoimmunity as the outcome have been published. Some have supported previous findings in case–control studies [210], whereas others did not find any significant association [211]. A recent advanced analysis of a cohort of more than 3500 children with risk-associated HLA genes, in which 111 cases positive for multiple autoantibodies (ICA plus at least one out of insulin, IA-2 and GAD autoantibodies) in the Finnish DIPP study concluded that there was no significant association between the duration of exclusive or total breast-feeding and risk of advanced islet autoimmunity [212], but this study did not have data on clinical type 1 diabetes. A randomized controlled trial initiated in Finland might provide an answer in the near future on whether delayed introduction of cow's milk protein can reduce the risk of islet autoimmunity and type 1 diabetes [213], but it will not give the answer to the question about the possible benefit of breast-feeding.

24.5.3.2 Age at Introduction of Cereals

Two cohort studies of islet autoimmunity have provided some evidence for a role of age at introduction of cereals or gluten [214, 215], although the relation is complex and difficult to interpret. Again, no data exist to say that such cereals would actually be related to clinical type 1 diabetes. Also, it must be noted that the genetic susceptibility of gluten-related celiac disease is related primarily to HLA-DR3, and some haplotypes carrying HLA-DR3 are also susceptibility haplotypes for type 1 diabetes. Therefore, it may be that a common genetic constellation rather than a specific environmental exposure may play a role in this possible association.

24.5.3.3 Vitamin D

Vitamin D status, as indicated by serum 25-hydroxy-vitamin D concentrations, has been found to be decreased in patients with type 1 diabetes compared with that in control subjects in a few studies [216–218], but the possibility that this was a consequence of disease or selection bias cannot be ruled out. Another similar study found no difference in serum 25-hydroxy-vitamin D or the active form 1,25-dihydroxy-vitamin D [219]. A European multicenter case–control study reported an association between use of vitamin D supplements in the first year of life and lower risk of type 1 diabetes in children [220], a finding later supported by a prospective Finnish study [221]. Maternal intake of vitamin D via food during pregnancy was associated with a reduced risk of islet autoimmunity in children in the DAISY study [222], but there were no association of maternal intake of vitamin D from food or supplements with advanced islet cell autoimmunity in the DIPP study [275]. Prospective studies using biomarkers of vitamin D have not yet (as of 2007) been published.

24.5.3.4 Omega-3 Fatty Acids

Maternal use of cod-liver oil was associated with lower risk of type 1 diabetes, while there was a suggested association for children's use of cod liver oil in the first year of life in a pilot case–control study from Norway [223]. In a much larger independent study, the association with maternal use of cod-liver oil in pregnancy disappeared after adjustment for potential confounders, while there was a significantly lower risk in children who used cod-liver oil in the first year of life [224]. Cod-liver oil, which is commonly used in Norway, is an important source of both vitamin D and long chain n-3 fatty acids (docosahexaenoic acid and eicosapentaenoic acid) in this population. The lack of association with other vitamin D supplements in these studies supports a role of n-3 fatty acids rather than vitamin D. Although recall bias cannot be entirely ruled out, a similar effect for other dietary supplements would have been expected if recall bias were present. One recent clinic-based cross-sectional study found that docosahexaenoic acid was significantly lower in children with type 1 diabetes than in controls [225]. Other studies support a role of inflammatory prostaglandins that are known to be influenced by dietary long-chain n-3 fatty acids [226]. Recently, evidence from the prospective DAISY study using both dietary intake data and biomarkers of omega-3 fatty acids early in life showed a significant relation between higher intake and lower risk of islet autoimmunity [276].

24.5.3.5 Vitamin E

Hypothesizing that antioxidants may protect against destruction of β-cells, Finnish investigators measured serum alpha-tocopherol concentration in frozen sera from 19 individuals who developed diabetes and in about 60 individually matched controls from a prospective cohort of individuals aged above 20 years [227]. Higher alpha-tocopherol was associated with a significantly lower risk of type 1 diabetes [227]. Another study from Finland attempted to replicate this finding in siblings of persons with type 1 diabetes, and found partial support, although the results were not significant [228]. There was no significant difference in serum vitamin E concentration between patients with insulin-dependent diabetes and nondiabetic controls in a cross-sectional study of prevalent cases [229], but we cannot exclude the possibility that the disease has influenced the serum level of vitamin E. Recently, the DIPP study reported no significant association between serum alpha- or gamma-tocopherol and risk of advanced islet cell autoimmunity or type 1 diabetes [277]. Since there are many much stronger antioxidants than vitamin E, this theory may not be proven with vitamin E. Moreover, the European Nicotinamide Diabetes Intervention Trial that used nicotinic acid (also an antioxidant) to prevent type 1 diabetes in children with ICA antibodies was clearly negative [278].

24.5.4 Perinatal Factors

24.5.4.1 Parental Age at Birth and Birth Order

Several studies have found an approximately 30–50% increased risk of type 1 diabetes in children associated with maternal age of 35 years or more at birth [230–235]. Both significantly higher [232, 236] and lower risks [234] among first-born compared with second or later born children have been found, and there was evidence of heterogeneity between centers in two of these studies [232, 234]. Some studies have not found any significant association between birth order and type 1 diabetes [68, 233, 237] or islet autoimmunity [238]. One study found the effect of maternal age to be dependent on birth order and vice versa [235]. Naturally, birth order and maternal age at birth of a child are highly correlated and it may not be easy to find out which one is the true etiological factor; biologically, both of them could be plausible.

24.5.4.2   Size at Birth

Some large studies have found a statistically significant association between higher birth weight or birth weight for gestational age and risk for type 1 diabetes, but the magnitude of the relative risk seems small [234, 239–242], and some have not found any significant association [68, 243]. Genetic factors could potentially influence both size at birth and risk of type 1 diabetes, and studies in nondiabetic children indicated that genotypes known to confer reduced risk for type 1 diabetes tended to be associated with larger size at birth [244–247], and a recent very large study also found evidence for the association between high-risk HLA genotypes and larger size at birth [247]. In a direct test, the association between size at birth and type 1 diabetes was not influenced by adjustment for genetic polymorhisms in the insulin gene and HLA genes, indicating that the associations, if any, are probably too weak to have important clinical implications [248], or the potential association is more complex.

24.5.4.3   Other Perinatal Factors

Maternal preeclampsia has been associated with childhood-onset type 1 diabetes in some studies [231, 233, 234, 237], whereas other studies found no association [68, 232, 249]. Caesarean section has been associated with an increased risk of type 1 diabetes in some studies [231, 232], but the majority of large studies found no association [68, 197, 233, 234, 249, 250]. However, the pooled estimate from a recent meta-analysis of twenty observational studies indicated an approximately 20% increased risk of childhood-onset type 1 diabetes in children born by Caesarean section compared to others [251]. Blood group incompatibility has been

associated with an increased risk of type 1 diabetes, but Rhesus-factor incompatibility less so than ABO incompatibility [231, 234, 237], if at all [249]. A Swedish study recently suggested that association may be with the associated phototherapy [252].

24.5.4.4   Socioeconomic Status

Because many variables, such as infant feeding practices, hygiene and living standards, obesity, diet and various other lifestyle factors, are related to socioeconomic status, the relation between socioeconomic status and type 1 diabetes or lack thereof can be instructive in evaluating putative etiological factors.

Many of the studies with the main focus on socioeconomic status as predictors of type 1 diabetes have used ecologic design, with inherent weaknesses. Some have found higher average socioeconomic status to be associated with higher incidence of type 1 diabetes [253, 254], and some found no association [255]. One area in Denmark with lower average socioeconomic status had a higher incidence than another area with higher status [74]. Lower socioeconomic status was associated with increased incidence in an ecologic study from northern England [256].

Results from individual level case–control studies have been similarly inconsistent. Studies in which parental education was determined indicated mostly an increased risk among those with lower parental education [197, 224, 233, 250, 257], but the opposite was indicated in one study from the United States [243] and in one cohort study from Finland involving only families with type 1 diabetes [258]. Low socioeconomic status parental occupations have been associated with both an increased [197, 233, 237] and a reduced risk of type 1 diabetes [236, 259], while opposing trends were seen in Northern Ireland and Scotland [232]. Low family income has also been associated with both an increased [260] and a reduced risk [243]. Nevertheless, in many populations it has been true that more-affluent families have been able to cover the costs of the care of type 1 diabetes in the past, and such a situation still exists in many populations today. Thus, in such families, children with type 1 diabetes had a better survival and a higher chance to reproduce, and to transmit their susceptibility genes to the next generation, compared with families with a lower socioeconomic status.

24.5.4.5 Gene–Environment Interactions

The current concept of etiology of type 1 diabetes involves both genes and environment, but notions about interaction between the two are often vague. The terms *effect modification* and *synergy* are sometimes used to describe 'epidemiological' or statistical interaction, which are known to be dependent on the scale on which association is measured [261]. Biological interpretations of such interactions should, therefore, be made with great caution, including for gene–gene interactions [261].

Whether putative contributory environmental factors have stronger effects in individuals with or without specific risk-conferring genotypes remains an open question. For instance, an increasing proportion of patients without the high-risk HLA–DR4–DQ8/DR3–DQ2 genotype over time [262, 263] indicates that environmental factors may have contributed to development of type 1 diabetes in more children with moderate risk ('permissive' genotypes) in recent years. Among the few population-based studies of type 1 diabetes that have looked at genetic markers and environmental exposure simultaneously are those of Kostraba *et al.* [264] and Pérez-Bravo *et al.* [265]. Both these studies indicated that the odds ratio conferred by short duration of breast-feeding was similar among those carrying the HLA-risk genotype and others [264, 265], but both may have been influenced by recall bias [207].

It has been suggested that all case–control studies of putative risk factors of type 1 diabetes must match control subjects for known HLA genes [266, 267], but lack of matching cannot lead to confounding unless there is an association between HLA genotype and the new putative risk factor [261]. In many early case–control studies of viral infections and type 1 diabetes, HLA typing was done only for cases and not controls [268]. Associations between HLA genotype and infections among cases reflect a mix of potential deviations from multiplicative effects of HLA and infection on development of type 1 diabetes and potential associations between HLA genotype and infections in the background population [269]. Without knowledge of the magnitude of each component, these results are impossible to interpret.

In summary, despite the biologic plausibility for gene–environment interactions, when using operational definitions, there is little direct evidence for a gene–environment interaction in type 1 diabetes from epidemiological studies.

24.6 CONCLUSION

One of the most striking issues in type 1 diabetes epidemiology is the very wide, over 400-fold difference in incidence of childhood-onset type 1 diabetes worldwide. The highest incidence is in Finland, which has been leading the rank ever since the population-based incidence data have been available. The reasons for the large geographic differences in incidence, besides the HLA genetics, are still mostly unknown. It is nevertheless obvious that much of the variation among populations observed is related to their HLA-haplotype distributions. The contributions of other (non-HLA) genes and proposed environmental factors to the large variation in type 1 diabetes incidence still remain to be confirmed. Second, it is clear that the incidence is increasing globally, both in low-incidence and high-incidence populations. The rate of increase has been relatively constant among the different populations, at around 3% per year globally, and observed now for many decades. The increase in incidence is neither unique to certain populations nor to a specific time period. Since the 1920–1930s, when insulin was introduced in industrialized countries, the number of cases of type 1 diabetes has been growing continuously. Despite many efforts to identify environmental risk factors for type 1 diabetes, the results have been disappointingly scarce. Type 1 diabetes is not a disease of children only. It has been estimated that more than half of the cases of type 1 are diagnosed at the age of 15 or older; and owing to increased survival, most patients with type 1 diabetes live long lives until older ages. Thus, the main health care requirements for type 1 diabetes deal with adults with the disease.

References

1. Foulis, A.K., Liddle, C.N., Farquharson, M.A. *et al.* (1986) The histopathology of the pancreas in type 1 (insulin-dependent) diabetes mellitus: a 25-year review of deaths in patients under 20 years of age in the United Kingdom. *Diabetologia*, **29**, 267–74.

2. Atkinson, M.A. (2005) ADA Outstanding Scientific Achievement Lecture 2004. Thirty years of investigating the autoimmune basis for type 1

diabetes: why can't we prevent or reverse this disease? *Diabetes*, **54**, 1253–63.

3. Mølbak, A.G., Christau, B., Marner, B. *et al.* (1994) Incidence of insulin-dependent diabetes mellitus in age groups over 30 years in Denmark. *Diabetic Medicine: A Journal of the British Diabetic Association*, **11**, 650–5.

4. Karjalainen, J., Salmela, P., Ilonen, J. *et al.* (1989) A comparison of childhood and adult type I diabetes mellitus. *The New England Journal of Medicine*, **320**, 881–6.

5. Dahlquist, G. and Mustonen, L.R. (1995) Clinical onset characteristics of familial versus nonfamilial cases in a large population-based cohort of childhood-onset diabetes patients. *Diabetes Care*, **18**, 852–4.

6. Bruno, G., Merletti, F., De Salvia, A. *et al.* (1997) Comparison of incidence of insulin-dependent diabetes mellitus in children and young adults in the Province of Turin, Italy, 1984–91. Piedmont Study Group for Diabetes Epidemiology. *Diabetic Medicine: A Journal of the British Diabetic Association*, **14**, 964–9.

7. Eberhardt, M.S., Wagener, D.K., Orchard, T.J. *et al.* (1985) HLA heterogeneity of insulin-dependent diabetes mellitus at diagnosis. The Pittsburgh IDDM study. *Diabetes*, **34**, 1247–52.

8. Atkinson, M.A. and Eisenbarth, G.S. (2001) Type 1 diabetes: new perspectives on disease pathogenesis and treatment. *Lancet*, **358**, 221–9.

9. Achenbach, P., Bonifacio, E., Koczwara, K. and Ziegler, A.G. (2005) Natural history of type 1 diabetes. *Diabetes*, **54** (Suppl 2), S25–31.

10. Eisenbarth, G.S., Moriyama, H., Robles, D.T. *et al.* (2002) Insulin autoimmunity: prediction/precipitation/prevention type 1A diabetes. *Autoimmunity Reviews*, **1**, 139–45.

11. Achenbach, P., Warncke, K., Reiter, J. *et al.* (2004) Stratification of type 1 diabetes risk on the basis of islet autoantibody characteristics. *Diabetes*, **53**, 384–92.

12. Fourlanos, S., Dotta, F., Greenbaum, C.J. *et al.* (2005) Latent autoimmune diabetes in adults (LADA) should be less latent. *Diabetologia*, **48**, 2206–12.

13. Adojaan, B., Knip, M., Vähäsalo, P. *et al.* (1996) Relationship between the incidence of childhood IDDM and the frequency of ICA positivity in nondiabetic children in the general population (Letter). *Diabetes Care*, **19**, 1452–4.

14. Marciulionyte, D., Williams, A.J., Bingley, P.J. *et al.* (2001) A comparison of the prevalence of islet autoantibodies in children from two countries with differing incidence of diabetes. *Diabetologia*, **44**, 16–21.

15. Rewers, M. (2002) Islet autoantibodies in cord blood: maternal, fetal, or neither? *Diabetes/Metabolism Research and Reviews*, **18**, 2–4.

16. Barker, J.M., Barriga, K.J., Yu, L. *et al.* (2004) Prediction of autoantibody positivity and progression to type 1 diabetes: Diabetes Autoimmunity Study in the Young (DAISY). *The Journal of Clinical Endocrinology and Metabolism*, **89**, 3896–902.

17. Achenbach, P., Koczwara, K., Knopff, A. *et al.* (2004) Mature high-affinity immune responses to (pro)insulin anticipate the autoimmune cascade that leads to type 1 diabetes. *The Journal of Clinical Investigation*, **114**, 589–97.

18. Kukko, M., Virtanen, S.M., Toivonen, A. *et al.* (2004) Geographical variation in risk *HLA-DQB1* genotypes for type 1 diabetes and signs of beta-cell autoimmunity in a high-incidence country. *Diabetes Care*, **27**, 676–81.

19. Williams, A.J., Bingley, P.J., Moore, W.P.T. and Gale, E.A.M. (2002) Islet autoantibodies, nationality and gender: a multinational screening study in first-degree relatives of patients with type I diabetes. *Diabetologia*, **45**, 217–23.

20. Gale, E.A. (2005) Spring harvest? Reflections on the rise of type 1 diabetes. *Diabetologia*, 1–6.

21. Kimpimäki, T., Kupila, A., Hämäläinen, A.M. *et al.* (2001) The first signs of beta-cell autoimmunity appear in infancy in genetically susceptible children from the general population: the Finnish Type 1 Diabetes Prediction and Prevention Study. *The Journal of Clinical Endocrinology and Metabolism*, **86**, 4782–8.

22. Knip, M., Veijola, R., Virtanen, S.M. *et al.* (2005) Environmental triggers and determinants of type 1 diabetes. *Diabetes*, **54** (Suppl 2), S125–36.

23. Diabetes Epidemiology Research International Group (1988) Geographic patterns of childhood insulin-dependent diabetes mellitus. *Diabetes*, **37**, 1113–19.

24. Karvonen, M., Viik-Kajander, M., Moltchanova, E. *et al.* (2000) Incidence of childhood type 1 diabetes worldwide. Diabetes Mondiale (DiaMond) Project Group. *Diabetes Care*, **23**, 1516–26.

25. EURODIAB ACE Study Group (2000) Variation and trends in incidence of childhood diabetes in Europe. *Lancet*, **355**, 873–6.

26. Green, A. and Patterson, C.C. (2001) Trends in the incidence of childhood-onset diabetes in Europe 1989–1998. *Diabetologia*, **44** (Suppl 3), B3–8.

27. LaPorte, R.E., McCarty, D., Bruno, G. *et al.* (1993) Counting diabetes in the next millennium. Application of capture–recapture technology. *Diabetes Care*, **16**, 528–34.

28. Chao, A., Tsay, P.K., Lin, S.H. *et al.* (2001) The applications of capture–recapture models to epidemiological data. *Statistics in Medicine*, **20**, 3123–57.

29. Karvonen, M., Tuomilehto, J., Libman, I. and LaPorte, R. (1993) A review of the recent epidemiological data on the worldwide incidence of type 1 (insulin-dependent) diabetes mellitus. World Health Organization DIAMOND Project Group. *Diabetologia*, **36**, 883–92.

30. Onkamo, P., Väänänen, S., Karvonen, M. and Tuomilehto, J. (1999) Worldwide increase in incidence of type 1 diabetes – the analysis of the data on published incidence trends. *Diabetologia*, **42**, 1395–403.

31. The DIAMOND Project Group (2006) Incidence and trends of type 1 diabetes worldwide in 1990–1999. *Diabetic Medicine: A Journal of the British Diabetic Association*, **23**, 857–66.

32. Joner, G., Stene, L.C. and Søvik, O. (2004) Nationwide, prospective registration of type 1 diabetes in children aged <15 years in Norway 1989–1998: no increase but significant regional variation in incidence. *Diabetes Care*, **27**, 1618–22.

33. Joner, G., Stene, L.C., Njølstad, P.R. and Søvik, O. (2005) Marked jump in incidence of childhood onset diabetes in Norway after ten years of stable incidence: prospective nationwide study 1999–2003 (Abstract). *Diabetologia*, **48** (Suppl 1), A103.

34. Cinek, O., Sumnik, Z. and Vavrinec, J. (2003) Continuing increase in incidence of childhood-onset type 1 diabetes in the Czech Republic 1990–2001. *European Journal of Pediatrics*, **162**, 428–9.

35. Newhook, L.A., Curtis, J., Hagerty, D. *et al.* (2004) High incidence of childhood type 1 diabetes in the Avalon Peninsula, Newfoundland, Canada. *Diabetes Care*, **27**, 885–8.

36. Campbell-Stokes, P.L. and Taylor, B.J. (2005) Prospective incidence study of diabetes mellitus in New Zealand children aged 0 to 14 years. *Diabetologia*, **48**, 643–8.

37. Swai, A.B., McLarty, D.G. and Alberti, K.G. (1993) IDDM in sub-Saharan Africa (Letter). *Diabetic Medicine: A Journal of the British Diabetic Association*, **10**, 188.

38. Svensson, J., Carstensen, B., Mølbak, A. *et al.* (2002) Increased risk of childhood type 1 diabetes in children born after 1985. *Diabetes Care*, **25**, 2197–201.

39. Van Wouwe, J.P., Verkerk, P.H., Mattiazzo, G.F. *et al.* (2002) Variation by ethnicity in incidence of diabetes type 1 and clinical condition at onset in the Netherlands. *European Journal of Pediatrics*, **161**, 559–60.

40. Ajlouni, K., Qusous, Y., Khawaldeh, A.K. *et al.* (1999) Incidence of insulin-dependent diabetes mellitus in Jordanian children aged 0–14 yr during 1992–1996. *Acta Paediatrica. Supplement*, **88**, 11–13.

41. Pishdad, G.R. (2005) Low incidence of type 1 diabetes in Iran. *Diabetes Care*, **28**, 927–8.

42. Rosenbauer, J., Icks, A. and Giani, G. (2002) Incidence and prevalence of childhood type 1 diabetes mellitus in Germany – model-based national estimates. *Journal of Pediatric Endocrinology and Metabolism*, **15**, 1497–504.

43. Bartsocas, C.S., Dacou-Voutetakis, C., Damianaki, D. *et al.* (1998) Epidemiology of childhood IDDM in Athens: trends in incidence fo the years 1989–1995 (Letter). *Diabetologia*, **41**, 245–8.

44. Cotellessa, M., Barbieri, P., Mazzella, M. *et al.* (2003) High incidence of childhood type 1 diabetes in Liguria, Italy, from 1989 to 1998. *Diabetes Care*, **26**, 1786–9.

45. Jarosz-Chobot, P., Otto-Buczkowska, E. and Koehler, B. (2000) The increased trend of type 1 diabetes mellitus in children (0–14 years) in the Upper Silesia region of Poland (Letter). *Acta Paediatrica*, **89**, 120.

46. Lora-Gómez, R.E., Morales-Pérez, F.M., Arroyo-Díez, F.J. and Barquero-Romero, J. (2005) Incidence of type 1 diabetes in children in Caceres, Spain, during 1988–1999. *Diabetes Research and Clinical Practice*, **69**, 169–74.

47. Haynes, A., Bower, C., Bulsara, M.K. *et al.* (2004) Continued increase in the incidence of childhood type 1 diabetes in a population-based Australian sample (1985–2002). *Diabetologia*, **47**, 866–70.

48. Joner, G. and Søvik, O. (1989) Increasing incidence of diabetes mellitus in Norwegian children 0–14 years of age 1973–1982. *Diabetologia*, **32**, 79–83.

49. Tzaneva, V., Iotova, V. and Yotov, Y. (2001) Significant urban/rural differences in the incidence of type 1 (insulin-dependent) diabetes mellitus among Bulgarian children (1982–1998). *Pediatric Diabetes*, **2**, 103–8.

50. Neu, A., Kehrer, M., Hub, R. and Ranke, M.B. (1997) Incidence of IDDM in German children aged 0–14 years. A 6-year population-based study (1987–1993). *Diabetes Care*, **20**, 530–3.

51. Nyström, L., Dahlquist, G., Östman, J. *et al.* (1992) Risk of developing insulin-dependent diabetes mellitus (IDDM) before 35 years of age:

indications of climatological determinants for age at onset. *International Journal of Epidemiology*, **21**, 352–8.

52. Bloom, A., Hayes, T.M. and Gamble, D.R. (1975) Register of newly diagnosed diabetic children. *British Medical Journal*, **3**, 580–3.

53. Rytkönen, M., Ranta, J., Tuomilehto, J. and Karvonen, M. (2001) Bayesian analysis of geographical variation in the incidence of type I diabetes in Finland. *Diabetologia*, **44** (Suppl 3), B37–44.

54. Casu, A., Pascutto, C., Bernardinelli, L. and Songini, M. (2004) Bayesian approach to study the temporal trend and the geographical variation in the risk of type 1 diabetes. The Sardinian Conscript Type 1 Diabetes Registry. *Pediatric Diabetes*, **5**, 32–8.

55. Aamodt, G., Stene, L.C., Njølstad, P.R. *et al.* (2007) Spatiotemporal trends and age–period–cohort modeling of the incidence of type 1 diabetes among children aged <15 years in Norway 1973–1982 and 1989–2003. *Diabetes Care*, **30**, 884–9.

56. Samuelsson, U. and Löfman, O. (2004) Geographical mapping of type 1 diabetes in children and adolescents in south east Sweden. *Journal of Epidemiology and Community Health*, **58**, 388–92.

57. Staines, A., Bodansky, H.J., Lilley, H.E. *et al.* (1993) The epidemiology of diabetes mellitus in the United Kingdom: the Yorkshire Regional Childhood Diabetes Register. *Diabetologia*, **36**, 1282–7.

58. Pundziute-Lyckå, A., Urbonaite, B., Ostrauskas, R. *et al.* (2003) Incidence of type 1 diabetes in Lithuanians aged 0–39 years varies by the urban–rural setting, and the time change differs for men and women during 1991–2000. *Diabetes Care*, **26**, 671–6.

59. Feltbower, R.G., McKinney, P.A. and Bodansky, H.J. (2000) Rising incidence of childhood diabetes is seen at all ages and in urban and rural settings in Yorkshire, United Kingdom (Letter). *Diabetologia*, **43**, 682–4.

60. Rytkönen, M., Moltchanova, E., Ranta, J. *et al.* (2003) The incidence of type 1 diabetes among children in Finland – rural–urban difference. *Health and Place*, **9**, 315–25.

61. Patterson, C.C., Carson, D.J. and Hadden, D.R. (1996) Epidemiology of childhood IDDM in Northern Ireland 1989–1994: low incidence in areas with highest population density and most household crowding. Northern Ireland Diabetes Study Group. *Diabetologia*, **39**, 1063–9.

62. Staines, A., Bodansky, H.J., McKinney, P.A. *et al.* (1997) Small area variation in the incidence of childhood insulin-dependent diabetes mellitus in Yorkshire, UK: links with overcrowding and population density. *International Journal of Epidemiology*, **26**, 1307–13.

63. Karvonen, M., Pitkaniemi, M., Pitkaniemi, J. *et al.* (1997) Sex difference in the incidence of insulin-dependent diabetes mellitus: an analysis of the recent epidemiological data. World Health Organization DIAMOND Project Group. *Diabetes/Metabolism Reviews*, **13**, 275–91.

64. Weets, I., Van Autreve, J., van der Auwera, B.J. *et al.* (2001) Male-to-female excess in diabetes diagnosed in early adulthood is not specific for the immune-mediated form nor is it *HLA-DQ* restricted: possible relation to increased body mass index. Belgian Diabetes Registry. *Diabetologia*, **44**, 40–7.

65. Kyvik, K.O., Nystrom, L., Gorus, F. *et al.* (2004) The epidemiology of type 1 diabetes mellitus is not the same in young adults as in children. *Diabetologia*, **47**, 377–84.

66. Pundziute-Lyckå, A., Dahlquist, G., Nyström, L. *et al.* (2002) The incidence of type I diabetes has not increased but shifted to a younger age at diagnosis in the 0–34 years group in Sweden 1983 to 1998. *Diabetologia*, **45**, 783–91.

67. Helgason, T. and Jonasson, M.R. (1981) Evidence for a food additive as a cause of ketosis-prone diabetes. *Lancet*, **2**, 716–20.

68. Bache, I., Bock, T., Vølund, A. and Buschard, K. (1999) Previous maternal abortion, longer gestation, and younger maternal age decease the risk of type 1 diabetes among male offspring. *Diabetes Care*, **22**, 1063–5.

69. Stene, L.C., Barriga, K., Norris, J.M. *et al.* (2003) Symptoms of common maternal infections in pregnancy and risk of islet autoimmunity in early childhood. *Diabetes Care*, **26**, 3136–41.

70. Svensson, J., Carstensen, B., Mortensen, H.B. and Borch-Johnsen, K. (2003) Gender-associated differences in type 1 diabetes risk factors? (Letter). *Diabetologia*, **46**, 442–3.

71. Gamble, D.R. (1980) The epidemiology of insulin dependent diabetes, with particular reference to the relationship of virus infection to its etiology. *Epidemiologic Reviews*, **2**, 49–70.

72. Siemiatycki, J., Colle, E., Aubert, D. *et al.* (1986) The distribution of type I (insulin-dependent) diabetes mellitus by age, sex, secular trend, seasonality, time clusters, and space-time clusters: evidence from Montreal, 1971–1983. *American Journal of Epidemiology*, **124**, 545–60.

73. Joner, G. and Søvik, O. (1991) The incidence of type 1 (insulin-dependent) diabetes mellitus 15–29 years in Norway 1978–1982. *Diabetologia*, **34**, 271–4.

74. Christau, B., Kromann, H., Andersen, O.O. *et al.* (1977) Incidence, seasonal and geographical patterns of juvenile-onset insulin-dependent diabetes mellitus in Denmark. *Diabetologia*, **13**, 281–4.

75. Weets, I., De Leeuw, I.H., Du Caju, M.V. *et al.* (2002) The incidence of type 1 diabetes in the age group 0–39 years has not increased in Antwerp (Belgium) between 1989 and 2000: evidence for earlier disease manifestation. *Diabetes Care*, **25**, 840–6.

76. Bruno, G., Runzo, C., Cavallo-Perin, P. *et al.* (2005) Incidence of type 1 and type 2 diabetes in adults aged 30–49 years: the population-based registry in the province of Turin, Italy. *Diabetes Care*, **28**, 2613–19.

77. Melton, L.J., Palumbo, P. and Chu-Pin, C. (1983) Incidence of diabetes mellitus by clinical type. *Diabetes Care*, **6**, 75–86.

78. Levy-Marchal, C., Patterson, C. and Green, A. (1995) Variation by age group and seasonality at diagnosis of childhood IDDM in Europe. *Diabetologia*, **38**, 823–30.

79. Shaltout, A.A., Moussa, M.A., Qabazard, M. *et al.* (2002) Further evidence for the rising incidence of childhood type 1 diabetes in Kuwait. *Diabetic Medicine: A Journal of the British Diabetic Association*, **19**, 522–5.

80. Yang, Z., Long, X., Shen, J. *et al.* (2005) Epidemics of type 1 diabetes in China. *Pediatric Diabetes*, **6**, 122–28.

81. Bingley, P.J. and Gale, E.A.M. (1989) Rising Incidence of IDDM in Europe. *Diabetes Care*, **12**, 289–95.

82. Diabetes Epidemiology Research International Group (1990) Secular trends in incidence of childhood IDDM in 10 countries. *Diabetes*, **39**, 858–64.

83. Tuomilehto, J., Karvonen, M., Pitkäniemi, J. *et al.* (1999) Record high incidence of type 1 (insulin-dependent) diabetes mellitus in Finnish children. *Diabetologia*, **42**, 655–60.

84. Gale, E.A. (2002) The rise of childhood type 1 diabetes in the 20th century. *Diabetes*, **51**, 3353–61.

85. Hanssen, P. (1946) Diabetes mellitus in Bergen 1925–41. A study of morbidity, mortality, causes of death and complications. *Acta Medica Scandinavica*, **125** (Suppl 178), 19–50.

86. Westlund, K. (1966) Incidence of diabetes mellitus in Oslo, Norway 1925 to 1954. *British Journal of Preventive and Social Medicine*, **20**, 105–16.

87. Ustvedt, H.J. and Olsen, E. (1977) Incidence of diabetes mellitus in Oslo, Norway 1956–65. *British Journal of Preventive and Social Medicine*, **31**, 251–7.

88. Zhao, H.X., Stenhouse, E., Soper, C. *et al.* (1999) Incidence of childhood-onset type 1 diabetes mellitus in Devon and Cornwall, England, 1975–1996. *Diabetic Medicine: A Journal of the British Diabetic Association*, **16**, 1030–5.

89. Shamis, I., Gordon, O., Albag, Y. *et al.* (1997) Ethnic differences in the incidence of childhood IDDM in Israel (1965–1993). Marked increase since 1985, especially in Yemenite Jews. *Diabetes Care*, **20**, 504–8.

90. Willis, J.A., Scott, R.S., Darlow, B.A. *et al.* (2005) Prospective incidence study of diabetes mellitus in New Zealand children aged 0 to 14 years (Letter). *Diabetologia*, **48**, 643–8, 2442–3.

91. Nyström, L., Dahlquist, G., Rewers, M. and Wall, S. (1990) The Swedish childhood diabetes study. An analysis of the temporal variation in diabetes incidence 1978–1987. *International Journal of Epidemiology*, **19**, 141–6.

92. Harjutsalo, V., Sjöberg, L. and Tuomilehto, J. (2008) Time trends in the incidence of type 1 diabetes in Finnish children: a cohort study. *Lancet*, **371**, 1777–1782.

93. Charkaluk, M.L., Czernichow, P. and Levy-Marchal, C. (2002) Incidence data of childhood-onset type I diabetes in France during 1988–1997: the case for a shift toward younger age at onset. *Pediatric Research*, **52**, 859–62.

94. Feltbower, R.G., McKinney, P.A., Parslow, R.C. *et al.* (2003) Type 1 diabetes in Yorkshire, UK: time trends in 0–14 and 15–29-year-olds, age at onset and age–period–cohort modelling. *Diabetic Medicine: A Journal of the British Diabetic Association*, **20**, 437–41.

95. Bruno, G., Merletti, F., Biggeri, A. *et al.* (2001) Increasing trend of type I diabetes in children and young adults in the Province of Turin (Italy). Analysis of age, period and birth cohort effects from 1984 to 1996. *Diabetologia*, **44**, 22–5.

96. Moltchanova, E., Penttinen, A. and Karvonen, M. (2005) A hierarchical Bayesian birth cohort analysis from incomplete registry data: evaluating the trends in the age of onset of insulin-dependent diabetes mellitus (T1DM). *Statistics in Medicine*, **24**, 2989–3004.

97. Kurtz, Z., Peckham, C.S. and Ades, A.E. (1988) Changing prevalence of juvenile-onset diabetes mellitus. *Lancet*, **2**, 88–90.

98. Lammi, N., Blomstedt, P.A., Moltchanova, E. *et al.* (2008) Marked temporal increase in the incidence of type 1 and type 2 diabetes among young adults in Finland. *Diabetologia*, **51**, 897–899.

99. Clayton, D. and Schifflers, E. (1987) Models for temporal variation in cancer rates. I: Age–period

and age–cohort models. *Statistics in Medicine*, **6**, 449–67.

100. Clayton, D. and Schifflers, E. (1987) Models for temporal variation in cancer rates. II: Age–period–cohort models. *Statistics in Medicine*, **6**, 469–81.

101. Holford, T.R. (1991) Understanding the effects of age, period, and cohort on incidence and mortality rates. *Annual Review of Public Health*, **12**, 425–57.

102. Rewers, M., Stone, R.A., LaPorte, R.E. *et al.* (1989) Poisson regression modeling of temporal variation in incidence of childhood insulin-dependent diabetes mellitus in Allegheny County, Pennsylvania, and Wielkopolska, Poland, 1970–1985. *American Journal of Epidemiology*, **129**, 569–81.

103. Tuomilehto, J., Rewers, M., Reunanen, A. *et al.* (1991) Increasing trend in type 1 (insulin-dependent) diabetes mellitus in childhood in Finland. Analysis of age, calendar time and birth cohort effects during 1965 to 1984. *Diabetologia*, **34**, 282–7.

104. Dahlquist, G. and Mustonen, L. (2000) Analysis of 20 years of prospective registration of childhood onset diabetes time trends and birth cohort effects. Swedish Childhood Diabetes Study Group. *Acta Paediatrica*, **89**, 1231–7.

105. Drykoningen, C.E., Mulder, A.L., Vaandrager, G.J. *et al.* (1992) The incidence of male childhood type 1 (insulin-dependent) diabetes mellitus is rising rapidly in the Netherlands. *Diabetologia*, **35**, 139–42.

106. Songini, M., Loche, M., Muntoni, S. *et al.* (1993) Increasing prevalence of juvenile onset type 1 (insulin-dependent) diabetes mellitus in Sardinia: the military service approach. *Diabetologia*, **36**, 547–52.

107. Schoenle, E.J., Molinari, L., Bagot, M. *et al.* (1994) Epidemiology of IDDM in Switzerland. Increasing incidence rate and rural-urban differences in Swiss men born 1948–1972. *Diabetes Care*, **17**, 955–60.

108. Redondo, M.J., Yu, L., Hawa, M. *et al.* (2001) Heterogeneity of type I diabetes: analysis of monozygotic twins in Great Britain and the United States. *Diabetologia*, **44**, 354–62.

109. Kyvik, K.O., Green, A. and Beck-Nielsen, H. (1995) Concordance rates of insulin dependent diabetes mellitus: a population based study of young Danish twins. *British Medical Journal*, **311**, 913–17.

110. Hyttinen, V., Kaprio, J., Kinnunen, L. *et al.* (2003) Genetic liability of type 1 diabetes and the onset age among 22,650 young Finnish twin pairs: a nationwide follow-up study. *Diabetes*, **52**, 1052–5.

111. Tillil, H. and Köbberling, J. (1987) Age-corrected empirical genetic risk estimates for first-degree relatives of IDDM patients. *Diabetes*, **36**, 93–9.

112. Lorenzen, T., Pociot, F., Hougaard, P. and Nerup, J. (1994) Long-term risk of IDDM in first-degree relatives of patients with IDDM. *Diabetologia*, **37**, 321–7.

113. Steck, A.K., Barriga, K.J., Emery, L.M. *et al.* (2005) Secondary attack rate of type 1 diabetes in Colorado families. *Diabetes Care*, **28**, 296–300.

114. Harjutsalo, V., Podar, T. and Tuomilehto, J. (2005) Cumulative incidence of type 1 diabetes in 10,168 siblings of Finnish young-onset type 1 diabetic patients. *Diabetes*, **54**, 563–9.

115. The Eurodiab Ace Study Group and The Eurodiab Ace Substudy 2 Study Group (1998) Familial risk of type I diabetes in European children. *Diabetologia*, **41**, 1151–56.

116. Warram, J.H., Krolewski, A.S., Gottlieb, M.S. and Kahn, C.R. (1984) Differences in risk of insulin-dependent diabetes in offspring of diabetic mothers and diabetic fathers. *The New England Journal of Medicine*, **311**, 149–52.

117. Tuomilehto, J., Podar, T., Tuomilehto-Wolf, E. and Virtala, E. (1995) Evidence for importance of gender and birth cohort for risk of IDDM in offspring of IDDM parents. *Diabetologia*, **38**, 975–82.

118. Harjutsalo, V., Reunanen, A. and Tuomilehto, J. (2006) Differential transmission of type 1 diabetes from diabetic fathers and mothers to their offspring. *Diabetes*, **55**, 1517–24.

119. Guo, S.W. and Tuomilehto, J. (2002) Preferential transmission of type 1 diabetes from parents to offspring: fact or artifact? *Genetic Epidemiology*, **23**, 323–34.

120. Douek, I.F., Gillespie, K.M., Bingley, P.J. and Gale, E.A. (2002) Diabetes in the parents of children with type I diabetes. *Diabetologia*, **45**, 495–501.

121. Ten, S., Kukreja, A. and Maclaren, N. (2003) Associations between immune-mediated (type 1) diabetes and other autoimmune diseases, in *Diabetes Mellitus: A Fundamental and Clinical Text* (eds D. LeRoith, S.I. Taylor and J.M. Olefsky), Lippincott, Williams & Wilkins, Philadelphia, PA, pp. 557–74.

122. Barker, J.M., Yu, J., Yu, L. *et al.* (2005) Autoantibody 'subspecificity' in type 1 diabetes: risk for organ-specific autoimmunity clusters in distinct groups. *Diabetes Care*, **28**, 850–5.

123. Rewers, M., Liu, E., Simmons, J. *et al.* (2004) Celiac disease associated with type 1 diabetes

mellitus. *Endocrinology and Metabolism Clinics of North America*, **33**, 197–214.

124. Mattila, P.S., Tarkkanen, J., Saxen, H. *et al.* (2002) Predisposition to atopic symptoms to inhaled antigens may protect from childhood type 1 diabetes. *Diabetes Care*, **25**, 865–8.

125. Olesen, A.B., Juul, S., Birkebaek, N. and Thestrup-Pedersen, K. (2001) Association between atopic dermatitis and insulin-dependent diabetes mellitus: a case–control study. *Lancet*, **357**, 1749–52.

126. Stene, L.C., Joner, G. and Norwegian Childhood Diabetes Study Group (2004) Atopic disorders and risk of childhood-onset type 1 diabetes in individuals. *Clinical and Experimental Allergy: Journal of the British Society for Allergy and Clinical Immunology*, **34**, 201–6.

127. Cardwell, C.R., Shields, M.D., Carson, D.J. and Patterson, C.C. (2003) A meta-analysis of the association between childhood type 1 diabetes and atopic disease. *Diabetes Care*, **26**, 2568–74.

128. Stene, L.C. and Nafstad, P. (2001) Relation between occurrence of type 1 diabetes and asthma. *Lancet*, **357**, 607–8.

129. Serrano-Rios, M., Goday, A. and Martinez, L.T. (1999) Migrant populations and the incidence of type 1 diabetes mellitus: an overview of the literature with a focus on the Spanish-heritage countries in Latin America. *Diabetes/Metabolism Research and Reviews*, **15**, 113–32.

130. Rønningen, K.S., Keiding, N. and Green, A. (2001) Correlations between the incidence of childhood-onset type I diabetes in Europe and HLA genotypes. *Diabetologia*, **44** (Suppl 3), B51–9.

131. Backman, V.M., Thorsson, A.V., Fasquel, A. *et al.* (2002) HLA class II alleles and haplotypes in Icelandic type I diabetic patients: comparison of Icelandic and Norwegian populations (Letter). *Diabetologia*, **45**, 452–8.

132. Tuomilehto, J., Podar, T., Reunanen, A. *et al.* (1991) Comparison of incidence of IDDM in childhood between Estonia and Finland, 1980–1988. *Diabetes Care*, **14**, 982–8.

133. Kondrashova, A., Reunanen, A., Romanov, A. *et al.* (2005) A six-fold gradient in the incidence of type 1 diabetes at the eastern border of Finland. *Annals of Medicine*, **37**, 67–72.

134. Rewers, M., LaPorte, R., Walczak, M. *et al.* (1987) Apparent epidemic of insulin-dependent diabetes mellitus in midwestern Poland. *Diabetes*, **36**, 106–13.

135. Lipman, T.H., Chang, Y. and Murphy, K.M. (2002) The epidemiology of type 1 diabetes in children in Philadelphia 1990–1994: evidence of an epidemic. *Diabetes Care*, **25**, 1969–75.

136. Samuelsson, U. and Carstensen, J. (2003) Space–time clustering at birth and at diagnosis of type 1 diabetes mellitus in relation to early clinical manifestation. *The Journal of Pediatric Endocrinology and Metabolism*, **16**, 859–67.

137. Dahlquist, G. and Källén, B. (1996) Time–space clustering of date at birth in childhood-onset diabetes. *Diabetes Care*, **19**, 328–32.

138. Zhao, H.X., Moyeed, R.A., Stenhouse, E.A. *et al.* (2002) Space–time clustering of childhood type 1 diabetes in Devon and Cornwall, England. *Diabetic Medicine: A Journal of the British Diabetic Association*, **19**, 667–72.

139. McNally, R.J., Feltbower, R.G., Parker, L. *et al.* (2006) Space–time clustering analyses of type 1 diabetes among 0- to 29-year-olds in Yorkshire, UK. *Diabetologia*, **49**, 900–4.

140. McKinney, P.A. (2001) Seasonality of birth in patients with childhood type I diabetes in 19 European regions. *Diabetologia*, **44** (Suppl 3), B67–74.

141. Morgenstern, H. (1995) Ecologic studies in epidemiology: concepts, principles, and methods. *Annual Review of Public Health*, **16**, 61–81.

142. Greenland, S. and Robins, J. (1994) Ecologic studies – biases, misconceptions, and counterexamples. *American Journal of Epidemiology*, **139**, 747–60.

143. Hyöty, H. and Taylor, K.W. (2002) The role of viruses in human diabetes. *Diabetologia*, **45**, 1353–61.

144. Jun, H.S. and Yoon, J.W. (2003) A new look at viruses in type 1 diabetes. *Diabetes/Metabolism Research and Reviews*, **19**, 8–31.

145. Kolb, H. and Elliott, R.B. (1994) Increasing incidence of IDDM a consequence of improved hygiene? *Diabetologia*, **37**, 729.

146. Bach, J.F. (2002) The effect of infections on susceptibility to autoimmune and allergic diseases. *The New England Journal of Medicine*, **347**, 911–20.

147. Kaila, B. and Taback, S.P. (2001) The effect of day care exposure on the risk of developing type 1 diabetes: a meta-analysis of case-control studies. *Diabetes Care*, **24**, 1353–8.

148. Wucherpfennig, K.W. (2001) Mechanisms for the induction of autoimmunity by infectious agents. *The Journal of Clinical Investigation*, **108**, 1097–104.

149. Varela-Calvino, R. and Peakman, M. (2003) Enteroviruses and type 1 diabetes. *Diabetes/Metabolism Research and Reviews*, **19**, 431–41.

150. Fujinami, R.S., von Herrath, M.G., Christen, U. and Whitton, J.L. (2006) Molecular mimicry, by-stander activation, or viral persistence: infections and autoimmune disease. *Clinical Microbiology Reviews*, **19**, 80–94.

151. Forrest, J.M., Menser, M.A. and Burgess, J.A. (1971) High frequency of diabetes mellitus in young adults with congenital rubella. *Lancet*, **2**, 332–4.

152. Forrest, J.M., Turnbull, F.M., Sholler, G.F. *et al.* (2002) Gregg's congenital rubella patients 60 years later. *The Medical Journal of Australia*, **177**, 664–7.

153. Smithells, R.W., Sheppard, S., Marshall, W.C. and Peckham, C. (1978) Congenital rubella and diabetes mellitus (Letter). *Lancet*, **1**, 439.

154. Viskari, H., Paronen, J., Keskinen, P. *et al.* (2003) Humoral beta-cell autoimmunity is rare in patients with the congenital rubella syndrome. *Clinical and Experimental Immunology*, **133**, 378–83.

155. Takasu, N., Ikema, T., Komiya, I. and Mimura, G. (2005) Forty-year observation of 280 Japanese patients with congenital rubella syndrome (Letter). *Diabetes Care*, **28**, 2331–2.

156. DePrins, F., Van Assche, F.A., Desmyter, J. and De Groote, G. (1978) Congenital rubella and diabetes mellitus. *Lancet*, **1**, 439–40.

157. Jenson, A.B., Rosenberg, H.S. and Notkins, A.L. (1980) Pancreatic islet-cell damage in children with fatal viral infections. *Lancet*, **2**, 354–8.

158. Banatvala, J.E., Bryant, J., Schernthaner, G. *et al.* (1985) Coxsackie B, mumps, rubella, and cytomegalovirus specific IgM responses in patients with juvenile-onset insulin-dependent diabetes mellitus in Britain, Austria, and Australia. *Lancet*, **1**, 1409–12.

159. Bodansky, H.J., Dean, B.M., Grant, P.J. *et al.* (1990) Does exposure to rubella virus generate endocrine autoimmunity? *Diabetic Medicine: A Journal of the British Diabetic Association*, **7**, 611–14.

160. Menser, M.A., Forrest, J.M., Honeyman, M.C. and Burgess, J.A. (1974) Diabetes, HL-A antigens, and congenital rubella (Letter). *Lancet*, **2**, 1508–9.

161. Rubinstein, P., Walker, M.E., Fedun, B. *et al.* (1982) The HLA system in congenital rubella patients with and without diabetes. *Diabetes*, **31**, 1088–91.

162. Menser, M.A., Forrest, J.M. and Bransby, R.D. (1978) Rubella infections and diabetes mellitus. *Lancet*, **1**, 57–60.

163. Ginsberg-Fellner, F., Witt, M.E., Fedun, B. *et al.* (1985) Diabetes mellitus and autoimmunity in patients with the congenital rubella syndrome. *Reviews of Infectious Diseases*, **7** (Suppl 1), S170–6.

164. McIntosh, E.D.G. and Menser, M.A. (1992) A fifty-year follow-up of congenital rubella. *Lancet*, **340**, 414–15.

165. Pallansch, M.A. and Roos, R.P. (2001) Enteroviruses: polioviruses, Coxsackieviruses, echoviruses, and newer enteroviruses, in *Fields Virology* (eds D.M. Knipe and P.M. Howley), Lippincott Williams & Wilkins, Philadelphia, PA, pp. 723–75.

166. Yoon, J.W., Austin, M., Onodera, T. and Notkins, A.L. (1979) Virus-induced diabetes mellitus: isolation of a virus from the pancreas of a child with diabetic ketoacidosis. *The New England Journal of Medicine*, **300**, 1173–9.

167. Foulis, A.K., McGill, M., Farquharson, M.A. and Hilton, D.A. (1997) A search for evidence of viral infection in pancreases of newly diagnosed patients with IDDM. *Diabetologia*, **40**, 53–61.

168. Dotta, F., Censini, S., van Halteren, A.G. *et al.* (2007) Coxsackie B4 virus infection of b cells and natural killer cell insulitis in recent-onset type 1 diabetic patients. *Proc Natl Acad Sci U S A*, **104**, 5115–5120.

169. Green, J., Casabonne, D. and Newton, R. (2004) Coxsackie B virus serology and type 1 diabetes mellitus: a systematic review of published case–control studies. *Diabetic Medicine: A Journal of the British Diabetic Association*, **21**, 507–14.

170. Hyöty, H., Hiltunen, M., Knip, M. *et al.* (1995) A prospective study of the role of Coxsackie B and other enterovirus infections in the pathogenesis of IDDM. *Diabetes*, **44**, 652–7.

171. Dahlquist, G., Ivarsson, S., Lindberg, B. and Forsgren, M. (1995) Maternal enteroviral infection during pregnancy as a risk factor for childhood IDDM. *Diabetes*, **44**, 408–13.

172. Dahlquist, G., Boman, J.E. and Juto, P. (1999) Enteroviral RNA and IgM antibodies in early pregnancy and risk for childhood-onset IDDM in offspring (Letter). *Diabetes Care*, **22**, 364–5.

173. Viskari, H.R., Roivainen, M., Reunanen, A. *et al.* (2002) Maternal first-trimester enterovirus infection and future risk of type 1 diabetes in the exposed fetus. *Diabetes*, **51**, 2568–71.

174. Sadeharju, K., Hamalainen, A.M., Knip, M. *et al.* (2003) Enterovirus infections as a risk factor for type I diabetes: virus analyses in a dietary intervention trial. *Clinical and Experimental Immunology*, **132**, 271–7.

175. Füchtenbusch, M., Irnstetter, A., Jäger, G. and Ziegler, A.G. (2001) No evidence for an association of Coxsackie virus infections during

pregnancy and early childhood with development of islet autoantibodies in offspring of mothers or fathers with type 1 diabetes. *Journal of Autoimmunity*, **17**, 333–40.

176. Dahlquist, G.G., Forsberg, J., Hagenfeldt, L. *et al.* (2004) Increased prevalence of enteroviral RNA in blood spots from newborn children who later developed type 1 diabetes: a population-based case-control study (Letter). *Diabetes Care*, **27**, 285–6.

177. Lönnrot, M., Salminen, K., Knip, M. *et al.* (2000) Enterovirus RNA in serum is a risk factor for beta-cell autoimmunity and clinical type 1 diabetes: a prospective study. Childhood Diabetes in Finland (DiMe) Study Group. *Journal of Medical Virology*, **61**, 214–20.

178. Salminen, K., Sadeharju, K., Lönnrot, M. *et al.* (2003) Enterovirus infections are associated with the induction of beta-cell autoimmunity in a prospective birth cohort study. *Journal of Medical Virology*, **69**, 91–8.

179. Graves, P.M., Rotbart, H.A., Nix, W.A. *et al.* (2003) Prospective study of enteroviral infections and development of beta-cell autoimmunity. Diabetes Autoimmunity Study in the Young (DAISY). *Diabetes Research and Clinical Practice*, **59**, 51–61.

180. Hyöty, H. (2002) Enterovirus infections and type 1 diabetes. *Annals of Medicine*, **34**, 138–47.

181. Hyöty, H., Leinikki, P., Reunanen, A. *et al.* (1988) Mumps infections in the etiology of type 1 (insulin-dependent) diabetes. *Diabetes Research*, **9**, 111–16.

182. Pak, C.Y., Eun, H.-M., McArthur, R.G. and Yoon, J.W. (1988) Association of cytomegalovirus infection with autoimmune type 1 diabetes. *Lancet*, **2**, 1–4.

183. Ivarsson, S.A., Lindberg, B., Nilsson, K.O. *et al.* (1993) The prevalence of type 1 diabetes mellitus at follow-up of Swedish infants congenitally infected with cytomegalovirus. *Diabetic Medicine: A Journal of the British Diabetic Association*, **10**, 521–3.

184. Hiltunen, M., Hyöty, H., Karjalainen, J. *et al.* (1995) Serological evaluation of the role of cytomegalovirus in the pathogenesis of IDDM: a prospective study. *Diabetologia*, **38**, 705–10.

185. Hiemstra, H.S., Schloot, N.C., van Veelen, P.A. *et al.* (2001) Cytomegalovirus in autoimmunity: T cell crossreactivity to viral antigen and autoantigen glutamic acid decarboxylase. *Proceedings of the National Academy of Sciences of the United States of America*, **98**, 3988–91.

186. Conrad, B., Weidmann, E., Trucco, G. *et al.* (1994) Evidence for superantigen involvement in insulin-dependent diabetes mellitus aetiology. *Nature*, **371**, 351–5.

187. Conrad, B., Weissmahr, R.N., Boni, J. *et al.* (1997) A human endogenous retroviral superantigen as candidate autoimmune gene in type I diabetes. *Cell*, **90**, 303–13.

188. Lower, R., Tonjes, R.R., Boller, K. *et al.* (1998) Development of insulin-dependent diabetes mellitus does not depend on specific expression of the human endogenous retrovirus HERV-K. *Cell*, **95**, 11–14.

189. Muir, A., Ruan, Q.G., Marron, M.P. and She, J.X. (1999) The IDDMK(1,2)22 retrovirus is not detectable in either mRNA or genomic DNA from patients with type 1 diabetes. *Diabetes*, **48**, 219–22.

190. Honeyman, M.C., Coulson, B.S., Stone, N.L. *et al.* (2000) Association between rotavirus infection and pancreatic islet autoimmunity in children at risk of developing type 1 diabetes. *Diabetes*, **49**, 1319–24.

191. Blomqvist, M., Juhela, S., Erkkilä, S. *et al.* (2002) Rotavirus infections and development of diabetes-associated autoantibodies during the first 2 years of life. *Clinical and Experimental Immunology*, **128**, 511–15.

192. Gibbon, C., Smith, T., Egger, P. *et al.* (1997) Early infection and subsequent insulin dependent diabetes. *Archives of Disease in Childhood*, **77**, 384–5.

193. The EURODIAB Substudy 2 Study Group (2000) Infections and vaccinations as risk factors for childhood type I (insulin-dependent) diabetes mellitus: a multicentre case-control investigation. *Diabetologia*, **43**, 47–53.

194. Pundziute-Lyckå, A., Urbonaite, B. and Dahlquist, G. (2000) Infections and risk of type I (insulin-dependent) diabetes mellitus in Lithuanian children. *Diabetologia*, **43**, 1229–34.

195. McKinney, P.A., Okasha, M., Parslow, R.C. *et al.* (2000) Early social mixing and childhood type 1 diabetes mellitus: a case-control study in Yorkshire, UK. *Diabetic Medicine: A Journal of the British Diabetic Association*, **17**, 236–42.

196. Hummel, M., Fuchtenbusch, M., Schenker, M. and Ziegler, A.G. (2000) No major association of breast-feeding, vaccinations, and childhood viral diseases with early islet autoimmunity in the German BABYDIAB Study. *Diabetes Care*, **23**, 969–74.

197. Blom, L., Dahlquist, G., Nyström, L. *et al.* (1989) The Swedish childhood diabetes study – social and perinatal determinants for diabetes in childhood. *Diabetologia*, **32**, 7–13.

198. Viskari, H.R., Koskela, P., Lönnrot, M. *et al.* (2000) Can enterovirus infections explain the increasing incidence of type 1 diabetes? (Letter). *Diabetes Care*, **23**, 414–16.

199. Viskari, H., Ludvigsson, J., Uibo, R. *et al.* (2004) Relationship between the incidence of type 1 diabetes and enterovirus infections in different European populations: results from the EPIVIR project. *Journal of Medical Virology*, **72**, 610–17.

200. Viskari, H., Ludvigsson, J., Uibo, R. *et al.* (2005) Relationship between the incidence of type 1 diabetes and maternal enterovirus antibodies: time trends and geographical variation. *Diabetologia*, **48**, 1280–7.

201. The Institute for Vaccine Safety Diabetes Workshop Panel (1999) Childhood immunizations and type 1 diabetes: summary of an Institute for Vaccine Safety Workshop. *The Pediatric Infectious Disease Journal*, **18**, 217–22.

202. DeStefano, F., Mullooly, J.P., Okoro, C.A. *et al.* (2001) Childhood vaccinations, vaccination timing, and risk of type 1 diabetes mellitus. *Pediatrics*, **108**, E112.

203. Hviid, A., Stellfeld, M., Wohlfahrt, J. and Melbye, M. (2004) Childhood vaccination and type 1 diabetes. *The New England Journal of Medicine*, **350**, 1398–404.

204. Wraith, D.C., Goldman, M. and Lambert, P.H. (2003) Vaccination and autoimmune disease: what is the evidence? *Lancet*, **362**, 1659–66.

205. Schattner, A. (2005) Consequence or coincidence? The occurrence, pathogenesis and significance of autoimmune manifestations after viral vaccines. *Vaccine*, **23**, 3876–86.

206. Borch-Johnsen, K., Joner, G., Mandrup-Poulsen, T. *et al.* (1984) Relation between breast-feeding and incidence rates of insulin-dependent diabetes mellitus: a hypothesis. *Lancet*, **2**, 1083–6.

207. Norris, J.M. and Scott, F.W. (1996) A meta-analysis of infant diet and insulin-dependent diabetes mellitus: do bias play a role? *Epidemiology (Cambridge, Mass.)*, **7**, 87–92.

208. Virtanen, S.M. and Knip, M. (2003) Nutritional risk predictors of cell autoimmunity and type 1 diabetes at a young age. *The American Journal of Clinical Nutrition*, **78**, 1053–67.

209. Harrison, L.C. and Honeyman, M.C. (1999) Cow's milk and type 1 diabetes: the real debate is about mucosal immune function. *Diabetes*, **48**, 1501–7.

210. Kimpimäki, T., Erkkola, M., Korhonen, S. *et al.* (2001) Short-term exclusive breastfeeding predisposes young children with increased genetic risk of type I diabetes to progressive beta-cell autoimmunity. *Diabetologia*, **44**, 63–9.

211. Hummel, M., Schenker, M. and Ziegler, A.G. (2001) Influence of perinatal factors on the appearance of islet autoantibodies in offspring of parents with type 1 diabetes. *Pediatric Diabetes*, **2**, 40–2.

212. Virtanen, S.M., Kenward, M.G., Erkkola, M. *et al.* (2006) Age at introduction of new foods in infancy and advanced beta-cell autoimmunity in young children with HLA-conferred susceptibility to type 1 diabetes. *Diabetologia*, **49**, 1512–21.

213. Åkerblom, H.K., Virtanen, S.M., Ilonen, J. *et al.* (2005) Dietary manipulation of beta cell autoimmunity in infants at increased risk of type 1 diabetes: a pilot study. *Diabetologia*, **48**, 829–37.

214. Norris, J.M., Barriga, K., Klingensmith, G. *et al.* (2003) Timing of initial cereal exposure in infancy and risk of islet autoimmunity. *The Journal of the American Medical Association*, **290**, 1713–20.

215. Ziegler, A.G., Schmid, S., Huber, D. *et al.* (2003) Early infant feeding and risk of developing type 1 diabetes-associated autoantibodies. *The Journal of the American Medical Association*, **290**, 1721–8.

216. Rødland, O., Markestad, T., Aksnes, L. and Aarskog, D. (1985) Plasma concentrations of vitamin D metabolites during puberty of diabetic children. *Diabetologia*, **28**, 663–6.

217. Baumgartl, H.J., Standl, E., Schmidt-Gayk, H. *et al.* (1991) Changes of vitamin D3 serum concentrations at the onset of immune-mediated type 1 (insulin-dependent) diabetes mellitus. *Diabetes Research (Edinburgh, Lothian)*, **16**, 145–8.

218. Pozzilli, P., Manfrini, S., Crino, A. *et al.* (2005) Low levels of 25-hydroxyvitamin D3 and 1,25-dihydroxyvitamin D3 in patients with newly diagnosed type 1 diabetes. *Hormone and Metabolic Research*, **37**, 680–3.

219. Heath, H., Lambert, P.W., Service, F.J. and Arnaud, S.B. III (1979) Calcium homeostasis in diabetes mellitus. *The Journal of Clinical Endocrinology and Metabolism*, **49**, 462–6.

220. EURODIAB Substudy 2 Study Group (1999) Vitamin D supplement in early childhood and risk for type 1 (insulin-dependent) diabetes mellitus. *Diabetologia*, **42**, 51–4.

221. Hyppönen, E., Läärä, E., Reunanen, A. *et al.* (2001) Intake of vitamin D and risk of type 1 diabetes: a birth–cohort study. *Lancet*, **358**, 1500–3.

222. Fronczak, C.M., Baron, A.E., Chase, H.P. *et al.* (2003) *In utero* dietary exposures and risk of islet autoimmunity in children. *Diabetes Care*, **26**, 3237–42.

223. Stene, L.C., Ulriksen, J., Magnus, P. and Joner, G. (2000) Use of cod liver oil during pregnancy

associated with lower risk of type I diabetes in the offspring. *Diabetologia*, **43**, 1083–92.

224. Stene, L.C., Joner, G. and Norwegian Childhood Diabetes Study Group (2003) Use of cod liver oil during the first year of life is associated with lower risk of childhood-onset type 1 diabetes: a large, population based, case–control study. *The American Journal of Clinical Nutrition*, **78**, 1128–34.

225. Decsi, T., Minda, H., Hermann, R. *et al.* (2002) Polyunsaturated fatty acids in plasma and erythrocyte membrane lipids of diabetic children. *Prostaglandins, Leukotrienes, and Essential Fatty Acids*, **67**, 203–10.

226. Litherland, S.A., Xie, X.T., Hutson, A.D. *et al.* (1999) Aberrant prostaglandin synthase 2 expression defines an antigen-presenting cell defect for insulin-dependent diabetes mellitus. *The Journal of Clinical Investigation*, **104**, 515–23.

227. Knekt, P., Reunanen, A., Marniemi, J. *et al.* (1999) Low vitamin E status is a potential risk factor for insulin-dependent diabetes mellitus. *Journal of Internal Medicine*, **245**, 99–102.

228. Uusitalo, L., Knip, M., Kenward, M.G. *et al.* (2005) Serum α-tocopherol concentrations and risk of type 1 diabetes mellitus: a cohort study in siblings of affected children. *Journal of Pediatric Endocrinology and Metabolism*, **18**, 1409–16.

229. Basu, T.K., Tze, W.J. and Leichter, J. (1989) Serum vitamin A and retinol-binding protein in patients with insulin-dependent diabetes mellitus. *The American Journal of Clinical Nutrition*, **50**, 329–31.

230. Flood, T.M., Brink, S.J. and Gleason, R.E. (1982) Increased incidence of type I diabetes in children of older mothers. *Diabetes Care*, **6**, 571–3.

231. Dahlquist, G. and Källén, B. (1992) Maternal–child blood group incompatibility and other perinatal events increase the risk for early-onset type 1 (insulin-dependent) diabetes mellitus. *Diabetologia*, **35**, 671–5.

232. Patterson, C.C., Carson, D.J., Hadden, D.R. *et al.* (1994) A case–control investigation of perinatal risk factors for childhood IDDM in Northern Ireland and Scotland. *Diabetes Care*, **17**, 376–81.

233. McKinney, P.A., Parslow, R., Gurney, K.A. *et al.* (1999) Perinatal and neonatal determinants of childhood type 1 diabetes: a case–control study in Yorkshire, U.K. *Diabetes Care*, **22**, 928–32.

234. Dahlquist, G., Patterson, C. and Stoltesz, G. (1999) Perinatal risk factors for childhood type 1 diabetes in Europe: the EURODIAB Substudy 2 Study Group. *Diabetes Care*, **22**, 1698–702.

235. Stene, L.C., Magnus, P., Lie, R.T. *et al.* (2001) Maternal and paternal age at delivery, birth order, and risk of childhood onset type 1 diabetes: population based cohort study. *British Medical Journal*, **323**, 369–71.

236. Wadsworth, E.J.K., Shield, J.P.H., Hunt, L.P. and Baum, J.D. (1997) A case–control study of environmental factors associated with diabetes in the under 5s. *Diabetic Medicine: A Journal of the British Diabetic Association*, **14**, 390–6.

237. Jones, M.E., Swerdlow, A.J., Gill, L.E. and Goldacre, M.J. (1998) Pre-natal and early life risk factors for childhood onset diabetes mellitus: a record linkage study. *International Journal of Epidemiology*, **27**, 444–9.

238. Stene, L.C., Barriga, K., Norris, J.M. *et al.* (2004) Perinatal factors and development of islet autoimmunity in early childhood: the Diabetes Autoimmunity Study In the Young. *American Journal of Epidemiology*, **160**, 3–10.

239. Dahlquist, G., Bennich, S.S. and Källén, B. (1996) Intrauterine growth pattern and risk of childhood onset insulin dependent (type 1) diabetes: population based case–control study. *British Medical Journal*, **313**, 1174–7.

240. Podar, T., Onkamo, P., Forsen, T. *et al.* (1999) Neonatal anthropometric measurements and risk of childhood-onset type 1 diabetes. DiMe Study Group (Letter). *Diabetes Care*, **22**, 2092–4.

241. Stene, L.C., Magnus, P., Lie, R.T. *et al.* (2001) Birth weight and childhood onset type 1 diabetes: population based cohort study. *British Medical Journal*, **322**, 889–92.

242. Dahlquist, G.G., Pundziute-Lyckå, A. and Nyström, L. (2005) Birthweight and risk of type 1 diabetes in children and young adults: a population-based register study. *Diabetologia*, **48**, 1114–17.

243. Lawler-Heavner, J., Cruickshanks, K.J., Hay, W.W. *et al.* (1994) Birth size and risk of insulin-dependent diabetes mellitus (IDDM). *Diabetes Research and Clinical Practice*, **24**, 153–9.

244. Dunger, D.B., Ong, K.K., Huxtable, S.J. *et al.* (1998) Association of the INS VNTR with size at birth. ALSPAC Study Team. Avon Longitudinal Study of Pregnancy and Childhood. *Nature Genetics*, **19**, 98–100.

245. Ong, K.K., Petry, C.J., Barratt, B.J. *et al.* (2004) Maternal–fetal interactions and birth order influence insulin variable number of tandem repeats allele class associations with head size at birth and childhood weight gain. *Diabetes*, **53**, 1128–33.

246. Stene, L.C., Magnus, P., Rønningen, K.S. and Joner, G. (2001) Diabetes-associated *HLA-DQ* genes and birth weight. *Diabetes*, **50**, 2879–82.

247. Larsson, H.E., Lynch, K., Lernmark, B. *et al.* (2005) Diabetes-associated *HLA* genotypes affect

birthweight in the general population. *Diabetologia*, **48**, 1484–91.

248. Stene, L.C., Thorsby, P.M., Berg, J.P. *et al.* (2006) The relation between size at birth and risk of type 1 diabetes is not influenced by adjustment for the insulin gene (-23 HphI) polymorphism or *HLA-DQ* genotype. *Diabetologia*, **49** (9), 2068–73).

249. Stene, L.C., Magnus, P., Lie, R.T. *et al.* (2003) No association between pre-eclampsia or cesarean section and incidence of type 1 diabetes among children: a large population based cohort study. *Pediatric Research*, **54**, 487–90.

250. Soltesz, G., Jeges, S. and Dahlquist, G. (1994) Non-genetic risk determinants for type 1 (insulin-dependent) diabetes mellitus in childhood. *Acta Paediatrica*, **83**, 730–5.

251. Cardwell, C.R., Stene, L.C., Joner, G. *et al.* (2008) Caesarean section is associated with an increased risk of childhood onset type 1 diabetes: A meta-analysis of observational studies. *Diabetologia*, **51**, 726–735.

252. Dahlquist, G. and Källén, B. (2003) Indications that phototherapy is a risk factor for insulin-dependent diabetes (Letter). *Diabetes Care*, **26**, 247–8.

253. Colle, E., Siemiatycki, J., West, R. *et al.* (1981) Incidence of juvenile onset diabetes in Montreal – demonstration of ethnic differences and socio-economic class differences. *Journal of Chronic Diseases*, **34**, 611–16.

254. Siemiatycki, J., Cole, E., Campbell, S. *et al.* (1988) Incidence of IDDM in Montreal by ethnic group and by social class and comparisons with ethnic groups living elsewhere. *Diabetes*, **37**, 1096–102.

255. LaPorte, R.E., Orchard, T.J., Kuller, L.H. *et al.* (1981) The Pittsburgh Insulin Dependent Diabetes Mellitus Registry: the relationship of insulin dependent diabetes mellitus incidence to social class. *American Journal of Epidemiology*, **114**, 379–84.

256. Crow, Y.J., Alberti, K.G. and Parkin, J.M. (1991) Insulin dependent diabetes in childhood and material deprivation in northern England, 1977–86. *British Medical Journal*, **303**, 158–60.

257. Verge, C.F., Joward, N.J., Irwig, L. *et al.* (1994) Environmental factors in childhood IDDM. *Diabetes Care*, **17**, 1381–9.

258. Virtanen, S.M., Hyppönen, E., Läärä, E. *et al.* (1998) Cow's milk consumption, disease-associated autoantibodies and type 1 diabetes mellitus: a follow up study in siblings of diabetes children. *Diabetic Medicine: A Journal of the British Diabetic Association*, **15**, 730–8.

259. Metcalfe, M.A. and Baum, J.D. (1992) Family characteristics and insulin dependent diabetes. *Archives of Disease in Childhood*, **67**, 731–6.

260. Tai, T.Y., Wang, C.Y., Lin, L.L. *et al.* (1998) A case–control study on risk factors for type 1 diabetes in Taipei City. *Diabetes Research and Clinical Practice*, **42**, 197–203.

261. Rothman, K.J. and Greenland, S. (1998) *Modern Epidemiology*, 2nd edn, Lippincott Williams & Wilkins, Philadelphia, PA.

262. Hermann, R., Knip, M., Veijola, R. *et al.* (2003) Temporal changes in the frequencies of *HLA* genotypes in patients with type 1 diabetes – indication of an increased environmental pressure? *Diabetologia*, **46**, 420–5.

263. Gillespie, K.M., Bain, S.C., Barnett, A.H. *et al.* (2004) The rising incidence of childhood type 1 diabetes and reduced contribution of high-risk *HLA* haplotypes. *Lancet*, **364**, 1699–700.

264. Kostraba, J., Cruickshanks, K.J., Lawler-Heavner, J. *et al.* (1993) Early exposure to cow's milk and solid foods in infancy, genetic predisposition, and risk of IDDM. *Diabetes*, **42**, 288–95.

265. Pérez-Bravo, F., Carrasco, E., Gutierrez-López, M.D. *et al.* (1996) Genetic predisposition and environmental factors leading to the development of insulin-dependent diabetes mellitus in Chilean children. *Journal of Molecular Medicine*, **74**, 105–9.

266. Pozzilli, P., Buzzetti, R., Bottazzo, G.F. and Tosi, R. (1993) The selection of control subjects for case/control analysis of susceptibility of type 1 (insulin-dependent) diabetes mellitus. *Diabetologia*, **36**, 1208–9.

267. Petrovsky, N. and Harrison, L.C. (1995) *HLA*-matched control subjects are essential in studies of susceptibility to IDDM (Letter). *Diabetologia*, **38**, 125–6.

268. Schernthaner, G., Banatvala, J.E., Scherbaum, W. *et al.* (1985) Coxsackie-B-virus-specific IgM responses, complement-fixing islet-cell antibodies, HLA DR antigens, and C-peptide secretion in insulin-dependent diabetes mellitus. *Lancet*, **2**, 630–2.

269. Piegorsch, W.W., Weinberg, C.R. and Taylor, J.A. (1994) Non-hierarchical logistic models and case-only designs for assessing susceptibility in population-based case-control studies. *Statistics in Medicine*, **13**, 153–62.

270. Wenzlau, J.M., Juhl, K., Yu, L. *et al.* (2007) The cation efflux transporter ZnT8 (Slc30A8) is a major autoantigen in human type 1 diabetes. *Proceedings of the National Academy of Sciences of the United States of America*, **104**, 17040–5.

271. Karvonen, M., Tuomilehto, J., Virtala, E. *et al.* (1996) Seasonality in the clinical onset of insulin-dependent diabetes mellitus in Finnish children. Childhood Diabetes in Finland (DiMe) Study Group. *American Journal of Epidemiology*, **143**, 167–76.

272. Tuomilehto-Wolf, E., Tuomilehto, J., Cepaitis, Z. and Lounamaa, R. (1989) New susceptibility haplotype for type 1 diabetes. DIME Study Group. *Lancet*, **2**, 299–302.

273. Muntoni, S., Fonte, M.T., Stoduto, S. *et al.* (1997) Incidence of insulin-dependent diabetes mellitus among Sardinian-heritage children born in Lazio region, Italy. *Lancet*, **349**, 160–2.

274. Rewers, M. and Zimmet, P. (2004) The rising tide of childhood type 1 diabetes – what is the elusive environmental trigger? *Lancet*, **364**, 1645–7.

275. Niinistö, S., Virtanen, S.M., Kenward, M.G. *et al.* (2007) Maternal intake of vitamin D during pregnancy and risk of advanced beta-cell autoimmunity in the offpring (Abstract). *Acta Diabetologica*, **44** (Suppl 1), S35–6.

276. Norris, J.M., Yin, X., Lamb, M.M. *et al.* (2007) Omega-3 polyunsaturated fatty acid intake and islet autoimmunity in children at increased risk for type 1 diabetes. *Journal of the American Medical Association*, **298**, 1420–8.

277. Uusitalo, L., Nevalainen, J., Niinistö, S. *et al.* (2008) Serum α- and γ-tocopherol concentrations and risk of advanced beta cell autoimmunity in children with HLA-conferred susceptibility to type 1 diabetes mellitus. *Diabetologia*, **51**, 773–80.

278. European Nicotinamide Diabetes Intervention Trial (ENDIT) Group (2004) European Nicotinamide Diabetes Intervention Trial (ENDIT): a randomised controlled trial of intervention before the onset of type 1 diabetes. *Lancet*, **363**, 925–31.

25

Epidemiology of Childhood Diabetes Mellitus in Non-Caucasian Populations

Rebecca B. Lipton

Section of Pediatric Endocrinology and Department of Health Studies, University of Chicago, Chicago, IL, USA

25.1 INTRODUCTION

The descriptive epidemiology of diabetes in non-European-origin children is limited by the paucity of population-based data collection outside Europe, as well as because studies with sufficiently large samples in multiethnic populations are rare. This is unfortunate, because interethnic comparisons offer the chance to understand genetic risk factors [1]; and specifically in the case of migrant studies, the role of the environment in disease etiology. Fortunately, the establishment of the World Health Organization DiaMond collaboration two decades ago [2] provided a framework, including standardized protocols, for childhood diabetes data collection across the world.

Examining diabetes as it occurs in children from a variety of ethnic backgrounds is also significant in providing the opportunity to unravel the etiology of the mixed forms of diabetes that are increasingly being described in children and adolescents. Historically, the incidence of type 1 diabetes has been low in non-Caucasian populations, while in many of these same populations the risk for type 2 diabetes in adults is extremely high. For a quarter of a century there have been reports of atypical diabetic syndromes among young people of Asian, African and Latin American origin [3–6]. Type 2 diabetes is now purportedly occurring at 'epidemic' rates among children in the United States and other westernized societies [7]. Careful examination of the data, however, indicates that the majority of children with diabetes have classical, autoimmune type 1 diabetes, and that others demonstrate a mixed form of diabetes with both type 1 and type 2 features, often in association with obesity. Key research questions in this area focus on how best to describe early-onset diabetes along the continuum of glucose tolerance in terms of descriptive epidemiology and etiology (i.e. metabolic, behavioral, genetic and immunologic risk factors).

25.2 DESCRIPTIVE EPIDEMIOLOGY OF CHILDHOOD-ONSET DIABETES: PREVALENCE AND INCIDENCE ACROSS THE WORLD

The small amount of data available on non-European populations worldwide demonstrates that type 1 diabetes rates are generally lower than those for European-origin children, and that, for many years, type 2 diabetes or mixed phenotypes may have comprised a large fraction of youth-onset diabetes.

25.2.1 Eastern Asia

Kitagawa and co-workers [8–10] have been screening Tokyo schoolchildren for glycosuria each year since 1974. Using glucose and tolbutamide tolerance tests in combination with data from other sources, they estimated that the yearly incidence of type 2 diabetes among elementary and junior high school students was 2.6 per 10^5 per year. These investigators reported that type 2 diabetes incidence increased, particularly among older

The Epidemiology of Diabetes Mellitus, second edition   Edited by Jean-Marie Ekoé, Marian Rewers, Rhys Williams and Paul Zimmet
© 2008 John Wiley & Sons, Ltd

children, in 1991–1995, but then stabilized through 2002. Nearly one-fourth (23%) of girls with presumed type 2 diabetes were not obese (greater than 20% above ideal body weight), compared with just 8.5% of male patients. A majority of these children reported a diagnosis of diabetes in a first- or second-degree relative, even though the absolute prevalence of diabetes in the Japanese population is much lower than in other industrialized nations. The incidence of type 1 diabetes during this period was about 2 per 10^5 [11], indicating that, in Japan, the risk for type 2 diabetes in childhood is greater than for type 1 diabetes, although the absolute risk is 5–10-fold lower than for European-origin children. Prevalence estimates from Osaka for type 2 diabetes in elementary and junior high school students during 1997 were obtained by combining data from a school screening program, hospital records and a government-supported medical benefits database [12]. Using the capture–mark–recapture method [13], they reported a prevalence rate of 21.1 per 10^5, which is much higher than had been previously reported. They speculated that because the school urine screening program in Osaka accounted for only about 20% of the cases, studies based primarily on this method of case-finding may be severely underascertained.

An incidence registry in Hong Kong demonstrated rates of 1.4 per 10^5 for type 1 diabetes, and 0.1 per 10^5 for type 2 diabetes, in children aged 0–14 years during 1984–1996 [14]. A collaborative study in the People's Republic of China demonstrated an overall type 1 diabetes incidence rate of 0.59 per 10^5 for ages 0–14 years during the years 1988–1996, with considerable geographic and ethnic variation in risk [15]. The risk for diabetes was 27% higher for girls than for boys, and there was a statistically significant increase in risk over the study interval, but data on the incidence of type 2 diabetes were not provided. An incidence study in northern Thailand during the same period reported a similar pattern of extremely low incidence of type 1 diabetes, with a higher risk for girls [16], but again no data on type 2 diabetes in children.

Population-based data from India are rare. In the southern city of Madras, incidence of type 1 diabetes during the years 1991–1994 averaged 10.5 per 10^5 among children aged 0–14 years [17], using a standard definition of type 1 diabetes based on clinical diagnosis and treatment with insulin.

This rate, 4–10-times higher than the incidence in Japan and China, may reflect a true increased risk based on greater genetic load, or some artifact such as undercount of the denominator (total child population-at-risk), or misclassification of some non-type 1 diabetes as type 1. Although no population-based incidence or prevalence rates are available for childhood type 2 diabetes in India, Mohan *et al.* [18] described 219 patients from a total clinic population of >4500 in southern India (~5%) who were ketosis resistant, had onset <25 years of age and were controlled without insulin treatment for at least 5 years.

25.2.2   New Zealand

Epidemiologic research on childhood diabetes has been ongoing in New Zealand for four decades. The mean annual incidence in the first published report, 1968–1972, was 8.9 per 10^5 in children aged 0–15 years, using a case-definition of 'type 1 diabetes' [19]. The most recent data, from 1999 to 2000, included all New Zealand residents aged 0–14 years with a diabetic blood glucose using standard cutoffs [20]. Clinical data were then requested from physicians to assist in determining the diabetic phenotype, resulting in the characterization of 94.6% of cases as type 1 diabetes, 3.8% with type 2 diabetes and 1.6% of other etiologies (Prader–Willi, cystic fibrosis, maturity-onset diabetes of the young (MODY), etc.). Type 1 diabetes incidence among children of Maori (indigenous) origin was 5.6 per 10^5 per annum, compared with 21.7 per 10^5 in European-origin children. The average annual incidence rates for type 2 diabetes in Maori- and European-origin children were 1.8 per 10^5 and 0.4 per 10^5 respectively; all type 2 cases occurred in children >10 years of age.

25.2.3   Africa and the Middle East

There is very little information on childhood diabetes incidence in sub-Saharan Africa. A registry active from 1982 to 1991 in Tanzania [21] reported the very low rate of 1.5 per 10^5 in children of Bantu origin ages 0–19 years. A mortality study in the early 1990s by this same group of investigators documented no deaths related to diabetes in children <15 years of age [22]. Among adolescent and young adult Tanzanians aged 15–24 years, the prevalence of type 2 diabetes was estimated in the late 1980s as 0.4 per 10^3 based on five subjects [23].

In contrast to sub-Saharan Africa, several groups have been investigating childhood diabetes in the Middle East over the past two decades. In the Benghazi, Libya Registry, incidence rates were 7.0 per 10^5 among children aged 0–14 years during 1981–1990, and 7.8 per 10^5 in 1991–2000 [24]. A registry in Saudi Arabia reported incidence of 12.3 per 10^5 among children aged 0–14 during 1986–1997 [25]. In both Libya and Saudi Arabia, incidence was higher for girls, and for those aged 10–14 years, compared with younger children. The Kuwaiti Registry demonstrated an extremely high incidence rate for this same age group, 0–14 years, of 20.1 per 10^5 in 1992–1997, with no gender difference in risk. In Israel, type 1 diabetes incidence rates for children aged 0–17 years were determined for the 28 years 1965–1993 [26]: marked ethnic differences began to appear after the mid 1980s. In the most recent period, from 1990 to 1993, children of Yemenite origin demonstrated an incidence rate of 18.5 per 10^5 compared with 10.0 per 10^5 among Ashkenazi (European-origin) children. Israeli Jewish, Israeli Arab and non-Yemenite Jewish children of Middle Eastern origin demonstrated a lower risk of type 1 diabetes, ranging from 2.9 per 10^5 to 7.3 per 10^5 per annum.

25.2.4 Non-Caucasian Children in the Americas

Few population-based incidence and prevalence data are available on the situation in North America. In the third National Health and Nutrition Examination Survey (NHANES) study, conducted between 1988 and 1994, 13 of 2867 subjects aged 12–19 years were considered to have diabetes based on insulin treatment ($n = 9$), treatment with oral agents ($n = 2$), or elevated fasting glucose levels ($n = 2$). The overall prevalence of diabetes in this age group, therefore, was calculated to be 4.1 per 10^3, with an estimate that 31% of these subjects had type 2 [7]. A similar analysis of data collected for NHANES in 1999–2002 demonstrated roughly equivalent findings: of 4370 adolescents aged 12–19 years, 18 reported having diabetes (prevalence 5.0 per 10^3); no undiagnosed diabetes was discovered [27]. Of those with diabetes, 29% ($n = 8$) were categorized as type 2. Despite being

based on an extremely small number of cases, the NHANES data are useful because they include three major ethnic groups in the sampling frame, allowing estimates of total diabetes prevalence of 3.1 per 10^3 among Mexican American, 4.2 per 10^3 among non-Hispanic Black and 5.6 per 10^3 among non-Hispanic White adolescents. The corresponding prevalence rate estimates for type 2 diabetes by ethnicity were 1.9 per 10^3, 1.6 per 10^3 and 1.35 per 10^3 among Mexican American, non-Hispanic Black, and non-Hispanic White adolescents respectively. Dolan *et al.* [28] reported in 2004 that the prevalence of any diabetes was 3.6 per 10^3 among 2501 Ohio students aged 10–18 years, roughly one-third of whom were of non-Hispanic Black origin. There were nine participants with diabetes, six of whom had type 1, two with known type 2 diabetes, and one young man whose type 2 diabetes was discovered on screening.

Of the limited population-based data extant, some of the most valuable come from the longitudinal study of the Pima Indians. An analysis over 30 years in this extremely high-risk population demonstrated increasing rates of overt type 2 diabetes among children [29]; it is generally assumed that type 1 diabetes does not occur among Pimas. The prevalence of diabetes was determined in 5274 Pima Indian children using oral glucose tolerance tests (OGTTs) for three 10-years intervals between 1967 and 1996; increases over time were seen in both boys and girls. For boys aged 10–14 years, prevalence rose from 0% in 1967–1976 to 1.4% in 1987–1996; it rose from 2.4% to 3.8% among boys 15–19-years-old. In girls the prevalence rate increased from 0.7% in 1967–1976 to 2.9% in 1987–1996 in the 10–14-year-old age group, and from 2.7% to 5.3% for girls aged 15–19 years. There was a concurrent increase in body weight among young Pimas over time, as well as an increase in the frequency of exposure to diabetes *in utero*; these variables accounted for much of the increase in prevalence over the 30 years.

Heather Dean, a pediatric endocrinologist practicing in Manitoba, Canada, reported on Native American children aged 6–17 years referred for type 2 diabetes treatment [30]. The first case was referred in 1985; by 1994–1998 there were on average 12 cases being diagnosed per year. She estimated minimum annual incidence and prevalence rates based on her patient load alone at 41 per 10^5 incident cases and 1.7 per 10^3 prevalent cases among Native American children aged 5–19 years. An analysis of the US Indian Health Service outpatient database revealed a 45% increase in the prevalence of diabetes between 1988 and 1996 for persons aged 15–24 years, from 4.8 per 10^3 to 7.0 per 10^3 per year [31]. During the same period, the prevalence rate for those <15-years-old remained stable and relatively low at 1.3 per 10^3.

Most Hispanic populations in the Americas have substantial Amerindian admixture [32], but it is not clear that genetic differences are at the root of the large gradient of risk in this area of the world. Among Puerto Rican children aged 0–14 years, the incidence rate of type 1 diabetes (using the standard definition of physician diagnosis and insulin treatment) was 17.4 per 10^5 in 1990–1994. In contrast, the annual type 1 incidence estimate for Cuban children during the same years was just 2.9 per 10^5 [2], despite nearly identical climates and roughly similar genetic admixture. Investigators in Santiago de Chile reported an increasing rate of presumed type 1 diabetes among children 0–14-years-old [33], with an overall rate of 4.0 per 10^5 per annum over the period 1986–2003. Higher rates were observed during more recent years in this population of mixed Caucasian and Amerindian descent; girls and older children were at greater risk.

In the United States there are just a few population-based registries that have been established with access to substantial numbers of non-Caucasian children. In Allegheny County, Pennsylvania, there were only 45 cases of type 1 diabetes in African Americans aged 0–19 years for the years 1990–1994, resulting in an incidence rate estimate of 17.6 per 10^5 per annum [34]. Type 1 diabetes incidence for African American children aged 0–14 years in Philadelphia, based on 98 subjects, was estimated at 12.8 per 10^5 per annum for 1990–1994 [35]. During the same period there were just 21 Latino patients in Philadelphia, mainly of Puerto Rican origin, for an incidence point estimate of 15.5 per 10^5 per annum. In contrast, the Latino population of Colorado is primarily of Mexican ancestry, demonstrating a state-wide incidence rate for type 1 diabetes in ages 0–17 years of 9.5 per 10^5 in 1980–1985 [36].

25.2.5 Incidence of Childhood Diabetes in Diverse Ethnic Groups in Chicago

The population-based Chicago Childhood Diabetes Registry has been ascertaining diabetes in the City of Chicago, Illinois, USA, since 1985 among African-American and Latino children with onset ages 0–17 years [37]. Initially, diabetes was defined by a record of insulin treatment. However, children with any diagnosis of diabetes, and those from all ethnic backgrounds, have been included if their diagnosis was made on or after 1 January 1992. We ascertained 1366 incident cases during the 10 years 1994–2003. Of these, 53% occurred in African Americans, 28% in Latinos and 17% in non-Hispanic White children, producing average 10-year incidence rates of 21.6 per 10^5 (95% confidence interval (CI): 19.3–24.2) for African American, 14.6 per 10^5 (95% CI: 13.0–16.4) for Latino, and 18.1 per 10^5 (95% CI: 15.9–20.2) for non-Hispanic White children [38]. Rates for non-Hispanic Whites and African Americans were thus significantly higher than for Latino patients.

25.2.6 Data-based Classification of Non-type 1 Diabetes in the Chicago Registry

Using medical records, and, when available, questionnaire responses, we were able to distinguish a group of non-type 1 subjects from the body of registered cases as follows. On the medical records, those with any mention of obesity, 'possible type 2' or 'atypical' diabetes, acanthosis nigricans, polycystic ovary syndrome or those with a body mass index (BMI) >95th age- and sex-specific percentile at onset were selected; in addition, those who responded to certain questions during the interview were considered likely to be non-type 1. (Interviews were conducted, on average, 6 years after the patients were first diagnosed.) These questions elicit information on cessation of insulin use after the 'honeymoon' period and on current treatment with oral agents. Those who did not meet one or more of these criteria were considered to have type 1 diabetes. It is important to note that none of the typical onset symptoms (polyuria, polydipsia, polyphagia, weight loss, diabetic ketoacidosis (DKA)) is used in the algorithm for distinguishing non-type 1 diabetes.

In Chicago, between 1994 and 2003, 61.8% (n = 844) of patients were classified as type 1 and

38.2% ($n = 522$) were classified as non-type 1 [38]. Type 1 diabetes incidence was predominant in all ethnic groups, although in African Americans the rate of non-type 1 was not significantly lower than for type 1. Specifically, for non-type 1 in African Americans the rate for type 1 was 11.6 per 10^5 (95% CI: 10.3–13.0) compared with 10.0 per 10^5 (95% CI: 8.9–11.2), for non-type 1 in Latinos it was 9.1 per 10^5 (95% CI: 8.1–10.2) for type 1 compared with 5.5 per 10^5 (95% CI: 4.6–6.6) and

for non-type 1 in non-Hispanic Whites it was 15.3 per 10^5 (95% CI: 3.0–18.1) compared with 2.8 per 10^5 (95% CI: 2.0–3.9) (**Figure 25.1**).

25.2.7   *Case Series*

A number of clinic-based studies in the United States demonstrate an increasing rate of diagnosis of type 2 diabetes among children. At the Cincinnati (Ohio) Children's Hospital, the major pediatric referral hospital in the region, 54 of 1027 diabetic

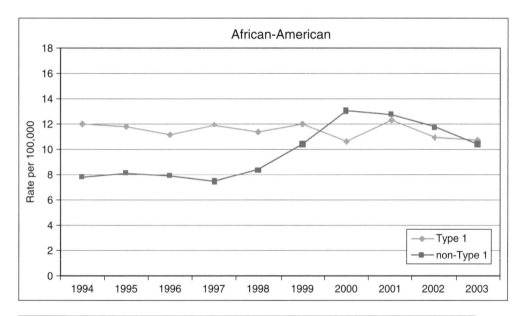

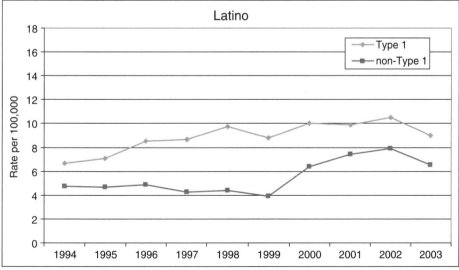

Figure 25.1 Incidence of childhood diabetes in Chicago by ethnicity, year, and diabetic phenotype: 3-year moving average rates in children ages 0–17 years.

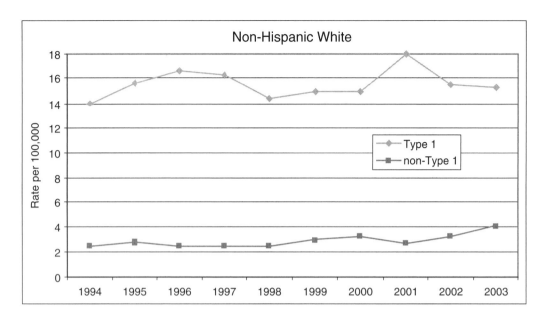

Figure 25.1 *(continued)*

patients aged 0–19 years (5.3%) met criteria for type 2 diabetes over a 13-year period [5]. Type 2 diabetes accounted for 2–4% of all diabetes diagnosed before 1992; in 1992–1994, the proportion increased to 8–17% of all incident cases. Most patients were diagnosed during a routine physical examination rather than by demonstrating the classic symptoms of diabetes onset. Diagnosis of type 2 diabetes was more frequent in African Americans and in females; the majority of these patients were obese (mean BMI was $37.7\,\mathrm{kg}\ \mathrm{m}^{-2}$) and had a first- or second-degree relative with diabetes. The investigators pointed to the rising prevalence of obesity among young people as a likely etiologic factor. Interestingly, there was also a concurrent and significant increase in type 1 diabetes in this population observed over the same period of time.

Similar data were reported from Arkansas in a retrospective chart review of 50 cases of childhood type 2 diabetes diagnosed over 8 years [6]. Again, a striking increase in the frequency of the diagnosis was observed, particularly in the last years of the study. Compared with 50 type 1 diabetes patients from the same hospital, young type 2 diabetes patients were more likely to be African American (74%), female, and older at diagnosis. In Cincinnati, young African American patients could be distinguished from non-Hispanic White youngsters with similar diagnoses by the severity

of presentation: fully 25% were in DKA at onset, compared with none of the Whites [39].

25.2.8 Summary

In general, we see that, among non-Europeans, the occurrence of early onset type 2 diabetes may not have been as rare as supposed prior to 1995. In the United States, insulin remained the only government-approved treatment for diabetes in patients aged 0–21 years until 2004, so ascertainment based on treatment with insulin most certainly would have led to at least some degree of misclassification. While an important component of the current 'epidemic' of type 2 diabetes in children may be attributed to misclassification of youth-onset type 2 as type 1 diabetes, real increases in incidence are likely to be occurring as well, in association with increases in childhood obesity and physical inactivity.

25.3 DESCRIPTIVE EPIDEMIOLOGY OF CHILDHOOD-ONSET DIABETES: TEMPORAL TRENDS AND MIGRANT STUDIES

As suggested by the above discussion, the incidence (and therefore prevalence) of type 1 and type 2 diabetes has been rising among children across the world over the past two decades. In New South Wales, Australia, the incidence of type 1 diabetes among children aged 0–14 years increased by 17% between 1990–1996 and 1997–2002 [40]. In the Franche-Comté region of France, there was a 50% increase in type 1 diabetes in this age group between the 1980s and 1990–1998 [41]. In the Australian study there was no definition of type 1 diabetes specified, while in France it was based on diabetes symptoms and fasting plasma glucose or OGTT.

In Japan, the increase has been most striking for type 2 diabetes [10], while both type 1 and type 2 diabetes incidence in Israel rose among non-European-origin children from ethnic groups recently immigrated to Israel [26]. These observations illustrate two major epidemiologic patterns of childhood diabetes incidence: first, that migrants rapidly take on the risk associated with their new locales; second, that rates of childhood type 2 diabetes have risen in a period of changing diagnostic practice and exposure to diabetogenic environmental conditions.

Comparing the first 5 years of the Chicago Registry, 1985–1989, and the most recent years, 1999–2003, we observed an increase in the average annual risk of insulin-treated diabetes among African Americans of 5.5%, from 14.5 per 10^5 to 15.3 per 10^5, and an increase of 12.5% among Latinos, from 9.6 per 10^5 to 10.8 per 10^5 [37, 38]. The increase in non-type 1 diabetes was even more impressive, particularly among Latinos (**Figure 25.1**). Among Israeli children of European extraction, there was a 59% increase in type 1 diabetes incidence (ages 0–14 years) when over 20 years, from 6.3 per 10^5 in 1980–1984 to 10.0 per 10^5 in 1990–1993; the same comparisons among Israeli children of Yemenite origin showed a 203% increase, from 9.1 per 10^5 in 1980–1984 to 18.5 per 10^5 in 1990–1993 [26]. Comparing incidence in migrants versus rates in the corresponding home populations has demonstrated increases among children of Jewish and French extraction in Montreal [42] and children of South Asian origin in England [43]. In Bradford, England, the average annual percentage change in type 1 diabetes incidence between 1978 and 1998 was 2.4% per annum for non-South Asian and 5.6% per annum for South Asian children [44].

Clearly, one possible explanation for these observations is variation in the number of children with type 2 diabetes who are misclassified as type 1, as most published studies defined type 1 diabetes by the use of insulin therapy. Different proportions of childhood-onset type 2 subjects might be included in epidemiologic studies of type 1 diabetes, according to whether local standards permit oral hypoglycemic agents to be used in children. Alternatively, it is probable that real differences in the risk of non-type 1 diabetes exist among ethnic groups located in different geographic regions, potentially attributable to differences in genetic admixture, the population frequency of relevant genes and/or environmental determinants of risk. Sufficient data have accumulated on rapid secular changes in incidence and migrant risk differences to support hypotheses that environmental factors are key to the development of childhood diabetes.

25.4 THE RANGE OF DIABETES IN YOUTH ACROSS THE WORLD: THE QUESTION OF MIXED PHENOTYPE

Surveys for diabetes among children and young adults from many geographic locations reveal a spectrum of characteristics. Winter's classic case-series, published in 1987 [3], described 12 of 129 African American patients with an atypical disease course, an absence of the type 1 diabetes-associated human leukocyte antigen (HLA) variants and no detectable islet cell antibodies islet cell antibody (ICAs). C-peptide levels in these patients were intermediate between those of type 1 diabetes patients and nondiabetic subjects. Additional characteristics resembling type 2 diabetes were observed, such as obesity and a high prevalence of diabetes among relatives, and these patients were ultimately characterized as having 'atypical' disease. A cooperative study in Asian patients aged 12–40 years described a variety of clinical characteristics in patients of Chinese, Indian or Malay ancestry, although the vast majority fit the clinical definition of type 2 [45]. Type 2 diabetes may comprise the bulk of diabetes among young Asian Indian patients in South Africa: Asmal *et al.* [46] reported that 86% of Indian patients under 40 years of age attending a diabetes clinic had type 2 diabetes; the prevalence for African-origin diabetic patients under the age of 35 years at the same clinic was 16%.

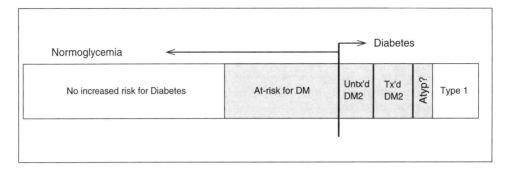

Figure 25.2 The continuum of glucose tolerance in young people.

Children with mixed phenotypes exhibit many of the classic symptoms of type 1 diabetes at onset (i.e. weight loss, polyphagia, polydipsia, polyuria, ketonuria or ketoacidosis), but the need for insulin diminishes with time. Most reports to date are simply case-series, but they have rekindled interest in clarifying the spectrum of diabetes mellitus among children and adolescents (**Figure 25.2**). In 2000, the US Centers for Disease Control and Prevention (CDC) established a collaboration of six population-based registries [47] to address this paucity of descriptive epidemiologic data on type 2 and mixed diabetes in children.

It may be that, compared with adults, glucose intoxication in young people at the outset of a type 2-like disease is generally more severe: marked hyperglycemia disrupts both the insulin secretory response and insulin signaling [48]. Once initial metabolic decompensation is resolved, β-cell function returns somewhat, allowing patients to avoid repeated bouts of ketosis despite, in many cases, poor glycemic control. In this scenario, the initial cause of metabolic disruption might be related to obesity, hormonal changes associated with puberty and/or genetic factors. The prognosis for these young patients would then be similar to that of adult type 2 diabetes, depending largely on the level of glycemic control and a gradual, long-term deterioration of β-cell function.

On the other end of the age range, Zimmet et al. [49] defined a syndrome, latent autoimmune diabetes of adults (LADA), to distinguish lean, ketosis-prone individuals with diabetes occurring in adulthood that progressed fairly quickly to insulin dependence. Taken as a whole, these developments undermine the conventional practice of categorizing diabetes as either autoimmune type 1 or

insulin-resistant type 2 diabetes. Aizawa et al. [50] suggest that a combination of many factors, including susceptibility genes, viral infections, immune attack, aging, variation in the β-cell mass at birth and glucose toxicity, can operate to cause β-cell damage and insulin resistance. They advocate a comprehensive view of the etiology of diabetes, taking these many potential risk factors into account for all patients.

Others refer to these mixed syndromes as 'double diabetes' in both adolescents and adults. Typically, 5–10% of most patients reported in clinic series have been unclassifiable into either major category of diabetes [51]. An incidence study of diabetes among Swedish youth aged 15–34 years demonstrated that, even in this relatively homogeneous population with few structural barriers to diagnosis and optimal treatment, confusion as to the clinical type and etiology of diabetes can occur [52]. Patients diagnosed in 1983–1984 ($n = 281$) were followed for 3 years. Initially, 75% were classified as type 1, 19% were thought to have type 2, and 6% were unclassifiable or their diabetes was secondary to another disease process. By 3 years' duration, 87% of the type 1 diabetes patients were still classified as type 1, and 72% of the initial type 2 diabetes patients were still in that category. Thus, 13% of type 1 diabetes and 28% of type 2 patients ($n = 43$ in all) exhibited an atypical clinical course. Of these, six patients were designated type 1 at onset on the basis of glycemia, ketonuria and other clinical characteristics. At follow-up, these patients remained lean, but had come off insulin without developing ketosis, and had C-peptide levels intermediate between those of the 'true' type 1 diabetics and the type 2 patients. Thus, even in a carefully defined population, correctly distinguishing type 1 from early onset type 2 diabetes can be difficult, particularly at the time of first diagnosis.

A case series following 89 young African American and Latino patients in New York City who were initially diagnosed with type 2 diabetes showed that, after 5 years, 18% were using insulin exclusively, while 37% used no medications at all and 45% were using pills. It is particularly important to note that patient characteristics at the time of diagnosis, such as obesity, insulin level or glycated hemoglobin, were not predictive of their long-term clinical course [53].

More than decade ago, two German clinicians proposed that a fraction of their type 1 patients were also affected by type 2 diabetes, based on clinical signs of the insulin resistance syndrome and a positive family history of type 2 diabetes [54]. Furthermore, they noted that, in any group of adult type 1 patients, this fraction with 'double diabetes' would be directly proportional to the prevalence of type 2 diabetes in the underlying population. Wilkin [55] proposed a related hypothesis, that early exposure to obesity can accelerate both autoimmune β-cell destruction as well as insulin resistance in genetically susceptible patients, engendering the onset of a mixed form of diabetes.

The prevalence of childhood overweight has increased dramatically across the developed world in recent years, accompanied by a marked increase in the diagnosis of type 2 diabetes in youth, disproportionately affecting non-Caucasian young people. However, many children who develop type 2 diabetes are severely ill at onset, and indistinguishable on clinical grounds from those with classic type 1 diabetes [39]. As described above, our group used available criteria to distinguish tentatively youth-onset type 2 diabetes patients in a population-based registry; clinical studies conducted on average at 8 years after diagnosis showed that a substantial fraction of those classified with type 2 displayed features of type 1 diabetes, that is absent β-cell function, autoantibodies and/or type 1 diabetes-related HLA-DQ alleles [56]. In addition, reports from Europe [57, 58] have linked early childhood obesity with type 1 diabetes, suggesting that youth-onset diabetes may often result from an interplay of autoimmunity and type 2 risk factors. Specifically, overnutrition may play a role in stimulating or prolonging autoimmune insulitis [55]. The likelihood that type 1 and type 2 diabetes coexist in the same patient is an attractive explanation for variant clinical manifestations of diabetes in young people.

25.5 RISK FACTORS FOR CHILDHOOD DIABETES IN NON-CAUCASIAN POPULATIONS

25.5.1 Islet Autoimmunity

The presence of one or another type of ICAs presumably indicates ongoing pancreatic autoimmunity and, therefore, ostensibly rules out an insulin-resistant or type 2 etiology in diabetes. ICAs are almost always found in newly diagnosed type 1 diabetes patients, and they are found in 3–5% of first-degree relatives of patients. They appear in <0.5% of the general population; when detected in nondiabetic individuals, the predictive value of ICAs for later developing type 1 diabetes is quite high: relative risks ranging from 50 to >200 have been reported by investigators from many parts of the world [59, 60]. This was explored in a large group of relatives of patients by Riley *et al.* [61], and the risk estimate among Blacks was actually somewhat higher than that among Whites. An analysis of islet cell autoimmunity among young insulin-treated patients, testing for ICAs on both human and rat pancreas substrates, demonstrated that 11.6% of 43 African American patients compared with just 4.1% of 394 non-Hispanic White patients were negative for all four major types of ICA [62].

Specific antibodies to glutamic acid decarboxylase (GAD) have been associated with pancreatic autoimmunity in more recent years [63, 64]. Like other kinds of ICA, they are found in 75–80% of newly diagnosed patients, and very rarely in nondiabetics. The presence of GAD antibodies is predictive of the development of type 1 diabetes in high-risk groups and population samples [65], and has been reported in subsets of type 2 diabetic patients as well. Ethnic differences in GAD antibody prevalence have also been demonstrated [66]. In Allegheny County, Pennsylvania, 71.7% of non-Hispanic White patients and 55.8% of the African American patients aged <19 years at onset were GAD antibody positive [62]; presumably, these were all type 1 patients. Compared with other kinds of ICA, GAD antibodies persist after the diagnosis of type 1 diabetes for an extended period: Rowley *et al.* [67] reported that 59% of type 2 diabetic adults with duration >3 years were GAD antibody positive, although just 13% were positive for conventional ICAs. This is a key advantage in studying autoimmunity among patients with diabetes of variable duration.

25.5.2 Residual β-Cell Function in Type 1 and Type 2 Diabetes

At the time of diagnosis, there is at least a small number of functioning β-cells in most patients, irrespective of the type and etiology of diabetes. Regulation of insulin release, as well as insulin signaling, is disturbed in response to prolonged hyperglycemia; once this glucose toxicity is resolved by treatment of the newly diagnosed disease, endogenous insulin secretion and insulin activity resume for at least a short interval in most patients [68]. The 'honeymoon' seen in the first few months of overt type 1 diabetes is a result of this sequence. Eventually, in type 1 diabetes patients, autoimmune β-cell destruction resumes until a complete loss of the ability to secrete insulin results. In contrast, type 2 diabetes patients continue to secrete insulin for a sustained period, although they, too, may eventually lose the capacity to produce insulin as their β-cells become exhausted. This pattern is seen in both youth-onset type 2 diabetes and the more common adult type. Thus, the measurement of C-peptide represents an obvious strategy for distinguishing type 1 from type 2 diabetes in questionable cases. If type 2 diabetic patients continue to secrete insulin (hence C-peptide) for an indefinite period, then the rate of fall in C-peptide might distinguish them from 'true' type 1 patients.

A number of investigators have addressed this question. Madsbad [69] reviewed the literature in preparation for the Diabetes Control and Complications Trial (DCCT), concluding that persistent secretors tended to be older at onset, but that the degree of metabolic control had no long-term association with C-peptide. He inferred that the evidence for a relationship with ICAs was inconsistent across studies, although a few years later Marner *et al.* [70] reported that those in whom ICAs were still present >30 months after diagnosis had a more rapid fall in β-cell function. Recruitment of potential DCCT subjects aged 13–39 years provided the opportunity to measure fasting and Sustacal-stimulated

C-peptide in large numbers of patients who had been classified as having type 1 diabetes on clinical grounds [71]. Average C-peptide levels declined from 0.2 pmol ml^{-1} (fasting) and 0.4 pmol ml^{-1} (stimulated) at 1 year to 0.05 pmol ml^{-1} (fasting) and <0.1 pmol ml^{-1} (stimulated) at 5 years. Importantly, a much more steep decline in residual β-cell function was observed for adolescents aged <18 years than for adults. Snorgaard *et al.* [72] tracked C-peptide levels from diagnosis to 6 years' duration in 124 patients under 30 years of age. Peak C-peptide reached a median level of 0.27 nmol l^{-1} at 6 months' duration; the median decline from the peak level was 0.08 nmol l^{-1} per year (fasting) and 0.03 nmol l^{-1} per year (postprandial). Median postprandial C-peptide was 0.06 nmol l^{-1} at 5 years' duration. These investigators also reported a more gradual decline among patients whose disease was diagnosed after age 30 years. Umpierrez *et al.* [73] studied a large series of African-American adults for β-cell function, genetic markers and autoantibodies, classifying these patients as lean with DKA ($n = 54$), obese with DKA ($n = 77$), obese without DKA ($n = 51$) and obese nondiabetics ($n = 25$). Obese patients presenting with DKA had fasting and stimulated C-peptide levels significantly higher than the lean DKA patients and significantly lower than the obese non-DKA group.

25.5.3 Genetic Associations with Type 1 and Type 2 Diabetes

Recent advances in the genetic epidemiology of type 1 diabetes, type 2 diabetes and MODY may soon make it possible to distinguish them based on genetic markers. Inheritance in European-origin MODY families usually follows that of an autosomal dominant pattern, with vertical transmission of disease from one generation to the next, and approximately 50% of siblings affected [74, 75]. Reports of non-type 1 diabetes in other ethnic groups show vertical transmission in only a subset of such families [18]. To date, associations of MODY with six specific mutations have been reported [76–79]; MODY3 is thought to account for about 65% of MODY cases, and along with MODY2, which is linked to about 15% of cases, has been found in all populations studied [75]. The other MODY genes have been found in only one or two ethnic groups and are related to a much smaller proportion of cases.

Among African-origin and US Hispanic patients with 'typical' type 1 diabetes, genetic similarities to European-origin type 1 diabetes patients have been demonstrated with a few notable exceptions [80, 81]. In a case–control study from Colorado, Mexican American children with type 1 diabetes were more likely than nondiabetic controls to have HLA-DR3, -DR4 and -DQ alleles which code for an amino acid other than aspartate at position 57 of the B1 subunit (non-Asp-57); similar findings were reported among non-Hispanic Whites [80]. The associated odds ratios (ORs) were not significantly different by ethnicity, although fewer Mexican American patients carried DR3. Among African-origin patients, similar strong associations with HLA-DR and -DQ alleles have been shown. Todd et al. [1] reported that the diabetes-associated DR9 haplotype among Afro-Caribbean type 1 diabetes patients in England carried a non-Asp codon at position 57 of DQB1, in contrast to DR9 among Whites, which appears to be protective against type 1 diabetes and codes for Asp at DQB1-57 [82]. A study of African-American women reported that HLA-B41 and -DR2 were positively associated with risk of insulin-requiring gestational diabetes mellitus, and with risk of developing type 2 diabetes in those with previous gestational diabetes [83]. This report is interesting in light of the findings that older, ketosis-prone Blacks with 'Flatbush' diabetes described by Banerji et al. [84] showed a higher than expected frequency of the type 1-associated HLA alleles.

While the strong association of HLA class II alleles with type 1 diabetes is not yet entirely understood, little attention has been given to the possibility that genetic variation with respect to insulin secretion and insulin signaling may modify risk for type 1 [85]. Edghill et al. [86] have determined that mutations in the KCNJ11 gene encoding the potassium channel subunit Kir6.2 are likely responsible for 45–64% of diabetes with onset in the first 6 months of life, children previously thought to have unambiguous type 1 diabetes. This insight has permitted these children to be transferred from insulin to sulfonylurea therapy.

There is widespread consensus that type 2 diabetes, in contrast to MODY, is a genetically heterogeneous condition. An array of polymorphisms have been linked to type 2 diabetes in single families or ethnic groups, but few associations have yet emerged that can be generalized to large groups of patients [87]. Genes linked to obesity may also provide clues to the role of heredity in the development of childhood type 2 diabetes. Thus far, genetic mutations affecting the melanocotin-4 receptor (MC4R), the small heterodimer partner (SHP) protein, the hormone leptin, the leptin receptor, the enzyme prohormone convertase-1 (PC1) and the amino acid proopiomelanocortin (POMC) have all been linked to obesity; POMC has been linked to obesity in people of European descent, African Americans, and Mexican Americans [88]. MC4R has also been well established in its relation to obesity and is currently thought to explain 3–4% of obesity cases [89]. The remaining associations with obesity have been shown in single groups or small numbers of cases, as is only to be anticipated for a polygenic trait such as obesity [90–92]. Among Amerindian children in Canada with type 2 diabetes, Sellars et al. [93] have determined that a mutant allele of the HNF-1α (hepatocyte nuclear factor) gene, G319S, is twice as common as among nondiabetic youth, and that its presence is associated with lower BMI and earlier age at onset, as well as more refractory disease.

25.5.4   Obesity and Physical Inactivity in Children

It is well accepted that being overweight as a child is a risk factor for obesity in adulthood. Using data from the Fels Longitudinal Study, Guo et al. [94] correlated girls' percentage ideal body weight aged 10–18 years with their percentage ideal weight at age 35 years; all coefficients exceeded 0.6. We know that obesity, impaired glucose tolerance and insulin resistance are important metabolic risk factors for type 2 diabetes mellitus in adults [95], and they are also suspected to be important etiologic components of youth-onset disease.

Defining obesity in growing children and adolescents is more problematic than in adults, and various investigators have relied on skinfolds, BMI (defined as weight/height^2), ponderosity (weight/height^3), and other methods [96]. Irrespective of which of these is used, most secular analyses indicate that adiposity has increased among youth in industrialized countries since 1960.

Comparing data from successive US national surveys beginning in 1963, Gortmaker et al. [97]

reported that, through 1980, the prevalence of obesity increased by 54% among children aged 6–11 years and by 39% in adolescents aged 12–17 years. These investigators defined obesity as triceps skinfold thickness >85th percentile of the 1963–1965 National Health Examination Survey 2 (NHES-2) distribution. Among young African Americans (age 6–11 years), the prevalence of obesity doubled, while fully 25.1% of Black females and 12.7% of Black males by 1980 were obese among African-American adolescents aged 12–17 years. More recently, the prevalence of obesity, defined by a BMI >95th age- and sex-specific percentile, increased yet again among children and adolescents during the 6-year period from 1999 to 2004. In 2003–2004, 17.1% of all US children and adolescents were obese. Tests for trend were significant for male and female children and adolescents, indicating a significant increase in the prevalence of obesity in female children and adolescents from 13.8% in 1999–2000 to 16.0% in 2003–2004 and in male children and adolescents from 14.0% to 18.2% [98]. Using logistic regression on national BMI data for 1999–2004, there was a 73% excess odds for obesity among Mexican-American boys compared with non-Hispanic Whites, with no increased risk for African-American boys. For girls there was an excess risk of obesity for both African Americans (OR = 1.46) and Mexican Americans (OR = 1.56) compared with non-Hispanic Whites aged 2–19 years [98].

Other investigators in the United States report similar high levels of overweight along with physical inactivity in children and adolescents in various geographic locations. A survey of 522 schoolgirls aged 10–18 years in 1991 recorded overweight (>85th percentile in NHANES-1) in 22% of non-Hispanic White, 38% of non-Hispanic Black and 27% of Hispanic girls in Lynn, Massachusetts [99]. More than 75% of these girls reported watching television >2 h per day, and only 13% participated in strenuous physical activity more than three times per week. In preparation for an intervention trial among 4th graders in Baltimore, Maryland, survey data were collected in 1995 from 785 students from primarily African-American, low-income schools. They reported, on average, watching more than 4 h of television per day [100].

A US national survey of adolescents conducted in 1996 demonstrated large ethnic differences in reported inactivity, but less of a disparity in moderate–vigorous physical activity [101]. Average television/video use was 20.4 h per week for non-Hispanic Blacks and 13.1 h for non-Hispanic Whites. Non-Hispanic Black and Asian girls had the lowest levels of physical activity. This increasing prevalence of obesity and physical inactivity among children provides a disconcerting glimpse of future generations, as recent longitudinal studies of the rate of fat accretion in children have revealed that a major determinant is parental fatness [102].

25.5.5 Insulin Resistance and Hyperinsulinemia in Healthy Children and Adolescents

A reasonably comprehensive literature is emerging on puberty and insulin metabolism. In a study of normal, European-origin children (14 prepubertal and 19 pubertal), Amiel *et al.* [103] showed them to exhibit selective insulin resistance which may have served to enhance the anabolic effect of insulin in proteins. A much larger study of insulin resistance (357 healthy children, ages 10–14 years; 73 were African American) demonstrated a significant decrease in insulin sensitivity through puberty, resolving to near-prepubertal levels by Tanner stage 5 [104]. Girls were more insulin resistant than boys at every pubertal stage; approximately 50% of this difference could be accounted for by adiposity as reflected by skinfold thickness. Non-Hispanic White boys were more insulin resistant than African Americans, and there was no significant ethnic difference among girls, controlled for BMI, adiposity and blood pressure. The initial reports of greater insulin resistance among Black compared with White children could have resulted from small numbers in these studies.

However, Black:White differences in insulin resistance and acute insulin response (AIR) were noted in a study of 95 prepubertal children [105]. Black children had higher vegetable/fruit and lower dairy intake than Whites, and they were more insulin resistant and had higher AIR. Dietary intake did not account for the ethnic differences in AIR, controlled for social class and adiposity. Using OGTTs, the Bogalusa (Louisiana) group demonstrated significantly higher 0–60 min insulin areas in nondiabetic Black children compared with

Whites aged 5–17 years, controlled for age, weight, height and Tanner stage [106].

An elevated fasting insulin concentration is recognized as a risk factor for type 2 diabetes. The longitudinal Pima Indian study provides information on the predictive value of obesity, family history and insulinemia in childhood for subsequent development of type 2 diabetes [107]. Overweight was closely correlated with fasting insulin levels and family history of diabetes; in those with a positive family history, obesity was the best predictor of diabetes risk. Compared with non-Hispanic White children, Pima children had consistently higher fasting insulin levels, despite similarities in age, height and fasting glucose concentration [108]. Multiple linear regression on (log) insulin demonstrated a significant interaction of race and relative weight; the models included age, age squared, and fasting glucose, and accounted for 49% of the variance in boys and 52% of the variance in girls. Fasting and 2 h insulin concentration were also higher among young Nauruans, ages 8–19 years, who developed impaired glucose tolerance or type 2 diabetes over the next 11 years, than among those who remained normoglycemic [109].

These studies corroborate other investigations of metabolic physiology that suggest that there are differences among racial groups in the anatomic and pathophysiologic correlates of glucose intolerance [73]. In particular, African-American children with equivalent body fatness to White children have less abdominal fat, higher insulin concentrations and lower insulin sensitivity [105, 110]. It is not clear whether these differences influence the clinical presentation of glucose intolerance in the different racial groups, but one would expect African-American children to be more vulnerable than White children to alterations in insulin secretion because of their dependence on elevated secretion to compensate for greater insulin resistance. Likewise, they would be more vulnerable than other groups to further decrements in insulin sensitivity, known to emerge during puberty.

25.5.6 Other Characteristics Associated with Insulin Resistance

Acanthosis nigricans is a skin condition characterized by raised, hyperpigmented areas that has been associated with obesity, lipid disturbances, hypertension and insulin resistance. This skin lesion is prevalent among non-White adults generally [111, 112], and among obese children. Polycystic ovary syndrome is typically diagnosed in patients with symptoms of androgen excess (i.e. infertility, hirsuitism or oligomenorrhea and elevated serum androgen levels) and is associated with insulin resistance. The prevalence of polycystic ovary syndrome was ~20% of asymptomatic Caucasian women in England, as detected by ultrasound [113, 114], but among 18–40-year-old Asian Indian women in England the prevalence was >50%. In these migrant women, polycystic ovary syndrome was significantly associated with acanthosis nigricans and elevated fasting blood glucose, in addition to the recognized symptoms of hirsuitism, infertility and menstrual irregularities [115]. Using a short intravenous glucose tolerance test, the presence of polycystic ovary syndrome in these women accounted for a reduction in insulin sensitivity comparable to that seen in women who had diagnosed type 2 diabetes without polycystic ovary syndrome (−60 mmol gluc/l per minute for polycystic ovary syndrome without diabetes versus −68 mmol gluc/l per minute for type 2 diabetes without polycystic ovary syndrome). There was no relationship to blood pressure, insulin sensitivity or lipids.

25.6 SUMMARY

In conclusion, the descriptive epidemiology of childhood diabetes shows evolving patterns consistent with changing environmental and clinical risk factors. The current status of research on childhood diabetes across the world demands a comprehensive study of variant types of youth-onset diabetes. Attempts to evaluate incidence or risk factors are frustrated where there is confusion regarding the case definition; this is a particular difficulty in those ethnic groups where youth-onset type 2 diabetes may be more prevalent. Adolescents and adults with intermediate clinical syndromes have been described, and may represent a group with features of both type 1 and type 2 diabetes. In short, much of the epidemiologic and clinical work on characterizing the range of childhood-onset diabetes and its risk factors is yet to be accomplished. Continuing to document the burden of diabetes in youth from diverse ethnic backgrounds is essential for improving the quality of diabetes care and addressing the public health needs of our society.

ACKNOWLEDGEMENT

This work was supported by NIH Grant Nos. M01RR0055 and R01DK44752.

References

1. Todd, J.A., Mijovic, C., Fletcher, J. *et al.* (1989) Identification of susceptibility loci for insulin-dependent diabetes mellitus by trans-racial gene mapping. *Nature*, **338**, 587–9.

2. Karvonen, M., Viik-Kajander, M., Moltchanova, E. *et al.* (2000) Incidence of childhood type 1 diabetes worldwide. Diabetes Mondiale (DiaMond) Project Group. *Diabetes Care*, **23**, 1516–26.

3. Winter, W.E., Maclaren, N.K. and Riley, W.J. (1987) Maturity-onset diabetes of youth in black Americans. *The New England Journal of Medicine*, **316**, 285–91.

4. Glaser, N., Araya, A., McFeely, M.E. and Jones, K.L. (1995) Non-insulin-dependent diabetes mellitus in childhood (Abstract). *Journal of Investigative Medicine*, **43**, 134a.

5. Pinhas-Hamiel, O., Dolan, L.M., Daniels, S.R. *et al.* (1996) Increased incidence of non-insulin-dependent diabetes mellitus among adolescents. *The Journal of Pediatrics*, **128**, 608–15.

6. Scott, C.R., Smith, J.M., Cradock, M.M. and Pihoker, C. (1997) Characteristics of youth-onset noninsulin-dependent diabetes mellitus and insulin-dependent diabetes mellitus at diagnosis. *Pediatrics*, **100**, 84–91.

7. Fagot-Campagna, A., Pettitt, D.J., Engelgau, M.M. *et al.* (2000) Type II diabetes among North American children and adolescents: an epidemiologic review and a public health perspective. *The Journal of Pediatrics*, **136**, 664–72.

8. Kitagawa, T., Mano, T. and Fujita, H. (1983) The epidemiology of childhood diabetes mellitus in Tokyo metropolitan area. *The Tohoku Journal of Experimental Medicine*, **141** (Suppl), 171–9.

9. Kitagawa, T., Owada, M., Urakami, T. and Yamauchi, K. (1998) Increased incidence of non-insulin-dependent diabetes mellitus among Japanese schoolchildren correlates with an increased intake of animal protein and fat. *Clinical Pediatrics*, **37**, 111–16.

10. Urakami, T., Kubota, S., Nitadori, Y. *et al.* (2005) Annual incidence and clinical characteristics of type 2 diabetes in children as detected by urine glucose screening in the Tokyo metropolitan area. *Diabetes Care*, **28**, 1876–81.

11. Kida, K., Mimura, G., Ito, T. *et al.* (2000) Incidence of type 1 diabetes in children aged 0–14 in Japan, 1986–1990, including an analysis for seasonality of onset and month of birth: JDS Study. *Diabetic Medicine*, **17**, 59–63.

12. Kwamura, T., Kadotani, S., Kimura, K. *et al.* (1999) The epidemiological study on the prevalence of childhood type 2 diabetes in Osaka City of Japan using capture–mark–recapture method (Abstract). *Diabetes*, **48** (Suppl 1), A168.

13. Sekar, C.C. and Deming, W.E. (1949) On a method of estimating birth and death rates and the extent of registration. *Journal of the American Statistical Association*, **44**, 101–115.

14. Huen, K.F., Low, L.C., Wong, G.W. *et al.* (2000) Epidemiology of diabetes mellitus in children in Hong Kong: the Hong Kong Childhood Diabetes Register. *Journal of Pediatric Endocrinology and Metabolism*, **13**, 297–302.

15. Li, X.H., Li, T.L., Yang, Z. *et al.* (2000) A nine-year prospective study on the incidence of childhood type 1 diabetes mellitus in China. *Biomedical and Environmental Sciences*, **13**, 263–70; Yang, Z., Wang, K., Li, T. *et al.* (1988) Childhood diabetes in China: enormous variation by place and ethnic group. *Diabetes Care*, **21**, 525–9.

16. Unachak, K. and Tuchinda, C. (2001) Incidence of type 1 diabetes in children under 15 years in northern Thailand, from 1991 to 1997. *Journal of the Medical Association of Thailand*, **84**, 923–8.

17. Ramachandran, A., Snehalatha, C. and Krishnaswami, C.V. (1996) Incidence of IDDM in children in urban population in southern India. *Diabetes Research and Clinical Practice*, **34**, 79–82.

18. Mohan, V., Ramachandran, A., Snehalatha, C. *et al.* (1985) High prevalence of maturity-onset diabetes of the young (MODY) among Indians. *Diabetes Care*, **8**, 371–4.

19. Crossley, J.R. and Upsdell, M. (1980) The incidence of juvenile diabetes mellitus in New Zealand. *Diabetologia*, **18**, 29–34.

20. Campbell-Stokes, P.L. and Taylor, B.J. (2005) Prospective incidence study of diabetes mellitus in New Zealand children aged 0 to 14 years. *Diabetologia*, **48**, 643–8.

21. Swai, A.B., Lutale, J.L. and McLarty, D.G. (1993) Prospective study of incidence of juvenile diabetes mellitus over 10 years in Dar es Salaam, Tanzania. *British Medical Journal*, **306**, 1570–2.

22. McLarty, D.G., Unwin, N., Kitange, H.M. and Alberti, K.G. (1996) Diabetes mellitus as a

cause of death in sub-Saharan Africa: results of a community-based study in Tanzania. The Adult Morbidity and Mortality Project. *Diabetic Medicine*, **13**, 990–4.

23. McLarty, D.G., Swai, A.B., Kitange, H.M. *et al.* (1989) Prevalence of diabetes and impaired glucose tolerance in rural Tanzania. *Lancet*, **1**, 871–5.

24. Kadiki, O.A. and Roaeid, R.B.M. (2002) Incidence of type 1 diabetes in children (0–14 years) in Benghazi, Libya (1991–2000). *Diabetes and Metabolism (Paris)*, **28**, 463–7.

25. Kulaylat, N.A. and Narchi, H. (2000) A twelve year study of the incidence of childhood type 1 diabetes mellitus in the Eastern Province of Saudi Arabia. *Journal of Pediatric Endocrinology and Metabolism*, **13**, 135–40.

26. Shamis, I., Gordon, O., Albag, Y. *et al.* (1997) Ethnic differences in the incidence of childhood IDDM in Israel (1965–1993). *Diabetes Care*, **20**, 504–8.

27. Duncan, G.E. (2006) Prevalence of diabetes and impaired fasting glucose levels among US adolescents: National Health and Nutrition Examination Survey, 1999–2002. *Archives of Pediatrics and Adolescent Medicine*, **160**, 523–8.

28. Dolan, L.M., Bean, J., D'Alessio, D. *et al.* (2005) Frequency of abnormal carbohydrate metabolism and diabetes in a population-based screening of adolescents. *The Journal of Pediatrics*, **146**, 751–8.

29. Dabelea, D., Hanson, R.L., Bennett, P.H. *et al.* (1998) Increasing prevalence of type II diabetes in American Indian children. *Diabetologia*, **41**, 904–10.

30. Dean, H. (1999) Incidence and prevalence of type 2 diabetes in youth in Manitoba, Canada, 1984–1998 (Abstract). *Diabetes*, **48** (Suppl 1), A168.

31. Burrows, N.R., Acton, K., Geiss, L. and Narayan, K.M.V. (1998) Trends in diabetes prevalence in American Indians and Alaskan Natives: an increasing burden among younger people (Abstract). *Diabetes*, **47** (Suppl 1), A187.

32. Hanis, C.L., Hewett-Emmett, D., Bertin, T.K. and Schull, W.J. (1991) Origins of U.S. Hispanics. Implications for diabetes. *Diabetes Care*, **14**, 618–27.

33. Carrasco, E., Pérez-Bravo, F., Dorman, J. *et al.* (2006) Increasing incidence of type 1 diabetes in population from Santiago of Chile: trends in a period of 18 years (1986–2003). *Diabetes/Metabolism Research and Reviews*, **22**, 34–7.

34. Libman, I.M., LaPorte, R.E., Becker, D. *et al.* (1998) Was there an epidemic of diabetes in nonwhite adolescents in Allegheny County, Pennsylvania? *Diabetes Care*, **21**, 1278–81.

35. Lipman, T.H., Chang, Y. and Murphy, K.M. (2002) The epidemiology of type 1 diabetes in children in Philadelphia 1990–1994: evidence of an epidemic. *Diabetes Care*, **25**, 1969–75.

36. Gay, E.C., Hamman, R.F., Carosone-Link, P.J. *et al.* (1989) Colorado IDDM registry: lower incidence of IDDM in Latinos: comparison of disease characteristics and care patterns in a biethnic community. *Diabetes Care*, **12**, 701–8.

37. Lipton, R., Keenan, H., Onyemere, K.U. and Freels, S. (2002) Incidence and onset features of diabetes in African American and Latino children, Chicago, 1985–1994. *Diabetes/Metabolism Research and Reviews*, **18**, 135–42.

38. Shaffer, T.L., Mencarini, M., Pourbovali, A. and Lipton, R. (2006) Did both type 1 and non-type 1 diabetes increase in Chicago children between 1994–2003 (Abstract)? In Endocrine Society Annual Meeting, June, 2006, Boston, MA.

39. Pinhas-Hamiel, O., Dolan, L.M. and Zeitler, P. (1997) Diabetic ketoacidosis among obese African-American adolescents with NIDDM. *Diabetes Care*, **20**, 484–6.

40. Taplin, C.E., Craig, M.E., Lloyd, M. *et al.* (2005) The rising incidence of childhood type 1 diabetes in New South Wales, 1990–2002. *The Medical Journal of Australia*, **183**, 243–6.

41. Mauny, F., Grandmottet, M., Lestradet, C. *et al.* (2005) Increasing trend of childhood type 1 diabetes in Franche-Comté (France): analysis of age and period effects from 1980–1998. *European Journal of Epidemiology*, **20**, 325–9.

42. Siemiatycki, J., Colle, E., Campbell, S. *et al.* (1988) Incidence of insulin-dependent (type I) diabetes by ethnic group and by social class in Montreal, and comparisons with comparable ethnic groups living elsewhere. *Diabetes*, **37**, 1096–102.

43. Raymond, N.T., Jones, J.R., Swift, P.G.F. *et al.* (2001) Comparative incidence of type 1 diabetes in children aged under 15 years from South Asian and White or other ethnic backgrounds in Leicestershire, UK, 1989–1998. *Diabetologia*, **44** (Suppl 3), B32–6.

44. Feltbower, R.G., Bodansky, H.J., Houghton, J. *et al.* (2002) Trends in incidence of childhood diabetes in South Asians and other children in Bradford, UK. *Diabetic Medicine*, **19**, 162–6.

45. Pan, C.Y., So, W.Y., Khalid, B.A. *et al.* (2004) Metabolic, immunological and clinical characteristics in newly diagnosed Asian diabetes patients aged 12–40 years. *Diabetic Medicine*, **21**, 1007–13.

46. Asmal, A.C., Dayal, B., Jialal, I. *et al.* (1981) Non-insulin-dependent diabetes mellitus with early onset in Blacks and Indians. *South African Medical Journal*, **60**, 93–6.

47. Dabelea, D., D'Agostino, R.B. Jr, Mayer-Davis, E.J. *et al.* (2006) Testing the accelerator hypothesis: body size, beta-cell function, and age at onset of type 1 (autoimmune) diabetes. *Diabetes Care*, **29**, 290–4.

48. Leahy, J.L., Bonner-Weir, S. and Weir, G.C. (1992) B-cell dysfunction induced by chronic hyperglycemia: current ideas on mechanism of impaired glucose-induced insulin secretion. *Diabetes Care*, **15**, 442–55.

49. Zimmet, P.Z., Tuomi, T., Mackay, I.R. *et al.* (1994) Latent autoimmune diabetes in adults (LADA): the role of antibodies to glutamic acid decarboxylase in diagnosis and prediction of insulin dependency. *Diabetic Medicine*, **11**, 299–303.

50. Aizawa, T., Funase, Y., Katakura, M. *et al.* (1997) Ketosis-onset diabetes in young adults with subsequent non-insulin-dependency, a link between IDDM and NIDDM? *Diabetic Medicine*, **14**, 989–91.

51. Harris, M.I. and Zimmet, P. (1992) Classification of diabetes mellitus and other categories of glucose intolerance, in *International Textbook of Diabetes Mellitus* (eds K.G.M.M. Alberti, R.A. DeFronzo, H. Keen and P. Zimmet), John Wiley & Sons, Ltd, Chichester, England, pp. 10–11.

52. Arnqvist, H.J., Littorin, B., Nystrom, L. *et al.* (1993) Difficulties in classifying diabetes at presentation in the young adult. *Diabetic Medicine*, **10**, 606–13.

53. Grinstein, G., Muzumdar, R., Aponte, L. *et al.* (2003) Presentation and 5-year follow-up of type 2 diabetes mellitus in African-American and Caribbean-Hispanic adolescents. *Hormone Research*, **60**, 121–6.

54. Teupe, B. and Bergis, K. (1991) Epidemiologic evidence for 'double diabetes' (Letter). *Lancet*, **337**, 361–2.

55. Wilkin, T.J. (2001) For debate – the accelerator hypothesis: weight gain as the missing link between type 1 and type 2 diabetes. *Diabetologia*, **44**, 914–22.

56. Lipton, R., Drum, M., Baumann, E. *et al.* (2005) Phenotyping minority young people: is it type 1 or type 2 diabetes (Abstract)? *Diabetes*, **54** (Suppl 1), A670.

57. Johansson, C., Samuelsson, U. and Ludvigsson, J. (1994) A high weight gain early in life is associated with an increased risk of type 1 (insulin-dependent) diabetes. *Diabetologia*, **37**, 91–4.

58. Hypponen, E., Virtanen, S.M., Kenward, M.G. *et al.* (2000) Obesity, increased linear growth, and risk of type 1 diabetes in children. *Diabetes Care*, **23**, 1755–60.

59. Lipton, R.B. and LaPorte, R.E. (1988) The epidemiology of islet cell antibodies. *Epidemiologic Reviews*, **11**, 182–203.

60. Bergau, M., Solé, J., Marion, G. *et al.* (1987) Prevalence of islet cell antibodies, insulin antibodies and hyperglycaemia in 2291 schoolchildren. *Diabetologia*, **30**, 724–6.

61. Riley, W.J., Maclaren, N.K., Krischer, J. *et al.* (1990) A prospective study of the development of diabetes in relatives of patients with insulin-dependent diabetes. *The New England Journal of Medicine*, **323**, 1167–72.

62. Libman, I.M., Pietropaolo, M., Trucco, M. *et al.* (1998) Islet cell autoimmunity in white and black children and adolescents with IDDM. *Diabetes Care*, **21**, 1824–7.

63. Baekkeskov, S., Aanstoot, H., Christgau, S. *et al.* (1990) Identification of the 64K autoantigen in insulin-dependent diabetes as the GABA-synthesizing enzyme glutamic acid decarboxylase. *Nature*, **347**, 151–6.

64. Christie, M.R., Tun, R.Y.M., Lo, S.S.S. *et al.* (1992) Antibodies to GAD and tryptic fragments of islet 64K antigen as distinct markers for development of IDDM. *Diabetes*, **41**, 782–7.

65. Atkinson, M.A., Maclaren, N.K., Scharp, D.W. *et al.* (1990) 64,000 Mr autoantibodies as predictors of insulin-dependent diabetes. *Lancet*, **335**, 1357–60.

66. Zimmet, P.Z., Rowley, M.J., Mackay, I.R. *et al.* (1993) The ethnic distribution of antibodies to glutamic acid decarboxylase: presence and levels in insulin-dependent diabetes mellitus in Europid and Asian subjects. *Journal of Diabetes and its Complications*, **7**, 1–7.

67. Rowley, M.J., Mackay, I.R., Chen, Q.Y. *et al.* (1992) Antibodies to glutamic acid decarboxylase discriminate major types of diabetes mellitus. *Diabetes*, **41**, 548–51.

68. Simonson, D.F., Rosetti, L., Giaccari, A. and DeFronzo, R.A. (1992) Glucose toxicity, in *International Textbook of Diabetes Mellitus*, (eds K.G.M.M. Alberti, R.A. DeFronzo, H. Keen and P. Zimmet), John Wiley & Sons, Ltd, Chichester, England, pp. 635–7.

69. Madsbad, S. (1983) Prevalence of residual β-cell function and its metabolic consequences in type I

(insulin-dependent) diabetes. *Diabetologia*, **24**, 141–7.

70. Marner, B., Agner, T., Binder, C. *et al.* (1985) Increased reduction in fasting C-peptide is associated with islet cell antibodies in type I (insulin-dependent) diabetic patients. *Diabetologia*, **28**, 875–80.

71. Klaff, L.J., Tamborlane, W.V., Cleary, P.A. *et al.* (1987) Effects of age, duration and treatment of insulin-dependent diabetes mellitus on residual β-cell function: observations during eligibility testing for the Diabetes Control and Complications Trial (DCCT). *The Journal of Clinical Endocrinology and Metabolism*, **65**, 30–6.

72. Snorgaard, O., Lassen, L.H. and Binder, C. (1992) Homogeneity in pattern of decline of β-cell function in IDDM: prospective study of 204 cases followed for 7.4 years. *Diabetes Care*, **15**, 1009–13.

73. Umpierrez, G.E., Woo, W., Hagopian, W.A. *et al.* (1999) Immunogenetic analysis suggests different pathogenesis for obese and lean African-Americans with diabetic ketoacidosis. *Diabetes Care*, **22** (9), 1517–23.

74. Fajans, S.S., Bell, G.I. and Polonsky, K.S. (2001) Molecular mechanisms and clinical pathophysiology of maturity-onset diabetes of the young. *Diabetes*, **345**, 971–80.

75. Owen, K. and Hattersley, A.T. (2001) Maturity-onset diabetes of the young: from clinical description to molecular genetic characterization. *Best Practice and Research Clinical Endocrinology and Metabolism*, **15**, 309–23.

76. Ryffel, G.U. (2001) Mutations in the human genes encoding the transcription factors of the hepatocyte nuclear factor (HNF)1 and HNF4 families: functional and pathological consequences. *Journal of Molecular Endocrinology*, **27**, 11–29.

77. Weng, J., Macfarlane, W.M., Lehto, M. *et al.* (2001) Functional consequences of mutations in the MODY4 gene (IPF1) and coexistence with MODY3 mutations. *Diabetologia*, **44**, 249–58.

78. Frayling, T.M., Evans, J.C., Bulman, M.P. *et al.* (2001) Beta-cell genes and diabetes: molecular and clinical characterization of mutations in transcription factors. *Diabetes*, **50**, S94–100.

79. Malecki, M.T., Jhala, U.S., Antonellis, A. *et al.* (1999) Mutations in NEUROD1 are associated with the development of type 2 diabetes mellitus. *Nature Genetics*, **23**, 323–8.

80. Cruickshanks, K.J., Jobim, L.F., Lawler-Heavner, J. *et al.* (1994) Ethnic differences in human leukocyte antigen markers of susceptibility to IDDM. *Diabetes Care*, **17**, 132–7.

81. Dorman, J.S., LaPorte, R.E., Stone, R.A. and Trucco, M. (1990) Worldwide differences in the incidence of type I diabetes are associated with amino acid variation at position 57 of the HLA-DQ beta chain. *Proceedings of the National Academy of Sciences of the United States of America*, **87**, 7370–4.

82. Tait, B.D. (1990) Genetic susceptibility to type I diabetes: a review. *Journal of Autoimmunity*, **3** (Suppl), 3–11.

83. Acton, R.T., Roseman, J.M., Bell, D.S.H. *et al.* (1994) Genes within the major histocompatibility complex predict NIDDM in African-American women in Alabama. *Diabetes Care*, **17**, 1491–4.

84. Banerji, M.A., Chaiken, R.L., Huey, H. *et al.* (1994) GAD antibody negative NIDDM in adult Black subjects with diabetic ketoacidosis and increased frequency of human leukocyte antigen DR3 and DR4: Flatbush diabetes. *Diabetes*, **43**, 741–5.

85. Pearson, E.R., Starkey, B.J., Powell, R.J. *et al.* (2003) Genetic aetiology of hyperglycemia determines response to treatment in diabetes. *Lancet*, **362**, 1275–81.

86. Edghill, E.L., Dix, R.J., Flanagan, S.E. *et al.* (2006) HLA genotyping supports a nonautoimmune etiology in patients diagnosed with diabetes under the age of 6 months. *Diabetes*, **55**, 1895–8.

87. Cox, N.J. (2001) Challenges in identifying genetic variation affecting susceptibility to type 2 diabetes: examples from studies of the calpain-10 gene. *Human Molecular Genetics*, **10**, 2301–5.

88. Wardlaw, S.L. (2001) Clinical review 127: obesity as a neuroendocrine disease: lessons to be learned from proopiomelanocortin and melanocortin receptor mutations in mice and men. *The Journal of Clinical Endocrinology and Metabolism*, **86**, 1442–6.

89. Farooqi, I., Yeo, G., Keogh, J. *et al.* (2000) Dominant and recessive inheritance of morbid obesity associated with melanocortin 4-receptor deficiency. *The Journal of Clinical Investigation*, **106**, 271–9.

90. Nishigori, H., Tomura, H., Tonooka, N. *et al.* (2001) Mutations in the small heterodimer partner gene are associated with mild obesity in Japanese subjects. *Proceedings of the National Academy of Sciences of the United States of America*, **98**, 575–80.

91. Montague, C.T., Farooqi, S.I., Whitehead, J.P. *et al.* (1997) Congenital leptin deficiency is associated with severe early-onset obesity in humans. *Nature*, **387**, 903–8.

92. Clement, K., Vaisse, C., Lahlou, N. *et al.* (1998) A mutation in the human leptin receptor gene

causes obesity and pituitary dysfunction. *Nature*, **392**, 398–401.

93. Sellars, E.A.C., Rockman-Greenberg, C., Triggs-Raine, B. and Dean, H.J. (2002) The prevalence of the HNF-1α G319S mutation in Canadian aboriginal youth with type 2 diabetes. *Diabetes Care*, **25**, 2202–6.

94. Guo, S.S., Roche, A.F., Chumlea, W.C. *et al.* (1994) The predictive value of childhood body mass index values for overweight at age 35 years. *The American Journal of Clinical Nutrition*, **59**, 810–19.

95. Haffner, S.M., Stern, M.P., Mitchell, B.D. *et al.* (1990) Incidence of type 2 diabetes in Mexican Americans predicted by fasting insulin and glucose levels, obesity, and body fat distribution. *Diabetes*, **39**, 283–8.

96. Flegal, K.M. (1993) Defining obesity in children and adolescents: epidemiologic approaches. *Critical Reviews in Food Science and Nutrition*, **33**, 307–12.

97. Gortmaker, S.L., Dietz, W.H., Sobol, A.M. and Wehler, C.A. (1987) Increasing pediatric obesity in the United States. *American Journal of Diseases of Children*, **141**, 535–40.

98. Ogden, C.L., Carroll, M.D., Curtin, L.R. *et al.* (2006) Prevalence of overweight and obesity in the United States, 1999–2004. *Journal of the American Medical Association*, **295**, 1549–55.

99. Wolf, A.M., Gortmaker, S.L., Cheung, L. *et al.* (1993) Activity, inactivity, and obesity: racial, ethnic, and age differences among schoolgirls. *American Journal of Public Health*, **83**, 1625–7.

100. Gortmaker, S.L., Cheung, L., Peterson, K. *et al.* (1999) Impact of a school-based interdisciplinary intervention on diet and physical activity among urban primary school children. *Archives of Pediatrics and Adolescent Medicine*, **153**, 975–83.

101. Gordon-Larsen, P., McMurray, R.G. and Popkin, B.M. (1999) Adolescent physical activity and inactivity vary by ethnicity: the National Longitudinal Study of Adolescent Health. *The Journal of Pediatrics*, **135**, 301–6.

102. Figueroa-Colon, R., Arani, B., Goran, M.I. and Weinsier, R.L. (2000) Paternal body fat is a longitudinal predictor of changes in body fat in premenarcheal girls. *The American Journal of Clinical Nutrition*, **71**, 829–34.

103. Amiel, S.A., Caprio, S., Sherwin, R.S. *et al.* (1991) Insulin resistance of puberty: a defect restricted to peripheral glucose metabolism. *The Journal of Clinical Endocrinology and Metabolism*, **72**, 277–82.

104. Moran, A., Jacobs, D.R., Steinberger, J. *et al.* (1999) Insulin resistance during puberty: results from clamp studies in 357 children. *Diabetes*, **48**, 2039–44.

105. Lindquist, C.H., Gower, B.A. and Goran, M.I. (2000) Role of dietary factors in ethnic differences in early risk of cardiovascular disease and type 2 diabetes. *The American Journal of Clinical Nutrition*, **71**, 725–32.

106. Svec, F., Nastasi, K., Hilton, C. *et al.* (1992) Black–White contrasts in insulin levels during pubertal development: The Bogalusa Heart Study. *Diabetes*, **41**, 313–17.

107. McCance, D.R., Pettitt, D.J., Hanson, R.L. *et al.* (1994) Glucose, insulin concentrations and obesity in childhood and adolescence as predictors of NIDDM. *Diabetologia*, **37**, 617–23.

108. Pettitt, D.J., Moll, P.P., Knowler, W.C. *et al.* (1993) Insulinemia in children at low and high risk of NIDDM. *Diabetes Care*, **16**, 608–15.

109. Zimmet, P.Z., Collins, V.R., Dowse, G.K. and Knight, L.T. (1992) Hyperinsulinaemia in youth is a predictor of type 2 (non-insulin-dependent) diabetes mellitus. *Diabetologia*, **35**, 534–41.

110. Arslanian, S.A. and Danadian, K. (1998) Insulin secretion, insulin sensitivity, and diabetes in Black children. *Trends in Endocrinology and Metabolism*, **9**, 194–9.

111. Stuart, C.A., Pate, C.J. and Peters, E.J. (1989) Prevalence of acanthosis nigricans in an unselected population. *The American Journal of Medicine*, **87**, 269–72.

112. Stuart, C.A., Smith, M.M., Gilkison, C.R. *et al.* (1994) Acanthosis nigricans among Native Americans: an indicator of high diabetes risk. *American Journal of Public Health*, **84**, 1839–42.

113. Polson, D.W., Adams, J., Wadsworth, J. and Franks, S. (1988) Polycystic ovaries – a common finding in normal women. *Lancet*, **1** (8590), 70–2.

114. Cresswell, J.L., Barker, D.J., Osmond, C. *et al.* (1997) Fetal growth, length of gestation, and polycystic ovaries in adult life. *Lancet*, **350**, 131–5.

115. Rodin, D.A., Bano, G., Bland, J.M. *et al.* (1998) Polycystic ovaries and associated metabolic abnormalities in Indian subcontinent Asian women. *Clinical Endocrinology*, **49**, 1–99.

26

Genetic Epidemiology of Type 1 Diabetes Mellitus

Kirsten O. Kyvik[1] and Anders Green[2]

[1]Institute of Regional Health Services Research and Epidemiology, Institute of Public Health, University of Southern Denmark, Odense, Denmark
[2]Department of Research and Applied Health Technology Assessment, Odense University Hospital and Epidemiology, Institute of Public Health, University of Southern Denmark, Odense, Denmark

26.1 INTRODUCTION

Genetic epidemiology is the research discipline that deals with the etiology, distribution and control of disease in groups of relatives and with inheritable causes of disease in populations. Epidemiologists, geneticists, statisticians and clinicians contribute to the task of unraveling the prime focus, namely the etiology of complex diseases. The outcome of this research can be distributed among the following categories: genetic information (inheritance patterns, heritability, recurrence risks within affected families, specific susceptibility genes) and epidemiological information (incidence, prevalence, nongenetic determinants of disease). In this chapter we will review the present knowledge of the genetic epidemiology of type 1 diabetes with special focus on important etiological factors and risk in relatives of patients.

26.2 EVIDENCE OF A GENETIC CONTRIBUTION TO TYPE 1 DIABETES

The etiological importance of genetic susceptibility to type 1 diabetes is clearly demonstrated by twin and family studies. It has been suggested that the concordance rate of type 1 diabetes in monozygotic twin pairs is 25–60%, against 7.5–15% in dizygotic twin pairs [1–3]. The heritability, namely the proportion of the total phenotypic variation of the liability to type 1 diabetes ascribable to genes, has been estimated to be 0.75–0.88 [2, 3]. Several family studies have found rather consistent estimates of recurrence risks of type 1 diabetes at about 5–10% among siblings and children of type 1 diabetes patients [4, 5]. Notably, these risk estimates are lower than the risk in dizygotic twin pairs, which could indicate that the environment shared by twins might be etiologically important as well.

It has been known for many years [6] that the quantitatively most important genetic locus influencing risk of type 1 diabetes is the *HLA* class II region, which explains approximately 40% of the familial aggregation of the disease [7]. The *HLA-DQB1*0602* allele has been found to be protective against type 1 diabetes, while the alleles *DQA1*03-DQB1*0302* and *DQA1*05-DQB1*0201* are associated with an increased risk [8, 9]. Another gene consistently found to be associated with type 1 diabetes is the insulin (*INS*) gene, where the VNTR class I allele confers increased risk and the class III allele confers reduced risk of type 1 diabetes [10, 11]. At least nine non-HLA-linked regions have been demonstrated to have some evidence of linkage to the disease [6].

The degree of haplotype sharing in siblings from type 1 diabetes families influences the recurrence

The Epidemiology of Diabetes Mellitus, second edition   Edited by Jean-Marie Ekoé, Marian Rewers, Rhys Williams and Paul Zimmet
© 2008 John Wiley & Sons, Ltd

risk considerably, with an estimated recurrence risk of about 15–20% for HLA-identical siblings, a risk of about 6% for haplo-identical sibs and close to 0% for nonidentical sibs. It is important to note that the estimated risk for HLA-identical siblings seems to be considerably lower than the concordance rate in monozygotic twins. On the other hand, the risk for HLA-identical siblings is considerably higher than the risk among unrelated individuals that carry high-risk HLA-markers.

The non-HLA-linked susceptibility to type 1 diabetes agrees with the higher concordance rate among monozygotic twins compared with HLA-identical siblings, although a higher degree of sharing of environment in twins also may contribute to this difference.

Although no definite models of the genetic susceptibility in type 1 diabetes have been obtained, simple dominance is unlikely, and that the frequency of the disease susceptibility gene(s) is rather high with a low penetrance [12, 13]. It is most likely that type 1 diabetes fits the 'Common disease, common variant' model [14]. Thus, the largest contribution to the pool of susceptibility genes originates from nonaffected individuals. This agrees well with the fact that 80–90% of newly diagnosed children represent single-case families; that is, those without prior known cases of type 1 diabetes among close relatives [15].

26.3 EVIDENCE OF ENVIRONMENTAL DETERMINANTS

The most striking evidence of a nongenetic contribution to type 1 diabetes relates to the fact that the concordance rate in monozygotic twins is far below unity [1–3]. Since monozygotic twin partners share all their segregating genes, this difference can be attributed to the influence of nongenetic exposures or epigenetic phenomena [16]. Here, we will concentrate on the first explanation, as very little research has been published on epigenetic phenomena and type 1 diabetes. Two additional lines of evidence provide support for the nongenetic contribution. First, the huge variation in the incidence of type 1 diabetes between Caucasian populations [17, 18] cannot be explained by the geographical distribution of susceptibility genes. Second, the rising incidence of type 1 diabetes, as observed

in many European populations [19], cannot possibly be explained by increased size of the pool of susceptibility genes [20] and must be attributed to increased susceptibility in individuals at genetic risk and/or the introduction of environmental causative agents in these populations [21].

The search for nongenetic determinants of type 1 diabetes has been intensified over the last 25 years and has focused on viral infections, nutritional factors, stressful life events, socioeconomic status and the intrauterine environment.

Virus infections have for a long time been implicated in the causation of type 1 diabetes [22]. It has been demonstrated that congenital rubella infection is associated with a high risk of subsequent development of type 1 diabetes [23]. The development of type 1 diabetes has also been associated with cytomegalovirus infection, mumps, Coxsackie B infections and enteroviruses [24, 25]. The importance of and the mechanisms by which infectious agents cause β-cell destruction by immune-mediated mechanisms are still debated [26–28].

Following the results from animal studies that dietary changes influence the incidence of diabetes [29], several studies in humans have focused on the possible role of dietary factors in type 1 diabetes.

A study from Iceland suggested that exposure to nitrosamines in women at the time of conception may increase the risk of type 1 diabetes in the male offspring [30], and this was supported by studies in Sweden [31, 32] and Finland [33]. The finding still needs confirmation and does not explain the high type 1 diabetes incidence level in populations where exposure to nitrosamines is less common than in Iceland.

The association between type 1 diabetes and breast feeding has been extensively studied since a Danish study [34] found that reduced length of breast feeding during infancy seems to be associated with increased risk of developing type 1 diabetes. The literature on cow's milk exposure and type 1 diabetes has also been reviewed extensively. The information is so far still controversial, but there seems to be some consensus that long breast feeding and supplementation with vitamin D in infancy partially protects against type 1 diabetes, while early exposure to cow's milk proteins, cereals and heavy weight in infancy are thought to be risk factors.

Birth weight has been extensively studied in the last 5–10 years [35–38] and most interesting birth weight has been reported to be associated to both the HLA and *INS VNTR* genes in nondiabetic populations [39–42]. Studies on the putative interaction between these genes, birth weight and diabetes are so far lacking.

A few studies have addressed the possible etiological role of psychological factors and stressful life events in the period preceding clinical onset of disease. Although with rather weak associations, several reports have provided consistent evidence of such possible influences [43–47]. It is possible that stressful life events and psychological dysfunction, through elevated stress hormone levels, increase the demand for endogeneous insulin production and thereby accelerate clinical precipitation of type 1 diabetes in individuals with ongoing β-cell destruction.

Conflicting results have been reported regarding the associations between socioeconomic status and type 1 diabetes. Some studies found higher incidence of type 1 diabetes in regions with relatively low average income level, whereas others found an opposite trend [48–51]. Such associations are probably explained by unknown events and factors in lifestyle that may influence the risk of developing type 1 diabetes and the socioeconomic status.

26.4 PREDICTING RISK OF TYPE 1 DIABETES: AVAILABLE MARKERS

The current appreciation of the etiology and pathogenesis of type 1 diabetes has important implications for predicting risk of developing the disease. Until immune markers appear in the circulation, the only available and reasonably well-established markers of type 1 diabetes are represented by genetic determinants (**Figure 26.1**). The appearance of immune markers signifies an activation of the immune system which, to a high degree, correlates with an ongoing destruction of the β-cells of the pancreas. When a sufficiently large part of the cells has been destroyed, metabolic decompensation develops, with clinical presentation of type 1 diabetes as the consequence. This may be preceded by the demonstration of reduced response in insulin secretion to a glucose challenge. This scenario provides for the establishment of several types of marker in predicting type 1 diabetes.

As mentioned above, type 1 diabetes tends to cluster in families due to sharing of genetic susceptibility factors. A positive family history (FH) of type 1 diabetes (e.g. the presence of type 1 diabetes among relatives of a subject) is, therefore, per se a marker for risk of type 1 diabetes. This is most strongly illustrated from estimation of probandwise concordance rates in twin studies, implying a long-term risk of type 1 diabetes mounting to 60% or even higher for monozygotic twin partners in some studies [3]. However, for first-degree relatives other than twins the long-term recurrence risks are considerably lower, and they are even further reduced when moving to more remote categories of relatives [4]. In spite of the genetic susceptibility to type 1 diabetes, the vast majority of newly diagnosed patients will have a negative family history [15]. Overall, when considering FH as the only marker, the ability to predict type 1 diabetes seems rather modest.

Since associations between type 1 diabetes and genetic markers from the HLA system were described more than 25 years ago, an increasing number of genetic susceptibility factors have been characterized [6]. Predicting risk of type 1 diabetes on the basis of the presence of genetic markers may thus supplement and enhance information from FH. However, currently defined genetic markers of type 1 diabetes occur frequently in unaffected subjects, and it can be calculated (as illustrated below) that the absolute cumulative lifetime risk in unrelated subjects carrying high-risk markers probably does not exceed 5–10%. These circumstances, combined with ethical and logistic problems, restrict the utilization of genetic markers for predictive purposes to individuals already classified as being at increased risk from a positive FH.

The presence of immune markers in the circulation, even years before clinical presentation of type 1 diabetes, has for decades been believed to signify an ongoing immune-mediated destruction of the β-cells [52]. Currently defined immune markers of type 1 diabetes include islet-cell antibodies (ICAs) [53], insulin autoantibodies [53] and autoantibodies to glutamic acid decarboxylase [54–58], as well as others. The utilization of immune marker assays, particularly when combined [59], has become particularly important as an instrument for identifying candidates at risk for developing type 1 diabetes and thus eligible for enrolment in intervention trials [60]. The prevalence of high-titer immune markers is relatively low in the

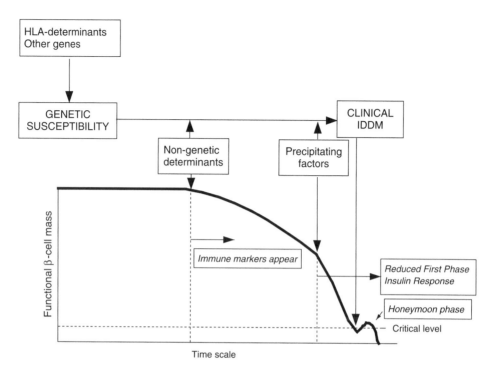

Figure 26.1 Graphic illustration of the disease process and development of type 1 diabetes (IDDM: insulin-dependent diabetes mellitus).

general population [60], thereby restricting their application to clinically unaffected relatives of patients with type 1 diabetes [61].

Assessment of β-cell function provides for the establishment of the class of metabolic markers of type 1 diabetes. Impaired secretion of C-peptide, with or without preceding glucagon stimulation, indicates severely impaired ability to produce insulin or respond to increased demands of insulin. Reduced first-phase insulin response to an intravenous glucose challenge predicts with a high power subsequent development of clinical type 1 diabetes and need of insulin treatment [62, 63]. Probably, both markers become positive very late in the prodromal (preclinical) phase (**Figure 26.1**) at a time where it may be too late to use them for intervention purposes.

26.5 PREDICTING RISK OF TYPE 1 DIABETES: METHODOLOGICAL CONSIDERATIONS

Predicting the risk of a chronic disease like type 1 diabetes involves a quantitative assessment of the risk of developing the disease over a specified period of time, usually an age span expressed in years. At the most basic level, ignoring specific markers, the disease risk may be estimated from the population incidence by the relationship

$$R_{t=1,2} 1 - \exp\{-[\text{INC}(t_2 - t_1)]\}$$

where $R_{t=1,2}$ represents the cumulative risk of developing type 1 diabetes during the time span from $t = 1$ to $t = 2$ in the general population and INC represents the population incidence rate (expressed as number of new cases per person-year at risk) applicable to this period and assumed constant. For a relatively rare disease like type 1 diabetes the quantity $\text{INC}(t_2 - t_1)$ is usually small (<0.05); under these circumstances, the relation approximates the more simple expression

$$R_{t=1,2} \approx \text{INC}(t_2 - t_1)$$

Thus, if the population incidence of type 1 diabetes among children aged 0–14 years is 16 per 100 000 person-years, then the cumulative risk of developing type 1 diabetes over a period of 5

Table 26.1 The 2 × 2 table illustrating the population distribution by marker status and disease.

	+ Type 1 diabetes	− Type 1 diabetes	Total
Marker +	a	b	$a + b$
Marker−	c	d	$c + d$
Total	$a + c$	$b + d$	$N = a + b + c + d$

General population risk $R = (a + c)/N$.

years may be estimated as 0.08% ($= 0.000\,16$/year $\times$ 5 years). Since no markers are involved, the estimated disease risk is applicable to all subjects at risk in the population concerned under the implicit assumption of equal risk for all such subjects.

Access to information of markers associated with the disease enhances risk assessment. Now, the population can be divided according to marker status and subsequent disease development. **Table 26.1** illustrates this for a cohort approach in which a out of $a + b$ marker-positive subjects develop disease within a given follow-up period, and c out of $c + d$ marker-negative subjects develop disease. The population risk R is $(a + c)/(a + b + c + d) = (a + c)/N$.

From the entries and totals of **Table 26.1**, the relevant measures of test performance can be derived immediately. These measures include the positive predictive value (PPV) of a test, the predictive value of a negative test, sensitivity (SENS) and specificity (SPEC); see **Table 26.2**, left and center columns. Whereas SENS and SPEC may be estimated from random samples of patients and unaffected subjects respectively, the direct estimation of the predictive values from the entries of **Table 26.1** requires that patients and unaffected subjects are represented

in numbers proportionate with the distribution in the general population. Formally, this is expressed in the following important relation, derived from combining and rearranging the estimates of the individual measures:

$$\text{PPV} = \frac{\text{SENS} \times R}{(\text{SENS} \times R) + (1 - \text{SPEC})(1 - R)}$$

This expression permits the estimation of PPV on the basis of the marker distributions in random samples of patients and unaffected subjects (**Tables 26.1** and **26.2**), if an estimate of the general population risk is available. The expression also illustrates the complicated relationship between, on the one hand, the PPV and, on the other hand, the general population risk, SENS and SPEC. The PPV will differ from population to population by differences in population risk, even should both SENS and SPEC be identical across populations. Accordingly, assessments of the performance of a given marker assay for predictive purposes are specific for a given population and cannot without due consideration to this fact be generalized to other populations.

The measures of test performance may be expressed in epidemiological terms as shown in

Table 26.2 Measures of test performance, their estimation and epidemiological correlates.

Measure of test performance	Estimation	Corresponding epidemiological measure
PPV	$a/(a + b)$	Disease risk among marker-positive subjects R_E
Predictive value of negative test	$d/(c + d)$	Disease-free survival in marker-negative subjects, $1 - R_0$
SENS	$a/(a + c)$	Proportion of marker-positive patients
SPEC	$d/(b + d)$	Proportion of marker-negative subjects remaining disease free

Table 26.2 (right column). For example, the PPV corresponds with the absolute disease risk among marker-positive subjects. This appreciation is important because the association between a disease and a marker is often summarized as the so-called relative risk (RR), from which the absolute risk among marker-positive subjects (PPV) may be estimated if knowledge of the population risk R is available. The RR contrasts in a ratio the disease risk in marker-positive subjects with that in marker-negative subjects; that is:

$$RR = \frac{R_E}{R_0}$$

With the definitions in **Table 26.1**, R_E (= PPV) is estimated from $a/(a + b)$ and R_0 from $c/(c + d)$. For a relatively rare disease like type 1 diabetes, the ratio R_E/R_0 approximates ad/bc, which is also known as the *cross-product ratio* or *odds ratio* of the 2 × 2 table, well-known from association studies.

Now, the population risk R represents the weighted average of R_E and R_0, the weights being provided by the population prevalence P_M of the marker:

$$R = P_M R_E + (1 - P_M) R_0$$

Using the relationship RR = R_E/R_0, the expression above can be rearranged to estimate R_E:

$$R_E = \frac{RR \times R}{1 + P_M(RR - 1)}$$

Let us assume that the population risk of type 1 diabetes over a period of 5 years is 0.08% (as before), and that a case-control study has found RR = 50 for a marker with a population prevalence of 0.20. These data yield an estimated value of R_E (and therefore also PPV) of 0.37%. In the same population, a marker conferring an RR = 50 but with a population marker prevalence as low as 0.01 would lead to an estimated value of R_E = 2.68%. For populations with lower general disease risk, the estimates would be correspondingly reduced.

As a contrast, let us consider a high-risk population; for example, unaffected first-degree relatives of type 1 diabetes patients. The incidence, and hence risk, may be assumed to be about 5–10 times higher than the risk in the general population; this corresponds with a cumulative risk over 3 years of, say, 0.5%. Let us further assume that the RR

of the marker remains at 50, but that the marker has a prevalence of 0.30 in this group of subjects. Now, the estimated R_E comes out at 1.59%. This figure may seem surprisingly low; nevertheless, the marker data have made it possible to classify the 70% marker-negative subjects in this prior defined high-risk group as having a negligible risk (R_E/RR = 1.59/50 = 0.03%).

The numerical data used in these examples are fairly representative for currently defined genetic and immune markers in societies at medium-to-high population risk of type 1 diabetes. The exercise demonstrates clearly that prediction of type 1 diabetes on the basis of any single marker leads to low PPVs. Even in subjects, classified as being at a high risk from a positive FH of type 1 diabetes, the performance, when assessed by estimated values of PPV, is rather modest. The main challenge in this respect involves the utilization of combined marker information as the basis of improved prediction of type 1 diabetes.

26.6 PREDICTING RISK OF TYPE 1 DIABETES: A HYPHOTHETICAL EXAMPLE

Numerous studies have illustrated how combined marker information enhances the prediction of type 1 diabetes [56], particularly in connection with preventive trials [46]. The approach is most conveniently illustrated by a numerical example. In this section we use a positive FH of type 1 diabetes as the first step marker which is combined with the presence of a genetic susceptibility marker (GM) as the second step marker. We apply hypothetical data which we, however, consider to be fairly representative for a country like England with well-established traditions in epidemiological and clinical diabetology [46, 52–54, 56].

First, we consider a population of unaffected children aged 0–14 years. For convenience, the population size will be fixed at 1 000 000 subjects whom we assume to follow as a cohort during a period of 5 years. The incidence of type 1 diabetes (ignoring marker status) may be set at 0.000 16 per person-year at risk, corresponding to an absolute cumulative disease risk of 0.08% over 5 years. Second, we assume that 1.0% of the subjects in this population have a positive FH; this is plausible considering the population

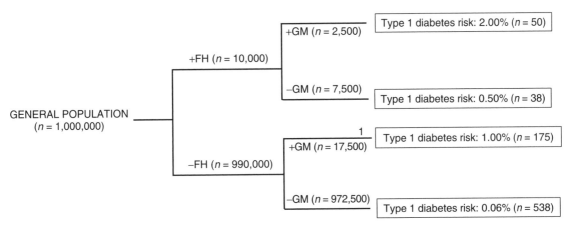

Figure 26.2 Distribution according to positive FH and presence of a GM in a population of 1 000 000 children. Assumptions: see text.

incidence level. A given GM has a population prevalence of 0.02 (2.0%), which is of the order of magnitude of the frequency of one of the currently defined genotypes conferring high risk of type 1 diabetes. However, within the FH-positive subjects the prevalence of GM is assumed to be 25% due to the prior probablity of sharing any given genotypes with a sibling. The presence of GM is assumed to confer an absolute risk of 1.0% over 5 years in FH-negative subjects; this agrees with estimated absolute risks at 5–10% over an extended period for unrelated subjects with a high-risk genetic marker of type 1 diabetes (as mentioned before). However, in FH-positive subjects, it is assumed that the disease risk over 5 years is 2% due to the effects of sharing additional risk factors with affected relatives. Under these

assumptions, the population distribution according to this dual marker system will be realized as shown in **Figure 26.2**. The absolute risks as obtained from assumptions and implications are also shown, together with the corresponding estimated number of new cases of type 1 diabetes over a period of 5 years.

The most important measures of test performance are presented in **Table 26.3**. The PPVs (and, thus, the marker-specific absolute risks of developing type 1 diabetes) are given by assumptions or implications in this example, but are realistic for the reasons given before. Their low level, even for the combined marker-positive category, indicates that the large majority of marker-positive subjects will remain disease free for a substantial period of

Table 26.3 PPV, SENS, SPEC and RR for markers in the prediction of type 1 diabetes (cf. Figure 26.2).[a]

Marker	PPV (%)	SENS (%)	SPEC (%)	RR (%)
Single markers				
FH alone	0.88[b]	10.94	99.01	12.16
GM alone	1.13[b]	28.13	98.02	19.17
Markers combined				
FH and GM	2.00[b]	6.25	99.75	36.47[c]

[a]FH: positive family history; GM: positive for genetic marker. Hypothetical data.
[b]Assumed values, expressed as estimated cumulative risk of type 1 diabetes over 5 years.
[c]Expressed relative to being negative for both markers.

time. Most importantly, this dual screening strategy, which in the first step is based on anamnestic information only, has allowed for the classification of more than 97% of the whole population as belonging to a very low-risk category. In spite of this, the estimated values of SENS in **Table 26.3** indicate that the majority of new cases of type 1 diabetes will not be predicted by these markers, whether applied as single markers or when combined.

It must be stressed that hypothetical examples like the one above are very sensitive to changes in the underlying assumptions, which, for the reasons mentioned above, most likely will differ from population to population. Until more precise population-based assessments of various strategies in the prediction of type 1 diabetes are available, different sets of assumptions should be explored in corresponding scenarios. The principles and methods illustrated above may be useful for such purposes. The methods may be further refined by stratification within a marker category, such as by distinguishing between subjects with low versus high ICA-titer.

26.7   CONCLUDING REMARKS

So far, there are no studies published of gene–environment interaction in type 1 diabetes. All currently available information considered together, there seems to be no doubt, though, that type 1 diabetes develops as the consequence of interaction(s) between genetic factors and nongenetic determinants, leading to an immune-mediated process of β-cell destruction which may be ongoing for several years before type 1 diabetes presents clinically. Many details of the etiological determinants remain to be established, particularly how genetic factors interact with nongenetic determinants in the activation of the immune system. Possibly, each of several distinct combinations of genetic markers may, when exposure to relevant environmental factors takes place, induce the disease process that represents the unique pathogenic feature of type 1 diabetes. Possibly, other factors (perhaps stress or infections) may accelerate the process to the precipitation of clinical disease. If so, this etiological heterogeneity implies severe difficulties in predicting the risk of developing type 1 diabetes in different subjects. As demonstrated above, our ability to predict risk

of developing type 1 diabetes is still limited, as available markers confer only a modest risk and most cases derive spontaneously without a known FH of the disease. To improve this situation, it is necessary to incorporate the influence of nongenetic etiological factors in the future methods of predicting type 1 diabetes, to develop strategies that apply to specific populations and to develop methods to study gene–environment interaction in type 1 diabetes.

References

1. Leslie, R.D.G., Lo, S.S.S., Hawa, M. and Tun, R.Y.M. (1992) Lessons on the etiology of insulin-dependent diabetes from twin studies, in *Epidemiology and Etiology of Insulin-Dependent Diabetes in the Young* (eds C. Levy-Marchal and P. Czernichow), Karger, Basel, pp. 91–106.
2. Hyttinen, V., Kaprio, J., Kinnunen, L. *et al.* (2003) Genetic liability of type 1 diabetes and the onset age among 22,650 young Finnish twin pairs: a nationwide follow-up study. *Diabetes*, **52** (4), 1052–5.
3. Kyvik, K.O., Green, A. and Beck-Nielsen, H. (1995) Concordance rates of insulin dependent diabetes mellitus: a population based study of young Danish twins. *British Medical Journal*, **311**, 913–17.
4. Degnbol, B. and Green, A. (1978) Diabetes mellitus among first and second degree relatives of early onset diabetics. *Annals of Human Genetics*, **42**, 25–47.
5. Tillil, H. and Köbberling, J. (1987) Age-corrected empirical genetic risk estimates for first-degree relatives of IDDM patients. *Diabetes*, **36**, 93–9.
6. Davies, J.L., Kawaguchi, Y., Bennett, S.T. *et al.* (1994) A genome-wide search for human type 1 diabetes susceptibility genes. *Nature*, **371**, 130–6.
7. Concannon, P., Erlich, H.A., Julier, C. *et al.* (2005) Type 1 diabetes: evidence for susceptibility loci from four genome-wide linkage scans in 1,435 multiplex families. *Diabetes*, **54**, 2995–3001.
8. Undlien, D.E., Lie, B.A. and Thorsby, E. (2001) HLA complex genes in type 1 diabetes and other autoimmune diseases. Which genes are involved? *Trends in Genetics*, **17**, 93–100.
9. Thorsby, E. and Rønningen, K.S. (1993) Particular HLA-DQ molecules play a dominant role in determining susceptibility or resistance to type 1 (insulin-dependent) diabetes mellitus. *Diabetologia*, **36**, 371–7.
10. Pugliese, A. and Miceli, D. (2002) The insulin gene in diabetes. *Diabetes/Metabolism Research and Reviews*, **18**, 13–25.

11. Barratt, B.J., Payne, F., Lowe, C.E. *et al.* (2004) Remapping the insulin gene/IDDM2 locus in type 1 diabetes. *Diabetes*, **53**, 1884–9.

12. Rich, S.S., Green, A., Morton, N.E. and Barbosa, J. (1987) A combined segregation and linkage analysis of insulin-dependent diabetes mellitus. *American Journal of Human Genetics*, **40**, 237–49.

13. Pascoe, L., Sherman, S., Wu, D. *et al.* (1989) Combined segregation and linkage analysis for IDDM and HLA-DR under several ascertainment assumptions. *Genetic Epidemiology*, **6**, 131–6.

14. Chakravarti, A. (1999) Population genetics–making sense out of sequence. Review. *Nature Genetics*, **21** (Suppl 1), 56–60.

15. Dahlquist, G., Blom, L., Tuvemo, T. *et al.* (1989) The Swedish Childhood Diabetes Study–results from a nine year case register and a one year case-referent study indicating that type 1 (insulin-dependent) diabetes mellitus is associated with both type 2 (non-insulin-dependent) diabetes mellitus and autoimmune disorders. *Diabetologia*, **32**, 2–6.

16. Wong, A.H., Gottesman, I.I. and Petronis, A. (2005) Phenotypic differences in genetically identical organisms: the epigenetic perspective. *Human Molecular Genetics*, **14** (Spec No. 1), R11–18.

17. Green, A., Gale, E.A.M. and Patterson, C.C. (1992) Incidence of childhood-onset insulin-dependent diabetes mellitus: the EURODIAB ACE study. *Lancet*, **339**, 905–9.

18. Karvonen, M., Viik-Kajander, M., Moltchanova, E. *et al.* (2000) Incidence of childhood type 1 diabetes worldwide. Diabetes Mondiale (DiaMond) Project Group. *Diabetes Care*, **23** (10), 1516–26.

19. Green, A. and Patterson, C.C. (2001) Trends in the incidence of childhood-onset diabetes in Europe 1989–1998. *Diabetologia*, **44**, (Suppl 3), B3–8.

20. Green, A. (1990) The role of genetic factors in the development of insulin-dependent diabetes mellitus, in *Current Topics in Microbiology and Immunology, vol. 164: Human Diabetes, Genetic, Environmental and Autoimmune Etiology*, (eds S. Bækkeskov and B. Hansen), Springer-Verlag, Berlin, pp. 3–16.

21. Patterson, C.C., Dahlquist, G., Soltész, G. and Green, A. (2001) Is childhood-onset type I diabetes a wealth-related disease? An ecological analysis of European incidence rates. *Diabetologia*, **44** (Suppl 3), B9–16.

22. Yoon, J-W., Pak, C.Y., Lee, M. and MacArthur, R.G. (1992) Is viral infection an initiating factor for insulin-dependent diabetes mellitus? in *Epidemiology and Etiology of Insulin-Dependent Diabetes in the Young* (eds C. Levy-Marchal and P. Czernichow), Karger, Basel, pp. 218–31.

23. Menser, M.S., Forrest, J.M. and Bransky, R.O. (1978) Rubella infection and diabetes mellitus. *Lancet*, **i**, 57–60.

24. Yoon, J.W. and Jun, H.S. (2004) Viruses in type 1 diabetes: brief review. *ILAR Journal*, **45** (3), 343–8.

25. Hyoty, H. and Taylor, K.W. (2002) The role of viruses in human diabetes. *Diabetologia*, **45** (10), 1353–61.

26. Honeyman, M. (2005) How robust is the evidence for viruses in the induction of type 1 diabetes? *Current Opinion in Immunology*, **17** (6), 616–23.

27. Filippi, C. and von Herrath, M. (2005) How can the innate immune system influence autoimmunity in type 1 diabetes and other autoimmune disorders? *Critical Reviews in Immunology*, **25** (3), 225–50.

28. Lammi, N., Karvonen, M. and Tuomilehto, J. (2005) Do microbes have a causal role in type 1 diabetes? *Medical Science Monitor*, **11** (3), RA63–9.

29. Elliott, R.B. and Martin, J.M. (1984) Dietary protein: a trigger of insulin-dependent diabetes in the BB rat? *Diabetologia*, **26**, 297–9.

30. Helgason, T. and Jonasson, M.R. (1981) Evidence for a food additive as a cause of ketosis-prone diabetes. *Lancet*, **ii**, 716–20.

31. Dahlquist, G., Blom, L.G., Persson, L.-Å. *et al.* (1989) Dietary factors and the risk of developing insulin dependent diabetes in childhood. *British Medical Journal*, **300**, 1302–6.

32. Dahlquist, G., Blom, L. and Lönnberg, G. (1991) The Swedish Childhood Diabetes Study–a multivariate analysis of risk determinants for diabetes in different age groups. *Diabetologia*, **34**, 757–62.

33. Virtanen, S.M., Jaakkola, L., Räsänen, L. *et al.* (1994) Nitrate and nitrite intake and the risk for type 1 diabetes in Finnish children. Childhood Diabetes in Finland Study Group. *Diabetic Medicine*, **11**, 656–62.

34. Borch-Johnsen, K., Joner, G., Mandrup-Poulsen, T. *et al.* (1984) Relation between breast-feeding and incidence rates of insulin-dependent diabetes. A hypothesis. *Lancet*, **ii**, 1083–6.

35. Dahlquist, G., Patterson, C. and Stoltesz, G. (1999) Perinatal risk factors for childhood type 1 diabetes in Europe: the EURODIAB substudy 2 study group. *Diabetes Care*, **22**, 1698–702.

36. Dahlquist, G.G., Pundziute-Lyckå, A. and Nyström, L. (2005) Birth weight and risk of type 1 diabetes in children and young adults: a population-based register study. *Diabetologia*, **48**, 1114–17.

37. Stene, L.C., Magnus, P., Lie, R.T. *et al.* (2001) Birth weight and childhood onset type 1 diabetes: population based cohort study. *British Medical Journal*, **322**, 889–92.

38. Kyvik, K.O., Bache, I., Green, A. *et al.* (2000) No association between birth weight and type 1 diabetes mellitus–a twin-control study. *Diabetic Medicine*, **17**, 158–62.

39. Dunger, D.B., Ong, K.K., Huxtable, S.J. *et al.* (1998) Association of the INS VNTR with size at birth. ALSPAC Study Team. Avon Longitudinal Study of Pregnancy and Childhood. *Nature Genetics*, **19**, 98–100.

40. Ong, K.K., Petry, C.J., Barratt, B.J. *et al.* (2004) Maternal–fetal interactions and birth order influence insulin variable number of tandem repeats allele class associations with head size at birth and childhood weight gain. *Diabetes*, **53**, 1128–33.

41. Stene, L.C., Magnus, P., Rønningen, K.S. and Joner, G. (2001) Diabetes-associated HLA-DQ genes and birth weight. *Diabetes*, **50**, 2879–82.

42. Larsson, H.E., Lynch, K., Lernmark, B. *et al.* (2005) Diabetes-associated HLA genotypes affect birth weight in the general population. *Diabetologia*, **48**, 1484–91.

43. Robinson, N. and Fuller, J.H. (1985) Role of life events and difficulties in the onset of diabetes mellitus. *Journal of Psychosomatic Research*, **29**, 583–91.

44. Siemiatycki, J., Colle, E., Campbell, S. *et al.* (1989) Case-control study of IDDM. *Diabetes Care*, **12**, 209–16.

45. Hägglöf, B., Blom, L., Dahlquist, G. *et al.* (1991) The Swedish childhood diabetes study: indications of severe psychological stress as a risk factor for type 1 (insulin-dependent) diabetes mellitus in childhood. *Diabetologia*, **34**, 579–83.

46. Sepa, A., Frodi, A. and Ludvigsson, J. (2005) Mothers' experiences of serious life events increase the risk of diabetes-related autoimmunity in their children. *Diabetes Care*, **28** (10), 2394–9.

47. Sepa, A., Wahlberg, J., Vaarala, O. *et al.* (2005) Psychological stress may induce diabetes-related autoimmunity in infancy. *Diabetes Care*, **28** (2), 290–5.

48. Christau, B., Kromann, H., Andersen, O.O. *et al.* (1977) Incidence, seasonal and geographic patterns of juvenile-onset insulin-dependent diabetes mellitus in Denmark. *Diabetologia*, **13**, 281–4.

49. Siemiatycki, J., Colle, E., Campbell, S. *et al.* (1988) Incidence of IDDM in Montreal by ethnic group and by social class and comparisons with ethnic groups living elsewhere. *Diabetes*, **37**, 1096–102.

50. Kaila, B., Dean, H.J., Schroeder, M. and Taback, S.P. (2003) HLA, day care attendance, and socio-economic status in young patients with type 1 diabetes. *Diabetic Medicine*, **20** (9), 777–9.

51. Blom, L., Dahlquist, G., Nyström, L. *et al.* (1989) The Swedish childhood diabetes study–social and perinatal determinants for diabetes in childhood. *Diabetologia*, **32**, 7–13.

52. Bottazzo, G.F., Florin-Christensen, A. and Doniach, D. (1974) Islet-cell antibodies in diabetes mellitus with polyendocrine disease. *Lancet*, **ii**, 1279–83.

53. Karjalainen, J.K. (1990) Islet cell antibodies as predictive markers for IDDM in children with high background incidence of disease. *Diabetes*, **39**, 1140–50.

54. Greenbaum, C.J. and Palmer, J.P. (1991) Insulin antibodies and insulin autoantibodies. *Diabetic Medicine*, **8**, 97–105.

55. Rowley, M.J., MacKay, I.R., Chen, Q.-Y. *et al.* (1992) Antibodies to glutamic acid decarboxylase discrimate major types of diabetes mellitus. *Diabetes*, **41**, 548–51.

56. Clare-Salzler, M.J., Tobin, A.J. and Kaufman, D.L. (1992) Glutamate decarboxylase: an autoantigen in IDDM. *Diabetes Care*, **15**, 132–5.

57. Franke, B., Galloway, T.S. and Wilkin, T.J. (2005) Developments in the prediction of type 1 diabetes mellitus, with special reference to insulin autoantibodies. *Diabetes/Metabolism Research and Reviews*, **21** (5), 395–415.

58. Schmidt, K.D., Valeri, C. and Leslie, R.D. (2005) Autoantibodies in type 1 diabetes. *Clinica Chimica Acta*, **354** (1–2), 35–40.

59. Bingley, P.J., Christie, M.R., Bonifacio, E. *et al.* (1994) Combined analysis of autoantibodies improves prediction of IDDM in islet cell antibody-positive relatives. *Diabetes*, **43**, 1304–10.

60. Bingley, P.J., Bonifacio, E. and Gale, E.A.M. (1993) Can we really predict IDDM? *Diabetes*, **42**, 213–20.

61. Achenbach, P. and Ziegler, A.G. (2005) Diabetes-related antibodies in euglycemic subjects. *Best Practice and Research. Clinical Endocrinology and Metabolism*, **19** (1), 101–17.

62. Vardi, P., Crisa, L. and Jackson, R.A. (1991) Predictive value of intravenous glucose tolerance test insulin secretion less than or greater than the first percentile in islet cell antibody positive relatives of type 1 (insulin-dependent) diabetic patients. *Diabetologia*, **34** (2), 93–102.

63. Keskinen, P., Korhonen, S., Kupila, A. *et al.* (2002) First-phase insulin response in young healthy children at genetic and immunological risk for type I diabetes. *Diabetologia*, **45** (12), 1639–48.

Recent Trends in Screening and Prevention of Type 1 Diabetes

Marian Rewers

Barbara Davis Center for Childhood Diabetes, University of Colorado School of Medicine, Aurora, CO, USA

27.1 INTRODUCTION

In the traditional view, acute onset of type 1 diabetes (T1D) renders screening unnecessary. However, recent studies have demonstrated a long preclinical period T1D that offers opportunities for screening and prevention (**Figure 27.1**). In most patients, diagnosis of T1D is preceded by several years of asymptomatic islet autoimmunity, marked by the presence of autoantibodies to pancreatic β-cell antigens, such as insulin, glutamic acid decarboxylase (GAD$_{65}$), IA-2 or ZnT8 [1–8].

Since islet autoimmunity develops predominantly in young children who carry high-risk HLA-DR, DQ genotypes, primary prevention trials are attempting modification of environmental exposures in infants identified as at risk by genetic screening. Recent examples include trials of elimination of cow's milk (Trial to Reduce Insulin-dependent Diabetes Mellitus in the Genetically at Risk (TRIGR)) [9], supplementation of diet with omega-3 fatty acids, Nutritional Intervention to Prevent Type 1 Diabetes (NIP)) [10], or immunomodulation with human oral insulin (Pre-POINT) [11]. While these approaches may eventually succeed, the design of primary prevention trials is hampered by a lack of convincing evidence about which environmental factor(s) initiates islet autoimmunity. A number of environmental exposures have been proposed, including exposures during pregnancy, infancy and later in life (for review, please see Chapter 24 by Stene *et al.*). The National Institutes of Health have established an international consortium The Environmental Determinants of Type 1 Diabetes in the Young (TEDDY) to evaluate the leading environmental candidate agents [12]. While significant β-cell damage present in persons with islet autoimmunity suggests that earlier interventions could be more effective, islet autoantibody-positive persons are ideal target for secondary prevention. Large randomized trials, such as the Diabetes Prevention Trial 1 (DPT-1), the European Nicotinamide Diabetes Intervention Trial (ENDIT) and the Diabetes Prediction and Prevention Project (DIPP) have attempted to prevent progression from islet autoimmunity to T1D [13–15]. These trails have not been successful, so far, but have shown [16, 17] similar to cohort studies [18] that a variable period of mild asymptomatic hyperglycemia precedes by months or years overt insulin dependence among persons with islet autoantibodies. While none of the available screening tests (random blood glucose, HbA$_{1c}$ or oral glucose tolerance test (OGTT)) is perfect, our ability to detect this prediabetic phase and implement early treatment may have important implications for preservation of endogenous insulin secretion and prevention of acute and long-term complications of the disease [19–21]. While screening for pre-T1D and prevention is currently the realm of research studies, our greatly improved understanding of the natural history of T1D holds promise for preventing T1D in high-risk-groups, for instance relatives of T1D patients, in the near future. After diagnosis of diabetes, preservation of residual insulin secretion and

The Epidemiology of Diabetes Mellitus, second edition Edited by Jean-Marie Ekoé, Marian Rewers, Rhys Williams and Paul Zimmet

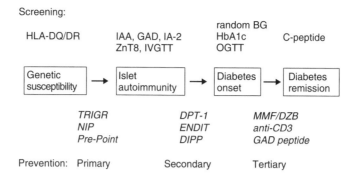

Figure 27.1 Opportunities for T1D screening and prevention.

induction of lasting remission, measured by the plasma levels of C-peptide, continues to attract interest of the research community. Recent tertiary prevention trials have used immunomodulatory agents (e.g. mycophenolate mofetil (MMF)/daclizumab (DZB), anti-CD3 antibody or GAD_{65} peptide).

27.2   RISK PREDICTION

The risk of T1D can be estimated by taking into the account factors summarized below.

27.2.1   The Family History of T1D

Monozygotic twins are 30–50% concordant for T1D, suggesting that both genetic and environmental factors strongly contribute to the pathogenesis of T1D. Among the first-degree relatives (FDRs), siblings are at a higher risk (5–10% risk by age 20 years) than offspring; offspring of diabetic fathers are at a higher risk (~12%) than offspring of diabetic mothers (~6%) [22–24]. In addition, persons sharing both human leukocyte antigen (HLA) haplotypes with a diabetic sibling are at a higher risk than those sharing one or none [25].

27.2.2   The Susceptibility Genotypes

The strongest genetic associations for T1D are with the *HLA* genes. Approximately 95% of the patients, compared with 50% of the general population, have either the HLA-DRB1*03 or DRB1*04, DQB1*0302 alleles and 30–53% of the patients, compared with 2.4% of the general population, have the DRB1*03/*04, DQB1*0302 genotype [1]. While this genotype confers extremely high risk, there is a wide and continuous spectrum of risk

associated with HLA-DR, DQ genotypes—from elevated, to neutral and protective. For instance, the HLA-DQA1*0102 DQB1*0602 haplotype confers dominant protection from T1D, even in the presence of islet autoantibodies [26].

The HLA-DRB1*04 subtypes influence the risk; for example, DRB1*0403 or *0406 decrease risk even on the haplotypes containing DQB1*0302 [27]. Lack of the aspartic acid at position 57 of the DQB1 chain (the Asp-negative status) is associated with high risk [28]. In Finland, Asp-negativity was found in 75% of patients with T1D, compared with 18% of controls, but for the most part this simply reflects the presence of the highest risk HLA-DQ alleles DQB1*0201 and DQB1*0302 [29]. It is important to realize that some high-risk alleles, such as the DQB1*0401, are Asp-positive, so typing for full DQB1 allele sequences is important.

HLA typing has predictive value independent of family history: 4% of siblings with either HLA-DR3 or DR4 develop T1D, compared with 10% of siblings HLA identical with the probands, and 16% of siblings with the HLA-DR3/DR4 genotype [30].

For screening purposes, a compromise has to be made between sensitivity (i.e. the proportion of future T1D cases that carry certain genotypes) and the population frequencies of these genotypes or the number of subjects that would require follow-up for islet autoantibodies and T1D. The Diabetes Autoimmunity Study in the Young (DAISY) selected the six highest-risk genotypes summarized in **Table 27.1** for research screening of the general population newborns.

In combination, these six genotypes are present in 10% of Colorado non-Hispanic White children and account for about 60% of T1D cases in this

Table 27.1 The population frequencies of the HLA genotypes associated with T1D susceptibility in non-Hispanic Whites and Hispanics (DAISY).[a]

HLA-DR,DQB1	Non-Hispanic Whites			Hispanics		
	T1D patients (%) N = 999	Population controls (%) N = 1661	OR (95% CI)	T1DM patients (%) N = 124	Population controls (%) N = 1032	OR (95% CI)
High risk						
3/4,*0302	31.7	2.5	17.9 (12.3–25)	31.5	2.8	15.9 (9.4–27)
Moderate risk						
4/4,*0302	10.2	3.0	3.7 (2.6–5.2)	15.3	4.1	4.3 (2.4–7.6)
1/4,*0302	7.2	2.2	3.4 (2.3–5.1)	6.5	3.1	2.2 (1.0–4.8)
8/4,*0302	1.9	0.9	2.1 (1.1–4.2)	4.8	2.9	1.7 (0.7–4.2)
9/4,*0302	1.0	0.1	8.4 (1.8–38)	0.8	0.6	1.4 (0.2–11)
3/3	8.4	1.9	4.8 (3.2–7.3)	3.2	0.3	11.4 (2.5–52)
All above						
	60.4	10.6	PPV = 1.7%	62.1	13.8	PPV = 0.9%
All other low/average risk						
	39.6	89.4		37.9	86.2	

[a]Modified from [31]. OR: odds ratio; PPV: positive predictive value.

population or 2 cases per 1000 general population children, by the age for 20 years. A screening program based on these six genotypes would require one to follow 100 out of each 1000 children, with only two of those children developing T1D and 98 not. The positive predictive value (PPV) of such a screening would be only 2% (1.7% exact value from data in **Table 27.1**).The PPV would be even lower (0.9%) in Hispanics–a population with lower prevalence of T1D and higher frequency of the six HLA risk genotypes. For this reason, genetic screening of the general population for T1D is currently limited to research projects.

On the other hand, in populations with higher prevalence of T1D (e.g. siblings of T1D patients) the predictive value of genetic screening increases, according to Bayes' theorem. The six high-risk HLA genotypes are present in 33% of siblings in Colorado and account for about 80% of T1D cases in this population or 4 cases per 100 by the age of 20 years [23]. The PPV of the screening would be 12%—perhaps high enough to justify screening with intent to enroll into a primary prevention trial. The PPV would increase to 50–80% if HLA-DR3/4 siblings or children sharing two haplotypes with a diabetic sibling were selected [25].

However, over 90% of T1Ds have no affected relative; so, to have a major impact, preventive efforts will require inclusion of the general population. Genetic screening will have to be followed up using islet autoantibodies or other markers, as described in the next section.

A number of non-HLA susceptibility gene markers have been confirmed [32–36] (for details, see Chapter 26byKyvik and Green). At present, polymorphisms of the insulin gene, PTPN22, CTLA-4 and IL2RA appear to contribute most to diabetes risk; however, there is little evidence that adding these genetic markers to HLA Class II genotyping can increase specificity or PPV of the general population screening. It is important, however, to include these markers into the prevention trial protocols to make sure that randomization is balanced with respect to relevant genetic markers.

27.2.3 The Islet Autoantibodies

Early studies of the prediction of T1D utilized islet cell autoantibody (ICA) assays based on indirect immunofluorescence. High-titer ICAs usually reflects the presence of multiple islet autoantibodies (GAD65, IA-2) and predicts progression to diabetes [37]. However, ICA assays were hard to standardize and were replaced by radioimmunoassays for autoantibodies to specific islet autoantigens that are now the mainstay of screening for pre-T1D [37, 38]. These include insulin autoantibodies insulin autoantibody (IAAs) [39], GAD [40], IA-2 [41] and most recently ZnT8 [42]. The presence of two or more of these autoantibodies, especially on multiple tests over time, is the best predictor of T1D risk currently available [43]. These radioassays are typically performed in 96-well filtration plates and are also commercially available. A high-throughput laboratory can perform each assay for less than $20 per sample, making large-scale screening feasible. However, after many rounds of proficiency workshops, standardization of these assays is still work in progress. The Diabetes Autoantibody Standardization Program (DASP) conducted workshop evaluations of key international diabetes laboratories in 2000, 2002, 2003, 2005 and 2007. DASP has validated ongoing improvement of radiobinding and enzyme-linked immunosorbent assay (ELISA) technologies for measuring autoantibodies [44, 45]. The Autoantibody Harmonization Group supported by the National Institute of Diabetes and Digestive and Kidney Diseases (NIDDK) has created reference sera from T1D patients and people with prediabetes that are available to ensure comparability of assays and expression of autoantibody levels in standard units, rather than laboratory-specific indices.

27.2.3.1   Screening among FDRs

The initial large screening studies found approximately 3% of the FDRs to be positive for ICAs [46, 47], with siblings more often being positive than parents and ICAs more frequent among younger relatives. The presence of IAAs was found to be an independent risk factor for T1D [48, 49]. The main limitation of ICA screening was that one-third of the relatives progressing to diabetes were ICA negative on the first test and, of these, 62% remained ICA negative at the onset of diabetes. As expected, with increasing ICA levels the PPV for future diabetes rose and the sensitivity fell. Later, multiple studies showed that the presence of ICAs in the absence of GAD65 or IA-2 autoantibodies does not predict diabetes [43, 50–52]. For instance, the cumulative 15-year risk of developing diabetes was 2.8% for

persons with ICAs without GAD or IA-2 autoantibodies versus 66% for those with ICAs and either or both of GAD or IA-2 autoantibodies [53].

The DAISY has demonstrated that the incidence of islet autoimmunity is much higher in FDRs (**Figure 27.2**) than inthe general population (**Figure 27.3**). The incidence is particularly high in the HLA-DR3/4, DQB1*0302 positive siblings (43%) and offspring (34%) and moderate-risk siblings (19%) (for risk definitions, see **Table 27.1**). The HLA genotype and having a diabetic relative, but not gender or ethnicity, predicted development of islet autoimmunity in proportional hazard analyses. Among children with the HLA-DR3/4,DQB1*0302 genotype, those with a diabetic relative had 10 times higher risk of islet autoimmunity (95% confidence interval (CI) 3.6–28) than those without; the hazard ratio was higher in siblings (16-fold) than in offspring (fivefold). In contrast, among children with other HLA genotypes, having a diabetic relative increased the risk only 1.5-fold.

Islet autoantibodies appear early in life. The BABYDIAB study and DAISY have demonstrated that a significant proportion of FDRs progressing to T1D developed islet autoantibodies before their second birthday, with IAAs usually being the first autoantibodies detected [5, 54, 55]. While islet autoantibodies are often found in cord blood samples from FDRs, they are nearly always transferred transplacentally from a diabetic or prediabetics mother [56, 57] and are not predictive of future diabetes. Transplacental insulin antibodies are usually of the IgG4 isotype; in contrast, IAAs are usually IgG1 [58]. A rising level of autoantibodies in an infant is almost always associated with spontaneous autoantibodies.

Once the persistent islet autoantibodies are present, the risk of progression to diabetes does not differ between FDRs and children from the general population. The cumulative 5-year risk of developing diabetes was 68% for relatives positive for two or more of islet autoantibodies [43].

27.2.3.2   Screening in the General Population Children

While most of the islet autoantibody screening studies included only FDRs, 90% of T1D cases occur in person with no family history of T1D. There have been a number of cross-sectional studies

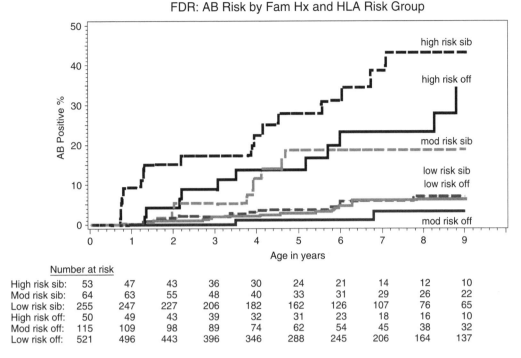

FDR: AB Risk by Fam Hx and HLA Risk Group

Number at risk									
High risk sib:	53	47	43	36	30	24	21	14	12	10
Mod risk sib:	64	63	55	48	40	33	31	29	26	22
Low risk sib:	255	247	227	206	182	162	126	107	76	65
High risk off:	50	49	43	39	32	31	23	18	16	10
Mod risk off:	115	109	98	89	74	62	54	45	38	32
Low risk off:	521	496	443	396	346	288	245	206	164	137

Figure 27.2 Cumulative incidence of islet autoimmunity in the first-degree relatives, by HLA-DR,DQ genotypes. DAISY 1994–2005.

that screened for islet autoantibodies in large groups of general population children of school age. Early surveys used ICAs and reported prevalence of ICAs among schoolchildren between 0.4% in Japan and 4.1% in Finland [59–69], with the prevalence of ICA generally in parallel with the incidence of T1D in the population.

It was noted that ICA was only two to three times more prevalent in siblings of diabetic probands than in the general population, compared with a 13 times greater risk of diabetes in the siblings [60]. In an analysis combining cross-sectional data from schoolchildren screened for islet autoantibodies and unrelated children diagnosed with T1D in the same population, the estimated risks of progression to diabetes within 10 years were 6.7% for ICAs, 6.6% for GAD autoantibody (GADA), 5.6% for IA-2 autoantibody (IA-2A), and 4.8% for IAA levels above the 97.5th centile, increasing to 20%, 23%, 24% and 11% respectively for antibody levels >99.5th centile. Having two or more autoantibodies above the 97.5th centile (0.7% of schoolchildren) conferred a 27% 10-year estimated risk of T1D. Such simulation analyses, while helpful, had to be

confirmed in prospective studies. It became obvious that a single 'snapshot' screening for autoantibodies will not be sufficient to refine the predictive values of genetic and autoantibody screening and optimize the methods for preventive trials. DAISY [1, 55], DIPP [8, 70] and most recently the TEDDY Study [12] have provided opportunities to fill important gaps in our understanding of the natural history of T1D by studying, with serial measurements from birth, high-risk general population children identified by newborn screening. While the risk of developing islet autoantibodies is three to five times higher in relatives than in the general population with the same HLA-DR/DQ genotypes, the persistent presence of islet autoantibodies portends similar high risk of progression to diabetes for both relatives and the general population. Higher titer and higher affinity of the autoantibodies, as well as a broader immune response (autoantibodies to multiple autoantigens), predict higher risk of diabetes. As summarized in **Figure 27.3**, in the DAISY population, the incidence of persistent islet autoantibodies by the age of 9 years was 10.6%, 5.5% and 3.4% respectively in high-,

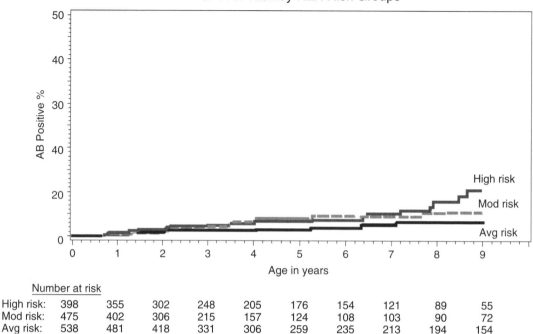

GP: AB Risk by HLA Risk Groups

Number at risk									
High risk:	398	355	302	248	205	176	154	121	89	55
Mod risk:	475	402	306	215	157	124	108	103	90	72
Avg risk:	538	481	418	331	306	259	235	213	194	154

Figure 27.3 Cumulative incidence of islet autoimmunity in the general population, by HLA-DR,DQ genotypes. DAISY 1994–2005.

moderate- and average-risk groups (defined in **Table 27.1**). Interestingly, the seroconversion to autoantibodies appears to continue unabated beyond early childhood and, in the high-risk group, apparently picks up after age 7 years. By back-calculating the incidence rates to the overall screened population, we estimated that 1.2% of Denver general population children develop islet autoantibodies by 6 years of age.

27.2.3.3 Measurement of Islet Autoantibodies in Patients with Adult-onset Diabetes

It has been estimated that at least 37% of T1D is diagnosed after the age of 19 years and 15% after the age of 30 years [71]. Islet autoantibodies and T1D can develop at any age [72], but in older persons the progression to diabetes is less rapid and C-peptide levels at diagnosis are higher than those in children [73], suggesting a slower rate of β-cell destruction. However, C-peptide levels in islet-autoantibody-positive adult diabetic patients are still significantly lower than in those with type 2 diabetes [74]. The GAD autoantibodies

have proved to be helpful in identifying latent autoimmune diabetes in adults (LADA); that is, T1D masquerading as type 2 diabetes [75]. Among adults diagnosed with type 2 diabetes and participating in the UKPDS, the proportion of patients with ICAs and GADA decreased with increasing age at diagnosis: from 21% in patients aged 25–34 years to 4% in those aged 55–65 years for ICA and from 34% to 7% for GADA [76]. The presence of GADA increased fivefold the risk of requiring insulin therapy within 6 years (PPV 33%). IA-2A was present in 2.2% of the patients, and further increased the risk of insulin dependency [77]. Between 5 and 10% of patients with gestational diabetes have islet autoantibodies and the great majority progress to T1D [78].

In summary, the presence of two or more of the islet autoantibodies indicates a high risk of progression to T1D. The risk exceeds 50% in 5 years even without the additional information provided by genetic or metabolic testing. However, metabolic tests described below may help to determine the rate of progression to diabetes.

27.2.4   Estimation of the β-cell Function and Mass

Direct measurement of the functional mass of islet cells is currently not possible; however, the first-phase insulin response (FPIR) to intravenous glucose predicts, to some extent, progression to diabetes among islet-autoantibody-positive persons [79–84]. The FPIR is the sum of the 1- and 3-min insulin levels measured after glucose is administered i.v. at 0.5 g per kilogram body weight, infused as a 20–25% solution over 2–4 min. Low FPIR has been defined as below the first or fifth percentile of the distribution in nonobese healthy subjects. The FPIR is severely depressed at the time of detection of islet autoantibodies in many young children [83]. In a study of FDRs with high-titer ICAs, those with FPIR below the first percentile on the first test had a 3-year diabetes-free survival of 13% (95% CI 0–30%) compared with 78% (95% CI 63–93%) in those with higher FPIR [85]. In the DPT-1, loss of the FPIR was strongly associated with diabetes [82]; however, a significant proportion of prediabetic individuals had normal FPIR within 1 year of diabetes. The average time from the fall of FPIR below the first percentile to the onset of diabetes was 1.8 years.

The interpretation of serial FPIR data is complicated by significant within-subject variability. The test needs to be performed with consistency and utmost accuracy in timing [86]. It should be performed after an overnight fast of uniform duration. The results are age dependent, particularly in prepubertal versus pubertal children [87, 88]. The results vary with insulin sensitivity according to age, physical fitness, body mass index (BMI), pubertal status and physical or psychological stress [87–91]. Different protocols for the intravenous glucose tolerance test (IVGTT) give different results [92], and the studies used different control groups to define the cutoffs. Several centers have performed duplicate IVGTTs, spaced weeks apart, on healthy volunteers. The reported group median within-subject coefficients of variation varied from 4 to 36% [87, 93, 94] but were as high as 56% for some subjects. Calculating the area under the curve for insulin release and adjustments for insulin sensitivity may improve reproducibility, compared with a sum of the 1- and 3-min insulin levels [87, 88, 93, 94]. Retrograde venous cannulation and arterialization of the samples drawn increased reproducibility

in some studies [93], but not in other studies [95, 96]. Placement of the intravenous line 1 h before the test to minimize the effects of stress hormones was reported to improve reproducibility. However, most subjects had a significant 'first test effect' with a higher FPIR on the second test [87]. Despite these limitations, the FPIR test is of value in predicting time to insulin dependence in persons who are islet autoantibody positive, and a standard protocol has been developed to allow comparisons [86].

The OGTT, performed in clinical trials of T1D prevention largely to formalize the diagnosis of clinical diabetes, has long been known to have some value in predicting progression to T1D among subjects with islet autoantibodies [16, 17]. However, a recent analysis of the DPT-1 data concluded rather unexpectedly that a risk score based on BMI, age, fasting C-peptide and post-challenge glucose and C-peptide from a 2 h OGTT predicted T1D as well as a risk score including, in addition, FPIR. The change in the risk score from baseline to 1 year was in itself also highly predictive of T1D. In light of that finding, the interest in performing the cumbersome IVGTT may wane.

In 1993, preliminary data from the Washington State Diabetes Prediction Study suggested that HbA_{1c} measured by high-performance liquid chromatography may be slightly but significantly higher in nondiabetic ICA-positive teenagers than in ICA-negative controls [97]. Recently, the DAISY has demonstrated that HbA_{1c} steadily increases within the normal range over a few years and may be useful in early detection of T1D [18]. Among 92 children who have developed persistent islet autoantibodies, HbA_{1c} measured using a point-of-care DCA2000 system predicted development of T1D, (hazard ratio 4.8, 95% CI 3.0–7.7, for each 0.4% (standard deviation (SD)) increase of HbA_{1c}) independent of random glucose and number of autoantibodies. Increase in random plasma glucose levels only marginally predicted the progression (hazard ratio 1.4, 95% CI 1.0–1.8, per SD of 1.1 mmol l^{-1}).

In addition to the FPIR, a measure of β-cell function, assessment of β-cell mass might also provide useful information. Approaches to β-cell mass assessment include nuclear magnetic resonance imaging (MRI) and isotopic scans. For years, MRI has been used to detect pancreatic graft rejection [98–100]. With refinements in MRI techniques it may be possible in the near future to detect insulitis and to approximate the β-cell mass [101, 102]. Pancreatic scintigraphy with ^{99m}Tc-interleukin-2 can identify pancreatic inflammation at diagnosis of T1D. In a series of 42 patients, significant pancreatic accumulation of ^{99m}Tc-interleukin-2 was found in 31% of the patients at the time of diagnosis. Interestingly, positive patients showed higher C-peptide values at 3 months and lower insulin requirement at 1 year, compared with negative patients. After 1 year, all the positive patients showed a significant decrease in pancreatic uptake of ^{99m}Tc-interleukin-2 [103].

In summary, despite its cumbersome nature, the FPIR test is of value in predicting time to insulin dependence in persons who are islet autoantibody positive. Among relatives with two or more antibodies, those with an FPIR less than the first percentile have a 50% risk of diabetes within 1 year; those with higher FPIR have a 50% risk within 3 years [43]. Newer and simpler methods are needed to enhance our ability to monitor β-cell function and mass longitudinally, as an intermediate endpoint in follow-up and intervention studies.

27.3 PREVENTION

It is not easy to prevent disease of unknown etiology, such as T1D. While a lot has been learned concerning the immunological mechanisms of islet autoimmunity, it is not known what triggers the destruction of β-cells and where the point of no return is. While hundreds of preventive modalities have succeeded in animal models of T1D [104], prevention of human T1D remains elusive as of late 2007. The attempts to prevent T1D have included:

- Antigen-specific 'vaccination' using islet autoantigens; for example, intact insulin, altered insulin or proinsulin peptides, GAD65 or heat shock protein HSP60 peptide. The goal is to induce autoantigen-specific tolerance by induction of regulatory T-cells that down-regulate immunity to a specific autoantigen as well as promote tolerance to additional autoantigens [105].
- Nonantigen-specific systemic immune modulation that ranges from mild modulation with oral nicotinamide or bacille Calmette–Guerin (BCG) vaccination to heavy immunosupression (reviewed in [105]).

- Avoidance of candidate environmental triggers of islet autoimmunity such as cow's milk [9] or gluten [106]. Celiac disease and rheumatic fever provide encouraging examples of autoimmune diseases that can be prevented this way. Alternatively, diet is supplemented with nutrients whose deficiency presumably triggers or promotes islet autoimmunity; for example, omega-3 fatty acids [10, 107] or vitamin D [108, 109].
- Metabolic modifications, such as weight loss and maintenance or increased physical activity [110], to neutralize the powerful effect of insulin resistance on progression to T1D [111, 112] and meticulous blood glucose control after diabetes onset [110, 113].
- Stimulation of β-cell regeneration in conjunction with suppression of apoptosis that is increased in islet autoimmunity [114] to overcome the relapsing-remitting course of prediabetes [115]. This new area of research has so far included GLP-1 and gastrin analogues alone or in combination with immunosupression [116, 117]

In addition to finding the specific cause(s) of T1D, multiple logistic issues remain; for example, the anticipated duration, toxicity and complexity of the prophylaxis. Unless tolerance can be established or restored permanently in a limited time period, intervention may need to be life-long, like a gluten free diet or penicillin prophylaxis for rheumatic fever. It is currently impossible to compare the cost/benefit ratio of such efforts with established and emerging insulin treatment regimens that, while not easy or complication free, have led to a dramatic improvement of mortality and morbidity associated with T1D over the past 20–30 years [118–120].

27.3.1 Primary Prevention of Islet Autoimmunity

As reviewed above, current technology to ascertain people at high risk of T1D before they develop islet autoantibodies is based on genetic screening for susceptible HLA-DR, DQ genotypes. Such screening of the general population is hampered by low specificity of these genotypes. However, the specificity is much higher in populations with higher *a priori* risk of T1D; that is, first-degree relatives, especially siblings.

TRIGR is currently the best example of a primary prevention trial. This international, randomized, double-blinded trial is evaluating the effect of hydrolyzed infant formula compared with cow's milk-based formula in decreasing the risk of islet autoimmunity and diabetes in infant relatives with increased genetic susceptibility [9]. The TRIGR trial will determine whether delayed exposure to intact food proteins will reduce the chances of developing T1D later in life. Eligible to participate are newborns who have first-degree relatives with T1D and one of the HLA genotypes listed below:

(a)   DQB1*0302/DQA1*05-DQB1*02;
(b)   DQB1*0302/x (x not DQB1*02, DQB1* 0301, or DQB1*0602);
(c)   DQA1*05-DQB1*02/y (y not DQA1*0201-DQB1*02, DQB1*0301, DQB1*0602, or DQB1*0603);
(d)   DQA1*03-DQB1*02/y (y not DQA1*0201-DQB1*02, DQB1*0301, DQB1*0602, or DQB1*0603).

All babies in the study receive the recommendation to breast-feed for at least the first 6 months of life. If a mother is unable to breast-feed exclusively before the baby is 8 months of age, her child will be randomly assigned to one of two groups. One group of these babies will receive breast-feeding supplements of a trial formula based on extensively hydrolyzed protein; the other group will receive a special trial formula containing a smaller amount of hydrolyzed protein. In hydrolyzed protein, the big protein molecules have been split into very small fragments to provide a source of nutritional amino acids, but the fragments are likely too small to stimulate the immune system. The recruitment of 2160 children from 77 centers in 15 countries for the trial was completed at the end of 2006. The main endpoint of the trial is development of diabetes by the age of 10 years.

The Nutritional Intervention to Prevent Type 1 Diabetes Study, or NIP Pilot Study, is part of the Type 1 Diabetes TrialNet [107]. This pilot, to include 90 infant FDRs with high-risk HLA-DR, DQ genotypes, is not powered to test the hypothesis formally, but rather to pilot the feasibility of a definitive trial of dietary supplementation with docosahexaenoic acid (DHA) before 6 months of age or even before birth. As of January 2008, nine NIP clinical centers have enrolled 60 infants.

The Pre-POINT trial will determine the feasibility of performing a primary autoantigen vaccination trial in high-risk children and will determine the dose and route of insulin administration that is safe and is bioavailable to the immune system [11]. The study will give oral or intranasal insulin to high-risk FDRs who have not yet developed islet autoantibodies in order to provide protection before islet autoimmunity starts. Eligible are children who have multiple first-degree relatives with T1D or those who have the HLA-DR3/DR4-DQ8 genotype inherited identical by descent with a sibling proband; such siblings have a T1D risk as high as 80% [25]. This multicenter, placebo-controlled, double-blinded trial will enroll up to 40 children randomized to increasing doses of oral insulin (2.5, 7.5, 22.5 or 67.5 mg per day) or intranasal insulin (0.28, 0.84, 2.5, 7.5 mg per day) to determine a dose and route that is safe and bioavailable to the immune system. Children will be monitored for the development of islet autoantibodies, diabetes and protective immune responses to insulin. Depending upon the outcome of Pre-POINT, the study will continue to the phase II POINT study, which will determine the efficacy of mucosal insulin administration in autoantibody-negative high-risk children.

27.3.2 Secondary Prevention of Clinical Diabetes

Approximately 1 in 20 first-degree relatives and one in 300 of the general population has multiple islet autoantibodies; that is, one million individuals in the United States alone are currently at a high risk of developing T1D. An intervention allowing the maintenance of insulin production and a life free of insulin treatment in a large proportion of these subjects would be a major public health achievement. However, identifying these high-risk subjects is expensive (according to the DPT-1 experience, $\sim$\$1200 per subject), and four large prevention trials targeting this population have found no effect on the rate of progression to clinical T1D of insulin administered parenterally [13], orally [15], or intranasally [121] as well as oral nicotinamide [14]. Smaller studies have evaluated other agents, also with little success.

The ENDIT screened nearly 30 000 relatives for ICAs and randomized 552 to placebo oral modified release nicotinamide (1.2 g m^{-2}). There was no decrease in diabetes incidence in the nicotinamide versus placebo group over 5 years of follow-up [14]. Subgroup analysis by age, gender, oral glucose tolerance status and FPIR was unable to identify a subgroup that responded to therapy.

The DPT-1, designed in the early 1990s, has screened more than 100 000 relatives of patients with T1D in the United States and Canada. Approximately 4% of the screened subjects were ICA positive. One-half of the ICA-positive individuals, however, did not express either GAD65 or IA-2 autoantibodies, and these individuals had only rarely lost the FPIR. There were two separate trials in DPT-1: parenteral insulin administration and a trial of oral insulin.

The parenteral insulin trial randomized 339 subjects, who had a projected 5-year risk of T1D greater than 50%, to either close observation or intravenous insulin for 4 days once a year and 0.125 U per kilogram body weight of subcutaneous ultralente insulin twice daily. Median follow-up was 3.7 years. Analysis of progression to diabetes, with OGTT performed every 6 months, indicated that the insulin therapy did not delay progression to diabetes [13].

The oral insulin trial randomized 372 relatives, who had a projected 5-year risk of diabetes of 26–50%, into double-blind intervention with oral insulin (7.5 mg per day) or placebo. OGTTs were performed every 6 months. The median follow-up was 4.3 years and the primary end point was diagnosis of diabetes. Oral insulin did not delay or prevent T1D. However, in a *post hoc* analysis of relatives with high levels of insulin autoantibodies, oral insulin appeared to delay progression to diabetes by about 4 years [15]. This has been used as the rationale for a repeat study conducted by the Type 1 Diabetes TrialNet Consortium. The study is currently enrolling FDRs of ages 1–45 years and second-degree relatives of ages 1–20 years (the relative with diabetes needs to have been diagnosed before the age of 40 years and started on insulin within the first year of diagnosis). Eligible subjects have to be IAA positive on two samples and meet additional criteria for other islet autoantibodies and FPIR characteristics. As of September 2007, the initial 30 subjects have been randomized.

Despite the lack of therapeutic benefit, the DPT-1 data have provided a wealth of information concerning prediction of T1D and trial design. In October 2001, the DPT-1 trial centers expanded and formed the Type 1 Diabetes TrialNet Consortium (www.diabetestrialnet.org) for conducting trials for

the prevention of T1D. TrialNet systematically evaluates therapies in new-onset patients, as well as in prediabetic subjects, and invites proposals from the research community at large. The Immune Tolerance Network (ITN; www.immunetolerance.org) is also accepting applications to support therapies aimed at tolerance induction and assays of tolerance.

Even though the secondary prevention trials have failed so far to prevent or delay the onset of diabetes, a growing body of evidence suggests that primary prevention of diabetic ketoacidosis (DKA) and hospitalization in newly diagnosed children is possible and should be a major goal of diabetes care systems. The DAISY has demonstrated that DKA can be prevented by periodic testing for diabetes autoantibodies, HbA_{1c} and random blood glucose of children at genetically high risk for T1D [122]. Similarly, in the DPT-1, awareness of increased level of risk and close biochemical monitoring made early diagnosis and prevention of DKA possible [13]. Early diagnosis and treatment not only eliminates mortality and greatly reduces the cost of initial treatment, but also has important implications for preservation of endogenous insulin secretion and prevention of acute and long-term complications of the disease [19–21].

27.3.3 Tertiary Prevention after Diagnosis of Diabetes

In the past several years, trials at the onset of T1D became the main focus of the research community. This shift away from primary or secondary prevention was due partially to the ease of finding and retaining trial participants, the availability of the TrialNet and ITN infrastructures, as well as the realization of how difficult and expensive are trials of the magnitude of TRIGR, ENDIT or DPT-1. The goal is preservation of remaining islet β-cells to induce and prolong partial remission. Unfortunately, 80–90% of islets have already been destroyed by the time diabetes is diagnosed [123]. Autoimmune β-cell destruction continues after the diagnosis of diabetes. A temporary remission from insulin dependency may occur in up to 27% of patients, soon after diagnosis [124], and is attributed to the β-cell rest caused by insulin treatment [21]. Younger age at onset, male sex, high titer of islet autoantibodies, severe ketoacidosis at diagnosis, and a short duration of symptoms prior to diagnosis are associated with a more rapid loss of C-peptide secretion [125]. There are conflicting reports concerning the effect of the HLA-DR, DQ genotypes [124–126]. The residual β-cell function can be retained for decades after the onset of diabetes in a subset of patients; however, very little of the normal function is retained, β-cell apoptosis continues and there is little spontaneous β-cell regeneration [127]. Complete remission of T1D is extremely rare [128].

The realistic outcome of the tertiary prevention trials is prolongation of residual insulin secretion, rather than complete reversal of diabetes. Benefits may include simpler insulin regimen, lower HbA$_{1c}$, and reduced risk of hypoglycemia and microvascular complications. Success is usually measured by higher fasting and stimulated C-peptide secretion in the treatment versus placebo arm, with both groups of patients maintaining good glycemic control. Preserved C-peptide secretion is associated with better glycemic control despite use of less insulin. Lower insulin dose, longer remission, lower HbA$_{1c}$, decreased variance of glucose and decreased rates of hypoglycemia have been used as secondary endpoints. In an effort to standardize clinical trials in this area, Greenbaum and Harrison [129], on behalf of the Immunology of Diabetes Society, have proposed guidelines for intervention trials in subjects with newly diagnosed T1D.

27.3.3.1 Antigen-specific Immunomodulators

An altered peptide ligand of the immunodominant insulin peptide B:9–23 [130] has completed phase I/II trials (Neurocrine) [131, 132]. This peptide could, by multiple routes of administration, prevent diabetes in animal models, and no severe adverse effects have been reported so far from human trials. However, the important caveat is anaphylaxis observed in the nonobese diabetic (NOD) mice with the native B:9–23 peptide [133] and activation of disease, marked by insulin autoantibodies in normal Balb/c mice and NOD mice with the insulin B:9–23 peptide [131, 134].

The whole GAD65 molecule produced by Diamyd has entered clinical trails in Scandinavia, encouraged by studies in animal models [135, 136]. A phase II placebo-controlled trial included 47 LADA patients with dose-escalation of alum-formulated recombinant human GAD65 injected subcutaneously at weeks 1 and 4 at doses of 4, 20, 100 or 500 μg. Fasting C-peptide levels at

24 weeks were increased compared with placebo only in the 20 μg group, not in the other dose groups. The apparent beneficial effects were not explained by changes in the GAD65Ab epitope pattern [137]. GAD65 autoantibody levels have clearly increased in response to the 500 μg dose, however, no serious side effects were observed during the ensuing 24 weeks, and in particular there has been no evidence of stiff man syndrome. However, patients with LADA (a slowly progressing form of diabetes) may not be the optimal therapeutic target. The second trial enrolled 70 T1D patients aged 10–18 years, within 18 months from diagnosis, with fasting C-peptide >0.10 pmol ml^{-1} and positive for GAD autoantibodies [138]. Participants were randomly assigned to receive either 20 μg GAD-alum or placebo administered subcutaneously at day 1 and 1 month later. At day 1 and at months 3, 9 and 15, a mixed meal tolerance test (MMTT; Sustacal) was performed to evaluate the impact of treatment on residual β-cell function. Change in fasting serum C-peptide was not significantly different between treatment groups, but the rate of decline in stimulated C-peptide secretion, measured as area under the curve, in the GAD-alum was approximately one-half of that in the placebo group. Maximum stimulated C-peptide at 15 months also decreased less in the GAD-alum group compared with the placebo group. The protective effect was most pronounced in patients treated within 3 months of diagnosis. These patients preserved their endogenous insulin secretion over 15 months, while the placebo patients lost a considerable portion of their stimulated C-peptide response. The incidence of clinical adverse events did not differ between GAD-alum and placebo groups. Treatment with GAD65 seemed to induce a specific T-cell population, with a subsequent deviation of a GAD65-specific immune response, toward a protective immune profile [139].

The p277 peptide of heat shock protein 60 (Peptor) [140, 141] has been reported to preserve C-peptide in a small trial of LADA patients with relatively short follow-up [142]. Phase II trials in children showed no effect [143]. A difficulty with the p277 peptide therapy is the lack of evidence that HSP60 is an autoantigen in the animal model and conflicting reports for therapeutic efficacy even in the NOD mouse [144].

27.3.3.2   Systemic Immunomodulators

Numerous nonantigen-specific immunomodulators have been tried in newly diagnosed patients. In early 2007, an excellent review by Staeva-Vieira *et al.* [105] listed at least 50 completed, ongoing and planned interventions, and this list will likely be seriously out of date when you read this chapter. Some immunosuppressive agents, such as cyclosporine A (CyA), azatiopirine and antithymocyte globulin + prednisolone, have unattractive side effects: weakening of immunity to infections, renal and pancreatic toxicity and potential long-term risk of malignancies. Others, such as nicotinamide, BCG vaccine, vitamin D supplementation or elimination of dietary gluten, while safer, have shown no efficacy [106, 145–147]. The interventions reviewed below illustrate, on selected examples, past milestones and current trends in this area.

Trials of CyA have demonstrated efficacy in prolonging insulin production [148]. However, the treatment had to be continued for at least 6–12 months to show benefit and the effect was lost when the drug was discontinued. In addition, the patients would progress to insulin dependency within 3 years even if CyA was continued and C-peptide secretion maintained. Renal and pancreatic β-cell toxicity of CyA, as well as the costs of the drug and monitoring of its blood levels, led to a consensus that the risks outweigh the benefits and this agent has been long abandoned. Nevertheless, CyA trials provided a proof of principle that immunosupression can slow the destruction of the β-cells, even if not stop it [149]. The trials also showed that the effect of CyA was greatest if the intervention was started within 6 weeks of diabetes diagnosis, suggesting that β-cell mass at the initiation of immunotherapy may by a key predictor of success.

Antithymocyte globulin (ATG) has been used in organ transplantation, but has not yet been shown to be effective in inducing immune tolerance. ATG is produced by isolating patient's T-lymphocytes and injecting them into an animal such as a rabbit or horse. The animal makes several antibodies to the T-cell antigens that are purified as ATG. Injected back into the subject, ATG attaches to T-cells, causing the host to see their own T-cells as foreign because of the attached antibodies and eliminating the potentially harmful T-cells. One clinical trial showed a reduction of HbA_{1c} levels and lower insulin requirements [150]. However, two patients developed severe thrombocytopenia. Upcoming trials of ATG will need to examine these risks carefully, particularly in children. The ITN is enrolling new-onset T1D patients, aged 12–35 years and within 6 weeks of diagnosis, to assess the effects of one course of ATG on preserving β-cell function. This is a multicenter, blinded, and randomized (2:1) phase II study. Participants have to be positive for one or more islet autoantibodies, have peak stimulated C-peptide >4.0 pmol ml^{-1} in an MMTT at least 3 weeks post-diagnosis, and evidence of prior Epstein–Barr virus infection. Enrolled subjects will be hospitalized for 5–8 days to receive four intravenous doses of ATG or placebo, and then followed for at least 2 years post-treatment. The primary endpoint is the 2 hC-peptide area under the curve in response to an MMTT at 1 year.

MMF (Cellcept) [151], an inhibitor of the synthesis of the purine guanosine monophosphate, prevents diabetes in BioBreeding rats [152]. In January 2007, TrialNet completed randomization of 126 new-onset T1D patients into a double-masked and placebo-controlled three-arm trail of MMF in combination with DZB (Zenapax), an immunosuppressive humanized IgG1 recombinant monoclonal antibody that binds to CD25, the p55 alpha subunit of the interleukin-2 receptor expressed on the surface of activated lymphocytes. Because T- and B-lymphocytes are dependent upon *de novo* synthesis of purines, MMF inhibits proliferation of lymphocytes. DZB competitively binds the CD25 (IL-2) receptor. Because these two drugs work at different targets, the combination therapy may be synergistic while minimizing toxicity. Participants will be followed for 2 years.

Rituximab (Rituxan) is a monoclonal antibody which targets the CD20 receptor unique to B-lymphocytes. Rituximab inhibits the B-lymphocyte function, thus reducing presentation of free antigen to T-cells, and theoretically secondarily preventing B-cell expansion and antibody production. This medication is approved for the treatment of B-cell non-Hodgkin's lymphoma and has shown success in treatment of patients with rheumatoid arthritis. By September 2007, TrialNet had enrolled the target group of 66 patients aged 12–45 years, with T1D of less than 12 weeks duration, into a two-arm, randomized, double-blinded, placebo-controlled trial of four doses of intravenous rituximab 375 mg m^{-2}, each a week apart. Participants will be followed for 2 years.

Monoclonal antibody to the CD3 receptor transiently activates the receptor, causes cytokine release and ultimately blocks T-cell proliferation and differentiation. Humanized hOKT3 anti-CD3 monoclonals, engineered to abrogate complement Fc binding, do not induce severe cytokine release syndromes, in contrast to standard OKT3, but have been associated with fever, rash and, in some patients, adenopathy, depending upon dose [153]. A randomized, placebo-controlled phase I–II trial with hOKT3 in 12 patients suggested less of a decline in stimulated C-peptide, lower HbA$_{1c}$ levels and lower insulin requirements in 9/12 of patients receiving hOKT3 compared with 2/12 controls. Toxicity was limited to a subset of patients developing anti-idiotypic antibodies [153]. The C-peptide levels held for approximately 18 months, followed by recurrence of progressive loss of C-peptide. A concern is the reactivation of Epstein–Barr virus infection in the European studies, but it was self-limiting with a single course of therapy [154]. Animal data and limited human data suggest that the effects of anti-CD3 is due to induction of regulatory T-cells [155–157]. However, it is likely that this form of therapy will require repeated administration of the monoclonal antibody, and the next trials will include repeated courses of therapy. The ITN/National Institutes of Health are currently enrolling into trials of hOKT3γ1 (Ala–Ala) patients 8–30 years old with new onset (<6 weeks) or recent onset T1D (4–12 months of diagnosis). The study will compare efficacy of two cycles of hOKT3γ1 infusion versus no infusion (new onset) or placebo infusions (recent onset). There will be two infusion cycles, 12 months apart. The treatment group will be hospitalized for 5 of the 14 days for the daily 15–30 min i.v. infusions. The subjects must remain under close observation for about 6 h post-infusion. Duration of study is 2 years. The anti-CD3 therapy protocols represent the most aggressive end of the spectrum of immunomodulation for tertiary prevention of T1D today with a very significant burden on the participants.

Additional interesting trials on the horizon include an ITN trial of aldesleukin, a recombinant human interleukin-2 (Proleukin) for 4 weeks and sirolimus (Rapamune) for 12 weeks in T1D patients with residual C-peptide within 4 years of diagnosis. The TrialNet is beginning enrollment into a trail of CTLA-Ig and a high-affinity variant (LEA29Y) is also available.

27.4 CONCLUSIONS

Development of safe and effective prevention of T1D is a major public health goal in industrialized countries today, as evidenced by strong legislative support in the United States in the form of the Special Statutory Funding Program http://www.t1diabetes.nih.gov. Genetic and environmental factors are being discovered that determine the relapsing–remitting course of β-cell destruction culminating in full insulin dependence. In the long run, the primary prevention of islet autoimmunity will likely be the optimal approach to the prevention of T1D, especially in high-risk groups, such as the FDRs. However, it is currently hampered by lack of convincing evidence about which environmental factor(s) initiates islet autoimmunity, and much more work is needed in this area. Poor predictive value of the existing genetic tests for T1D means also that the number of children to intervene on will remain high in relation to the number of T1D cases prevented.

Once tolerance is broken to more than one of islet autoantigen, the levels of islet autoantibodies may fluctuate, but most individuals progress to diabetes in 5–10 years. The presence of more than one of the autoantibodies (to insulin, GAD65, IA-2 or ZnT8), combined with low FPIR, mild glucose intolerance or/and presence of susceptible HLA-DR, DQ genotypes helps to identify persons with sufficiently high risk of disease to attempt prevention. However, the screening tools need further improvement to discern the individuals with loss of β-cells so slow that overt diabetes will not occur during the person's lifetime and no intervention is warranted. As patients develop autoimmunity, the β-cell mass declines, resulting in potentially decreased therapeutic benefit of secondary intervention. Additionally, it might be quite difficult to alter the autoimmune process once it has begun. In retrospect, the DPT-1 and ENDIT secondary prevention trials seem very speculative when viewed in the context of the knowledge at the time of their conception and the complexity of immunoregulation and autoimmunity. It will be very important to sharpen the predictive tools and potential interventions before they are applied to the general population, where the majority of T1D cases occur. Mass screening for islet autoantibodies and secondary prevention may be needed, if a primary prevention is not feasible at the level of the general population.

T1D can be successfully managed and complications delayed or avoided by intensive insulinotherapy with technological advantages of insulin pumps and continuous glucose monitoring. This has placed significant constraints on the tertiary prevention trials after diagnosis of diabetes. In my opinion, the systemic immunomodulators currently explored carry an unacceptable risk of long-term complications to be the main answer to T1D prevention. Despite the enthusiasm of the researchers evaluating systematically the newest immunosupression drugs in the context of new-onset T1D, this is still a sledgehammer approach in most cases. However, this work is incredibly important, because even with successful primary or secondary prevention programs there will always be patients that manifest with full-blown diabetes.

Diabetes prevention research is expanding at an unprecedented rate. The history of diabetes is filled with many ground-breaking discoveries. If the past performance predicts future returns, then the prevention of T1D diabetes has a bright future.

References

1. Rewers, M., Bugawan, T.L., Norris, J.M. *et al.* (1996) Newborn screening for HLA markers associated with IDDM: Diabetes Autoimmunity Study in the Young (DAISY). *Diabetologia*, **39** (7), 807–12.

2. Norris, J.M., Barriga, K., Klingensmith, G. *et al.* (2003) Timing of initial cereal exposure in infancy and risk of islet autoimmunity. *The Journal of the American Medical Association*, **290** (13), 1713–20.

3. Bingley, P.J., Bonifacio, E., Williams, A.J. *et al.* (1997) Prediction of IDDM in the general population: strategies based on combinations of autoantibody markers. *Diabetes*, **46** (11), 1701–10.

4. Bingley, P.J., Williams, A.J. and Gale, E.A. (1999) Optimized autoantibody-based risk assessment in family members. Implications for future intervention trials. *Diabetes Care*, **22** (11), 1796–801.

5. Ziegler, A.G., Hillebrand, B., Rabl, W. *et al.* (1993) On the appearance of islet associated autoimmunity in offspring of diabetic mothers: a prospective study from birth. *Diabetologia*, **36** (5), 402–8.

6. Achenbach, P., Warncke, K., Reiter, J. *et al.* (2006) Type 1 diabetes risk assessment: improvement by follow-up measurements in young islet autoantibody-positive relatives. *Diabetologia*, **49** (12), 2969–76.

7. Kimpimaki, T., Kupila, A., Hamalainen, A.M. *et al.* (2001) The first signs of beta-cell autoimmunity appear in infancy in genetically susceptible children from the general population: the Finnish type 1 diabetes prediction and prevention study. *The Journal of Clinical Endocrinology and Metabolism*, **86** (10), 4782–8.

8. Kupila, A., Muona, P., Simell, T. *et al.* (2001) Feasibility of genetic and immunological prediction of type I diabetes in a population-based birth cohort. *Diabetologia*, **44** (3), 290–7.

9. TRIGR Study Group (2007) Study design of the trial to reduce IDDM in the genetically at risk (TRIGR). *Pediatric Diabetes*, **8** (3), 117–37.

10. Norris, J.M., Yin, X., Lamb, M.M. *et al.* (2007) Omega-3 polyunsaturated fatty acid intake and islet autoimmunity in children at increased risk for type 1 diabetes. *The Journal of the American Medical Association*, **298** (12), 1420–8.

11. Pre-POINT (2008) http://onlineapps.jdfcure.org /AbstractReport.cfm?grant_id = 26014&abs_type = LAY. Last accessed 1 January 2008.

12. The TEDDY Study Group (2007) The environmental determinants of diabetes in the young (TEDDY) study: study design. *Pediatric Diabetes*, **8** (5), 286–98.

13. Diabetes Prevention Trial–Type 1 Diabetes Study Group (2002) Effects of insulin in relatives of patients with type 1 diabetes mellitus. *The New England Journal of Medicine*, **346** (22), 1685–91.

14. Gale, E.A., Bingley, P.J., Emmett, C.L. and Collier, T. (2004) European Nicotinamide Diabetes Intervention Trial (ENDIT): a randomised controlled trial of intervention before the onset of type 1 diabetes. *Lancet*, **363** (9413), 925–31.

15. Skyler, J.S., Krischer, J.P., Wolfsdorf, J. *et al.* (2005) Effects of oral insulin in relatives of patients with type 1 diabetes: the Diabetes Prevention Trial–Type 1. *Diabetes Care*, **28** (5), 1068–76.

16. Sosenko, J.M., Palmer, J.P., Greenbaum, C.J. *et al.* (2006) Patterns of metabolic progression to type 1 diabetes in the Diabetes Prevention Trial–Type 1. *Diabetes Care*, **29** (3), 643–9.

17. Sosenko, J.M., Palmer, J.P., Greenbaum, C.J. *et al.* (2007) Increasing the accuracy of oral glucose tolerance testing and extending its application

to individuals with normal glucose tolerance for the prediction of type 1 diabetes: the diabetes prevention trial-type 1. *Diabetes Care*, **30** (1), 38–42.

18. Stene, L.C., Barriga, K., Hoffman, M. *et al.* (2006) Normal but increasing hemoglobin A1c levels predict progression from islet autoimmunity to overt type 1 diabetes: Diabetes Autoimmunity Study in the Young (DAISY). *Pediatric Diabetes*, **7** (5), 247–53.

19. Steffes, M.W., Sibley, S., Jackson, M. and Thomas, W. (2003) Beta-cell function and the development of diabetes-related complications in the diabetes control and complications trial. *Diabetes Care*, **26** (3), 832–6.

20. Palmer, J.P., Fleming, G.A., Greenbaum, C.J. *et al.* (2004) C-peptide is the appropriate outcome measure for type 1 diabetes clinical trials to preserve beta-cell function: report of an ADA Workshop, 21–22 October 2001. *Diabetes*, **53** (1), 250–64.

21. Sherry, N.A., Tsai, E.B. and Herold, K.C. (2005) Natural history of beta-cell function in type 1 diabetes. *Diabetes*, **54** (Suppl 2), S32–9.

22. Warram, J.H., Krolewski, A.S., Gottlieb, M.S. and Kahn, C.R. (1984) Differences in risk of insulin-dependent diabetes in offspring of diabetic mothers and diabetic fathers. *The New England Journal of Medicine*, **311** (3), 149–52.

23. Steck, A.K., Barriga, K.J., Emery, L.M. *et al.* (2005) Secondary attack rate of type 1 diabetes in Colorado families. *Diabetes Care*, **28** (2), 296–300.

24. Harjutsalo, V., Reunanen, A. and Tuomilehto, J. (2006) Differential transmission of type 1 diabetes from diabetic fathers and mothers to their offspring. *Diabetes*, **55** (5), 1517–24.

25. Aly, T.A., Ide, A., Jahromi, M.M. *et al.* (2006) Extreme genetic risk for type 1A diabetes. *Proceedings of the National Academy of Sciences of the United States of America*, **103** (38), 14074–9.

26. Pugliese, A., Gianani, R., Moromisato, R. *et al.* (1995) HLA-DQB1*0602 is associated with dominant protection from diabetes even among islet cell antibody-positive first-degree relatives of patients with IDDM. *Diabetes*, **44** (6), 608–13.

27. Rewers, A., Babu, S., Wang, T.B. *et al.* (2003) Ethnic differences in the associations between the HLA-DRB1*04 subtypes and type 1 diabetes. *Annals of the New York Academy of Sciences*, **1005**, 301–9.

28. Morel, P.A., Dorman, J.S., Todd, J.A. *et al.* (1988) Aspartic acid at position 57 of the HLA-DQ beta chain protects against type I diabetes: a family study. *Proceedings of the National Academy of Sciences of the United States of America*, **85** (21), 8111–15.

29. Reijonen, H., Ilonen, J., Knip, M. and Akerblom, H.K. (1991) HLA-DQB1 alleles and absence of Asp 57 as susceptibility factors of IDDM in Finland. *Diabetes*, **40** (12), 1640–4.

30. Deschamps, I. and Khalil, I. (1993) The role of DQ alpha–beta heterodimers in genetic susceptibility to insulin-dependent diabetes. *Diabetes/Metabolism Reviews*, **9** (2), 71–92.

31. Emery, L.M., Babu, S., Bugawan, T.L. *et al.* (2005) Newborn HLA-DR, DQ genotype screening: age- and ethnicity-specific type 1 diabetes risk estimates. *Pediatric Diabetes*, **6** (3), 136–44.

32. The Wellcome Trust Case Control Consortium (2007) Genome-wide association study of 14,000 cases of seven common diseases and 3,000 shared controls. *Nature*, **447** (7145), 661–78.

33. Todd, J.A., Walker, N.M., Cooper, J.D. *et al.* (2007) Robust associations of four new chromosome regions from genome-wide analyses of type 1 diabetes. *Nature Genetics*, **39** (7), 857–64.

34. Lowe, C.E., Cooper, J.D., Brusko, T. *et al.* (2007) Large-scale genetic fine mapping and genotype-phenotype associations implicate polymorphism in the IL2RA region in type 1 diabetes. *Nature Genetics*, **9** (9), 1074–82.

35. Hakonarson, H., Grant, S.F., Bradfield, J.P. *et al.* (2007) A genome-wide association study identifies KIAA0350 as a type 1 diabetes gene. *Nature*, **448** (7153), 591–4.

36. Steck, A.K., Bugawan, T.L., Zhang, W. *et al.* (2007) Do non-HLA genes influence progression to persistent islet autoimmunity and type 1 diabetes? (Abstract). *Acta Diabetologica*, **44** (Suppl 1), S50.

37. Yu, L., Cuthbertson, D.D., Maclaren, N. *et al.* (2001) Expression of GAD65 and islet cell antibody (ICA512) autoantibodies among cytoplasmic ICA+ relatives is associated with eligibility for the diabetes prevention trial-type 1. *Diabetes*, **50** (8), 1735–40.

38. Krischer, J.P., Cuthbertson, D.D., Yu, L. *et al.* (2003) Screening strategies for the identification of multiple antibody-positive relatives of individuals with type 1 diabetes. *The Journal of Clinical Endocrinology and Metabolism*, **88** (1), 103–8.

39. Palmer, J.P., Asplin, C.M., Clemons, P. *et al.* (1983) Insulin antibodies in insulin-dependent diabetics before insulin treatment. *Science*, **222** (4630), 1337–9.

40. Baekkeskov, S., Aanstoot, H.J., Christgau, S. *et al.* (1990) Identification of the 64K autoantigen in insulin-dependent diabetes as the GABA-synthesizing enzyme glutamic acid decarboxylase. *Nature*, **347** (6289), 151–6.

41. Rabin, D.U., Pleasic, S.M., Palmer-Crocker, R. and Shapiro, J.A. (1992) Cloning and expression of IDDM-specific human autoantigens. *Diabetes*, **41** (2), 183–6.

42. Wenzlau, J.M., Juhl, K., Yu, L. *et al.* (2007) The cation efflux transporter ZnT8 (Slc30A8) is a major autoantigen in human type 1 diabetes. *Proceedings of the National Academy of Sciences of the United States of America*, **104** (43), 17040–5.

43. Verge, C.F., Gianani, R., Kawasaki, E. *et al.* (1996) Prediction of type I diabetes in first-degree relatives using a combination of insulin, GAD, and ICA512bdc/IA-2 autoantibodies. *Diabetes*, **45** (7), 926–33.

44. Bingley, P.J., Bonifacio, E. and Mueller, P.W. (2003) Diabetes antibody standardization program: first assay proficiency evaluation. *Diabetes*, **52** (5), 1128–36.

45. Bingley, P.J. and Williams, A.J. (2004) Validation of autoantibody assays in type 1 diabetes: workshop programme. *Autoimmunity*, **37** (4), 257–60.

46. Riley, W.J., Maclaren, N.K., Krischer, J. *et al.* (1990) A prospective study of the development of diabetes in relatives of patients with insulin-dependent diabetes. *The New England Journal of Medicine*, **323** (17), 1167–72.

47. Bonifacio, E., Bingley, P.J., Shattock, M. *et al.* (1990) Quantification of islet-cell antibodies and prediction of insulin-dependent diabetes. *Lancet*, **335** (8682), 147–9.

48. Ziegler, A.G., Ziegler, R., Vardi, P. *et al.* (1989) Life-table analysis of progression to diabetes of anti-insulin autoantibody-positive relatives of individuals with type I diabetes. *Diabetes*, **38** (10), 1320–5.

49. Krischer, J.P., Schatz, D., Riley, W.J. *et al.* (1993) Insulin and islet cell autoantibodies as time-dependent covariates in the development of insulin-dependent diabetes: a prospective study in relatives. *The Journal of Clinical Endocrinology and Metabolism*, **77** (3), 743–9.

50. Maclaren, N., Lan, M., Coutant, R. *et al.* (1999) Only multiple autoantibodies to islet cells (ICA), insulin, GAD65, IA-2 and IA-2beta predict immune-mediated (type 1) diabetes in relatives. *Journal of Autoimmunity*, **12** (4), 279–87.

51. Verge, C.F., Stenger, D., Bonifacio, E. *et al.* (1998) Combined use of autoantibodies (IA-2 autoantibody, GAD autoantibody, insulin autoantibody, cytoplasmic islet cell antibodies) in type 1 diabetes: Combinatorial Islet Autoantibody Workshop. *Diabetes*, **47** (12), 1857–66.

52. Eisenbarth, G.S. (2004) Prediction of type 1 diabetes: the natural history of the prediabetic period. *Advances in Experimental Medicine and Biology*, **552**, 268–90.

53. Bingley, P.J., Christie, M.R., Bonifacio, E. *et al.* (1994) Combined analysis of autoantibodies improves prediction of IDDM in islet cell antibody-positive relatives. *Diabetes*, **43** (11), 1304–10.

54. Rewers, M., Norris, J.M., Eisenbarth, G.S. *et al.* (1996) Beta-cell autoantibodies in infants and toddlers without IDDM relatives: Diabetes Autoimmunity Study in the Young (DAISY). *Journal of Autoimmunity*, **9** (3), 405–10.

55. Barker, J.M., Barriga, K.J., Yu, L. *et al.* (2004) Prediction of autoantibody positivity and progression to type 1 diabetes: diabetes autoimmunity study in the young (DAISY). *The Journal of Clinical Endocrinology and Metabolism*, **89** (8), 3896–902.

56. Stanley, H.M., Norris, J.M., Barriga, K. *et al.* (2004) Is presence of islet autoantibodies at birth associated with development of persistent islet autoimmunity? The Diabetes Autoimmunity Study in the Young (DAISY). *Diabetes Care*, **27** (2), 497–502.

57. Naserke, H.E., Bonifacio, E. and Ziegler, A.G. (2001) Prevalence, characteristics and diabetes risk associated with transient maternally acquired islet antibodies and persistent islet antibodies in offspring of parents with type 1 diabetes. *The Journal of Clinical Endocrinology and Metabolism*, **86** (10), 4826–33.

58. Ziegler, A.G., Hummel, M., Schenker, M. and Bonifacio, E. (1999) Autoantibody appearance and risk for development of childhood diabetes in offspring of parents with type 1 diabetes: the 2-year analysis of the German BABYDIAB Study. *Diabetes*, **48** (3), 460–8.

59. Schatz, D., Krischer, J., Horne, G. *et al.* (1994) Islet cell antibodies predict insulin-dependent diabetes in United States school age children as powerfully as in unaffected relatives. *The Journal of Clinical Investigation*, **93** (6), 2403–7.

60. Bingley, P.J., Bonifacio, E., Shattock, M. *et al.* (1993) Can islet cell antibodies predict IDDM in the general population? *Diabetes Care*, **16** (1), 45–50.

61. Notsu, K., Oka, N., Note, S. *et al.* (1985) Islet cell antibodies in the Japanese population and

subjects with type 1 (insulin-dependent) diabetes. *Diabetologia*, **28** (9), 660–2.

62. Boehm, B.O., Manfras, B., Seissler, J. *et al.* (1991) Epidemiology and immunogenetic background of islet cell antibody–positive nondiabetic schoolchildren. Ulm–Frankfurt Population Study. *Diabetes*, **40** (11), 1435–9.

63. Levy-Marchal, C., Tichet, J., Fajardy, I. *et al.* (1992) Islet cell antibodies in normal French schoolchildren. *Diabetologia*, **35** (6), 577–82.

64. Bruining, G.J., Molenaar, J.L., Grobbee, D.E. *et al.* (1989) Ten-year follow-up study of islet-cell antibodies and childhood diabetes mellitus. *Lancet*, **1** (8647), 1100–3.

65. Bergua, M., Sole, J., Marion, G. *et al.* (1987) Prevalence of islet cell antibodies, insulin antibodies and hyperglycaemia in 2291 schoolchildren. *Diabetologia*, **30** (9), 724–6.

66. Elliott, R.B., Pilcher, C.C., Stewart, A. *et al.* (1993) The use of nicotinamide in the prevention of type 1 diabetes. *Annals of the New York Academy of Sciences*, **696**, 333–41.

67. LaGasse, J.M., Brantley, M.S., Leech, N.J. *et al.* (2002) Successful prospective prediction of type 1 diabetes in schoolchildren through multiple defined autoantibodies: an 8-year follow-up of the Washington State diabetes prediction study. *Diabetes Care*, **25** (3), 505–11.

68. Colman, P.G., McNair, P., King, J. *et al.* (2000) Screening for preclinical type 1 diabetes in a discrete population with an apparent increased disease incidence. *Pediatric Diabetes*, **1** (4), 193–8.

69. Karjalainen, J.K. (1990) Islet cell antibodies as predictive markers for IDDM in children with high background incidence of disease. *Diabetes*, **39** (9), 1144–50.

70. Kimpimaki, T., Kulmala, P., Savola, K. *et al.* (2002) Natural history of beta-cell autoimmunity in young children with increased genetic susceptibility to type 1 diabetes recruited from the general population. *The Journal of Clinical Endocrinology and Metabolism*, **87** (10), 4572–9.

71. Laakso, M. and Pyorala, K. (1985) Age of onset and type of diabetes. *Diabetes Care*, **8** (2), 114–17.

72. Harjutsalo, V., Podar, T. and Tuomilehto, J. (2005) Cumulative incidence of type 1 diabetes in 10,168 siblings of Finnish young-onset type 1 diabetic patients. *Diabetes*, **54** (2), 563–9.

73. Karjalainen, J., Salmela, P., Ilonen, J. *et al.* (1989) A comparison of childhood and adult type I diabetes mellitus. *The New England Journal of Medicine*, **320** (14), 881–6.

74. Tuomi, T., Groop, L.C., Zimmet, P.Z. *et al.* (1993) Antibodies to glutamic acid decarboxylase reveal latent autoimmune diabetes mellitus in adults with a non-insulin-dependent onset of disease. *Diabetes*, **42** (2), 359–62.

75. Zimmet, P.Z., Tuomi, T., Mackay, I.R. *et al.* (1994) Latent autoimmune diabetes mellitus in adults (LADA): the role of antibodies to glutamic acid decarboxylase in diagnosis and prediction of insulin dependency. *Diabetic Medicine*, **11** (3), 299–303.

76. Turner, R., Stratton, I., Horton, V. *et al.* (1997) UKPDS 25: autoantibodies to islet-cell cytoplasm and glutamic acid decarboxylase for prediction of insulin requirement in type 2 diabetes. UK Prospective Diabetes Study Group. *Lancet*, **350** (9087), 1288–93.

77. Bottazzo, G.F., Bosi, E., Cull, C.A. *et al.* (2005) IA-2 antibody prevalence and risk assessment of early insulin requirement in subjects presenting with type 2 diabetes (UKPDS 71). *Diabetologia*, **48** (4), 703–8.

78. Fuchtenbusch, M., Ferber, K., Standl, E. and Ziegler, A.G. (1997) Prediction of type 1 diabetes postpartum in patients with gestational diabetes mellitus by combined islet cell autoantibody screening: a prospective multicenter study. *Diabetes*, **46** (9), 1459–67.

79. Srikanta, S., Ganda, O.P., Jackson, R.A. *et al.* (1983) Type I diabetes mellitus in monozygotic twins: chronic progressive beta cell dysfunction. *Annals of Internal Medicine*, **99** (3), 320–6.

80. Knip, M., Vahasalo, P., Karjalainen, J. *et al.* (1994) Natural history of preclinical IDDM in high risk siblings. Childhood Diabetes in Finland Study Group. *Diabetologia*, **37** (4), 388–93.

81. Bingley, P.J. (1996) Interactions of age, islet cell antibodies, insulin autoantibodies, and first-phase insulin response in predicting risk of progression to IDDM in ICA+ relatives: the ICARUS data set. Islet Cell Antibody Register Users study. *Diabetes*, **45** (12), 1720–8.

82. Chase, H.P., Cuthbertson, D.D., Dolan, L.M. *et al.* (2001) First-phase insulin release during the intravenous glucose tolerance test as a risk factor for type 1 diabetes. *The Journal of Pediatrics*, **138** (2), 244–9.

83. Keskinen, P., Korhonen, S., Kupila, A. *et al.* (2002) First-phase insulin response in young healthy children at genetic and immunological risk for type I diabetes. *Diabetologia*, **45** (12), 1639–48.

84. Barker, J.M., McFann, K., Harrison, L.C. *et al.* (2007) Pre-type 1 diabetes dysmetabolism: maximal sensitivity achieved with both oral and intravenous glucose tolerance testing. *The Journal of Pediatrics*, **150** (1), 31–6.

85. Eisenbarth, G.S., Verge, C.F., Allen, H. and Rewers, M.J. (1993) The design of trials for prevention of IDDM. *Diabetes*, **42** (7), 941–7.

86. Bingley, P.J., Colman, P., Eisenbarth, G.S. *et al.* (1992) Standardization of IVGTT to predict IDDM. *Diabetes Care*, **15** (10), 1313–16.

87. Allen, H.F., Jeffers, B.W., Klingensmith, G.J. and Chase, H.P. (1993) First-phase insulin release in normal children. *The Journal of Pediatrics*, **123** (5), 733–8.

88. Cutfield, W.S., Menon, R.K., Bright, G.N. and Sperling, M.A. (2000) Limitations of first-phase insulin response to evaluate insulin secretion in children. *Pediatric Diabetes*, **1** (1), 3–9.

89. Carel, J.C., Boitard, C. and Bougneres, P.F. (1993) Decreased insulin response to glucose in islet cell antibody-negative siblings of type 1 diabetic children. *The Journal of Clinical Investigation*, **92** (1), 509–13.

90. Cutfield, W.S., Bergman, R.N., Menon, R.K. and Sperling, M.A. (1990) The modified minimal model: application to measurement of insulin sensitivity in children. *The Journal of Clinical Endocrinology and Metabolism*, **70** (6), 1644–50.

91. Smith, C.P., Williams, A.J., Thomas, J.M. *et al.* (1988) The pattern of basal and stimulated insulin responses to intravenous glucose in first degree relatives of type 1 (insulin-dependent) diabetic children and unrelated adults aged 5 to 50 years. *Diabetologia*, **31** (7), 430–4.

92. Colman, P.G., Stewart, V., Kean, J. *et al.* (1992) Comparison of two commonly used standard IVGTTs. *Diabetes Care*, **15** (8), 1053–5.

93. Rayman, G., Clark, P., Schneider, A.E. and Hales, C.N. (1990) The first phase insulin response to intravenous glucose is highly reproducible. *Diabetologia*, **33** (10), 631–4.

94. Smith, C.P., Tarn, A.C., Thomas, J.M. *et al.* (1988) Between and within subject variation of the first phase insulin response to intravenous glucose. *Diabetologia*, **31** (2), 123–5.

95. McNair, P.D., Colman, P.G., Alford, F.P. and Harrison, L.C. (1995) Reproducibility of the first-phase insulin response to intravenous glucose is not improved by retrograde cannulation and arterialization or the use of a lower glucose dose. *Diabetes Care*, **18** (8), 1168–73.

96. Rowe, R.E., Leech, N.J., Finegood, D.T. and McCulloch, D.K. (1994) Retrograde versus antegrade cannulation in the intravenous glucose tolerance test. *Diabetes Research and Clinical Practice*, **25** (2), 131–6.

97. Leech, N.J., Rowe, R.E., Bucksa, J. and McCulloch, D.K. (1993) HbA1c may be an early indicator of islet cell dysfunction (Abstract). *Autoimmunity*, **15** (Suppl), 75.

98. Yuh, W.T., Wiese, J.A., bu-Yousef, M.M. *et al.* (1988) Pancreatic transplant imaging. *Radiology*, **167** (3), 679–83.

99. Kelcz, F., Sollinger, H.W. and Pirsch, J.D. (1991) MRI of the pancreas transplant: lack of correlation between imaging and clinical status. *Magnetic Resonance in Medicine*, **21** (1), 30–8.

100. Fernandez, M.P., Bernardino, M.E., Neylan, J.F. and Olson, R.A. (1991) Diagnosis of pancreatic transplant dysfunction: value of gadopentetate dimeglumine-enhanced MR imaging. *American Journal of Roentgenology*, **156** (6), 1171–6.

101. Turvey, S.E., Swart, E., Denis, M.C. *et al.* (2005) Noninvasive imaging of pancreatic inflammation and its reversal in type 1 diabetes. *The Journal of Clinical Investigation*, **115** (9), 2454–61.

102. Moore, A., Grimm, J., Han, B. and Santamaria, P. (2004) Tracking the recruitment of diabetogenic CD8+ T-cells to the pancreas in real time. *Diabetes*, **53** (6), 1459–66.

103. Chianelli, M., Parisella, M.G., Visalli, N. *et al.* (2008) Pancreatic scintigraphy with ^{99m}Tc-interleukin-2 at diagnosis of type 1 diabetes and after 1 year of nicotinamide therapy. *Diabetes/Metabolism Research and Reviews*, **24** (2), 115–22.

104. Atkinson, M.A. (2005) Thirty years of investigating the autoimmune basis for type 1 diabetes: why can't we prevent or reverse this disease? *Diabetes*, **54** (5), 1253–63.

105. Staeva-Vieira, T., Peakman, M. and von, H.M. (2007) Translational mini-review series on type 1 diabetes: immune-based therapeutic approaches for type 1 diabetes. *Clinical and Experimental Immunology*, **148** (1), 17–31.

106. Pastore, M.R., Bazzigaluppi, E., Belloni, C. *et al.* (2003) Six months of gluten-free diet do not influence autoantibody titers, but improve insulin secretion in subjects at high risk for type 1 diabetes. *The Journal of Clinical Endocrinology and Metabolism*, **88** (1), 162–5.

107. The Nutritional Intervention to Prevent Type 1 Diabetes (NIP) Pilot Study (2008) http://www2.diabetestrialnet.org/nip. Last accessed January 1, 2008.

108. Wicklow, B.A. and Taback, S.P. (2006) Feasibility of a type 1 diabetes primary prevention trial using

108. 2000 IU vitamin D3 in infants from the general population with increased HLA-associated risk. *Annals of the New York Academy of Sciences*, **1079**, 310–12.

109. Brekke, H.K. and Ludvigsson, J. (2007) Vitamin D supplementation and diabetes-related autoimmunity in the ABIS study. *Pediatric Diabetes*, **8** (1), 11–14.

110. Baughcum, A.E., Johnson, S.B., Carmichael, S.K. *et al.* (2005) Maternal efforts to prevent type 1 diabetes in at-risk children. *Diabetes Care*, **28** (4), 916–21.

111. Fourlanos, S., Narendran, P., Byrnes, G.B. *et al.* (2004) Insulin resistance is a risk factor for progression to type 1 diabetes. *Diabetologia*, **47** (10), 1661–7.

112. Xu, P., Cuthbertson, D., Greenbaum, C. *et al.* (2007) Role of insulin resistance in predicting progression to type 1 diabetes. *Diabetes Care*, **30** (9), 2314–20.

113. Type 1 Diabetes TrialNet Multi-center Clinical Trial of the Effects of Metabolic Control on Progression of Type 1 Diabetes (2008) http://techdev.niddk.nih.gov/_PDFs/TrialNetMCS.pdf. Last accessed January 1, 2008.

114. Butler, P.C., Meier, J.J., Butler, A.E. and Bhushan, A. (2007) The replication of beta cells in normal physiology, in disease and for therapy. *Nature Clinical Practice Endocrinology and Metabolism*, **3** (11), 758–68.

115. Von Herrath, M., Sanda, S. and Herold, K. (2007) Type 1 diabetes as a relapsing-remitting disease? *Nature Reviews Immunology*, **7** (12), 988–94.

116. Clinical Trial of Diabetes Regenerative Therapy (2008) http://www.jdrf.org/index.cfm?page_id = 106725. Last accessed January 1, 2008.

117. Type 1 Diabetes (T1D) Clinical Trail of the Effects of Anti-CD3 and Exenatide on Loss of Insulin Production in Patients with Recent Onset T1D and Individuals at High Risk (2008) http://www.govcb.com/A-TYPE-DIABETES-T-D-CLINICAL-ADP11447883610001858.htm. Last accessed January 1, 2008.

118. Pambianco, G., Costacou, T., Ellis, D. *et al.* (2006) The 30-year natural history of type 1 diabetes complications: the Pittsburgh Epidemiology of Diabetes Complications Study experience. *Diabetes*, **55** (5), 1463–9.

119. Nishimura, R., LaPorte, R.E., Dorman, J.S. *et al.* (2001) Mortality trends in type 1 diabetes. The Allegheny County (Pennsylvania) Registry 1965–1999. *Diabetes Care*, **24** (5), 823–7.

120. Hovind, P., Tarnow, L., Rossing, K. *et al.* (2003) Decreasing incidence of severe diabetic microangiopathy in type 1 diabetes. *Diabetes Care*, **26** (4), 1258–64.

121. Simell, O. (2008) Results of the DIPP Study. In 9th International Congress of the Immunology of Diabetes Society and American Diabetes Association Research Symposium, November 14–18, 2007, Miami Beach, FL, USA.

122. Barker, J.M., Goehrig, S.H., Barriga, K. *et al.* (2004) Clinical characteristics of children diagnosed with type 1 diabetes through intensive screening and follow-up. *Diabetes Care*, **27** (6), 1399–1404.

123. Gepts, W. and De Mey, J. (1978) Islet cell survival determined by morphology. An immunocytochemical study of the islets of langerhans in juvenile diabetes mellitus. *Diabetes*, **27** (Suppl 1), 251–61.

124. Martin, S., Pawlowski, B., Greulich, B. *et al.* (1992) Natural course of remission in IDDM during 1st yr after diagnosis. *Diabetes Care*, **15** (1), 66–74.

125. Schiffrin, A., Suissa, S., Weitzner, G. *et al.* (1992) Factors predicting course of beta-cell function in IDDM. *Diabetes Care*, **15** (8), 997–1001.

126. Knip, M., Ilonen, J., Mustonen, A. and Akerblom, H.K. (1986) Evidence of an accelerated B-cell destruction in HLA-Dw3/Dw4 heterozygous children with type 1 (insulin-dependent) diabetes. *Diabetologia*, **29** (6), 347–51.

127. Meier, J.J., Bhushan, A., Butler, A.E. *et al.* (2005) Sustained beta cell apoptosis in patients with long-standing type 1 diabetes: indirect evidence for islet regeneration? *Diabetologia*, **48** (11), 2221–8.

128. Karges, B., Durinovic-Bello, I., Heinze, E. *et al.* (2004) Complete long-term recovery of beta-cell function in autoimmune type 1 diabetes after insulin treatment. *Diabetes Care*, **27** (5), 1207–8.

129. Greenbaum, C.J. and Harrison, L.C. (2003) Guidelines for intervention trials in subjects with newly diagnosed type 1 diabetes. *Diabetes*, **52** (5), 1059–65.

130. Daniel, D. and Wegmann, D.R. (1996) Protection of nonobese diabetic mice from diabetes by intranasal or subcutaneous administration of insulin peptide B-(9-23). *Proceedings of the National Academy of Sciences of the United States of America*, **93** (2), 956–60.

131. Abiru, N., Maniatis, A.K., Yu, L. *et al.* (2001) Peptide and major histocompatibility complex-specific breaking of humoral tolerance

to native insulin with the B9-23 peptide in diabetes-prone and normal mice. *Diabetes*, **50** (6), 1274–81.

132. Alleva, D.G., Crowe, P.D., Jin, L. *et al.* (2001) A disease-associated cellular immune response in type 1 diabetics to an immunodominant epitope of insulin. *The Journal of Clinical Investigation*, **107** (2), 173–80.

133. Liu, E., Moriyama, H., Abiru, N. *et al.* (2002) Anti-peptide autoantibodies and fatal anaphylaxis in NOD mice in response to insulin self-peptides B:9-23 and B:13-23. *The Journal of Clinical Investigation*, **110** (7), 1021–7.

134. Moriyama, H., Wen, L., Abiru, N. *et al.* (2002) Induction and acceleration of insulitis/diabetes in mice with a viral mimic (polyinosinic-polycytidylic acid) and an insulin self-peptide. *Proceedings of the National Academy of Sciences of the United States of America*, **99** (8), 5539–44.

135. Tisch, R., Wang, B. and Serreze, D.V. (1999) Induction of glutamic acid decarboxylase 65-specific Th2 cells and suppression of autoimmune diabetes at late stages of disease is epitope dependent. *Journal of Immunology*, **163** (3), 1178–87.

136. Tisch, R., Liblau, R.S., Yang, X.D. *et al.* (1998) Induction of GAD65-specific regulatory T-cells inhibits ongoing autoimmune diabetes in nonobese diabetic mice. *Diabetes*, **47** (6), 894–9.

137. Bekris, L.M., Jensen, R.A., Lagerquist, E. *et al.* (2007) GAD65 autoantibody epitopes in adult patients with latent autoimmune diabetes following GAD65 vaccination. *Diabetic Medicine*, **24** (5), 521–6.

138. Ludvigsson, J., Vaarala, O., Forsander, G. *et al.* (2008) GAD65-vaccination preserves residual insulin secretion in children and adolescents with recent onset type 1 diabetes: Results of a randomized controlled phase II trial (Abstract). *Pediatric Diabetes*, **8** (Suppl 7), 12.

139. Ludvigsson, J., Casas, R., Hedman, M. *et al.* (2008) Specific immune response to GAD65 in type 1 diabetic children treated with GAD65 (DiamydTM) (Abstract). *Pediatric Diabetes*, **8** (Suppl 7), 12.

140. Elias, D. and Cohen, I.R. (1995) Treatment of autoimmune diabetes and insulitis in NOD mice with heat shock protein 60 peptide p277. *Diabetes*, **44** (9), 1132–8.

141. Ablamunits, V., Elias, D., Reshef, T. and Cohen, I.R. (1998) Islet T cells secreting IFN-gamma in NOD mouse diabetes: arrest by p277 peptide treatment. *Journal of Autoimmunity*, **11** (1), 73–81.

142. Raz, I., Elias, D., Avron, A. *et al.* (2001) Beta-cell function in new-onset type 1 diabetes and immunomodulation with a heat-shock protein peptide (DiaPep277): a randomised, double-blind, phase II trial. *Lancet*, **358** (9295), 1749–53.

143. Lazar, L., Ofan, R. and Weintrob, N. Heat-shock protein peptid DiaPep277 treatment in children with newly diagnosed type 1 diabetes: a randomised, double-blind phase II study. (2006) *Diabetes/Metabolism Research and Reviews*, **23** (4), 286–91 DOI: 10.1002/dmdd.711.

144. Bowman, M. and Atkinson, M.A. (2002) Heat shock protein therapy fails to prevent diabetes in NOD mice. *Diabetologia*, **45** (9), 1350–51.

145. Allen, H.F., Klingensmith, G.J., Jensen, P. *et al.* (1999) Effect of bacillus Calmette–Guerin vaccination on new-onset type 1 diabetes. A randomized clinical study. *Diabetes Care*, **22** (10), 1703–7.

146. Lampeter, E.F., Klinghammer, A., Scherbaum, W.A. *et al.* (1998) The Deutsche Nicotinamide Intervention Study: an attempt to prevent type 1 diabetes. DENIS Group. *Diabetes*, **47** (6), 980–84.

147. Pitocco, D., Crino, A., Di Stasio, E. *et al.* (2006) The effects of calcitriol and nicotinamide on residual pancreatic beta-cell function in patients with recent-onset Type 1 diabetes (IMDIAB XI). *Diabetic Medicine*, **23** (8), 920–23.

148. Stiller, C.R., Dupre, J., Gent, M. *et al.* (1984) Effects of cyclosporine immunosuppression in insulin-dependent diabetes mellitus of recent onset. *Science*, **223** (4643), 1362–7.

149. Carel, J.C., Boitard, C., Eisenbarth, G. *et al.* (1996) Cyclosporine delays but does not prevent clinical onset in glucose intolerant pre-type 1 diabetic children. *Journal of Autoimmunity*, **9** (6), 739–45.

150. Eisenbarth, G.S., Srikanta, S., Jackson, R. *et al.* (1985) Anti-thymocyte globulin and prednisone immunotherapy of recent onset type 1 diabetes mellitus. *Diabetes Research*, **2** (6), 271–6.

151. Vu, M.D., Qi, S., Xu, D. *et al.* (1998) Synergistic effects of mycophenolate mofetil and sirolimus in prevention of acute heart, pancreas, and kidney allograft rejection and in reversal of ongoing heart allograft rejection in the rat. *Transplantation*, **66** (12), 1575–80.

152. Hao, L., Chan, S.M. and Lafferty, K.J. (1993) Mycophenolate mofetil can prevent the development of diabetes in BB rats. *Annals of the New York Academy of Sciences*, **696**, 328–32.

153. Herold, K.C., Hagopian, W., Auger, J.A. *et al.* (2002) Anti-CD3 monoclonal antibody in

new-onset type 1 diabetes mellitus. *The New England Journal of Medicine* **346** (22), 1692–8.

154. Keymeulen, B., Vandemeulebroucke, E., Ziegler, A.G. *et al.* (2005) Insulin needs after CD3-antibody therapy in new-onset type 1 diabetes. *The New England Journal of Medicine*, **352** (25), 2598–608.

155. Chatenoud, L. and Bach, J.F. (2005) Regulatory T cells in the control of autoimmune diabetes: the case of the NOD mouse. *International Reviews of Immunology*, **24** (3–4), 247–67.

156. Belghith, M., Bluestone, J.A., Barriot, S. *et al.* (2003) TGF-beta-dependent mechanisms mediate restoration of self-tolerance induced by antibodies to CD3 in overt autoimmune diabetes. *Nature Medicine*, **9** (9), 1202–8.

157. Herold, K.C., Gitelman, S.E., Masharani, U. *et al.* (2005) A single course of anti-CD3 monoclonal antibody hOKT3gamma1(Ala–Ala) results in improvement in C-peptide responses and clinical parameters for at least 2 years after onset of type 1 diabetes. *Diabetes*, **54** (6), 1763–9.

28

Non pharmacological Prevention of Type 2 Diabetes

Jaakko Tuomilehto

Department of Epidemiology and Health Promotion, National Public Health Institute, Helsinki, Finland

28.1 INTRODUCTION

The primary prevention of type 2 diabetes (T2D) was first proposed by Dr E. Joslin in 1921 [1], but only after decades was its importance slowly recognized by others [2]. To be able to prevent a chronic disease such as T2D it is necessary to have knowledge about its natural history with a preclinical phase, modifiable risk factors, an effective and simple screening tool to identify high-risk subjects and an effective intervention that is affordable and acceptable and proven under a clinical trial setting. It is well known that obesity, unbalanced diet and physical inactivity are the major risk factors, and in people genetically predisposed to the disease the probability of developing T2D is very high once exposed to an 'unhealthy' lifestyle. In understanding the potential for prevention of T2D it is important to know what may be the magnitude of effects of a preventive lifestyle intervention. The development of T2D is a slow process that will take a long time, involving both genetic and environmental effects [3, 4]. It is commonly agreed that T2D may develop only in subjects who carry a genetic predisposition to the disease; but, based on epidemiological observations, about half the population [5, 6], or even more in some populations [7], will have T2D during their lifetime. Therefore, it is likely that probably more than half of the population carry genes that permit T2D to develop. Even though

genetic effects are important for the development of the disease, it is not possible to modify them in order to prevent T2D.

Dr Joslin wrote in 1921 [1]:

> There are entirely too many diabetic patients in the country. Statistics for the last thirty years show so great an increase in the number that, unless this were in part explained by a better recognition of the disease, the outlook for the future would be startling. Therefore, it is proper at the present time to devote attention not alone to treatment, but still more, as in the campaign against the typhoid fever, to prevention. The results may not be quite so striking or as immediate, but they are sure to come and to be important.

Until recently, proper evidence regarding the prevention of T2D tested and confirmed under a randomized clinical trial setting has been virtually missing.

28.2 WHY PRIMARY PREVENTION OF T2D?

T2D is a very expensive disease: about 10–15% of the total health care costs in developed countries are spent on treating T2D and, in particular, its complications [8, 9]. Therefore, prevention of T2D itself is desirable to avoid late complications of T2D and related costs. Efficacy of prevention in

The Epidemiology of Diabetes Mellitus, second edition   Edited by Jean-Marie Ekoé, Marian Rewers, Rhys Williams and Paul Zimmet
© 2008 John Wiley & Sons, Ltd

subjects with impaired glucose tolerance (IGT) has been tested and currently the evidence that we can prevent or delay the onset of T2D is unequivocal and strong.

There are some 'natural' experiments available in which ethnic groups have experienced rapid westernization and with it a rapid increase in the rates of obesity and T2D [10]. Therefore, it is logical to assume that by reversing these lifestyle changes it would be possible to prevent the development of the disease. Such a potential for the reversibility has been shown among Australian Aboriginals by O'Dea [11]. In these experiments, hyperglycemic people returned back to nature living in a traditional hunter–gatherer way of life. As a result, hyperglycemia reversed.

T2D develops as a result of complex multi-factorial process with both lifestyle and genetic origins. The main risk factors for T2D are obesity and sedentary lifestyle [12]. A 'westernized' dietary pattern with low fiber [13–15] and high saturated [16] and trans fats [17], refined carbohydrates [18], sweetened beverages [19], sodium [20] and red meat [21, 22] intake has been shown to be associated with increased T2D risk. Another feature of modern lifestyle, voluntary sleep deprivation, also increases diabetes risk [23, 24]. Fortunately, there are also protective factors in the modern lifestyle: the data are accumulating on decreased T2D risk associated with coffee [25–27] and moderate alcohol, particularly wine consumption [28].

It is a well-known fact that antidiabetic drug treatment in T2D has only a limited effect on glycemic control, which deteriorates with diabetes duration despite intensive treatment, as demonstrated, for instance, in the United Kingdom Prospective Diabetes Study [29]. Thus, it is obvious that interventions to prevent increase in blood glucose must start much earlier than at the time when clinical symptoms of diabetes occur, ideally before glucose levels reach the values considered as diabetes or clinical symptoms due to the disease. Of the people with IGT, approximately half have T2D during a 10-year follow-up [30, 31], and the rate of progression in Asian populations seems to be even faster [32, 33]. It is well known that the risk of complications begins in the prediabetic phase prior to the glucose levels reaching diagnostic cut-points for T2D [8, 34, 35]. Thus, waiting until individuals attain the

diagnostic criteria for T2D will result in significant morbidity and mortality from cardiovascular disease (CVD).

Another very important reason for the primary prevention of T2D is the high costs related to the disease. It is estimated that, currently, 10–15% of the entire health care expenditure goes on the treatment of diabetes, and the vast majority of it on the secondary and tertiary care of T2D patients who have late complications, primarily CVD [36, 37]. With increasing numbers of diabetic patients worldwide, this proportion will inevitably rise. The only logical way to prevent this projected increase in health care costs is to prevent or postpone the onset of T2D.

28.3 MAJOR LIFESTYLE TRIALS IN PREVENTION OF T2D

One of the early randomized intervention studies was the Malmöhus study in Sweden [38] comprised 267 men. A significant difference in the rates of development of T2D was found between IGT subjects randomized to dietary intervention compared with those randomized to no therapy. Unclear is what kind of dietary advice was actually given and how well the men randomized to the diet group followed this advice. Nevertheless, this trial suggested that the worsening from IGT to T2D could be prevented or delayed. More recently, a few trials have tested this hypothesis: we may call them the 'major lifestyle trials in prevention of T2D'. A summary of the randomized controlled trials (RCTs) in the prevention of T2D using lifestyle intervention is given in **Table 28.1**.

28.3.1 The Malmö Feasibility Study

The feasibility of diet and exercise intervention in 217 men with IGT was assessed in the Malmö feasibility study [41]. The effect of exercise and diet ($n = 161$) was compared to a reference group ($n = 56$) with no intervention. The reference group consisted of men who themselves decided not to join the intervention program. Thus, the groups were not assigned at random. The lifestyle intervention was delivered in group sessions, aiming at reduction in the intake of refined sugar, simple carbohydrates, fat, saturated fat, energy and alcohol (if relevant)

Table 28.1 Summary of randomized clinical trials using lifestyle intervention in the prevention of T2D.

Study	No. of participants	Study participants	Mean age (years)	Duration (years)	Adherence (%)	Incidence in control group (%/year)	RRR (%)[b]
DPS (Finland) [41]	522	IGT; BMI >25 kg m^{-2}	55	3.2	92	6	58
DPP (United States) [39]	3234	IGT; BMI >24 kg m^{-2} FPG > 5.3 mmol l	51	3	92.5	10	58
Pan et al. (China)[a] [32]	577	IGT	45	6	92	15.7	38
Kosaka et al. (Japan) [40]	458	IGT (men); BMI > 24 kg m^{-2}	55	4	91.5	9.3	67
Indian DPP [33]	531	IGT	46	3	92.3	18.3	29

[a] Group randomization.
[b] RRR: relative risk reduction.

and increase in the intake of complex carbohydrates and vegetables. Physical activity training consisted of two weekly 60 min sessions with various dynamic activities.

By the end of the 5-year study period 11% of the intervention group and 29% of the reference group had developed diabetes. This study is important in demonstrating the feasibility of carrying out a diet–exercise program for 5 years among the volunteers and, furthermore, suggests that the incidence of T2D might be reduced by approximately 50%. Overall, the progression to diabetes in these Swedish men was relatively low even in the reference group compared with the data from the observational studies [3]. Even for those men who did not want to join the intervention program, some of them may have changed their lifestyle as a result of the screening program. Thus, these results based on intention-to-treat analysis may underestimate the true effect of lifestyle changes. The intervention resulted in significant changes in lifestyle and physiological parameters. While the results on diabetes risk in the Malmö feasibility study are likely to be due to the effects on diet and exercise, the nonrandomized study design limits the generalizability of the results.

28.3.2 The Da-Qing Study

Data on the preventive effect of a diet and exercise intervention have been reported in a cluster-randomized clinical trial in Da-Qing, China [32]. Altogether, 577 subjects (mean age 45.0 years, mean body mass index (BMI) 25.8 kg m^{-2}) with IGT were assigned to the control, exercise alone, diet alone or exercise plus diet groups. In clinics assigned to dietary intervention, the participants were encouraged to reduce weight if their BMI $\geq$ 25 kg m^{-2} (61% of all participants), aiming at 23 kg m^{-2}, otherwise a high-carbohydrate (55–65% of energy) and moderate-fat (25–30% of energy) diet was recommended. Counseling was done individually by physicians, and group sessions were also organized weekly for the first month, monthly for 3 months and every 3 months thereafter. In clinics assigned to physical exercise, counseling sessions were arranged at a similar frequency. The participants were encouraged to increase their level of leisure-time physical activity by at least 1–2 'units' per day. One unit would correspond, for instance, to 30 min slow walking, 10 min slow running or 5 min swimming.

The cumulative 6-year incidence of T2D was lower in each of the three intervention groups (41–46%) than with the control group (68%). In this study, the relative risk reduction was approximately 40% and the absolute risk reduction was 22–26% during the 6-year period. The progression from IGT to diabetes was high: more than 10% per year in the control group, which is more than usually reported in observational studies.

The study did not apply an individual allocation of study subjects to the intervention and control groups, but the participating clinics were assigned. Furthermore, the study subjects were relatively lean, making inferences, for instance, to European obese IGT subjects difficult. Body weight did not change in lean subjects, and there was a modest (~1 kg m^{-2}) reduction in subjects with baseline BMI > 25 kg m^{-2}.

28.3.3 The Finnish Diabetes Prevention Study

The results of the Diabetes Prevention Study (DPS) conducted in Finland provided the first convincing evidence from a proper randomized controlled trial that T2D can be prevented by lifestyle modification [42, 43]. A total of 522 persons (mean age 55 years, all with IGT) were randomized to either an intensive lifestyle or a control intervention. During an average of 3.2 years of follow-up, T2D incidence was reduced by 58% in the lifestyle group compared with the control group. The subjects in the intervention group had frequent consultation visits with a nutritionist (seven times during the first year and every 3 months thereafter). They received individual advice about how to achieve the intervention goals. These goals were (i) reduction in weight of ≥5%, (ii) total fat intake less than 30% of energy consumed, (iii) saturated fat intake less

than 10% of energy consumed, (iv) fiber intake of at least 15 g per 1000 kcal and (v) moderate exercise for 30 min per day or more. During the first year of the study, body weight decreased on average 4.5 kg in the intervention group and 1.0 kg in the control group subjects ($p < 0.0001$). Indicators of central adiposity and fasting glucose and insulin, 2 h post-challenge glucose and insulin, and HbA1c reduced significantly more in the intervention group than in the control group at the 1-year examination (**Figure 28.1**).

28.3.4 The Diabetes Prevention Program

The US Diabetes Prevention Program (DPP) [39] was completed 1 year after the DPS. In the DPP, 3234 individuals (mean age 51 years, mean BMI = 34.0 kg m^{-2}, all with IGT and fasting glucose ≥95 mg dl^{-1}) were randomized to receive intensive dietary and exercise counseling, metformin or placebo. The lifestyle intervention included a 16-session (individual and/or group) core curriculum for 24 weeks and a maintenance period thereafter, with monthly contacts between the case manager and participant [44]. Furthermore, many different exercise activities were offered. The main aims of the intervention were 7% weight reduction and 150 min of moderate physical activity in a week. The relative risk reduction after 2.8 years of follow-up in the lifestyle intervention

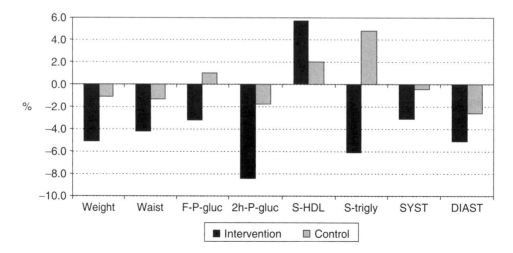

Figure 28.1 Changes in clinical and metabolic characteristics among the intervention and control group participants of the DPS.

group compared with the placebo control group was exactly as in the DPS, namely 58%. The effect of lifestyle was higher than the effect of metformin, which showed a 35% relative risk reduction compared with the placebo control group. During the first year of the intervention, weight reduction was 5.6 kg (~6%), with slight, gradual regain to the end of the study at year 4 [42].

28.3.5 Indian Diabetes Prevention Program

The Indian Diabetes Prevention Program (IDPP) [33] required 531 subjects with IGT (mean age 45.9 ± 5.7 years, BMI 25.8 ± 3.5 kg m^{-2}) who were randomized into four groups (control, lifestyle modification, metformin, and combined lifestyle modification and metformin). Lifestyle modification included advice on physical activity (30 min of brisk walking per day) and reduction in total calories, refined carbohydrates and fats, avoidance of sugar and inclusion of fiber-rich foods. The intervention included personal sessions at baseline and six-monthly, and monthly telephone contacts. The intensity of the intervention was thus lower than in the DPP and DPS. After median follow-up of 30 months, the relative risk reduction was 28.5% with lifestyle modification, 26.4% with metformin and 28.2% with lifestyle modification and metformin, compared with the control group. Thus, there was no added benefit from combining the drug and lifestyle interventions. In the control group, diabetes incidence was high (55.0% in 3 years) and comparable to the findings from the Chinese study [32]. These populations apparently have high rates of insulin resistance and IGT and lower thresholds for the risk factors for diabetes [45].

28.3.6 Japanese Prevention Trial

The Japanese trial with IGT males [40] included 458 men who were diagnosed with IGT in health screening and allocated randomly to receive either intensive lifestyle intervention ($n = 102$) or standard intervention ($n = 356$). The participants in the intensive intervention group visited hospital every 3–4 months, where they were given detailed, repeated advice to reduce body weight if BMI was ≥ 22 kg m^{-2} (otherwise, to maintain present weight) by consuming large amounts of vegetables and reducing the total amount of other food by 10% by, for example, using a smaller rice bowl. Intakes

of fat (<50 g per day) and alcohol (<50 g per day) were limited, as was eating out (no more than once a day), and physical activity was recommended (e.g. 30–40 min per day of walking). The participants in the control group visited hospital every 6 months and were given standard advice to eat smaller meals and increase physical activity.

The cumulative 4-year incidence of diabetes was 3% in the intervention group and 9.3% in the control group, with 67.4% risk reduction ($p < 0.001$). BMI at baseline was 23.8 ± 2.1 kg m^{-2} in the intervention group and 24.0 ± 2.3 kg m^{-2} in the control group. Body weight decreased by 2.18 kg in the intervention group and by 0.39 kg in the control group during the 4 years ($p < 0.001$). Thus, there was a remarkable reduction in diabetes risk despite the relatively modest weight reduction. Post hoc analyses in the control group revealed that diabetes incidence was positively correlated with change in body weight in this population; however, weight loss apparently was not the sole explanator of diabetes risk reduction.

28.4 LONG-TERM EFFECTIVENESS OF LIFESTYLE PREVENTION OF T2D

Several studies have demonstrated the benefit of healthy lifestyle on delaying the deterioration of glucose tolerance to manifest T2D, at least as long as the intervention continues [33, 39, 40, 43]. However, data on whether the risk reduction achieved during active counseling for lifestyle changes will last in the long term are scarce. The 12-year follow-up of the Malmö study [41, 46] revealed that the mortality rate among men in the former IGT intervention group was lower than among the men in the nonrandomized IGT group who received 'routine care' only (6.5 per 1000 person-years versus 14.0 per 1000 person-years, $p = 0.009$). The findings suggest that a long-term intervention program including dietary counseling and physical exercise will reduce mortality in subjects with IGT who are at an increased risk of premature death due to ischemic heart disease and other causes.

In a recent analysis using the data collected during the extended follow-up of the DPS we were able to show that, after a median of 7 years total follow-up, a marked reduction in the cumulative incidence of diabetes was sustained

[31]. The relative risk reduction during the total follow-up was 43%. More importantly, the effect of intervention on diabetes risk was maintained among those who after the intervention period were without diabetes: after median post-intervention follow-up time of 3 years, the number of incident new cases of T2D was 31 in the intervention group among 221 people at risk, and 38 in the control group among 185 people at risk. The corresponding incidence rates were 4.6 per 100 person-years and 7.2 per 100 person-years respectively (log-rank test $p = 0.0401$); that is, a 36% relative risk reduction. Thus, the absolute risk difference between groups increased slightly during the post-intervention period.

There is an important message from the public-health point of view: an intensive lifestyle intervention lasting for a limited time can yield long-term benefits in reducing the risk of T2D in high-risk individuals.

28.5 CLINICAL TRIAL EVIDENCE OF THE EFFECT OF LIFESTYLE FACTORS ON T2D RISK

In most of the published prevention trials the main aim was to see whether comprehensive lifestyle intervention reduces T2D risk. In the Chinese prevention study [32], an attempt to determine whether a diet or exercise intervention was more effective by randomizing the participating centers to diet only, physical activity only or diet plus physical activity intervention revealed no difference in outcome between the two interventions.

In the DPS, the risk of being diagnosed with diabetes was strongly associated with the number of lifestyle goals achieved [31]. Success in achieving the intervention goals in the DPS was estimated from the food records and exercise questionnaires. The success score (from 0 to 5) was calculated as the sum of lifestyle goals achieved. There was a strong inverse correlation between the success score and the incidence of diabetes during the total follow-up. This was especially apparent when the success in achieving the goals was assessed at year 3, which probably reflects the importance of sustained lifestyle changes. The hazard ratios were 1.00, 0.87, 0.67, 0.70 and 0.23, for success scores from 0 to 4–5 respectively (p for trend <0.001).

Because the question about the effects of different components of intervention is interesting, we did complete some post hoc analyses related to this issue. The independent effects of achieving the success score components at the 3-year examination was assessed by including each of the five lifestyle goal variables individually in a Cox model. Univariate hazard ratios for diabetes incidence (95% confidence interval (CI)) were 0.45 (0.31–0.64) for weight reduction from baseline, 0.65 (0.45–0.95) for intake of fat, 0.59 (0.31–1.13) for intake of saturated fat, 0.69 (0.49–0.96) for intake of fiber and 0.62 (0.46–0.84) for physical activity, comparing those who did or did not achieve the respective goal. When all the five success score components were simultaneously included in the Cox model, the multivariate-adjusted hazard ratios for diabetes (95% CI) were 0.43 (0.30–0.61) for weight reduction, 0.80 (0.48–1.34) for intake of fat, 0.55 (0.26–1.16) for intake of saturated fat, 0.97 (0.63–1.51) for intake of fiber and 0.80 (0.57–1.12) for physical activity. Furthermore, weight change was significantly associated with the achievement of each of the other four lifestyle goals; consequently, success score was strongly and inversely correlated with weight reduction [31].

Correspondingly, the reduction in body weight was reported to be the main determinant of risk reduction in the US DPP [47]. After adjustment for other components of the intervention, there was a 16% reduction in diabetes risk per 1 kg weight lost during the first year of the intervention. Furthermore, a lower percentage of calories from fat and increased physical activity predicted weight loss, and increased physical activity was important to help sustain weight loss. Achieving the physical activity goal of 150 min per week reduced diabetes risk, especially among those participants who did not achieve the weight reduction goal of 7%, with risk reduction of 44% compared with those who achieved neither the weight reduction nor the physical activity goal.

The findings suggest that dietary composition and physical activity are important in diabetes prevention, but their effect on diabetes risk is, in large part, although not entirely, mediated through resulting weight reduction. Nevertheless, due to multicollinearity, the interpretation of the results should be done cautiously. Also, it should be noted that in the IDPP [33] and Chinese prevention study [32] the participants were relatively lean and there was no large change in body weight; but despite that, a remarkable reduction in diabetes risk was apparent. Thus, in these studies, other components of the intervention than weight control were responsible for the beneficial effects on diabetes risk.

28.6 DOES THE RISK REDUCTION WORK IN THE ENTIRE POPULATION?

While we still await results from various actions that have been initiated to prevent T2D at the population level, we can use epidemiological data to estimate the potential for prevention under the scenario applied in the lifestyle intervention trials.

A recent prospective study based on the data from EPIC-Norfolk, United Kingdom, comprising 24 155 individuals at the baseline survey, estimated the association between the achievement of the five lifestyle goals used in the Finnish DPS (BMI $< 25 \, \text{kg m}^{-2}$, fat intake $<30\%$ of energy intake, saturated fat intake $<10\%$ of energy intake, fiber intake $\geq 15 \, \text{g}$ per 1000 kcal, and physical activity $>4 \, \text{h}$ per week) and the risk of developing diabetes during a follow-up (mean 4.6 years) [48]. The incidence of T2D was inversely related to the number of goals achieved ($p < 0.001$). None of the participants who met all five of the goals (0.8% of the total population) developed diabetes, whereas the risk of diabetes was highest in those who did not meet any of these goals. If the entire population were able to meet one more goal, then the total incidence of diabetes would be predicted to fall by 20%. This finding suggests that health promotion interventions that result in an increase in healthy lifestyle in the general population might significantly reduce the growing burden of T2D.

28.7 COSTS ASSOCIATED WITH LIFESTYLE INTERVENTION TO PREVENT T2D

Statistical simulation based on the DPP data [49] indicated that the DPP intervention in high-risk individuals would result in reduced lifetime cumulative incidence of microvascular, neuropathic and cardiovascular complications and improved survival

by 0.5 years (lifestyle) and 0.2 years (metformin). Cost-effectiveness would be improved if the interventions were implemented as they might be in routine clinical practice, with group intervention and generic medication. The DPP included a cost–benefit analysis that estimated that the per capita costs of the lifestyle intervention exceeded that of the usual care group by USD 3450 which translated to a cost of USD 15 700 per case of T2D prevented [50]. Lifetime cost–utility analysis showed an overall cost of USD 1100 per quality-adjusted life year gained by the lifestyle intervention [49]. Thus, these results unequivocally demonstrate that the lifestyle intervention is cost-effective from both short-term and lifetime perspectives. In the Finnish DPS, the lifestyle intervention was far less manpower intensive, but the benefits were identical to those attained in the DPP. Currently, the economic data are not available from the DPS.

A Dutch modeling study recently explored the health benefits and cost-effectiveness of both an intensive lifestyle intervention implemented in high-risk individuals (health care intervention) and community-based lifestyle program in the general population (community intervention) [51]. The results showed that both kinds of interventions to reduce the risk of T2D were cost-effective. Although the average lifetime benefit per individual for the community intervention is relatively low, gains on a population level may be substantial.

These long-term cost-effectiveness assessments have been based on the assumption that the lifestyle intervention will last with a similar intensity. However, the extended follow-up of the DPS demonstrated that the long-term health benefits may be obtained by a relatively short-term intensive intervention lasting a few years only [31]. When these results are taken into account in the economic analyses, the true long-term cost-effectiveness of the lifestyle intervention in the prevention of T2D is in reality much more favorable than estimated by the previous analyses of the DPP data.

The changes in the costs of an actual self-selected diet among the participants of the DPS were assessed based on the dietary intakes recorded with 3-day food diaries at the baseline and after the first year of intervention [52]. Food costs were obtained by using retail prices, and individual diet costs were calculated in euros by multiplying the weight of each food item consumed by its unit cost and summing overall foods and beverages consumed by each person over the 3-day period. At baseline, mean daily diet costs per individual were similar in the lifestyle intervention and the control groups. During the first year of the intervention, diet costs decreased slightly both in the intervention group and in the control group, with no difference between the groups. The only dietary determinant that was associated with change in diet costs was fiber density. Increase in dietary fiber density was related with a decrease in dietary costs. Thus, it seems that adopting a health-promoting diet in T2D prevention does not increase the diet costs.

28.8   DETECTION OF PEOPLE AT HIGH RISK FOR DEVELOPING T2D

By definition, people at high risk for developing T2D have no symptoms of diabetes and most of them are not aware of their high-risk status. Thus, even though they may have sufficient general knowledge about T2D prevention, they may not know that they could effectively reduce their own T2D risk with lifestyle changes. Some individuals at high risk, such as the offspring of T2D patients and women with previous gestational diabetes, may be generally aware of their risk status, but until now it has not been possible to quantify the level of risk. Without such quantitative information it is difficult for a lay person to take appropriate action. While much attention has been directed at detecting undiagnosed T2D in the past [53], only recently has attention turned to those with prediabetes and risk assessment.

In the detection of subject at high risk for T2D, two approaches may be applied. The first includes measuring blood glucose levels to explicitly determine prevalent prediabetes. This strategy results in detecting undiagnosed T2D, too. The second approach is to rely on demographic and clinical characteristics and previous laboratory tests (avoiding the need for new laboratory or glycemic tests) to determine the likelihood of future incident T2D. This strategy leaves current glycemic status and previously unrecognized T2D ambiguous.

While choosing among various tests and strategies, there will be a trade-off between sensitivity and specificity among the strategies, and the choice will depend on the goal and on relative health liabilities, such as false positive versus false negatives. A higher false positive rate of a test may be tolerable, if the burden imposed by confirmatory testing is not great and the treatment is relatively harmless and inexpensive. On the other hand, if the consequences of not treating in a timely manner are not great, then a higher false negative rate of the screening test may be acceptable. If a strategy does not use determination of an oral glucose tolerance test (OGTT) or fasting blood glucose, then an individual's glucose tolerance status cannot be explicitly determined. However, it should be noted that the level of risk of having or developing future T2D can be assessed.

Most strategies use risk factors and biochemical testing with three approaches: combinations of risk factors with various cut-points, and statistical models that incorporate risk factors as discrete or as continuous values. Diabetes 'risk scores,' where each risk factor is assigned a weight or score derived from a comprehensive risk factor model, have received increasing attention [54]. Different approaches all tend to perform in a moderately effective range, although formal comparisons have not been made.

It is necessary to separate three different scenarios: (i) general population; (ii) subjects with assumed metabolic abnormalities (obese, hypertensive, family history of diabetes); and (iii) patients with prevalent CVD. The general population may be dealt with applying the strategy that uses the assessment of the future risk of T2D as the primary screening tool combined with subsequent glucose testing in those identified with a high risk. For public health purposes, a risk assessment tool for T2D was developed in Finland [55]. This Finnish Diabetes Risk Score (FINDRISC) is based on easily available information and it uses eight parameters (**Figure 28.2**; **Table 28.2**). The FINDRISC was shown to predict the 10-year risk of (drug-treated) T2D with 78–81% sensitivity and 76–77% specificity, and it also detects asymptomatic T2D and abnormal glucose tolerance [56] reasonably well. It was recently validated in the Italian population with identical results [57]. In addition to the prediction of T2D, FINDRISC also predicts the incidence of myocardial infarction and stroke [58]. In addition to the FINDRISC, there are similar types of diabetes risk assessment tools in other countries [59–61].

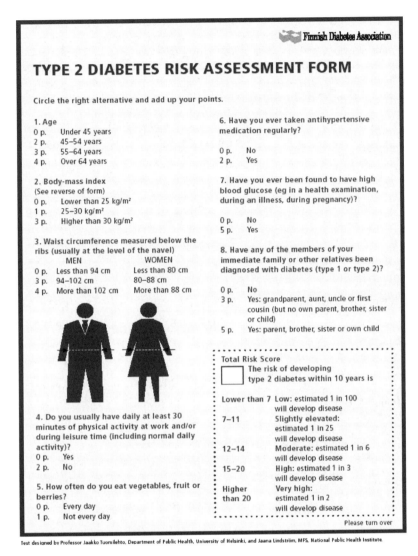

Figure 28.2 The Finnish Diabetes Risk Score (FINDRISC) [55, 56], www.diabetes.fi.

28.9 CONCLUSION

With compelling evidence that T2D can be prevented or delayed, strategies to implement the primary prevention of T2D both in high-risk subjects and at the population level are urgently needed. While the T2D prevention trials rigorously defined populations by explicitly characterizing their glycemic status, these studies did not include all groups at risk of developing T2D. Methods that can also define other groups at high risk for developing T2D have recently been developed and are increasingly being used in several countries, but direct evidence that these groups will benefit from the prevention interventions is thus far lacking.

Groups that will be the targets for prevention efforts can be identified though several reasonably effective strategies. However, there is no universal well-tested method that will identify all those at high risk of developing T2D, and there may be some variation in the optimal strategies for different populations and regions around the world. It is also important to realize that the identification of people having a high risk of T2D or asymptomatic T2D is not identical with the diagnosis of T2D. In practice, we can identify people at high risk with simple and

Table 28.2 Multivariate logistic regression model to predict diabetes during 10-year follow-up.

	Odds ratio (95% CI)	Coefficient β	Score*
Intercept	–	−5.658	
Age (years)			
<45	1	0	0
45–54	1.92 (1.13–3.25)	0.650	2
55–64	2.56 (1.53–4.28)	0.940	3
BMI (kg m^{-2})			
≤25	1	0	0
>25 to 30	1.02 (0.48–2.15)	0.015	1
>30	2.55 (1.10–5.92)	0.938	3
Waist circumference (cm)			
Men <94, women <80	1	0	0
Men 94 to <102, women 80 to <88	2.78 (1.43–5.40)	1.021	3
Men ≥102, women ≥ 88	4.16 (2.00–8.63)	1.424	4
Blood pressure medication			
No	1	0	0
Yes	2.04 (1.45–2.88)	0.714	2
History of high blood glucose			
No	1	0	0
Yes	9.61 (6.31–14.63)	2.263	5
Physical activity			
4 h per week or more	1	0	0
<4 h per week	1.31 (0.88–1.95)	0.268	2
Consumption of vegetables, fruits or berries			
Every day	1	0	0
Less often than once a day	1.18 (0.85–1.64)	0.165	1
Area under the ROC curve		0.860	0.852

cost-efficient tools. The main question, however, is how to implement an efficient preventive strategy in those identified to be at high risk; that is, how to translate the results of the recent successful T2D prevention trials to a real-life setting. Regarding the early diagnosis of T2D, a lot of attention has been paid to the methodology for the assessment of glycemia, and less on the coverage of the detection of T2D, that is asymptomatic for a long time. The evidence is compelling that, without applying an OGTT or an assessment of postprandial glucose, a large proportion of early cases of T2D will remain unrecognized.

References

1. Joslin, E. (1921) The prevention of diabetes mellitus. *The Journal of the American Medical Association*, **76**, 79–84.
2. WHO Study Group (1994) Primary Prevention of Diabetes Mellitus. Tech. Rep. Ser. 844, WHO, Geneva.

3. Knowler, W., Narayan, K., Hanson, R. *et al.*
    (1995) Perspectives in diabetes. Preventing
    non-insulin-dependent diabetes. *Diabetes*, **44**,
    483–8.
4. Neel, J.V. (1962) Diabetes mellitus: a "thrifty"
    genotype rendered detrimental by progress? *American Journal of Human Genetics*, **14**, 353–62.
5. The DECODA Study Group (2003) Age- and
    sex-specific prevalence of diabetes and impaired
    glucose regulation in 11 Asian cohorts. *Diabetes
    Care*, **26**, 1770–80.
6. The DECODE Study Group (2003) Age- and
    sex-specific prevalences of diabetes and impaired
    glucose regulation in 13 European cohorts. *Diabetes
    Care*, **26**, 61–9.
7. Bennett, P.H., Bogardus, C., Tuomilehto, J. and
    Zimmet, P. (1992) Epidemiology and natural
    history of NIDDM: non-obese and obese, in
    International Textbook of Diabetes, John Wiley
    & Sons, Ltd.
8. Haffner, S.M., Stern, M.P., Hazuda, H.P. *et al.*
    (1990) Cardiovascular risk factors in confirmed
    prediabetic individuals. Does the clock for coronary
    heart disease start ticking before the onset of clinical
    diabetes? *The Journal of the American Medical
    Association*, **263**, 2893–8.
9. Harris, M., Klein, R., Welborn, T. and Knuiman, M.
    (1992) Onset of NIDDM occurs at least 4–7
    years before clinical diagnosis. *Diabetes Care*, **15**,
    815–19.
10. Zimmet, P., Alberti, K.G. and Shaw, J. (2001)
    Global and societal implications of the diabetes
    epidemic. *Nature*, **414**, 782–7.
11. O'Dea, K. (1980) Marked improvement in carbo-
    hydrate and lipid metabolism in diabetic Australian
    Aborigines after temporary reversion to traditional
    lifestyle. *Diabetes*, **33** (6), 596–603.
12. WHO Study Group (1985) Diabetes Mellitus. Tech.
    Rep. Ser. 727, WHO, Geneva.
13. Salmeron, J., Manson, J.E., Stampfer, M.J. *et al.*
    (1997) Dietary fiber, glycemic load, and risk of
    non-insulin-dependent diabetes mellitus in women.
    The Journal of the American Medical Association,
    277, 472–7.
14. Schulze, M.B., Liu, S., Rimm, E.B. *et al.* (2004)
    Glycemic index, glycemic load, and dietary fiber
    intake and incidence of type 2 diabetes in younger
    and middle-aged women. *The American Journal of
    Clinical Nutrition*, **80**, 348–56.
15. Montonen, J., Knekt, P., Järvinen, R. *et al.* (2003)
    Whole-grain and fiber intake and the incidence of
    type 2 diabetes. *The American Journal of Clinical
    Nutrition*, **77**, 622–9.
16. Feskens, E.J., Virtanen, S.M., Räsänen, L. *et al.*
    (1995) Dietary factors determining diabetes and

impaired glucose tolerance. A 20-year follow-up
    of the Finnish and Dutch cohorts of the Seven
    Countries Study. *Diabetes Care*, **18**, 1104–12.
17. Salmeron, J., Hu, F.B., Manson, J.E. *et al.* (2001)
    Dietary fat intake and risk of type 2 diabetes
    in women. *The American Journal of Clinical
    Nutrition*, **73**, 1019–26.
18. Hodge, A.M., English, D.R., O'Dea, K. and Giles,
    G.G. (2004) Glycemic index and dietary fiber and
    the risk of type 2 diabetes. *Diabetes Care*, **27**,
    2701–6.
19. Schulze, M.B., Manson, J.E., Ludwig, D.S. *et al.*
    (2004) Sugar-sweetened beverages, weight gain,
    and incidence of type 2 diabetes in young and
    middle-aged women. *The Journal of the American
    Medical Association*, **292**, 927–34.
20. Hu, G., Jousilahti, P., Peltonen, M. *et al.* (2005)
    Urinary sodium and potassium excretion and the
    risk of type 2 diabetes: a prospective study in
    Finland. *Diabetologia*, **48**, 1477–83.
21. Fung, T.T., Schulze, M., Manson, J.E. *et al.* (2004)
    Dietary patterns, meat intake, and the risk of type 2
    diabetes in women. *Archives of Internal Medicine*,
    164, 2235–40.
22. Song, Y., Manson, J.E., Buring, J.E. and Liu, S.
    (2004) A prospective study of red meat consump-
    tion and type 2 diabetes in middle-aged and elderly
    women: the women's health study. *Diabetes Care*,
    27, 2108–15.
23. Ayas, N.T., White, D.P., Al-Delaimy, W.K. *et al.*
    (2003) A prospective study of self-reported sleep
    duration and incident diabetes in women. *Diabetes
    Care*, **26**, 380–4.
24. Mallon, L., Broman, J.-E. and Hetta, J. (2005) High
    incidence of diabetes in men with sleep complaints
    or short sleep duration: a 12-year follow-up study
    of a middle-aged population. *Diabetes Care*, **28**,
    2762–7.
25. Salazar-Martinez, E., Willett, W.C., Ascherio, A.
    et al. (2004) Coffee consumption and risk for type 2
    diabetes mellitus. *Annals of Internal Medicine*, **140**,
    1–8.
26. Tuomilehto, J., Hu, G., Bidel, S. *et al.* (2004) Coffee
    consumption and risk of type 2 diabetes mellitus
    among middle-aged Finnish men and women. *The
    Journal of the American Medical Association*, **291**,
    1213–19.
27. Van Dam, R.M., Willett, W.C., Manson, J.E. and
    Hu, F.B. (2006) Coffee, caffeine, and risk of type 2
    diabetes: a prospective cohort study in younger
    and middle-aged U.S. women. *Diabetes Care*, **29**,
    398–403.
28. Hodge, A.M., English, D.R., O'Dea, K. and Giles,
    G.G. (2006) Alcohol intake, consumption pattern
    and beverage type, and the risk of type 2 diabetes.

Diabetic Medicine: A Journal of the British Diabetic Association, **23**, 690–7.

29. UK Prospective Diabetes Study (UKPDS) Group (1995) UK prospective diabetes study 16: overview of six years' therapy of type 2 diabetes – a progressive disease. *Diabetes*, **44**, 1249–58.

30. Knowler, W.C., Narayan, K.M., Hanson, R.L. *et al.* (1995) Preventing non-insulin-dependent diabetes. *Diabetes*, **44**, 483–8.

31. Lindström, J., Ilanne-Parikka, P., Peltonen, M. *et al.* (2006) Sustained reduction in the incidence of type 2 diabetes by lifestyle intervention: the follow-up results of the Finnish Diabetes Prevention Study. *Lancet*, **368**, 1673–9.

32. Pan, X.R., Li, G.W., Hu, Y.H. *et al.* (1997) Effects of diet and exercise in preventing NIDDM in people with impaired glucose tolerance. The Da Qing IGT and Diabetes Study. *Diabetes Care*, **20**, 537–44.

33. Ramachandran, A., Snehalatha, C., Mary, S. *et al.* (2006) The Indian Diabetes Prevention Programme shows that lifestyle modification and metformin prevent type 2 diabetes in Asian Indian subjects with impaired glucose tolerance (IDPP-1). *Diabetologia*, **49**, 289–97.

34. The DECODE Study Group (2001) Glucose tolerance and cardiovascular mortality: comparison of fasting and 2-hour diagnostic criteria. *Archives of Internal Medicine*, **161**, 397–405.

35. Qiao, Q., Jousilahti, P., Eriksson, J. and Tuomilehto, J. (2003) Predictive properties of impaired glucose tolerance for cardiovascular risk are not explained by the development of overt diabetes during follow-up. *Diabetes Care*, **26**, 2910–14.

36. Henriksson, F., Agardh, C.D., Berne, C. *et al.* (2000) Direct medical costs for patients with type 2 diabetes in Sweden. *Journal of Internal Medicine*, **248**, 387–96.

37. Williams, R., Van Gaal, L. and Lucioni, C. (2002) Assessing the impact of complications on the costs of type II diabetes. *Diabetologia*, **45**, S13–17.

38. Sartor, G., Schersten, B., Carlstrom, S. *et al.* (1980) Ten-year follow-up of subjects with impaired glucose tolerance. Prevention of diabetes by tolbutamide and diet regulation. *Diabetes*, **29**, 41–9.

39. The Diabetes Prevention Program Research Group (2002) Reduction in the incidence of type 2 diabetes with lifestyle intervention or metformin. *The New England Journal of Medicine*, **346**, 393–403.

40. Kosaka, K., Noda, M. and Kuzuya, T. (2005) Prevention of type 2 diabetes by lifestyle intervention: a Japanese trial in IGT males. *Diabetes Research and Clinical Practice*, **67**, 152–62.

41. Eriksson, K.F. and Lindgärde, F. (1991) Prevention of type 2 (non-insulin-dependent) diabetes mellitus by diet and physical exercise. The 6-year Malmö feasibility study. *Diabetologia*, **34**, 891–8.

42. Lindström, J., Louheranta, A., Mannelin, M. *et al.* (2003) The Finnish Diabetes Prevention Study (DPS): lifestyle intervention and 3-year results on diet and physical activity. *Diabetes Care*, **26**, 3230–6.

43. Tuomilehto, J., Lindström, J., Eriksson, J.G. *et al.* (2001) Prevention of type 2 diabetes mellitus by changes in lifestyle among subjects with impaired glucose tolerance. *The New England Journal of Medicine*, **344**, 1343–50.

44. The Diabetes Prevention Program Research Group (2002) The Diabetes Prevention Program (DPP): description of lifestyle intervention. *Diabetes Care*, **25**, 2165–71.

45. Ramachandran, A., Snehalatha, C. and Vijay, V. (2004) Low risk threshold for acquired diabetogenic factors in Asian Indians. *Diabetes Research and Clinical Practice*, **65**, 189–95.

46. Eriksson, K.F. and Lindgarde, F. (1998) No excess 12-year mortality in men with impaired glucose tolerance who participated in the Malmö preventive trial with diet and exercise. *Diabetologia*, **41**, 1010–16.

47. Hamman, R.F., Wing, R.R., Edelstein, S.L. *et al.* (2006) Effect of weight loss with lifestyle intervention on risk of diabetes. *Diabetes Care*, **29**, 2102–7.

48. Simmons, R.K., Harding, A.H., Jakes, R.W. *et al.* (2006) How much might achievement of diabetes prevention behaviour goals reduce the incidence of diabetes if implemented at the population level? *Diabetologia*, **49**, 905–11.

49. Herman, W.H., Hoerger, T.J., Brandle, M. *et al.* (2005) The cost-effectiveness of lifestyle modification or metformin in preventing type 2 diabetes in adults with impaired glucose tolerance. *Annals of Internal Medicine*, **142**, 323–32.

50. The Diabetes Prevention Program Research Group (2003) Costs associated with the primary prevention of type 2 diabetes mellitus in the Diabetes Prevention Program. *Diabetes Care*, **26**, 36–47.

51. Jacobs-van der Bruggen, M.A.M., Bos, G., Bemelmans, W.J. *et al.* (2007) Lifestyle interventions are cost-effective in people with different levels of diabetes risk: results from a modeling study. *Diabetes Care*, **30**, 128–34.

52. Ottelin, A.M., Lindström, J., Peltonen, M. *et al.* (2007) Costs of a self-selected, health-promoting

diet among the participants of the Finnish Diabetes Prevention Study. *Diabetes Care* **30**, 1275–7.

53. Harris, M.I. (1993) Undiagnosed NIDDM: clinical and public health issues. *Diabetes Care*, **16**, 642–52.

54. Engelgau, M.M., Colagiuri, S., Ramachandran, A. *et al.* (2004) Prevention of type 2 diabetes: issues and strategies for identifying persons for interventions. *Diabetes Technology and Therapeutics*, **6**, 874–82.

55. Lindström, J. and Tuomilehto, J. (2003) The diabetes risk score: a practical tool to predict type 2 diabetes risk. *Diabetes Care*, **26**, 725–31.

56. Saaristo, T., Peltonen, M., Lindström, J. *et al.* (2005) Cross-sectional evaluation of the Finnish Diabetes Risk Score: a tool to identify undetected type 2 diabetes, abnormal glucose tolerance and metabolic syndrome. *Diabetes and Vascular Disease Research*, **2**, 67–72.

57. Franciosi, M., De Berardis, G., Rossi, M.C. *et al.* (2005) Use of the diabetes risk score for opportunistic screening of undiagnosed diabetes and impaired glucose tolerance: the IGLOO (Impaired Glucose Tolerance and Long-Term Outcomes Observational) study. *Diabetes Care*, **28**, 1187–94.

58. Silventoinen, K., Pankow, J., Lindström, J. *et al.* (2005) The validity of the Finnish Diabetes Risk Score for the prediction of the incidence of coronary heart disease and stroke, and total mortality. *European Journal of Cardiovascular Prevention and Rehabilitation*, **12**, 451–8.

59. Glümer, C., Carstensen, B., Sandbaek, A. *et al.* (2004) A Danish diabetes risk score for targeted screening: the Inter99 study. *Diabetes Care*, **27**, 727–33.

60. Griffin, S.J., Little, P.S., Hales, C.N. *et al.* (2000) Diabetes risk score: towards earlier detection of type 2 diabetes in general practice. *Diabetes/Metabolism Research and Reviews*, **16**, 164–71.

61. Ruige, J.B., de Neeling, J.N., Kostense, P.J. *et al.* (1997) Performance of an NIDDM screening questionnaire based on symptoms and risk factors. *Diabetes Care*, **20**, 491–6.

29

Pharmacological Prevention of Type 2 Diabetes

André J. Scheen

Division of Diabetes, Nutrition and Metabolic Disorders, Department of Medicine, CHU Sart Tilman, University of Liège, Liège, Belgium

29.1 INTRODUCTION

Type 2 diabetes mellitus (T2DM) is associated with excess morbidity and mortality, and is considered as one of the most costly and burdensome chronic diseases of our time [1–3]. It is a dynamic disease with dual defects, that is it is a progressive insulin secretory defect combined with insulin resistance [4–6], and is intimately linked to the so-called metabolic syndrome and an increased risk of cardiovascular disease [7]. It is well established that the development of T2DM results from an interaction of a subject's genetic makeup and their environment [6]. With the increasing prevalence of obesity, the prevalence of diabetes is reaching epidemic proportions [3, 8]. The development of obesity seems to be an important factor portending the development of insulin resistance [9], which in the presence of a genetically determined propensity to β-cell dysfunction results in alterations in glucose tolerance, leading to impaired glucose tolerance (IGT), impaired fasting glucose (IFG) and T2DM [6, 10]. Several risk factors have been identified, allowing the screening of so-called high-risk individuals [11, 12]. On the basis of an expert consensus, the American Diabetes Association recommends clinicians consider screening for T2DM individuals with such risk factors as family history, overweight/obesity and hypertension [13].

Prevention programs of T2DM depend on the identification of potentially modifiable risk factors

[14]. Recently, a great deal of effort has been made on slowing or even preventing the development of T2DM in high-risk subjects [15, 16]. In this context, a lifestyle intervention, typically comprising a combination of diet and exercise, can reduce the risk of progression from IGT to T2DM by up to 58% [17, 18]. The precise mechanisms by which lifestyle changes reduce the rate of development of T2DM in these prevention studies have yet to be reported. However, one can anticipate that the resultant weight loss, although rather modest, was associated with improved insulin sensitivity [19]. While lifestyle modifications are clearly beneficial in reducing the risk of developing T2DM, they cannot be implemented in all clinical settings and are not practical for all subjects [20–22]. In addition to lifestyle strategies, various pharmacological approaches have already proven their efficacy in preventing or delaying T2DM [23, 24]. Therefore, drug therapy targeting insulin resistance, β-cell function or both may be considered to prevent T2DM [25]. Primary prevention may be important in the pediatric population because of the rapidly increasing risk in adolescents due to the obesity epidemics, although no long-term clinical trial is available in this population yet [26]. Almost all antihyperglycemic agents used for the treatment of T2DM [27] have been assessed or are currently evaluated in clinical trials aiming to prevent the development of T2DM in high-risk patients: insulin

The Epidemiology of Diabetes Mellitus, second edition Edited by Jean-Marie Ekoé, Marian Rewers, Rhys Williams and Paul Zimmet
© 2008 John Wiley & Sons, Ltd

Table 29.1 Placebo-controlled randomized clinical trials assessing the effect of metformin, acarbose and thiazolidinediones on the incidence of new-onset diabetes in patients with impaired glucose tolerance.

Trial (Reference)	Drug	Daily dose (mg)	F-U (years)	N	RR (95% CI)	P
US DPP [18]	Metformin	850 b.i.d.	2.8	2155	0.69 (0.57–0.83)	0.001
CDPS [44]	Metformin	250 t.i.d.	3	261	0.23 (NA)	0.0002
EDIT [45]	Metformin	500 t.i.d.	6	631	0.99 (NA)	0.94
Indian DPP [46]	Metformin	250 b.i.d.	2.5	531	0.74 (0.65–0.81)	0.029
TRIPOD [61]	Troglitazone	400 o.d.	2.5	236	0.45 (0.25–0.83)	0.01
US DPP [65]	Troglitazone	400 o.d.	0.9	585	0.25 (NA)	0.02
DREAM [66]	Rosiglitazone	8 o.d.	3.0	5269	0.40 (0.35–0.46)	0.0001
STOP-NIDDM [71]	Acarbose	100 t.i.d.	3.2	1368	0.75 (0.63–0.90)	0.0015
CDPS [44]	Acarbose	50 t.i.d.	3	261	0.12 (NA)	0.00001
EDIT [45]	Acarbose	50 t.i.d.	6	631	1.04 (NA)	0.81
	Acarbose	50 t.i.d.	6	?[a]	0.66 (NA)	0.046
ACT-NOW	Pioglitazone	45 o.d.	2.6	602	0.19 (0.09-0.39)	0.00001

F-U: follow-up; RR: relative risk of developing diabetes versus placebo; 95% CI, 95% confidence interval; NA, not available.

[a] Subgroup of patients (n = NA) with impaired glucose tolerance (IGT) at baseline.

secretagogues (sulfonylureas and glinides), metformin, thiazolidinediones (glitazones), acarbose and even insulin (**Table 29.1**) [28, 29]. One key question when analyzing the results of these trials is to be able to distinguish between a true preventing, a delaying or only a masking effect of diabetes by the antihyperglycemic effect of the drug [30, 31]. As obesity plays a crucial role in the pathophysiology of T2DM, antiobesity agents may be considered for the prevention of diabetes in overweight/obese patients, especially those with abdominal obesity [9]. Various antiobesity compounds, such as orlistat, sibutramine and rimonabant, have been or are currently evaluated to prove their efficacy in preventing the development of T2DM [28, 29]. Because of the complex pathophysiology of T2DM [5, 6, 10], other pharmacological strategies have also been considered. On the one hand, lipotoxicity has been shown to promote both insulin resistance and defect in insulin secretion [32]. Therefore, lipid-lowering agents may theoretically be used in an attempt to prevent T2DM, although observational data in clinical trials with statins and fibrates gave rather disappointing results [28, 29]. On the other hand, activation of the rennin–angiotensin–aldosterone

system (RAAS) appears to have deleterious effects on glucose metabolism, and numerous trials have analyzed the potential beneficial effects of angiotensin-converting enzyme (ACE) inhibitors or of angiotensin receptor blockers (ARBs), especially in patients with cardiovascular disease [33]. In postmenopausal women, combined therapy with estrogen and progestin has also been shown to be associated with a reduction in the incidence of T2DM, despite a negative effect on cardiovascular risk [34]. A major objective in the future will be to compare the clinical outcomes and cost-effectiveness of all these strategies for managing people at high risk for diabetes, especially pharmacological approaches with intensive lifestyle intervention [35].

The aim of the present review chapter is to describe and discuss the results of clinical trials demonstrating a preventive effect of various pharmacological compounds in the development of T2DM in at-risk individuals. We will successively consider the effects of various glucose-lowering agents, antiobesity drugs, lipid-lowering agents and inhibitors of the RAAS, to end up with various agents (estrogens) and new perspectives (anti-inflammatory compounds).

29.2 PREVENTION BY GLUCOSE-LOWERING AGENTS

29.2.1 Metformin

Metformin is now considered as the first-line drug for the treatment of T2DM [36] and appears to exert several metabolic effects that may be favorable in patients with abdominal obesity and IGT [37, 38]. Metformin primarily reduces glucose output from the liver, despite no reduction in liver fat [39], and could also increase (although to a rather small extent) glucose uptake in the peripheral tissues in the presence of insulin, thereby reducing demand on the beta cell. Interestingly, favorable effects of metformin on body mass index (BMI) and glucose tolerance have also been observed in obese adolescents with fasting hyperinsulinemia and a family history of T2DM, a subgroup of individuals who are known to be at high risk of later developing diabetes [40]. A few old studies investigating biguanides (metformin) found no significant reduction in the incidence of T2DM compared with placebo using intention-to-treat analyses. However, all of these studies had very low diabetes incidence and were likely underpowered [28].

The largest and most methodologically rigorous trial was the Diabetes Prevention Program (DPP) performed in the United States [18]. It randomized 2155 individuals (age 51 years, BMI $34\,kg\,m^{-2}$, 45% high-risk minority groups) with IGT to metformin (850 mg twice a day (b.i.d.)) or placebo (another arm assessed the effect of intensive lifestyle intervention). After a mean follow-up period of 2.8 years, the incidence of new diabetes was 7.8% in the placebo-treated patients versus 4.8% in those treated with metformin (relative risk (RR) = 0.69, 95% confidence interval (CI) 0.57–0.83). To prevent one case of diabetes during a period of 3 years (number needed to treat (NNT)), 14 would have to receive metformin. In post hoc subgroup analyses, the benefits of metformin were primarily observed in young patients (>60 years) and in obese patients (BMI > $35\,kg\,m^{-2}$). In order to avoid a direct metabolic effect of the drug [41], subjects were submitted to a final investigation after a 1–2 weeks washout period. In the 79% of eligible patients who completed this last visit, the incidence of diabetes increased from 25.2 to 30.6% in the metformin group and from 33.4 to

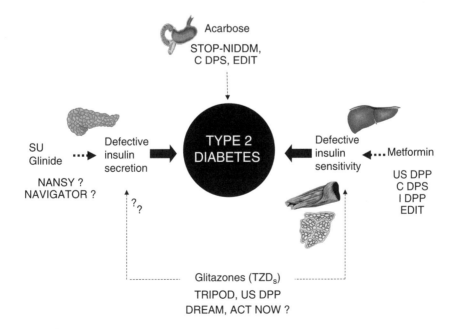

Figure 29.1 Illustration of the sites of action of oral glucose-lowering agents used in the various clinical trials of prevention of type 2 diabetes in high-risk patients (mainly because of impaired glucose tolerance). ? = results not available yet.

36.7% in the placebo group [42]. When results of the washout period were included in the overall analysis, metformin still significantly decreased diabetes incidence (RR = 0.75, 95% CI 0.62–0.92). However, as pointed out [31], the washout period was rather short (1–2 weeks only), which could not definitely exclude a partial masking effect [43]. Moreover, because type 2 diabetes is a progressive disease [4, 5, 10] and because the study was rather short (2.8 years), it remains to demonstrate whether the effect attributed to metformin is really a true preventing effect rather than only a delaying effect [30]. Finally, it should be pointed out that the reduction in the incidence of T2DM with metformin (31%) was lower than that obtained with intensive lifestyle intervention (58%) [18].

In the Chinese Diabetes Prevention Study, subjects with mild overweight (BMI = $25 \, \text{kg m}^{-2}$; age 50 years) and IGT were divided into a control group ($n = 85$) which received conventional education, a metformin group ($n = 88$, 250 mg three times a day (t.i.d.)) and an acarbose group ($n = 88$, 50 mg t.i.d.) (see Section 29.2.4) [44]. Over a 3-year period, 34.9% in the control group versus 12.4% in the metformin group progressed to diabetes. This represents an impressive risk reduction of 76.8% for metformin, despite the absence of significant weight loss. Unfortunately, the procedure of randomization was not described in the paper.

The Early Diabetes Intervention Trial (EDIT) was a 6-year, prospective, randomized, double-blind, placebo-controlled study in subjects thought to be at increased risk of developing diabetes, and who had two consecutive fasting plasma glucose levels in the range $5.5–7.7 \, \text{mmol} \, \text{l}^{-1}$. The primary aim of this UK trial was to determine whether deterioration in glucose tolerance toward diabetes could be delayed or prevented using a biguanide (metformin, 500 mg t.i.d.) or an alpha-glucosidase inhibitor (acarbose, 50 mg t.i.d.) (see Section 29.2.4) [45]. The 2×2 factorial design of this study has the potential to reveal a synergistic effect between metformin and acarbose on diabetes prevention. However, the double intervention group is small, with just over 160 patients, and may be underpowered to find such synergy. Six-year results for both arms have been published only as abstracts, and primary analyses showed no significant difference between groups [45]. Of the initial cohort, 31% became diabetic

and 14% discontinued follow-up. No differences were seen in RR for diabetes by 6 years with metformin (RR = 0.99; $p = 0.94$) or combination metformin–acarbose therapy (RR = 1.02; $p = 0.91$) compared with placebo. Similarly, nonsignificant differences were observed versus placebo in those patients with IGT at baseline.

More recently, the Indian Diabetes Prevention Programme (IDPP-1) randomized 531 individuals with IGT in four groups: control, lifestyle alone, metformin alone (250 mg b.i.d.) and combined lifestyle plus metformin. This trial confirmed that lifestyle modification and metformin prevent T2DM in Asian Indian subjects with IGT [46]. However, there was no added benefit from combining the two approaches after a median follow-up period of 30 months. Of note is that the average dose of metformin was only 250 mg b.i.d., which is much lower than that used in the US DPP [18]. The 3-year cumulative incidences of diabetes were 55.0% in the control group, 39.3% in the group with lifestyle modification, 40.5% in the group treated with metformin and 39.5% in the group given lifestyle advice plus metformin. Thus, the relative reduction was 26.4% with metformin alone (95% CI 19.1–35.1%, $p = 0.029$), and 28.2% with combined approach lifestyle plus metformin (95% CI 20.3–37.0%, $p = 0.022$). The NNT to prevent one incident case of diabetes was 6.4 for lifestyle alone, 6.9 for metformin and 6.5 for lifestyle plus metformin. The absence of synergistic effect may be disappointing, especially because the RR reduction of diabetes with lifestyle modification was less in the IDPP-1 than the 58% reduction in previous trials, especially the US DPP [18]. In this latter trial, part of the metformin effect was attributed to a modest weight loss, which was not observed with metformin in the Indian trial, possibly because of the lower daily metformin dose used.

Thus, most of the trials performed with metformin gave positive results, despite some heterogeneity. As metformin benefits from a long-lasting clinical experience, is generally well tolerated and is a rather cheap drug, it should be considered not only as the first choice drug for the management of hyperglycemia in patients with type 2 diabetes [36], but also as a valuable option for the prevention of type 2 diabetes in high-risk individuals, especially those with IGT [35].

29.2.2 Sulfonylureas/Glinides

While defective insulin secretion has been long considered as a rather late event in the natural history of T2DM, recent studies have clearly demonstrated that there is an early defect in beta-cell function [47], even in individuals with IGT [48], especially when insulin secretion is evaluated in comparison with concomitant insulin resistance [5]. Therefore, the use of insulin secretagogue agents might be considered as a potential alternative to prevent progression to T2DM, even if the risk of hypoglycemia may be a serious limitation in clinical practice [49]. As reviewed by Alberti [50], the first-generation compound tolbutamide showed positive results in five out of seven intervention trials. However, data interpretation is complicated by the fact that these trials preceded the modern definition of IGT and studied 'borderline' or 'chemical' or 'latent' diabetes. Two old studies examined the effect of tolbutamide therapy (1000–1500 mg per day) on diabetes incidence in patients with IGT or high–normal/elevated fasting glucose levels [51, 52]. Neither study reported a statistically significant decrease in the incidence of T2DM compared with control or placebo, although both studies were small ($n = 97$ and $n = 248$) and potentially underpowered. These negative results were confirmed in a larger and more recent trial (Fasting Hyperglycemia Study, reported only in an abstract form) showing that sulfonylurea therapy (gliclazide) over 6 years does not delay progression to diabetes [53]. In this trial, hypoglycemia was a potentially limiting side effect of sulfonylurea therapy, occurring at a frequency of 3% in nondiabetic patients. Perhaps an ongoing trial should provide more definitive evidence of the potential interest of sulfonylureas. Indeed, the Network for Pharmacoepidemiology Antidiabetes Study (NANSY) has recruited almost 2000 individuals with fasting glucose levels of 5.6–6.0 mmol l^{-1}, who will be randomized to glimepiride or placebo and followed for 5 to 7 years with diabetes as primary endpoint [54].

Because new insulin-secreting agents of the meglitinide family (repaglinide, nateglinide) have a more favorable pharmacokinetic profile that allows better control of postprandial hyperglycemia while reducing the risk of late hypoglycemia [55], they represent a possible alternative to sulfonylurea for the prevention of T2DM. No such demonstration is available yet, neither with repaglinide nor nateglinide. However, a large trial (NAVIGATOR: 'Nateglinide and Valsartan in Impaired Glucose Tolerance Outcomes Research') is currently investigating the effect of nateglinide in high-risk subjects [56]. This multinational, randomized, double-blind, placebo-controlled, forced-titration, 2×2 factorial design trial assessed the effect of nateglinide (30–60 mg t.i.d.) and valsartan (80–160 mg once a day) (see Section 29.6.2) on the prevention of diabetes and cardiovascular events in approximately 7500 subjects with IGT and increased risk for a cardiovascular event. The delay or prevention of progression to diabetes will be evaluated in the core phase of the study (3 years), whereas the prevention of cardiovascular events will be evaluated during an extension phase in the same patients. The efficacy of nateglinide and valsartan will be determined prospectively using validated measures of diagnosis of diabetes, namely oral glucose tolerance tests (OGTTs) and/or fasting glucose levels [56].

Thus, the place of insulin secretagogues in the prevention of T2DM is not obvious yet. In this respect, data from the NAVIGATOR trial are awaited with interest. If positive (that is, a reduced incidence of new-onset diabetes with a good safety profile), this approach will offer a new alternative for the prevention of T2DM in high-risk individuals. New agents capable of stimulating insulin secretion and possibly protecting and even regenerating beta cells as well, such as GLP-1 analogues and DDP-IV inhibitors, offer new exciting perspectives [57]. However, the cost of the new drugs will be higher and there are no clinical trials available (or ongoing) demonstrating their interest in the prevention of T2DM yet.

29.2.3 Glitazones

Thiazolidinediones (glitazones) are insulin sensitizers with glucose-lowering effects, which are widely used for the treatment of T2DM, especially in the United States [58]. These agents increase insulin sensitivity, both in the peripheral tissues (muscle and fat) and liver (reducing hepatic fat depot), thereby decreasing the glucose load on the B cell [39]. Besides this classical effect, thiazolidinediones may exert protection of B cells, by preserving cell mass and improving insulin secretory function [59, 60]. The Troglitazone Prevention of Diabetes (TRIPOD) study reported a marked reduction in the incidence of T2DM from 45% with placebo to 20% with troglitazone (RR = 0.45, 95% CI 0.25–0.83) in 236 overweight Hispanic women with previous gestational diabetes (age 35 years, BMI 30.5 kg m^{-2}) [61]. This effect was observed after a 2.5 year follow-up and occurred despite a modest and nonsignificant weight gain of 0.3 kg compared with placebo. However, the nearly 33% attrition rate during follow-up is a major limitation of this study. In addition, troglitazone has been withdrawn from the market because of liver toxicity [62]. The Pioglitazone in Prevention of Diabetes (PIPOD) study was conducted to evaluate β-cell function, insulin resistance, and the incidence of diabetes during treatment with pioglitazone in Hispanic women with prior gestational diabetes who had completed participation in the TRIPOD study [63]. Women were offered participation in an open study with pioglitazone (30 mg per day, uptitrated to 45 mg per day) treatment for 3 years and for 6 months of postdrug washout. Metabolic investigation includes both oral and intravenous glucose tolerance tests. The similarity of findings between the PIPOD and TRIPOD studies supports a class effect of thiazolidinediones to enhance insulin sensitivity, reduce insulin secretory demands and preserve pancreatic β-cell function, all in association with a relatively low rate of T2DM. The lowest rate of diabetes occurred in association with the greatest reduction in insulin secretory demands during the first year of treatment. Taken together, findings from these two trials support a role for thiazolidinediones in modifying the natural history of progression to T2DM in high-risk Hispanic patients. The generalizability to other high-risk groups will require additional studies.

In a small cohort study on 172 patients with IGT and insulin resistance, a significant reduction in diabetes incidence was observed with thiazolidinedione therapy (troglitazone followed by either rosiglitazone 4 mg o.d. or pioglitazone 30 mg o.d.) versus a untreated comparison group after a 3-year follow-up (RR = 0.11, 95% CI 0.03–0.36) [64]. It was concluded that progression of insulin resistance and IGT to T2DM appears to be delayed or prevented with early thiazolidinedione treatment.

In the US DPP, troglitazone (400 mg o.d.) was used initially but was discontinued during the trial for safety reason [18]. During the mean 0.9 year

(range 0.5–1.5 years) of troglitazone treatment, the diabetes incidence rate was 3.0 cases per 100 person-years, compared with 12.0, 6.7 and 5.1 cases per 100 person-years in the placebo, metformin and intensive lifestyle participants respectively ($p < 0.001$, troglitazone versus placebo and $p = 0.02$ troglitazone versus metformin) [65]. However, during the 3 years after troglitazone withdrawal, the diabetes incidence rate was almost identical to that in the placebo group. It was concluded that troglitazone markedly reduces the incidence of diabetes during its limited period of use, but that this action does not persist after drug withdrawal. Whether other thiazolidinedione drugs used for longer periods can safely prevent diabetes remains to be determined.

The DREAM ('Diabetes Reduction Assessment with ramipril and rosiglitazone Medication') randomized clinical trial evaluated the effect of rosiglitazone versus placebo to prevent T2DM in a large cohort of 5269 individuals with IFG and/or IGT [66]. Rosiglitazone (at a maximal daily dose of 8 mg) for 3 years substantially reduced incident T2DM (RR = 0.39; 95% CI 0.34–0.45; $p < 0.0001$) and increased the likelihood of regression to normoglycemia in adults with mild dysglycemia at baseline (RR = 1.70; 95% CI 1.56–1.86; $p < 0.0001$) compared with placebo. However, as for the first report of the DPP on metformin [18], results recently published in the original paper [66] were obtained on treatment with rosiglitazone. In the US DPP, part of the prevention effect of metformin disappeared after a short period of washout of only 1 to 2 weeks [42]. Thus, the question of whether the remarkable effect obtained with rosiglitazone in the DREAM study is a true preventing effect or only a delaying effect, or even simply a masking effect, remains an open question [67]. Data from a previous troglitazone trial suggested that the benefit of a thiazolidinedione persists several months after the drug is stopped [61], although this durable effect was not seen in another trial [65]. Therefore, the post-trial washout data of the DREAM study are expected with great interest [67].

ACT NOW (Actos Now for Prevention of Diabetes) is a smaller ongoing study ($n = 692$) assessing the efficacy of pioglitazone (45 mg once a day) compared with placebo on the prevention of T2DM as the primary objective in subjects with IGT. The diagnosis is based on two OGTTs as recommended [12] and the subjects were be treated for approximately 3 years. The results were reported at the recent American Diabetes Association Congress in June 2008. After a mean follow-up of 2.6 years, the incidence of new onset diabetes was remarkably lower in the pioglitazone group as compared to the placebo group (HR = 0.19; 95% CI 0.09-0.39; p < 0.00001). It means that only 3.5 patients with IGT should be treated for 1 year to prevent 1 case of T2DM. It should be noted, however, that these results were obtained when the patients were still on treatment. A follow-up is scheduled after a 6-month wash out period in order to verify that pioglitazone is really able to modify the natural history of the disease, presumably by protecting the beta-cell function (results unknown yet).

Currently available data suggest that glitazones are the most promising drugs for the prevention of T2DM. However, the rather high cost of such a pharmacological approach and the possible occurrence of adverse effects (weight gain, fluid retention, congestive heart failure) may limit the use of thiazolidinediones in this indication in the future, especially if high dosage (as in the DREAM trial) is recommended [67]. One alternative to increase the efficacy while improving the cost-effectiveness might be to use a combination pharmacological therapy, such as rosiglitazone plus metformin, in addition to a healthy lifestyle program, as currently evaluated in the moderately sized Canadian Normoglycemia Outcomes Evaluation (CANOE) study in subjects with IGT [68].

29.2.4 Acarbose

Antidiabetic drugs of the family of α-glucosidase inhibitors comprise three compounds: acarbose, miglitol and voglibose. Their mechanism of action is to retard carbohydrate absorption and reduce postprandial glucose responses by inhibiting α-glucosidase enzymes present on the brush border of the small intestine which hydrolyze di- and oligo-saccharides into their component monosaccharides [69]. Of the three α-glucosidase inhibitors, only acarbose has been specifically evaluated in its ability to prevent or delay the progression from IGT to T2DM [70]. Acarbose, although almost not absorbed from the gut, has been reported to reduce insulin resistance, perhaps through lower postprandial plasma glucose concentrations reducing both glucose toxicity and demand on the B cells, and to

have the potential of preventing diabetes in patients with IGT.

The Study to Prevent Non-Insulin-Dependent Diabetes Mellitus (STOP-NIDDM) trial is an international multicenter, placebo-controlled study on the efficacy of the α-glucosidase inhibitor acarbose in preventing or delaying the development of T2DM in a population with IGT [71]. A total of 1429 subjects (age 55 years, BMI 31 kg m^{-2}) diagnosed with IGT and having a fasting plasma glucose concentration ≥ 5.6 mmol l^{-1} were randomized in a double-blind fashion to receive either acarbose (100 mg t.i.d., $n = 714$) or placebo ($n = 715$) for a predictive median follow-up period of 3.9 years. The primary outcome was the development of T2DM diagnosed using a 75 g OGTT. The final analysis of the data regarding primary endpoint showed that 221 (32%) patients randomized to acarbose versus 285 (42%) randomized to placebo developed diabetes (RR = 0.75; 95% CI 0.63–0.90; $p = 0.0015$). The small weight loss in the acarbose group probably contributed to delaying onset of diabetes; however, acarbose was still effective after adjustment for weight loss ($p = 0.0063$). The results suggest that 11 patients with IGT would need to be treated for 3.3 years to prevent one event of development of diabetes. They also suggest that acarbose effectively reduced the risk of developing T2DM irrespective of age, sex and BMI. If the diagnosis of diabetes was based on two OGTTs as recommended by the Expert Committee of the American Diabetes Association [12], then acarbose treatment resulted in a 36.4% reduction in the incidence of diabetes ($p = 0.0003$). Furthermore, acarbose significantly increased reversion of IGT to normal glucose tolerance ($p < 0.0001$). At the end of the study, treatment with placebo for 3 months was associated with an increase in conversion of IGT to diabetes, an observation which again suggests that long-term treatment may be mandatory to prevent diabetes in such at-risk patients. It is noteworthy that almost a quarter of patients discontinued early, of whom 48% discontinued during the first year, mostly because of gastrointestinal side effects. Although the molecular mechanisms still need investigation, it was concluded that acarbose could be used, either as an alternative or in addition to changes in lifestyle, to delay development of T2DM in patients with IGT, especially since the drug has no toxic effects. These conclusions were challenged in a 'for debate' paper suggesting that the validity of the results of the STOP-NIDDM trial is seriously flawed, because of selection bias, inadequate blinding and bias in data analysis and reporting [72]. However, the authors confirmed that the trial results are scientifically sound and credible. The investigators stand strongly behind these results demonstrating that acarbose treatment is associated with a delay in the development of T2DM (as well as hypertension and cardiovascular complications) in a high-risk population with IGT [73].

In the Chinese Diabetes Prevention Study (DPS), subjects with mild overweight (BMI: $25 \, kg \, m^{-2}$) and IGT were divided into a control group ($n = 85$) which received conventional education, a metformin group ($n = 88$; see above) and an acarbose group ($n = 88$) [44]. Over a 3-year period, 34.9% in the control group versus 6.0% in the acarbose group progressed to diabetes. This represents an impressive risk reduction of 87.8% for acarbose. However, these remarkable results were only partially confirmed in a UK trial, the Early Diabetes Intervention Trial (EDIT) [45]. Indeed, primary analyses showed no significant difference in relative risk for T2DM between the control group and the acarbose group after a mean 6-year follow-up ($RR = 1.04; p = 0.81$). However, in those patients with IGT at baseline, RR of conversion to T2DM was reduced significantly with acarbose ($RR = 0.66; p = 0.046$) [45]. Even if the number of patients in the treatment group was rather small and might be underpowered to show a significant difference, it was not smaller, but rather slightly higher, than the Chinese DPS [44]. As already mentioned, a similar discrepancy between the two trials was observed as far as the effect of metformin on diabetes prevention is concerned. The reasons for such discrepancies are not clear, but may result from the different designs of the two studies; that is, a randomized controlled trial (RCT) in EDIT versus a cohort study in the Chinese DPS.

Thus, acarbose, because of its absence of toxicity and its efficacy to prevent T2DM in individuals with IGT in the STOP-NIDDM trial, appears to be a valuable alternative, although not all clinical trials provided clear-cut results. In addition, the cost of the drug, although considered as acceptable when considering the prevention of both diabetes and cardiovascular events [74], and its rather poor gastrointestinal tolerance may represent limitations

to use acarbose only for prevention, so that the drug should probably considered only for high-risk individuals.

29.2.5 Insulin

The Outcome Reduction with an Initial Glargine Intervention (ORIGIN) study is an international randomized placebo-controlled trial examining the efficacy of glargine insulin (and/or omega 3 in a 2×2 factorial design) in decreasing the risk of cardiovascular events in 12 500 subjects followed for 3.5 years [75]. As a secondary objective, investigators will look at the effect of glargine (and/or omega 3) on the development of T2DM, whose diagnosis will be based on OGTT (however, only 19% of the population have IFG and/or IGT at baseline). The results should be available in 2009.

29.3 PREVENTION BY ANTIOBESITY AGENTS

Obesity is strongly associated with T2DM [9, 19]. Minor long-term changes in body weight have beneficial effects on insulin sensitivity and beta-cell function in obese subjects [76], which may retard or prevent the progression to T2DM in at risk individuals. Weight loss strategies using dietary, physical activity or behavioral interventions produced significant improvements in weight among persons with prediabetes and a significant decrease in T2DM incidence [77]. A recent post hoc analysis of the DPP revealed that, for every kilogram of weight loss, there was a 16% reduction in risk of T2DM, adjusted for changes in diet and physical activity, and concluded that interventions to reduce diabetes risk should primarily target weight reduction [78]. However, the rate of responders is rather low, the degree of weight loss is generally disappointing and the long-term weight maintenance is questionable with lifestyle changes. Therefore, various antiobesity drugs have been developed in order to improve these outcomes [79, 80].

29.3.1 Orlistat

Orlistat is a gastric and pancreatic lipase inhibitor that blocks the absorption of about one-third of the fat contained in a meal and thus promotes fecal

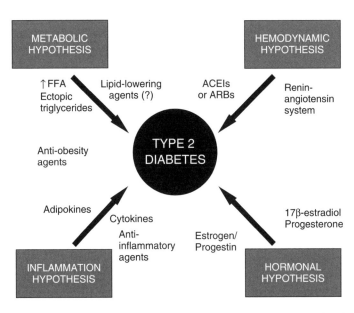

Figure 29.2 Various hypothetical mechanisms implicated in the pathogenesis of type 2 diabetes and illustration of the sites of action of non-glucose-lowering agents considered for the prevention of type 2 diabetes in high-risk patients.

excretion of undigested fat [81]. In a meta-analysis summarizing the results of 29 randomized placebo-controlled studies of orlistat (usual dosage of 120 mg t.i.d.), the pooled random-effects estimate of the mean weight loss for orlistat-treated patients compared with placebo recipients was 2.89 kg (95% CI 2.27–3.51 kg) after 12 months [80]. The placebo-subtracted weight reduction induced by orlistat was even less impressive in adults with type 2 diabetes (2.0 kg; 95% CI 1.3–2.8 kg) at 12–57 weeks follow-up [82]. Despite this modest weight loss, a significant reduction in HbA_{1c} levels was consistently reported [82]. This suggests that orlistat may enhance insulin sensitivity [83, 84], although controversial results have been reported in nondiabetic individuals [85]. A pooled analysis of three 2-year randomized clinical trials enrolling 642 obese patients reported a nonsignificant reduction in the incidence of T2DM from 2.0 to 0.6% with orlistat therapy (RR = 0.25, 95% CI 0.05–1.2) [86]. The CIs were wide, reflecting the low absolute incidence of diabetes within these trials, and attrition rates averaged >30%. Nevertheless, these observations lead to the concept that orlistat may prevent T2DM in at-risk obese patients [87] and lead to the initiation of the Xenical in the Prevention of Diabetes in Obese Subjects (XENDOS) trial.

XENDOS is the most important RCT performed with orlistat until now, as far as the number of subjects (mean age 43 years, BMI 37.4 kg m^{-2}) enrolled ($n = 3277$) and the duration of the trial (4 years) are concerned [88]. It demonstrates that the beneficial effects of orlistat on body weight persisted up to 4 years (–6.9 kg with orlistat versus–4.1 kg with placebo; $p < 0.001$), although the difference between orlistat and placebo group tended to attenuate over time. The most striking finding of XENDOS is that such a modest difference in weight reduction (mean of 2.8 kg) was sufficient to reduce the cumulative incidence of T2DM significantly (6.2% with orlistat versus 9.0% with placebo; RR = 0.63, 95% CI 0.46–0.86; $p = 0.0032$). The annual incidence of T2DM in XENDOS was four to five times lower than in previously mentioned trials, mainly because only 21% of enrolled subjects had IGT. The reduction in the incidence of T2DM was especially remarkable in those obese patients with IGT at baseline, with a reduction of conversion to T2DM after 4 years decreasing from 28.8% in the placebo group to 18.8% in the orlistat group ($p < 0.005$) and an NNT to avoid one event of 11 only. However, the attrition rate was 57%, partly due to a higher incidence of gastrointestinal side effects with orlistat. XENDOS is the first study demonstrating that an antiobesity agent, like orlistat, is able to reduce the progression to T2DM in obese subjects compared with lifestyle changes alone.

29.3.2 Sibutramine

Sibutramine is a combined norepinephrine and serotonin reuptake inhibitor [89]. At a daily dosage of 10–20 mg, it is associated with increased satiation and a resulting reduction in food intake (although some thermogenic effects may exist as well) [89]. Weight changes were associated with various favorable metabolic effects [90]. A meta-analysis included 44 trials with sibutramine that were considered of sufficiently high quality for inclusion in the analysis [91]. Sibutramine was more effective than placebo in promoting weight loss in overweight and obese adults at all time points assessed, from 8 weeks up to 54 weeks. A Cochrane systematic review included five high-quality sibutramine weight loss studies over 1 year (three weight loss and two weight maintenance trials) [79]. Attrition rates averaged 43% during the weight loss phase. Compared with placebo, sibutramine-treated patients lost 4.3 kg (95% CI 3.6–4.9 kg). The number of patients achieving 10% or greater weight loss was 15% (95% CI 4–27%) higher with sibutramine than with placebo. In the STORM (Sibutramine Trial of Obesity Reduction and Maintenance) study, an individualized management program combining restricted diet and sibutramine achieved weight loss in almost 75% of obese patients after 6 months and sustained weight loss in around 50% of patients continuing therapy for 2 years [92]. A Cochrane review on the use of pharmacotherapy for weight loss in adults with T2DM revealed that sibutramine produced significant reductions in body weight (5.1 kg; 95% CI 3.2–7.0 kg) at 12–52 weeks follow-up [82]. However, despite this weight reduction, the average impact on HbA_{1c} was rather modest [93], except in patients with the largest weight reduction, possibly because of drug-associated sympathetic activation [83].

There is no direct evidence that sibutramine reduces the incidence of new-onset diabetes in overweight/obese patients. A long-term large-scale prospective trial (Sibutramine Cardiovascular and Diabetes Outcome Study (SCOUT)) has been designed to determine whether weight management

with a novel lifestyle intervention plus either sibutramine (10–15 mg per day) or placebo in cardiovascular high-risk overweight and obese patients can impact upon cardiovascular endpoints [94]. To be eligible for inclusion, patients must have experienced a cardiovascular event or have diagnosed T2DM and another cardiovascular risk factor. The primary endpoint of the trial will include a composite cardiovascular endpoint. Because of the size of the study (almost 9000 patients followed for at least 3 years), informative data on the effect of sibutramine on the risk of developing T2DM might also be obtained from this trial.

29.3.3 Rimonabant

Rimonabant is the first selective cannabinoid type 1 (CB_1) receptor antagonist launched for the treatment of overweight/obese subjects with risk factor(s), such as T2DM and dyslipidemia. The endocannabinoid (EC) system, consisting of the CB_1 receptor and endogenous lipid-derived ligands, appears to modulate energy homeostasis as well as glucose and lipid metabolism, both through central orexigenic effects and peripheral metabolic effects in adipose tissue, liver, skeletal muscle and pancreas [95, 96]. In nondiabetic overweight/obese patients, rimonabant 20 mg, compared with placebo, has been shown to produce significant weight loss and waist circumference reduction, the latter being a key marker of intra-abdominal adiposity, and improvements in multiple cardiometabolic risk factors. Besides a significant increase in high-density lipoprotein (HDL)-cholesterol and a significant decrease in triglyceride levels, improvements in glucose metabolism have been described, with a reduction in high fasting insulin levels and homeostasis model assessment (HOMA) insulin resistance index [97–99]. In a 1-year trial performed in overweight/obese patients with diabetes, all these effects were confirmed and, in addition, a placebo-subtracted 0.7% reduction in HbA_{1c} levels was observed [100]. Almost half of these metabolic effects occur beyond weight loss [101]. Part of these metabolic improvements may be attributed to a significant increase in plasma adiponectin levels [98]. Rimonabant also improves glucose tolerance and reduces postglucose load plasma insulin response in both RIO-Europe [97] and RIO-Lipids [98]. The favorable effects on plasma glucose and insulin levels observed with rimonabant 20 mg after 1 year persisted after 2 years in the RIO-Europe trial [102]. In a pooled post hoc analysis of the three RCTs performed in nondiabetic patients, more obese subjects improved glucose tolerance and fewer individuals progressed toward T2DM in the rimonabant 20 mg group than in the placebo group [103]. The ongoing RAPSODI (Rimonabant in Prediabetic Subjects to Delay Onset of Type 2 Diabetes) 2-year trial has enrolled 2100 participants, with researchers specifically focusing on whether rimonabant 20 mg helps prevent T2DM in patients with prediabetes in the form of IFG and/or IGT.

29.4 PREVENTION BY LIPID-LOWERING AGENTS

There is an intimate relationship between glucose and lipid metabolism [104]. In particular, high circulating levels of free fatty acid [105] and ectopic depots of triglycerides in various organs, such as liver, skeletal muscle and pancreas [106], have been shown to be associated with increased insulin resistance and impaired insulin secretion, leading to the concept of lipotoxicity [33]. Therefore, drugs interfering with lipid metabolism may exert favorable effects on glucose metabolism and possibly prevent the progression from IGT to T2DM. However, despite some anecdotal small-sized trials, there is no convincing and consistent evidence of a favorable effect of statins [107] or fibrates [108, 109] on insulin sensitivity, and nicotinic acid has been shown to be associated with impaired rather than improved insulin sensitivity [110].

29.4.1 Statins

Statins act by inhibiting 3-hydroxy-3-methyl-glutaryl coenzyme A (HMG-CoA) reductase, a key enzyme in the synthesis of cholesterol in the hepatocytes. Besides the remarkable reduction in total and low-density lipoprotein (LDL)-cholesterol levels, they exert numerous pleiotropic effects, which may explain their favorable effect of prevention of cardiovascular events [111]. Even if they are recognized to improve endothelial function and to reduce low-grade inflammation, statins do not exert strong beneficial effects on insulin sensitivity, although some studies reported a significant reduction of insulin resistance after statin therapy [107]. In a post

hoc analysis from the West of Scotland Coronary Prevention Study (WOSCOPS), diabetes incidence was significantly lower with pravastatin treatment than with placebo (1.9% versus 2.8%, RR = 0.70, 95% CI 0.50–0.99) [112]. However, the rate of progression to T2DM was low in this trial, leading to a low number of events, the prevalence of IGT at entry into the study was unknown and the diagnosis of diabetes was only based on self-reporting or a fasting glucose level ≥ 7.0 mmol l^{-1}. In three other post hoc analyses of large placebo-controlled statin cardiovascular trials, no significant reduction in the incidence of new T2DM was observed with the cholesterol-lowering drug: with simvastatin in the Heart Protection Study (HPS) (4.6% versus 4.0%, RR = 1.15, 95% CI 0.99–1.34) [113], with pravastatin in the Long-Term Intervention with Pravastatin in Ischemic Disease (LIPID) study (4.0% versus 4.5%, RR = 0.89, 95% CI 0.70–1.13) [114], and with atorvastatin in the Anglo-Scandinavian Cardiac Outcomes Trial-Lipid Lowering Arm (ASCOT-LLA) (3.0% versus 2.6%, RR = 1.15, 95% CI 0.91–1.44) [115]. Therefore, there is no current evidence supporting a significant effect of a statin therapy to prevent the development of T2DM.

A retrospective cohort study using Saskatchewan health databases to identify subjects newly started on oral antidiabetic agents from 1991 to 1996 showed that the use of statins is associated with an average 10-month delay in starting insulin treatment in 10 996 patients with T2DM initially treated with oral antidiabetic agents [116]. However, after 7 years of follow-up, there were no differences between the statin and control groups in their requirements for insulin therapy. The authors asked whether this protection also exists for patients at high-risk of developing diabetes. A nested case-control study based on data from the UK-based General Practice research database concluded that there is little if any protective effect of statins on the development of T2DM [117].

29.4.2 Fibrates

Because of their specific mechanism of action on peroxisome proliferator-activated receptor (PPAR)-alpha receptors and their effects on circulating triglyceride and free fatty acid (FFA) levels, fibrate derivatives may exert more favorable effects on glucose metabolism than statins [118].

However, previous studies have yielded conflicting results for effects of fibrates on glycemic control, and both bezafibrate [108] and gemfibrozil [109] were reported to have no effect on insulin resistance. Nevertheless, in the Bezafibrate Infarction Prevention (BIP) trial, a post hoc analysis of 303 patients with IGT showed that bezafibrate therapy was associated with a significant reduction in T2DM incidence compared with placebo (hazard ratio (HR) = 0.70, 95% CI 0.49–0.99) [119]. However, no other trials reported similar favorable results with other fibrates, either gemfibrozil or fenofibrate, so that such possible effects of fibrates to avoid progression to T2DM require further confirmation.

29.4.3 Nicotinic Acid

Unexpectedly, despite its inhibitory effect on lipolysis and its lowering action on FFA levels, nicotinic acid has been shown to be associated with increased insulin resistance rather than improved insulin sensitivity. This effect, probably due to a marked rebound in plasma FFA concentrations, requires increased insulin secretion to maintain normal glucose tolerance and may lead to IGT [110]. Prolonged-release nicotinic acid has improved tolerability compared with nicotinic acid and exerts less deterioration of insulin sensitivity and glucose tolerance, presumably because a less marked rebound in plasma FFA levels [120]. Although it may be used in the management of dyslipidemia associated with diabetes and metabolic syndrome [121], there is no evidence that nicotinic acid may prevent T2DM in patients with IGT and there is no ongoing trial trying to demonstrate such a protective effect.

29.5 EFFECTS OF RAAS INHIBITION ON DEVELOPMENT OF DIABETES

During recent years, there has been a growing interest for the ability to prevent T2DM by inhibition of the RAAS [33, 122–124]. It is well known that the risk of new-onset diabetes is increased in patients with arterial hypertension. The risk is even greater in patients receiving antihypertensive therapy, although this may largely vary according to the type of antihypertensive agents used. In this respect, old antihypertensive medications, such as diuretics and beta-blockers,

are more deleterious than new agents, such as calcium-channel antagonists and RAAS inhibitors [125–128].

The inhibition of the RAAS has been shown to be associated with various metabolic effects that may contribute to protecting against the development of T2DM [129]. It resulted in improvement of insulin sensitivity in some studies [33, 130]. However, the data were heterogeneous across the trials and tended to be less consistent with ARBs than with ACE inhibitors. In fact, the effects of ACE inhibition on glucose tolerance are more consistent than those on insulin sensitivity. Many reports in nondiabetic patients have found some improvement in glucose tolerance, whether assessed by the OGTT or judged from fasting plasma glucose or glycated hemoglobin levels (review in [33]). Recent data brought support for a positive effect of RAAS inhibition on B-cell function and insulin secretion as well [131, 132]. It remains to be established the extent to which these metabolic effects will influence the long-term consequences for future risk of T2DM, especially in at-risk populations, such as in patients with arterial hypertension, congestive heart failure or coronary heart disease treated with either ACE inhibitors or ARBs [133].

29.5.1 ACE Inhibitors

At least nine trials have examined as a secondary outcome the effect of ACE inhibitors on the prevention of T2DM in a high-risk population [33, 122–124]. Most studies were performed in patients with arterial hypertension. Except in the STOP-Hypertension-2 study [134] comparing enalapril/lisinopril with beta-blocker, a significant reduction in the incidence of new-onset diabetes was observed in patients receiving an ACE inhibitor versus patients receiving a comparator, either placebo or an active drug (**Table 29.2**): the Captopril Prevention Project (CAPPP) comparing captopril with conventional treatment with beta-blockers or diuretics [135]; the Antihypertensive and Lipid-Lowering Treatment to Prevent Heart Attack Trial (ALLHAT) comparing lisinopril with chlorthalidone or lisinopril with amlodipine [136]; the 2nd Australian National Blood Pressure Study' (ANBP2) comparing enalapril with hydrochlorothiazide [137]; the Anglo-Scandinavian Cardiac Outcomes Trial (ASCOT) comparing perindopril (added as required to amlodipine) with

Table 29.2 Randomized clinical trials assessing the effect of ACE inhibitors on the incidence of diabetes in high-risk patients with hypertension, congestive heart failure and coronary artery disease. In the bottom, results of the DREAM study performed in patients without high cardiovascular risk.

Trial (Reference)	n	ACE inhibitor	Comparator	F-U (years)	RR (95% CI)	p
STOP-HTN2 [134]	6 614	Enalapril/lisinopril	β-blocker	5.0	0.96 (0.72–1.27)	NS
CAPPP [135]	10 985	Captopril	β-blocker-diuretic	6.1	0.79 (0.67–0.94)	0.039
ALLHAT [136]	33 357	Lisinopril	Chlorthalidone	4.9	0.70 (0.56–0.86)	0.001
ALLHAT [136]	33 357	Lisinopril	Amlodipine	4.9	0.83 (0.74–0.93)	0.001
ANBP2 [138]	6 083	Enalapril[a]	HCTZ	4.1	0.66 (0.54–0.85)	0.001
ASCOT [137]	19 257	Perindopril	Atenolol	5.5	0.70 (0.63–0.78)	0.001
PEACE [139]	8 290	Trandolapril[a]	Placebo	4.8	0.83 (0.72–0.96)	0.001
INVEST [140]	16 176	Trandolapril	HCTZ	2.7	0.85 (0.77–0.95)	0.001
EUROPA [141]	12 228	Perindopril[a]	Placebo	4.2	0.97 (NA)	NS
HOPE [142, 143]	9 297	Ramipril	Placebo	5.0	0.66 (0.51–0.85)	0.001
SOLVD [145][b]	4 228	Enalapril	Placebo	3.4	0.26 (0.13–0.53)	0.0001
DREAM [146][c]	5 269	Ramipril	Placebo	3.0	0.91 (0.80–1.03)	NS

F-U: follow-up; RR: relative risk of developing diabetes versus comparator; HCTZ: hydrochlorothiazide; NA: not available; NS, not significant.

[a] ACE inhibitor as add-on therapy.

[b] Patients with congestive heart failure.

[c] Individuals without cardiovascular disease.

atenolol (added as required to bendroflumethiazide) [138]. Three studies [139–141] were performed in patients with coronary heart disease, with a significant reduction of new-onset T2DM in two out of them [139, 140]: Prevention of Events with Angiotensin-Converting Enzyme Inhibition (PEACE) comparing trandolapril with placebo [139], the International Verapamil–Trandolapril Study (INVEST) comparing a verapamil sustained release/trandolapril (trandolapril as add-on therapy) strategy with an atenolol/hydrochlorothiazide strategy [140], the 'EUropean trial on Reduction Of cardiac events with Perindopril in patients with stable coronary Artery disease' (EUROPA) comparing perindopril with placebo [141]. The Heart Outcomes Prevention Evaluation (HOPE) trial recruited patients with high cardiovascular risk, because of arterial hypertension or the presence of other cardiovascular risk factors, and compared ramipril with placebo [142, 143]. A post hoc analysis reported a remarkable 35% relative risk reduction (RRR) of new-onset T2DM with ramipril compared with placebo at the end of a 4.5-year follow-up. Interestingly, during a 2.6-year

extension study, there was a significant further reduction in risk of diabetes for patients in the ramipril group versus in the placebo group (RR = 0.66; 95% CI 0.46–0.95) [144]. Thus, the benefits observed during the HOPE trial were sustained during passive follow-up despite late similar rates of ACE inhibitor use in the two randomized groups. Considering the combined in-trial period and post-trial follow-up of 7.2 years, there was a 31% RRR in new diagnoses of T2DM in the ramipril group compared with the placebo group. Only one study concerned patients with congestive heart failure. In a retrospective study assessing the effect of the ACE inhibitor enalapril on the incidence of diabetes in a small subgroup of the Studies Of Left Ventricular Dysfunction (SOLVD) [145], a dramatic reduction of new cases of T2DM was noticed in patients treated with enalapril compared with those receiving placebo. By multivariate analysis, enalapril was the most powerful predictor for risk reduction of developing T2DM (RR = 0.22; 95 % CI 0.10–0.46; $p < 0.0001$). Despite this almost remarkable consistency of the observations, it should be pointed out, however, that all these results were the product of a post hoc analysis or the secondary results of trials projected for a different scope (i.e. cardiovascular protection) and obtained using heterogeneous criteria for diabetes diagnosis. Unfortunately, the prevalence of IGT is unknown in those study populations. Thus, the consistent positive findings that ACE inhibitors may prevent T2DM should receive a definite answer after completion of large-scale trials specifically devoted to answer this important question.

As already mentioned, the DREAM trial was designed to evaluate prospectively whether ramipril 15 mg o.d. prevents T2DM among individuals at high risk because of IGT or IFG [146]. After a median follow-up of 3 years in 5269 participants, the incidence of the primary outcome (effects of ramipril on the development of T2DM or death) did not differ significantly between the ramipril group (18.1%) and the placebo group (19.5%; HR = 0.91, 95% CI 0.81–1.03; $p = 0.15$). However, participants receiving ramipril were more likely to have regression to normoglycemia (a prespecified secondary outcome) than those receiving placebo (HR = 1.16, 95% CI 1.07–1.27; $p = 0.001$). Thus, among persons with IGT or IFG, the use of ramipril for 3 years does not significantly reduce the incidence of T2DM or death but does significantly increase regression to normoglycemia. There may be several reasons why the results of DREAM differ from the reductions in the rates of newly diagnosed diabetes reported previously with ACE inhibitors. Besides the use of a more rigorous protocol concerning the definition of diabetes and its screening at baseline and during the study, it is of note that participants of DREAM differed from those of previous studies, who were older and primarily had known cardiovascular disease, heart failure, hypertension or a combination thereof. It is possible, therefore, that the degree of activation of the RAAS is higher in the latter patients and that the ACE inhibition may have a greater effect in these people than in others such as those recruited in DREAM. Thus, ACE inhibitors are not recommended to prevent T2DM in the absence of other cardiovascular risk factors [147]. Nevertheless, the results of DREAM suggest that ramipril may have favorable effects on glucose metabolism (mild reduction in glucose levels and higher conversion rate to normal glucose tolerance),

a finding that is consonant with other reports on studies of ACE inhibitors.

29.5.2 ARBs

At least four studies assessed the efficacy of an ARB, and three of them demonstrated a significant reduction in new cases of T2DM in hypertensive patients compared with a placebo or an other active antihypertensive drug (**Table 29.3**) [33, 122–124]: the 'Losartan Intervention For Endpoint reduction in hypertension study' (LIFE) comparing losartan with atenolol [148, 149]; the 'Antihypertensive treatment and Lipid Profile In a North of Sweden Efficacy Evaluation' (ALPINE) comparing candesartan with hydrochlorothiazide [150]; the 'Valsartan Amlodipine Long-term Use Evaluation' (VALUE) comparing valsartan with amlodipine [151]. Only the 'Study on Cognition and Prognosis in the Elderly' (SCOPE), comparing candesartan with placebo, showed a 25% difference that did not reach statistical significance [152]. These observations in hypertensive individuals were confirmed in one trial in patients with congestive heart failure, the 'Candesartan in Heart failure Assessment of Reduction in Mortality and morbidity' (CHARM) study [153, 154]. After a mean follow-up of 37.7 months, the number of newly diagnosed patients as having diabetes was significantly lower with candesartan (6%) than with placebo (7%): HR = 0.78; 95% CI 0.64–0.96; $p = 0.020$. There is, therefore, enough circumstantial evidence to justify a prospective study on the effect of ARBs on the prevention of T2DM in a high-risk population.

The NAVIGATOR trial is an international randomized placebo-controlled 2×2 factorial design to assess the effect of nateglinide (see Section 29.3.2) and/or valsartan on the prevention of T2DM and cardiovascular events as primary outcomes in subjects with IGT and high risk for cardiovascular disease [56]. The diagnosis of diabetes is based on the OGTT. More than 9500 individuals were recruited and will be followed for 3 years. The results should be available in 2009.

ONTARGET ('Telmisartan Alone and in combination with Ramipril Global Endpoint trial') is a three-arm study testing telmisartan, ramipril and telmisartan plus ramipril on cardiovascular events in a high-risk population of 25 620 subjects [155].

Table 29.3 Randomized clinical trials assessing the effect of angiotensin receptor blockers (ARB) on the incidence of diabetes in high-risk patients with hypertension, congestive heart failure and coronary artery disease.

Trial (reference)	n	ARB	Comparator	F-U (years)	RR (95% CI)	p
LIFE [148, 149]	9 193	Losartan	Atenolol	4.8	0.75 (0.63–0.88)	0.001
ALPINE [150]	392	Candesartan	Atenolol	1.0	0.13 (0.03–0.99)	0.03
VALUE [151]	15 245	Valsartan	Amlodipine	4.2	0.77 (0.69–0.86)	0.0001
SCOPE [152]	4 937	Candesartan	Placebo	3.7	0.81 (0.61–1.02)	0.09
CHARM [153, 154][a]	7 599	Candesartan	Placebo	3.2	0.78 (0.64–0.96)	0.02

F-U: follow-up; RR: relative risk of developing diabetes versus comparator.
[a]Patients with congestive heart failure.

Those individuals who cannot tolerate ACE inhibitors will be enrolled in a parallel study, TRANSCEND ('Telmisartan RANdomized assessment Study in angiotensin inhibitor intolerant patients with cardiovascular Disease'), which will compare telmisartan with placebo in almost 5000 individuals. The ONTARGET–TRANSCEND studies will also look at the effect of those treatments on the development of T2DM based on fasting plasma glucose as a prespecified secondary outcome. ONTARGET offers the unique opportunity to compare the effects of an ACE inhibitor and an ARB in a head-to-head trial and to investigate the potential of any additional effect of an ACE inhibitor–ARB combination to prevent T2DM compared with monotherapy. The use of telmisartan is also of special interest, as this highly lipophilic ARB has been shown to exert partial PPAR-γ activity (selective PPAR modulator or SPPARM), thus an effect related to glitazones, which may bring an add-on value for the prevention of T2DM [156, 157]. The results of ONTARGET were recently reported (155). After a median follow-up of 56 months, the percentage of patients with new diagnosis of diabetes was almost similar in the telmisartan group (399/5294 patients, 7.5%) and in the ramipril group (366/5427 patients, 6.7%), with a RR of 1.12 (CI 0.97-1.29). The incidence of new onset diabetes tended to be slightly but not significantly lower in the combined telmisartan + ramipiril group (323/5280, 6.3%) than in the group treated by ramipril alone (RR = 0.91, CI 0.78 = 1.06). Thus, the available results of ONTARGET could not demonstrate a greater preventive effect against the development of diabetes

of telmisartan as compared to ramipril or of the combination telmisartan-ramipril versus ramipril alone in non-diabetic patients who have vascular disease.

In conclusion, there is growing and consistent evidence that RAAS inhibition may prevent the development of T2DM in high-risk individuals. Indirect comparison suggests that ACE inhibitors and ARBs have a similar and significant ability to reduce the occurrence of new-onset T2DM among subjects with arterial hypertension, congestive heart failure and coronary heart disease [33, 122–124, 133]. Therefore, an ACE inhibitor or ARB is a logical first-line antihypertensive therapy in patients with IFG or metabolic syndrome for multiple reasons, including the reduction of risk of progression to overt T2DM. Obviously, part of the antidiabetic mechanisms occurs beyond the RAAS [158]. However, as shown recently by the results of DREAM, the routine use of ACE inhibitors such as ramipril for the express purpose of preventing diabetes, in the absence of cardiovascular disease, is not indicated. Furthermore the recent results of ONTARGET do not support the use of a combination ramipril-telmisartan in order to optimize the protective effect against diabetes in patients with vascular disease (155).

29.6 PREVENTION BY VARIOUS DRUGS

29.6.1 Estrogen

There is increasing evidence, both in rodents and in humans, linking the endogenous estrogen 17β-estradiol (E2) to the maintenance of glucose homeostasis [159, 160]. Five cohort studies, which have examined the association between estrogen use and T2DM incidence, reported controversial results [28]. However, several trials failed to adjust for potentially important covariates, such as family history of T2DM, body weight, or baseline glucose measurements. The Nurses Health Study, the largest of the cohort studies, found that, over 12 years, current estrogen use was associated with a significant reduction in T2DM incidence compared with never users, but no difference between former estrogen users and never users [161] (**Table 29.4**). In the Strong Heart Study in American Indian post-menopausal women, the risk of T2DM was not significantly increased when comparing current users with past or never users, but increased modestly with increasing duration of estrogen use among current users, with an odds ratio of 1.10 per year of use [162]. In contrast, a recent study revealed that transdermal 17-β-estradiol significantly reduced the risk of developing T2DM in healthy, nonobese, postmenopausal women [163] (**Table 29.4**).

The two most important data result from post hoc analysis of the Heart and Estrogen/Progestin Replacement Study (HERS) [164] and the Women's Health Initiative Hormone Trial (WHI) studies [165, 166]. In HERS, combination estrogen and progesterone therapy was associated with a significant reduction in the incidence of T2DM from 9.0% to 6.2% compared with placebo (RR = 0.65) [164]. In the WHI trial, the cumulative incidence of treated diabetes after 5.6 years of follow-up was 3.5% in the hormone therapy group (daily 0.625 mg conjugated equine estrogens plus 2.5 mg medroxyprogesterone acetate) and 4.2% in the placebo group (HR = 0.79) [165]. However, there was little change in the HR after adjustment for changes in BMI and waist circumference. During the first year of follow-up, changes in fasting insulin levels indicated a significant fall in insulin resistance in actively treated women compared with the control group. In a substudy of this large trial, the effect of daily 0.625 mg conjugated equine estrogen alone was compared with placebo in women who had previously had a hysterectomy [166]. After a mean 7.1-year follow-up, the cumulative incidence of treated T2DM was 8.3% in the estrogen-alone group and 9.3% in the placebo group (HR 0.88, $p = 0.072$) (**Table 29.4**). A significant reduction in insulin resistance assessed by the HOMA model was observed after 1 year, but not after 3 and 6 years of follow-up. Therefore, the effect appears to be smaller with estrogen alone than that seen with estrogen plus progestin.

These recent data suggest that combined therapy with estrogen and progestin reduces the incidence of T2DM, possibly by a decrease in insulin resistance unrelated to body size. However, in view of the overall adverse effects of this combination, especially the increased risk of cardiovascular disease, it is not justified to use combined estrogen plus progestin therapy for the prevention of T2DM in postmenopausal women. Nevertheless, further study of mechanisms seems warranted to explore

Table 29.4 Clinical studies assessing the effect of estrogen replacement therapy on the incidence of new-onset diabetes in postmenopausal women[a].

Reference	n	F-U (years)	RR	95% CI	p
Manson *et al* [161]	21 028	12.0	0.80	0.67–0.96	0.005
Zhang *et al.* [162]	857	4.0	1.11	0.62–1.97	NS
Kanaya *et al.* [164]	2 029	4.1	0.65	0.48–0.89	0.006
Margolis *et al.* [165]	15 641	5.6	0.79	0.67–0.93	0.004
Rossi *et al.* [163][b]	673	3.7	0.45	0.29–0.56	0.001
Bonds *et al.* [166][c]	10 739	7.1	0.88	0.77–1.01	0.072

[a]In this study, the risk of D2TM increased with increasing duration of estrogen use among current users.

[b]Only trial performed with transdermal 17-β-estradiol instead of oral conjugated estrogen therapy.

[c]Estrogen alone (without progestin).

the role of hormonal factors in diabetes prevention. Recent data from the Rancho Bernardo Study showed that proinsulin, but not insulin, levels were significantly lower in current hormone replacement therapy users than in previous and never hormone replacement therapy users [167]. Proinsulin reflects insulin resistance more than intact insulin, and hyperproinsulinemia may be a sign of a pancreatic B-cell defect, augmented by an increased demand placed on the B cells. The effects of estrogen on insulin secretion merit further investigation and might lead to new therapies [168]. Further studies of alternative postmenopausal hormone therapy regimens and selective estrogen agonists and/or antagonists should consider the effects of these regimens on insulin resistance, insulin secretion and new-onset T2DM.

29.6.2 Anti-inflammatory Drugs

There is a growing body of evidence for the role of inflammation in insulin resistance and T2DM [169–171]. More than 15 studies in different ethnic groups have shown a remarkable consistency in demonstrating that high sensitive C-reactive protein (hs-CRP), interleukin-6 (Il-6) and some other inflammatory markers predict the development of T2DM [172–176]. For example, an overall inflammation score based on four inflammatory markers plus white cell count and fibrinogen predicted diabetes in the Atherosclerosis Risk in Communities Study participants [177]. In general, the predictive power of hs-CRP, the most widely used marker, was somewhat stronger than that of Il-6. However, it was reduced after adjustment for BMI or other factors related to insulin resistance, although it remained a significant independent risk marker in most studies. In addition, almost 10 prospective studies have demonstrated that low adiponectin levels predict an increased incidence of T2DM [178]. For instance, in the Atherosclerosis Risk in Communities Study, a case-cohort study representing the approximately 9-year experience of 10 275 middle-aged US participants, HRs (95% CIs) for developing T2DM, for those in the second, third and fourth (versus the first) quartiles of adiponectin were 0.72 (0.48–1.09), 0.67 (0.43–1.04) and 0.58 (0.34–0.99) respectively, after extensive adjustments for all known confounding risk factors [179]. Thus, there is accumulating evidence suggesting that inflammation

is the bridging link between obesity, T2DM and atherosclerosis. Therefore, interventions using agents with anti-inflammatory properties may reduce the risk of both conditions.

Evidence is emerging that many drugs that may reduce the incidence and/or delay the onset of T2DM have apparent 'anti-inflammatory' properties [180]. It is the case for thiazolidinediones, metformin, ACE inhibitors, ARBs, fibrates and statins, which all are able to reduce hs-CRP levels and other inflammatory markers [181]. However, although all these drugs with potential anti-inflammatory properties reduce the risk of developing T2DM, it is difficult to prove whether such anti-inflammatory properties contribute to their diabetes prevention effect and, if yes, to what extent. Indeed, nearly all drugs have other, often more pronounced, metabolic actions that can explain the prevention effect of T2DM. Thus, only specific trials with drugs exerting specific anti-inflammatory effects may answer the question. High-dose aspirin inhibits cyclooxygenase and IkappaB kinase-beta and reduces fasting plasma glucose concentration in patients with T2DM [182]. While controversial results about the effect of acetylsalicylic acid on insulin resistance have been reported, a recent study in healthy men showed that acetylsalicylic acid specifically attenuates the lipid-induced insulin resistance, but not insulin resistance in absence of high lipid levels [183]. However, this beneficial effect of acetylsalicylic acid was not accompanied by any changes in inflammatory markers. Unfortunately, there has not, as yet, been a large-scale trial to examine the effect of aspirin on the risk of developing T2DM. Clinical trials to test efficacy, tolerability and durability of salsalate (nonacetylated salicylate) are currently being undertaken in the NIH-funded trials Targeting Inflammation with Salsalate (TINSAL) in T2DM and in cardiovascular disease. Other more specific anti-inflammatory strategies (JNK or IKKβ inhibitors, compounds that block TNF-a, Il-6, TLR or chemokine signaling) are being considered, but these studies are at much earlier stages [171]. Studies with these novel inhibitors of inflammatory pathways will help determine whether targeting the inflammation axis is a fertile mechanism to prevent (or treat) T2DM [181].

Succinobucol (AGI-1067), the monosuccinic acid ester of probucol, is a metabolically stable compound that has greater antioxidant efficacy in vitro than probucol and has also anti-inflammatory properties. A recent large randomised, double-blind, placebo-controlled trial testing the effects of succinobucol on cardiovascular outcomes in patients with recent acute coronary syndromes evaluated as a tertiary endpoint the occurrence of new-onset diabetes [184]. After a mean follow-up of 24 months, fewer patients without diabetes at baseline progressed to diabetes in the succinobucol group than in such patients in the placebo group (30 of 1923 vs 82 of 1950 patients; HR = 0.37, 95% CI 0.24-0.56; p < 0.0001). Similar protection was observed in patients who had impaired fasting glucose at baseline. Interestingly enough, among the 2271 patients with diabetes at baseline, glycated haemoglobin and fasting plasma glucose levels were significantly lower in those given succinobucol than in those on placebo. These results occur without significant changes in body weight or waist circumference. The magnitude of the preventive effect of succinobucol on new-onset diabetes was greater than that seen with acarbose and metformin and comparable to the effect of thiazolidinidiones [67]. As discussed by Tardiff et al [184], the anti-diabetic effect of succinobucol is consistent with the role of oxidative stress and inflammation in diabetes and with preclinical studies showing that probucol prevented diabetes by preserving beta-cell function, possibly as a result of its antioxidant and anti-inflammatory effects in the pancreas. These promising results must be confirmed in further studies before considering succinobucol as a new antidiabetic agent.

29.7   CONCLUSION

The goal of ultimately reducing the population burden of diabetes by early treatment and prevention is clearly of pivotal importance. Obviously, intensive lifestyle intervention is the mainstay for the prevention of T2DM, given the remarkable reduction in the incidence of T2DM, the prolonged benefits, the demonstrable cost-effectiveness and the absence of adverse events. Unfortunately, intensive lifestyle intervention is difficult to implement and to sustain in most individuals, and many subjects will still progress to T2DM. Besides lifestyle modifications, pharmacological strategies using various glucose-lowering agents, antiobesity drugs and

compounds that inhibit RAAS activity might be considered as a valuable alternative. Owing to the pathophysiology of T2DM, these drugs must act either by reducing insulin resistance and/or by improving insulin secretion, with a special interest in the protection of β-cells. The effects of lipid-lowering agents are more controversial, so that these compounds should be used for their cardiovascular protection but not for diabetes prevention. Although estrogen use is controversial as far as cardiovascular prevention is concerned, increasing evidence suggests that estrogen may prevent T2DM in postmenopausal women. As chronic inflammation seems to play a role in the pathophysiology of T2DM, it is plausible that new compounds will emerge in the near future targeting this abnormality. As far as glucose-lowering agents are concerned, an at least partial masking effect should be excluded, because most results were obtained either when subjects were still on the drug or after a rather short washout period. In addition, because T2DM is a progressive disease, it remains to be established in long-term studies whether the so-called preventing effect is not simply a postponing effect.

It is of note that no pharmacological agent is currently approved for the particular indication of diabetes prevention. However, because so many different pharmacological approaches may be theoretically used, a practical key question would be which one should be chosen for each patient. Besides the phenotype of the patient, it is expected that genotype studies will help in the selection in the near future. Another interesting question is whether combined drug therapy may add further protection against new-onset diabetes. Although no additive protection was observed neither in the DREAM study with the rosiglitazone–ramipril combination compared with rosiglitazone alone nor in the ONTARGET trial with the telmisartan-ramipril combination compared to ramipril alone, new ongoing trials assessing the potential of various other combinations (metformin + rosiglitazone, nateglinide + valsartan, + ramipril) would provide a partial answer to this last question. Finally, all available data and ongoing trials are limited to the middle-aged or elderly population. The prevalence of diabetes is growing rapidly in adolescents, so that preventive measures, including pharmacological approaches when necessary, should be implemented rapidly among pediatric patients and presumably should target first overweight/obese young people with a family history of T2DM. However, long-term benefits from preventing new-onset diabetes, although easily conceivable, remain to be demonstrated in the future.

ACKNOWLEDGMENTS

No sources of funding were used to assist in the preparation of this manuscript. The author has no conflicts of interest that are directly relevant to the content of this manuscript.

References

1. Harris, M.I. (2000) Health care and health status and outcomes for patients with type 2 diabetes. *Diabetes Care*, **23**, 754–8.

2. Massi-Benedetti, M. (ed) (2002) The cost of diabetes type II in Europe. The CODE-2 study. *Diabetologia*, **45** (Suppl 1), S1–28.

3. International Diabetes Forum (2006) Prevalence of Diabetes, http://www.idf.org/home/index.cfm (accessed 14 March 2006), International Diabetes Forum.

4. Scheen, A.J. and Lefèbvre, P.J. (2000) Insulin resistance versus insulin deficiency: which one comes first? The old question revisited in *Diabetes in the New Millennium* (eds U. Di Mario, F. Leonetti, G. Pugliese, *et al.*), John Wiley & Sons, Ltd, New York, pp. 101–13.

5. Kahn, S.E. (2003) The relative contributions of insulin resistance and beta-cell dysfunction to the pathophysiology of type 2 diabetes. *Diabetologia*, **46**, 3–19.

6. Stumvoll, M., Goldstein, B.J. and van Haeften, T.W. (2005) Type 2 diabetes: principles of pathogenesis and therapy. *Lancet*, **365**, 1333–46.

7. Grundy, S.M., Cleeman, J.I., Daniels, S.R. *et al.* (2005) Diagnosis and management of the metabolic syndrome. An American Heart Association/National Heart, Lung, and Blood Institute Scientific Statement. *Circulation*, **112**, 2735–52.

8. King, H., Aubert, R.E. and Herman, W.H. (1998) Global burden of diabetes, 1995–2025: prevalence, numerical estimates, and projections. *Diabetes Care*, **21**, 1414–31.

9. Scheen, A.J. (2001) Obesity and diabetes in *The Management of Obesity and Related Disorders* (ed P.G. Kopelman), Martin Dunitz, London, UK, pp. 11–44.

10. Scheen, A.J. and Lefèbvre, P.J. (1996) Pathophysiology of type 2 diabetes in *Handbook of Experimental Pharmacology, Oral Antidiabetics*, (eds J. Kuhlmann and W. Puls), Springer-Verlag, Berlin, pp. 7–42.

11. Edelstein, S.L., Knowler, W.C. Bain, R.P. *et al.* (1997) Predictors of progression from impaired glucose tolerance to NIDDM. An analysis of six prospective studies. *Diabetes*, **46**, 701–10.

12. Harris, R., Donahue, K., Rathore, S.S. *et al.* (2003) Screening adults for type 2 diabetes: a review of the evidence for the U.S. Preventive Services Task Force. *Annals of Internal Medicine*, **138**, 215–29.

13. The Expert Committee on the Diagnosis and Classification of Diabetes Mellitus (1997) Report on the Expert Committee on the Diagnosis and Classification of Diabetes Mellitus. *Diabetes Care*, **20**, 1183–97.

14. WHO Study Group (1994) *Prevention of diabetes mellitus: report of WHO study group*. WHO Technical Report Series, 844, WHO, Geneva, pp. 1–100.

15. Donelly, R. and Garber, A. (eds) (2001) Progression of type 2 diabetes–inevitable or preventable? *Diabetes, Obesity and Metabolism*, **3** (Suppl 1), S1–43.

16. American Diabetes Association and National Institute of Diabetes, Digestive and Kidney Diseases (2002) The prevention or delay of type 2 diabetes. *Diabetes Care*, **25**, 742–9.

17. Tuomilehto, J., Lindström, J., Eriksson J.G. *et al.* (2001) Prevention of type 2 diabetes mellitus by changes in lifestyle among subjects with impaired glucose tolerance. *New England Journal of Medicine*, **344**, 1343–50.

18. Knowler, W.C., Barrett-Connor, E., Fowler, S.E. *et al.* (2002) Reduction in the incidence of type 2 diabetes with lifestyle intervention or metformin. *New England Journal of Medicine*, **346**, 393–403.

19. Scheen, A.J. (2003) Current management strategies for coexisting diabetes mellitus and obesity. *Drugs*, **63**, 1165–84.

20. Zimmet, P., Shaw, J. and Alberti, K.G.M.M. (2003) Preventing type 2 diabetes and the dysmetabolic syndrome in the real world: a realistic view. *Diabetic Medicine: A Journal of the British Diabetic Association*, **20**, 693–702.

21. Davies, M.J., Tringham, J.R., Troughton, J. and Khunti, K.K. (2004) Prevention of type 2 diabetes mellitus: a review of the evidence and its application in a UK setting. *Diabetic Medicine: A Journal of the British Diabetic Association*, **21**, 403–14.

22. Schulze, M.B. and Hu, F.B. (2005) Primary prevention of diabetes: what can be done and how much can be prevented? *Annual Review of Public Health*, **26**, 445–67.

23. Simpson, R.W., Shaw, J.E. and Zimmet, P.Z. (2003) The prevention of type 2 diabetes–lifestyle change or pharmacotherapy? *Diabetes Research and Clinical Practice*, **103**, 357–62.

24. Liberopoulos, E.N., Tsouli, S., Mikhailidis, D.P. and Elisaf, M.S. (2006) Preventing type 2 diabetes in high risk patients: an overview of lifestyle and pharmacological measures. *Current Drug Targets*, **7**, 211–28.

25. Chiasson, J.L. and Rabasa-Lhoret, R. (2004) Prevention of type 2 diabetes: insulin resistance and beta-cell function. *Diabetes*, **53** (Suppl 3), S34–8.

26. Freemark, M. (2003) Pharmacologic approaches to the prevention of type 2 diabetes in high risk pediatric patients. *The Journal of Clinical Endocrinology and Metabolism*, **88**, 3–13.

27. Krentz, A.J. and Bailey, C.J. (2005) Oral antidiabetic agents: current role in type 2 diabetes mellitus. *Drugs*, **65**, 385–411.

28. Padwal, R., Majumdar, S.R., Johnson, J.A. *et al.* (2005) A systematic review of drug therapy to delay or prevent type 2 diabetes. *Diabetes Care*, **28**, 736–44.

29. Anderson, D.C. Jr (2005) Pharmacologic prevention or delay of type 2 diabetes mellitus. *The Annals of Pharmacotherapy*, **39**, 102–9.

30. Buchanan, T.A. (2003) Prevention of type 2 diabetes. What is it really? *Diabetes Care*, **26**, 1306–8.

31. Scheen, A.J. (2003) Preventing, delaying or masking type 2 diabetes with metformin in the Diabetes Prevention Program? *Diabetes Care*, **26**, 2701.

32. McGarry, J.D. and Dobbins, R.L. (1999) Fatty acids, lipotoxicity and insulin secretion. *Diabetologia*, **42**, 128–38.

33. Scheen, A.J. (2004) Prevention of type 2 diabetes mellitus through inhibition of the renin–angiotensin system. *Drugs*, **64**, 2537–65.

34. Barrett-Connor, E., Grady, D. and Stefanick, M.L. (2005) The rise and fall of menopausal hormone therapy. *Annual Review of Public Health*, **26**, 115–40.

35. Eddy, D.M., Schlessinger, L. and Kahn, R. (2005) Clinical outcomes and cost-effectiveness of strategies for managing people at high risk for diabetes. *Annals of Internal Medicine*, **143**, 251–64.

36. Nathan, D.M., Buse, J.B., Davidson, M.B. *et al.* (2006) Management of hyperglycemia in type 2 diabetes: a consensus algorithm for the initiation and adjustment of therapy. A consensus statement from the American Diabetes Association and the European Association for the Study of Diabetes. *Diabetes Care*, **29**, 1963–72; and (2006) *Diabetologia*, **49**, 1711–21.

37. Cusi, K. and DeFronzo, R.A. (1998) Metformin: a review of its metabolic effects. *Diabetes Forecast*, **6**, 89–131.

38. Fontbonne, A., Charles, M.A. and Juhan-Vague, I. (1994) The effect of metformin on the metabolic abnormalities associated with upper body fat distribution. BIGPRO Study Group. *Diabetes Care*, **19**, 920–6.

39. Tiikkainen, M., Häkkinen, A.-M. and Korsheninnikova, E. *et al.* (2004) Effects of rosiglitazone and metformin on liver fat content, hepatic insulin resistance, insulin clearance, and gene expression in adipose tissue in patients with type 2 diabetes. *Diabetes*, **53**, 2169–76.

40. Freemark, M. and Bursey, D. (2001) The effects of metformin on body mass index and glucose tolerance in obese adolescents with fasting hyperinsulinemia and a family history of type 2 diabetes. *Pediatrics*, **107**, 1–7.

41. Scheen, A.J., Letiexhe, M.R. and Lefèbvre, P.J. (1995) Short administration of metformin improves insulin sensitivity in obese android subjects with impaired glucose tolerance. *Diabetic Medicine: A Journal of the British Diabetic Association*, **12**, 985–9.

42. Diabetes Prevention Program Research Group (2003) Effects of withdrawal from metformin on the development of diabetes in the Diabetes Prevention Program. *Diabetes Care*, **26**, 977–80.

43. Scheen, A.J., Letiexhe, M.R. and Lefèbvre, P.J. (1995) Effects of metformin in obese patients with impaired glucose tolerance. *Diabetes/Metabolism Reviews*, **11**, S69–80.

44. Yang, W., Lin, L. and Qi, J. (2001) The preventive effect of acarbose and metformin on the IGT population from becoming diabetes mellitus: a 3-year multicentre prospective study. *Chinese Journal of Endocrinology and Metabolism*, **17**, 131–6.

45. Holman, R.R., Blackwell, L. Stratton, I.M. *et al.* (2003) Six-year results from the early diabetes intervention trial (abstract). *Diabetic Medicine: A Journal of the British Diabetic Association*, **20** (Suppl 2), S15.

46. Ramachandran, A., Snehalatha, C., Mary, S. *et al.* (2006) The Indian Diabetes Prevention Programme shows that lifestyle modification and metformin prevent type 2 diabetes in Asian Indian subjects with impaired glucose tolerance (IDPP-1). *Diabetologia*, **49**, 289–97.

47. Scheen, A.J. (2004) Pathophysiology of insulin secretion. *Annales d'endocrinologie*, **65**, 29–36.

48. Ferrannini, E., Gastaldelli, A. Miyazaki, Y. *et al.* (2005) β-Cell function in subjects spanning the range from normal glucose tolerance to overt diabetes: a new analysis. *The Journal of Clinical Endocrinology and Metabolism*, **90**, 493–500.

49. Rendell, M. (2004) The role of sulphonylureas in the management of type 2 diabetes mellitus. *Drugs*, **64**, 1339–58.

50. Alberti, K.G.M.M. (1996) The clinical implications of impaired glucose tolerance. *Diabetic Medicine: A Journal of the British Diabetic Association*, **13**, 927–37.

51. Keen, H., Jarrett, R.J., Ward, J.D. and Fuller, J.H. (1973) Boderline diabetics and their response to tolbutamide. *Advances in Metabolic Disorders*, **2** (Suppl 2), 521–31.

52. Sartor, G., Schersten, B. Carlstrom, S. *et al.* (1980) Ten-year follow-up of subjects with impaired glucose tolerance: prevention of diabetes by tolbutamide and diet regulation. *Diabetes*, **29**, 41–9.

53. Herlihy, O.M., Morris, R.J., Karunakaran, S. and Holman, R. (2000) Sulphonylurea therapy over six years does not delay progression to diabetes (abstract). *Diabetologia*, **43** (Suppl 1), A73.

54. Lindblad, U., Lindwall, K., Sjostrand, A. *et al.* (2001) The NEPI Antidiabetes Study (NANSY). 1. Short-term dose–effect relations of glimepiride in subjects with impaired fasting glucose. *Diabetes, Obesity and Metabolism*, **3**, 443–51.

55. Dornhorst, A. (2001) Insulinotropic meglitinide analogues. *Lancet*, **358**, 1709–16.

56. The NAVIGATOR Trial Steering Committee (2002) Nateglinide and valsartan in impaired glucose tolerance outcomes research, rationale and design of the NAVIGATOR trial (abstract). *Diabetes*, **51** (Suppl 2), A116.

57. Gautier, J.F., Fetita, S., Sobngwi, E. and Salaun-Martin, C. (2005) Biological actions of the incretins GIP and GLP-1 and therapeutic perspectives in patients with type 2 diabetes. *Diabetes and Metabolism*, **31**, 233–42.

58. Yki-Järvinen, H. (2004) Thiazolidinediones. *New England Journal of Medicine*, **351**, 1106–18.

59. Leiter, L.A. (2005) beta-cell preservation: a potential role for thiazolidinediones to improve clinical care in type 2 diabetes. *Diabetic Medicine: A Journal of the British Diabetic Association*, **22**, 963–72.

60. Walter, H. and Lubben, G. (2005) Potential role of oral thiazolidinedione therapy in preservation of beta-cell function in type 2 diabetes mellitus. *Drugs*, **65**, 1–13.

61. Buchanan, T.A., Xiang, A.H., Peters, R.K. *et al.* (2002) Preservation of pancreatic beta-cell function and prevention of type 2 diabetes by pharmacological treatment of insulin resistance in high-risk Hispanic women. *Diabetes*, **51**, 2796–803.

62. Scheen, A.J. (2001) Hepatotoxicity with thiazolidinediones. Is it a class effect? *Drug Safety: An International Journal of Medical Toxicology and Drug Experience*, **24**, 873–88.

63. Xiang, A.H., Peters, R.K., Kjos, S.L. *et al.* (2006) Effect of pioglitazone on pancreatic β-cell function and diabetes risk in Hispanic women with prior gestational diabetes. *Diabetes*, **55**, 517–22.

64. Durbin, R.J. (2004) Thiazolidinedione therapy in the prevention/delay of type 2 diabetes in patients with impaired glucose tolerance and insulin resistance. *Diabetes, Obesity and Metabolism*, **6**, 280–5.

65. The Diabetes Prevention Program Research Group (2005) Prevention of type 2 diabetes with troglitazone in the Diabetes Prevention Program. *Diabetes*, **54**, 1150–6.

66. The DREAM (Diabetes Reduction Assessment with Ramipril and Rosiglitazone Medication) Trials Investigators (2006) Effect of rosiglitazone on the frequency of diabetes in patients with impaired glucose tolerance or impaired fasting glucose: a randomised controlled trial. *Lancet*, **368**, 1096–105.

67. Scheen, A.J. (2007) Antidiabetic agents in patients with mild dysglycaemia: prevention or early treatment of type 2 diabetes? *Diabetes and Metabolism*, **33**, 3–12.

68. Zinman, B., Harris, S.B., Gerstein, H.C. *et al.* (2006) Preventing type 2 diabetes using combination therapy: design and methods of the Canadian Normoglycaemia Outcomes Evaluation (CANOE) trial. *Diabetes, Obesity and Metabolism*, **8**, 531–7.

69. Lebovitz, H.E. (1998) α-Glucosidase inhibitors as agents in the treatment of diabetes. *Diabetes Forecast*, **6**, 132–45.

70. Scheen, A.J. (2003) Is there a role to α-glucosidase inhibitors in the prevention of type 2 diabetes? *Drugs*, **63**, 933–51.

71. Chiasson, J.-L., Josse, R.G., Gomis, R. *et al.* (2002) Acarbose for prevention of type 2 diabetes mellitus: the STOP-NIDDM randomised trial. *Lancet*, **359**, 2072–7.

72. Kaiser, T. and Sawicki, P.T. (2004) For debate. Acarbose for prevention of diabetes, hypertension and cardiovascular events? A critical analysis of the STOP-NIDDM data. *Diabetologia*, **47**, 575–80.

73. Chiasson, J-L., Josse, R.G., Gomis, R. *et al.* (2004) Acarbose for the prevention of type 2 diabetes, hypertension and cardiovascular disease in subjects with impaired glucose tolerance: facts and interpretations concerning the critical analysis of the STOP-NIDDM trial data. *Diabetologia*, **47**, 969–75.

74. Josse, R.G., McGuire, A.J. and Saal, G.B. (2006) A review of the economic evidence for acarbose in the prevention of diabetes and cardiovascular events in individuals with impaired glucose tolerance. *International Journal of Clinical Practice*, **60**, 847–55.

75. Gerstein, H.C. and Rosenstock, J. (2005) Insulin therapy in people who have dysglycemia and type 2 diabetes mellitus: can it offer both cardiovascular protection and beta-cell preservation? *Endocrinology and Metabolism Clinics of North America*, **34**, 137–54.

76. Rosenfalck, A.M., Hendel, H., Rasmussen, M.H. *et al.* (2002) Minor long-term changes in weight have beneficial effects on insulin sensitivity and beta-cell function in obese subjects. *Diabetes, Obesity and Metabolism*, **4**, 19–28.

77. Norris, S.L., Zhang, X., Avenell, A. *et al.* (2005) Long-term non-pharmacological weight loss interventions for adults with prediabetes. *Cochrane Database of Systematic Reviews (Online: Update Software)*, 3 (Art. No.: CD005270), DOI: 10.1002/14651858.CD005270.

78. Hamman, R.F., Wing, R.R., Edelstein, S.L. *et al.* (2006) Effect of weight loss with lifestyle intervention on risk of diabetes. *Diabetes Care*, **29**, 2102–7.

79. Padwal, R., Li, S.K. and Lau, D.C. (2004) Long-term pharmacotherapy for obesity and overweight. *Cochrane Database of Systematic Reviews (Online: Update Software)*, 3 (Art. No.: CD004094), DOI: 10.1002/14651858. CD004094.pub2.

80. Li, Z., Maglione, M., Tu, W. *et al.* (2005) Meta-analysis: pharmacologic treatment of obesity. *Annals of Internal Medicine*, **142**, 532–46.

81. Curran, M.P. and Scott, L.J. (2004) Orlistat: a review of its use in the management of patients with obesity. *Drugs*, **64**, 2845–64.

82. Norris, S.L., Zhang, X., Avenell, A. *et al.* (2005) Pharmacotherapy for weight loss in adults with type 2 diabetes. *Cochrane Database of Systematic Reviews (Online: Update Software)*, 1 (Art. No.: CD004096), DOI: 10.1002/ 14651858.CD004096.pub2.

83. Scheen, A.J. and Ernest, P. (2002) Antiobesity treatment in type 2 diabetes: results of clinical trials with orlistat and sibutramine. *Diabetes and Metabolism*, **28**, 437–45.

84. Kelley, D.E., Kuller, L.H., McKolanis, T.M. *et al.* (2004) Effects of moderate weight loss and orlistat on insulin resistance, regional adiposity, and fatty acids in type 2 diabetes. *Diabetes Care*, **27**, 33–40.

85. Tiikkainen, M., Bergholm, R., Rissanen, A. *et al.* (2004) Effects of equal weight loss with orlistat and placebo on body fat and serum fatty acid composition and insulin resistance in obese women. *The American Journal of Clinical Nutrition*, **79**, 22–30.

86. Heysmfield, S.B., Segal, K.R., Hauptman, J. *et al.* (2000) Effects of weight loss with orlistat on glucose tolerance and progression to type 2 diabetes in obese adults. *Archives of Internal Medicine*, **160**, 1321–6.

87. Keating, G.M. and Jarvis, B. (2001) Orlistat in the prevention and treatment of type 2 diabetes mellitus. *Drugs*, **61**, 2107–19.

88. Torgerson, J.S., Hauptman, J., Boldrin, M.N. and Sjöström, L. (2004) Xenical in the Prevention of Diabetes in Obese Subjects (XENDOS) study. A randomised study of orlistat as an adjunct to lifestyle for the prevention of type 2 diabetes in obese patients. *Diabetes Care*, **27**, 155–61.

89. McNeely, W. and Goa, K.L. (1998) Sibutramine. A review of its contribution in the management of obesity. *Drugs*, **56**, 1093–124.

90. Filippatos, T.D., Kiotsis, D.N., Liberopoulos, E.N. *et al.* (2005) A review of the metabolic effects of sibutramine. *Current Medical Research and Opinion*, **21**, 457–68.

91. Arterburn, D.E., Crane, P.K. and Veenstra, D.L. (2004) The efficacy and safety of sibutramine for weight loss: a systematic review. *Archives of Internal Medicine*, **164**, 994–1003.

92. Vettor, R., Serra, R., Fabris, R. *et al.* (2005) Effect of sibutramine on weight management and metabolic control in type 2 diabetes: a meta-analysis of clinical studies. *Diabetes Care*, **28**, 942–9.

93. James, W.P.T., Astrup, A., Fier, N. *et al.* (2000) Effect of sibutramine on weight maintenance after weight loss: a randomised trial. *Lancet*, **356**, 2119–25.

94. James, W.P.T. (2005) The SCOUT study: risk-benefit profile of sibutramine in overweight high-risk cardiovascular patients. *European Heart Journal*, **7** (Suppl L), L44–8.

95. Di Marzo, V., Bifulco, M. and De Petrocellis, L. (2004) The endocannabinoid system and its

therapeutic exploitation. *Nature Reviews. Drug Discovery*, **3**, 771–84.

96. Pagotto, U., Marsicano, G., Cota, D. *et al.* (2006) The emerging role of the endocannabinoid system in endocrine regulation and energy balance. *Endocrine Reviews*, **27**, 73–100.

97. Van Gaal, L.F., Rissanen, A.M., Scheen, A.J. *et al.* (2005) Effects of the cannabinoid-1 receptor blocker rimonabant on weight reduction and cardiovascular risk factors in overweight patients: 1-year experience from the RIO-Europe study. *Lancet*, **365**, 1389–97.

98. Després, J.P., Golay, A. and Sjöström, L. (2005) Effect of rimonabant on body weight and the metabolic syndrome in overweight patients. *New England Journal of Medicine*, **353**, 2121–34.

99. Pi-Sunyer, F.X., Aronne, L.J., Heshmati, H.M. *et al.* (2006) Effect of rimonabant, a cannabinoid-1 receptor blocker, on weight and cardiometabolic risk factors in overweight or obese patients. RIO-North America: a randomized controlled trial. *The Journal of the American Medical Association*, **295**, 761–75.

100. Scheen, A.J., Finer, N., Hollander, P. *et al.* (2006) Effects of rimonabant on body weight, glucose control, and cardiometabolic risk factors in patients with type 2 diabetes. *Lancet*, **368**, 1660–73.

101. Van Gaal, L.F., Pi-Sunyer, X., Després, J.P. *et al.* (2008) Efficacy and safety of rimonabant for improvement of multiple cardiometabolic risk factors in overweight/obese patients: pooled 1-year data from the RIO program. *Diabetes Care*, **31** (Suppl 2), S229–40.

102. Van Gaal, L.F., Scheen, A.J., Rissanen, A.M. *et al.* (2008) RIO-Europe 2-year. Long-term effect of CB1 blockade with rimonabant on cardiometabolic risk factors: two-year results from the RIO-Europe study. *European Heart Journal*, DOI: 10.1093/eurheart/ehn076.

103. Rosenstock, J. (2005) The potential of rimonabant in prediabetes: pooled 1-year results from the RIO-Lipids, RIO-Europe and RIO-North America studies (abstract). *Diabetologia*, **48** (Suppl 1), A16.

104. Taskinen, M.R. (2005) Type 2 diabetes as a lipid disorder. *Current Molecular Medicine*, **5**, 297–308.

105. Boden, G. (1997) Role of fatty acids in the pathogenesis of insulin resistance and NIDDM. *Diabetes*, **45**, 3–10.

106. Lewis, G.F., Carpentier, A., Adeli, K. and Giacca, A. (2002) Disordered fat storage and mobilization in the pathogenesis of insulin resistance and type 2 diabetes. *Endocrine Reviews*, **23**, 201–29.

107. Paolisso, G., Barbagallo, M., Petrella, G. *et al.* (2000) Effects of simvastatin and atorvastatin administration on insulin resistance and respiratory quotient in aged dyslipidemic non-insulin dependent diabetic patients. *Atherosclerosis*, **150**, 121–7.

108. Karhapää, P., Uusitupa, M., Voutilainen, E. and Laakso, M. (1992) Effect of bezafibrate on insulin sensitivity and glucose tolerance in subjects with combined hyperlipidaemia. *Clinical Pharmacology and Therapeutics*, **52**, 620–6.

109. Vuorinen-Markkola, H., Yki-Järvinen, H. and Taskinen, M.-R. (1993) Lowering of triglycerides by gemfibrozil affects neither the glucoregulatory nor antipolytic effect of insulin in type 2 (non-insulin-dependent) diabetic patients. *Diabetologia*, **36**, 161–9.

110. Kahn, S.E., Beard, J.C., Schwartz, M.W. *et al.* (1989) Increased beta-cell secretory capacity as mechanism for islet adaptation to nicotinc acid-induced insulin resistance. *Diabetes*, **38**, 562–8.

111. Bonetti, P.O., Lerman, L.O., Napoli, C. and Lerman, A. (2003) Statin effects beyond lipid lowering–are they clinically relevant? *European Heart Journal*, **24**, 225–48.

112. Freeman, D.J., Norrie, J., Sattar, N. *et al.* (2001) Pravastatin and the development of diabetes mellitus: evidence for a protective treatment effect in the West of Scotland Coronary Prevention Study. *Circulation*, **103**, 357–62.

113. Heart Protection Study Collaborative Group (2002) MRC/BHF Heart Protection Study of cholesterol lowering with simvastatin in 20,536 high risk individuals. *Lancet*, **360**, 7–22.

114. Keech, A., Colquhoun, D., Best, J. *et al.* (2003) Secondary prevention of cardiovascular events with long-term pravastatin in patients with diabetes or impaired fasting glucose. *Diabetes Care*, **26**, 2713–21.

115. Sever, P.S., Dahlof, B., Poulter, N.R. *et al.* (2003) Prevention of coronary and stroke events with atorvastatin in hypertensive patients who have average or lower-than-average cholesterol concentrations in the Anglo-Scandinavian Cardiac Outcomes Trial-Lipid Lowering Arm (ASCOT-LLA): a multicentre randomised controlled trial. *Lancet*, **361**, 1149–58.

116. Yee, A., Majumdar, S.R., Simpson, S.H. *et al.* (2004) Statin use in type 2 diabetes mellitus is associated with a delay in starting insulin. *Diabetic Medicine: A Journal of the British Diabetic Association*, **21**, 962–7.

117. Jick, S.S. and Bradbury, B.D. (2004) Statins and newly diagnosed diabetes. *British Journal of Clinical Pharmacology*, **58**, 303–9.

118. Staels, B. and Fruchart, J.C. (2005) Therapeutic roles of peroxisome proliferator-activated receptor agonists. *Diabetes*, **54**, 2460–70.

119. Tenenbaum, A., Motro, M., Fisman, E.Z. *et al.* (2004) Peroxisome proliferator-activated receptor ligand bezafibrate for prevention of type 2 diabetes mellitus in patients with coronary artery disease. *Circulation*, **109**, 2197–202.

120. Vega, G.L., Cater, N.B., Meguro, S. and Grundy, S.M. (2005) Influence of extended-release nicotinic acid on nonesterified fatty acid flux in the metabolic syndrome with atherogenic dyslipidemia. *The American Journal of Cardiology*, **95**, 1309–13.

121. Shepherd, J., Betteridge, J. and Van Gaal, L. (2005) Nicotinic acid in the management of dyslipidaemia associated with diabetes and metabolic syndrome: a position paper developed by a European Consensus Panel. *Current Medical Research and Opinion*, **21**, 665–82.

122. Abuissa, H., Jones, P.G., Marso, S.P. and O'Keefe, J.H. (2005) Angiotensin-converting enzyme inhibitors or angiotensin receptor blockers for prevention of type 2 diabetes. A meta-analysis of randomized clinical trials. *Journal of the American College of Cardiology*, **46**, 821–6.

123. Gillespie, E.L., White, C.M., Kardas, M. *et al.* (2005) The impact of ACE inhibitors or angiotensin II type 1 receptor blockers on the development of new-onset type 2 diabetes. *Diabetes Care*, **28**, 2261–6.

124. Vijayaraghavan, K. and Deedwania, P.C. (2005) The renin angiotensin system as a therapeutic target to prevent diabetes and its complications. *Cardiology Clinics*, **23**, 165–83.

125. Gress, T.W., Nieto, F.J., Shahar, E. *et al.* (2000) Hypertension and antihypertensive therapy as risk factors for type 2 diabetes mellitus. *New England Journal of Medicine*, **342**, 905–12.

126. Padwal, R. and Laupacis, A. (2004) Antihypertensive therapy and incidence of type 2 diabetes. A systematic review. *Diabetes Care*, **27**, 247–55.

127. Pepine, C.J. and Cooper-DeHoff, R.M. (2004) Cardiovascular therapies and risk for development of diabetes. *Journal of the American College of Cardiology*, **44**, 509–12.

128. Stump, C.S., Hamilton, M.T. and Sowers, J.R. (2006) Effect of antihypertensive agents on the development of type 2 diabetes mellitus. *Mayo Clinic Proceedings*, **81**, 796–806.

129. Jandeleit-Dahm, K.A., Tikellis, C., Reid, C.M. *et al.* (2005) Why blockade of the rennin–angiotensin system reduces the incidence of new-onset diabetes. *Journal of Hypertension*, **23**, 463–73.

130. Scheen, A.J. (2004) Renin–angiotensin system inhibition prevents type 2 diabetes mellitus. Part 2. Overview of physiological and biochemical mechanisms. *Diabetes and Metabolism*, **30**, 498–505.

131. Leiter, L.A. and Lewanczuk, R.Z. (2005) Of the renin–angiotensin system and reactive oxygen species. Type 2 diabetes and angiotensin II inhibition. *American Journal of Hypertension*, **18**, 121–8.

132. Tikellis, C., Cooper, M.E. and Thomas, M.C. (2006) Role of the renin–angiotensin system in the endocrine pancreas: implications for the development of diabetes. *The International Journal of Biochemistry and Cell Biology*, **38**, 737–51.

133. Scheen, A.J. (2004) Renin–angiotensin system inhibition prevents type 2 diabetes mellitus. Part 1. A meta-analysis of randomised clinical trials. *Diabetes and Metabolism*, **30**, 487–96.

134. Hansson, L., Lindholm, L.H., Ekblom, T. *et al.* (1999) Randomised trial of old and new antihypertensive drugs in elderly patients: cardiovascular mortality and morbidity the Swedish Trial in Old Patients with Hypertension-2 study. *Lancet*, **354**, 1751–6.

135. Hansson, L., Lindholm, L.H., Niskanen, L. *et al.* (1999) Effect of angiotensin-converting-enzyme inhibition compared with conventional therapy on cardiovascular morbidity and mortality in hypertension: the Captopril Prevention Project (CAPPP) randomised trial. *Lancet*, **353**, 611–16.

136. The ALLHAT Officers and Coordinators for the ALLHAT Collaborative Research Group (2002) Major outcomes in high-risk hypertensive patients randomized to angiotensin-converting enzyme inhibitor or calcium channel blocker vs diuretic. The Antihypertensive and Lipid-Lowering Treatment to Prevent Heart Attack Trial (ALLHAT). *The Journal of the American Medical Association*, **288**, 2981–97.

137. Reid, C.M., Johnston, C.I., Ryan, P. *et al.* (2003) Diabetes and cardiovascular outcomes in elderly subjects treated with ACE-inhibitors or diuretics: findings from the 2nd Australian National Blood Pressure Study (abstract). *American Journal of Hypertension*, **16**, 11A.

138. Dahlof, B., Sever, P.S., Poulter, N.R. *et al.* (2005) Prevention of cardiovascular events with an antihypertensive regimen of amlodipine adding perindopril as required versus atenolol adding bendroflumethiazide as required, in the Anglo-Scandinavian Cardiac Outcomes Trial-Blood Pressure Lowering Arm (ASCOT-BPLA):

a multicentre randomised controlled trial. *Lancet*, **366**, 895–906.

139. Braunwald, E., Domanski, M.J., Fowler, S.E. *et al.* (2004) Angiotensin-converting-enzyme inhibition in stable coronary artery disease. *New England Journal of Medicine*, **351**, 2058–68.

140. Pepine, C.J., Handberg, E.M., Cooper-DeHoff, R.M. *et al.* (2003) A calcium antagonist vs a non-calcium antagonist hypertension treatment strategy for patients with coronary artery disease. The International Verapamil-Trandolapril Study (INVEST): a randomized controlled trial. *The Journal of the American Medical Association*, **290**, 2805–16.

141. The European Trial on Reduction of Cardiac Events with Perindopril in Patients with Stable Coronary Artery Disease Investigators (EUROPA) (2003) Efficacy of perindopril in reduction of cardiovascular events among patients with stable coronary artery disease: randomised, double-blind, placebo-controlled, multicentre trial (the EUROPA study). *Lancet*, **362**, 782–8.

142. Yusuf, S., Sleight, P., Pogue, J. *et al.* (2000) Effects of an angiotensin-converting-enzyme inhibitor, ramipril, on cardiovascular events in high-risk patients: the Heart Outcomes Prevention Evaluation Study Investigators. *New England Journal of Medicine*, **342**, 145–53.

143. Yusuf, S., Gerstein, H., Hoogwerf, B. *et al.* (2001) Ramipril and the development of diabetes. *The Journal of the American Medical Association*, **286**, 1882–5.

144. HOPE/HOPE-TOO Study Investigators (2005) Long-term effects of ramipril on cardiovascular events and on diabetes. Results of the HOPE study extension. *Circulation*, **112**, 1339–46.

145. Vermes, E., Ducharme, A., Bourassa, M.G. *et al.* (2003) Enalapril reduces the incidence of diabetes in patients with chronic heart failure. Insight from the Studies Of Left Ventricular Dysfunction (SOLVD). *Circulation*, **107**, 1291–6.

146. The DREAM Trial Investigators (2006) Effect of ramipril on the incidence of diabetes. *New England Journal of Medicine*, **355**, 1551–62.

147. Ingelfinger, J.R. and Solomon C.G. (2006) Angiotensin-converting-enzyme inhibitors for impaired glucose tolerance—is there still hope? *New England Journal of Medicine*, **355** (15), 1551–62.

148. Dahlöf, B., Devereux, R.B., Kjeldsen S.E. *et al.* (2002) Cardiovascular morbidity and mortality in the Losartan Intervention For Endpoint reduction in hypertension study (LIFE): a randomised trial against atenolol. *Lancet*, **359**, 995–1003.

149. Lindholm, L.H., Ibsen, H., Borch-Johnsen, K. *et al.* (2002) Risk of new onset-diabetes in the Losartan Intervention for Endpoint reduction in hypertension study. *Journal of Hypertension*, **20**, 1879–86.

150. Lindholm, L.H., Persson, M., Alaupovic, P. *et al.* (2003) Metabolic outcome during 1 year in newly detected hypertensives: results of the Antihypertensive Treatment and Lipid Profile in a North of Sweden Efficacy Evaluation (ALPINE study). *Journal of Hypertension*, **21**, 1563–74.

151. Julius, S., Kjeldsen, S.E. Weber, M. *et al.* (2004) Outcomes in hypertensive patients at high cardiovascular risk treated with regimens based on valsartan or amlodipine: the VALUE randomised trial. *Lancet*, **363**, 2022–31.

152. Lithell, H., Hansson, L., Skoog, I. *et al.* (2003) The Study on Cognition and Prognosis in the Elderly (SCOPE): principal results of a randomized double-blind intervention trial. *Journal of Hypertension*, **21**, 875–86.

153. Pfeffer, M.A., Swedberg, K., Granger, C.B. *et al.* (2003) Effects of candesartan on mortality and morbidity in patients with chronic heart failure: the CHARM-Overall programme. *Lancet*, **362**, 759–66.

154. Yusuf, S., Ostergren, J.B. Gerstein, H.C. *et al.* (2005) Effects of candesartan on the development of a new diagnosis of diabetes mellitus in patients with heart failure. *Circulation*, **112**, 48–53.

155. The ONTARGET Investigators (2008) Telmisartan, ramipril, or both in patients at high risk for vascular events. *New Engl J Med*, **358**, 1547–59.

156. Schupp, M., Clemenz, M., Gineste, R. *et al.* (2005) Molecular characterization of new selective peroxisome proliferators-activated receptor γ modulators with angiotensin receptor blocking activity. *Diabetes*, **54**, 3442–52.

157. Pershadsingh, H.A. (2006) Treating the metabolic syndrome using angiotensin receptor antagonists that selectively modulate peroxisome proliferators-activated receptor-γ. *The International Journal of Biochemistry and Cell Biology*, **38**, 766–81.

158. Kurtz, T.W. and Pravenec, M. (2004) Antidiabetic mechanisms of angiotensin-converting enzyme inhibitors and angiotensin II receptor antagonists: beyond the renin–angiotensin system. *Journal of Hypertension*, **22**, 2253–61.

159. Louet, J.F., LeMay, C. and Mauvais-Jarvis, F. (2004) Antidiabetic actions of estrogen: insight from human and genetic mouse models. *Current Atherosclerosis Reports*, **6**, 180–5.

160. Barros, R.P., Machado, U.F. and Gustafsson, J.A. Estrogen receptors: new players in diabetes mellitus. (2006) *Trends in Molecular Medicine*, **12**, 425–31.

161. Manson, J.E., Rimm, E.B., Colditz, G.A. *et al.* (1992) A prospective study of postmenopausal estrogen therapy and subsequent incidence of non-insulin-dependent diabetes mellitus. *Annals of Epidemiology*, **2**, 665–73.

162. Zhang, Y., Howard, B.V., Cowan, L.D. *et al.* (2002) The effect of estrogen use on levels of glucose and insulin and the risk of type 2 diabetes in America Indian postmenopausal women: the Strong Heart Study. *Diabetes Care*, **25**, 500–4.

163. Rossi, R., Origliani, G. and Modena, M.G. (2004) Transdermal 17-β-estradiol and risk of developing type 2 diabetes in a population of healthy, non-obese postmenopausal women. *Diabetes Care*, **27**, 645–9.

164. Kanaya, A.M., Herrington, D., Vittinghoff, E. *et al.* (2003) Glycemic effects of postmenopausal hormone therapy: the heart and estrogen/progestin replacement study. *Annals of Internal Medicine*, **138**, 1–9.

165. Margolis, K.L., Bonds, D.E., Rodabough, R.J. *et al.* (2004) Effect of oestrogen plus progestin on the incidence of diabetes in postmenopausal women: results from the Women's Health Initiative Hormone Trial. *Diabetologia*, **47**, 1175–87.

166. Bonds, D.E., Lasser, N., Qi, L. *et al.* (2006) The effect of conjugated equine oestrogen on diabetes incidence: the Women's Health Initiative randomised trial. *Diabetologia*, **49**, 459–68.

167. Kim, D.-J. and Barrett-Conor, E. (2006) Association of serum proinsulin with hormone replacement therapy in nondiabetic older women. The Rancho Bernardo Study. *Diabetes Care*, **29**, 618–24.

168. Godsland, I.F. (2005) Oestrogens and insulin secretion. *Diabetologia*, **48**, 2213–20.

169. Pickup, J.C. and Crook, M.A. (1998) Is type 2 diabetes mellitus a disease of the innate immune system? *Diabetologia*, **41**, 1241–8.

170. Helmersson, J., Vessby, B., Larsson, A. and Basu, S. (2004) Association of type 2 diabetes with cyclooxygenase-mediated inflammation and oxidative stress in an elderly population. *Circulation*, **109**, 1729–34.

171. Shoelson, S.E., Lee, J. and Goldfine, A.B. (2006) Inflammation and insulin resistance. *The Journal of Clinical Investigation*, **116**, 1793–801.

172. Schmidt, M.I., Duncan, B.B., Sharrett, A.R. *et al.* (1999) Markers of inflammation and prediction of diabetes mellitus in adults (Atherosclerosis Risk in Communities Study): a cohort study. *Lancet*, **353**, 1649–52.

173. Pradhan, A.D., Manson, J., Rifai, N. *et al.* (2001) C-reactive protein, interleukin 6, and risk of developing type 2 diabetes mellitus. *The Journal of the American Medical Association*, **286**, 327–34.

174. Barzilay, J.I., Araham, L., Heckbert, S.R. *et al.* (2001) The relation of markers of inflammation to the development of glucose disorders in the elderly: the Cardiovascular Health Study. *Diabetes*, **50**, 2384–9.

175. Freeman, D.J., Norrie, J., Caslake, M.J. *et al.* (2002) C-reactive protein is an independent predictor of risk for the development of diabetes in the West of Scotland Coronary Prevention Study. *Diabetes*, **51**, 1596–600.

176. Festa, A., D'Agostino, R. Jr, Tracy R.P. *et al.* (2002) Elevated levels of acute-phase proteins and plasminogen activator inhibitor-1 predict the development of type 2 diabetes: the Insulin Resistance Atherosclerosis Study. *Diabetes*, **51**, 1131–7.

177. Duncan, B.B., Schmidt, M.I., Pankow, J.S. *et al.* (2003) Low-grade systemic inflammation and the development of type 2 diabetes: the Atherosclerosis Risk in Communities Study. *Diabetes*, **52**, 1799–805.

178. Spranger, J., Kroke, A., Mohlig, M. *et al.* (2003) Adiponectin and protection against type 2 diabetes. *Lancet*, **361**, 226–8.

179. Duncan, B.B., Schmidt, M.I., Pankow, J.S. *et al.* (2004) Adiponectin and the development of type 2 diabetes: the Atherosclerosis Risk in Communities Study. *Diabetes*, **53**, 2473–8.

180. Haffner, S. (2001) Do interventions to reduce coronary heart disease reduce the incidence of type 2 diabetes? A possible role for inflammatory factors. *Circulation*, **103**, 346–7.

181. Deans, K.A. and Sattar, N. (2006) ''Anti-inflammatory'' drugs and their effects on type 2 diabetes. *Diabetes Technology and Therapeutics*, **8**, 18–27.

182. Hundal, R.S., Petersen, K.F., Mayerson, A.B. *et al.* (2002) Mechanism by which high-dose aspirin improves glucose metabolism in type 2 diabetes. *The Journal of Clinical Investigation*, **109**, 1321–6.

183. Möhlig, M., Freudenberg, M., Bobbert, T. *et al.* (2006) Acetylsalicylic acid improves lipid-induced insulin resistance in healthy men. *The Journal of Clinical Endocrinology and Metabolism*, **91**, 964–7.

184. Tardiff, J.C., McMurray, J.J.V., Klug, E. *et al.* (2008) Effects of succinobucol (AGI-1067) after an acute coronary syndrome : a randomised, double-blind, placebo-controlled trial. *Lancet*, **371**, 1761–8.

30

The Epidemiology of Eye Diseases in Diabetes

Tien Y. Wong[1] and Ron Klein[2]

[1]Centre for Eye Research Australia, University of Melbourne, Melbourne, Victoria, Australia

[2]Department of Ophthamology and Visual Sciences, University of Wisconsin School of Medicine and Public Health, Madison, WI, USA

30.1 INTRODUCTION

Diabetes mellitus has profound effects on the structure and function of the eye. First, the primary microvascular complication of diabetes in the eye, diabetic retinopathy, is the leading cause of blindness among persons aged 20–64 years in the United States [1]. A recent study suggest that up to 4 million Americans 40 years and older with diabetes have retinopathy, with nearly 1 million having retinopathy that is sight threatening [2]. Each year, it has been estimated nearly 100 000 Americans will develop proliferative retinopathy and 120 000 will develop macular edema.

In addition to retinopathy, diabetes is a major risk factor for the development of other vascular diseases in the eye, such as retinal vein and artery occlusion and ischemic optic neuropathy. Diabetes is also associated with several nonvascular ocular diseases, including cataract and glaucoma, two important causes of visual impairment. This chapter will review the epidemiology and risk factors of these ocular conditions in people with diabetes.

30.2 DIABETIC RETINOPATHY

30.2.1 Classification of Diabetic Retinopathy

Diabetic retinopathy can be broadly divided into an early stage of nonproliferative diabetic retinopathy

(NPDR) and a later stage of proliferative diabetic retinopathy (PDR). NPDR includes a spectrum of retinal vascular signs, such as microaneurysms, retinal hemorrhages, cotton wool spots and hard exudates. With increasing severity, retinal venous beading and intraretinal microvascular abnormalities may develop. These signs usually precede frank new vessel formation, heralding the onset of PDR. Although numerous classifications of diabetic retinopathy have been developed, principally for use in clinical trials, the American Academy of Ophthalmology has adopted a new, simplified classification for use in routine clinical practice [3]. In this system, diabetic retinopathy is simply divided into none, mild, moderate, severe and proliferative (**Table 30.1**).

30.2.2 Prevalence of Diabetic Retinopathy

Epidemiological studies in the United States have provided data on the prevalence and risk factors of diabetic retinopathy [4–14]. The Wisconsin Epidemiologic Study of Diabetic Retinopathy (WESDR) reported both the prevalence and incidence of diabetic retinopathy in a community-based cohort of White persons with diabetes in Wisconsin [15–17]. Using stereoscopic fundus photographs of seven fields to define retinopathy, the WESDR has shown that in persons with type 1 diabetes (younger-onset diabetes who were

The Epidemiology of Diabetes Mellitus, second edition   Edited by Jean-Marie Ekoé, Marian Rewers, Rhys Williams and Paul Zimmet
© 2008 John Wiley & Sons, Ltd

Table 30.1 International clinical diabetic retinopathy disease severity scale.

Proposed disease severity level	Retinal findings
No apparent retinopathy	No abnormalities
Mild NPDR	Microaneurysms only
Moderate NPDR	More than just microaneurysms but less than severe NPDR
Severe NPDR	Any of the following with no signs of PDR: • More than 20 intraretinal hemorrhages in each of four quadrants • Definite venous beading in ≥ 2 quadrants • Prominent intra-retinal microvascular abnormalities in ≥ 1 quadrant
PDR	One or more of the following: • Neovascularization • Vitreous/preretinal hemorrhage

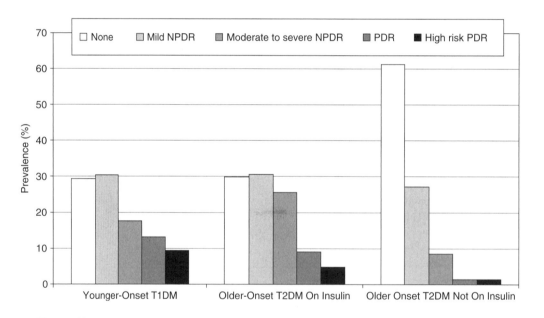

Figure 30.1 Prevalence of diabetic retinopathy at baseline (1980–1982), the WESDR.

on insulin treatment), about 71% had retinopathy at diagnosis, with 23% having PDR and 6% having clinically significant macular edema (CSME) [16]. In persons with type 2 diabetes (older-onset diabetes) who were not on insulin treatment, 39% had retinopathy at diagnosis, with 3% having PDR and 4% having CSME. In persons with type 2 diabetes who were on insulin treatment, the prevalence of diabetic retinopathy was higher, with 70% having some retinopathy,

14% PDR and 11% CSME [18]. These are shown in **Figure 30.1**. A more recent meta-analysis of eight population-based studies that included the WESDR that had used standardized photographic methods to grade retinopathy estimated that, in the United States, 40% of persons with type 2 diabetes aged 40 years and older have diabetic retinopathy, with 8% having sight-threatening disease (either severe NPDR, PDR or macular edema) [2].

There have also been several epidemiological studies on the prevalence of diabetic retinopathy in other countries around the world [19–29]. In general, whilst direct comparisons between reports are limited by differences in participant characteristics and assessment of retinopathy, these studies show that diabetic retinopathy is common. For example, one study in England in Melton Mowbray showed that retinopathy was present in 41% of participants with type 1 diabetes [25] and 52% in those with type 2 diabetes [26]. In Australia, three population-based studies have assessed diabetic retinopathy from standardized assessments of retinal photographs. The Visual Impairment Project in Melbourne reported a retinopathy prevalence of 29% among persons aged 40 years or older with self-reported diabetes [20]. The Blue Mountains Eye Study in Sydney found a similar overall retinopathy prevalence of 32% among a slightly older population 49 years and older with known or newly diagnosed diabetes [22]. The Australian Diabetes Obesity and Lifestyle (AusDiab) study, which examined adults 25 years and older from urban and rural communities in Australia found a retinopathy prevalence of 25% among participants with known diabetes [29].

There are fewer epidemiological data of diabetic retinopathy in Asia, although the prevalence of diabetes seems to have increased substantially in the last few decades [30–33]. In Singapore, serial population surveys have documented an increase in diabetes prevalence of 2% in 1975, 4.7% in 1985 and 8.6% in 1992 in people between 15 and 69 years [33, 34]. Two population-based studies in India reported diabetic retinopathy prevalence of 27% and 22% in southern Indian persons with type 2 diabetes [35, 36]. There are few reliable data from other Asian countries.

30.2.3 Incidence of Diabetic Retinopathy

In contrast to the abundance of studies on the prevalence of diabetic retinopathy, there are fewer long-term data on the incidence and natural history of this diabetic condition [37–44]. In the WESDR, Klein and colleagues has reported on the incidence of retinopathy in type 1 and type 2 diabetes [45–47]. The overall 4-year incidence of any diabetic retinopathy in the WESDR was 40% [45, 46], but incidence and progression rates were generally higher in participants with younger-onset type 1 diabetes than those with older-onset type 2 diabetes (**Figure 30.2**).

In the WESDR, the 10-year incidence of diabetic retinopathy was 75% in the younger-onset type 1 diabetes group, 70% in the older-onset type 2

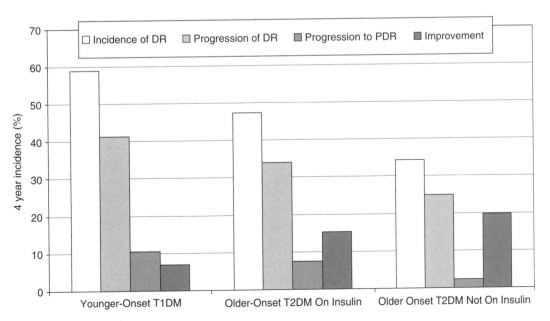

Figure 30.2 Four-year incidences of retinopathy, progression of retinopathy, progression to PDR and improvement in retinopathy, the WESDR.

diabetes group on insulin treatment and 50% in those not on insulin treatment [47]. The WESDR showed that, amongst those with retinopathy, progression to proliferative retinopathy occurred in nearly a third of the participants with younger-onset type 1 diabetes, and between 10 and 25% in participants with older-onset type 2 diabetes [47]. The 10-year incidence of macular edema was 20% in the type 1 diabetes and between 15 and 25% in the type 2 diabetes [48].

There are few other studies on the incidence of diabetic retinopathy. In the Pittsburgh Epidemiology of Diabetes Complications Study, the 2-year incidence of retinopathy was 33% in type 1 diabetes [49]. Among persons with retinopathy at baseline, 23% progressed by two or more steps on the early treatment for diabetic retinopathy study (ETDRS) scale and 10% developed PDR. For type 2 diabetes, the Liverpool Diabetic Eye Study showed that the annual incidence of sight-threatening retinopathy was 0.3% in the first year and 1.8% in the fifth year [44].

30.2.4 Time Trends in the Epidemiology of Diabetic Retinopathy

There are expectations that rates of diabetic blindness may have declined with better screening, recognition and management of diabetic retinopathy and its risk factors. Studies conducted in contemporary populations indicate lower rates of retinopathy in later studies than in earlier studies, although comparisons with older studies are typically hampered by differences in study design, participant characteristics and changing diabetes definition. Nonetheless, in the meta-analysis of eight population-based studies, estimates of retinopathy prevalence were about 10–20% lower in the seven later studies conducted in the 1990s compared with the WESDR, which was conducted in the early 1980s [2]. Furthermore, prospective data from both the United Kingdom Prospective Diabetes Study (UKPDS) [43] and the Liverpool Diabetic Eye Study [44] show lower incidence rates for retinopathy, particularly severe or sight-threatening retinopathy, than was reported previously in the WESDR [15–17] and other studies in the early 1980s [50]. Serial data from Sweden have indicated that the prevalence of retinopathy may have decreased in the past decade [38]. One recent study showed that the median diabetes duration before the onset of retinopathy was 17 years in patients with type 1 diabetes [51], which was longer than reported in previous studies. These observations suggest that advances in diabetes management and improved levels of metabolic and blood pressure control may have had a positive impact in reducing the prevalence and incidence of retinopathy.

30.2.5 Demographic Variations in Diabetic Retinopathy

The relationship of diabetic retinopathy with age, gender and race has been extensively analyzed. In type 1 diabetes, the prevalence and incidence of diabetic retinopathy increases with age. In the WESDR, prior to 13 years of age, diabetic retinopathy was infrequent, irrespective of the duration of the disease [16]. In the WESDR, the 4-year incidence of retinopathy increased with age and was highest in persons 15–19 years of age, after which there was a gradual decline [45]. The 4-year progression to PDR was low among younger type 1 WESDR diabetes participants and there no participant younger than 13 years of age who developed PDR at the 4-year follow-up examination. These data are supported by similar observations in other cohorts with type 1 diabetes [52, 53]. Therefore, it has been recommended that retinopathy screening may not be necessary in young children with type 1 diabetes [54].

In contrast to type 1 diabetes, the risk of retinopathy appears to be lower with age in persons with type 2 diabetes. In the older-onset type 2 diabetes participants using insulin in WESDR, the 4-year incidence and progression of retinopathy were lower while the 4-year rate of improvement was higher in older than in younger people [46]. In fact, few participants 75 years or older developed PDR after 10 years of follow-up [47]. Other studies indicate similar results [37, 48]. In a study in Rochester, Minnesota, a lower incidence of retinopathy with increasing age was seen in people with type 2 diabetes 60 years and older [5]. The explanation for this age pattern is unknown. While it is possible that older persons have less severe diabetes (less likely to require insulin), these findings may reflect selective mortality (i.e. older persons with severe retinopathy are more likely to die).

Epidemiological studies have not shown a consistent pattern of gender variation in either the prevalence or incidence of retinopathy. In the WESDR, younger-onset men were more likely to have PDR than younger women [16], but there were no significant differences in the incidence or progression of diabetic retinopathy by gender [45, 47]. In older-onset diabetes participants in the WESDR, there were no significant gender differences in either the prevalence or incidence of retinopathy [17, 46, 47].

There is an abundance of data that show the prevalence of diabetic retinopathy varies between racial/ethnic groups. Compared with Caucasian White populations, Native Americans have long been known to have a higher prevalence of type 2 diabetes and a higher prevalence of retinopathy for a given duration of diabetes [55–59]. Studies comparing rates of retinopathy between racial/ethnic groups in the United States have consistently shown a higher prevalence of diabetic retinopathy in African-Americans [10, 13, 14] and Hispanics [2, 9, 60] than in Whites. In one study, Haffner et al. [6] showed that retinopathy prevalence was about two times higher in Hispanics living in San Antonio than non-Hispanic Whites in the WESDR. Varma et al. [60] found Mexican Americans living in Los Angeles to have a higher prevalence of proliferative retinopathy and macular edema than Whites living in Beaver Dam, Wisconsin.

Fewer studies have examined the epidemiology of retinopathy in Asian Americans [61, 62], but one study reported that the prevalence of retinopathy was significantly lower in second-generation Japanese American males than native Japanese people in Tokyo [63]. One of the few studies to compare rates of retinopathy among different racial/ethnic groups directly was the Multiethnic Study of Atherosclerosis (MESA), which examined the prevalence of diabetic retinopathy in a US population of Whites, African-Americans, Hispanics and Chinese-Americans aged 45 years and older [64]. This study showed that the prevalence of retinopathy was similar between African-Americans (37%) and Hispanics (37%) and was lower in Whites (25%) and Chinese-Americans (26%).

The underlying reasons for these racial/ethnic differences are complex, and likely to reflect a combination of variations in health care access, genetic susceptibility and other risk factors for retinopathy, such as duration of diabetes, levels of glycemia

and blood pressure. Harris et al. [10] showed that in the National Health and Nutrition Examination Survey III (NHANES III) that the higher prevalence of retinopathy in African-Americans compared with Whites disappeared once these common risk factors were controlled for. Likewise, in the Atherosclerosis Risk in Communities (ARIC) Study, the higher prevalence of retinopathy in African-Americans (28%) than Whites (17%) was largely explained by Black–White differences in glycemic control, duration of diabetes and blood pressure [13]. These data reinforce the need to achieve tight glycemic and blood pressure control in African Americans and other groups with a higher prevalence of retinopathy. Nonetheless, it is worth noting that controlling for these known risk factors had no appreciable effect on the higher retinopathy prevalence among Hispanic Whites compared with non-Hispanic Whites in NHANES III [10], suggesting other unmeasured possible risk factors (genetic or otherwise) may account for other racial/ethnic variations in retinopathy prevalence.

30.2.6 Diabetes Duration and Diabetic Retinopathy

The strongest risk factor for prevalent diabetic retinopathy in persons with both type 1 and type 2 diabetes is the duration of diabetes. In the WESDR, the prevalence of retinopathy ranged from 2% among type 1 diabetes participants with less than 2 years of diabetes to 98% in those with 15 years or more of disease, and the prevalence of PDR ranged from 4% among participants with 10 years of diabetes to 56% in those with 20 or more years of disease [16]. This pattern has been observed in virtually all epidemiological studies on diabetic retinopathy. In the AusDiab Study, the prevalence of retinopathy was 9.2% among participants with duration of less than 5 years, 23% for those with duration between 5 and 9 years, 33% for duration between 10 and 19 years and 57% for duration 20 years or longer [29]. A Swedish study of type 1 diabetes showed an increased in prevalence of retinopathy from 4% in those with duration of diabetes less than 2 years to 32% among those with diabetes duration of 10–12 years [65].

In fact, it is recognized that one of the explanations for the higher prevalence of retinopathy in people with type 2 compared with type 1 diabetes is a reflection of longer diabetes duration prior to diagnosis in type 2 diabetes. Harris *et al.* [66] showed that, by extrapolating data of retinopathy prevalence by diabetes duration, the onset of detectable retinopathy occurred approximately from 4 to 7 years before the clinical diagnosis of type 2 diabetes.

Likewise, the incidence of retinopathy also increases with increasing diabetes duration [45–47, 67]. Among type 1 diabetes participants in the WESDR, the 4-year incidence of PDR was 0% for those with a duration of 5 years and 28% for those with a duration of 13 years.

30.2.7 Hyperglycemia and Diabetic Retinopathy

The most consistent risk factor for diabetic retinopathy is hyperglycemia [5, 7, 8, 13, 16, 17, 23, 24, 26, 29, 68–77]. In the WESDR, participants with mean glycosylated hemoglobin levels above 12% had a threefold higher risk of retinopathy than those with HbA1c levels under 12%, independent of diabetes duration and other risk factors [76].

Two large clinical trials have confirmed the importance of glycemic control in reducing the risk of retinopathy. The Diabetes Control and Complications Trial (DCCT) was a multicentered trial that assessed the effect of intensive glycemic control on the development and progression of diabetic retinopathy and other vascular complications in 1441 patients with type 1 diabetes [78–80]. After a follow-up of 6.5 years, patients randomized to tight glycemic control (with an average glycosylated hemogloblin of 7%) had a 75% lower incidence of retinopathy and 50% lower rate of progression to more severe retinopathy than patients randomized to conventional treatment (glycosylated hemogloblin of 9%) [78].

There were several clinically important observations from the DCCT regarding the relationship of glycemic control and the risk of diabetic retinopathy. First, the DCCT confirmed observations from other studies that tight glycemic control may lead to an early worsening of retinopathy [73, 81]. The DCCT showed that early worsening occurred in the first year of the trial in the intensive glycemic control group and reversed after 18 months, with the beneficial effect of intensive glycemic control increasing over time. Second, the DCCT demonstrated that there was no threshold glycosylated hemoglobin level above which the risk of

retinopathy would increased markedly [82]. This is supported by data from more recent studies, such as the EURODIAB prospective complications study which showed no glycemic threshold for the development of retinopathy in 764 patients with type 1 diabetes followed for 7 years [83]. Thus, the relationship of glycemia and retinopathy was graded and continuous. Third, the DCCT showed that the beneficial effects of intensive glycemic control were more pronounced when instituted earlier in the development of retinopathy, with progression rates of retinopathy noted to be 7% for patients who had retinopathy for less than 2.5 years and 20% for those who had retinopathy for more than 2.5 years [80]. Finally, ongoing observational follow-up of the cohort via the Epidemiology of Diabetes Interventions and Complications (EDIC) study showed that the effects of tight glycemic control persisted over time, with retinopathy progression remaining low in DCCT patients who were originally randomized to tight glycemic control, despite an increase in the levels of glycosylated hemoglobin levels to that found in the conventionally randomized group [84].

It has been estimated that, based on the DCCT findings, tight glycemic control may result in a gain of nearly 1 million years of sight for patients with type 1 diabetes in the United States who meet the study criteria [1].

The UKPDS examined the effect of tight glycemic control on the development and progression of diabetic retinopathy and other complications in 3867 patients with newly diagnosed type 2 diabetes [85]. After 12 years of follow-up, the UKPDS showed that tight glycemic control (with an overall lowering of mean glycosylated hemoglobin levels of 1%) was associated with a 21% reduction in progression of retinopathy, a 29% reduction in the need for laser treatment, and a 37% reduction in the risk of any microvascular complications [43, 85].

In summary, there is a substantial body of evidence from epidemiological and clinical trials data that hyperglycemia is an important risk factor for the development and progression of diabetic retinopathy, and that this relationship has no threshold levels. It is important to know that retinopathy risk is not greatly affected by short-term improvements in glycemic control, as there is a lag between metabolic control and changes to the risk of retinopathy.

30.2.8 Hypertension and Diabetic Retinopathy

Epidemiological studies have not shown a consistent relationship between elevated blood pressure and risk of diabetic retinopathy [5, 7, 8, 16–18, 37, 55, 56, 58, 59, 86, 87]. In the WESDR, elevated blood pressure was associated with an increased 14-year incidence of diabetic retinopathy in type 1 diabetes [67], independent of glycemia levels and duration of diabetes. However, in participants with type 2 diabetes, blood pressure was not related to the 10-year incidence of retinopathy [86]. Two other prospective studies in type 1 diabetes did not find an association between blood pressure and incident retinopathy in persons with type 1 diabetes [83, 88].

The UKPDS, however, has provided much stronger clinical trial evidence regarding the importance of hypertension as a risk factor in diabetic retinopathy development and progression. In the UKPDS, patients with hypertension randomized tight blood pressure control with atenolol or captopril had a 37% reduction in the risk of any microvascular disease, a 34% reduction in progression of retinopathy and a 47% reduction in the deterioration of visual acuity compared with patients with less tight blood pressure control [89]. These effects were independent glycemic control in the UKPDS. Additionally, atenolol and captopril were equally effective in reducing the risk of microvascular complications, suggesting that blood pressure reduction was more important than the type of medication used to reduce it. In a later report, subjects with systolic blood pressure 140 mmHg or greater were nearly three times as likely to develop retinopathy as those with systolic blood pressure less than 125 mmHg [43]. No threshold systolic blood pressure and risk of retinopathy was evident in the UKPDS [90]. It has been estimated that each 10 mmHg reduction in systolic blood pressure may reduce the risk of diabetic retinopathy by 10% [43]. Another clinical trial, the Appropriate Blood Pressure Control in Diabetes trial, showed benefit in retinopathy risk reduction in normotensive patients with type 2 diabetes who were randomly assigned to intensive blood pressure control [91, 92]. Based on these studies, clinical guidelines recommend adequate control of blood pressure in patients with type 2 diabetes as a means of preventing visual loss from diabetic retinopathy [93, 94].

30.2.9 Dyslipidemia and Diabetic Retinopathy

There is increasing evidence that dyslipidemia is an important risk factor for retinopathy and macular edema [13, 95–102]. In the WESDR, higher total serum cholesterol was associated with retinal hard exudates in participants with type 1 diabetes and type 2 diabetes using insulin, but not in those with type 2 diabetes using oral hypoglycemic agents [103]. In ETDRS, higher levels of triglycerides, low-density lipoproteins and very low-density lipoproteins at baseline were associated with an increased risk of hard exudates and decreased visual acuity [104].

A recent large clinical trial has provided the initial evidence that lipid-lowering therapy may prevent visual loss from diabetic retinopathy. In the Fenofibrate Intervention and Event Lowering in Diabetes (FIELD) study, the effect of fenofibrate on vascular events was examined in 9795 participants with type 2 diabetes who were not taking statin therapy at study entry [105]. Patients had a total cholesterol concentration of $3.0–6.5 \, \text{mmol} \, \text{l}^{-1}$ and a total cholesterol/high-density lipoprotein (HDL)-cholesterol ratio of 4.0 or more, or plasma triglyceride of $1.0–5.0 \, \text{mmol} \, \text{l}^{-1}$. After 5 years, participants treated on fenofibrate were less likely to have retinopathy needing laser treatment (5.2% versus 3.6%, $p = 0.0003$). However, the severity of retinopathy, the indication of laser treatment and the type of laser treatment (focal or panretinal) were not reported in the FIELD study. This study is supported by smaller clinical case series [106–108] that suggest lipid-lowering therapy with statins could be a useful as an adjunct therapy to laser treatment. Thus, lipid-lowering therapy may be beneficial for patients with diabetes and dyslipidemia not only for its effects on cardiovascular morbidity, but also for its possible effects on retinopathy.

30.2.10 Nephropathy and Diabetic Retinopathy

Diabetic retinopathy and nephropathy frequently coexist as microvascular complications in diabetic patients, reflecting common risk factors (e.g. hyperglycemia and hypertension) and pathogenic mechanisms [109]. Studies have shown that retinopathy is associated with preclinical morphological changes in the kidneys in normotensive diabetic patients [110], and may precede the subsequent development of clinical nephropathy [111]. The presence of diabetic nephropathy is also a risk factor for the development and progression of retinopathy [112, 113]. In the WESDR, participants with type 1 diabetes with gross proteinuria at baseline were two times more likely to develop PDR after 4 years [112] and macular edema after 14 years [67] than participants without gross proteinuria at baseline. Some of these associations reached only borderline significance when other retinopathy risk factors were controlled for, suggesting that similar processes, such as poor glycemic and blood pressure control, may explain both microvascular complications.

There are no clinical trial data to show that interventions that prevent or slow diabetic nephropathy will reduce the incidence and progression of retinopathy. However, there are small series that show kidney dialysis in diabetic patients with renal failure may reduce the severity of macular edema [114, 115].

30.2.11   Obesity and Diabetic Retinopathy

The association between obesity and diabetic retinopathy has been investigated in several studies. Some [5, 53, 64, 116–120], but not others [17, 59, 61, 121, 122], have documented a relationship between larger body mass index (BMI) and risk of retinopathy. Few of these studies, however, have prospective data [5, 17, 38, 83]. A study in Sweden showed that in young patients with diabetes (80% type 1) higher BMI at baseline was associated with an earlier onset of retinopathy [38]. The EURODIAB Prospective Complications Study of 764 individuals with type 1 diabetes showed that waist/hip ratio (WHR) was an independent risk factor for diabetic retinopathy [83]. However, conflicting data were observed in the WESDR [17, 120]. Although obesity (BMI $> 31.0\,\mathrm{kg\,m^{-2}}$ for men and $32.1\,\mathrm{kg\,m^{-2}}$ for women) was found to associate with progression and severity of retinopathy, these associations were not statistically significant and were limited to only individuals with type 2 diabetes [120]. In contrast, participants who were underweight (BMI $< 20\,\mathrm{kg\,m^{-2}}$) had a threefold higher risk of developing retinopathy [17], which has been suggested to reflect a more 'severe' phase of diabetes or a marker of late-onset type 1 diabetes [120].

The underlying pathophysiological mechanisms of the possible association between obesity and retinopathy are not well understood [123]. Obesity shares many common risk factors for diabetic retinopathy, including hyperglycemia, hypertension and dyslipidemia. However, there is some evidence that obesity may have a more direct role in the development of retinopathy. For example, systemic levels of vascular endothelial growth factor have been reported to be higher in obese patients [124], and may provide a potential link between obesity and development of PDR. Patients who are obese also have higher levels of plasma leptin, which has been linked with diabetic retinopathy development [116, 125].

Whether weight loss reduces the risk of diabetic retinopathy is uncertain [126, 127], although weight reduction has a proven cardiovascular benefit in obese diabetic individuals.

30.2.12   Pregnancy, Puberty and Diabetic Retinopathy

Pregnancy is known to affect retinal hemodynamics [128, 129], and associated hormonal changes, such as progesterone, may induce the production of vascular endothelial growth factor [130]. It is well recognized that diabetic retinopathy may progress rapidly during pregnancy [131], but this is usually a transient effect that resolves after delivery. There are fewer studies on whether pregnancy is a risk factor for the long-term development of retinopathy [132–134]. In a case–control study in Wisconsin, when compared with nonpregnant type 1 diabetic women of similar age and duration of diabetes, pregnant women participants were more likely to develop retinopathy, when the groups were followed for a time interval about equal to the length of the pregnancy, independent of other risk factors [132]. Others have shown that progression of retinopathy is increased only in diabetic women with pre-eclampsia [135].

In type 1 diabetic women who are pregnant, the risk factors for retinopathy progression are no different to nonpregnant diabetic individuals [133, 135, 136]. The Diabetes in Early Pregnancy Study, a prospective study of 140 pregnant type 1 diabetic patients, showed that women with the poorest glycemic control at baseline, but with the greatest reduction in HbA1c in the first trimester, were at increased risk of retinopathy progression

[133]. These findings underscore the importance of good glycemic and blood pressure control in female diabetic patients who are pregnant.

Like pregnancy, puberty may be a risk factor for retinopathy development. In the WESDR, menarchal status at the baseline examination was related to the prevalence of retinopathy [137]. Use of oral contraceptives and hormone replacement therapy does not appear to increase the risk of retinopathy [138, 139].

30.2.13 Inflammation and Diabetic Retinopathy

Chronic inflammation and dysfunction of the vascular endothelium have been proposed as possible pathogenic factors in type 2 diabetes development [140, 141]. There is increasing evidence from animal models, and human studies, that chronic inflammation and glucose-induced arteriolar endothelial dysfunction are related to development, severity and progression of diabetic retinopathy [142–144]. Studies have shown that inflammatory protein levels of cytokines, chemokines and adhesion molecules are elevated in both the vitreous [145] and serum [146] of patients with diabetic retinopathy. Epidemiological studies have provided further support. In the Hoorn Study and the EURO-DIAB Prospective Complications Study, systemic markers of inflammation and endothelial activation (e.g. C-reactive protein, soluble intercellular adhesion molecule-1 and von Willebrand factor) were associated with retinopathy, independent of other risk factors [147, 148]. However, whether anti-inflammatory treatment can delay the onset or progression of retinopathy is unclear. In the ETDRS, patients with mild-to-severe NPDR or early PDR were assigned randomly to either aspirin (650 mg per day) or placebo. Aspirin did not prevent the development of high-risk PDR and did not reduce the risk of visual loss, or increase the risk of vitreous hemorrhage [149].

30.2.14 Other Risk Factors for Diabetic Retinopathy

Whether cigarette smoking and alcohol consumption are risk factors for diabetic retinopathy is unclear. Most epidemiological studies have not found a consistent pattern of association of retinopathy with either smoking [5, 8, 59, 150, 151] or alcohol consumption [22, 151–153]. Some studies, in fact, have shown somewhat paradoxical results, with cigarette smoking associated with a lower risk of retinopathy, suggesting a possible beneficial component of smoking on the retinal vasculature in persons with diabetes [154]. It is likely that these are not significant factors in retinopathy development.

Physical activity and exercise have a positive effect in reducing the risk of diabetes development and possibly its complications, either directly by improving glycemic control, or indirectly by improved cardiovascular health. The few epidemiologic data available have produced mixed results regarding an association between physical exercise and risk of diabetic retinopathy [155, 156]. In the WESDR, for example, physical exercise was not associated with incidence or progression of retinopathy [156].

30.2.15 Retinopathy in Persons without Clinical Diabetes

There is increasing recognition that typical lesions of early diabetic retinopathy (microaneurysms, hemorrhages and cotton wool spots) are commonly seen in persons without clinically diagnosed diabetes [157]. Studies using fundus photographs to evaluate retinopathy have reported prevalence rates of up to 14% in some populations (**Figure 30.3**) [23, 29, 158–162]. Prospective data from the Beaver Dam and Blue Mountains Eye Studies show that these retinopathy signs developed in 6–10% of non-diabetic persons over a 5-year period [154, 163].

The pathogenesis of retinopathy signs in nondiabetic persons remains uncertain. Various studies show that these retinopathy signs may be related to impaired glucose tolerance [164–166], to components related to metabolic syndrome [119] or to other risk factors, such as hypertension [167–169]. However, population-based studies in nondiabetic adult patients show that while hypertension is strongly associated with prevalence of retinal hemorrhages and microaneurysms [157, 158, 160], higher blood pressure is not associated with the incidence of these retinopathy signs [39, 163].

Few studies have investigated if these retinopathy signs are preclinical markers of diabetes. In the ARIC Study, retinopathy signs in nondiabetic persons were not significantly associated with the subsequent incidence of diabetes, except among individuals with a positive family history of diabetes [170]. This suggests that, in persons with underlying

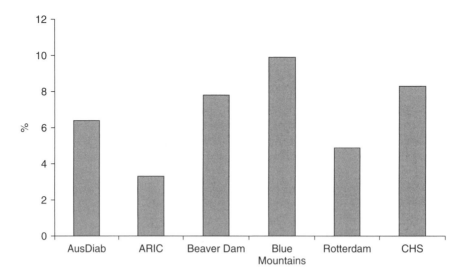

Figure 30.3 Prevalence of retinopathy signs in persons without diabetes, selected population-based studies. ARIC: Atherosclerosis Risk in Communities Study, USA; AusDiab: the Australian Diabetes Obesity and Lifestyle Study, Australia; Beaver Dam: Beaver Dam Eye Study, Wisconsin, USA; Blue Mountains: Blue Mountains Eye Study, Sydney, Australia; Rotterdam: Rotterdam Eye Study, the Netherlands; CHS: the Cardiovascular Health Study, USA.

predisposition to diabetes, retinopathy signs may markers of underlying abnormalities in glucose metabolism or microvascular disease.

30.2.16 Relationship of Diabetic Retinopathy with Cardiovascular Morbidity and Mortality

Retinopathy in persons with diabetes may be a marker of systemic vascular diseases and has been linked with cardiovascular diseases and mortality [157]. In the WESDR, participants with proliferative retinopathy had higher risk of incident myocardial infarction, stroke, nephropathy and lower leg amputation than those with no or minimal retinopathy at baseline [171]. In type 1 diabetes participants, after adjusting for age and sex, retinopathy severity was associated with all-cause and coronary heart disease mortality, and in type 2 diabetes participants it was associated with all-cause, coronary heart disease mortality and stroke [171]. The associations of retinopathy with all-cause and stroke mortality in type 2 diabetes persisted after controlling for systemic risk factors. In the ARIC Study, the presence of retinopathy was associated with a fourfold risk of congestive heart failure among diabetic participants without previous coronary heart disease or hypertension, independent of standard

risk factors [172]. Several large epidemiological studies, such as the Hoorn Study, the EURODIAB Prospective Complications Study and the ETDRS, have also reported associations between retinopathy severity and all-cause and cardiovascular mortality [173–176].

New epidemiological studies further indicate that retinopathy signs predict cardiovascular diseases even in persons without diabetes. In the ARIC Study and the Blue Mountains Eye Study, retinopathy was associated with higher risk of stroke events and stroke deaths, independent of blood pressure, cigarette smoking and other risk factors [168, 177]. Among participants without stroke or transient ischaemic attack, retinopathy was correlated with magnetic resonance image (MRI)-defined cerebral infarctions and white matter lesions [169, 178]. These data, therefore, suggest that the presence of retinopathy in both diabetic and nondiabetic patients may be an indicator for increased risk of stroke and other cardiovascular diseases.

30.3 RETINAL VASCULAR DISEASES

Diabetes has been linked to the development of a range of retinal vascular conditions, including retinal vein occlusion (RVO), retinal arteriolar emboli, retinal artery occlusion (RAO) and the ocular ischemic syndrome. RVO is a potentially sight-threatening condition commonly seen in patients with diabetes, and is characterized clinically by dilated and tortuous retinal veins and the presence of hemorrhages, cotton wool spots and macular edema. These signs can be seen in all four quadrants (central RVO) or in one quadrant (branch RVO). Central RVO occurs in 0.1–0.4% and branch RVO in 0.6–1.1% of adults aged 40 years and older with and without diabetes [179, 180]. Epidemiological studies have not shown consistently a relationship between diabetes and RVO, with some studies finding a positive association [181–183], particularly with ischemic central RVO [184, 185], but others reporting no associations with either central or branch RVO [179, 185, 186]. There is some evidence that persons with diabetes with RVO may have a poorer visual prognosis, with reports that these patients are more likely to develop retinal neovascularization than patients without diabetes [187].

Retinal arteriolar emboli are discrete plaque-like lesions lodged in the lumen of retinal arterioles. These emboli are heterogeneous and may be composed of cholesterol crystals (reflective emboli) or fibrin, platelets, calcium and other materials (non-reflective emboli). Epidemiological studies report that asymptomatic retinal emboli occur in 1.3–1.4% of adult persons aged 40 years and older [188, 189]. Diabetes has been found to be a risk factor for emboli in some [189], but not all [186, 188, 190–192], studies. In the Beaver Dam Eye Study, after controlling for age and gender, the presence of type 2 diabetes at baseline was associated with a twofold higher prevalence of retinal emboli [189], but was not significantly associated with either the 5-year [189] or 10-year incidence of emboli [190]. The Blue Mountains Eye Study did not find an association between diabetes and either prevalent or incident emboli [188, 192].

RAO occurs commonly in patients with cardiovascular disease. Retinal emboli may be visible in the vessels at the point of occlusion or further downstream. Although RAO has been associated with diabetes in small series [193, 194], there are few large epidemiological studies to confirm this association.

Ocular ischemic syndrome is an uncommon condition that arises secondary to chronic ocular hypoperfusion caused by severe carotid artery obstruction. Studies have suggested that more than half of patients with this condition have diabetes [195]. Ocular ischemic syndrome has also been suggested to explain asymmetry in the risk of PDR in patients with diabetes [196–198].

30.4 NEURO-OPHTHALMIC MANIFESTATIONS

The neuro-ophthalmic manifestations of diabetes are diverse, and include disorders of the afferent visual system (optic nerve), the efferent system (III, IV and VI cranial nerves) and the orbit and its associated structures. Ischemic optic neuropathy is typically divided into anterior ischemic optic neuropathy (AION) and the rarer form of posterior ischemic optic neuropathy [199]. AION is further subdivided into arteritic and nonarteritic subtypes, the former classically due to giant cell temporal arteritis but not diabetes. Several studies have reported that diabetes is a risk factor for nonarteritic AION, particularly in younger patients with this condition [199–201]. Data from one study showed that up to 25% of patients with nonarteritic AION had a history of diabetes [201].

Another common neuro-ophthalmic problem in the diabetic patient is ocular motility disorders. Diabetes is a risk factor for complete or partial paresis of cranial nerves III, IV or VI. In one population-based case–control study of isolated VI cranial nerve palsy (76 cases, and 76 controls matched for age, gender and length of medical follow-up), patients with VI cranial nerve palsy were six times more likely to have diabetes than controls [202].

30.5 CATARACT

Persons with both types 1 and 2 diabetes are at higher risk for the development of cataracts. This association is supported by an abundance of data from clinical, epidemiological and basic science studies [203–220].

Population-based studies have shown that diabetes is associated most strongly with posterior subcapsular (PSC) cataract and, to a lesser extent, cortical cataract, but not nuclear cataract [203–216]. In White populations, cross-sectional and prospective data from three population-based studies, the

Beaver Dam Eye Study, the Blue Mountains Eye Study and the Visual Impairment Project, have reported associations between diabetes with prevalent and incident PSC, and less consistently with prevalent and incident cortical cataract [206–211]. In the Beaver Dam Eye Study, baseline diabetes status and higher glycated hemoglobin levels were associated with both incidence and progression of PSC and cortical cataracts [207]. The Blue Mountains Eye Study showed that impaired fasting glucose in the absence of clinical diabetes was an additional risk factor for the development of cortical cataract [208]. The associations of diabetes with PSC and cortical cataract have been confirmed in other racial/ethnic groups around the world, including Chinese people in Singapore [214] and Taiwan [215] and in southern Indians [216].

In persons with diabetes, the risk of cataract increases with longer duration of disease and poorer glycemic control. There is a greater severity of lens opacities in patients with diabetes than age-matched controls [221]. Patients with diabetes have also been reported to have higher rates of cataract surgery and to require surgery at an early age [222]. In the WESDR, the 10-year cumulative incidence of cataract surgery was 8% in participants with type 1 diabetes and 25% in type 2 diabetes. Predictors of cataract surgery include increasing age, severity of diabetic retinopathy and baseline proteinuria in type 1 diabetes, and increasing age and use of insulin in type 2 diabetes [222].

The association between diabetes and cataract has been examined in numerous experimental studies [220, 223–226]. Cataractogenesis has been hypothesized to be due to increased oxidative stress, sorbitol accumulation and deposition of advanced glycated end products in the lens of people with diabetes. In animal studies, inhibition of glycation and oxidative stress has been shown to delay the development of cataract [227]. Other studies suggest that genetic factors (e.g. the aldose reductase gene) may play a role in cataract formation in patients with diabetes [228].

30.6   GLAUCOMA

Diabetes has been suggested as a major risk factor for the development of glaucoma [229–233]. A number of population-based studies have found a positive association between diabetes and glaucoma

[230, 231, 234, 235] or between diabetes and raised intraocular pressure, the major risk factor for glaucomatous optic nerve damage [236, 237]. In the Blue Mountains Study and Beaver Dam Eye Study, people with diabetes were two times more likely to have glaucoma than those without diabetes [231, 234]. However, not all population-based studies have found this association [238, 239].

Several pathophysiological mechanisms have been proposed to explain a possible association between diabetes and glaucoma. Direct microvascular damage from diabetes could impair blood flow to the anterior optic nerve, resulting in ischemic optic nerve damage [240, 241]. This is supported by data from studies showing associations between glaucoma and abnormal ocular blood flow [242]. Diabetes could interfere with the autoregulation of the posterior ciliary circulation, and this may exacerbate glaucomatous neuropathy [243]. Finally, persons with diabetes often have concomitant cardiovascular risk factors (e.g. hypertension) that may also affect vascular perfusion of the optic nerve head [244].

30.7   CONCLUSION

Diabetes mellitus is associated with a range of eye diseases, many of which are sight threatening. Retinopathy, the most serious ocular complication, affects a substantial number of persons with diabetes. Although clinical trials show that prevention of diabetic retinopathy through risk factor reduction (controlling hyperglycemia, hypertension and hyperlipidemia) will decrease the incidence and impact of this complication, diabetic retinopathy remains the leading cause of severe visual impairment (legal blindness) among working-age adults in the United States and other countries around the world. Thus, intensive glycemic, blood pressure, and possibly lipid level control and early detection of retinopathy and other conditions through regular eye examinations, along with timely treatment, remains an important public health strategy in the prevention of visual loss in patients with diabetes.

ACKNOWLEDGEMENT

This work was partially supported by National Eye Institute grant RO1 EY 016379.

References

1. Congdon, N., Friedman, D.S. and Lietman, T. (2003) Important causes of visual impairment in the world today. *The Journal of the American Medical Association*, **290** (15), 2057–60.

2. Kempen, J.H., O'Colmain, B.J., Leske, M.C. *et al.* (2004) The prevalence of diabetic retinopathy among adults in the United States. *Archives of Ophthalmology*, **122** (4), 552–63.

3. Wilkinson, C.P., Ferris, F.L. III, Klein, R.E. *et al.* (2003) Proposed international clinical diabetic retinopathy and diabetic macular edema disease severity scales. *Ophthalmology*, **110** (9), 1677–82.

4. Kahn, H.A., Leibowitz, H.M., Ganley, J.P. *et al.* (1977) The Framingham Eye Study. I. Outline and major prevalence findings. *American Journal of Epidemiology*, **106** (1), 17–32.

5. Ballard, D.J., Melton, L.J. III, Dwyer, M.S. *et al.* (1986) Risk factors for diabetic retinopathy: a population-based study in Rochester, Minnesota. *Diabetes Care*, **9** (4), 334–42.

6. Haffner, S.M., Fong, D., Stern, M.P. *et al.* (1988) Diabetic retinopathy in Mexican Americans and non-Hispanic whites. *Diabetes*, **37** (7), 878–84.

7. Hamman, R.F., Mayer, E.J., Moo-Young, G.A. *et al.* (1989) Prevalence and risk factors of diabetic retinopathy in non-Hispanic whites and Hispanics with NIDDM. San Luis Valley Diabetes Study. *Diabetes*, **38** (10), 1231–7.

8. Kostraba, J.N., Klein, R., Dorman, J.S. *et al.* (1991) The epidemiology of diabetes complications study. IV. Correlates of diabetic background and proliferative retinopathy. *American Journal of Epidemiology*, **133** (4), 381–91.

9. West, S.K., Klein, R., Rodriguez, J. *et al.* (2001) Diabetes and diabetic retinopathy in a Mexican-American population: proyecto VER. *Diabetes Care*, **24** (7), 1204–9.

10. Harris, M.I., Klein, R., Cowie, C.C. *et al.* (1998) Is the risk of diabetic retinopathy greater in non-Hispanic blacks and Mexican Americans than in non-Hispanic whites with type 2 diabetes? A U.S. population study. *Diabetes Care*, **21** (8), 1230–5.

11. Klein, R., Klein, B.E., Moss, S.E. and Linton, K.L. (1992) The Beaver Dam Eye Study. Retinopathy in adults with newly discovered and previously diagnosed diabetes mellitus. *Ophthalmology*, **99** (1), 58–62.

12. Roy, M.S. (2000) Diabetic retinopathy in African Americans with type 1 diabetes: The New Jersey 725: I. Methodology, population, frequency of retinopathy, and visual impairment. *Archives of Ophthalmology*, **118** (1), 97–104.

13. Klein, R., Sharrett, A.R., Klein, B.E. *et al.* (2002) The association of atherosclerosis, vascular risk factors, and retinopathy in adults with diabetes: the atherosclerosis risk in communities study. *Ophthalmology*, **109** (7), 1225–34.

14. Klein, R., Marino, E.K., Kuller, L.H. *et al.* (2002) The relation of atherosclerotic cardiovascular disease to retinopathy in people with diabetes in the cardiovascular health study. *The British Journal of Ophthalmology*, **86** (1), 84–90.

15. Klein, R., Klein, B.E., Moss, S.E. *et al.* (1984) Prevalence of diabetes mellitus in southern Wisconsin. *American Journal of Epidemiology*, **119** (1), 54–61.

16. Klein, R., Klein, B.E., Moss, S.E. *et al.* (1984) The Wisconsin Epidemiologic Study of Diabetic Retinopathy. II. Prevalence and risk of diabetic retinopathy when age at diagnosis is less than 30 years. *Archives of Ophthalmology*, **102** (4), 520–6.

17. Klein, R., Klein, B.E., Moss, S.E. *et al.* (1984) The Wisconsin Epidemiologic Study of Diabetic Retinopathy. III. Prevalence and risk of diabetic retinopathy when age at diagnosis is 30 or more years. *Archives of Ophthalmology*, **102** (4), 527–32.

18. Klein, R., Klein, B.E., Moss, S.E. *et al.* (1984) The Wisconsin Epidemiologic Study of Diabetic Retinopathy. IV. Diabetic macular edema. *Ophthalmology*, **91** (12), 1464–74.

19. Broadbent, D.M., Scott, J.A., Vora, J.P. and Harding, S.P. (1999) Prevalence of diabetic eye disease in an inner city population: the Liverpool Diabetic Eye Study. *Eye*, **13** (Pt 2), 160–5.

20. McKay, R., McCarty, C.A. and Taylor, H.R. (2000) Diabetic retinopathy in Victoria, Australia: the Visual Impairment Project. *The British Journal of Ophthalmology*, **84** (8), 865–70.

21. Leske, M.C., Wu, S.Y., Hyman, L. *et al.* (1999) Diabetic retinopathy in a black population: the Barbados Eye Study. *Ophthalmology*, **106** (10), 1893–99; [erratum: (2000) *Ophthalmology*, **107** (3), 412].

22. Mitchell, P., Smith, W., Wang, J.J. and Attebo, K. (1998) Prevalence of diabetic retinopathy in an older community. The Blue Mountains Eye Study. *Ophthalmology*, **105** (3), 406–11.

23. Stolk, R.P., Vingerling, J.R., de Jong, P.T. *et al.* (1995) Retinopathy, glucose, and insulin in an elderly population. The Rotterdam Study. *Diabetes*, **44** (1), 11–15.

24. Van Leiden, H.A., Dekker, J.M., Moll, A.C. *et al.* (2003) Risk factors for incident retinopathy in a diabetic and nondiabetic population: the Hoorn Study. *Archives of Ophthalmology*, **121** (2), 245–51.

25. McLeod, B.K., Thompson, J.R. and Rosenthal, A.R. (1988) The prevalence of retinopathy in the insulin-requiring diabetic patients of an English country town. *Eye*, **2** (Pt 4), 424–30.

26. Sparrow, J.M., McLeod, B.K., Smith, T.D. *et al.* (1993) The prevalence of diabetic retinopathy and maculopathy and their risk factors in the non-insulin-treated diabetic patients of an English town. *Eye*, **7** (Pt 1), 158–63.

27. Foulds, W.S., McCuish, A., Barrie, T. *et al.* (1983) Diabetic retinopathy in the west of Scotland: its detection and prevalence, and the cost-effectiveness of a proposed screening programme. *Health Bulletin*, **41** (6), 318–26.

28. Sjolie, A.K. (1985) Ocular complications in insulin treated diabetes mellitus. An epidemiological study. *Acta Ophthalmologica, Supplementum*, **172**, 1–77.

29. Tapp, R.J., Shaw, J.E., Harper, C.A. *et al.* (2003) The prevalence of and factors associated with diabetic retinopathy in the Australian population. *Diabetes Care*, **26** (6), 1731–7.

30. Zimmet, P., Alberti, K.G. and Shaw, J. (2001) Global and societal implications of the diabetes epidemic. *Nature*, **414** (6865), 782–7.

31. Pan, X.R., Yang, W.Y., Li, G.W. and Liu, J. (1997) Prevalence of diabetes and its risk factors in China, 1994. National Diabetes Prevention and Control Cooperative Group. *Diabetes Care*, **20** (11), 1664–9.

32. Ramachandran, A., Snehalatha, C., Latha, E. *et al.* (1997) Rising prevalence of NIDDM in an urban population in India. *Diabetologia*, **40** (2), 232–7.

33. Tan, C.E., Emmanuel, S.C., Tan, B.Y. and Jacob, E. (1999) Prevalence of diabetes and ethnic differences in cardiovascular risk factors. The 1992 Singapore National Health Survey. *Diabetes Care*, **22** (2), 241–7.

34. Cheah, J.S., Yeo, P.P., Thai, A.C. *et al.* (1985) Epidemiology of diabetes mellitus in Singapore: comparison with other ASEAN countries. *Annals of the Academy of Medicine, Singapore*, **14** (2), 232–9.

35. Narendran, V., John, R.K., Raghuram, A. *et al.* (2002) Diabetic retinopathy among self reported diabetics in southern India: a population based assessment. *The British Journal of Ophthalmology*, **86** (9), 1014–18.

36. Dandona, L., Dandona, R., Naduvilath, T.J. *et al.* (1999) Population based assessment of diabetic retinopathy in an urban population in southern India. *The British Journal of Ophthalmology*, **83** (8), 937–40.

37. Teuscher, A., Schnell, H. and Wilson, P.W. (1988) Incidence of diabetic retinopathy and relationship to baseline plasma glucose and blood pressure. *Diabetes Care*, **11** (3), 246–51.

38. Henricsson, M., Nystrom, L., Blohme, G. *et al.* (2003) The incidence of retinopathy 10 years after diagnosis in young adult people with diabetes: results from the nationwide population-based Diabetes Incidence Study in Sweden (DISS). *Diabetes Care*, **26** (2), 349–54.

39. Klein, R., Palta, M., Allen, C. *et al.* (1997) Incidence of retinopathy and associated risk factors from time of diagnosis of insulin-dependent diabetes. *Archives of Ophthalmology*, **115** (3), 351–56.

40. Tudor, S.M., Hamman, R.F., Baron, A. *et al.* (1998) Incidence and progression of diabetic retinopathy in Hispanics and non-Hispanic whites with type 2 diabetes. San Luis Valley Diabetes Study, Colorado. *Diabetes Care*, **21** (1), 53–61.

41. Porta, M., Sjoelie, A.K., Chaturvedi, N. *et al.* (2001) Risk factors for progression to proliferative diabetic retinopathy in the EURODIAB prospective complications study. *Diabetologia*, **44** (12), 2203–9.

42. Nielsen, N.V. (1984) Diabetic retinopathy I. The course of retinopathy in insulin-treated diabetics. A one year epidemiological cohort study of diabetes mellitus. The Island of Falster, Denmark. *Acta Ophthalmologica*, **62** (2), 256–65.

43. Stratton, I.M., Kohner, E.M., Aldington, S.J. *et al.* (2001) UKPDS 50: risk factors for incidence and progression of retinopathy in type II diabetes over 6 years from diagnosis. *Diabetologia*, **44** (2), 156–63.

44. Younis, N., Broadbent, D.M., Vora, J.P. *et al.* (2003) Incidence of sight-threatening retinopathy in patients with type 2 diabetes in the Liverpool Diabetic Eye Study: a cohort study. *Lancet*, **361** (9353), 195–200.

45. Klein, R., Klein, B.E., Moss, S.E. *et al.* (1989) The Wisconsin Epidemiologic Study of Diabetic Retinopathy. IX. Four-year incidence and progression of diabetic retinopathy when age at diagnosis is less than 30 years. *Archives of Ophthalmology*, **107** (2), 237–43.

46. Klein, R., Klein, B.E., Moss, S.E. *et al.* (1989) The Wisconsin Epidemiologic Study of Diabetic Retinopathy. X. Four-year incidence and progression of diabetic retinopathy when age at diagnosis is 30 years or more. *Archives of Ophthalmology*, **107** (2), 244–9.

47. Klein, R., Klein, B.E., Moss, S.E. and Cruickshanks, K.J. (1994) The Wisconsin Epidemiologic Study of Diabetic Retinopathy. XIV. Ten-year incidence and progression of diabetic retinopathy

[see comment]. *Archives of Ophthalmology*, **112** (9), 1217–28.

48. Klein, R., Moss, S.E., Klein, B.E. *et al.* (1989) The Wisconsin Epidemiologic Study of Diabetic Retinopathy. XI. The incidence of macular edema. *Ophthalmology*, **96** (10), 1501–10.

49. Lloyd, C.E., Klein, R., Maser, R.E. *et al.* (1995) The progression of retinopathy over 2 years: the Pittsburgh Epidemiology of Diabetes Complications (EDC) Study. *Journal of Diabetes and its Complications*, **9** (3), 140–8.

50. Mitchell, P. (1980) The prevalence of diabetic retinopathy: a study of 1300 diabetics from Newcastle and the Hunter Valley. *Australian Journal of Ophthalmology*, **8** (3), 241–6.

51. Holl, R.W., Lang, G.E., Grabert, M. *et al.* (1998) Diabetic retinopathy in pediatric patients with type-1 diabetes: effect of diabetes duration, prepubertal and pubertal onset of diabetes, and metabolic control. *The Journal of Pediatrics*, **132** (5), 790–4.

52. Fairchild, J.M., Hing, S.J., Donaghue, K.C. *et al.* (1994) Prevalence and risk factors for retinopathy in adolescents with type 1 diabetes. *The Medical Journal of Australia*, **160** (12), 757–62.

53. Zhang, L., Krzentowski, G., Albert, A. and Lefebvre, P.J. (2001) Risk of developing retinopathy in diabetes control and complications trial type 1 diabetic patients with good or poor metabolic control. *Diabetes Care*, **24** (7), 1275–9.

54. Maguire, A., Chan, A., Cusumano, J. *et al.* (2005) The case for biennial retinopathy screening in children and adolescents. *Diabetes Care*, **28** (3), 509–13.

55. Dorf, A., Ballintine, E.J., Bennett, P.H. and Miller, M. (1976) Retinopathy in Pima Indians. Relationships to glucose level, duration of diabetes, age at diagnosis of diabetes, and age at examination in a population with a high prevalence of diabetes mellitus. *Diabetes*, **25** (7), 554–60.

56. Bennett, P.H., Rushforth, N.B., Miller, M. and LeCompte, P.M. (1976) Epidemiologic studies of diabetes in the Pima Indians. *Recent Progress in Hormone Research*, **32**, 333–76.

57. Berinstein, D.M., Stahn, R.M., Welty, T.K. *et al.* (1997) The prevalence of diabetic retinopathy and associated risk factors among Sioux Indians. *Diabetes Care*, **20** (5), 757–9.

58. Lee, E.T., Lee, V.S., Lu, M. and Russell, D. (1992) Development of proliferative retinopathy in NIDDM. A follow-up study of American Indians in Oklahoma. *Diabetes*, **41** (3), 359–67.

59. Lee, E.T., Lee, V.S., Kingsley, R.M. *et al.* (1992) Diabetic retinopathy in Oklahoma Indians with NIDDM. Incidence and risk factors. *Diabetes Care*, **15** (11), 1620–7.

60. Varma, R., Torres, M., Pena, F. *et al.* (2004) Prevalence of diabetic retinopathy in adult Latinos: the Los Angeles Latino eye study. *Ophthalmology*, **111** (7), 1298–306.

61. Dowse, G.K., Humphrey, A.R., Collins, V.R. *et al.* (1998) Prevalence and risk factors for diabetic retinopathy in the multiethnic population of Mauritius. *American Journal of Epidemiology*, **147** (5), 448–57.

62. Collins, V.R., Dowse, G.K., Plehwe, W.E. *et al.* (1995) High prevalence of diabetic retinopathy and nephropathy in Polynesians of Western Samoa. *Diabetes Care*, **18** (8), 1140–9.

63. Fujimoto, W. and Fukuda, M. (1976) Natural history of diabetic retinopathy and its treatment in Japan, in *Diabetes Mellitus in Asia* (eds S. Baba, Y. Goto, I. Fukui), Excerpta Medica, Amsterdam, pp. 225–31.

64. Wong, T.Y., Klein, R., Islam, F.M. *et al.* (2006) Diabetic retinopathy in a multi-ethnic cohort in the United States. *American Journal of Ophthalmology*, **141** (3), 446–55.

65. Kernell, A., Dedorsson, I., Johansson, B. *et al.* (1997) Prevalence of diabetic retinopathy in children and adolescents with IDDM. A population-based multicentre study. *Diabetologia*, **40** (3), 307–10.

66. Harris, M.I., Klein, R., Welborn, T.A. and Knuiman, M.W. (1992) Onset of NIDDM occurs at least 4–7 yr before clinical diagnosis. *Diabetes Care*, **15** (7), 815–19.

67. Klein, R., Klein, B.E., Moss, S.E. and Cruickshanks, K.J. (1998) The Wisconsin Epidemiologic Study of Diabetic Retinopathy: XVII. The 14-year incidence and progression of diabetic retinopathy and associated risk factors in type 1 diabetes. *Ophthalmology*, **105** (10), 1801–15.

68. Krolewski, A.S., Warram, J.H., Rand, L.I. *et al.* (1986) Risk of proliferative diabetic retinopathy in juvenile-onset type I diabetes: a 40-yr follow-up study. *Diabetes Care*, **9** (5), 443–52.

69. Colwell, J.A. (1966) Effect of diabetic control on retinopathy. *Diabetes*, **15** (7), 497–9.

70. Miki, E., Fukuda, M., Kuzuya, T. *et al.* (1969) Relation of the course of retinopathy to control of diabetes, age, and therapeutic agents in diabetic Japanese patients. *Diabetes*, **18** (11), 773–80.

71. Doft, B.H., Kingsley, L.A., Orchard, T.J. *et al.* (1984) The association between long-term diabetic control and early retinopathy. *Ophthalmology*, **91** (7), 763–9.

72. Friberg, T.R., Rosenstock, J., Sanborn, G. *et al.* (1985) The effect of long-term near normal glycemic control on mild diabetic retinopathy. *Ophthalmology*, **92** (8), 1051–8.

73. The Kroc Collaborative Study Group (1984) Blood glucose control and the evolution of diabetic retinopathy and albuminuria. A preliminary multicenter trial. The Kroc Collaborative Study Group. *The New England Journal of Medicine*, **311** (6), 365–72.

74. Lauritzen, T., Frost-Larsen, K., Larsen, H.W. and Deckert, T. (1983) Effect of 1 year of near-normal blood glucose levels on retinopathy in insulin-dependent diabetics. *Lancet*, **1** (8318), 200–4.

75. Klein, R. (1987) The epidemiology of diabetic retinopathy: findings from the Wisconsin Epidemiologic Study of Diabetic Retinopathy. *International Ophthalmology Clinics*, **27** (4), 230–8.

76. Klein, R., Klein, B.E., Moss, S.E. *et al.* (1988) Glycosylated hemoglobin predicts the incidence and progression of diabetic retinopathy. *The Journal of the American Medical Association*, **260** (19), 2864–71.

77. Klein, R., Klein, B.E., Moss, S.E. and Cruickshanks, K.J. (1994) Relationship of hyperglycemia to the long-term incidence and progression of diabetic retinopathy. *Archives of Internal Medicine*, **154** (19), 2169–78.

78. The Diabetes Control and Complications Trial Research Group (1993) The effect of intensive treatment of diabetes on the development and progression of long-term complications in insulin-dependent diabetes mellitus. *The New England Journal of Medicine*, **329** (14), 977–86.

79. The Diabetes Control and Complications Trial (1995) The effect of intensive diabetes treatment on the progression of diabetic retinopathy in insulin-dependent diabetes mellitus. The Diabetes Control and Complications Trial. *Archives of Ophthalmology*, **113** (1), 36–51.

80. Diabetes Control and Complications Trial Research Group (1995) Progression of retinopathy with intensive versus conventional treatment in the diabetes control and complications trial. Diabetes Control and Complications Trial Research Group. *Ophthalmology*, **102** (4), 647–61.

81. Dahl-Jorgensen, K., Brinchmann-Hansen, O., Hanssen, K.F. *et al.* (1986) Effect of near normoglycaemia for two years on progression of early diabetic retinopathy, nephropathy, and neuropathy: the Oslo study. *British Medical Journal*, **293** (6556), 1195–9.

82. The Diabetes Control and Complications Trial (1996) The absence of a glycemic threshold for the development of long-term complications: the perspective of the Diabetes Control and Complications Trial. *Diabetes*, **45** (10), 1289–98.

83. Chaturvedi, N., Sjoelie, A.K., Porta, M. *et al.* (2001) Markers of insulin resistance are strong risk factors for retinopathy incidence in type 1 diabetes. *Diabetes Care*, **24** (2), 284–9.

84. The Diabetes Control and Complications Trial (2000) Retinopathy and nephropathy in patients with type 1 diabetes four years after a trial of intensive therapy. The Diabetes Control and Complications Trial/Epidemiology of Diabetes Interventions and Complications Research Group. *The New England Journal of Medicine*, **342** (6), 381–9; [erratum: (2000) *The New England Journal of Medicine*, **342** (18), 1376].

85. UK Prospective Diabetes Study (UKPDS) Group (1998) Intensive blood-glucose control with sulphonylureas or insulin compared with conventional treatment and risk of complications in patients with type 2 diabetes (UKPDS 33). *Lancet*, **352** (9131), 837–53.

86. Klein, R., Klein, B.E., Moss, S.E. *et al.* (1989) Is blood pressure a predictor of the incidence or progression of diabetic retinopathy? *Archives of Internal Medicine*, **149** (11), 2427–32.

87. Klein, B.E., Klein, R., Moss, S.E. and Palta, M. (1995) A cohort study of the relationship of diabetic retinopathy to blood pressure. *Archives of Ophthalmology*, **113** (5), 601–6 [erratum: (1996) *Archives of Ophthalmology*, **114** (1), 109].

88. Olsen, B.S., Sjolie, A., Hougaard, P. *et al.* (2000) A 6-year nationwide cohort study of glycaemic control in young people with type 1 diabetes. Risk markers for the development of retinopathy, nephropathy and neuropathy. Danish Study Group of Diabetes in Childhood. *Journal of Diabetes and its Complications*, **14** (6), 295–300.

89. UK Prospective Diabetes Study Group (1998) Tight blood pressure control and risk of macrovascular and microvascular complications in type 2 diabetes: UKPDS 38. *British Medical Journal*, **317** (7160), 703–13.

90. Adler, A.I., Stratton, I.M., Neil, H.A. *et al.* (2000) Association of systolic blood pressure with macrovascular and microvascular complications of type 2 diabetes (UKPDS 36): prospective observational study. *British Medical Journal*, **321** (7258), 412–19.

91. Schrier, R.W., Estacio, R.O., Esler, A. and Mehler, P. (2002) Effects of aggressive blood pressure control in normotensive type 2 diabetic patients on albuminuria, retinopathy and strokes. *Kidney International*, **61** (3), 1086–97.

92. Estacio, R.O., Jeffers, B.W., Gifford, N. and Schrier, R.W. (2000) Effect of blood pressure control on diabetic microvascular complications

in patients with hypertension and type 2 diabetes. *Diabetes Care*, **23** (Suppl 2), B54–64.

93. Fong, D.S., Aiello, L., Gardner, T.W. *et al.* (2003) Diabetic retinopathy. *Diabetes Care*, **26** (1), 226–29.

94. McCarty, C.A., McKay, R. and Keeffe, J.E. (2000) Management of diabetic retinopathy by Australian ophthalmologists. Working Group on evaluation of the NHMRC retinopathy guideline distribution. National Health and Medical Research Council. *Clinical and Experimental Ophthalmology*, **28** (2), 107–12.

95. Ferris, F.L. III, Chew, E.Y. and Hoogwerf, B.J. (1996) Serum lipids and diabetic retinopathy. Early Treatment Diabetic Retinopathy Study Research Group. *Diabetes Care*, **19** (11), 1291–3.

96. Lyons, T.J., Jenkins, A.J., Zheng, D. *et al.* (2004) Diabetic retinopathy and serum lipoprotein subclasses in the DCCT/EDIC cohort. *Investigative Ophthalmology and Visual Science*, **45** (3), 910–18.

97. Chew, E.Y. (1997) Diabetic retinopathy and lipid abnormalities. *Current Opinion in Ophthalmology*, **8** (3), 59–62.

98. Su, D.H. and Yeo, K.T. (2000) Diabetic retinopathy and serum lipids. *Singapore Medical Journal*, **41** (6), 295–7.

99. Cusick, M., Chew, E.Y., Chan, C.C. *et al.* (2003) Histopathology and regression of retinal hard exudates in diabetic retinopathy after reduction of elevated serum lipid levels. *Ophthalmology*, **110** (11), 2126–33.

100. Curtis, T.M. and Scholfield, C.N. (2004) The role of lipids and protein kinase Cs in the pathogenesis of diabetic retinopathy. *Diabetes/Metabolism Research and Reviews*, **20** (1), 28–43.

101. Cohen, R.A., Hennekens, C.H., Christen, W.G. *et al.* (1999) Determinants of retinopathy progression in type 1 diabetes mellitus. *American Journal of Medicine*, **107** (1), 45–51.

102. Nazimek-Siewniak, B., Moczulski, D. and Grzeszczak, W. (2002) Risk of macrovascular and microvascular complications in type 2 diabetes: results of longitudinal study design. *The Journal of Diabetic Complications*, **16** (4), 271–6.

103. Klein, B.E., Moss, S.E., Klein, R. and Surawicz, T.S. (1991) The Wisconsin Epidemiologic Study of Diabetic Retinopathy. XIII. Relationship of serum cholesterol to retinopathy and hard exudate. *Ophthalmology*, **98** (8), 1261–5.

104. Chew, E.Y., Klein, M.L., Ferris, F.L. III *et al.* (1996) Association of elevated serum lipid levels with retinal hard exudate in diabetic retinopathy. Early Treatment Diabetic Retinopathy Study

(ETDRS) report 22. *Archives of Ophthalmology*, **114** (9), 1079–84.

105. Keech, A., Simes, R.J., Barter, P. *et al.* (2005) Effects of long-term fenofibrate therapy on cardiovascular events in 9795 people with type 2 diabetes mellitus (the FIELD study): randomised controlled trial. *Lancet*, **366** (9500), 1849–61.

106. Gupta, A., Gupta, V., Thapar, S. and Bhansali, A. (2004) Lipid-lowering drug atorvastatin as an adjunct in the management of diabetic macular edema. *American Journal of Ophthalmology*, **137** (4), 675–82.

107. Sen, K., Misra, A., Kumar, A. and Pandey, R.M. (2002) Simvastatin retards progression of retinopathy in diabetic patients with hypercholesterolemia. *Diabetes Research and Clinical Practice*, **56** (1), 1–11.

108. Gordon, B., Chang, S., Kavanagh, M. *et al.* (1991) The effects of lipid lowering on diabetic retinopathy. *American Journal of Ophthalmology*, **112** (4), 385–91.

109. Root, H., Pote, W.H. and Frehner, H. (1954) Triopathy of diabetes; sequence of neuropathy, retinopathy and nephropathy in one hundred fifty-five patients. *Archives of Internal Medicine*, **94** (6), 931–41.

110. Klein, R., Zinman, B., Gardiner, R. *et al.* (2005) The relationship of diabetic retinopathy to preclinical diabetic glomerulopathy lesions in type 1 diabetic patients: the rennin–angiotensin system study. *Diabetes*, **54** (2), 527–33.

111. Ballone, E., Colagrande, V., Di Nicola, M. *et al.* (2003) Probabilistic approach to developing nephropathy in diabetic patients with retinopathy. *Statistics in Medicine*, **22** (24), 3889–97.

112. Cruickshanks, K.J., Ritter, L.L., Klein, R. and Moss, S.E. (1993) The association of microalbuminuria with diabetic retinopathy. The Wisconsin Epidemiologic Study of Diabetic Retinopathy. *Ophthalmology*, **100** (6), 862–7.

113. Klein, R., Moss, S.E. and Klein, B.E. (1993) Is gross proteinuria a risk factor for the incidence of proliferative diabetic retinopathy? *Ophthalmology*, **100** (8), 1140–6.

114. Bresnick, G.H. (1983) Diabetic maculopathy. A critical review highlighting diffuse macular edema. *Ophthalmology*, **90** (11), 1301–17.

115. Perkovich, B.T. and Meyers, S.M. (1988) Systemic factors affecting diabetic macular edema. *American Journal of Ophthalmology*, **105** (2), 211–12.

116. Uckaya, G., Ozata, M., Bayraktar, Z. *et al.* (2000) Is leptin associated with diabetic retinopathy? *Diabetes Care*, **23** (3), 371–6.

117. Van Leiden, H.A., Dekker, J.M., Moll, A.C. *et al.* (2002) Blood pressure, lipids, and obesity are associated with retinopathy: the Hoorn Study. *Diabetes Care*, **25** (8), 1320–5.

118. De Block, C.E., De Leeuw, I.H. and Van Gaal, L.F. (2005) Impact of overweight on chronic microvascular complications in type 1 diabetic patients. *Diabetes Care*, **28** (7), 1649–55.

119. Wong, T.Y., Duncan, B.B., Golden, S.H. *et al.* (2004) Associations between the metabolic syndrome and retinal microvascular signs: the atherosclerosis risk in communities study. *Investigative Ophthalmology and Visual Science*, **45** (9), 2949–54.

120. Klein, R., Klein, B.E. and Moss, S.E. (1997) Is obesity related to microvascular and macrovascular complications in diabetes? The Wisconsin Epidemiologic Study of Diabetic Retinopathy. *Archives of Internal Medicine*, **157** (6), 650–6.

121. Chaturvedi, N. and Fuller, J.H. (1995) Mortality risk by body weight and weight change in people with NIDDM. The WHO multinational study of vascular disease in diabetes. *Diabetes Care*, **18** (6), 766–74.

122. Nelson, R.G., Wolfe, J.A., Horton, M.B. *et al.* (1989) Proliferative retinopathy in NIDDM. Incidence and risk factors in Pima Indians. *Diabetes*, **38** (4), 435–40.

123. Dorchy, H., Claes, C. and Verougstraete, C. (2002) Risk factors of developing proliferative retinopathy in type 1 diabetic patients: role of BMI. *Diabetes Care*, **25** (4), 798–9.

124. Aiello, L.P., Avery, R.L., Arrigg, P.G. *et al.* (1994) Vascular endothelial growth factor in ocular fluid of patients with diabetic retinopathy and other retinal disorders. *New England Journal of Medicine*, **331** (22), 1480–7.

125. Gariano, R.F., Nath, A.K., D'Amico, D.J. *et al.* (2000) Elevation of vitreous leptin in diabetic retinopathy and retinal detachment. *Investigative Ophthalmology and Visual Science*, **41** (11), 3576–81.

126. Sheard, N.F. (2003) Moderate changes in weight and physical activity can prevent or delay the development of type 2 diabetes mellitus in susceptible individuals. *Nutrition Reviews*, **61** (2), 76–9.

127. Tamburrino, M.B. and McGinnis, R.A. (2002) Anorexia nervosa. A review. *Panminerva Medica*, **44** (4), 301–11.

128. Chen, H.C., Newsom, R.S., Patel, V. *et al.* (1994) Retinal blood flow changes during pregnancy in women with diabetes. *Investigative Ophthalmology and Visual Science*, **35** (8), 3199–208.

129. Schocket, L.S., Grunwald, J.E., Tsang, A.F. and DuPont, J. (1999) The effect of pregnancy on retinal hemodynamics in diabetic versus nondiabetic mothers. *American Journal of Ophthalmology*, **128** (4), 477–84.

130. Sone, H., Okuda, Y., Kawakami, Y. *et al.* (1996) Progesterone induces vascular endothelial growth factor on retinal pigment epithelial cells in culture. *Life Sciences*, **59** (1), 21–5.

131. Moloney, J.B. and Drury, M.I. (1982) The effect of pregnancy on the natural course of diabetic retinopathy. *American Journal of Ophthalmology*, **93** (6), 745–56.

132. Klein, B.E., Moss, S.E. and Klein, R. (1990) Effect of pregnancy on progression of diabetic retinopathy. *Diabetes Care*, **13** (1), 34–40.

133. Chew, E.Y., Mills, J.L., Metzger, B.E. *et al.* (1995) Metabolic control and progression of retinopathy. The diabetes in early pregnancy study. National Institute of Child Health and Human Development Diabetes in Early Pregnancy Study. *Diabetes Care*, **18** (5), 631–7.

134. Hemachandra, A., Ellis, D., Lloyd, C.E. and Orchard, T.J. (1995) The influence of pregnancy on IDDM complications. *Diabetes Care*, **18** (7), 950–4.

135. Lovestam-Adrian, M., Agardh, C.D., Aberg, A. and Agardh, E. (1997) Pre-eclampsia is a potent risk factor for deterioration of retinopathy during pregnancy in type 1 diabetic patients. *Diabetic Medicine*, **14** (12), 1059–65.

136. Rosenn, B., Miodovnik, M., Kranias, G. *et al.* (1992) Progression of diabetic retinopathy in pregnancy: association with hypertension in pregnancy. *American Journal of Obstetrics and Gynecology*, **166** (4), 1214–18.

137. Klein, B.E., Moss, S.E. and Klein, R. (1990) Is menarche associated with diabetic retinopathy? *Diabetes Care*, **13** (10), 1034–8.

138. Klein, B.E., Moss, S.E. and Klein, R. (1990) Oral contraceptives in women with diabetes. *Diabetes Care*, **13** (8), 895–8.

139. Klein, B.E., Klein, R. and Moss, S.E. (1999) Exogenous estrogen exposures and changes in diabetic retinopathy. The Wisconsin Epidemiologic Study of Diabetic Retinopathy. *Diabetes Care*, **22** (12), 1984–7.

140. Meigs, J.B., Hu, F.B., Rifai, N. and Manson, J.E. (2004) Biomarkers of endothelial dysfunction and risk of type 2 diabetes mellitus. *The Journal of the American Medical Association*, **291** (16), 1978–86.

141. Pradhan, A.D., Manson, J.E., Rifai, N. *et al.* (2001) C-reactive protein, interleukin 6, and risk of developing type 2 diabetes mellitus. *The Journal*

of the American Medical Association, **286** (3), 327–34.

142. Miyamoto, K., Khosrof, S., Bursell, S.E. et al. (1999) Prevention of leukostasis and vascular leakage in streptozotocin-induced diabetic retinopathy via intercellular adhesion molecule-1 inhibition. *Proceedings of the National Academy of Sciences of the United States of America*, **96** (19), 10836–41.

143. Izuora, K.E., Chase, H.P., Jackson, W.E. et al. (2005) Inflammatory markers and diabetic retinopathy in type 1 diabetes. *Diabetes Care*, **28** (3), 714–15.

144. Joussen, A.M., Poulaki, V., Le, M.L. et al. (2004) A central role for inflammation in the pathogenesis of diabetic retinopathy. *FASEB Journal*, **18** (12), 1450–2.

145. Mitamura, Y., Takeuchi, S., Yamamoto, S. et al. (2002) Monocyte chemotactic protein-1 levels in the vitreous of patients with proliferative vitreoretinopathy. *Japanese Journal of Ophthalmology*, **46** (2), 218–21.

146. Meleth, A.D., Agron, E., Chan, C.C. et al. (2005) Serum inflammatory markers in diabetic retinopathy. *Investigative Ophthalmology and Visual Science*, **46** (11), 4295–301.

147. Van Hecke, M.V., Dekker, J.M., Nijpels, G. et al. (2005) Inflammation and endothelial dysfunction are associated with retinopathy: the Hoorn Study. *Diabetologia*, **48** (7), 1300–6.

148. Schram, M.T., Chaturvedi, N., Schalkwijk, C.G. et al. (2005) Markers of inflammation are cross-sectionally associated with microvascular complications and cardiovascular disease in type 1 diabetes – the EURODIAB Prospective Complications Study. *Diabetologia*, **48** (2), 370–8.

149. Early Treatment Diabetic Retinopathy Study Research Group (1991) Effects of aspirin treatment on diabetic retinopathy. ETDRS report number 8. Early Treatment Diabetic Retinopathy Study Research Group. *Ophthalmology*, **98** (Suppl 5), 757–65.

150. Moss, S.E., Klein, R. and Klein, B.E. (1991) Association of cigarette smoking with diabetic retinopathy. *Diabetes Care*, **14** (2), 119–26.

151. Moss, S.E., Klein, R. and Klein, B.E. (1996) Cigarette smoking and ten-year progression of diabetic retinopathy. *Ophthalmology*, **103** (9), 1438–42.

152. Moss, S.E., Klein, R. and Klein, B.E. (1992) Alcohol consumption and the prevalence of diabetic retinopathy. *Ophthalmology*, **99** (6), 926–32.

153. Moss, S.E., Klein, R. and Klein, B.E. (1994) The association of alcohol consumption with the incidence and progression of diabetic retinopathy. *Ophthalmology*, **101** (12), 1962–8.

154. Klein, R., Klein, B.E. and Moss, S.E. (1997) The relation of systemic hypertension to changes in the retinal vasculature: the Beaver Dam Eye Study. *Transactions of the American Ophthalmological Society*, **95**, 329–48; discussion 348–50.

155. Kriska, A.M., LaPorte, R.E., Patrick, S.L. et al. (1991) The association of physical activity and diabetic complications in individuals with insulin-dependent diabetes mellitus: the Epidemiology of Diabetes Complications Study – VII. *Journal of Clinical Epidemiology*, **44** (11), 1207–14.

156. Cruickshanks, K.J., Moss, S.E., Klein, R. and Klein, B.E. (1992) Physical activity and proliferative retinopathy in people diagnosed with diabetes before age 30 yr. *Diabetes Care*, **15** (10), 1267–72.

157. Wong, T.Y., Klein, R., Klein, B.E. et al. (2001) Retinal microvascular abnormalities and their relationship with hypertension, cardiovascular disease, and mortality. *Survey of Ophthalmology*, **46** (1), 59–80.

158. Wong, T.Y., Hubbard, L.D., Klein, R. et al. (2002) Retinal microvascular abnormalities and blood pressure in older people: the cardiovascular health study. *The British Journal of Ophthalmology*, **86** (9), 1007–13.

159. Wong, T.Y., Klein, R., Sharrett, A.R. et al. (2003) The prevalence and risk factors of retinal microvascular abnormalities in older persons: the cardiovascular health study. *Ophthalmology*, **110** (4), 658–66.

160. Yu, T., Mitchell, P., Berry, G. et al. (1998) Retinopathy in older persons without diabetes and its relationship to hypertension. *Archives of Ophthalmology*, **116** (1), 83–9.

161. Klein, R., Klein, B.E., Moss, S.E. and Wang, Q. (1994) Hypertension and retinopathy, arteriolar narrowing, and arteriovenous nicking in a population. *Archives of Ophthalmology*, **112** (1), 92–8.

162. Klein, R., Sharrett, A.R., Klein, B.E. et al. (2000) Are retinal arteriolar abnormalities related to atherosclerosis? The Atherosclerosis Risk in Communities Study. *Arteriosclerosis, Thrombosis and Vascular Biology*, **20** (6), 1644–50.

163. Cugati, S., Cikamatana, L., Wang, J.J. et al. (2005) Five-year incidence and progression of vascular retinopathy in persons without diabetes: the Blue Mountains Eye Study. *Eye*, **20** (11), 1239–45.

164. Wong, T.Y., Barr, E.L., Tapp, R.J. et al. (2005) Retinopathy in persons with impaired glucose

metabolism: the Australian Diabetes Obesity and Lifestyle (AusDiab) Study. *American Journal of Ophthalmology*, **140** (6), 1157–9.

165. Rajala, U., Laakso, M., Qiao, Q. and Keinanen-Kiukaanniemi, S. (1998) Prevalence of retinopathy in people with diabetes, impaired glucose tolerance, and normal glucose tolerance. *Diabetes Care*, **21** (10), 1664–9.

166. Singleton, J.R., Smith, A.G., Russell, J.W. and Feldman, E.L. (2003) Microvascular complications of impaired glucose tolerance. *Diabetes*, **52** (12), 2867–73.

167. Wong, T.Y. and Mitchell, P. (2004) Hypertensive retinopathy. *New England Journal of Medicine*, **351** (22), 2310–17.

168. Wong, T.Y., Klein, R., Couper, D.J. *et al.* (2001) Retinal microvascular abnormalities and incident stroke: the Atherosclerosis Risk in Communities Study. *Lancet*, **358** (9288), 1134–40.

169. Wong, T.Y., Klein, R., Sharrett, A.R. *et al.* (2002) Cerebral white matter lesions, retinopathy, and incident clinical stroke. *The Journal of the American Medical Association*, **288** (1), 67–74.

170. Wong, T.Y., Mohamed, Q., Klein, R. and Couper, D.J. (2006) Do retinopathy signs in non-diabetic individuals predict the subsequent risk of diabetes? *The British Journal of Ophthalmology*, **90** (3), 301–3.

171. Klein, R., Klein, B.E. and Moss, S.E. (1992) Epidemiology of proliferative diabetic retinopathy. *Diabetes Care*, **15** (12), 1875–91.

172. Wong, T.Y., Rosamond, W., Chang, P.P. *et al.* (2005) Retinopathy and risk of congestive heart failure. *The Journal of the American Medical Association*, **293** (1), 63–9.

173. Van Hecke, M.V., Dekker, J.M., Nijpels, G. *et al.* (2003) Retinopathy is associated with cardiovascular and all-cause mortality in both diabetic and nondiabetic subjects: the Hoorn Study. *Diabetes Care*, **26** (10), 2958.

174. Van Hecke, M.V., Dekker, J.M., Stehouwer, C.D. *et al.* (2005) Diabetic retinopathy is associated with mortality and cardiovascular disease incidence: the EURODIAB Prospective Complications Study. *Diabetes Care*, **28** (6), 1383–9.

175. Cusick, M., Meleth, A.D., Agron, E. *et al.* (2005) Associations of mortality and diabetes complications in patients with type 1 and type 2 diabetes: Early Treatment Diabetic Retinopathy Study report no. 27. *Diabetes Care*, **28** (3), 617–25.

176. Miettinen, H., Haffner, S.M., Lehto, S. *et al.* (1996) Retinopathy predicts coronary heart disease events in NIDDM patients. *Diabetes Care*, **19** (12), 1445–8.

177. Mitchell, P., Wang, J.J., Wong, T.Y. *et al.* (2005) Retinal microvascular signs and risk of stroke and stroke mortality. *Neurology*, **65** (7), 1005–9.

178. Cooper, L.S., Wong, T.Y., Klein, R. *et al.* (2006) Retinal microvascular abnormalities and MRI-defined subclinical cerebral infarction: the Atherosclerosis Risk in Communities Study. *Stroke*, **37** (1), 82–6.

179. Klein, R., Klein, B.E., Moss, S.E. and Meuer, S.M. (2000) The epidemiology of retinal vein occlusion: the Beaver Dam Eye Study. *Transactions of the American Ophthalmological Society*, **98**, 133–41; discussion 141–43.

180. Mitchell, P., Smith, W. and Chang, A. (1996) Prevalence and associations of retinal vein occlusion in Australia. The Blue Mountains Eye Study. *Archives of Ophthalmology*, **114** (10), 1243–7.

181. Shahsuvaryan, M.L. and Melkonyan, A.K. (2003) Central retinal vein occlusion risk profile: a case–control study. *European Journal of Ophthalmology*, **13** (5), 445–52.

182. Sperduto, R.D., Hiller, R., Chew, E. *et al.* (1998) Risk factors for hemiretinal vein occlusion: comparison with risk factors for central and branch retinal vein occlusion: the eye disease case–control study [see comment]. *Ophthalmology*, **105** (5), 765–71.

183. Rath, E.Z., Frank, R.N., Shin, D.H. and Kim, C. (1992) Risk factors for retinal vein occlusions. A case–control study. *Ophthalmology*, **99** (4), 509–14.

184. Hayreh, S.S., Zimmerman, B., McCarthy, M.J. and Podhajsky, P. (2001) Systemic diseases associated with various types of retinal vein occlusion. *American Journal of Ophthalmology*, **131** (1), 61–77.

185. The Eye Disease Case–Control Study Group (1996) Risk factors for central retinal vein occlusion. *Archives of Ophthalmology*, **114** (5), 545–54.

186. Wong, T.Y., Larsen, E.K., Klein, R. *et al.* (2005) Cardiovascular risk factors for retinal vein occlusion and arteriolar emboli: the Atherosclerosis Risk in Communities & Cardiovascular Health Studies. *Ophthalmology*, **112** (4), 540–7.

187. Funderburk, R.L. and Feinberg, E.B. (1989) Diabetes as a risk factor for retinal neovascularization in retinal vein occlusion. *Annals of Ophthalmology*, **21** (2), 65–6.

188. Mitchell, P., Wang, J.J., Li, W. *et al.* (1997) Prevalence of asymptomatic retinal emboli in an Australian urban community. *Stroke*, **28** (1), 63–6.

189. Klein, R., Klein, B.E., Jensen, S.C. *et al.* (1999) Retinal emboli and stroke: the Beaver Dam

Eye Study. *Archives of Ophthalmology*, **117** (8), 1063–8.

190. Klein, R., Klein, B.E., Moss, S.E. and Meuer, S.M. (2003) Retinal emboli and cardiovascular disease: the Beaver Dam Eye Study. *Archives of Ophthalmology*, **121** (10), 1446–51.

191. Wong, T.Y. and Klein, R. (2002) Retinal arteriolar emboli: epidemiology and risk of stroke. *Current Opinion in Ophthalmology*, **13** (3), 142–6.

192. Cugati, S., Wang, J.J., Rochtchina, E. and Mitchell, P. (2006) Ten-year incidence of retinal emboli in an older population. *Stroke*, **37** (3), 908–10.

193. Recchia, F.M. and Brown, G.C. (2000) Systemic disorders associated with retinal vascular occlusion. *Current Opinion in Ophthalmology*, **11** (6), 462–7.

194. Wilson, L.A., Warlow, C.P. and Russell, R.W. (1979) Cardiovascular disease in patients with retinal arterial occlusion. *Lancet*, **1** (8111), 292–4.

195. Mizener, J.B., Podhajsky, P. and Hayreh, S.S. (1997) Ocular ischemic syndrome. *Ophthalmology*, **104** (5), 859–64.

196. Dogru, M., Inoue, M., Nakamura, M. and Yamamoto, M. (1998) Modifying factors related to asymmetric diabetic retinopathy. *Eye*, **12** (Pt 6), 929–33.

197. Duker, J.S., Brown, G.C., Bosley, T.M. *et al.* (1990) Asymmetric proliferative diabetic retinopathy and carotid artery disease. *Ophthalmology*, **97** (7), 869–74.

198. Moss, S.E., Klein, R. and Klein, B.E. (1994) Ocular factors in the incidence and progression of diabetic retinopathy. *Ophthalmology*, **101** (1), 77–83.

199. Hayreh, S.S., Joos, K.M., Podhajsky, P.A. and Long, C.R. (1994) Systemic diseases associated with nonarteritic anterior ischemic optic neuropathy. *American Journal of Ophthalmology*, **118** (6), 766–80.

200. Jacobson, D.M., Vierkant, R.A. and Belongia, E.A. (1997) Nonarteritic anterior ischemic optic neuropathy. A case–control study of potential risk factors. *Archives of Ophthalmology*, **115** (11), 1403–7.

201. The Ischemic Optic Neuropathy Decompression Trial Research Group (1996) Characteristics of patients with nonarteritic anterior ischemic optic neuropathy eligible for the Ischemic Optic Neuropathy Decompression Trial. *Archives of Ophthalmology*, **114** (11), 1366–74.

202. Patel, S.V., Holmes, J.M., Hodge, D.O. and Burke, J.P. (2005) Diabetes and hypertension in isolated sixth nerve palsy: a population-based study. *Ophthalmology*, **112** (5), 760–3.

203. Hiller, R., Sperduto, R.D. and Ederer, F. (1986) Epidemiologic associations with nuclear, cortical, and posterior subcapsular cataracts. *American Journal of Epidemiology*, **124** (6), 916–25.

204. Miglior, S., Marighi, P.E., Musicco, M. *et al.* (1994) Risk factors for cortical, nuclear, posterior subcapsular and mixed cataract: a case–control study. *Ophthalmic Epidemiology*, **1** (2), 93–105.

205. Delcourt, C., Cristol, J.P., Tessier, F. *et al.* (2000) Risk factors for cortical, nuclear, and posterior subcapsular cataracts: the POLA study. Pathologies Oculaires Liées à l'Age. *American Journal of Epidemiology*, **151** (5), 497–504.

206. Klein, B.E., Klein, R., Wang, Q. and Moss, S.E. (1995) Older-onset diabetes and lens opacities. The Beaver Dam Eye Study. *Ophthalmic Epidemiology*, **2** (1), 49–55.

207. Klein, B.E., Klein, R. and Lee, K.E. (1998) Diabetes, cardiovascular disease, selected cardiovascular disease risk factors, and the 5-year incidence of age-related cataract and progression of lens opacities: the Beaver Dam Eye Study. *American Journal of Ophthalmology*, **126** (6), 782–90.

208. Rowe, N.G., Mitchell, P.G., Cumming, R.G. and Wans, J.J. (2000) Diabetes, fasting blood glucose and age-related cataract: the Blue Mountains Eye Study. *Ophthalmic Epidemiology*, **7** (2), 103–14.

209. Saxena, S., Mitchell, P. and Rochtchina, E. (2004) Five-year incidence of cataract in older persons with diabetes and pre-diabetes. *Ophthalmic Epidemiology*, **11** (4), 271–7.

210. McCarty, C.A., Mukesh, B.N., Fu, C.L. and Taylor, H.R. (1999) The epidemiology of cataract in Australia. *American Journal of Ophthalmology*, **128** (4), 446–65.

211. Mukesh, B.N., Le, A., Dimitrov, P.N. *et al.* (2006) Development of cataract and associated risk factors: the visual impairment project. *Archives of Ophthalmology*, **124** (1), 79–85.

212. Leske, M.C., Chylack, L.T. Jr and Wu, S.Y. (1991) The lens opacities case–control study. Risk factors for cataract. *Archives of Ophthalmology*, **109** (2), 244–51.

213. Hennis, A., Wu, S.Y., Nemesure, B. *et al.* (2004) Risk factors for incident cortical and posterior subcapsular lens opacities in the Barbados Eye Studies. *Archives of Ophthalmology*, **122** (4), 525–30.

214. Foster, P.J., Wong, T.Y., Machin, D. *et al.* (2003) Risk factors for nuclear, cortical and posterior subcapsular cataracts in the Chinese population of Singapore: the Tanjong Pagar survey. *British Journal of Ophthalmology*, **87** (9), 1112–20.

215. Tsai, S.Y., Hsu, W.M., Cheng, C.Y. *et al.* (2003) Epidemiologic study of age-related cataracts among an elderly Chinese population in Shih-Pai, Taiwan. *Ophthalmology*, **110** (6), 1089–95.

216. Nirmalan, P.K., Robin, A.L., Katz, J. *et al.* (2004) Risk factors for age related cataract in a rural population of southern India: the Aravind Comprehensive Eye Study. *The British Journal of Ophthalmology*, **88** (8), 989–94.

217. Leske, M.C., Wu, S.Y., Hennis, A. *et al.* (1999) Diabetes, hypertension, and central obesity as cataract risk factors in a black population. The Barbados Eye Study. *Ophthalmology*, **106** (1), 35–41.

218. Harding, J.J., Harding, R.S. and Egerton, M. (1989) Risk factors for cataract in Oxfordshire: diabetes, peripheral neuropathy, myopia, glaucoma and diarrhoea. *Acta Ophthalmologica*, **67** (5), 510–17.

219. Harding, J.J., Egerton, M., van Heyningen, R. and Harding, R.S. (1993) Diabetes, glaucoma, sex, and cataract: analysis of combined data from two case control studies. *The British Journal of Ophthalmology*, **77** (1), 2–6.

220. Bron, A.J., Sparrow, J., Brown, N.A. *et al.* (1993) The lens in diabetes. *Eye*, **7** (Pt 2), 260–75.

221. Kato, S., Shiokawa, A., Fukushima, H. *et al.* (2001) Glycemic control and lens transparency in patients with type 1 diabetes mellitus. *American Journal of Ophthalmology*, **131** (3), 301–4.

222. Klein, B.E., Klein, R. and Moss, S.E. (1995) Incidence of cataract surgery in the Wisconsin Epidemiologic Study of Diabetic Retinopathy. *American Journal of Ophthalmology*, **119** (3), 295–300.

223. Lee, A.Y. and Chung, S.S. (1999) Contributions of polyol pathway to oxidative stress in diabetic cataract. *FASEB Journal*, **13** (1), 23–30.

224. Kinoshita, J.H., Merola, L.O., Satoh, K. and Dimak, E. (1962) Osmotic changes caused by the accumulation of dulcitol in the lenses of rats fed with galactose. *Nature*, **194**, 1085–7.

225. Van Heyningen, R. (1959) Formations of polyols by the lens of the rat with sugar cataract. *Nature*, **184**, 194–5.

226. Dvornik, E., Simard-Duquesne, N., Krami, M. *et al.* (1973) Polyol accumulation in galactosemic and diabetic rats: control by an aldose reductase inhibitor. *Science*, **182** (117), 1146–8.

227. Agardh, E., Hultberg, B. and Agardh, C. (2000) Effects of inhibition of glycation and oxidative stress on the development of cataract and retinal vessel abnormalities in diabetic rats. *Current Eye Research*, **21** (1), 543–9.

228. Lee, S.C., Wang, Y., Ko, G.T. *et al.* (2001) Risk factors for cataract in Chinese patients with type 2 diabetes: evidence for the influence of the aldose reductase gene. *Clinical Genetics*, **59** (5), 356–9.

229. Becker, B. (1971) Diabetes mellitus and primary open-angle glaucoma. The XXVII Edward Jackson Memorial Lecture. *American Journal of Ophthalmology*, **1** (1 Pt 1), 1–16.

230. Kahn, H.A. and Milton, R.C. (1980) Revised Framingham Eye Study prevalence of glaucoma and diabetic retinopathy. *American Journal of Epidemiology*, **111** (6), 769–76.

231. Klein, B.E., Klein, R. and Moss, S.E. (1984) Intraocular pressure in diabetic persons. *Ophthalmology*, **91** (11), 1356–60.

232. Mapstone, R. and Clark, C.V. (1985) Prevalence of diabetes in glaucoma. *British Medical Journal (Clinical Research Education)*, **291** (6488), 93–5.

233. Nakamura, M., Kanamori, A. and Negi, A. (2005) Diabetes mellitus as a risk factor for glaucomatous optic neuropathy. *Ophthalmologica*, **219** (1), 1–10.

234. Mitchell, P., Smith, W., Chey, T. and Healey, P.R. (1997) Open-angle glaucoma and diabetes: the Blue Mountains Eye Study, Australia. *Ophthalmology*, **104** (4), 712–18.

235. Dielemans, I., de Jong, P.T., Stolk, R. *et al.* (1996) Primary open-angle glaucoma, intraocular pressure, and diabetes mellitus in the general elderly population. The Rotterdam Study. *Ophthalmology*, **103** (8), 1271–5.

236. Hennis, A., Wu, S.Y., Nemesure, B. *et al.* (2003) Hypertension, diabetes, and longitudinal changes in intraocular pressure. *Ophthalmology*, **110** (5), 908–14.

237. Lin, H.Y., Hsu, W.M., Chou, P. *et al.* (2005) Intraocular pressure measured with a noncontact tonometer in an elderly Chinese population: the Shihpai Eye Study. *Archives of Ophthalmology*, **123** (3), 381–6.

238. Tielsch, J.M., Katz, J., Quigley, H.A. *et al.* (1995) Diabetes, intraocular pressure, and primary open-angle glaucoma in the Baltimore Eye Survey. *Ophthalmology*, **102** (1), 48–53.

239. Vijaya, L., George, R., Paul, P.G. *et al.* (2005) Prevalence of open-angle glaucoma in a rural south Indian population. *Investigative Ophthalmology and Visual Science*, **46** (12), 4461–7.

240. Flammer, J., Orgul, S., Costa, V.P. *et al.* (2002) The impact of ocular blood flow in glaucoma. *Progress in Retinal and Eye Research*, **21** (4), 359–93.

241. Piltz-seymour, J.R., Grunwald, J.E., Hariprasad, S.M. and Dupont, J. (2001) Optic nerve blood flow is diminished in eyes of primary open-angle

glaucoma suspects. *American Journal of Ophthalmology*, **132** (1), 63–9.

242. Logan, J.F., Rankin, S.J. and Jackson, A.J. (2004) Retinal blood flow measurements and neuroretinal rim damage in glaucoma. *British Journal of Ophthalmology*, **88** (8), 1049–54.

243. Grunwald, J.E., Riva, C.E., Stone, R.A. *et al.* (1984) Retinal autoregulation in open-angle glaucoma. *Ophthalmology*, **91** (12), 1690–4.

244. Hayreh, S.S. (1999) The role of age and cardiovascular disease in glaucomatous optic neuropathy. *Survey of Ophthalmology*, **43** (Suppl 1), S27–42.

31

The Epidemiology of Diabetic Kidney Disease

Anne T. Reutens, Louise Prentice and Robert C. Atkins

Department of Epidemiology and Preventive Medicine, Monash University, Alfred
Hospital, Melbourne, Australia

31.1 INTRODUCTION

The International Diabetes Federation predicts that the number of people with diabetes in the world will rise from 194 million today to 333 million in 2025 [1]. The next 25–50 years will see a rapid increase in prevalence of diabetic kidney disease. A recent global study of 24 151 patients in 33 countries showed that 30–50% of people with type 2 diabetes have evidence of kidney damage [2]. Multiple factors will influence changes in prevalence of diabetes over the next few decades: ageing of Western populations; dietary changes with increased consumption of energy-dense foods; increasing urbanization with associated sedentary lifestyle; a rise in prevalence of obesity at an earlier age with an associated secondary increase in insulin resistance syndrome, hypertension and type 2 diabetes.

If there is a major increase in the prevalence of diabetes, it is likely there will be a concurrent increase in the prevalence of diabetic kidney disease or diabetic nephropathy (DN). This will result in a rapidly increasing burden on renal replacement services with an increased incidence of end-stage renal disease (ESRD) due to diabetes.

This chapter aims to examine three main areas in the epidemiology of diabetic kidney disease:

1. Current prevalence and future trends in prevalence.
2. Epidemiology of risk factors for DN.
3. The epidemiology of prevention.

31.2 DEFINITION

The definition of overt DN is generally accepted as persistent proteinuria (more than 500 mg of protein or 300 mg of albumin per 24 h) in the presence of diabetes and the absence of any other cause of proteinuria. Overt DN correlates with the pathological lesions described by Kimmelsteil and Wilson [3]. By the time this stage is reached, progression to ESRD is usually the case, although there is some evidence for slowing or even reversal of the process with intensive treatment [4].

Persistent microalbuminuria is accepted as the preclinical stage of overt nephropathy (ON). *Microalbuminuria* refers to detection of intact albumin in the urine. Note that in addition to intact albumin, low-molecular-weight albumin fragments are renally excreted, but these are not detected by the usual immunochemical assays for urinary albumin [5]. The definition of microalbuminuria is still a source of some dispute, with several different definitions used in the literature. Tests and definitions used for diagnosis are not necessarily suitable for screening. The generally accepted diagnostic definition is an albumin excretion of 30–300 mg per 24 h [6, 7]. This requires a 24 h urine collection, which is not always feasible, particularly since at least two out of three positive specimens are required for a definite diagnosis. An alternative commonly used is a spot urine specimen, preferably from the first morning void, with calculation of

The Epidemiology of Diabetes Mellitus, second edition   Edited by Jean-Marie Ekoé, Marian Rewers, Rhys Williams and Paul Zimmet
© 2008 John Wiley & Sons, Ltd

the albumin:creatinine ratio (ACR). The sensitivity and specificity of the morning ACR to predict a 24 h urinary albumin excretion within the microalbuminuric range is >85% [8]. The ACR range for microalbuminuria is 30–300 mg g^{-1} for females and 20–200 mg g^{-1} for males [9, 10].

The pathological changes of DN are likely to be present before microalbuminuria develops in type 1 diabetes. In a study of 29 patients with type 1 diabetes, renal biopsies were performed 6 years apart. Nineteen of these patients remained normoalbuminuric and normotensive. However, they all showed progression in the morphological parameters of diabetic glomerulopathy [11]. Usually, by the time microalbuminuria is present, glomerular hyperfiltration has also developed. A prospective study of 308 patients with type 1 diabetes showed that, in the group that was initially normoalbuminuric, development of hyperfiltration was predictive of subsequent development of microalbuminuria [12].

In addition, a correlation between development of nephropathy and the level of albuminuria within the normal range has been documented [13]. Reduced glomerular filtration may be present without occurrence of microalbuminuria. In a study of 105 normoalbuminuric patients with long-standing type 1 diabetes, reduced estimated glomerular filtration rate (eGFR) (<90 ml min^{-1} per 1.73 m^2) was present in 22% and correlated with more severe glomerular structural changes [14]. These patients were more likely to be female. In type 2 diabetes, the prevalence of reduced glomerular filtration rate (GFR) (<60 ml min^{-1} per 1.73 m^2) in the presence of normoalbuminuria was 23%. (This analysis excluded patients on renin-angiotensin inhibition.) These patients tended to be older women [15]. This suggests that for some patients, even when the albuminuria is within the currently accepted normal range, glomerulopathy is developing.

31.3 INCIDENCE AND PREVALENCE OF DIABETIC KIDNEY DISEASE

Three aspects to need to be considered when interpreting prevalence data and predicting future changes:

- the prevalence of DN in patients with diabetes;
- the prevalence of DN in the general population;

- changes in the survival of patients with established nephropathy.

31.3.1 Prevalence of Nephropathy in Patients with Established Diabetes

Epidemiological studies undertaken before the current acceptance of intensive therapy (IT) showed that around 30% of patients with type 1 diabetes mellitus (DM) will develop nephropathy after 20 years [16, 17]. However, a recent review of the literature showed a decline in the incidence of DN [18]. A study in the Swedish population, reported in 1994 [19], showed that the 20-year cumulative incidence in type 1 patients in who first developed diabetes in 1961–1965 was 28%, whereas in those first diagnosed in 1971–1975 the incidence was 5.8%. A similar study was undertaken at the Steno Centre, finding the 20-year cumulative incidence of DN to be 31.1% for patients diagnosed with diabetes in 1965–1969, falling to 13.7% for those diagnosed in 1979–1984 [20]. Nishimura et al. [21] did the same study on patients in the United States, with 20-year cumulative incidence falling from 9.1% to 3.6% when comparing patients diagnosed in 1965–1969 with those diagnosed in 1975–1979. He also reported an increase in the time to development of ESRD comparing the two groups. It is likely that the trend to reduced incidence of DN relates to the introduction of IT for type 1 diabetes, and earlier and more aggressive treatment of hypertension over the time period studied. It is also important to note that many of these studies are from patients treated at referral centers and may not be applicable to the general population of type 1 diabetics. However, the 25-year follow-up of type 1 diabetics in the Pittsburgh Epidemiology of Diabetes Complications (EDC) Study did not show any significant difference in the cumulative incidence of overt DN between the cohorts diagnosed in 1965–1974 and 1975–1980 [22]. The cumulative incidence was 32%.

Data are available from the United States regarding rate of presentation for renal replacement therapy (RRT) among diabetics [23]. RRT refers to hemodialysis, peritoneal dialysis or renal transplantation. In 1996, the age-adjusted rates were 590.3 per 100 000 diabetics for blacks and 312.1 per 100 000 diabetics for whites. Type 2 diabetes predominated amongst all age groups for the black population. Between 1984 and 1996, the population of individuals in the United States with diabetes increased 40%. In contrast, the number of persons initiating treatment for ESRD due to diabetes increased more than 300%. Therefore, in patients with diabetes, the risk of ESRD (measured by acceptance into an RRT programme) had increased. Similar data are available for southwestern American Indian populations [24], where the age-adjusted rate in 1993 was 804 per 10 000 diabetics, falling to 558 per 100 000 diabetics in 2001. The fall in this initially high rate was attributed to monitoring and treatment of risk factors, with increased use of angiotensin-converting enzyme inhibitors (ACEis) and angiotensin II receptor blockers (ARBs) (an increase of 35% in use of these medications). A similar improvement in renal failure rate was noted in the Pittsburgh observational study of type 1 diabetics [22]. The renal failure rate at 30 years duration fell from 31% in those diagnosed in the 1950s to 18% in those diagnosed from 1965–1969.

The prevalence of albuminuria in diabetic populations has been measured in various studies. In the Pittsburgh EDC Study [25], a large clinic-based study of type 1 diabetes, the prevalence of macroalbuminuria and microalbuminuria was 27% and 22% respectively. In EURODIAB [26], a study of a similar population of type 1 diabetics, the prevalence of macroalbuminuria and microalbuminuria was 12% and 21% respectively, while Esmatjes et al. [27] found the prevalence

of microalbuminuria to be 23.1% and 5.4% for macroalbuminuria in a type 2 diabetic population. Similar levels of microalbuminuria were found in other European countries, varying from 17% in the United Kingdom to 30% in Denmark. A surprisingly high incidence of macroalbuminuria (23.5%) and microalbuminuria (48.5%) was found in a survey of hypertensive patients with type 2 diabetes in 10 Asian countries [28]. Microalbuminuria has been documented to predate the diagnosis of type 2 diabetes in some studies [28].

31.3.2 Prevalence of DN in the General Population

Table 31.1 lists the published proportion of patients registered with ESRD with diabetes as the etiology in different populations [27, 29–34]. As would be expected, in populations where there is a high prevalence of diabetes, such as the Northern Mariana Islands and Pima Indians, DN represents a high proportion of cases presenting for RRT.

Data from the Diabetes Surveillance Program of the Centers for Disease Control and Prevention [23] in the United States found that the number of individuals initiating treatment for newly diagnosed ESRD grew dramatically over the two decades from 1980 to 1999. The rapid increase was accounted for by cases where the primary diagnosis was either hypertension or diabetes. The rate of increase for hypertension was greatest in the early and mid 1980s and abated thereafter. The steep rate of

Table 31.1 Proportion of patients with ESRD with diabetes as the etiology in different populations. Population prevalence of diabetes (where available) is also listed in parentheses.

	Percentage ESRD due to diabetic nephropathy (%)
Australia	25 (7.4)
France (Ile de France region)	20.6
USA	44.5 (incident)
Spain	19
Pima Indians	92
Czech Republic	31
Poland	12 prevalence
	17 incident
Northern Mariana Islands	76 incident (11)
USA Southwest American Indians	—
Hong Kong	38 (incident)

increase due to diabetes continued throughout the study period.

Data from the European Renal Association–European Dialysis and Transplant Association (ERA–EDTA) show the highest incidence for RRT for type 1 diabetes occurs in Denmark, Sweden and Finland. There has been a significant increase with time in Greece and Scotland and a decrease in Belgium. For type 2 diabetes, the highest incidence is in Austria, Belgium and Greece. Presentation has increased markedly over time in all countries, with a mean annual rise of 11.9% [34].

Data from the AusDiab study, a longitudinal Australian population-based study, show the incidence of albuminuria in the whole population was 0.83%, with the incidence of albuminuria in males almost double that of females [35]. Annual incidence was increased in older people. People with prediabetes (impaired fasting glucose or impaired glucose tolerance) at baseline had an annual incidence of albuminuria that was 1.5–2 times higher than people with normal glucose tolerance at baseline. People with diabetes at baseline had an incidence of albuminuria of 3.1% per year, which is almost five times the rate of people with normal glucose tolerance at baseline.

In Australia, the number of people with diabetes accepted to dialysis has doubled in the last 7 years. Currently, around 10% of patients on dialysis in Australia are indigenous [36]. Interestingly, in a study by Hoy *et al.* [37] set in an outreach program for Aboriginal communities, diabetes was generally a late development after the onset of chronic kidney disease (CKD), suggesting other factors in the etiology of CKD to be of greater significance.

The frequency of CKD in Australian patients with type 2 diabetes seen in the general practice clinic setting was determined in the NEFRON (National Evaluation of the Frequency of Renal impairment cO-existing with Noninsulin-dependent diabetes mellitus) study [38]. CKD in this study was defined as eGFR < 60 ml min^{-1} per 1.73 m^2, or the presence of microalbuminuria or macroalbuminuria. Almost one in two (47%) patients with type 2 diabetes consulting their General Practioners had evidence of kidney disease: 23% had an eGFR < 60 ml min^{-1} per 1.73 m^2, 35% had an elevated ACR and there was ~10% overlap between these two groups.

31.3.3 Survival of Patients with Established Nephropathy

Historically, ON had a poor prognosis, with relentless decline in GFR of 10–15 ml min^{-1} year^{-1} [16, 39, 40]. When ESRD was reached, the median survival was 6–7 years after onset of nephropathy. Therefore, the perception arose that ON was irreversible, relentless in progression and fatal. However, the natural history has changed dramatically with improved management. Reversal of nephropathy was observed after prolonged normoglycemia in recipients of pancreas transplants [4], and aggressive antihypertensive treatment to achieve normotensive levels slowed the rate of decline of GFR to 1.9 ml min^{-1} year^{-1} in type 1 diabetic patients with DN [41]. A study of 125 patients with overt DN and albuminuria in the nephrotic range (>2.5 g per 24 h) who were followed-up for 12.4 years showed that, in the 26% of patients able to achieve remission of the proteinuria (to <0.6 g per 24 h for at least 1 year), the rate of decline of GFR slowed from 7.4 to 3.2 ml min^{-1} year^{-1}, with a 60% reduction in the percentage of those reaching the composite end point of ESRD or death [42].

The prevalence of renal morbidity and mortality in type 2 diabetes has been shown to differ around the world, and these variations are probably not just due to differences in availability of treatment. In a comparison of data derived from the EURODIAB and Pittsburgh EDC studies, the United States cohort had a significantly increased rate of macroalbuminuria (and hence more advanced renal disease), which was not explained by differences in blood pressure (BP) control, duration of diabetes, glycemic control or smoking. Hypertension was actually better controlled in the American group although there was a lower rate of ACEi usage [43].

It is worth noting that CKD patients are dying before entering RRT. Keith *et al.* [44] studied 30 000 people in the United States with a GFR of <90 ml min^{-1}. The patients were stratified according to stage of renal disease and followed for 6 years. Of the group with stage 1 renal failure, there was a mortality of 10% with no patients entering RRT. However, for patients with stage 4 renal failure, 20% had entered RRT but 46% had died. Congestive cardiac failure, coronary artery disease, diabetes and anemia were all more prevalent in those who died before receiving RRT.

Although major advances have been made in the primary and secondary prevention of cardiovascular disease (CVD) in the last 15 years, there is little evidence that this has improved the survival from CVD in DN. In the United States, population data do not support significant change in cardiovascular mortality in a diabetic population. In the National Health and Nutrition Examination Survey (NHANES) study, 8–9-year follow-up data showed that age-adjusted heart disease mortality fell 13% in diabetic men and rose 23% in diabetic women, at the same time falling by 36% and 27% in non-diabetic men and women [45]. In the Framingham study, it was found that increased prevalence of diabetes and improved myocardial infarction and stroke survival were insufficient to account for the increase in diabetes-related ESRD [46].

31.4 ASSOCIATION WITH CVD

31.4.1 Albuminuria and Vascular Disease

Association of ON with CVD in type 1 diabetes is stronger than would be explained by increased cardiovascular risk factors in this population. In a 12-year observational study of 462 patients with type 1 diabetes without prior history of heart disease at baseline, the risk for cardiovascular (coronary, stroke or other vascular) death in patients with macroalbuminuria was 18.3 (95% confidence interval (CI) 5.2–64.1) times higher than in patients with normoalbuminuria (adjusted for age and gender) [47]. After adjustment for diabetes duration, HbA_{1c} level and BP, the relative risk (RR) was attenuated (RR 8.2, 95% CI 2.1–31.7) but still significantly elevated. Furthermore, in univariate analyses, the presence of retinopathy was not associated with increased cardiovascular mortality; but, after adjustment for albuminuria, the association was no longer significant. In the IDNT (Irbesartan in Diabetic Nephropathy Trial), in which patients with type 2 diabetes had proteinuria $\geq 900\,mg\;day^{-1}$ at baseline, every natural log increase in baseline albumin excretion increased cardiovascular risk by 29%.

31.4.2 Microalbuminuria and Vascular Disease

In the HOPE (Heart Outcomes Prevention Evaluation) study, which followed a cohort of patients aged 55 years or more (5545 with known CVD and 3498 with diabetes and at least one other cardiovascular risk factor) for 4.5 years, baseline microalbuminuria increased the risk of major cardiovascular events: RR 1.83 (95% CI 1.64–2.05) [48]. A relationship between ACR and CVD was also present at ACR levels below thresholds for microalbuminuria. With each ACR increase of $0.4\,mg\;mmol^{-1}$, the risk of myocardial infarction, stroke or cardiovascular death increased by 5.9%.

31.4.3 Microalbuminuria, Albuminuria and Insulin Resistance

Microalbuminuria is associated with insulin resistance in the type 1 diabetic population. Yip et al. [49], using clamp studies in a cross-sectional analysis, showed that microalbuminuria in type 1 diabetics was associated with insulin resistance. De Cosmo et al. [50] demonstrated an increased prevalence of CVD in parents of type 1 diabetics with microalbuminuria. The relationship between insulin resistance and microalbuminuria in type 2 diabetes is less clear because of conflicting results. Recently, De Cosmo et al. used the homeostasis model assessment of insulin resistance to determine its relationship with urinary albumin excretion in a large cohort of type 2 diabetic patients. A significant correlation was found in men but not in women [51]. In a case–control study using insulin clamps to examine insulin sensitivity in matched pairs of type 2 diabetic patients with normo- or micro-albuminuria [52], there was no significant difference between the groups in duration of diabetes. For each decrease in glucose disposal rate (GDR), the prevalence of microalbuminuria increased by 40%. Using 10-year follow-up data from the Pittsburgh EDC study, Orchard et al. [53] showed that insulin sensitivity was a powerful predictor of early onset (within 5 years) and later onset of ON. In this study, the measurement of insulin resistance was estimated GDR (eGDR), a calculation previously validated by clamp studies.

It is not clear whether the increased cardiovascular risk associated with DN arises from the effect of renal disease on BP and lipid metabolism or because DN and coronary artery disease share the same risk factors and genetic susceptibility. A common mechanism (e.g. endothelial dysfunction or inflammation) may explain the increased cardiovascular risk and the microalbuminuria. Potential mechanisms have been recently reviewed [54, 55]. Microalbuminuria has emerged as an independent predictor of CVD. This raises the issue of whether all patients with microalbuminuria should undergo further definitive investigation for vascular disease, particularly CVD.

31.5 ETIOLOGICAL FACTORS: MARKERS OF RISK FOR DEVELOPMENT OF DN

Established risk factors for development of nephropathy in diabetes are glycemic control, duration of diabetes, proteinuria, hypertension and hyperlipidemia. In the next section, the evidence for the importance of these risk factors will be reviewed, as well as discussion of merging evidence for roles of novel or related risk factors.

31.5.1 Glycemic Control

The Diabetes Control and Complications Trial (DCCT) documented that the level of glycemic control was associated with the incidence of microvascular complications in diabetes [56]. At the end of the DCCT study (mean follow-up 6.5 years), significant differences were observed between the IT and conventional therapy (CT) groups, the IT group having a lower HbA_{1c} (7.1% versus 9.0%) and a lower incidence of microalbuminuria (reduced by 39%). IT led to a risk reduction of 84% for development of new cases of microalbuminuria, and 83% reduction for progression from microalbuminuria to overt albuminuria. There was a continuous relationship between the risks of diabetic microvascular complications and glycemia, with no evidence of any glycemic threshold.

The DCCT cohort was studied for a further 8 years in the Epidemiology of Diabetes Interventions and Complications (EDIC) trial [57]. Patients previously on IT were encouraged to continue and patients in the CT group were encouraged to commence IT. At the end of 8 years, the two groups were similar in level of glycemic control (HbA_{1c} 8.0% versus 8.2%). Despite this, there was a significant difference in the rate of conversion from normoalbuminuria to microalbuminuria. In the IT group, 6.8% progressed to microalbuminuria, compared with 15.8% of the CT group (odds reduction of 84%). The incidence of severe renal outcomes

was too low to give the study adequate power to detect treatment differences. Protection initiated by IT persisted even after levels of glycemic control deteriorated.

The Stockholm Diabetes Intervention Study followed 91 patients with type 1 diabetes randomized to IT or CT for 10 years [58]. IT was associated with a significant decrease in nephropathy (26% in the CT group versus 7% in the IT group).

Similar findings in type 2 diabetes have emerged from the UK Prospective Diabetes Study (UKPDS) [59–61]. Over 10 years of follow-up, IT with sulfonylurea or insulin reduced HbA_{1c} (7.0% compared with 7.9% in the CT group) and reduced microvascular endpoints by 25% (RR 0.75, 95% CI 0.60–0.93). Treatment with metformin in overweight patients reduced median HbA_{1c} by 0.6%, with a trend to reduced microvascular complications which did not reach statistical significance (RR 0.77, 95% CI 0.51–1.15). There was no glycemic threshold of risk in this study. The smaller Kumamoto study, a prospective study with 8 years of follow-up which compared the effect of IT with a multidose insulin regimen versus conventional insulin regimen in patients with type 2 diabetes, demonstrated that improved glycemic control (HbA_{1c} 7.2% versus 9.4%) significantly reduced the development of nephropathy (74% reduction in microalbuminuria and 100% reduction in microalbuminuria respectively) [62]. No worsening of nephropathy was observed in patients with $HbA_{1c} < 6.5\%$. An observational study in Japanese patients with type 2 diabetes associated remission or regression of microalbuminuria with $HbA_{1c} < 6.95\%$ [63]. Similar findings have been demonstrated in the Steno type 2 study, where the target level proposed to prevent progression of DN was $<6.5\%$ [64].

Finally, the fact that morphological lesions of DN can be reversed by normoglycemia following pancreas transplantation provides evidence that supports the clinical observations that even established nephropathy can be significantly reversed with intensive management [4].

31.5.2 Microalbuminuria and Proteinuria

The presence of microalbuminuria may precede both diabetes and hypertension [65, 66] and may be considered one of the earliest components to appear of the insulin resistance syndrome. Albuminuria may be marker of vascular inflammation and endothelial dysfunction, with albumin leakage occurring as a consequence. For this reason, some have advocated screening the general population. Screening studies have shown a high incidence of undiagnosed disease (diabetes and hypertension) in those positive for microalbuminuria.

Multiple studies have documented the association of microalbuminuria and proteinuria with the subsequent risk of developing overt DN:

- A large-scale Japanese study, screened 100 000 individuals with dipstick proteinuria. After 17 years the risk of being on dialysis increased with the degree of proteinuria [67].
- The Pittsburgh EDC study results were analyzed using a nested case–control study [68]. Analysis showed baseline log albumin excretion rate (AER) predicted subsequent development of ON.
- In the Prevention of Renal and Vascular End-Stage Disease study [69], after 4.2 years of follow-up, the risk of stage 3 or worse CKD was related to baseline albuminuria. Individuals with albuminuria were at increased risk of all-cause death as well as cardiovascular mortality.
- The Reduction of Endpoints in NIDDM with the Angiotensin II Antagonist Losartan (RE-NAAL) study [70] measured multiple baseline risk factors. Of all these, albuminuria was by far the strongest predictor of ESRD and the composite renal endpoint (doubling of serum creatinine, ESRD or death). Development of the renal endpoint was 5.2-fold higher in the high versus low albuminuria group. ESRD was 8.1-fold higher in the high versus low albuminuria. When multivariate analysis was performed controlling for other factors, an almost linear relationship between albuminuria and risk of renal endpoint/ESRD became apparent. Similarly, an almost linear relationship was observed between the reduction in albuminuria and reduction in ESRD/renal endpoint risk. The authors argued that the antiproteinuric effect of losartan appeared to explain almost all of the renoprotection by this agent, beyond that which could be attributable to lowering of BP alone. The RENAAL study observed that the greater the reduction in albuminuria

in the first 6 months and the lower the albuminuria after the first 6 months, the less likely the patient would have ESRD or the renal endpoint. The RENAAL study also showed that albuminuria risk was independent of whether a patient was on albuminuria-lowering therapy; for example, 2 g albuminuria conferred the same risk whether on losartan or not. This was a novel finding, that both baseline and residual albuminuria (albuminuria after 6 months of therapy) were powerful predictors of outcome. Therefore, further lowering of the residual albuminuria to the lowest achievable level by additional treatments has been suggested.
- The IDNT [71] was a large randomized double-blind trial comparing the effect of irbesartan with amlodipine and conventional treatment alone on renal outcomes in type 2 diabetes. Baseline proteinuria and changes in proteinuria during follow-up were strong independent predictors of the renal outcomes measured.

Cross-sectional studies have shown an association between microalbuminuria and other risk factors. In Pima Indians with diabetes, patients with microalbuminuria were more likely to be male, have higher systolic BP (SBP) and diastolic BP (DBP), more complications of diabetes and higher body mass index (BMI). Smokers were more prevalent amongst those with microalbuminuria [72]. Similar associations were found in the AusDiab study [73]. Microalbuminuria was found to have a prevalence of 6.0% in a general population survey. In those with microalbuminuria, hypertension and diabetes were the most common associated risk factors. However, 25.9% of those with microalbuminuria had neither diabetes nor hypertension. In these subjects, microalbuminuria was associated with obesity in 13.5%, smoking in 20.7% and low GFR in 12.3%.

31.5.3 Hypertension
31.5.3.1 SBP
There have been several studies specifically addressing the question of which component of BP (i.e. SBP versus DBP versus pulse pressure (PP)) is associated with development of DN. The strongest evidence is for SBP. One of the largest studies to

examine the relationship between BP and development of ESRD was the Veterans Affairs study of approximately 10 000 hypertensive men followed for a minimum of 13.9 years: 901 patients had diabetes. In this study, pretreatment SBP, but not DBP, was an independent risk factor for renal disease progression [74]. Interestingly, ESRD risk was decreased in patients in whom SBP was reduced by 2–20 mmHg with treatment, but was increased in those in whom SBP decreased by more than 20 mmHg. In type 2 diabetes, the UKPDS demonstrated that a decrease of 10 mmHg in SBP was associated with a 13% risk reduction for development of microvascular complications [75]. This study did not show any J-shaped association between SBP achieved on treatment and subsequent complications.

SBP was found to be independently associated with nephropathy in the IDNT [76, 77] in patients who already had overt proteinuria. On univariate analysis, baseline SBP but not DBP correlated significantly with renal outcome (doubling of creatinine or ESRD). On multivariate analysis, SBP achieved on treatment (but not follow-up DBP, mean arterial BP or PP) predicted renal outcome. A decrease of 20 mmHg in SBP resulted in a 47% decrease in risk. The risk for mortality increased in patients with follow-up SBP < 120 mmHg.

Analysis of the RENAAL data [78] provided several important findings with regard to BP in patients with overt proteinuria:

- Baseline SBP was an independent risk factor for ESRD and death.
- SBP and PP had similar predictive value for ESRD alone.
- Baseline DBP did not predict outcome in this cohort.
- Those with the greatest baseline PP had the greatest benefit from treatment for slowing nephropathy progression. Of significance, there was no J-curve noted for renal outcomes in the lower BP range.

31.5.3.2 Does BP Predict Subsequent Development of DN?

Several studies examined the importance of BP control in subsequent development of DN. Whether hypertension precedes microalbuminuria is not certain, as prospective studies to date have yielded conflicting results [79].

- In a study of the Pima Indian population, the level of BP at time of diagnosis of diabetes was associated with subsequent development of DN [80].
- The Natural History Study, a 5-year prospective study in normoalbuminuric young type 1 diabetic patients, did not show an association between clinic BP and subsequent AER [81].
- Lurbe et al. [82] showed that an increase in nocturnal SBP preceded the development of microalbuminuria in type 1 diabetes.
- Mean BP predicted decline in renal function and increase in albuminuria in a prospective study of newly diagnosed patients with type 2 diabetes [83].
- Mean SBP predicted incidence of microalbuminuria in Korean patients with type 2 diabetes [84].
- Development of albuminuria or renal impairment in the UKPDS were independently associated with increased baseline SBP [85].

31.5.3.3 Hypertension and Glycemic Control

Several studies have observed the association between glycemic control and hypertension. A study from the Joslin Clinic in the United States enrolled Caucasian subjects with type 2 diabetes. The development of DN among those with hypertension was conditional on poor glycemic control. Those with hypertension alone and no nephropathy had the best glycemic control [79]. The association between glycemic control and hypertension was also noted in the DCCT/EDIC in type 1 diabetes. Interestingly, the positive effect of intensive control carried over throughout the EDIC period where the level of glycemic control was significantly worse. A retrospective study conducted in 148 children with type 1 diabetes of average duration 4.5 years found that poor glycemic control was associated with increased DBP [86]. It has been demonstrated in patients with early type 1 diabetes that moderate hyperglycemia without glycosuria has a pressor effect, elevating mean arterial pressure [87, 88]. Type 2 diabetes and impaired glucose tolerance are associated with elevated BP. NHANES II data demonstrated that those individuals with diabetes or impaired glucose tolerance had twice the prevalence of hypertension compared with the rest of the population studied [89].

31.5.3.4 Inherited Factors

The association of hypertension with DN is complicated by inherited factors, both in type 1 and type 2 diabetes. Barzilay *et al.* [90] found that subjects with type 1 diabetes who developed nephropathy were more likely to have parents with hypertension and higher SBP during adolescence and early adulthood. In the Joslin Centre study in type 2 diabetes [91], the risk of hypertension was strongly related to degree of obesity before diabetes had been diagnosed and the risk was significantly higher in those with parental hypertension.

In summary, the relationship between hypertension and nephropathy is a complex one. Familial factors contribute to both nephropathy and hypertension. There is also an interrelationship between hypertension and glycemic control. Predisposition to hypertension and hyperglycemia is likely to act synergistically in the development of nephropathy.

31.6 LIPIDS

Hyperlipidemia is a recognized risk factor for DN. Lipid lowering with medication has been shown to ameliorate renal damage [92]. The relationship with lipids was studied in detail in the cohort from the DCCT/EDIC [93]. A multivariate analysis of the association of AER with various lipid parameters yielded a complex list of associations, including: positive associations with intermediate-density lipoprotein (IDL) and small high-density lipoprotein (HDL) in males, medium and small very low-density lipoprotein (VLDL) in both sexes, and a borderline negative association with large HDL. There was no association between AER and the oxidizability of low-density lipoprotein (LDL). Similar associations were also found with the development of retinopathy, suggesting that dyslipidemia may contribute to and not just result from diabetic microvascular disease.

Analysis of the RENAAL study found that baseline levels of total cholesterol, LDL and triglycerides were associated with significantly increased prevalence of the primary composite endpoint. Total cholesterol and LDL were strongly associated with risk of ESRD. It was also found, in a post hoc analysis of RENAAL, that losartan therapy was associated with a lower total cholesterol level at 12 and 36 months, despite similar use of lipid-lowering drugs in the treatment and placebo groups [94].

Other studies have also shown the association between dyslipidemia and nephropathy. Total cholesterol, triglyceride and ApoB have been demonstrated to be significant predictors of subsequent nephropathy [95]. Triglycerides and LDL cholesterol were identified as predictors of microalbuminuria in the EDC. Thomas *et al.* [96] demonstrated that different lipid variables were associated with progression at different disease stages in kidney disease of type 1 diabetes. Progression from normo- to micro-albuminuria was associated with LDL-free cholesterol, whereas progression was associated with triglyceride content of VLDL and IDL in established microalbuminuria [96].

Lipid-lowering treatment for dyslipidemia is part of standard therapy in DN. A decrease in LDL cholesterol was shown to be associated with regression of proteinuria in subjects with type 1 diabetes [97] and slowing of progression of renal disease in both type 1 and 2 diabetes [98].

31.7 FAMILIAL PREDISPOSITION

31.7.1 Type 1 Diabetes

Studies have shown familial clustering of DN [99–101]. An inherited susceptibility to DN has been proposed in type 1 diabetes. Evidence for this came from a large study with 110 families including at least two siblings with type 1 diabetes [101]. The families were followed for 15 years or more. The cumulative incidence at 25 years for DN was 71.5% for siblings of individuals with DN and 25.4% in siblings of individuals without DN, a nearly 50% difference in risk. It has also been postulated that an autosomal dominant major gene exists which may predispose individuals with insulin-dependent diabetes mellitus (IDDM) to DN [102].

The DCCT showed increased risk of microalbuminuria in relatives of mi croalbuminuria-positive subjects. The *ACE* (angiotensin-I converting enzyme) gene has been proposed as a mediator of nephropathy. Increased ACE activity increases intraglomerular pressure and can lead to glomerular sclerosis. Many polymorphisms have been documented which can result in variation in ACE activity. The DCCT/EDIC Genetics Study provided strong evidence that, in Caucasians, genetic variation at the *ACE* gene was associated with onset of albuminuria as well as with development of severe DN in type 1 diabetes [103]. Variable results were found in earlier studies. In 1994, Marre *et al.* [104] reported *ACE*-D had an odds ratio of 3.88 for development of DN in IDDM. (ACE-D has been implicated in myocardial infarction, ventricular hypertrophy and stroke.) Since then, numerous inconsistent results have been published. A meta-analysis [105] of these earlier studies failed to confirm an association. However, methodological problems in the studies were noted by the authors.

31.7.2   Type 2 Diabetes

Familial aggregation of DN in Pima Indians and other populations with increased prevalence of type 2 diabetes suggests that there are additional genes determining susceptibility to nephropathy. Members of the Gila River community have participated in a longitudinal study since 1965 [106]. An oral glucose tolerance test (OGTT) is performed on all members every 2 years. The heritability of ACR was 21% among 767 diabetic siblings after adjusting for age, sex and duration of diabetes. A subsequent linkage analysis in a subset of individuals suggested a nephropathy susceptibility locus on chromosome 18q.

Polymorphisms at the *ACE* gene have been examined in type 2 diabetes to determine their relationship to nephropathy. A more recent meta-analysis of studies concluded that in Asian (Chinese, Japanese, Korean) type 2 diabetics, those with the II genotype had a reduced risk of DN compared with those with the D genotype (odds ratio 0.65, 95% CI 0.51–0.83) [107].

31.8   SMOKING

Prospective trials have demonstrated an association between cigarette smoking and development of nephropathy in type 1 diabetes. Cigarette smoking was correlated with development of persistent microalbuminuria in previously normoalbuminuric subjects in a 4-year prospective study [108]. A 24-month Australian study showed a significant correlation between smoking and AER, independent of age and other variables, in cross-sectional and longitudinal analyses [109]. In a 4-year study at the Joslin Clinic, current smokers had an adjusted odds ratio of 3.1 (95% CI 1.9–5.1) of developing microalbuminuria, and the effect of smoking was enhanced, especially in those with $HbA_{1c} > 8.0\%$ [110]. Rossing *et al.* [13] found in a 10-year study that smoking was a significant predictor of progression from normoalbuminuria to microalbuminuria or microalbuminuria: RR 1.461 (95% CI 1.1–2.3). A shorter and smaller study in type 1 diabetes with follow-up over 1 year also demonstrated that cigarette consumption expressed as pack years was an independent predictor for progression of DN [111]. A contradictory result was published by the Steno group on progression from overt albuminuria to ESRD in a prospective 3-year study. Smoking status (nonsmoker, former smoker or current smoker) had no statistically significant effect on progression [112].

In type 2 diabetes, Gambaro *et al.* [113] conducted a retrospective study in 273 patients with long duration of diabetes and at least 3 years of follow-up. At baseline, microalbuminuria and proteinuria were more frequent in current smokers than nonsmokers or former smokers. Logistic regression analysis showed that current smoking was the most important factor associated with the progression of nephropathy during the study [113]. Biesenbach *et al.* [114] prospectively followed smoking and nonsmoking patients with type 2 diabetes for approximately 62 months. There were no statistically significant differences between the two groups in HbA_{1c}, BPs or lipids. A significant difference was found in the rate of decline of the creatinine clearance: smokers 1.24 ± 0.34 ml min^{-1} per $1.73\,m^2$ versus nonsmokers 0.99 ± 0.35 ml min^{-1} per $1.73\,m^2$. Similar results were found in another small prospective study in type 2 diabetes with follow-up for 64 months [115]. Cigarette smoking in this study remained a risk factor for renal function decline in type 2 DN despite treatment of BP (mean BP reduction to 92 ± 1 mmHg) and use of ACEis.

31.9   FIBRINOGEN

Studies in the general population show an association between fibrinogen levels and subsequent major cardiovascular events [116]. Elevated fibrinogen levels indicate inflammation and endothelial dysfunction and serve as a marker of unstable vascular lesions. Elevated fibrinogen levels are also associated with smoking. Several studies have shown an association between hyperfibrinogenemia and microalbuminuria in type 1 diabetes. It is uncertain as to whether increased fibrinogen is a primary abnormality or secondary to nephropathy. A study in 957 patients from the DCCT/EDIC cohort [117] measured fibrinogen level and assessed genotype. In the total group, significant correlations were found between fibrinogen and age, BMI, triglycerides, total and LDL cholesterol, current HbA_{1c}, DBP, AER and average ankle/brachial ratio. Fibrinogen tended to increase with microalbuminuria; however, there was a marked 1.5-fold elevation with development of proteinuria. It was suggested that fibrinogen contributes to the accelerated atherosclerosis that accompanies proteinuria. Beta gene polymorphism of the fibrinogen gene did not contribute to the genetic effects for development of DN. In type 2 diabetes, the Casale Monferrato Study, a prospective Italian study with 7 years of follow-up, demonstrated that fibrinogen $>3.49\,\mathrm{g\,l^{-1}}$ was a predictor of progression to ON, independent of the presence of microalbuminuria or BP [118].

31.10 KALLIKREIN

Kallikrein is present in tissue and plasma and acts on forms of kininogen to release bradykinin. Bradykinin in turn acts systemically and locally in vessel wall, influencing tone and vessel structure. It has been suggested that this system is the physiological counterbalance to the renin–angiotensin system. The association of development of nephropathy with levels of kallikrein was studied in the DCCT/EDIC cohort [119]. Results of this study showed plasma prekallikrein (PK) levels correlated with both SBP and DBP. Patients with BP > 140/90 mmHg had higher levels then patients with BP < 140/90 mmHg. A significant correlation was found with log AER in both micro and macro-albuminuric ranges, but not in normoalbuminuria. This correlation was still present after multivariate analysis. The authors concluded that augmented PK levels in type 1 diabetes independently associate with hypertension and albuminuria, an association that could contribute to the development of vascular disease in type 1 diabetics.

31.11 NOVEL CARDIOVASCULAR RISK FACTORS

Yishak et al. [68], using a nested case–control study from the Pittsburgh EDC study, examined the association of ON with novel cardiovascular risk markers measured at baseline. Oxidative damage, circulating immune complexes that contain oxidized LDL, and adhesion molecules were measured in subjects that subsequently developed ON and controls matched for age, sex and duration of diabetes. The results were subdivided according to baseline AER. In those with lowest AER, immune complexes, eGDR (a derived measure of insulin resistance), HbA_{1c} and retinol were most predictive of ON. In the group with high AER, lipids and BP were the predominant predictive factors of ON. The authors postulated that, in the early stages of nephropathy, glycemic exposure, insulin resistance and possibly oxidative damage are 'initiators' and that BP and lipids act as 'accelerators' once nephropathy is established.

Beisswenger et al. [120] examined whether dicarbonyl and oxidative stress generated by hyperglycemia correlated with susceptibility to nephropathy in two groups of patients with type 1 diabetes and one group of Pima Indians with type 2 diabetes. The type 1 diabetics formed two cohorts: the first consisted of a group of complication-resistant diabetics (nonprogressors) and complication-susceptible diabetics (progressors); the second group had renal biopsies taken at 5-year intervals. The Pima Indians had a baseline renal biopsy and urine ACR. Dicarbonyl stress and oxidative stress were measured by cross-sectional assays using the patients' erythrocytes and urine. Dicarbonyl stress, reflected by higher methylgloxal level (a precursor of advanced glycation end products which contribute to diabetes complications), was higher in progressors, correlated with morphologic and clinical measurements of nephropathy progression and showed a cross-sectional relationship with severity of nephropathy in the type 2 diabetics. Higher oxidative stress was also observed in the progressors than in nonprogressors.

31.12   THE EPIDEMIOLOGY OF PREVENTION

31.12.1   Primary Prevention

Primary prevention of diabetes will be discussed in another chapter. In summary, several recent studies have shown that a significant reduction in the development of diabetes in those at risk can be made with lifestyle intervention and pharmacological intervention [121–123]. Lifestyle measures have also been shown to have some effect in prevention of development of hypertension, although not directly in the diabetic population.

Primary prevention of DN addresses prevention of progression from normoalbuminuria to microalbuminuria. There have been relatively few studies. In type 1 diabetes, the EURODIAB Controlled Trial of Lisinopril in Insulin-Dependent Diabetes Mellitus study examined the effect of the ACEi lisinopril on progression from either normo- or micro-albuminuric baseline in normotensive subjects. Lisinopril treatment produced a $1.0 \ \mu g \min^{-1}$ lowering in AER ($p = 0.1$) [124]. The Bergamo Nephrologic Diabetes Complications Trial was a primary prevention study in type 2 diabetes and hypertension [125]. This prospective trial of 1204 subjects over 3 years examined the effect of the ACEi trandalopril compared with placebo, verapamil alone or combination of trandalopril with verapamil. Both arms with trandalopril treatment reduced the onset of microalbuminuria comparably (2.1–2.6-fold). Verapamil had a similar effect to placebo. All arms achieved similar BPs on treatment. The Randomised Olmesartan and Diabetes Microalbuminuria Prevention (ROADMAP) study is an ongoing trial studying the effects of olmesartan versus placebo in the prevention of development of microalbuminuria [126].

A recent meta-analysis on the use of antihypertensives for primary prevention of DN concluded that only ACEi had demonstrated effects in reducing progression to microalbuminuria, the effect appeared to be independent of baseline BP, renal function and type of diabetes, but more studies were needed to be confident that the latter factors were not important modifiers [127].

31.12.2   Secondary and Tertiary Prevention

It is beyond the scope of this chapter to discuss in detail the studies of various interventions in secondary and tertiary prevention of DN. Secondary prevention trials focus on preventing progression from microalbuminuria to overt proteinuria. A criticism of this group of trials to date is that the effect on clinical outcomes (e.g. progression to ESRD, time to doubling of serum creatinine, death) has so far not been assessed. Tertiary prevention trials aimed at slowing progression of decline in renal function once the patient has developed overt proteinuria have addressed these clinical outcomes.

In addition to maintenance of good glycemic control, antihypertensive therapy is the second mainstay of prevention. Older studies demonstrated a decline in GFR of $10–15 \ ml \ min^{-1} \ year^{-1}$ in established DN. With antihypertensive treatment, this has been documented at $3.7 \ ml \ min^{-1} \ year^{-1}$ (for comparison, the normal decline in otherwise healthy individuals is $1 \ ml \ min^{-1} \ year^{-1}$). The DETAIL study (a comparison of telmisartan and enalapril in hypertensive type 2 diabetics with early-stage nephropathy) demonstrated that, after an initial decline in GFR in the first 2 years, there was almost complete stabilization of renal function at 3 years or longer in both treatment groups. Over 5 years, there were no increases in AER or increase in creatinine beyond $200 \ \mu mol \ l^{-1}$ [128]. Hovind et al. [41] demonstrated in a long-term prospective observational study that aggressive antihypertensive therapy in albuminuric patients with type 1 diabetes was able to induce remission in 31% (reduction in albuminuria $<200 \ \mu g \ min^{-1}$ and $\geq 30\%$ reduction from baseline) and regression in 22% (reduction in rate of GFR decline to that of natural ageing).

The effects of agents blocking the renin–angiotensin system on mortality and renal outcomes were recently reviewed in DN [129] and in hypertensive renal disease in general [130]. In DN [129], ACEis:

- significantly reduced mortality (RR 0.79, 95% CI 0.63–0.99);
- significantly reduced risk of progression from micro- to macro-albuminuria (RR 0.45, 95% CI 0.28–0.71);
- significantly increased rate of regression from macro- to micro-albuminuria (RR 3.42, 95% CI 1.95–5.99);
- there was weak evidence for reduction in ESRD or doubling of serum creatinine concentration

(RR 0.64, 95% CI 0.40–1.03; RR 0.60, 95% CI 0.34–1.05 respectively).

In DN [129], ARBs:

- did not significantly affect mortality;
- significantly reduced risk of progression from micro- to macro-albuminuria (RR 0.49, 95% CI 0.32–0.75);
- significantly increased rate of regression from macro- to micro-albuminuria (RR 1.42, 95% CI 1.05–1.93);
- significantly reduced risk of ESRD (RR 0.78, 95% CI 0.67–0.91);
- significantly reduced risk of doubling of serum creatinine concentration (RR 0.79, 95% CI 0.67–0.93).

The relative roles of BP lowering and reduction in albuminuria on the overall treatment effect in DN remain unclear. Analysis of the IDNT and RENAAL studies suggests that reduction of albuminuria has a separate effect to that of BP lowering. However, a meta-analysis recently published [130] suggested all benefit on renal outcomes is explicable on the basis of BP lowering, and that the agent used was not significant. The role of dual ACE inhibition and ARB therapy is another area that needs clarification. Studies to date have used small numbers with variable or poorly defined degrees of inhibition of the renin–angiotensin axis achieved.

31.12.3 Prevention in Practice

There remains a significant gap between what is proven to be effective for prevention of CKD and what is currently being achieved. In the AusDiab study [131], of those with renal insufficiency, only 58% of those with hypertension were being treated and only 32% of those with hyperlipidemia were on treatment. For both risk factors, only a small proportion of those treated achieved target levels (14% for hypertension and 7% for hyperlipidemia). Of the 439 subjects with previously diagnosed type 2 diabetes, the mean HbA$_{1c}$ level was 7.3 ± 1.8%.

The US JNC7 recommendations for those with diabetes are an SBP goal of <130 mmHg and DBP < 80 mmHg [132]. These goals are supported by the National Kidney Foundation, the American Diabetes Association and the Canadian Hypertension Society. A recent retrospective medical record review of 4814 diabetic patients in managed care organizations showed that more than two-thirds of the patients did not have controlled BP [133]. Of those with albuminuria or nephropathy, 35.4% were not taking either an ACEi or ARB.

A recent study demonstrated that early referral to a nephrologist resulted in slower progression of diabetic kidney disease as measured by GFR and albuminuria. Better control of SBP and DBP was achieved by nephrologists when compared with family doctors [134].

If current trends continue, there will be a massive increase in the demand for RRT over the next few decades. This demand will be beyond the means of even relatively affluent economies. Prevention, through primary prevention of diabetes and secondary/tertiary preventive measures in established diabetes remains the highest priority. Screening for albuminuria of the general population needs further consideration, as many of those at risk are currently not recognized.

References

1. Sicree, R., Shaw, J. and Zimmet, P. (2003) The global burden of diabetes, in *Diabetes Atlas*, (ed D. Gan), International Diabetes Federation, Brussels, pp. 15–71.
2. Parving, H., Lewis, J., Ravid, M. *et al.* (2006) Prevalence and risk factors for microalbuminuria in a referred cohort of type II diabetic patients: a global perspective. *Kidney International*, **69**, 2057–63.
3. Kimmelstiel, P. and Wilson, C. (1936) Intercapillary lesions in glomeruli of the kidney. *American Journal of Pathology*, **12**, 82–97.
4. Fioretto, P., Steffes, M., Sutherland, D. *et al.* (1998) Reversal of lesions of diabetic nephropathy after pancreas transplantation. *The New England Journal of Medicine*, **339**, 69–75.
5. Russo, L., Bakris, G. and Comper, W. (2002) Renal handling of albumin: a critical review of basic concepts and perspective. *American Journal of Kidney Diseases*, **39**, 899–919.
6. Mogensen, C. and Christensen, C. (1984) Predicting diabetic nephropathy in insulin-dependent patients. *The New England Journal of Medicine*, **311**, 89–93.
7. Mogensen, C. (1986) Microalbuminuria predicts clinical proteinuria and early mortality in maturity

onset diabetes. *The New England Journal of Medicine*, **310**, 356–60.

8. Eshoj, O., Feldt-Rasmussen, B., Larsen, M. and Mogensen, E. (1987) Comparison of overnight, morning and 24-hour urine collections in the assessment of diabetic microalbuminuria. *Diabetic Medicine*, **4**, 531–3.

9. Levey, A., Eckardt, K. and Tsukumato, Y. *et al.* (2005) Definition and classification of chronic kidney disease: a global position statement from Kidney Disease: Improving Global Outcome (KDIGO). *Kidney International*, **67**, 2098–100.

10. National Kidney Foundation (2002) K/DOQI clinical practice guidelines for chronic kidney disease: evaluation, classification and stratification. *American Journal of Kidney Diseases*, **39** (2 Suppl 1), S1–266.

11. Perrin, N., Torbjornsdotter, T., Jaremko, G. and Berg, U. (2006) The course of diabetic glomerulopathy in patients with type 1 diabetes: a 6-year follow-up with serial biopsies. *Kidney International*, **69**, 699–705.

12. Amin, R., Turner, C., Van Aken, S. *et al.* (2005) The relationship between microalbuminuria and glomerular filtration rate in young type 1 diabetic subjects: the Oxford Regional Prospective Study. *Kidney International*, **68**, 1740–9.

13. Rossing, P., Hougaard, P. and Parving, H. (2002) Risk factors for development of incipient and overt diabetic nephropathy in type 1 diabetic patients: a 10-year prospective observational study. *Diabetes Care*, **25**, 859–64.

14. Caramori, M., Fioretto, P. and Mauer, M. (2003) Low glomerular filtration rate in normoalbuminuric type 1 diabetic patients. *Diabetes*, **52**, 1036–40.

15. MacIsaac, R., Tsalamandris, C., Panagiotopoulos, S. *et al.* (2004) Nonalbuminuric renal insufficiency in type 2 diabetes. *Diabetes Care*, **27**, 195–200.

16. Andersen, A., Christiansen, J., Andersen, J. *et al.* (1983) Diabetic nephropathy in type 1 (insulin-dependent) diabetes: an epidemiological study. *Diabetologia*, **25**, 496–501.

17. Krolewski, A., Warram, J., Christlieb, A. *et al.* (1985) The changing natural history of nephropathy in type 1 diabetes. *The American Journal of Medicine*, **78**, 785–94.

18. Rossing, P. (2005) The changing epidemiology of diabetic microangiopathy in type 1 diabetes. *Diabetologia*, **48**, 1439–44.

19. Bojestig, M., Arnqvist, H., Hermansson, G. *et al.* (1994) Declining incidence of nephropathy in insulin-dependent diabetes mellitus. *The New England Journal of Medicine*, **330**, 15–18.

20. Hovind, P., Tarnow, L., Rossing, K. *et al.* (2003) Decreasing incidence of severe diabetic microangiopathy in type 1 diabetes. *Diabetes Care*, **26**, 1258–64.

21. Nishimura, R., Dorman, J., Bosnyak, Z. *et al.* (2003) Incidence of ESRD and survival after renal replacement therapy in patients with type 1 diabetes: a report from the Allegheny County Registry. *American Journal of Kidney Diseases*, **42**, 117–24.

22. Pambianco, G., Costacou, T., Ellis, D. *et al.* (2006) The 30-year natural history of type 1 diabetes complications. The Pittsburgh Epidemiology of Diabetes Complications Study experience. *Diabetes*, **55**, 1463–9.

23. Jones, C., Krolewski, A., Rogus, J. *et al.* (2005) Epidemic of end-stage renal disease in people with diabetes in the United States population: do we know the cause? *Kidney International*, **67**, 1684–91.

24. Burrows, N., Narva, A., Geiss, L. *et al.* (2005) End-stage renal disease due to diabetes among southwestern American Indians, 1990–2001. *Diabetes Care*, **28**, 1041–4.

25. Orchard, T., Dorman, J., Maser, R. *et al.* (1990) Prevalence of complications in IDDM by sex and duration: Pittsburgh Epidemiology of Diabetes Complications Study II. *Diabetes*, **39**, 1116–24.

26. Stephensen, J. and Fuller, J. (1994) Microvascular and acute complications in IDDM patients: the EURODIAB IDDM Complications Study. *Diabetologia*, **37**, 278–85.

27. Esmatjes, E., Castell, C., Gonzalez, T. *et al.* (1996) Epidemiology of renal involvement in type II diabetics (NIDDM) in Catalonia. The Catalan Diabetic Nephropathy Study Group. *Diabetes Research and Clinical Practice*, **32**, 157–63.

28. Wu, A., Tan, C., Eng, P. *et al.* (2006) Microalbuminuria prevalence study in hypertensive patients with type 2 diabetes mellitus in Singapore. *Singapore Medical Journal*, **47**, 315–20.

29. International Diabetes Institute (2001) Diabetes and Associated Disorders in Australia: the Accelerating Epidemic. Australian Diabetes, Obesity and Lifestyle Report, 1–46.

30. Atkins, R. (2005) The epidemiology of chronic kidney disease. *Kidney International. Supplement*, **94**, S14–18.

31. Jungers, P., Choukroun, G., Robino, C. *et al.* (2000) Epidemiology of end-stage renal failure in the Ile-de-France area: a prospective study in 1998. *Nephrology, Dialysis, Transplantation*, **15**, 2000–6.

32. Rutkowski, B. (2000) Changing patterns of end-stage renal disease in central and eastern Europe. *Nephrology, Dialysis, Transplantation*, **15**, 156–60.

33. Abidi, S., Negrete, H., Zahid, I. *et al.* (2005) Diabetic end-stage renal disease in the indigenous population of the Commonwealth of the Northern Mariana Islands. *Nephrology*, **10**, 291–5.

34. Van Dijk, P., Jager, K., Stengel, B. *et al.* (2005) Renal replacement therapy for diabetic end-stage renal disease: data from 10 registries in Europe (1991–2000). *Kidney International*, **67**, 1489–99.

35. Barr, E., Magliano, D. and Zimmet, P. *et al.* (2006) *AusDiab 2005, The Australian Diabetes and Lifestyle Study. Tracking the Accelerating Epidemic: Its Causes and Outcomes*, International Diabetes Institute, Melbourne, Australia.

36. Mathew, T. (2004) Addressing the epidemic of chronic kidney disease in Australia. *Nephrology*, **9**, S109–12.

37. Hoy, W., Kondalsamy-Chennakesavan, S., Scheppingen, J. *et al.* (2005) A chronic disease outreach program for Aboriginal communities. *Kidney International. Supplement*, **68**, S76–82.

38. Thomas, M., Weekes, A., Broadley, O. *et al.* (2006) The burden of chronic kidney disease in Australian patients with type 2 diabetes (the NEFRON study). *The Medical Journal of Australia*, **185**, 140–4.

39. Rossing, P., Hommel, E., Smidt, U. and Parving, H.-H. (1993) Impact of arterial blood pressure and albuminuria on the progression of diabetic nephropathy in IDDM patients. *Diabetes*, **42**, 715–19.

40. Kussman, M., Goldstein, H. and Gleason, R. (1976) The clinical course of diabetic nephropathy. *The Journal of the American Medical Association*, **236**, 1861–3.

41. Hovind, P., Rossing, P., Tarnow, L. *et al.* (2001) Remission and regression in the nephropathy of type 1 diabetes when blood pressure is controlled aggressively. *Kidney International*, **60**, 277–83.

42. Hovind, P., Tarnow, L., Rossing, P. *et al.* (2004) Improved survival in patients obtaining remission of nephrotic range albuminuria in diabetic nephropathy. *Kidney International*, **66**, 1180–6.

43. Lloyd, C., Stephenson, J., Fuller, J. and Orchard, T. (1996) A comparison of renal disease across two continents: the Epidemiology of Diabetes Complications Study and the EURODIAB IDDM Complications Study. *Diabetes Care*, **19**, 219–25.

44. Keith, D., Nichols, G., Gullion, C. *et al.* (2004) Longitudinal follow-up and outcomes among a population with chronic kidney disease in a large managed care organization. *Archives of Internal Medicine*, **164**, 559–63.

45. Gu, K., Cowie, C. and Harris, M. (1999) Diabetes and decline in heart disease mortality in US adults. *The Journal of the American Medical Association*, **281**, 1291–7.

46. Larson, T., Santanello, N. and Shahinfar, S. (2000) Trends in persistent proteinuria in adult-onset diabetes. A population study. *Diabetes Care*, **23**, 51–6.

47. Torffvit, O., Lovestam-Adrian, M., Agardh, E. and Agardh, C. (2005) Nephropathy, but not retinopathy, is associated with the development of heart disease in type 1 diabetes: a 12-yera observation study of 462 patients. *Diabetic Medicine*, **22**, 723–9.

48. Gerstein, H., Mann, J., Yi, Q. *et al.* (2001) Albuminuria and risk of cardiovascular events, death, and heart failure in diabetic and nondiabetic individuals. *The Journal of the American Medical Association*, **286**, 421–6.

49. Yip, J., Matlock, M. and Morocutti, A. (1993) Insulin resistance in insulin-dependent diabetic patients with microalbuminuria. *Lancet*, **342**, 883–7.

50. De Cosmo, S., Bacci, S. and Piras, G. (1997) High prevalence of risk factors for cardiovascular disease in parents of IDDM patients with albuminuria. *Diabetologia*, **40**, 1191–6.

51. De Cosmo, S., Minenna, A., Ludovico, O. *et al.* (2005) Increased urinary albumin excretion, insulin resistance, and related cardiovascular risk factors in patients with type 2 diabetes. *Diabetes Care*, **28**, 910–15.

52. Parvanova, A., Trevisan, R., Iliev, I. *et al.* (2006) Insulin resistance and microalbuminuria: a cross-sectional, case-control study of 158 patients with type 2 diabetes and different degrees of urinary albumin excretion. *Diabetes*, **55**, 1456–62.

53. Orchard, T., Chang, Y.-F., Ferrell, R. *et al.* (2002) Nephropathy in type 1 diabetes: a manifestation of insulin resistance and multiple genetic susceptibilities? Further evidence from the Pittsburgh Epidemiology of Diabetes Complication Study. *Kidney International*, **62**, 963–70.

54. Stehouwer, C. and Smulders, Y. (2006) Microalbuminuria and risk for cardiovascular disease: analysis of potential mechanisms. *Journal of the American Society of Nephrology*, **17**, 2106–11.

55. Basi, S. and Lewis, J. (2006) Microalbuminuria as a target to improve cardiovascular and renal outcomes. *American Journal of Kidney Diseases*, **47**, 927–46.

56. The Diabetes Control and Complications Trial Research Group (1993) The effect of intensive treatment of diabetes on the development and progression of long-term complications in insulin-dependent diabetes mellitus. *New England Journal on Criminal and Civil Confinement*, **329**, 977–86.

57. Writing Team for the Diabetes Control and Complications Trial/Epidemiology of Diabetes Interventions and Complications Research Group (2003) Sustained effect of intensive treatment of type 1 diabetes mellitus on development and progression of diabetic nephropathy: the Epidemiology of Diabetes Interventions and Complications (EDIC) study. *The Journal of the American Medical Association*, **290**, 2159–67.

58. Reichard, P., Pihl, M., Rosenqvist, U. and Sule, J. (1996) Complications in IDDM are caused by elevated blood glucose level: The Stockholm Diabetes Intervention Study (SDIS) at 10-year follow up. *Diabetologia*, **39**, 1483–8.

59. UK Prospective Diabetes Study Group (1998) Intensive blood-glucose control with sulphonylureas or insulin compared with conventional treatment and risk of complications in patients with type 2 diabetes (UKPDS 33). *Lancet*, **352**, 837–53.

60. Stratton, I., Adler, A., Neil, H. *et al.* (2000) Association of glycaemia with macrovascular and microvascular complications of type 2 diabetes (UKPDS 35): prospective observational study. *British Medical Journal*, **321**, 405–512.

61. UK Prospective Diabetes Study Group (1998) Effect of intensive blood-glucose control with metformin on complications in overweight patients with type 2 diabetes (UKPDS 34). UK Prospective Diabetes Study (UKPDS) Group. *Lancet*, **352**, 854–65.

62. Shichiri, M., Kishikawa, H., Ohkubo, Y. and Wake, N. (2000) Long-term results of the Kumamoto study on optimal diabetes control in type 2 diabetic patients. *Diabetes Care*, **23**, B21–9.

63. Araki, S., Haneda, M., Sugimoto, T. *et al.* (2005) Factors associated with frequent remission of microalbuminuria in patients with type 2 diabetes. *Diabetes*, **54**, 2983–7.

64. Gaede, P., Vedel, P., Parving, H.-H. and Pedersen, O. (1999) Intensified multifactorial intervention in patients with type 2 diabetes mellitus and microalbuminuria: the Steno type 2 randomised study. *Lancet*, **353**, 617–22.

65. Brantsma, A., Bakker, S., Hillege, H. *et al.* (2005) Urinary albumin excretion and its relation with C-reactive protein and the metabolic syndrome in the prediction of type 2 diabetes. *Diabetes Care*, **28**, 2525–30.

66. Brantsma, A., Bakker, S., de Zeeuw, D. *et al.* (2006) Urinary albumin excretion as a predictor of the development of hypertension in the general population. *Journal of the American Society of Nephrology*, **17**, 331–5.

67. Iseki, K., Ikemiya, Y., Iseki, C. and Takishita, S. (2003) Proteinuria and the risk of developing end-stage renal disease. *Kidney International*, **63**, 1468–74.

68. Yishak, A., Costacou, T., Virella, G. *et al.* (2006) Novel predictors of overt nephropathy in subjects with type 1 diabetes. A nested case control study from the Pittsburgh Epidemiology of Diabetes Complications cohort. *Nephrology, Dialysis, Transplantation*, **21**, 93–100.

69. Pinto-Sietsma, S., Janssen, W., Hillege, H. *et al.* (2000) Urinary albumin excretion is associated with renal functional abnormalities in a nondiabetic population. *Journal of the American Society of Nephrology*, **11**, 1882–8.

70. Keane, W., Brenner, B., de Zeeuw, D. *et al.* (2003) The risk of developing end-stage renal disease in patients with type 2 diabetes and nephropathy: the RENAAL study. *Kidney International*, **63**, 1499–507.

71. Lewis, E., Hunsicker, L., Clarke, W. *et al.* (2001) Renoprotective effect of the angiotensin-receptor antagonist irbesartan in patients with nephropathy due to type 2 diabetes. *The New England Journal of Medicine*, **345**, 851–60.

72. Nelson, R., Bennett, P., Beck, G. *et al.* (1996) Development and progression of renal disease in Pima Indians with non-insulin-dependent diabetes mellitus. Diabetic Renal Disease Study Group. *The New England Journal of Medicine*, **335**, 1636–42.

73. Atkins, R., Polkinghorne, K., Briganti, E. *et al.* (2004) Prevalence of albuminuria in Australia: the AusDiab Kidney Study. *Kidney International. Supplement*, **92**, S22–4.

74. Perry, H.J., Miller, J., Fornoff, J. *et al.* (1995) Early predictors of 15-year end-stage renal disease in hypertensive patients. *Hypertension*, **25**, 587–94.

75. Adler, A., Stratton, I., Neil, H. *et al.* (2000) Association of systolic blood pressure with macrovascular and microvascular complications of type 2 diabetes (UKPDS 36): prospective observational study. *British Medical Journal*, **321**, 412–19.

76. Atkins, R., Briganti, E., Lewis, J. *et al.* (2005) Proteinuria reduction and progression to renal failure in patients with type 2 diabetes mellitus and overt nephropathy. *American Journal of Kidney Diseases*, **45**, 281–7.

77. Pohl, M., Blumenthal, S., Cordonnier, D. *et al.* (2005) Independent and additive impact of blood pressure control and angiotensin II receptor

blockade on renal outcomes in the Irbesartan Diabetic Nephropathy Trial: clinical implications and limitations. *Journal of the American Society of Nephrology*, **16**, 3027–37.

78. Bakris, G., Weir, M., Shanifar, S. *et al.* (2003) Effects of blood pressure level on progression of diabetic nephropathy: results from the RENAAL study. *Archives of Internal Medicine*, **163**, 1555–65.

79. Krolewski, A., Fogarty, D. and Warram, J. (1998) Hypertension and nephropathy in diabetes mellitus: what is inherited and what is acquired? *Diabetes Research and Clinical Practice*, **39** (Suppl 1), S1–14.

80. Nelson, R., Pettitt, D., Baird, H. *et al.* (1993) Pre-diabetic blood pressure predicts urinary albumin excretion after the onset of type 2 (non-insulin-dependent) diabetes mellitus in Pima Indians. *Diabetologia*, **36**, 998–1001.

81. Steinke, J., Sinaiko, A., Kramer, M. *et al.* (2005) The early natural history of nephropathy in type 1 diabetes: III. Predictors of 5-year urinary albumin excretion rate patterns in initially normoalbuminuric patients. *Diabetes*, **54**, 2164–71.

82. Lurbe, E., Redon, J., Pascual, J. *et al.* (2001) The spectrum of circadian blood pressure changes in type I diabetic patients. *Journal of Hypertension*, **19**, 1421–8.

83. Ravid, M., Brosh, D., Ravid-Safran, D. *et al.* (1998) Main risk factors for nephropathy in type 2 diabetes mellitus are plasma cholesterol levels, mean blood pressure, and hyperglycemia. *Archives of Internal Medicine*, **158**, 998–1004.

84. Park, J., Kim, H., Chung, Y. *et al.* (1998) Incidence and determinants of microalbuminuria in Koreans with type 2 diabetes. *Diabetes Care*, **21**, 530–4.

85. Retnakaran, R., Cull, C., Thorne, K. *et al.* (2006) Risk factors for renal dysfunction in type 2 diabetes: U.K. Prospective Diabetes Study 74. *Diabetes*, **55**, 1832–9.

86. Torchinsky, M., Gomez, R., Rao, J. *et al.* (2004) Poor glycemic control is associated with increased diastolic blood pressure and heart rate in children with type 1 diabetes. *Journal of Diabetes and its Complications*, **18**, 220–3.

87. Miller, J., Floras, J., Zinman, B. *et al.* (1996) Effect of hyperglycaemia on arterial pressure, plasma renin activity and renal function in early diabetes. *Clinical Science (London, England)*, **90**, 189–95.

88. Miller, J. (1999) Impact of hyperglycemia on the renin angiotensin system in early human type 1 diabetes mellitus. *Journal of the American Society of Nephrology*, **10**, 1778–85.

89. Harris, M. (1989) Impaired glucose tolerance in the U.S. population. *Diabetes Care*, **12**, 464–74.

90. Barzilay, J., Warram, J., Bak, M. *et al.* (1992) Predisposition to hypertension: risk factor for nephropathy and hypertension in IDDM. *Kidney International*, **41**, 723–30.

91. Warram, J., Weijnen, C., Friere, M. and Krolewski, A. (1997) Epidemiology of Hypertension in NIDDM. 16th International Diabetes Federation Congress, Helsinki, Finland.

92. Attman, P., Samuelsson, O. and Alaupovic, P. (1997) Progression of renal failure: role of apolipoprotein B-containing lipoproteins. *Kidney International. Supplement*, **63**, S98–101.

93. Jenkins, A., Lyons, T., Zheng, D. *et al.* (2003) Lipoproteins in the DCCT/EDIC cohort: associations with diabetic nephropathy. *Kidney International*, **64**, 817–28.

94. Appel, G., Radhakrishnan, J., Avram, M. *et al.* (2003) Analysis of metabolic parameters as predictors of risk in the RENAAL study. *Diabetes Care*, **26**, 1402–7.

95. Mulec, H., Johnsen, S., Wiklund, O. and Bjorck, S. (1993) Cholesterol: a renal risk factor in diabetic nephropathy? *American Journal of Kidney Diseases*, **22**, 196–201.

96. Thomas, M., Rosengard-Barlund, M., Mills, V. *et al.* (2006) Serum lipids and the progression of nephropathy in type 1 diabetes. *Diabetes Care*, **29**, 317–22.

97. Ellis, D., Lloyd, C., Becker, D. *et al.* (1996) The changing course of diabetic nephropathy: low-density lipoprotein cholesterol and blood pressure correlate with regression of proteinuria. *American Journal of Kidney Diseases*, **27**, 809–18.

98. Bonnet, F. and Cooper, M. (2000) Potential influence of lipids in diabetic nephropathy: insights from experimental data and clinical studies. *Diabetes and Metabolism*, **26**, 254–64.

99. Quinn, M., Angelico, M., Warram, J. and Krolewski, A. (1996) Familial factors determine the development of diabetic nephropathy in patients with IDDM. *Diabetologia*, **39**, 940–5.

100. Seaquist, E., Goetz, F., Rich, S. and Barbosa, J. (1989) Familial clustering of diabetic kidney disease. Evidence for genetic susceptibility to diabetic nephropathy. *The New England Journal of Medicine*, **320**, 1161–5.

101. Borch-Johnsen, K., Norgaard, K., Hommel, E. *et al.* (1992) Is diabetic nephropathy an inherited complication? *Kidney International*, **41**, 719–22.

102. Krolewski, A. (1999) Genetics of diabetic nephropathy: evidence for major and minor gene effects. *Kidney International*, **55**, 1582–96.

103. Boright, A., Paterson, A., Mirea, L. *et al.* (2005) Genetic variation at the *ACE* gene is associated with persistent microalbuminuria and severe nephropathy in type 1 diabetes: the DCCT/EDIC Genetics Study. *Diabetes*, **54**, 1238–44.

104. Marre, M., Bernadet, P., Gallois, Y. *et al.* (1994) Relationships between angiotensin I converting enzyme gene polymorphism, plasma levels, and diabetic retinal and renal complications. *Diabetes*, **43**, 384–8.

105. Kunz, R., Bork, J., Fritsche, L. *et al.* (1998) Association between the angiotensin-converting enzyme-insertion/deletion polymorphism and diabetic nephropathy: a methodologic appraisal and systematic review. *Journal of the American Society of Nephrology*, **9**, 1653–63.

106. Imperatore, G., Knowler, W., Pettitt, D. *et al.* (2000) Segregation analysis of diabetic nephropathy in Pima Indians. *Diabetes*, **49**, 1049–56.

107. Ng, D., Tai, B., Koh, D. *et al.* (2005) Angiotensin-I converting enzyme insertion/deletion polymorphism and its association with diabetic nephropathy: a meta-analysis of studies reported between 1994 and 2004 and comprising 14,727 subjects. *Diabetologia*, **48**, 1008–16.

108. Microalbuminuria Collaborative Study Group UK (1993) Risk factors for development of microalbuminuria in insulin dependent diabetic patients: a cohort study. Microalbuminuria Collaborative Study Group, United Kingdom. *British Medical Journal*, **306**, 1235–9.

109. Couper, J., Staples, A., Cocciolone, R. *et al.* (1994) Relationship of smoking and albuminuria in children with insulin-dependent diabetes. *Diabetic Medicine*, **11**, 666–9.

110. Scott, L., Warram, J., Hanna, L. *et al.* (2001) A nonlinear effect of hyperglycemia and current cigarette smoking are major determinants of the onset of microalbuminuria in type 1 diabetes. *Diabetes*, **50**, 2842–9.

111. Sawicki, P., Didjurgeit, U., Muhlhauser, I. *et al.* (1994) Smoking is associated with progression of diabetic nephropathy. *Diabetes Care*, **17**, 126–31.

112. Hovind, P., Rossing, P., Tarnow, L. and Parving, H. (2003) Smoking and progression of diabetic nephropathy in type 1 diabetes. *Diabetes Care*, **26**, 911–16.

113. Gambaro, G., Bax, G., Fusaro, M. *et al.* (2001) Cigarette smoking is a risk factor for nephropathy and its progression in type 2 diabetes mellitus. *Diabetes, Nutrition and Metabolism*, **14**, 337–42.

114. Biesenbach, G., Grafinger, P., Janko, O. and Zazgornik, J. (1997) Influence of cigarette-smoking on the progression of clinical diabetic nephropathy in type 2 diabetic patients. *Clinical Nephrology*, **48**, 146–50.

115. Chuahirun, T. and Wesson, D. (2002) Cigarette smoking predicts faster progression of type 2 established diabetic nephropathy despite ACE inhibition. *American Journal of Kidney Diseases*, **39**, 376–82.

116. Ernst, E. and Resch, K. (1993) Fibrinogen as a cardiovascular risk factor: a meta-analysis and review of the literature. *Annals of Internal Medicine*, **118**, 956–63.

117. Klein, R., Hunter, S., Jenkins, A. *et al.* (2003) Fibrinogen is a marker for nephropathy and peripheral vascular disease in type 1 diabetes: studies of plasma fibrinogen and fibrinogen gene polymorphism in the DCCT/EDIC cohort. *Diabetes Care*, **26**, 1439–48.

118. Bruno, G., Merletti, F., Biggeri, A. *et al.* (2003) Progression to overt nephropathy in type 2 diabetes: the Casale Monferrato Study. *Diabetes Care*, **26**, 2150–5.

119. Jaffa, A., Durazo-Arvizu, R., Zheng, D. *et al.* (2003) Plasma prekallikrein: a risk marker for hypertension and nephropathy in type 1 diabetes. *Diabetes*, **52**, 1215–21.

120. Beisswenger, P., Drummond, K., Nelson, R. *et al.* (2005) Susceptibility to diabetic nephropathy is related to dicarbonyl and oxidative stress. *Diabetes*, **54**, 3274–81.

121. Padwal, R., Majumdar, S., Johnson, J. *et al.* (2005) A systematic review of drug therapy to delay or prevent type 2 diabetes. *Diabetes Care*, **28**, 736–55.

122. Gerstein, H., Yusuf, S., Bosch, J. *et al.* (2006) Effect of rosiglitazone on the frequency of diabetes in patients with impaired glucose tolerance or impaired fasting glucose: a randomised controlled trial. *Lancet*, **368**, 1096–105.

123. The Diabetes Prevention Program Research Group (2002) Reduction in the incidence of type 2 diabetes with lifestyle intervention or metformin. *The New England Journal of Medicine*, **346**, 393–403.

124. The EUCLID Study Group (1997) Randomised placebo-controlled trial of lisinopril in normotensive patients with insulin-dependent diabetes and normoalbuminuria or microalbuminuria. *Lancet*, **349**, 1787–92.

125. Ruggenenti, P., Fassi, A., Ilieva, A. *et al.* (2004) Preventing microalbuminuria in type 2 diabetes. *The New England Journal of Medicine*, **351**, 1941–51.

126. Haller, H., Viberti, G., Mimran, A. *et al.* (2006) Preventing microalbuminuria in patients with diabetes: rationale and design of the Randomised

Olmesartan and Diabetes Microalbuminuria Prevention (ROADMAP) study. *Journal of Clinical Hypertension*, **24**, 403–8.

127. Strippoli, G., Craig, M. and Craig, J. (2005) Antihypertensive agents for preventing diabetic kidney disease. *Cochrane Database of Systematic Reviews*, 4 (Art. No.: CD004136), DOI: 10.1002/14651858.CD004136.pub2.

128. Barnett, A. (2005) Preventing renal complications in diabetic patients: the Diabetics Exposed to Telmisartan And enalapriL (DETAIL) study. *Acta Diabetologica*, **42**, S42–9.

129. Strippoli, G., Craig, M., Deeks, J. *et al.* (2004) Effects of angiotensin converting enzyme inhibitors and angiotensin II receptor antagonists on mortality and renal outcomes in diabetic nephropathy: systematic review. *British Medical Journal*, **329**, 828–31.

130. Casas, J., Chua, W., Loukogeorgakis, S. *et al.* (2005) Effect of inhibitors of the renin–angiotensin system and other antihypertensive drugs on renal outcomes: systematic review and meta-analysis. *Lancet*, **366**, 2026–33.

131. Briganti, E., Kerr, P., Shaw, J. *et al.* (2005) Prevalence and treatment of cardiovascular disease and traditional risk factors in Australian adults with renal insufficiency. *Nephrology (Carlton, Vic.)*, **10**, 40–7.

132. Chobanian, A., Bakris, G., Black, H., *et al.* (2003) The Seventh Report of the Joint National Committee on Prevention, Detection, Evaluation, and Treatment of High Blood Pressure: the JNC7 report. *The Journal of the American Medical Association*, **289**, 2560–72.

133. Andros, V., Egger, A. and Dua, U. (2006) Blood pressure goal attainment according to JNC7 guidelines and utilization of antihypertensive drug therapy in MCO patients with type 1 or type 2 diabetes. *Journal of Managed Care Pharmacy*, **12**, 303–9.

134. Martinez-Ramirez, H., Jalomo-Martinez, B., Cortes-Sanabria, L. *et al.* (2006) Renal function preservation in type 2 diabetes mellitus patients with early nephropathy: a comparative prospective cohort study between primary health care doctors and a nephrologist. *American Journal of Kidney Diseases*, **47**, 78–87.

32

Epidemiology of Large-vessel Disease in Diabetes: Coronary Heart Disease and Stroke

Elizabeth Barrett-Connor

Division of Epidemiology/Department of Family and Preventive Medicine, University of California, San Diego, La Jolla, CA, USA

32.1 INTRODUCTION

Cardiovascular disease (CVD), which includes coronary heart disease (CHD) and stroke, is the major cause of morbidity and mortality in patients with insulin-dependent (type 1) or noninsulin-dependent (type 2) diabetes. Although diabetes is as powerful a risk factor as cholesterol, blood pressure or cigarette smoking, the diabetes–CVD association received relatively little systematic study until the publication of Kelly West's monumental book *Epidemiology of Diabetes Mellitus and Its Vascular Complications* [1] and the development of standard World Health Organization [2] and National Diabetes Data Group [3] criteria for the definition of diabetes in the 1980s. Since then the literature on the association between diabetes and CVD has increased exponentially. This review considers evidence from prospective cohort studies and randomized clinical trials, beginning with common risk factors for CHD and concluding with studies of specific CVD outcomes.

32.2 RISK FACTORS

32.2.1 Glucose

Because a diagnosis of diabetes requires hyperglycemia, it has been difficult to separate the effect of diabetes *per se* on CVD risk from the effect of covariates and glycemia below diabetes-diagnostic levels. An early attempt was made by Epstein [4], who reviewed 29 prospective studies of glycemia and CHD to determine whether any observed association was independent of cholesterol, blood pressure and cigarette smoking. In 5 of 13 studies of postchallenge glucose there was a positive association that remained significant after adjusting for the other risk factors; no studies of fasting or casual glucose showed an independent association with CHD, nor did any of the four studies that included women. In 1999, Coutinho *et al.* [5] examined the association between glucose and incident CVD in a meta-analysis of 20 published studies, which included 95 783 individuals followed for about 12 years. Only two of these 20 studies included women. The authors found a progressive association with a risk that extended below the diabetic threshold, but no adjustment for other risk factors was made.

The Diabetes Epidemiology: Collaborative analysis Of Diagnostic criteria in Europe (DECODE) study group analyzed individual data from 22 European cohort studies, which included 29 714 adults followed for an average of 11 years, to determine whether the glucose association with CVD was linear or had a threshold effect, and whether it was independent of classic CHD risk factors [6]. Most studies allowed adjustment for blood pressure, cholesterol and cigarette smoking. In the pooled analysis for fatal CVD, there was a J-shaped association with a threshold effect for

The Epidemiology of Diabetes Mellitus, second edition   Edited by Jean-Marie Ekoé, Marian Rewers, Rhys Williams and Paul Zimmet
© 2008 John Wiley & Sons, Ltd

fasting plasma glucose (FPG; 5.4 mmol l^{-1}) and a linear association with 2 h postchallenge glucose. Although hazard ratios were higher in those with diabetes, risks were increased below glucose levels diagnostic of diabetes. In DECODE, the 2 h postchallenge glucose was a stronger CVD risk factor than FPG, and impaired glucose tolerance (IGT) was a stronger CVD risk factor than impaired fasting glucose (IFG).

The European Prospective Investigation into Cancer–Norfolk cohort (EPIC–Norfolk study), the first large cohort study of glycated hemoglobin and CVD risk in a cohort unselected for diabetes, showed a graded association between HbA$_{1c}$ levels and the risk for CVD and death [7]. This association was present in both sexes and was not materially changed after the exclusion of participants with known diabetes. The quarter of the cohort with an HbA$_{1c}$ concentration <5% had the lowest risk of death and CVD.

In patients with diabetes, the level of glucose is an independent CVD risk factor, as shown in a meta-analysis of three cohort studies of patients with type 1 diabetes, and 10 cohort studies of patients with type 2 diabetes published from 1966 to July 2003 [8]. Based on the most fully adjusted models, the risk of CVD increased to a similar degree with increasing levels of glycated hemoglobin in type 1 and type 2 patients. In type 2 diabetes, the pooled relative risk (RR) for total CVD was 1.18 (1.10–1.26) for each percentage point increase in glycated hemoglobin.

In patients with diabetes, the variability of glucose (glucose spikes) is also a strong risk factor for CVD. In an Italian study of patients 75 years and older, both the 3-year average and the 3-year variability of fasting glucose were significantly associated with the 5-year mortality – with the highest mortality rates in the highest tertile for glucose variability [9, 10]. In younger patients, the mean glucose was no longer predictive of mortality after adjusting for glucose variability [11]. A review of postprandial and postchallenge glucose [12] emphasized the CVD risk of nonfasting hyperglycemia in patients with a normal fasting glucose. Interest in controlling postprandial hyperglycemia is increasing [13].

32.2.1.1   Clinical Trials

Results of clinical trials designed to determine whether glycemic control prevents macrovascular

disease in patients with type 2 diabetes have been disappointing. The first large controlled clinical trial was the 13-year University Group Diabetes Program (UGDP) [14]. In the UGDP trial, variable insulin therapy lowered glucose levels more than standard insulin or placebo, without reducing the risk of fatal or nonfatal CVD risk. As reviewed by Genuth [15], 10% of participants in each of these three treatment groups experienced a myocardial infarction.

The UK Prospective Diabetes Study (UKPDS), a clinical trial of intensive control of blood glucose after diagnosis of type 2 diabetes, achieved a median HbA$_{1c}$ of 7.0%, compared with 7.9% in those allocated to conventional treatment over a median 10 years of follow-up [16]. The trial showed a substantial reduction in the risk of microvascular complications, but only a borderline significant reduction in the risk of myocardial infarction RR = 0.84, 95% confidence interval (CI) 0.71–1.00, $p = 0.052$. However, each 1% reduction in updated HbA$_{1c}$ during the follow-up was associated with 14% (8–21%, $p < 0.0001$) reduction in the risk of myocardial infarction [17].

A recent systematic review of glycemic control and macrovascular disease included eight randomized trials in 1800 patients with type 1 diabetes and six trials in 447 patients with type 2 diabetes. Combined incidence rate ratios for any macrovascular event were 0.38 (95% CI 0.26–0.56) in type 1 diabetes and 0.81 (95% CI 0.73–0.91) in type 2 diabetes. The benefit was mainly due to reduction of cardiac and peripheral vascular events in type 1 diabetes and due to reductions in stroke and peripheral vascular events in type 2 diabetes [18].

Hyperglycemia presumably contributes to CVD by gradual effects accumulated over decades. Difficulty showing the role of glucose control in prevention of CVD in clinical trials may reflect a too short follow up and/or inadequate glucose control. Bonora [19] has suggested that another reason clinical trials have failed to demonstrate that intensive glucose control prevents CVD may be because the treatment target has been fasting glucose, not glucose variation or postprandial glucose.

32.2.2   Hyperglycemia at the Time of a Heart Attack

An increased mortality rate in patients who have hyperglycemia at the time of a heart attack was the subject of a systematic review of 15 observational studies published in 2000; patients with or without diabetes who had hyperglycemia when hospitalized with acute myocardial infarction or acute coronary syndrome had a poorer outcome [20]. A more recent observational study of more than 140 000 elderly heart attack patients showed a graded increase in mortality with each higher quintile of baseline glucose [21]. Another observational study included 1469 patients whose glucose was measured at hospitalization for an acute myocardial infarction and 24 h later; in this study, every $0.6 \, \text{mmol} \, \text{l}^{-1}$ increase in baseline glucose in patients without diabetes was associated with a 12% increase in the risk of death by 30 days, while a fall in glucose within the first 24 h predicted a better prognosis [22]. Similar associations are reported for acute coronary syndrome. For example, there was a significant increase in 10-month mortality in patients with acute coronary syndrome who had a baseline random glucose in the top quartile, compared with patients in the lowest quartile [23]. This association was independent of comorbidity and history of diabetes.

These results are compatible with studies showing that postprandial hyperglycemia causes myocardial perfusion defects secondary to deterioration in vascular function [24], and led to recommendations in the United States and Europe that hyperglycemia be reduced as soon as possible after an acute myocardial infarction.

32.2.2.1 Clinical Trials

Many clinical trials have used insulin to treat hyperglycemia in patients having a heart attack, acute coronary syndrome or revascularization; most trials used an infusion of glucose–insulin–potassium (GIK). An early meta-analysis of GIK infusion studies including 1932 patients with acute myocardial infarction showed that 1-year mortality was reduced by 28% [25]. In a recent meta-analysis of GIK infusion during cardiac surgery, evidence for cardioprotection was mixed and the authors concluded that more research was necessary [26]. In yet another meta-analysis of 38 trials of insulin treatment for acutely ill hospitalized patients, statistically significant benefit was observed for patients on the surgical intensive care unit and for patients with diabetes, but not for patients with acute myocardial infarction [27].

Results from the best known clinical trials are mixed. Although GIK infusion controlled hyperglycemia and reduced long-term mortality in diabetic patients hospitalized with acute myocardial infarction in the first Diabetes Insulin–Glucose infusion in Acute Myocardial Infarction (DIGAMI) trial [28], the larger multicenter DIGAMI-2 trial found no benefit [29]. The insulin-treated patients in DIGAMI-2 did not achieve the protocol-planned reduction in glycated hemoglobin. In the first Estudios Cardiologicos Latinoamerica (ECLA) trial, high- or low-dose GIK therapy did not prevent major in-hospital events, but did significantly reduce mortality in patients treated by reperfusion [30]. The largest randomized trial of GIK following acute myocardial infarction, the Clinical Trial of Revirapine and Metabolic Modulation in Acute Myocardial Infarction Treatment Evaluation (CREATE–ECLA), showed no reduction in 30-day mortality, but specific glucose targets were not set and glucose levels were actually higher in the active treatment group [31]. The Hyperglycemia: Intensive Insulin Infusion In Infarction (HI-5) trial used a variable insulin and dextrose infusion to reduce hyperglycemia to $<10 \, \text{mmol} \, \text{l}^{-1}$ for 24 h after myocardial infarction: there was no reduction in 3- or 6-month mortality in patients with or without diabetes, but a subset analysis showed significantly less heart failure and reinfarction in those whose blood glucose was reduced to $\leq 8 \, \text{mmol} \, \text{l}^{-1}$ [32]. Most recently, an open-label randomized clinical trial in patients with or without diabetes undergoing on-pump cardiac surgery found that continuous insulin infusion targeted to maintain intraoperative glucose levels between 4.4 and $5.6 \, \text{mmol} \, \text{l}^{-1}$ increased the incidence of stroke and death [33]. The trial was too small ($n = 371$) to determine whether outcome differed by diabetes status. These trial differences may reflect differences in the patients or in the control of hyperglycemia.

32.2.3 Insulin

Insulin resistance, usually measured as the fasting insulin level in epidemiologic studies, precedes the development of diabetes by one or two decades. Insulin and insulin resistance have been implicated in the genesis of atherosclerotic disease since the hypotheses of Stout published in 1990 [34]. The atherogenic potential of insulin has been summarized by Ferrara *et al.* [35] and McKeigue and Davey [36]. Although early epidemiologic studies suggested that hyperinsulinemia was a precursor of CVD [37–39], this association has not been found in women or in ethnic groups other than Caucasians [35]. A meta-analysis [40] of 12 studies published through 1996 showed a weak but significant positive association of hyperinsulinemia with CVD; an increase of $50 \, pmol \, l^{-1}$ of fasting insulin yielded a summary RR of 1.18. There was a highly significant heterogeneity among studies, however, with data suggesting ethnicity or insulin assay methods as possible explanations for these differences. A more recent study in Finnish patients with type 2 diabetes found that hyperinsulinemia predicted CHD death in men, but not women, and the association in men was not independent of high-density lipoprotein (HDL) and triglycerides [41]. In Italian patients with type 2 diabetes, insulin resistance (based on a comparison of the lowest and highest quartiles of the homeostasis model assessment of insulin resistance (HOMA-IR) index) predicted an increased risk of CVD [42]. In contrast, neither hyperinsulinemia nor insulin sensitivity based on the HOMA-IR was independently associated with CVD in the UKPDS [43, 44]. However, a cross-sectional, four-center study in the United States found that low insulin sensitivity (assessed by a frequently sampled intravenous glucose tolerance test and minimal model analysis) was an independent risk factor for CHD, but fasting and 2 h insulin levels were not [45].

One reason for these contradictory results could be differences in poorly standardized insulin assays. Also, radioimmunoassays for insulin usually fail to discriminate between intact insulin and proinsulin-like molecules. Proinsulin is a marker for β-cell failure and appears to be an important risk factor for CVD. Although a 6.5 year follow-up study showed that the association between proinsulin and CHD was no longer significant after controlling for body weight [46], a 27-year follow up of Swedish men found that proinsulin, but not specific insulin or immunoreactive insulin, predicted fatal and non-fatal CHD independent of other risk factors [47]. A cross-sectional study of older North American men and women without diabetes also found that proinsulin was more strongly and consistently associated with CHD than intact insulin [48].

32.2.4 Exogenous Insulin

Although some epidemiological data suggest a higher risk for CHD in type 2 diabetic patients treated with higher doses of insulin [49, 50], these results likely reflect patients with longer diabetes duration or more severe diabetes. Neither the UGDP nor UKPDS trials showed increases in CVD event rates in insulin-treated versus placebo-treated patients [14, 51].

32.2.4.1 Clinical Trials

Thiazolidinediones are the only currently available drugs that primarily target insulin resistance and reduce hyperglycemia by binding to peroxisome proliferator-activated receptor gamma (PPAR-gamma) [52, 53]. The evidence that glitazones are cardioprotective is weak. The Diabetes REduction Assessment with ramipril and rosiglitazone Medication (DREAM) trial showed that rosiglitazone, compared with placebo, significantly reduced the incidence of new diabetes in patients with IGT [54]. Unfortunately, CVD results were not encouraging: rosiglitazone was associated with a significantly increased risk of heart failure, and every other cardiovascular outcome was (nonsignificantly) increased in the rosiglitazone group. The PROspective pioglitAzone Clinical Trial in macroVascular Events (PROactive) trial compared pioglitazone with placebo in prevention of CVD endpoints in diabetic patients, more than half of whom had already had macrovascular disease [55]. Pioglitazone showed no significant benefit for the prespecified composite endpoint of all-cause mortality, nonfatal myocardial infarction, stroke, acute coronary syndrome and vascular surgery. A significant benefit was observed for a prespecified secondary endpoint – the composite of death, nonfatal myocardial infarction and stroke – but the study design and analyses have met significant criticism.

32.2.5 Hypertension

Hypertension is common in patients with diabetes, and often precedes it [56, 57]. In the UKPDS [58], 38% of the newly diagnosed diabetic patients had systolic/diastolic blood pressures $\geq 160/90 \, mmHg$ or were being treated for hypertension. Because overweight and obesity are associated with both diabetes and high blood pressure, it is difficult to determine which plays a leading role, but it is clear that hypertension further increases the risk of CVD in the diabetic patient [51].

Some of the most informative data come from an epidemiologic analysis of the UKPDS data [59]. In this analysis, the risk of each of the macrovascular complications of type 2 diabetes was strongly associated with systolic blood pressure (SBP), with no evidence of a threshold effect. Myocardial infarction occurred about twice as frequently as microvascular endpoints at each level of blood pressure. The decrease in risk of macro- or micro-vascular disease for each 10 mmHg lower level of updated mean SBP was about 11% for myocardial infarction and 13% for microvascular complications.

32.2.5.1 Clinical Trials

The evidence that blood pressure control reduces stroke risk in patients with diabetes comes largely from the UKPDS clinical trial, in which 'tight control' of blood pressure substantially reduced the risk of microvascular disease, stroke and death due to diabetes, but not myocardial infarction [51]. However, longer follow-up of the UKPDS cohort clearly demonstrated a beneficial effect of lowering blood pressure on the risk of both myocardial infarction and stroke. A 10 mmHg decrement in updated mean SBP predicted 11% (7–15%, $p < 0.0001$) decrease in the risk of myocardial infarction and 18% (12–23%, $p < 0.0001$) decrease in the risk of stroke, adjusted for gender, age at diagnosis, ethnicity, smoking, HDL-cholesterol, low-density lipoprotein (LDL-cholesterol), triglycerides and albuminuria [60]. This beneficial effect of lowering SBP was independent and additive to the effect of lowering HbA_{1c}.

A systematic review (through April 2002) of eight randomized controlled trials of treatment of hypertension in patients with type 2 diabetes (four placebo controlled and four with other comparisons) showed a reduced risk of cardiovascular events and deaths [61]. In the same review, studies designed to compare the effects of specific classes of antihypertensives showed no evidence that newer agents were superior to diuretics. In the Anti-hypertensive and Lipid-Lowering Treatment to Prevent Heart Attack Trial (ALLHAT), one of the largest antihypertensive trials, thiazide diuretics reduced combined fatal and nonfatal CVD as well as

angiotensin-converting enzyme (ACE) inhibitors or calcium channel blocker therapy did, and prevented heart failure better than any other initial treatment in both diabetic and nondiabetic patients [62]. A recent Cochrane meta-analysis of 16 clinical trials conducted in normotensive and hypertensive diabetics without microalbuminuria found that only ACE inhibitors reduced the risk of developing microalbuminuria, independent of baseline blood pressure or type of diabetes [63], but none of the antihypertensive medications studied were shown to reduce all-cause mortality. In seven of eight trials in hypertensive patients (10–35% of whom had diabetes), no class of antihypertensive was superior to any other class in reducing all-cause or cardiovascular mortality.

It is now recognized that most patients with hypertension will require two or more antihypertensive agents to control blood pressure, making the choice of medication to prevent CVD less important than achieving target blood pressures [61].

32.2.6 Lipids

A majority of patients with type 2 diabetes have dyslipidemia. Unfavorable levels of lipids and lipoproteins are present years before the diagnosis of diabetes [56]. Because diabetic patients have LDL-cholesterol levels that are smaller and denser than nondiabetic persons [64], similar LDL levels in persons with diabetes versus without diabetes mask a higher number of LDL particles among diabetics. Individuals with diabetes also have lower HDL and higher triglyceride levels than persons without diabetes. Dyslipidemia characterized by high triglycerides and low HDL-cholesterol levels is called *pattern B dyslipidemia*, a marker for highly atherogenic small, dense LDL-cholesterol, and usually is associated with normal or only slightly elevated levels of LDL-cholesterol [65].

32.2.6.1 Clinical Trials

Many trials have compared lipid-lowering treatment effects in patients with and without diabetes; in most of these trials the patients with diabetes were a smaller subgroup of the participants. A meta-analysis of 14 clinical trials published through September 2002 showed that both statins and fibrates reduced the risk of CVD in diabetic participants at least as well as in nondiabetics [66].

This analysis was used in the United States as the basis for an LDL target $<100 \, \text{mg dl}^{-1}$ for patients with diabetes [67]. Another meta-analysis of 14 randomized controlled clinical trials with 90 056 participants showed that lowering cholesterol with statins reduced CHD mortality, myocardial infarction, coronary revascularization and stroke – overall by about one-fifth per millimole per liter reduction in LDL-cholesterol – without increasing all-cause mortality or nonvascular mortality [68]. The pooled benefit was similar in those with and without a history of diabetes.

Another meta-analysis of 12 controlled clinical trials of lipid-lowering therapy (10 statin trials and two gemfibrosil trials) published between 1996 and April 2004 also showed that lipid-lowering therapy was at least as effective in reducing CHD in diabetic patients as in nondiabetic patients [69]. Further, when results were adjusted for baseline risk, individuals with diabetes had a greater absolute risk reduction than those without diabetes. The risk reduction was similar for secondary prevention (eight trials) and primary prevention (six trials). In primary prevention, the risk reduction for a major coronary event was 21% in diabetic patients and 23% in nondiabetic patients treated with either statins or a fibrate (gemfibrosil). For secondary prevention the risk reduction was also 21% and 23% respectively. The number needed to treat was small (37 versus 15 in diabetics and 47 versus 17 in nondiabetics). Most of these trials showed total cholesterol decreases of 15–20% and HDL-cholesterol increases of 5–8%.

The Collaborative Atorvastatin Diabetes Study (CARDS) was the first large randomized controlled clinical trial designed specifically to determine the effect of cholesterol-lowering therapy on CVD in patients with type 2 diabetes and no known CVD [70]. After 4 years, atorvastatin reduced cardiovascular events 36% (95% CI -55 to -9%, $p = 0.001$) compared to placebo, with an overall reduction in mortality of 27% (95% CI -48 to 1%, $p = 0.059$). During the trial, atorvastatin reduced total- and LDL-cholesterol and triglycerides, with no change in HDL-cholesterol.

Fibrates reduce LDL-cholesterol by 10–15% (much less than statins) and triglycerides by 30% (much more than statins), and have been shown to reduce progression of coronary atherosclerosis in diabetic patients [71]. The second large clinical outcome trial in patients with type 2 diabetes was the 5-year Fenofibrate Intervention and Event Lowering in Diabetes (FIELD) trial, comparing fenofibrate with placebo [72]. In this trial there was no significant difference by treatment in the composite primary outcome of fatal and nonfatal CHD. In secondary analyses, however, those assigned to fenofibrate had a significantly reduced risk of nonfatal myocardial infarction and revascularization, but a (nonsignificant) increase in CHD mortality. Benefit was largely in participants who had no history of CVD at baseline, perhaps suggesting that fibrates might be beneficial for primary but not secondary prevention. However, the CARDS risk reduction was less than that observed for secondary prevention in the Veterans Affairs High-density lipoprotein cholesterol Intervention Trial (VA-HIT) [73].

No head-to-head comparisons of fibrates with statins have been reported. Patients with type 2 diabetes had similar CVD rates in the FIELD and CARDS trials.

Metformin also alters diabetic dyslipidemia, lowers insulin levels, and does not increase weight gain, unlike most other diabetes medications. In a meta-analysis of 41 trials conducted in 3074 patients with diabetes, metformin modestly but significantly reduced triglycerides and LDL and had minimal effects on HDL-cholesterol [74]. The UKPDS included 753 overweight patients with newly diagnosed type 2 diabetes who were assigned to metformin or conventional treatment. Despite the small number, after 10.7 years the metformin group had a 39% lower risk of myocardial infarction than the conventional group ($p = 0.01$) [58].

A large meta-analysis compared the effect of the insulin sensitizers rosiglitazone and pioglitazone treatment versus placebo on lipoproteins in 23 controlled clinical trials conducted in more than 8000 patients with diabetes [75]. In the pooled analysis, rosiglitazone increased LDL-cholesterol and pioglitazone did not, while pioglitazone reduced triglycerides but rosiglitazone did not. Both drugs increased HDL-cholesterol, but pioglitazone was twice as effective. In the first large head-to-head comparison trial of rosiglitazone and pioglitazone in patients with type 2 diabetes, there were striking differences in lipid effects despite similar effects on glycemia [76]. Pioglitazone significantly decreased triglyceride levels, while rosiglitazone increased triglycerides. LDL levels were increased with both glitazones, but the mean increase was about half as great with pioglitazone. Also, compared with rosiglitazone, pioglitazone significantly increased LDL particle size ($p = 0.005$) and reduced LDL particle concentration ($p = 0.001$), changes expected to be antiatherogenic.

32.2.7 Clustered Risk Factors (Metabolic Syndrome and Covariates)

Cohort studies such as those from Italy [77], Finland and Sweden [78] and the United States [79] have shown that adults with metabolic syndrome have more than a threefold increased risk of CVD. The Kuopio Ischemic Heart Study showed that this increased risk occurred in the absence of diabetes [80]. In contrast, the National Health and Nutrition Examination Survey II (NHANES II) Mortality Study, a cohort study of a representative sample of adults in the United States, did not find that metabolic syndrome significantly increased the risk of heart disease when participants with diabetes were excluded [81]. Further, metabolic syndrome was not as good a predictor of CVD as the Framingham cardiovascular score was [82].

Controversy over the scientific basis for the definition of this cluster of risk factors stems from the arbitrariness of the included (and excluded) variables and of their cutpoints, the loss of risk prediction when continuous risk factors are categorized and the unproven assumption that there is a single underlying biology [83, 84]. Nevertheless, the syndrome has become a useful common phenotype for clinicians, drawing attention to the importance of previously neglected risk factors such as central obesity and elevated triglycerides, and to the importance of multifactorial management when there are modest elevations in risk factors occurring in combination [85].

32.2.8 Obesity

Obesity, particularly central (upper body) obesity as assessed by waist girth, is a strong risk factor for both type 2 diabetes and for CVD [86]. About 10 years ago, a systematic review of clinical trials of weight loss by lifestyle intervention showed beneficial effects on heart disease risk factors, including blood pressure (35 clinical trials), serum triglycerides and HDL-cholesterol (14 trials), and

glucose (nine trials) [87]. In clinical trials such as the Finnish Diabetes Prevention Study [88] and the US Diabetes Prevention Program [89], weight loss by intensive lifestyle change reduced blood glucose and delayed or prevented the onset of diabetes by 58% in adults with IGT. There are no published clinical trials in persons with or without diabetes showing that lifestyle-induced weight loss prevents CVD.

32.2.9 Smoking

There is overwhelming epidemiologic evidence that smoking cessation decreases the risk of CHD and stroke. No clinical trials have randomized individuals with diabetes to smoking cessation (as the only intervention) versus no intervention, with incidence or progression of CVD outcomes. Yudkin [90] estimated the benefits of smoking cessation for persons with and without diabetes, using data from the Multiple Risk Factor Intervention Trial (MRFIT) [91]. He estimated that smoking cessation would prolong the life of a 45-year-old man with diabetes by a mean of 3 years, compared with 4 years in a 45-year-old man without diabetes [90].

32.2.10 Aspirin Prophylaxis

One meta-analysis and several clinical trials have demonstrated the efficacy of low-dose aspirin in prevention of myocardial infarction and stroke in patients with diabetes [92]. The largest randomized trial of low-dose aspirin in women was published after the above meta-analysis: in this large primary prevention trial, aspirin lowered the risk of stroke, with no effect on the risk of myocardial infarction or death from cardiovascular causes, leading to a nonsignificant finding with respect to the primary endpoint [93]. The American Diabetes Association recommends use of aspirin (75–162 mg per day) or clopidogrel as a secondary prevention of CVD in diabetic patients, as well as a primary prevention strategy in those who are older than 40 years and have additional risk factors (family history of CVD, hypertension, smoking, dyslipidemia or albuminuria) [94].

32.2.11 Novel Risk Factors

The last 10 years have seen an incremental increase in 'novel risk factors,' each claiming to add to the prediction of CVD and the identification of patients who need preventive intervention. Many of these markers are higher in overweight patients and in persons with diabetes. The evidence that they add predictive power to conventional risk factors is weak. In a recent report from the Atherosclerosis Risk in Communities cohort, 19 of the 'most exciting new' CVD risk markers added nothing of significance to the prediction of CVD beyond prediction afforded by the classical risk factors [95]. Similar results have been reported from the Framingham Heart Study [96]. The classical risk factors shown to be causal in clinical trials are the only appropriate targets of therapy at this time.

32.3 OUTCOMES

32.3.1 CHD

The incidence of fatal CHD in persons with diabetes is at least doubled, as clearly shown in US and UK population-based studies published in 1979 and 1983 [97, 98]. In the United States, CVD accounts for 80% of diabetic mortality and more than 75% of all hospitalizations for diabetic patients [99].

32.3.1.1 Sex Differences

Diabetes is known for reducing the usual female cardioprotection. Comprehensive data on the sex-specific epidemiology of diabetes and CHD come from a meta-analysis of 37 prospective cohort studies which include 447 064 men and women published between 1996 and March 2005 [100]. The pooled RR for fatal CHD in diabetic versus nondiabetic women (3.50; 95% CI 2.7–4.5) was greater than the risk in diabetic versus nondiabetic men (2.06; 95% CI 1.8–2.3). The pooled risk ratio of the 29 studies that provided multiply adjusted estimates was attenuated, but still almost 50% higher and still statistically significant (1.46; 95% CI 1.1–1.9). The attenuation after adjustment for risk factors was greater in women with diabetes than in men with diabetes. This suggests that the sex difference is mediated in large part by diabetic women's less favorable levels of several risk factors, as reported in a previous smaller pooled analysis [101].

Some of the sex difference could be explained by less aggressive treatment in women than men: several studies show that men with diabetes or CVD are more likely to be treated with aspirin, statins or antihypertensives than women with the same conditions [102–104].

32.3.1.2 Diabetes as a Heart Disease Equivalent

In 1998, Haffner *et al.* [105] reported that diabetes was a heart disease equivalent with regard to the risk of future CHD. Although this equivalency has not been consistently documented [106–112], this observation has had a useful impact on heart disease prevention in diabetics by alerting more of the medical community to the importance of treating patients with diabetes to prevent heart disease.

32.3.1.3 Clinical Differences in CHD by Diabetes Status

People with type 2 diabetes appear to have a higher incidence of silent myocardial infarction than people without diabetes [113] and a poorer prognosis after the first myocardial infarction [114, 115].

32.3.2 Heart Failure

There is now little doubt that diabetes increases the risk of heart failure secondary to hypertension or heart attack. The first strong epidemiologic evidence that diabetes is an independent predictor of heart failure probably came from the Framingham Heart Study, which reported in 1974 that this association was independent of age, blood pressure, cholesterol, weight or history of heart disease [116]. Studies have shown that the diabetes–heart failure association is stronger in women, possibly reflecting their better survival. National registry data show that approximately 40% of patients hospitalized for heart failure have diabetes [117]. Based on Framingham data from the pretreatment era, heart failure patients with diabetes had about three times the mortality risk than heart failure patients without diabetes [118]. Heart failure remains a neglected complication of diabetes, as reviewed elsewhere [119].

While the diabetes–heart failure association is usually attributed to prior myocardial infarction or hypertension, diabetes also affects cardiac structure and function independent of coronary artery disease (CAD) and high blood pressure [120]. The 22-year follow up of the Cardiovascular Health Study (CHS) confirmed a significant association between diabetes and diastolic dysfunction leading to heart failure in the absence of systolic dysfunction [121]. A US nationwide case–control study found that patients with idiopathic dilated cardiomyopathy were 75% more likely to have diabetes than age-matched controls, and the association was strongest in patients with diabetic microvascular complications, suggesting a role for longer duration of hyperglycemia [122]. Similarly, systolic dysfunction is most common in patients with type 1 diabetes who have microvascular complications [123]. On the other hand, clinical heart failure may precede the diagnosis of diabetes. In a 3-year follow-up study of nondiabetic subjects, heart failure was an independent risk factor for the development of diabetes [124].

Poornima *et al.* [120] have proposed that systolic dysfunction reflects the magnitude and duration of hyperglycemia, while diastolic dysfunction is a consequence of hypertrophy or hyperglycemia; if hypertrophy appears earlier, then this would explain why diastolic abnormalities dominate the clinical findings. Elevated free fatty acid (FFA) levels and increased myocardial uptake of FFA during stress and ischemia could be responsible for the increased susceptibility of the diabetic heart to myocardial ischemia, and to a larger decrease in myocardial performance for a given amount of ischemia than observed in the nondiabetic heart [125]. Impaired systolic and diastolic function of the diabetic heart may facilitate the development of overt heart failure in the presence of reduced coronary blood flow, as occurs at the time of myocardial infarction or with hypertension.

Some of the heart failure excess may be caused by diabetic cardiomyopathy, which often presents as diastolic dysfunction with the characteristics of a restrictive cardiomyopathy [126]. Epidemiologic studies of diabetic cardiomyopathy are few, in part because diabetic cardiomyopathy is a diagnosis of exclusion, made when heart failure occurs in the absence of (diagnosed) CHD and hypertension. Its clinical manifestations are similar in type 1 and type 2 diabetes [127, 128].

32.3.2.1 Clinical Trials

Beta-blocker therapy improves survival in patients with congestive heart failure, but was previously not recommended for patients with diabetes because of concerns about glucose control. A meta-analysis of published and individual data from the 12 largest randomized clinical trials of ACE inhibitors and beta-blockers for the management of heart failure showed reduced all-cause mortality for either treatment in patients with or without diabetes [129]. In this meta-analysis, ACE inhibitors (seven trials) may have been less effective in women with asymptomatic left ventricular dysfunction than in men, but there were fewer women than men and they had a shorter follow up. Beta-blockers (five studies) showed no sex difference and significant risk reduction in persons with and without diabetes; the latter comparison included only three studies, so a difference by diabetes status could not be excluded. Another meta-analysis restricted to six large trials that reported mortality outcomes of beta-blocker therapy in patients with heart failure (25% with diabetes) showed that beta-blockers reduced mortality in patients with diabetes (RR 0.84, 95% CI 0.73–0.96) and in patients without diabetes (RR 0.72, 95% CI 0.65–0.79), but the risk reduction was significantly greater in patients without diabetes [130]. A third meta-analysis of seven placebo-controlled clinical trials of the beta-blocker carvedilol showed similar survival benefits and a similar number needed to treat to prevent one death in patients with and without diabetes [131]. The pooled risk reduction was greater than that reported in other trials using different beta-blockers, but no head-to-head comparisons have been reported.

32.3.3 Stroke

Early epidemiologic studies showed that diabetes doubles or triples the risk of stroke [97, 132]. Diabetes is now recognized as one of the classic risk factors for ischemic stroke, along with hypertension, atrial fibrillation, myocardial infarction and heart failure. Hypertension, the strongest stroke risk factor, often coexists with diabetes, and adds to the stroke risk. A study showing that one-in-five stroke survivors admitted to stroke-related clinical trials had diabetes is likely to underestimate the true association, because clinical trials recruit patients who tend to be healthier than the general population with the same diagnosis [133]. In addition, older hypertensive adults who have diabetes are three times more likely to have single or multiple silent cerebral infarcts by brain magnetic resonance imaging (MRI) than hypertensives without diabetes [134]. In the UKPDS, tight control of blood pressure (a 10 mmHg reduction in SBP and a 5 mmHg reduction in diastolic blood pressure) resulted in a significant 44% reduction in cerebrovascular events [51].

Beyond hypertension, many other stroke risk factors are more common in persons with diabetes, including hyperinsulinemia (insulin resistance) [135], low HDL-cholesterol [136] and proteinuria [137]. Evidence for hyperglycemia as an independent risk factor for stroke is mixed [138]. In DECODE, a large collaborative analysis of data from 10 prospective European cohort studies [139], postchallenge hyperglycemia did not predict stroke, although it was a good predictor of total cardiovascular risk. In the 22-year follow up of the Helsinki Policemen Study, hyperinsulinemia was not a risk factor for stroke after controlling for upper body obesity [140].

Myocardial infarction is a strong stroke risk factor. A meta-analysis of 22 prospective studies published from 1978 to 2004, including 464 159 heart attack survivors, found 12.2 ischemic strokes per 1000 heart attacks within 30 days of hospitalization, and this rate was doubled in studies with 1-year follow up [141]. In the pooled analysis, age, diabetes, hypertension and heart failure were each associated with an increased risk of post-myocardial infarction stroke, but the authors provided no data on the amount of risk contributed by diabetes *per se*.

Strokes in patients with diabetes are associated with a worse outcome than strokes in persons without diabetes, which is apparently not explained by a larger area of infarction [134, 142]. As reviewed elsewhere, many studies have shown a higher mean admission glucose in nonstroke survivors than in stroke survivors [143, 144]. The prevalence of previously diagnosed diabetes in stroke survivors varies from 8 to 20%, an additional 28% may have IGT and between 10 and 20% of stroke patients have hyperglycemia but do not have an elevated glycated hemoglobin (suggesting they have stress hyperglycemia, not diabetes). Thus, 20 to 50% of stroke patients have hyperglycemia at the time of hospitalization.

In a long-term follow-up study of patients without diabetes admitted to an acute stroke unit, plasma glucose levels $>8\,\mathrm{mmol\,l^{-1}}$ had a poor prognosis independent of age, stroke severity and type of stroke [145]. In a systematic review of 26 studies, stroke patients who had hyperglycemia on admission to hospital had a nearly twofold increased risk of death (odds ratio (ORs) 1.93; 95%

CI 1.15–3.24) [144]. In this study, one-third of all stroke patients were hyperglycemic on admission but did not have a history of diabetes; they had a threefold higher risk of short-term mortality and a significantly increased risk of poststroke disability.

Many mechanisms have been proposed for the increased severity of stroke in patients with hyperglycemia, including direct glucose toxicity, change in the blood brain barrier or glucose-associated covariates, as reviewed elsewhere [133]. It is not clear whether the poor prognosis associated with admission hyperglycemia reflects stroke severity and stress, or an untoward effect of hyperglycemia *per se*.

32.3.3.1   Clinical Trials

The strong epidemiologic evidence that hyperglycemia worsens the prognosis in stroke patients led to recommendations to treat hyperglycemia ($>10\,\mathrm{mmol\,l^{-1}}$) with glucose potassium and insulin infusion. The small Glucose Insulin Stroke Trial (GIST) of GIK infusion in acute stroke patients with mild to moderate hyperglycemia showed no benefit, but there were no significant differences in plasma glucose levels throughout the 4-week trial [143].

Patients with diabetes are at increased risk of hemorrhagic transformation after ischemic stroke. In a pooled analysis of clinical trials in patients with acute ischemic stroke, streptokinase increased the risk of hemorrhagic transformation almost sixfold, but the second most powerful predictor of hemorrhagic transformation was diabetes; this risk was similar in patients receiving streptokinase (OR 3.0; 95% CI 1.1–7.9) or placebo (OR 3.7; 95% CI 1.3–10.6) [146]. This increased risk has been confirmed in other trials reviewed elsewhere [133].

32.4   TYPE 1 DIABETES RISK FACTORS

While type 1 and type 2 diabetes share most risk factors for CHD and stroke, there are notable differences reviewed below. The traditional cardiovascular risk factors of hyperglycemia, dyslipidemia, elevated blood pressure, smoking and metabolic syndrome are of importance, but do not explain the excess risk of CAD in type 1 diabetes patients. CVD prediction models that are valid in nondiabetic persons (Framingham score) or in persons with type 2 diabetes (the UKPDS risk engine) poorly predict CVD events in patients with type 1 diabetes [147]. This area is currently a subject of intensive investigation [148] and a comprehensive review is available [149].

32.4.1 Glucose

Until recently, the role of chronic hyperglycemia as a major CHD risk factor in type 1 diabetes has been questioned [150]. However, first observational studies using intermediate endpoint of coronary artery calcification [151] and later the Epidemiology of Diabetes Interventions and Complications (EDIC) Study [152] have provided strong evidence that hyperglycemia plays an important role in development of coronary atherosclerosis and disease in patients with type 1 diabetes.

32.4.1.1 Clinical Trials

The Diabetes Control and Complications Trial (DCCT) was the first trial of glycemic control and vascular outcomes in type 1 diabetes: 1441 patients, aged 13–40 years, were assigned to intensive care (≥3 daily insulin injections or an external insulin pump) or conventional insulin (one or two injections per day). After 6.5 years there was a 41% lower rate of CVD in the tighter control group, but events were few and these differences were not statistically significant [153]. More than 90% of the DCCT participants were followed (the EDIC study) for a cumulative follow up of 17 years [152]. By this time there were significantly fewer CVD events in the intensively treated group (46 events in 31 patients) than in the placebo group (98 events in 52 patients), and the risk of nonfatal myocardial infarction, stroke or death from CVD was reduced by 57% (95% CI 12–79%). The glycated hemoglobin value *during* the DCCT explained a large part of the delayed cardiovascular protection with intensive therapy.

32.4.2 Lipids

The relative importance of dyslipidemia differs between type 1 and type 2 diabetes; for instance, LDL- and HDL-cholesterol levels are generally more favorable in type 1 diabetes patients than in nondiabetic controls [154]. Elevated HDL-cholesterol levels in type 1 diabetes, compared with nondiabetic persons, may reflect enhanced lipoprotein lipase and reduced hepatic lipase activity due to systemic insulin administration [155]. Lower activity of paraoxonase, weakening HDLs ability to prevent LDL oxidation [156], may explain why higher HDL levels do not translate into protection from CHD. In a lipoprotein analysis using nuclear magnetic resonance, higher H_3 fraction levels predicted development of CHD and the H_4 and H_5 fractions were protective, as expected [157].

32.4.3 Nephropathy

The increased risk of CHD in type 1 diabetic patients who develop nephropathy has been widely reported [158–161]. However, CHD develops in many patients free of nephropathy [159].

32.5 OUTCOMES

The incidence of CHD is approximately 1–2% per year among young asymptomatic persons with type 1 diabetes mellitus [150, 162]. These rates have to be put in the appropriate context: the mean age at baseline for patients in these studies was only about 30 years. Over the next 10 years, a staggering 16% of the patients will have developed CHD in the Pittsburgh Epidemiology of Diabetes Complication study. By their mid 40s, over 70% of men and 50% of women with type 1 diabetes will develop coronary artery calcification [163] – a marker of atherosclerotic plaque burden. CAD is the main cause of death in persons with type 1 diabetes. Accelerated atherosclerosis and diabetic cardiomyopathy contribute to the excess mortality. In type 1 diabetes patients, atherosclerosis occurs earlier in life and is more diffuse [164, 165], leading to higher case fatality [166, 167], higher cardiac failure [168] and restenosis rates [169], and shorter survival [170–172], compared with the general population. Women with type 1 diabetes are affected as often as men and 9–29 times more likely to die of CAD than nondiabetic women; the risk for men is increased fourfold to ninefold [173–176]. By age 55, 35% of type 1 diabetes patients will have died of CAD, compared with only 8% of nondiabetic men and 4% of women [173].

32.6 SUMMARY

This short chapter cannot include all or even most of the remarkable advances in understanding the association between diabetes and CVD.

The number of cohort studies that include baseline glucose tolerance tests in addition to the classical heart disease risk factors has increased, as has the information derived from systematic reviews and meta-analyses showing that postprandial or postchallenge glucose is a stronger risk factor for macrovascular disease than fasting glucose, that proinsulin may be a stronger risk factor than total insulin, and that much of the increased cardiovascular risk is due to dyslipidemia and hypertension, which appear before hyperglycemia. Clinical trials have confirmed the clinical importance of these risk factors, with lipid-lowering and antihypertensive therapy usually as beneficial for diabetics as for nondiabetics. Hyperglycemia at the time of heart attack or stroke is associated with a poorer prognosis, but the cardiovascular benefit of insulin treatment and glucose control is less certain.

Many studies have confirmed that diabetes is an independent risk factor for stroke; antihypertensives are the most effective prevention in persons with and without diabetes.

References

1. West, K. (1978) *Epidemiology of Diabetes Mellitus and Its Vascular Complications*, Elsevier, New York.
2. WHO (1980) WHO Expert Committee on Diabetes Mellitus. 2nd report. WHO Tech. Rep. Ser. 646, World Health Organization, Geneva.
3. National Diabetes Data Group (1979) Classification and diagnosis of diabetes mellitus and other categories of glucose intolerance. *Diabetes*, **28** (12), 1039–57.
4. Epstein, F.H. (1985) Hyperglycaemia as a risk factor for coronary heart disease. *Monographs on Atherosclerosis*, **13**, 92–7.
5. Coutinho, M., Gerstein, H.C., Wang, Y. and Yusuf, S. (1999) The relationship between glucose and incident cardiovascular events. A metaregression analysis of published data from 20 studies of 95,783 individuals followed for 12.4 years. *Diabetes Care*, **22** (2), 233–40.
6. DECODE Study Group, European Diabetes Epidemiology Group (2003) Is the current definition for diabetes relevant to mortality risk from all causes and cardiovascular and noncardiovascular diseases? *Diabetes Care*, **26** (3), 688–96.
7. Khaw, K.T., Wareham, N., Bingham, S. *et al.* (2004) Association of hemoglobin A1c with cardiovascular disease and mortality in adults: the European prospective investigation into cancer in Norfolk. *Annals of Internal Medicine*, **141** (6), 413–20.
8. Selvin, E., Marinopoulos, S., Berkenblit, G. *et al.* (2004) Meta-analysis: glycosylated hemoglobin and cardiovascular disease in diabetes mellitus. *Annals of Internal Medicine*, **141** (6), 421–31.
9. Muggeo, M., Verlato, G., Bonora, E. *et al.* (1995) Long-term instability of fasting plasma glucose predicts mortality in elderly NIDDM patients: the Verona Diabetes Study. *Diabetologia*, **38** (6), 672–9.
10. Muggeo, M., Verlato, G., Bonora, E. *et al.* (1997) Long-term instability of fasting plasma glucose, a novel predictor of cardiovascular mortality in elderly patients with non-insulin-dependent diabetes mellitus: the Verona Diabetes Study. *Circulation*, **96** (6), 1750–4.
11. Muggeo, M., Zoppini, G., Bonora, E. *et al.* (2000) Fasting plasma glucose variability predicts 10-year survival of type 2 diabetic patients: the Verona Diabetes Study. *Diabetes Care*, **23** (1), 45–50.
12. Bonora, E. and Muggeo, M. (2001) Postprandial blood glucose as a risk factor for cardiovascular disease in type II diabetes: the epidemiological evidence. *Diabetologia*, **44** (12), 2107–14.
13. Ceriello, A. (2005) Postprandial hyperglycemia and diabetes complications: is it time to treat? *Diabetes*, **54** (1), 1–7.
14. Knatterud, G.L., Klimt, C.R., Levin, M.E. *et al.* (1978) Effects of hypoglycemic agents on vascular complications in patients with adult-onset diabetes. VII. Mortality and selected nonfatal events with insulin treatment. *Journal of the American Medical Association*, **240** (1), 37–42.
15. Genuth, S. (1996) Exogenous insulin administration and cardiovascular risk in non-insulin-dependent and insulin-dependent diabetes mellitus. *Annals of Internal Medicine*, **124** (1 Pt 2), 104–9.
16. UK Prospective Diabetes Study (UKPDS) Group (1998) Intensive blood-glucose control with sulphonylureas or insulin compared with conventional treatment and risk of complications in patients with type 2 diabetes (UKPDS 33). *Lancet*, **352** (9131), 837–53.
17. Stratton, I.M., Adler, A.I., Neil, H.A. *et al.* (2000) Association of glycaemia with macrovascular and microvascular complications of type 2 diabetes (UKPDS 35): prospective observational study. *British Medical Journal*, **321** (7258), 405–12.
18. Stettler, C., Allemann, S., Juni, P. *et al.* (2006) Glycemic control and macrovascular disease in types 1 and 2 diabetes mellitus: meta-analysis of randomized trials. *American Heart Journal*, **152**, 27–38.

19. Bonora, E. (2002) Postprandial peaks as a risk factor for cardiovascular disease: epidemiological perspectives. *International Journal of Clinical Practice. Supplement*, **129**, 5–11.

20. Capes, S.E., Hunt, D., Malmberg, K. and Gerstein, H.C. (2000) Stress hyperglycaemia and increased risk of death after myocardial infarction in patients with and without diabetes: a systematic overview. *Lancet*, **355** (9206), 773–8.

21. Kosiborod, M., Rathore, S.S., Inzucchi, S.E. *et al.* (2005) Admission glucose and mortality in elderly patients hospitalized with acute myocardial infarction: implications for patients with and without recognized diabetes. *Circulation*, **111** (23), 3078–86.

22. Goyal, A., Mahaffey, K.W., Garg, J. *et al.* (2006) Prognostic significance of the change in glucose level in the first 24h after acute myocardial infarction: results from the CARDINAL study. *European Heart Journal*, **27** (11), 1289–97.

23. Bhadriraju, S., Ray, K.K., DeFranco, A.C. *et al.* (2006) Association between blood glucose and long-term mortality in patients with acute coronary syndromes in the OPUS-TIMI 16 trial. *The American Journal of Cardiology*, **97** (11), 1573–7.

24. Scognamiglio, R., Negut, C., De Kreutzenberg, S.V. *et al.* (2005) Postprandial myocardial perfusion in healthy subjects and in type 2 diabetic patients. *Circulation*, **112** (2), 179–84.

25. Fath-Ordoubadi, F. and Beatt, K.J. (1997) Glucose–insulin–potassium therapy for treatment of acute myocardial infarction: an overview of randomized placebo-controlled trials. *Circulation*, **96** (4), 1152–6.

26. Schipke, J.D., Friebe, R. and Gams, E. (2006) Forty years of glucose–insulin–potassium (GIK) in cardiac surgery: a review of randomized, controlled trials. *European Journal of Cardio-Thoracic Surgery*, **29** (4), 479–85.

27. Pittas, A.G., Siegel, R.D. and Lau, J. (2006) Insulin therapy and in-hospital mortality in critically ill patients: systematic review and meta-analysis of randomized controlled trials. *JPEN: Journal of Parenteral and Enteral Nutrition*, **30** (2), 164–72.

28. Malmberg, K. (1997) Prospective randomised study of intensive insulin treatment on long term survival after acute myocardial infarction in patients with diabetes mellitus. DIGAMI (Diabetes Mellitus, Insulin Glucose Infusion in Acute Myocardial Infarction) Study Group [see comments]. *British Medical Journal*, **314** (7093), 1512–15.

29. Malmberg, K., Ryden, L., Wedel, H. *et al.* (2005) Intense metabolic control by means of insulin in patients with diabetes mellitus and acute myocardial infarction (DIGAMI 2): effects on mortality and morbidity. *European Heart Journal*, **26** (7), 650–61.

30. Diaz, R., Paolasso, E.A., Piegas, L.S. *et al.* (1998) Metabolic modulation of acute myocardial infarction. The ECLA (Estudios Cardiologicos Latinoamerica) Collaborative Group. *Circulation*, **98** (21), 2227–34.

31. Mehta, S.R., Yusuf, S., Diaz, R. *et al.* (2005) Effect of glucose–insulin–potassium infusion on mortality in patients with acute ST-segment elevation myocardial infarction: the CREATE-ECLA randomized controlled trial. *Journal of the American Medical Association*, **293** (4), 437–46.

32. Cheung, N.W., Wong, V.W. and McLean, M. (2006) The Hyperglycemia: Intensive Insulin Infusion In Infarction (HI-5) study: a randomized controlled trial of insulin infusion therapy for myocardial infarction. *Diabetes Care*, **29** (4), 765–70.

33. Gandhi, G.Y., Nuttall, G.A., Abel, M.D. *et al.* (2007) Intensive intraoperative insulin therapy versus conventional glucose management during cardiac surgery. *Annals of Internal Medicine*, **146**, 233–43.

34. Stout, R.W. (1990) Insulin and atheroma. 20-yr perspective. *Diabetes Care*, **13** (6), 631–54.

35. Ferrara, A., Barrett-Connor, E.L. and Edelstein, S.L. (1994) Hyperinsulinemia does not increase the risk of fatal cardiovascular disease in elderly men or women without diabetes: the Rancho Bernardo Study, 1984–1991. *American Journal of Epidemiology*, **140** (10), 857–69.

36. McKeigue, P. and Davey, G. (1995) Associations between insulin levels and cardiovascular disease are confounded by comorbidity. *Diabetes Care*, **18** (9), 1294–8.

37. Welborn, T.A. and Wearne, K. (1979) Coronary heart disease incidence and cardiovascular mortality in Busselton with reference to glucose and insulin concentrations. *Diabetes Care*, **2** (2), 154–60.

38. Pyorala, K. (1979) Relationship of glucose tolerance and plasma insulin to the incidence of coronary heart disease: results from two population studies in Finland. *Diabetes Care*, **2** (2), 131–41.

39. Ducimetiere, P., Eschwege, E., Papoz, L. *et al.* (1980) Relationship of plasma insulin levels to the incidence of myocardial infarction and coronary heart disease mortality in a middle-aged population. *Diabetologia*, **19** (3), 205–10.

40. Ruige, J.B., Assendelft, W.J., Dekker, J.M. *et al.* (1998) Insulin and risk of cardiovascular disease: a meta-analysis. *Circulation*, **97** (10), 996–1001.

41. Lehto, S., Ronnemaa, T., Pyorala, K. and Laakso, M. (2000) Cardiovascular risk factors clustering with endogenous hyperinsulinaemia predict death from coronary heart disease in patients with type II diabetes. *Diabetologia*, **43** (2), 148–55.

42. Bonora, E., Formentini, G., Calcaterra, F. *et al.* (2002) HOMA-estimated insulin resistance is an independent predictor of cardiovascular disease in type 2 diabetic subjects: prospective data from the Verona Diabetes Complications Study. *Diabetes Care*, **25** (7), 1135–41.

43. Adler, A.I., Neil, H.A., Manley, S.E. *et al.* (1999) Hyperglycemia and hyperinsulinemia at diagnosis of diabetes and their association with subsequent cardiovascular disease in the United Kingdom Prospective Diabetes Study (UKPDS 47). *American Heart Journal*, **138** (5 Pt 1), S353–9.

44. Adler, A.I., Levy, J.C., Matthews, D.R. *et al.* (2005) Insulin sensitivity at diagnosis of type 2 diabetes is not associated with subsequent cardiovascular disease (UKPDS 67). *Diabetic Medicine*, **22** (3), 306–11.

45. Rewers, M., Zaccaro, D., D'Agostino, R. *et al.* (2004) Insulin sensitivity, insulinemia, and coronary artery disease: the Insulin Resistance Atherosclerosis Study. *Diabetes Care*, **27** (3), 781–7.

46. Yudkin, J.S., Denver, A.E., Mohamed-Ali, V. *et al.* (1997) The relationship of concentrations of insulin and proinsulin-like molecules with coronary heart disease prevalence and incidence. A study of two ethnic groups. *Diabetes Care*, **20** (7), 1093–100.

47. Zethelius, B., Byberg, L., Hales, C.N. *et al.* (2002) Proinsulin is an independent predictor of coronary heart disease: report from a 27-year follow-up study. *Circulation*, **105** (18), 2153–8.

48. Oh, J.Y., Barrett-Connor, E. and Wedick, N.M. (2002) Sex differences in the association between proinsulin and intact insulin with coronary heart disease in nondiabetic older adults: the Rancho Bernardo Study. *Circulation*, **105** (11), 1311–16.

49. Janka, H.U., Ziegler, A.G., Standl, E. and Mehnert, H. (1987) Daily insulin dose as a predictor of macrovascular disease in insulin treated non-insulin-dependent diabetics. *Diabete and Metabolisme*, **13** (3 Pt 2), 359–64.

50. Nelson, R.G., Sievers, M.L., Knowler, W.C. *et al.* (1990) Low incidence of fatal coronary heart disease in Pima Indians despite high prevalence of non-insulin-dependent diabetes. *Circulation*, **81** (3), 987–95.

51. UK Prospective Diabetes Study Group (1998) Tight blood pressure control and risk of macrovascular and microvascular complications in type 2 diabetes: UKPDS 38. *British Medical Journal*, **317** (7160), 703–13.

52. Irons, B.K., Greene, R.S., Mazzolini, T.A. *et al.* (2006) Implications of rosiglitazone and pioglitazone on cardiovascular risk in patients with type 2 diabetes mellitus. *Pharmacotherapy*, **26** (2), 168–81.

53. Yki-Jarvinen, H. (2004) Thiazolidinediones. *The New England Journal of Medicine*, **351** (11), 1106–18.

54. Gerstein, H.C., Yusuf, S., Bosch, J. *et al.* (2006) Effect of rosiglitazone on the frequency of diabetes in patients with impaired glucose tolerance or impaired fasting glucose: a randomised controlled trial. *Lancet*, **368** (9541), 1096–105.

55. Dormandy, J.A., Charbonnel, B., Eckland, D.J. *et al.* (2005) Secondary prevention of macrovascular events in patients with type 2 diabetes in the PROactive Study (PROspective pioglitAzone Clinical Trial In macroVascular Events): a randomised controlled trial. *Lancet*, **366** (9493), 1279–89.

56. Haffner, S.M., Stern, M.P., Hazuda, H.P. *et al.* (1990) Cardiovascular risk factors in confirmed prediabetic individuals. Does the clock for coronary heart disease start ticking before the onset of clinical diabetes? *Journal of the American Medical Association*, **263** (21), 2893–8.

57. McPhillips, J.B., Barrett-Connor, E. and Wingard, D.L. (1990) Cardiovascular disease risk factors prior to the diagnosis of impaired glucose tolerance and non-insulin-dependent diabetes mellitus in a community of older adults. *American Journal of Epidemiology*, **131** (3), 443–53.

58. UK Prospective Diabetes Study (UKPDS) Group (1998) Effect of intensive blood-glucose control with metformin on complications in overweight patients with type 2 diabetes (UKPDS 34). *Lancet*, **352** (9131), 854–65.

59. Adler, A.I., Stratton, I.M., Neil, H.A. *et al.* (2000) Association of systolic blood pressure with macrovascular and microvascular complications of type 2 diabetes (UKPDS 36): prospective observational study. *British Medical Journal*, **321** (7258), 412–19.

60. Stratton, I.M., Cull, C.A., Adler, A.I. *et al.* (2006) Additive effects of glycaemia and blood pressure exposure on risk of complications in type 2 diabetes: a prospective observational study (UKPDS 75). *Diabetologia*, **49**, 1761–9.

61. Vijan, S. and Hayward, R.A. (2003) Treatment of hypertension in type 2 diabetes mellitus: blood

pressure goals, choice of agents, and setting priorities in diabetes care. *Annals of Internal Medicine*, **138** (7), 593–602.

62. The Antihypertensive and Lipid-Lowering Treatment to Prevent Heart Attack Trial (ALLHAT) (2002) Major outcomes in high-risk hypertensive patients randomized to angiotensin-converting enzyme inhibitor or calcium channel blocker vs diuretic. *Journal of the American Medical Association*, **288** (23), 2981–97.

63. Strippoli, G.F., Craig, M. and Craig, J.C. (2005) Antihypertensive agents for preventing diabetic kidney disease. *Cochrane Database of Systematic Reviews*, 4 (Art. No.: CD004136), DOI: 10.1002/14651858.CD004136.pub2.

64. Laakso, M., Voutilainen, E., Sarlund, H. *et al.* (1985) Serum lipids and lipoproteins in middle-aged non-insulin-dependent diabetics. *Atherosclerosis*, **56** (3), 271–81.

65. Austin, M.A. and Edwards, K.L. (1996) Small, dense low density lipoproteins, the insulin resistance syndrome and noninsulin-dependent diabetes. *Current Opinion in Lipidology*, **7** (3), 167–71.

66. Vijan, S. and Hayward, R.A. (2004) Pharmacologic lipid-lowering therapy in type 2 diabetes mellitus: background paper for the American College of Physicians. *Annals of Internal Medicine*, **140** (8), 650–8.

67. Snow, V., Aronson, M.D., Hornbake, E.R. *et al.* (2004) Lipid control in the management of type 2 diabetes mellitus: a clinical practice guideline from the American College of Physicians. *Annals of Internal Medicine*, **140** (8), 644–9.

68. Baigent, C., Keech, A., Kearney, P.M. *et al.* (2005) Efficacy and safety of cholesterol-lowering treatment: prospective meta-analysis of data from 90,056 participants in 14 randomised trials of statins. *Lancet*, **366** (9493), 1267–78.

69. Costa, J., Borges, M., David, C. and Vaz Carneiro, A. (2006) Efficacy of lipid lowering drug treatment for diabetic and non-diabetic patients: meta-analysis of randomised controlled trials. *British Medical Journal*, **332** (7550), 1115–24.

70. Colhoun, H.M., Betteridge, D.J., Durrington, P.N. *et al.* (2004) Primary prevention of cardiovascular disease with atorvastatin in type 2 diabetes in the Collaborative Atorvastatin Diabetes Study (CARDS): multicentre randomised placebo-controlled trial. *Lancet*, **364** (9435), 685–96.

71. Diabetes Atherosclerosis Intervention Study Investigators (2001) Effect of fenofibrate on progression of coronary-artery disease in type 2 diabetes: the Diabetes Atherosclerosis Intervention Study, a randomised study. *Lancet*, **357** (9260), 905–10.

72. Keech, A., Simes, R.J., Barter, P. *et al.* (2005) Effects of long-term fenofibrate therapy on cardiovascular events in 9795 people with type 2 diabetes mellitus (the FIELD study): randomised controlled trial. *Lancet*, **366** (9500), 1849–61.

73. Rubins, H.B., Robins, S.J., Collins, D. *et al.* (2002) Diabetes, plasma insulin, and cardiovascular disease: subgroup analysis from the Department of Veterans Affairs high-density lipoprotein intervention trial (VA-HIT). *Archives of Internal Medicine*, **162** (22), 2597–604.

74. Wulffele, M.G., Kooy, A., de Zeeuw, D. *et al.* (2004) The effect of metformin on blood pressure, plasma cholesterol and triglycerides in type 2 diabetes mellitus: a systematic review. *Journal of Internal Medicine*, **256** (1), 1–14.

75. Chiquette, E., Ramirez, G. and Defronzo, R. (2004) A meta-analysis comparing the effect of thiazolidinediones on cardiovascular risk factors. *Archives of Internal Medicine*, **164** (19), 2097–104.

76. Goldberg, R.B., Kendall, D.M., Deeg, M.A. *et al.* (2005) A comparison of lipid and glycemic effects of pioglitazone and rosiglitazone in patients with type 2 diabetes and dyslipidemia. *Diabetes Care*, **28** (7), 1547–54.

77. Trevisan, M., Liu, J., Bahsas, F.B. and Menotti, A. (1998) Syndrome X and mortality: a population-based study. Risk Factor and Life Expectancy Research Group. *American Journal of Epidemiology*, **148** (10), 958–66.

78. Isomaa, B., Almgren, P., Tuomi, T. *et al.* (2001) Cardiovascular morbidity and mortality associated with the metabolic syndrome. *Diabetes Care*, **24** (4), 683–9.

79. Hunt, K.J., Resendez, R.G., Williams, K. *et al.* (2004) National Cholesterol Education Program versus World Health Organization metabolic syndrome in relation to all-cause and cardiovascular mortality in the San Antonio Heart Study. *Circulation*, **110** (10), 1251–7.

80. Lakka, H.M., Laaksonen, D.E., Lakka, T.A. *et al.* (2002) The metabolic syndrome and total and cardiovascular disease mortality in middle-aged men. *Journal of the American Medical Association*, **288** (21), 2709–16.

81. Ford, E.S. (2004) The metabolic syndrome and mortality from cardiovascular disease and all-causes: findings from the National Health and Nutrition Examination Survey II Mortality Study. *Atherosclerosis*, **173** (2), 309–14.

82. Stern, M.P., Williams, K., Gonzalez-Villalpando, C. *et al.* (2004) Does the metabolic syndrome

improve identification of individuals at risk of type 2 diabetes and/or cardiovascular disease? *Diabetes Care*, **27** (11), 2676–81.

83. Kahn, R., Buse, J., Ferrannini, E. and Stern, M. (2005) The metabolic syndrome: time for a critical appraisal: joint statement from the American Diabetes Association and the European Association for the Study of Diabetes. *Diabetes Care*, **28** (9), 2289–304.

84. Grundy, S.M. (2006) Does the metabolic syndrome exist? *Diabetes Care*, **29** (7), 1689–92; discussion 1693–86.

85. Gotto, A.M. Jr, Blackburn, G.L., Dailey, G.E. III *et al.* (2006) The metabolic syndrome: a call to action. *Coronary Artery Disease*, **17** (1), 77–80.

86. Han, T.S., Sattar, N. and Lean, M. (2006) Assessment of obesity and its clinical implications. *British Medical Journal*, **333**, 695–8.

87. National Heart, Lung, and Blood Institute, National Institute of Diabetes and Digestive and Kidney Diseases (1998) *Clinical Guidelines on the Identification, Evaluation, and Treatment of Overweight and Obesity in Adults: The Evidence Report*, NIH Publication 98-4083, US Department of Health and Human Services, Bethesda, MD.

88. Tuomilehto, J., Lindstrom, J., Erikson, J.G. *et al.* (2001) Prevention of type 2 diabetes mellitus by changes in lifestyle among subjects with impaired glucose tolerance. *The New England Journal of Medicine*, **344**, 1343–50.

89. Knowler, W.C., Barrett-Connor, E., Fowler, S.E. *et al.* (2002) Reduction in the incidence of type 2 diabetes with lifestyle intervention or metformin. *The New England Journal of Medicine*, **346**, 393–403.

90. Yudkin, J.S. (1993) How can we best prolong life? Benefits of coronary risk factor reduction in non-diabetic and diabetic subjects. *British Medical Journal*, **306**, 1313–18.

91. Ockene, J.K., Kuller, L.H., Svendsen, K.H. and Meilahn, E. (1990) The relationship of smoking cessation to coronary heart disease and lung cancer in the Multiple Risk Factor Intervention Trial. *Journal of Public Health*, **80**, 954–8.

92. American Diabetes Association (2004) Aspirin therapy in diabetes (position statement). *Diabetes Care*, **27** (Suppl 1), S72–3.

93. Ridker, P.M., Cook, N.R., Lee, I.-M. *et al.* (2005) A randomized trial of low-dose aspirin in the primary prevention of cardiovascular disease in women. *The New England Journal of Medicine*, **352**, 1293–304.

94. American Diabetes Association (2007) Standards of medical care in diabetes – 2007 (position statement). *Diabetes Care*, **27** (Suppl 1), S4–41.

95. Folsom, A.R., Chambless, L.E., Ballantyne, C.M. *et al.* (2006) An assessment of incremental coronary risk prediction using C-reactive protein and other novel risk markers: the atherosclerosis risk in communities study. *Archives of Internal Medicine*, **166** (13), 1368–73.

96. Wang, T.J., Gona, P., Larson, M.G. *et al.* (2006) Multiple biomarkers for the prediction of first major cardiovascular events and death. *The New England Journal of Medicine*, **355**, 2631–9.

97. Kannel, W.B. and McGee, D.L. (1979) Diabetes and cardiovascular disease. The Framingham study. *Journal of the American Medical Association*, **241** (19), 2035–8.

98. Fuller, J.H., Shipley, M.J., Rose, G. *et al.* (1983) Mortality from coronary heart disease and stroke in relation to degree of glycaemia: the Whitehall study. *British Medical Journal (Clinical Research Edition)*, **287** (6396), 867–70.

99. National Diabetes Data Group (1995) *Diabetes in America*, 2nd edn, National Institutes of Health, National Institute of Diabetes and Digestive and Kidney Diseases, Bethesda, MD.

100. Huxley, R., Barzi, F. and Woodward, M. (2006) Excess risk of fatal coronary heart disease associated with diabetes in men and women: meta-analysis of 37 prospective cohort studies. *British Medical Journal*, **332** (7533), 73–8.

101. Kanaya, A.M., Grady, D. and Barrett-Connor, E. (2002) Explaining the sex difference in coronary heart disease mortality among patients with type 2 diabetes mellitus: a meta-analysis. *Archives of Internal Medicine*, **162** (15), 1737–45.

102. Tonstad, S., Rosvold, E.O., Furu, K. and Skurtveit, S. (2004) Undertreatment and overtreatment with statins: the Oslo Health Study 2000–2001. *Journal of Internal Medicine*, **255** (4), 494–502.

103. Cull, C.A., Neil, H.A. and Holman, R.R. (2004) Changing aspirin use in patients with type 2 diabetes in the UKPDS. *Diabetic Medicine*, **21** (12), 1368–71.

104. Wexler, D.J., Grant, R.W., Meigs, J.B. *et al.* (2005) Sex disparities in treatment of cardiac risk factors in patients with type 2 diabetes. *Diabetes Care*, **28** (3), 514–20.

105. Haffner, S.M., Lehto, S., Ronnemaa, T. *et al.* (1998) Mortality from coronary heart disease in subjects with type 2 diabetes and in nondiabetic subjects with and without prior myocardial infarction. *The New England Journal of Medicine*, **339** (4), 229–34.

106. Lee, C.D., Folsom, A.R., Pankow, J.S. and Brancati, F.L. (2004) Cardiovascular events in diabetic and nondiabetic adults with or without

history of myocardial infarction. *Circulation*, **109** (7), 855–60.

107. Whiteley, L., Padmanabhan, S., Hole, D. and Isles, C. (2005) Should diabetes be considered a coronary heart disease risk equivalent? Results from 25 years of follow-up in the Renfrew and Paisley Survey. *Diabetes Care*, **28** (7), 1588–93.

108. Malmberg, K., Yusuf, S., Gerstein, H.C. *et al.* (2000) Impact of diabetes on long-term prognosis in patients with unstable angina and non-Q-wave myocardial infarction: results of the OASIS (Organization to Assess Strategies for Ischemic Syndromes) Registry. *Circulation*, **102** (9), 1014–19.

109. Lotufo, P.A., Gaziano, J.M., Chae, C.U. *et al.* (2001) Diabetes and all-cause and coronary heart disease mortality among US male physicians. *Archives of Internal Medicine*, **161** (2), 242–7.

110. Wannamethee, S.G., Shaper, A.G. and Lennon, L. (2004) Cardiovascular disease incidence and mortality in older men with diabetes and in men with coronary heart disease. *Heart*, **90** (12), 1398–403.

111. Juutilainen, A., Lehto, S., Ronnemaa, T. *et al.* (2005) Type 2 diabetes as a 'coronary heart disease equivalent': an 18-year prospective population-based study in Finnish subjects. *Diabetes Care*, **28** (12), 2901–7.

112. Hu, G., Jousilahti, P., Qiao, Q. *et al.* (2005) Sex differences in cardiovascular and total mortality among diabetic and non-diabetic individuals with or without history of myocardial infarction. *Diabetologia*, **48** (5), 856–61.

113. Langer, A., Freeman, M.R., Josse, R.G. *et al.* (1991) Detection of silent myocardial ischemia in diabetes mellitus. *The American Journal of Cardiology*, **67** (13), 1073–8.

114. Miettinen, H., Lehto, S., Salomaa, V. *et al.* (1998) Impact of diabetes on mortality after the first myocardial infarction. The FINMONICA Myocardial Infarction Register Study Group. *Diabetes Care*, **21** (1), 69–75.

115. Mukamal, K.J., Nesto, R.W., Cohen, M.C. *et al.* (2001) Impact of diabetes on long-term survival after acute myocardial infarction: comparability of risk with prior myocardial infarction. *Diabetes Care*, **24** (8), 1422–7.

116. Kannel, W.B., Hjortland, M. and Castelli, W.P. (1974) Role of diabetes in congestive heart failure: the Framingham study. *The American Journal of Cardiology*, **34** (1), 29–34.

117. Funarow, G., Adams, K. and Strausser, B. (2002) ADHERE (Acute Decompensated Heart Failure National Registry): rationale, design, and subject population. *Journal of Cardiac Failure*, **8**, S49.

118. Garcia, M.J., McNamara, P.M., Gordon, T. and Kannel, W.B. (1974) Morbidity and mortality in diabetics in the Framingham population. Sixteen year follow-up study. *Diabetes*, **23** (2), 105–11.

119. Bell, D.S. (2003) Heart failure: the frequent, forgotten, and often fatal complication of diabetes. *Diabetes Care*, **26** (8), 2433–41.

120. Poornima, I.G., Parikh, P. and Shannon, R.P. (2006) Diabetic cardiomyopathy: the search for a unifying hypothesis. *Circulation Research*, **98** (5), 596–605.

121. Kitzman, D.W., Gardin, J.M., Gottdiener, J.S. *et al.* (2001) Importance of heart failure with preserved systolic function in patients > or = 65 years of age. Cardiovascular Health Study. *The American Journal of Cardiology*, **87** (4), 413–19.

122. Bertoni, A.G., Tsai, A., Kasper, E.K. and Brancati, F.L. (2003) Diabetes and idiopathic cardiomyopathy: a nationwide case–control study. *Diabetes Care*, **26** (10), 2791–5.

123. Huikuri, H.V., Airaksinen, J.K., Lilja, M. and Takkunen, J.T. (1986) Echocardiographic evaluation of left ventricular response to isometric exercise in young insulin-dependent diabetics. *Acta Diabetologica Latina*, **23** (3), 193–200.

124. Amato, L., Paolisso, G., Cacciatore, F. *et al.* (1997) Congestive heart failure predicts the development of non-insulin-dependent diabetes mellitus in the elderly. The Osservatorio Geriatrico Regione Campania Group. *Diabetes and Metabolism*, **23** (3), 213–18.

125. Rosano, G.M., Vitale, C., Sposato, B. *et al.* (2003) Trimetazidine improves left ventricular function in diabetic patients with coronary artery disease: a double-blind placebo-controlled study. *Cardiovascular Diabetology*, **2**, 16.

126. Bell, D.S. (1995) Diabetic cardiomyopathy. A unique entity or a complication of coronary artery disease? *Diabetes Care*, **18** (5), 708–14.

127. Raev, D.C. (1994) Left ventricular function and specific diabetic complications in other target organs in young insulin-dependent diabetics: an echocardiographic study. *Heart Vessels*, **9** (3), 121–8.

128. Sasso, F.C., Carbonara, O., Cozzolino, D. *et al.* (2000) Effects of insulin–glucose infusion on left ventricular function at rest and during dynamic exercise in healthy subjects and noninsulin dependent diabetic patients: a radionuclide ventriculographic study. *Journal of the American College of Cardiology*, **36** (1), 219–26.

129. Shekelle, P.G., Rich, M.W., Morton, S.C. *et al.* (2003) Efficacy of angiotensin-converting enzyme inhibitors and beta-blockers in the management of left ventricular systolic dysfunction according to

race, gender, and diabetic status: a meta-analysis of major clinical trials. *Journal of the American College of Cardiology*, **41** (9), 1529–38.

130. Haas, S.J., Vos, T., Gilbert, R.E. and Krum, H. (2003) Are beta-blockers as efficacious in patients with diabetes mellitus as in patients without diabetes mellitus who have chronic heart failure? A meta-analysis of large-scale clinical trials. *American Heart Journal*, **146** (5), 848–53.

131. Bell, D.S., Lukas, M.A., Holdbrook, F.K. and Fowler, M.B. (2006) The effect of carvedilol on mortality risk in heart failure patients with diabetes: results of a meta-analysis. *Current Medical Research and Opinion*, **22** (2), 287–96.

132. Kagan, A., Popper, J.S. and Rhoads, G.G. (1980) Factors related to stroke incidence in Hawaii Japanese men. The Honolulu Heart Study. *Stroke*, **11** (1), 14–21.

133. Lees, K.R. and Walters, M.R. (2005) Acute stroke and diabetes. *Cerebrovascular Diseases*, **20** (Suppl 1), 9–14.

134. Eguchi, K., Kario, K. and Shimada, K. (2003) Greater impact of coexistence of hypertension and diabetes on silent cerebral infarcts. *Stroke*, **34** (10), 2471–4.

135. Folsom, A.R., Rasmussen, M.L., Chambless, L.E. *et al.* (1999) Prospective associations of fasting insulin, body fat distribution, and diabetes with risk of ischemic stroke. *Diabetes Care*, **22** (7), 1077–83.

136. Sacco, R.L., Benson, R.T., Kargman, D.E. *et al.* (2001) High-density lipoprotein cholesterol and ischemic stroke in the elderly: the Northern Manhattan Stroke Study. *Journal of the American Medical Association*, **285** (21), 2729–35.

137. Guerrero-Romero, F. and Rodriguez-Moran, M. (1999) Proteinuria is an independent risk factor for ischemic stroke in non-insulin-dependent diabetes mellitus. *Stroke*, **30** (9), 1787–91.

138. Idris, I., Thomson, G.A. and Sharma, J.C. (2006) Diabetes mellitus and stroke. *International Journal of Clinical Practice*, **60** (1), 48–56.

139. The DECODE Study Group, European Diabetes Epidemiology Group (2001) Glucose tolerance and cardiovascular mortality: comparison of fasting and 2-hour diagnostic criteria. *Archives of Internal Medicine*, **161** (3), 397–405.

140. Pyorala, M., Miettinen, H., Laakso, M. and Pyorala, K. (1998) Hyperinsulinemia and the risk of stroke in healthy middle-aged men: the 22-year follow-up results of the Helsinki Policemen Study. *Stroke*, **29** (9), 1860–6.

141. Witt, B.J., Ballman, K.V., Brown, R.D. Jr *et al.* (2006) The incidence of stroke after myocardial infarction: a meta-analysis. *The American Journal of Medicine*, **119** (4), 354.e1–9.

142. Mankovsky, B.N., Patrick, J.T., Metzger, B.E. and Saver, J.L. (1996) The size of subcortical ischemic infarction in patients with and without diabetes mellitus. *Clinical Neurology and Neurosurgery*, **98** (2), 137–41.

143. Scott, J.F., Robinson, G.M., French, J.M. *et al.* (1999) Glucose potassium insulin infusions in the treatment of acute stroke patients with mild to moderate hyperglycemia: the Glucose Insulin in Stroke Trial (GIST). *Stroke*, **30** (4), 793–9.

144. Capes, S.E., Hunt, D., Malmberg, K. *et al.* (2001) Stress hyperglycemia and prognosis of stroke in nondiabetic and diabetic patients: a systematic overview. *Stroke*, **32** (10), 2426–32.

145. Weir, C.J., Murray, G.D., Dyker, A.G. and Lees, K.R. (1997) Is hyperglycaemia an independent predictor of poor outcome after acute stroke? Results of a long-term follow up study. *British Medical Journal*, **314** (7090), 1303–6.

146. Jaillard, A., Cornu, C., Durieux, A. *et al.* (1999) Hemorrhagic transformation in acute ischemic stroke. The MAST-E Study. *Stroke*, **30** (7), 1326–32.

147. Zgibor, J.C., Piatt, G.A., Ruppert, K. *et al.* (2006) Deficiencies of cardiovascular risk prediction models for type 1 diabetes. *Diabetes Care*, **29** (8), 1860–5.

148. Libby, P., Nathan, D.M., Abraham, K. *et al.* (2005) Report of the National Heart, Lung, and Blood Institute–National Institute of Diabetes and Digestive and Kidney Diseases Working Group on cardiovascular complications of type 1 diabetes mellitus. *Circulation*, **111** (25), 3489–93.

149. Orchard, T.J., Costacou, T., Kretowski, A. and Nesto, R.W. (2006) Type 1 diabetes and coronary artery disease. *Diabetes Care*, **29** (11), 2528–38.

150. Orchard, T.J., Olson, J.C., Erbey, J.R. *et al.* (2003) Insulin resistance-related factors, but not glycemia, predict coronary artery disease in type 1 diabetes: 10-year follow-up data from the Pittsburgh Epidemiology of Diabetes Complications Study. *Diabetes Care*, **26**, 1374–9.

151. Snell-Bergeon, J.K., Hokanson, J.E., Jensen, L. *et al.* (2003) Progression of coronary artery calcification in type 1 diabetes: the importance of glycemic control. *Diabetes Care*, **26**, 2923–8.

152. Nathan, D.M., Cleary, P.A., Backlund, J.Y. *et al.* (2005) Intensive diabetes treatment and

cardiovascular disease in patients with type 1 diabetes. *The New England Journal of Medicine*, **353** (25), 2643–53.

153. The Diabetes Control and Complications Trial Research Group (1993) The effect of intensive treatment of diabetes on the development and progression of long-term complications in insulin-dependent diabetes mellitus. *The New England Journal of Medicine*, **329** (14), 977–86.

154. Taskinen, M.R. (1992) Quantitative and qualitative lipoprotein abnormalities in diabetes mellitus. *Diabetes*, **41** (Suppl 2), 12–17.

155. Valabhji, J., Donovan, J., McColl, A.J. *et al.* (2002) Rates of cholesterol esterification and esterified cholesterol net mass transfer between high-density lipoproteins and apolipoprotein B-containing lipoproteins in type 1 diabetes. *Diabetic Medicine*, **19**, 424–8.

156. Mackness, B., Durrington, P.N., Boulton, A.J. *et al.* (2002) Serum paraoxonase activity in patients with type 1 diabetes compared to healthy controls. *European Journal of Clinical Investigation*, **32**, 259–64.

157. Soedamah-Muthu, S.S., Chang, Y.-F., Otvos, J. *et al.* (2003) Lipoprotein subclass measurements by nuclear magnetic resonance spectroscopy improve the prediction of coronary artery disease in type 1 diabetes: a prospective report from the Pittsburgh Epidemiology of Diabetes Complications Study. *Diabetologia*, **46**, 674–82.

158. Jensen, T., Borch-Johnsen, K., Kofoed-Enevoldsen, A. and Deckert, T. (1987) Coronary heart disease in young type 1 (insulin-dependent) diabetic patients with and without nephropathy: incidence and risk factors. *Diabetologia*, **30**, 144–8.

159. Krolewski, A.S., Warram, J.H., Christlieb, A.R. *et al.* (1985) The changing natural history of nephropathy in type I diabetes. *The American Journal of Medicine*, **78**, 785–94.

160. Tuomilehto, J., Borch-Johnsen, K., Molarius, A. *et al.* (1998) Incidence of cardiovascular disease in type 1 (insulin-dependent) diabetic subjects with and without diabetic nephropathy in Finland. *Diabetologia*, **41**, 784–90.

161. Torffvit, O., Lövestam-Adrian, M., Agardh, E. and Agardh, C.-D. (2005) Nephropathy, but not retinopathy, is associated with the development of heart disease in type 1 diabetes: a 12-year observation study of 462 patients. *Diabetic Medicine*, **22**, 723–9.

162. Soedamah-Muthu, S.S., Chaturvedi, N., Toeller, M. *et al.* (2004) Risk factors for coronary heart disease in type 1 diabetic patients in Europe. The EURODIAB Prospective Complications Study (PCS). *Diabetes Care*, **27**, 530–7.

163. Dabelea, D., Kinney, G., Snell-Bergeon, J.K. *et al.* (2003) Effect of type 1 diabetes on the gender difference in coronary artery calcification: a role for insulin resistance? The Coronary Artery Calcification in Type 1 Diabetes (CACTI) Study. *Diabetes*, **52**, 2833–9.

164. Crall, F.V. Jr and Roberts, W.C. (1978) The extramural and intramural coronary arteries in juvenile diabetes mellitus: analysis of nine necropsy patients aged 19 to 38 years with onset of diabetes before age 15 years. *The American Journal of Medicine*, **64**, 221–30.

165. Valsania, P., Zarich, S.W., Kowalchuk, G.J. *et al.* (1991) Severity of coronary artery disease in young patients with insulin-dependent diabetes mellitus. *American Heart Journal*, **122**, 695–700.

166. Chun, B.Y., Dobson, A.J. and Heller, R.F. (1997) The impact of diabetes on survival among patients with first myocardial infarction. *Diabetes Care*, **20**, 704–8.

167. Miettinen, H., Lehto, S., Salomaa, V. *et al.* (1998) Impact of diabetes on mortality after the first myocardial infarction. The FINMONICA Myocardial Infarction Register Study Group [see comments]. *Diabetes Care*, **21**, 69–75.

168. Savage, M.P., Krolewski, A.S., Kenien, G.G. *et al.* (1988) Acute myocardial infarction in diabetes mellitus and significance of congestive heart failure as a prognostic factor. *The American Journal of Cardiology*, **62**, 665–9.

169. Rozenman, Y., Sapoznikov, D., Mosseri, M. *et al.* (1997) Long-term angiographic follow-up of coronary balloon angioplasty in patients with diabetes mellitus: a clue to the explanation of the results of the BARI study. *Journal of the American College of Cardiology*, **30**, 1420–5.

170. Ferguson, J.J. (1995) NHLBI BARI clinical alert on diabetics treated with angioplasty. *Circulation*, **92**, 3371.

171. Portuese, E. and Orchard, T.J. (1995) Mortality in insulin-dependent diabetes, in *Diabetes in America* (ed National Diabetes Data Group), National Institutes of Health, Bethesda, MD.

172. Weintraub, W.S., Stein, B., Kosinski, A. *et al.* (1998) Outcome of coronary bypass surgery versus coronary angioplasty in diabetic patients with multivessel coronary artery disease. *Journal of the American College of Cardiology*, **31**, 10–19.

173. Krolewski, A.S., Kosinski, E.J., Warram, J.H. *et al.* (1987) Magnitude and determinants of coronary artery disease in juvenile-onset, insulin-dependent diabetes mellitus. *The American Journal of Cardiology*, **59**, 750–5.

174. Moss, S.E., Klein, R. and Klein, B.E. (1991) Cause-specific mortality in a population-based study of diabetes. *American Journal of Public Health*, **81**, 1158–62.

175. Dorman, J.S., LaPorte, R.E., Kuller, L.H. *et al.* (1984) The Pittsburgh insulin-dependent diabetes mellitus (IDDM) morbidity and mortality study. Mortality results. *Diabetes*, **33**, 271–6.

176. Laing, S.P., Swerdlow, A.J., Slater, S.D. *et al.* (2003) Mortality from heart disease in a cohort of 23,000 patients with insulin-treated diabetes. *Diabetologia*, **46**, 760–5.

33

The Epidemiology of Peripheral Vascular Disease[1]

Nalini Singh,[1] Stephanie Wheeler[2] and Edward J. Boyko[3]

[1]Healthcare Partners, Arcadia, CA, USA

[2]University of Washington School of Medicine, VA Puget Sound Health Care System, Seattle, WA, USA

[3]Department of Medicine, University of Washington School of Medicine, Epidemiologic Research and Information Center, VA Puget Sound Health Care System, Seattle, WA, USA

33.1 INTRODUCTION

This chapter will review the epidemiology of peripheral arterial disease (PAD) and its association with diabetes. Population-based studies have been selected to describe prevalence and incidence of PAD in the lower extremities, as well as risk factors and associated conditions. For conditions for which population-based studies do not exist, such as renal arterial stenosis and abdominal aortic aneurysm (AAA), studies using clinic-based samples are described and discussed.

33.2 MEASUREMENT AND VALIDITY

Multiple methods exist for the assessment of PAD ranging from those performed as part of the clinical exam to invasive methods requiring sophisticated technology and expense. An overview is provided in a recent American Diabetes Association consensus conference [1]. Aspects of the clinical examination that have proved valuable in identifying PAD

include abnormal pedal pulses, a unilaterally cool extremity, a prolonged venous filling time and a femoral bruit [2, 3]. The ankle–arm index (AAI), also referred to as the *ankle–brachial index*, can be easily performed and provides a direct measurement of lower limb perfusion. It has advantages over peripheral pulse palpation, in that the latter clinical method is subject to a high level of observer variability. The preferred method of the American Diabetes Association for measurement of the AAI and the one that is most reliable is to divide the higher of the dorsalis pedis or posterior tibial artery pressure as measured using a hand-held Doppler device by the higher of the right and left arm brachial systolic pressure [4]. Additional tests which might provide information about the presence of ischemia in uncertain cases are pulse volume waveform analysis and exercise treadmill testing [5]. Transcutaneous oximetry and laser Doppler measurements of the lower limb provide an assessment of skin oxygen delivery and microcirculation function, but the correlation with the AAI is low in the case of transcutaneous oximetry [6]. Nevertheless, transcutaneous oximetry has been shown to be an excellent predictor of diabetic foot ulcer healing [7]. X-ray contrast angiography should be used to provide an anatomic evaluation of a patient under evaluation for revascularization, and not as a diagnostic test

---

[1]Note to readers: we calculated *p* values and confidence intervals from the data presented in publications when these results were not provided in the publication. Such calculations are indicated by ** following the *p* value or confidence interval. In the absence of the double asterisk, the reader can presume that the numbers shown are those provided in the publications.

The Epidemiology of Diabetes Mellitus, second edition Edited by Jean-Marie Ekoé, Marian Rewers, Rhys Williams and Paul Zimmet
© 2008 John Wiley & Sons, Ltd

for PAD [1]. Given that epidemiologic research usually requires a large sample size of subjects, the method that provides the highest information content in relation to the costs of its performance is the AAI, and use of this method is predominant in the epidemiologic literature on PAD.

It is important to note that there may be considerable variability in the performance of the AAI across epidemiologic studies, which should be taken into account in their interpretation. For example, in the important 1999–2000 National Health and Nutrition Examination Survey (NHANES) conducted in the United States, the AAI was defined as the posterior tibial systolic pressure in a given limb divided by the right arm brachial pressure [8]. This methodology will likely overestimate the prevalence of PAD defined as AAI < 0.9, since the dorsalis pedis pressure was not measured, which potentially could have been higher and resulted in a higher AAI.

The problem of measurement error in the assessment of vascular disease is well recognized. Angiographic assessments of the coronary and carotid arteries result in some degree of misclassification [9, 10]. A similar situation holds for the diagnosis of PAD. Peripheral angiographic measurements have been shown to have less than perfect reliability and underestimate postmortem arterial diameter [11, 12]. Use of the AAI may be insensitive to the presence of poor limb perfusion. For example, claudication may occur even with normal or high AAI, if noncompressible, calcified distal vessels result in falsely high readings of the ankle systolic blood pressure [13]. Hallux toe blood pressure may be useful in this setting, but a strain gauge or photoplethysmograph is required for its measurement. This misclassification issue is even more problematic when a test result is used to formulate a clinical plan for an individual patient, compared with epidemiologic analysis where population statistics are the result of interest. When misclassification of PAD status occurs nondifferentially with regard to exposure (randomly), the net result is bias of any observed difference toward the null value [14]. The same holds true for exposures that are nondifferentially misclassified with regard to PAD. Therefore, observed differences found in an epidemiologic analysis of risk factors for PAD validly reflect potential causative factors for this complication, but probably underestimate the magnitude of the risk increase. Epidemiologic studies

may, therefore, draw valid conclusions regarding risk factors for PAD even if the techniques used to measure either vascular disease or the potential risk factor are prone to nondifferential misclassification.

33.3 PAD PREVALENCE

The true prevalence of PAD disease in people with diabetes is difficult to determine, since many patients are asymptomatic, do not report their symptoms or their pain perception is blunted by neuropathy. In addition, different methods have been used to estimate its presence. Claudication may be the most notable clinical symptom of PAD, but it is an insensitive measure of this condition, with symptomless diminished arterial flow estimated to occur at least two to five times as frequently as claudication [15]. The Rose questionnaire has been used by investigators to assess claudication prevalence, but it has been shown to have only moderate sensitivity (60–68%) in capturing persons with this clinical diagnosis [16]. The AAI is used most commonly, but various cutoffs have been used, leading to some difficulty with direct comparison of study findings. As mentioned previously, the American Diabetes Association produced a consensus statement in 2003 recommending the use of the AAI to screen for PAD in patients with diabetes over the age of 50 years [1]. The issues of screening and misclassification and the limitations of the AAI were acknowledged. However, the problems were not felt to detract from the clinical usefulness of the AAI in the screening and diagnosis of PAD in patients with diabetes. Recommended AAI cutpoints were:

normal if 0.91–1.30
mild obstruction if 0.70–0.90
moderate obstruction if 0.40–0.69
severe obstruction if < 0.40
poorly compressible if > 1.30.

Among population-based studies in which diabetes status was not assessed, asymptomatic PAD was found to be relatively common. Symptoms, such as claudication, were less common. Key features of studies of PAD prevalence are found in **Table 33.1**. In a population-based study in southern California by Criqui *et al.* [17] in 1985 in 613 subjects, 11.7% were found to have an AAI < 0.8, whereas 2.2% of the men and 1.7% of the women had claudication. The Edinburgh Artery

Table 33.1 Prevalence of peripheral arterial disease and claudication.[a]

Reference	Subjects	Subjects with diabetes	Prevalence AAI < 0.9	Prevalence of claudication	Notes
Orchard et al. [23]	788 with type 1 DM, ages 10–29 years	100% type 1	35% men[b] 26% women at 16 years' duration	Not assessed	Pittsburgh Epidemiology of Diabetes Complications Study II
Fowkes et al. [18]	1592 community-based subjects ages 55–74 years	—	9.0%	4.5%	Edinburgh Artery Study
Newman et al. [24]	Community-based subjects, 2214 men 2870 women ages 65 to >85 years	8.4% diabetes	13.8% men 11.4% women	2%	Cardiovascular Health Study
Beks et al. [25]	Population-based, cross-sectional survey of 2484 randomly selected adults living in Hoorn, ages 50–74 years	288 normal GT 170 impaired GT 106 new DM 67 known DM 4.9% total DM	7.0% 9.5% 15.1% 20.9%	3.1% 3.5% 3.9% 7.5%	The Hoorn Study
Hiatt et al. [20]	Community-based subjects, 1710 people ages 20–74 years	25.1% type 2 diabetes	1.6–4.3%[c]	Not assessed	The San Luis Valley Diabetes Study
Curb et al. [26]	3450 ambulatory, community-based Japanese-American men living on the island of Oahu, HI	Not described	12.6% without DM 16.7% with DM	Not assessed	The Honolulu Heart Study
Zheng et al. [27]	15 106 community-based subjects ages 45–64 years	AA men 16.0% AA women 18.5% White men 7.7% White women 6.4%	AA men 3.3% AA women 4.0% White men 2.3% White women 3.3%	AA men 0.6% AA women 0.5% White men 1.1% White women 0.6%	Atherosclerosis Risk in Communities (ARIC) Study

(continued overleaf)

Table 33.1 (*continued*)

Reference	Subjects	Subjects with diabetes	Prevalence AAI < 0.9	Prevalence of claudication	Notes
Meijer et al. [21]	Population-based cross-sectional study in 7715 subjects aged 55 years and over	9.9% diabetes	19%	1.6%	The Rotterdam Study
Hirsch et al. [22]	Clinic-based, multicenter, cross-sectional study of 6979 subjects, ages 50 to >90 years	41.3% diabetes	29%	8.7%	The PAD Awareness, Risk and Treatment: New Resources for Survival program
Murabito et al. [28]	Population-based study of 3313 subjects aged ≥ 40 years	Men 12.1 % DM Women 8.2% DM	3.6%	1.3%	Framingham Offspring Study
Gregg et al. [8]	Population-based study of 2873 subjects aged ≥ 40 years	14.6% with diabetes	4.5%	1.4%	1999–2000 National Health and Nutrition Examination Survey
Munter et al. [29]	Population-based study of 4526 subjects aged ≥ 40 years	19.3% with diabetes	5.1%Overall No DM, A_{1c}:<5.3, 3.1% 5.3–5.4, 4.8% 5.5–5.6, 4.7% 5.7–6.0, 6.4% DM A_{1c}:<7.0, 7.5% ≥7.0, 8.8%	Not assessed	National Health and Nutrition Survey 1999–2002

[a] AA: African American; DM: diabetes mellitus; GT: glucose tolerance.
[b] PAD defined as AAI < 0.8.
[c] PAD defined as the 1.0 or 5.0 percentile cutoff.

Study [18] evaluated 1592 men and women ages 55–74 years. They found 9% of the population had an AAI < 0.9 and 4.6% had claudication. The prevalence of claudication in men increased from 2.2% in the 50–59 years age category to 7.7% in the 70–74 years age category [19]. In the San Luis Valley Diabetes Study, a community-based study of 1710 people aged 20–74 years, 25.1% had type 2 diabetes [20]. This study used the 1.0 and 5.0 percentile cutoff points instead of an AAI of <0.9. The prevalence of a two-vessel abnormality on AAI testing, adjusted for diabetes status, was 1.6% at the 1.0 percentile cutoff and 4.3% at the 5.0 percentile cutoff. No data were presented on the prevalence among those without diabetes compared with those with diabetes. The Rotterdam Study enrolled 7715 subjects aged 55 years and over and found the prevalence of AAI < 0.9 to be 19.1% (16.9% in men, 20.5% in women) [21]. By contrast, 1.6% reported claudication (2.2% in men, 1.2% in women). The prevalence of AAI < 0.9 increased with age, ranging from 6.6% in men and 9.5% in women aged 55–59 years to 52% in men and 59.6% in women aged 85 years or older. Hirsch *et al.* [22] provided results from the PAD Awareness, Risk and Treatment: New Resources for Survival (PARTNERS) program, which was a clinic-based, large, multicenter, cross-sectional survey of 6979 patients chosen because they were over age 70 years or over age 50 years but with a history of tobacco use or diabetes. In this study, the prevalence of AAI < 0.9 was 29%. The prevalence of claudication ranged from 1.7% in the reference group that had no vascular disease to 15.3% in those with known prior PAD plus cerebrovascular disease.

Both asymptomatic PAD and claudication are more common among subjects with diabetes. PAD in people with diabetes is both morphologically and physiologically distinguished from nondiabetic atherosclerosis [30]. The femoropopliteal segments are most often affected, as in nondiabetic patients, but smaller vessels below the knee, such as the tibial and peroneal arteries, are more severely affected in diabetic patients than in nondiabetic patients [31, 32]. In practical terms, diabetes is associated with a high prevalence of distal arterial disease, a propensity to earlier calcification, increased thrombogenicity and generally poorer prognosis.

The Pittsburgh Epidemiology of Diabetes Complications Study II included 788 patients with type 1 diabetes for 16 years on average. Among these individuals, 35% of the men and 26% of the women had an AAI < 0.8. An interesting finding in this study was that cross-sectional prevalence of PAD was similar for men and women with 5–24 years' duration of diabetes, but after 25 years' duration, a higher prevalence of PAD was observed in women (65%) than in men (45%).

The Cardiovascular Health Study (CHS), a community-based investigation with 5084 participants aged 65 years or older at baseline, of whom 8.4% had diabetes, found that 12.4% had an AAI < 0.9 [24]. The prevalence of claudication overall was 2%. Among those in the study with diabetes, 7.2% had a normal AAI (AAI ≥ 1.0). However, 18.2% had an AAI ≥ 0.8–0.9 and 17.2% had an AAI < 0.8. The relative risk (RR) for 0.8 ≤ AAI < 0.9 associated with diabetes was 2.9 and for AAI < 0.8 was 2.6, after adjustment for age and sex.

The Hoorn Study investigated the cross-sectional association between PAD and glycemia in a random sample of people between ages 50–74 years who resided in the town of Hoorn, the Netherlands [25]. Among the 2484 subjects, the prevalence of AAI < 0.9 was 7.3%. The prevalence of an AAI < 0.9 increased according to glycemic level: it was 7.0% among those with normal glucose tolerance, 9.5% among those with impaired glucose tolerance, 15.1% among those with newly diagnosed diabetes and 20.9% among those with known diabetes. The same pattern was seen for claudication (3.1% normal glucose tolerance; 3.5% impaired glucose tolerance; 3.9% newly diagnosed diabetes; and 7.5% known diabetes).

The Honolulu Heart Study enrolled Japanese-American men living on the island of Oahu, Hawaii. Prevalence of PAD (AAI < 0.9) in the 3450 ambulatory subjects increased with age, ranging from 8.0% in those aged 71–74 years to 27.4% among those aged 85–93 years [26]. Among those without diabetes, 12.6% had an AAI < 0.9, compared with 16.7% of those with diabetes.

The Atherosclerosis Risk in Communities (ARIC) Study enrolled 15 106 middle-aged adults and examined the prevalence of PAD by ethnicity and diabetes status [27]. In African-American men the prevalence of diabetes was 16.0%, AAI < 0.9 was 3.3% and claudication was 0.6%. In African-American women the prevalence of diabetes, AAI < 0.9 and claudication was 18.5%,

4.0% and 0.5% respectively. White men, on the other hand, had a prevalence of diabetes of 7.7%, AAI < 0.9 was 2.3% and claudication was 1.1%. White women had the lowest prevalence of diabetes at 6.4%, but 3.3% had AAI < 0.9 and 0.6% had claudication.

The Framingham Offspring Study included 3313 men and women who were the children of the original cohort of the Framingham Heart Study. Subjects had a mean age of 59 years and a prevalence of diabetes of 12.1% in the men and 8.2% in the women [28]. Overall, 3.5% of the men and 3.3% of the women had an AAI < 0.9. Claudication was found in 1.9% of the men and 0.8% of the women. The odds ratio (OR) for PAD associated with diabetes was 2.3 (95% confidence interval (CI), 1.5–3.6).

The 1999–2000 NHANES included 2873 men and women aged 40 years or older, of whom 14.6% had diabetes [8]. PAD was present in 4.0% in those without diabetes and claudication was present in 1.5%. Among those with diabetes, 9.5% had PAD and 2.1% had claudication. Lower extremity ulcers were present in 2.2% of the population without diabetes but in 7.7% of the diabetic population.

Among studies that examined prevalence of PAD, this condition was found in general to be more frequent in persons with diabetes when a diabetes-specific rate was calculated, or the proportion of persons with diabetes among those with PAD was higher than in persons without this condition.

33.4 PAD INCIDENCE

A Finnish study by Uusitupa *et al.* [33] examined the 5-year incidence of claudication in a group of 133 middle-aged subjects with newly diagnosed type 2 diabetes compared with a control group of 144 people without diabetes. The age-adjusted incidence of claudication at 5 years was 20.3% in the diabetic men compared with 8.0% in the control group ($p = 0.06$). Among the women, 21.8% of the subjects with diabetes developed claudication compared with 4.2% of the controls ($p = 0.003$). Ankle–arm indices were not assessed in this study.

The Framingham Heart Study, a community-based project which began in 1948, enrolled 2336 men and 2873 women between the ages of 28 and 62 years. Claudication was identified using a physician-administered questionnaire at 2-year intervals for 38 years. Male sex and age were associated with an increased risk of claudication. The 4-year risks of intermittent claudication at ages 45–54 years were 0.9% for men and 0.4% for women, whereas at ages 65–74 years the risks were 2.5% for men and 1.5% for women. Among those with intermittent claudication, 20% were diabetic. Among those without claudication, only 6% had diabetes. The OR for claudication associated with diabetes was 2.6 (95% CI 2.0–3.4).

The CHS included 5888 men and women aged 65 years or over, measuring AAI at baseline and again 6 years later. At baseline, individuals with AAI < 0.9 or confirmed lower extremity arterial disease were excluded. The overall percentage of subjects with incident PAD was 9.5% over the 6 years of follow-up. Among the incident cases of PAD, 18.8% had diabetes, compared with the noncases, 10.5% of whom had diabetes.

33.5 PAD AND MORTALITY

PAD has been associated with a substantially increased risk of mortality. Criqui *et al.* [34] in 1992 reported on a cohort of 565 men and women, with an average age of 66 years, who were followed prospectively for 10 years. There were 67 subjects, or 11.9% of this population who were found to have PAD, which was defined by AAI < 0.8, abnormal Doppler flow in the femoral or posterior tibial arteries, or claudication. After adjusting for age, sex and risk factors for cardiovascular disease, including fasting plasma glucose, the RR of dying among subjects with PAD, compared with those without disease, was 3.1 (95% CI 1.9–4.9) for death from all causes, 5.9 (95% CI 3.0–11.4) for all deaths from cardiovascular disease and 6.6 (95% CI 2.9–14.9) for deaths from coronary heart disease. The RR of dying of coronary heart disease among those with claudication was 11.4 (95% CI 3.6–35.8).

The Edinburgh Artery Study enrolled 1592 men and women in 1988 from general medical practices in Edinburgh, Scotland, and followed them prospectively for 12 years [35]. When adjusted for age, sex, diabetes, prevalent coronary heart disease, systolic blood pressure, total and high-density lipoprotein (HDL)-cholesterol and smoking status, an AAI < 0.9 at baseline was associated with an RR of fatal myocardial infarction of 1.69 (95% CI 1.06–2.69). In this study, the authors found that low AAI was independently predictive of the risk of fatal myocardial infarction when traditional cardiovascular risk factors were included in the statistical model. They proposed that AAI be incorporated into routine screening and considered for inclusion into cardiovascular scoring systems.

More recently, Feringa *et al.* [36] in 2006 reported on a prospectively studied cohort of 3209 subjects with known or suspected PAD referred to a university-based vascular surgery clinic, and followed for 8 years. Mean age was 63 years. Resting and postexercise AAI values were measured, and the reduction of postexercise AAI over the baseline reading was calculated. During the follow-up period, 41.2% of the population died. After adjusting for clinical risk factors, the risk of overall mortality increased by 8% for every 0.10 decrease in the resting AAI (hazard ratio (HR) 1.08, 95% CI 1.06–1.10), and by 9% for every 0.10 decrease in the postexercise AAI (HR 1.09, 95% CI 10.8–1.11). The adjusted risk for cardiac death increased by 12% for every 0.10 decrease in the resting AAI (HR 1.12, 95% CI 1.09–1.14), and by 15% for every 0.10 decrease in the postexercise AAI (HR 1.15, 95% CI 1.12–1.17). In patients with normal resting AAI values, a reduction in the postexercise AAI by more than 55% was associated with an HR for death of 4.8 (95% CI 2.5–9.1).

PAD, a condition associated with diabetes, is related to a significantly higher risk of mortality in prospective research. This increase in risk appears to be independent of the presence of diabetes in several adjusted analyses. Whether the presence of both diabetes and PAD together result in a greater combined mortality than would be expected has not been examined.

33.6   RISK FACTORS FOR PAD

There are a number of risk factors that are associated with PAD (**Table 33.2**). Nearly every study reviewed found an association with age and cigarette smoking. The Framingham Heart Study found a strong relationship between the number of cigarettes smoked and the incidence of intermittent claudication, and a multivariate analysis identified smoking as the strongest single risk factor for development of symptomatic obstructive arterial disease, regardless of gender [37]. The occurrence of intermittent claudication is twice as frequent in smokers as nonsmokers. In the Edinburgh Artery Study, PAD prevalence was strongly and positively related to lifetime cigarette smoking [38]. Smoking was related to a higher relative prevalence of PAD (OR range 1.8–5.6) than heart disease (OR range 1.1–1.6). A prospective analysis of this cohort over 5 years revealed an incidence of new claudication of 2.6% among nonsmokers, 4.5% in moderate smokers (≤25 pack-years) and 9.8% in heavy smokers (>25 pack-years) [39].

Blood glucose levels have been shown to be associated with PAD. In the UK Prospective Diabetes Study (UKPDS), hyperglycemia was found to be associated with an increased risk of incident PAD, independent of other risk factors including age, elevated systolic blood pressure, low HDL, smoking, prior cardiovascular disease, peripheral sensory neuropathy and retinopathy. Each 1% increase in hemoglobin A_{1c} was associated with a 28% increased risk of peripheral vascular disease (PVD) (95% CI 12–46) [41]. Munter *et al.* [29] in 2005 found that the prevalence of PAD increased even among subjects with normal HbA_{1c} levels. Compared with subjects with an A_{1c} < 5.3%, subjects with an A_{1c} of 5.7–6.0% had an OR for PAD of 1.57 (95% CI 1.02–2.47). For those with diabetes and an A_{1c} < 7.0%, the OR of PAD was 2.33 (95% CI 1.15–4.70), and the OR was 2.74% (95% CI 1.25–6.02) for $A_{1c} \geq 7\%$.

Hypertensive patients show a threefold increased risk of intermittent claudication at a 16-year follow-up [42]. Limb arterial obstructive disease occurs twice as frequently as coronary artery disease (CAD) among hypertensive individuals and hypertension has been reported in 29–39% of patients with symptomatic PVD [43]. The CHS reported about a 50% higher prevalence of an AAI < 0.9 associated with hypertension in a multivariate analysis adjusted for age, smoking, diabetes and dyslipidemia [24]. Observational data analysis among 3642 patients in the UKPDS showed that the aggregate endpoint of amputation or death from PVD was associated with a 16% decrease per 10 mmHg reduction in systolic blood pressure,

Table 33.2 Risk factors associated with peripheral arterial disease.[a]

Reference	Risk factor	RR or OR (95% CI)	Notes
Newman et al. [40]	Age (per year)	RR 1.06 (0.0–3.08)	Systolic Hypertension in the Elderly Program
	Current smoking	RR 3.67 (0.3–7.04)	
Newman et al. [24]	Age (per 5 years)	RR 1.69 (1.50–1.92)	Cardiovascular Health Study
	Race (non-White)	RR 2.12 (1.31–3.44)	
	Total cholesterol (10 mg dl^{-1})	RR 1.10 (1.06–1.14)	
	HDL (1 mg dl^{-1})	RR .99 (0.98–1.00)	
	Creatinine (0.1 mg dl^{-1})	RR 1.07 (1.03–1.12)	
	BMI (kg m^{-2})	RR 0.94 (0.91–0.97)	
	FVC (l)	RR 0.63 (0.52–0.76)	
	DM	RR 4.05 (2.78–5.90)	
	Current smoking	RR 2.55 (1.76–3.68)	
	Pack-years	RR 1.01 (1.01–1.02)	
	Reported HTN	RR 1.51 (1.15–1.99)	
Beks et al. [25]	A$_{1c}$ (per %)	OR 1.32 (1.11–1.58)	The Hoorn Study
	Fasting glucose (mmol l^{-1})	OR 1.16 (1.05–1.28)	
	2-h glucose (mmol l^{-1})	OR 1.06 (1.02–1.10)	
	Age (per yr)	OR 1.09 (1.04–1.15)	
	Ever smoking	OR 3.53 (1.35–9.19)	
	HTN	OR 3.03 (1.59–5.77)	
Hiatt et al. [20]	Age	OR 2.00 (1.43–2.80)	The San Luis Valley Diabetes Study
	Diabetes	OR 3.09 (1.62–5.93)	
	Smoking (>5 pack-years)	OR 2.39 (1.43–4.00)	
	HTN	OR 3.12 (1.46–6.70)	
	Cholesterol (10 mg dl^{-1})	OR 1.08 (1.02–1.15)	
Curb et al. [26]	Cholesterol	OR 1.26 (1.07–1.49)	The Honolulu Heart Study
	Fibrinogen	OR 1.54 (1.34–1.78)	
	BMI	OR 0.72 (0.60–0.86)	
	Physical activity	OR 0.64 (0.63–0.78)	
	HDL	OR 0.74 (0.62–0.89)	
	Fasting insulin	OR 1.12 (1.06–1.19)	
	Fasting glucose	OR 1.18 (1.10–1.27)	
	Alcohol intake	OR 1.20 (1.08–1.33)	
	HTN	OR 1.80 (1.46–2.21)	
	Current smoker	OR 4.78 (3.35–6.81)	
	Past smoker	OR 1.46 (1.16–1.84)	
	Diabetes	OR 1.46 (1.16–2.84)	

Table 33.2 (*continued*)

Reference	Risk factor	RR or OR (95% CI)	Notes
Murabito *et al.* [28]	Age (10 years)	OR 2.6 (2.0–3.4)	Framingham Offspring
	HTN	OR 2.2 (1.4–3.5)	Study
	Smoking	OR 2.0 (1.1–3.4)	
	10 pack-years	OR 1.3 (1.2–1.4)	
	Fibrinogen (50 mg dl^{-1})	OR 1.2 (1.1–1.4)	
	CAD	OR 2.6 (1.6–4.1)	
Munter *et al.* [29][b]	HbA$_{1c}$		National Health and
	<5.3	OR 1.0	Nutrition Survey
	5.3–5.4	OR 1.43 (0.91–2.25)	1999–2002
	5.5–5.6	OR 1.50 (0.81–2.79)	
	5.7–6.0	OR 1.83 (1.22–2.75)	
	DMA$_{1c}$		
	<7.0	OR 2.54 (1.33–4.87)	
	≥7.0	OR 3.04 (1.50–6.15)	

[a]AA: African American; BMI: body mass index; DM: diabetes mellitus; HTN: hypertension; GT: glucose tolerance.
[b]Adjusted for age, race and sex.

adjusted for age at diagnosis of diabetes, ethnic group, smoking status, presence of albuminuria, hemoglobin A$_{1c}$, high- and low-density lipoprotein cholesterol and triglyceride [44].

The association of hypercholesterolemia with atherosclerosis of the lower extremities has been known for ~75 years [45]. The prevalence of claudication in patients with serum cholesterol levels over 260 mg dl^{-1} is on average over twice as high as in those with a concentration below this level. The prevalence of hyperlipidemia in patients with clinical manifestations of lower extremity arterial occlusive disease ranges in various studies from 31 to 57%. The Edinburgh Artery Study reported a higher prevalence of PAD in association with higher serum cholesterol and lower HDL-cholesterol in multiple logistic regression analysis [38]. The CHS reached similar conclusions among its sample of 5084 subjects aged 65 years or older, with PAD defined as an AAI < 0.9. [24].

Other risk factors have been shown to be associated with a higher prevalence of PVD. Increased levels of hemostatic factors, such as fibrinogen, von Willebrand factor, tissue plasminogen activator (t-PA), fibrin D-dimer and plasma viscosity

explained in part the higher prevalence of PAD in subjects with diabetes or impaired glucose tolerance in the Edinburgh Artery Study [39]. Higher circulating levels of homocysteine have been demonstrated in this condition [46], as have parallel low levels of folate in red blood cells and circulating vitamin B6, which raises the possibility that supplementation with these vitamins may reduce the incidence of PAD [47]. One small, randomized, placebo-controlled study of secondary prevention has shown that oral therapy with folic acid, vitamin B12 and vitamin B6 decreased the need for revascularization in patients receiving percutaneous coronary intervention [48]. Higher levels of various hemostatic factors have been demonstrated in persons with lower AAI, suggesting that a hypercoagulable state predisposes to the development of PAD [49, 50]. Infectious agents, such as *Chlamydia pneumoniae*, have been implicated in the development of atherosclerosis in several vascular beds [51, 52]. The prevalence of low AAI (<1.05) was highest among persons with a birthweight <6.6 lb, a demonstration of the 'thrifty phenotype' hypothesis that postulates fetal growth retardation as a cause of metabolic disorders and vascular disease in adult life [53, 54].

No study has directly compared the rate of PAD among patients with type 1 diabetes with those with type 2 diabetes, but it is possible to perform this comparison across studies that collected data at approximately similar time intervals. The Epidemiology of Diabetes and Complications (EDIC) study, the long-term follow-up of the Diabetes Control and Complications Trial (DCCT), identified those patients with AAI < 0.9 [15]. The EDIC study found that intensively treated participants, with an average duration of type 1 diabetes of about 14 years, had a prevalence of PAD of 8.8% among women and 4.6% among men. The conventionally treated participants had a prevalence of 8.7% among women and 6.9% among men. The Pittsburgh Epidemiology of Diabetes Study II was an observational study that did not include intensive control, and, in fact, did not describe the level of glycemic control [23]. The definition of probable PAD in this study was AAI < 0.9 or claudication. The rate of PAD at diagnosis was not reported. At 5 years' duration, the rate of PAD was approximately 17% and at 16 years' duration it was 30%. Patients with type 2 diabetes were enrolled in the UKPDS [41]. PAD in the UKPDS was defined as the presence of any two of the following: (i) AAI < 0.8, (ii) absence of both dorsalis pedis and posterior tibial pulses to palpation in at least one leg and (iii) claudication. The prevalence of PAD was 1.2% (95% CI 0.9–1.5%) at the time of diagnosis. After 6 years' follow-up, 2.7% of participants (95% CI 2.2–3.2%) had PAD according to these criteria that was not present at baseline and at least one of these three measures was abnormal in 10.6%. The prevalence of PAD increased to 12.5% in the smaller subgroup of participants followed for 18 years (95% CI 3.8–21.1%). **Figure 33.1** shows a comparison of the rates of PAD in subjects included in the Pittsburgh Study compared with those included in the UKPDS. This comparison suggests that, for a similar diabetes duration, the risk of PAD is higher in type 1 than type 2 disease, but this difference might also be potentially explained by discrepancies between these populations with regard to level of glycemic control, PAD definition and frequency of other PAD risk factors.

Diabetes is one of several independent risk factors that have been identified for the development

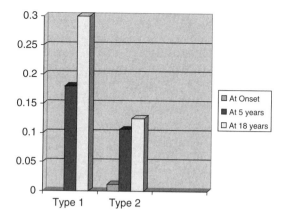

Figure 33.1 Prevalence of peripheral arterial disease at diagnosis and after approximately 5-years' and 18-years' duration, comparing diabetes type 1 and type 2 [23, 41].

of PAD. The evidence supports a key role for glycemia in this process, as risk of PAD increases in proportion to poorer glycemic control, although other evidence argues for a role for hemostatic factors in this process.

33.7 EPIDEMIOLOGY OF RENAL ARTERIAL STENOSIS AND DIABETES MELLITUS

There are almost no large population-based studies examining the epidemiology of renal artery stenosis (RAS). One of the largest is a cross-sectional study that included autopsy data from 5194 patients who died during an 8-year period at a university hospital [55]. A random sample of 300 patients without RAS and all 225 patients with RAS (defined as >50% stenosis of renal artery found at autopsy) were selected for further study. The prevalence of RAS was 4.3% in all autopsies and nearly twice as high (8.3%) in patients with diabetes mellitus in the random sample, and diabetes was significantly linked to RAS (OR = 3.5, 95% CI 2.6–4.6).

One cross-sectional population-based study invited participants in the Forsyth County cohort of the CHS to undergo renal duplex sonography to detect renovascular disease [56]. The CHS is a population-based prospective cohort study examining risk factors for CAD and cerebrovascular disease in men and women 65 years and older living in four US communities. Seventy percent of the Forsyth cohort was recruited by (i) randomly sampling Medicare eligibility lists of the Health Care Financing Administration to generate a group of 5000, (ii) then using a customized program to randomly select subjects from these groups to reproduce the gender and age distribution of the county and (iii) inviting subjects to participate; 61% joined the study. The other 30% of the Forsyth cohort were recruited from the households of the participants. Baseline intake included a home interview and clinical examination, with recording of cardiovascular risk factors. Eight hundred and seventy people had renal duplex sonography, and 96% were technically adequate. The overall prevalence of renovascular disease, which was defined as ≥60% diameter-reducing RAS or occlusion (no Doppler signal from imaged artery), was 6.8%. The 64 renal arteries with renovascular disease were divided into 57 kidneys with ≥60% RAS and seven with occlusion [56]. In multivariate analysis, independent risk factors for renovascular disease were age (OR 1.3, 95% CI 1.0–1.7), HDL-cholesterol levels <40 mg dl^{-1} (OR 2.6, 95% CI 1.4–4.9) and increasing systolic blood pressure (OR 1.4, 95% CI 1.1–1.9). Diabetes was not a risk factor. The strengths of this study were the size and diversity of the study population (with the same age and gender distribution as Forsyth County) and rigorous screening technique. The renal duplex studies consisted of multiple Doppler images and were performed by two skilled technicians. Although the recruitment process did include random selection, the inclusion of subjects in the same household may have contributed selection bias [56].

Most other studies on RAS focus on specific subsets of the population, such as patients with clinical suspicion for RAS or those undergoing evaluation for other suspected atherosclerotic disease. In a cross-sectional study of patients admitted for renal angiography at one hospital, RAS was detected in 36% of 28 patients with diabetes and hypertension and in 48% of 104 patients with hypertension but no diabetes [57]. In this specific group of patients with hypertension referred for renal angiography, diabetes did not carry an increased risk of RAS (OR 0.6, 95% CI 0.3–1.4**). In one recent large cross-sectional study at a university cardiovascular center in Korea, 1459 patients undergoing coronary angiography over a 16-month period because of suspicion of CAD also consented to abdominal aortography to detect RAS and to carotid angiography [58]. The prevalence of ≥50% RAS was 10.8% in the general cohort and 13.5% in the 994 patients found to have significant CAD. In multivariate logistic regression, significant risk factors for RAS were extracranial carotid artery stenosis (OR 4.9, 95% CI 2.6–9.3, $p < 0.001$), peripheral artery disease (OR 4.6, 95% CI 2.7–9.3, $p < 0.001$), renal insufficiency (OR 2.7, 95% 1.4–5.0, $p = 0.002$), significant CAD (OR 2.0, 95% CI 1.1–3.6), hypercholesterolemia (OR 1.9, 95% CI 1.1–3.4, $p = 0.028$), hypertension (OR 1.9, 95% 1.2–3.0, $p = 0.010$) and age >60 years (OR 1.6, 95% CI 1.0–2.6, $p = 0.044$). Diabetes was not a clinical predictor of RAS (OR 0.9, 95% CI 0.5–1.5) [58]. One Chinese hospital-based cross-sectional study included 141 patients with suspected CAD who underwent coronary and renal angiography [59]. Eighteen percent were found to have RAS (luminal narrowing of ≥50%), with a higher prevalence (31%) in the 52 patients with confirmed CAD (luminal narrowing of ≥50%) compared with those without CAD (11%). Univariate logistic regression revealed that the most important predictors of RAS were older age (RR 1.1, 95% CI 1.0–1.1), CAD (RR 3.6, 95% CI 1.2–10.8), hypertension (RR 17.0, 95% CI 4.1–69.9) and hyperlipidemia (RR 4.7, 95% CI 1.5–14.4); they did not examine diabetes as a predictor [59].

A few studies have examined the epidemiology of RAS specifically in patients with diabetes. One cross-sectional study included 44 patients with diabetes (19 insulin-dependent, 25 noninsulin-dependent) selected by age (<70 years old) and hypertension (diastolic blood pressure (DBP) >95 mmHg or on antihypertensive therapy) criteria from 465 patients chosen by random number allocation from a diabetes clinic population of 2093 being screened for hypertension [60]. The prevalence of RAS by intravenous digital subtraction angiography was 12% in the group as a whole, 0% in patients with noninsulin-dependent diabetes and 21% in those with insulin-dependent diabetes [60]. In another study, 208 outpatients or inpatients with type 2 diabetes and criteria worrisome for RAS (severe hypertension, ≥3 antihypertensives, creatinine clearance ≤60 ml per minute or macroangiography) were recruited during a 4-year period [61]. RAS, defined as ≥70% stenosis of the renal artery by Doppler with confirmation by arteriography or magnetic resonance angiography, was found in 16.3% of this high-risk group. Risk factors for RAS in patients with diabetes were smoking (OR 2.7, 95% CI 1.3–5.8**), insulin therapy (OR 2.5, 95% CI 1.2–5.5**) and coronary heart disease (OR 5.4, 95% CI 2.5–11.8**), but, surprisingly, not severe hypertension (OR 2.1, 95% CI 1.0–4.4**) [61]. A more recent study with a cross-sectional component focused on 45 patients with type 2 diabetes, diabetic nephropathy, uncontrolled hypertension and serum creatinine ≥ 1.8 mg dl^{-1} for women, ≥ 2.0 mg dl^{-1} for men recruited from outpatient medicine/nephrology clinics and the inpatient service over 2 years [62]. The prevalence of RAS ($\geq 10\%$ stenosis of renal artery by three-dimensional (3-D) gadolinium-enhanced magnetic resonance angiography) was 40%, and RAS was associated with current smoking (OR 10.0, 95% CI 1.1–94.7**) and claudication (OR 8.0, 95% CI 1.8–36.4**) [62].

These RAS studies share similar limitations, most notably small sample size, cross-sectional study design and lack of control groups. None of the studies was population based, and patients were recruited from outpatient clinics and hospitals. In a few, selection bias was readily apparent, because only patients suspected of having RAS were included. Although such studies may provide information on the predictive value of clinical characteristics, their results (in terms of prevalence and risk factors) cannot be extrapolated to the general population.

Different definitions and diagnostic methods for RAS created case ascertainment or detection bias. For example, the prevalence of RAS was higher in one study (40%) than another (16.3%), despite the inclusion of similar high-risk patient populations with diabetes [61, 62]. RAS was defined as $\geq 70\%$ stenosis of the renal artery by Doppler with confirmation by arteriography or magnetic resonance angiography in the first study, and as $\geq 10\%$ stenosis of renal artery by 3-D gadolinium-enhanced magnetic resonance angiography in the latter. In one cross-sectional clinic-based study, 269 patients > 50 years old with late-onset hypertension or chronic renal failure unexplained by known renal pathologies (patients with diabetic nephropathy in the presence of nonrenal atherosclerotic disease were allowed) consecutively referred to a nephrology outpatient

clinic were subjected to renal radionuclide scintigraphy ($n = 224$) and/or color-duplex ultrasonography ($n = 238$) of renal arteries [63]. Forty patients found to have RAS by one or both of these underwent 3-D contrast-enhancement magnetic resonance angiography and/or selective angiography. Twenty-three subjects with normal results on other studies had magnetic resonance angiography or selective angiography. Forty-nine out of 238 patients had $\geq 60\%$ RAS by duplex (systolic peak velocity > 180 cm s^{-1} or ratio between systolic peak velocity in renal artery and that in suprarenal abdominal aorta ≥ 3.5). Thirty-five of the 49 underwent magnetic resonance angiography or selective angiography, and the diagnosis was confirmed in 31 [63]. If magnetic resonance angiography or selective angiography is considered the gold standard for diagnosing RAS, then color duplex sonography has a positive predictive value (PPV) of 94.3% and negative predictive value (NPV) of 87.0%, and renal scintigraphy has a PPV of 72.2% and NPV of 29.4% [63].

The clinical evidence discussed here suggests that there is an increased risk of RAS in people with certain cardiovascular risk factors (increasing age, dyslipidemia, hypertension, smoking) or other evidence of vasculopathy (PVD, CAD). Most studies show that diabetes is not a significant risk factor for RAS.

33.8 EPIDEMIOLOGY OF ABDOMINAL AORTIC ANEURYSM AND DIABETES MELLITUS

In the 1990s, many cross-sectional studies addressed the epidemiology of AAA in the general population, including some subjects with diabetes (see **Table 33.3** for specific details of studies) [64–70]. Most studies recruited subjects ≥ 55–65 years old in one geographic locale in cooperation with their health care providers or a local health care organization. Risk factor information was collected by questionnaire or interview. AAA was most often regarded as ≥ 30 mm in diameter on ultrasound, which is a standard definition, and the prevalence of AAA in these studies ranged from 2.1 to 9.5%. The lowest prevalence was reported in the Rotterdam study, which used a slightly different definition of AAA (aortic diameter on ultrasound ≥ 35 mm or dilatation of distal part of abdominal aorta $\geq 50\%$) [66].

Table 33.3 Epidemiologic studies of abdominal aortic aneurysm.[a]

Reference and type of study	Population	AAA diagnostic criteria	Prevalence	Risk factors	OR (95% CI)
Krohn et al. [64] (cross-sectional)	500 men over age 60 enrolled in a Norwegian HMO	Ultrasound: *Small AAA*: either ↑aortic diameter distally and maximum diameter >1.5 × diameter of origin of superior mesenteric artery, or maximum diameter of >29 mm *Large AAA*: maximum diameter >39 mm	Overall: 8.2% (5.7–10.7) Small AAA: 5.8% Large AAA: 2.4%	History of smoking Poor health (HTN, CV disease or DM) Increasing age	Not provided by the authors and not calculable from information provided in the publication
Smith et al. [65] (cross-sectional)	2669 men recruited by letter from 3500 men aged 65–76 years from 20 urban general practices (participation rate of 76.3%, 2597 successfully imaged by u/s)	Ultrasound: aortic diameter >29 mm	Overall: 8.4% Aortic diameter of 29–40 mm: 5.4%	*Associations* Smoking Ischemic heart disease Previous MI PVD *No association:* HTN DM	2.1 (1.5–2.8)** 2.1 (1.5–3.0)** 2.8 (1.9–4.1)** 1.7 (1.2–2.7) 1.2 (0.9–1.8)** 0.8 (0.4–1.6)**
Pleumeekers et al. [66] (cross-sectional within a prospective study)	10 215 subjects ≥55 years old identified with help of local municipality invited to participate (attendance rate of 78%, 5283 successfully imaged by u/s)	Ultrasound: aortic diameter ≥35 mm or dilatation of distal part of abdominal aorta ≥50%	Overall: 2.1% (1.7–2.5) Men: 4.1% (3.2–4.9) Women: 0.7% (0.4–1.0)	*Associations* Smoking Previous MI *No association* DM	2.6 (1.8–3.8)** 2.4 (1.4–4.2)** 0.7 (0.3–1.5)**

(continued overleaf)

Table 33.3 (*continued*)

Reference and type of study	Population	AAA diagnostic criteria	Prevalence	Risk factors	OR (95% CI)
Scott *et al.* [67] Kanagasabay *et al.* [68] (cross-sectional and prospective study)	15 775 subjects aged 65–80 years on practice registers and Family Health Service lists in one district randomized to control or screening groups (attendance rate of 68%, 5394 imaged by u/s)	Ultrasound: aortic diameter ≥30 mm Screened subjects who met surgical criteria were repaired, and then screened and control patients were followed prospectively	Overall: 4.0%	*Associations at baseline* Previous MI Claudication *No association* DM	1.7 (1.1–2.6)* 1.7 (1.2–2.4)* 0.8 (0.4–1.6)*
Simoni *et al.* [69] (cross-sectional)	2734 subjects aged 65–75 years in one Health Service District in Italy invited by letter to participate (attendance rate of 59%, 1601 imaged by u/s)	Ultrasound: aortic diameter ≥29 mm or dilatation of distal part of abdominal aorta ≥50%	Overall: 4.4% Males: 8.8% Females: 0.6%	*Associations* Smoking Alcohol use Coronary heart disease COPD *No association* DM	10.1 (4.7–22.0)** 2.6 (1.5–4.2)** 2.9 (1.8–4.8)** 5.0 (2.9–8.6)** 1.0 (0.5–2.0)**
Mattes *et al.* [70] (cross-sectional study nested in	316 men ≥60 years old invited from the first 1000 participants in a	Ultrasound: aortic diameter ≥30 mm or history of AAA repair	Overall: 2.3% (0.6–4.0)	*Univariate analysis: No association* Duration of DM	

Study	Methods/population	Imaging/definition	Prevalence	Associations	OR (95% CI)
prospective DM cohort study) community-based DM study in one hospital's catchment area (recruited by hospital data review, involvement of providers and local ads) 303 imaged by u/s				Glycosylated hemoglobin	
				Glycosylated hemoglobin *Multivariate logistic regression analysis: Associations* Fasting triglycerides	1.3 (1.0–1.8)*
				Claudication	5.2 (1.1–25.3)*
Lederle et al. [71] (cross-sectional)	320 000 veterans, 50–79 years of age, without a previous history of AAA at 15 VA medical centers invited my mail to attend a screening clinic (attendance rate of 23%, 73 451 successfully imaged by u/s)	Ultrasound:AAA: infrarenal aortic diameter ≥30 mm	AAA ≥ 30 mm: 4.6% AAA ≥ 40 mm: 1.4%	*Associated with AAA ≥ 30 mm*	
				Smoking	2.7 (2.4–3.1)*
				Age (per 7 years increase)	1.5 (1.5–1.6)*
				FH AAA	2.0 (1.7–2.3)*
				HTN	1.3 (1.1–1.4)*
				High cholesterol	1.3 (1.2–1.5)*
				Coronary artery disease	1.4 (1.3–1.6)*
				Height (per 7 cm)	1.2 (1.1–1.3)*
				Negative association	
				DM	0.7 (0.6–0.8)*

(continued overleaf)

Table 33.3 (*continued*)

Reference and type of study	Population	AAA diagnostic criteria	Prevalence	Risk factors	OR (95% CI)
Lederle *et al.* [72] Aneurysm Detection and Management Study Screening Program (cross-sectional)	52 943 veterans aged 50–79 years without a previous history of AAA underwent screening (52 745 successfully imaged by u/s)	Ultrasound: AAA: infrarenal aortic diameter ≥30 mm	AAA ≥ 30 mm: 3.6% AAA ≥ 40 mm: 1.2%	*Associated with AAA ≥ 30 mm:*	
				Smoking	3.5 (2.9–4.2)*
				Age (per 7 years increase)	1.7 (1.6–1.8)*
				FH AAA	1.9 (1.6–2.4)*
				HTN	1.2 (1.1–1.4)*
				High cholesterol	1.5 (1.3–1.8)*
				Coronary artery disease	1.5 (1.3–1.7)*
				Height (per 7 cm)	1.2 (1.1–1.3) *
				Negative association	
				DM	0.6 (0.5–0.7)*
Blanchard *et al.* [73] (hospital-based case–control study)	98 subjects with AAA by u/s at two tertiary care hospitals over 3.5 years, 102 controls referred for u/s for reasons similar to cases (but no AAA found) Cases and controls further divided on basis of whether clinical suspicion of AAA was an indication for u/s	Ultrasound: definite focal widening of infrarenal aorta, 92% cases with maximum aortic diameter ≥30 mm	—	*Associations*	
				Smoking	
				1–19 pack-years	2.8 (0.9–8.9)*
				20–34 pack-years	7.3 (2.4–21.9)*
				35–49 pack-years	7.4 (2.4–22.5)*
				≥50 pack-years	9.5 (2.8–32.5)*
				Male gender	2.7 (1.3–5.7)*
				Diastolic blood pressure (per 10 mmHg)	1.9 (1.3–2.7)*
				FH AAA	4.8 (1.3–18.1)*
				Inverse association	
				DM	0.3 (0.1–0.9)*

				Associations	
Wanhainen et al. [74] (population-based case–control study) Wanhainen et al. [75]	35 pts found to have AAA at screening in a cross-sectional study of all men and women aged 65–75 years living in Norsjo municipality invited to a health exam, 140 age- and sex-matched controls. Risk factor data: current and historical (12 years prior)	Ultrasound and CT scan: mean maximal infrarenal aortic diameter ≥30 mm	Second study looked at the influence of diagnostic criteria on prevalence: AAA prevalence varied from 3.6–16.9% in men, 0.8–9.4% in women (see text for discussion)	Atherosclerotic disease	3.8 (1.7–8.5)
				FH AAA	4.4 (1.5–13.0)
				Smoking	5.2 (1.6–16.8)
				HDL	0.1 (0.02–0.7)
				hsCRP	1.1 (1.0–1.2)
				No association	
				DM	No results given or data provided for calculation
				HTN	

a AAA: abdominal aortic aneurysm; u/s: ultrasound; DM: diabetes mellitus; HTN: hypertension; CV: cardiovascular; MI: myocardial infarction; COPD: chronic obstructive pulmonary disease; hsCRP: highly sensitive C-reactive protein; HDL, high-density lipoprotein; FH, family history.

**Confidence interval not presented in the publication and calculated by the authors of this chapter.

*Confidence interval presented in the publication.

Recurrent risk factors for AAA were older age, male sex, smoking, hyperlipidemia, CAD and PVD. Diabetes was consistently not a risk factor for AAA.

Two large cross-sectional studies examined the prevalence and risk factors for AAA in veterans aged 50–79 years without a previous history of AAA enrolled at Veterans Affairs medical centers [71, 72]. In the first study spanning 2.5 years, 73 451 subjects, 30% of those invited by mail, filled out questionnaires about risk factors and had abdominal ultrasounds that successfully visualized the abdominal aorta [71]. The prevalence of AAA was 4.6% when AAA was defined as ≥3.0 cm and 1.4% for AAA ≥ 4.0 cm. The main risk factor for AAA ≥ 3.0 cm was smoking (OR 2.7, 95% CI 2.4–3.1), and diabetes was negatively associated (OR 0.7, 95% CI 0.6–0.8) with AAA. In the Aneurysm Detection and Management Study Screening Program, a second similar study of 52 745 veterans, AAA ≥ 3.0 cm was detected in 3.6% and AAA ≥ 4.0 cm in 1.2% [72]. Again, smoking conferred an increased risk of AAA (OR 3.5, 95% CI 2.9–4.2), and diabetes was linked to a reduced risk of this outcome (OR 0.6, 95% CI 0.5–0.7).

In a recent case–control study conducted at two tertiary care hospitals in Canada between June 1992 and December 1995, 98 patients were found to have AAA by ultrasound, which was defined as a definite focal widening of the infrarenal aorta [73]. Ninety percent of cases had a maximum aortic diameter ≥30 mm. Detection bias was minimized by designating two groups of cases and controls on the basis of the reason for the ultrasound. The first group included 60 cases and 67 controls, both suspected of having AAA. The second group consisted of 38 cases and 35 controls who were referred for ultrasound for reasons other than suspected AAA. Logistic regression with adjustment for covariates revealed the following AAA predictors: 20–34 pack-years smoking (OR 7.3, 95% CI 2.4–21.9), 35–49 pack-years smoking (OR 7.4, 95% CI 2.4–22.5), ≥50 pack-years smoking (OR 9.6, 95% CI 2.8–32.5), male gender (OR 2.7, 95% CI 1.3–5.7), DBP (OR per 10 mmHg increase 1.9, 95% CI 1.3–2.7) and family history of AAA (OR 4.8, 95% CI 1.3–18.1) [73]. Diabetes mellitus was inversely associated with odds of AAA (OR 0.3, 95% 0.1–0.9). Hyperlipidemia was not associated with AAA. Results were similar when analyses were stratified on the basis of whether there was a high suspicion of AAA prior to ultrasound [73].

In a population-based case–control and retrospective cohort study, all men and women aged 65–75 years of age living in one municipality in Sweden were invited to undergo baseline risk assessment (labs, questionnaire on lifestyle factors) and ultrasound screening for AAA [74]; 504 (91%) participated. Sixty-three subjects with a maximum aortic diameter ≥28 mm also had an abdominal computed tomography (CT) scan. The definition of AAA was a mean maximal infrarenal aortic diameter ≥30 mm on abdominal ultrasound and CT scan. The main risk factors for AAA were atherosclerotic disease (OR 3.8, 95% CI 1.7–8.5), having a first-degree relative with AAA (OR 4.4, 95% CI 1.5–13.0), current smoking (OR 5.2, 95% CI 1.6–16.8), HDL-cholesterol level (OR 0.1, 95% CI 0.02–0.7) and highly sensitive C-reactive protein (hsCRP) level (OR 1.1, 95% CI 1.01–1.2). There was not an association between AAA and diabetes or hypertension [74].

This study included a secondary analysis that examined the influence of diagnostic criteria on the prevalence of AAA [75]. AAA was defined in four different ways: (1) aortic diameter ≥30 mm, (2) aortic diameter ≥1.5 times suprarenal aortic diameter, (3) aortic diameter ≥40 mm or infrarenal aortic diameter exceeding suprarenal aortic diameter by at least 0.5 cm, and (4) aortic diameter ≥1.5 times normal infrarenal diameter. Depending on the diagnostic criteria, the AAA prevalence ranged from 4.8 to 16.9% in men and 0.8 to 9.4% in women, with the highest prevalence in men (16.9%) when AAA was defined as aortic maximum diameter ≥30 mm by ultrasound and the lowest when it was defined as aortic maximum diameter ≥50 mm by ultrasound [75]. Most of the other studies here used the standard definition: aortic diameter ≥30 mm.

In general, clinical studies suggest that increasing age, male sex, smoking, family history of AAA, hyperlipidemia, CAD and PVD are risk factors for AAA. Diabetes is not a risk factor for AAA, and available data suggest that the risk of AAA may be lower in persons with this metabolic disorder. Patients with diabetes have been shown to have increased aortic stiffness [76, 77]. One study in diabetic rats showed that advanced glycation end products accumulate in the collagen of blood vessels in diabetes, leading to altered biomechanics and increased aortic wall matrix stiffness [78]. Some have postulated that these changes may reduce the likelihood of aortic aneurysmal dilatation [79].

33.9 EPIDEMIOLOGY OF VENOUS THROMBOEMBOLIC DISEASE AND DIABETES

One large prospective cohort study examined risk factors for pulmonary embolism (PE) in 112 822 women aged 30–55 years followed for 16 years [80]. They were asked to fill out mailed questionnaires about their medical histories, cardiovascular risk factors and incident PE at baseline and every 2 years thereafter. Self-reported PE was confirmed by reviewing medical records (with subjects' consent). Relatives or postal authorities reported deaths in the cohort; and, if a cardiovascular cause or PE was suspected, permission to review medical records was also requested. The diagnosis of PE was confirmed by a positive pulmonary angiogram, a high-probability ventilation–perfusion scan, or an autopsy [80]. Overall, 280 cases of PE occurred, 125 defined as primary PE (no strong predisposing factor, such as cancer, surgery, trauma, immobilization) and 115 as secondary PE (presence of strong predisposing factor). In multivariate analysis, independent risk factors for PE included body mass index (BMI) $\geq 29.0\,\mathrm{kg\,m^{-2}}$ (RR 2.9, 95% CI 1.5–5.4), smoking 25–34 cigarettes per day (RR 1.9, 95% CI 0.9–3.7), smoking ≥ 35 cigarettes a day (RR 3.3, 95% CI 1.7–6.5) and hypertension (RR 1.9, 95% CI 1.2–2.8). Diabetes was not associated with primary PE (RR 0.7, 95% CI 0.3–1.9). The main strengths of the Nurses' Health Study were the prospective study design (which reduced recall bias), the large cohort size and the validation of incident cases. In many studies, the accuracy of risk factor data obtained by self-report may be questioned. This source of bias was minimized in the Nurses' Health Study because, in a sample of study subjects, self-reported weight and height correlated with measurements by trained personnel, and reported medical illnesses were verified by reviewing medical records [80].

One large retrospective cohort study examined risk factors for PE in 26 years of follow-up in the Framingham Health Study [81]. Of 3470 subjects who had baseline data about cardiovascular risk factors, 998 died and 46 were found to have autopsy confirmed or clinical significant PE. In multivariate

analysis of subjects with autopsy-confirmed major PE and all subjects who died, glucose level was not independently associated with PE, and the only significant risk factor for PE was metropolitan relative weight in women ($p < 0.001$). Case finding by autopsy excludes nonfatal PE and, thus, may not provide the most accurate information about risk factors [81].

Unlike the Framingham Study and the Nurses' Health Study, several other studies have linked diabetes to an increased risk of venous thromboembolic events. One prospective study, the Longitudinal Investigation of Thromboembolism Etiology, followed 19 293 men and women (15 792 men and women aged 45–64 years from the ARIC study, 5201 men and women ≥ 65 years from Medicare eligibility lists in the CHS without previous venous thromboembolism) in six US communities from 1987 to 1998 [82]. Baseline data collection for risk factor measurement entailed physical examination and extensive questionnaires. Hospitalizations were identified by participant report and surveillance of local discharge lists for cohort members, deep venous thrombosis (DVT) was diagnosed by Doppler or impedance plethysmography, and PE was diagnosed by ventilation–perfusion scan, angiogram or autopsy. The overall crude incidence rate of venous thromboembolism was 1.5 (95% CI 1.3–1.7) per 1000 person-years. In multivariate analysis, risk factors for DVT were increasing age (age 55–59: HR 2.1, 95% CI 1.5–3.1; age 65–74: HR 4.0, 95% CI 2.7–6.0; age 75–84: HR 5.7, 95% CI 3.4–9.3; age ≥ 85: HR 14.8, 95% CI 6.3–35.1), male sex (HR 1.4, 95% CI 1.1–1.9), BMI (BMI 25–29: HR 1.5, 95% 1.0–2.1; BMI 30–34: HR 2.2, 95% CI 1.5–3.1; BMI 35–39: HR 1.5, 95% CI 0.8–3.0; BMI ≥ 40: HR 2.7, 95% CI 1.3–5.8), African-American ancestry (HR 1.4, 95% CI 1.0–1.9) and diabetes (HR 1.5, 95% CI 1.0–2.1). The association between venous thromboembolism and diabetes was attenuated after adjustment for obesity (HR 1.5, 95% CI 1.0–2.0). The strengths of this study were its large sample size, prospective study design and the uniform validation of all venous thromboembolic events. The main weakness was that the two substudies, ARIC and CHS, utilized slightly different methods for measuring risk factors [82].

In one small prospective study of 83 consecutive patients undergoing kidney transplant for end-stage renal disease (ESRD) during a 2.3-year period, the frequency of DVT (detected by venous occlusion plethysmography and thermography on postoperative days 7 and 21) was greater in 33 patients with type 1 diabetes (40%) than in those without diabetes (14%) and the whole cohort (24%) [83]. The risk of DVT in renal transplant patients was 2.8 times higher (RR 2.8, 95% CI 1.3–6.3**) with concurrent type 1 diabetes [83]. A large retrospective cohort study followed a similar population, 1833 people who underwent kidney transplant and 276 people who underwent simultaneous kidney–pancreas transplant during a 10-year period [84]. Thromboembolic events were diagnosed by clinical assessment and imaging (venogram or duplex for DVT, and PE by ventilation–perfusion scans, angiogram or necropsy). DVT occurred in 6.2% of the cohort, 18.1% after simultaneous kidney–pancreas transplant and 4.5% after kidney transplant, and PE occurred in 2.1%, 4.7% after simultaneous kidney–pancreas transplant and 1.7% after kidney transplant. Multivariate analysis revealed that an increased risk of DVT was associated with age >40-years old (HR 2.2, $p < 0.001$), diabetes (HR 4.4, $p = 0.001$), previous DVT (HR 4.4, $p = 0.001$) and simultaneous kidney–pancreas transplant (HR 2.8, $p < 0.001$). The risk of PE was higher with diabetes (HR 2.6, $p = 0.005$) and recent DVT (HR 8.9, $p = 0.0001$) [84]. The results of these studies can only be applied to a very specific population: patients undergoing kidney transplant or simultaneous kidney–pancreas transplant. Nonetheless, they may have important implications for perioperative DVT prophylaxis for these high-risk groups.

A large retrospective cohort study examined the incidence of DVT or PE in 2.8 million members enrolled in 37 health plans in the United States continuously over 2 years with complete enrollment history records in the PharMetrics Integrated Outcomes Database [85]. Risk factor data were obtained from diagnoses recorded on hospital and professional claims, as well as the list of medications on pharmacy claims. One thousand three hundred and thirty cases of DVT or PE requiring hospitalization in 1999 were identified from principal diagnoses recorded on hospital claims. Specific diagnostic methods for DVT and PE were not mentioned. The crude annual incidence rate of DVT or PE was 47 per 100 000. Risk

factors for DVT in women included increasing age (age >64 years: OR = 3.9, $p = 0.0001$), prior DVT and/or PE (OR 13.9, $p = 0.0001$), major orthopedic procedure (OR 2.4, $p = 0.0001$), diabetes (OR 1.8, $p = 0.0001$), primary nonlymphatic neoplasm (OR 1.7, $p = 0.001$), primary lymphatic neoplasm (OR 2.0, $p = 0.01$) and cellulitis (OR 3.6, $p = 0.0001$). In men, the association between diabetes and DVT was not statistically significant (OR 1.3, $p = 0.08$). Risk factor information, such as the presence of diabetes, derived from diagnoses on claims may be inaccurate and is not standardized [85]. Case ascertainment bias was likely, as not all cases of DVT were included, since DVTs or PEs in already hospitalized patients or subjects treated as outpatients were excluded, diagnostic methods varied and were not discussed, and DVT rates may be underreported by physicians required to list only one diagnosis on the hospital claim for reimbursement.

In one cross-sectional study, 302 adult patients (56 with diabetes, 246 without diabetes) admitted to a university hospital with the diagnosis of venous thromboembolism during a 12-year period were identified by the World Health Organization's International Classification of Diseases ICD-9 codes (210 DVT of lower extremity, 7 DVT of upper extremity, 1 renal vein thrombosis, 1 vena cava thrombosis, 83 PE) [86]. DVTs were diagnosed by Doppler ultrasound (83.1%), phlebography (9.6%), both (3.2%), or clinical assessment only (3.2%), and diagnostic methods for PE included angiography (49.4%), ventilation–perfusion scan and chest X-ray (16.9%), autopsy (13.3%), or a combination (7.2%). Population data were derived from computerized registries in primary care centers and the university hospital, and the Swedish population registry. The annual incidence rate of venous thromboembolism was 91 (95% CI 81–102) per 100 000 in the general population, 432 (95% CI 375–496) per 100 000 in people with diabetes, and 78 (95% CI 68–88) per 100 000 in people without diabetes. The age-adjusted incidence rate in people with diabetes was 274 (95% CI 262–286) per 100 000, with diabetes doubling the risk of venous thromboembolism compared with the general population (standardized morbidity ratio (SMR) 2.3, 95% CI 1.8–3.0). This study was not truly population based because cases of venous thromboembolism were drawn from the main hospital in the catchment area, and cases of diabetes were identified from the registries of local primary health care centers and the hospital. The authors do mention that >95% of all patients with diabetes in the area received care at these medical facilities, and diabetes rates were consistent with the results of other studies in Sweden [86].

It is unclear why the results of the Nurses' Health Study and the Framingham Study do not correlate with those of the other studies, which support an association between diabetes and higher risk of venous thromoembolism. Some studies, such as the Longitudinal Investigation of Thromboembolism Etiology, may have enrolled a generally older population with other risk factors for venous thromboembolism. The studies on transplant patients focused on a higher risk population. Risk factors, such as diabetes, also may have been defined differently in these studies.

Nonetheless, the potential association between diabetes and venous thromboembolism is an intriguing one. Diabetes is clearly associated with other thrombotic complications, such as CAD and PVD, although these diseases involve the arterial side of the circulation. There may be an increased thrombogenic tendency in diabetes due to defects in fibrinolysis and coagulation. Fibrinolysis is impaired because of abnormal clot structures that resist degradation and elevated platelet activator inhibitor 1 [87]. Increased platelet aggregation and platelet hyperactivity contribute to hypercoagulability [88]. As mentioned previously, there also may be changes in collagen in blood vessels in diabetes. The relationship between diabetes and obesity may also partially explain the effect of diabetes on venous thromboembolism. This association deserves further investigation, since it may affect recommendations regarding the DVT prophylaxis of high-risk patients.

33.10   CONCLUSIONS

Diabetes mellitus plays an important role in the development of PAD affecting the lower limbs. PAD is an important predictor of mortality independent of diabetes, but it is not clear whether simultaneous presence of diabetes and PAD create a synergism that results in a greater than expected increase risk of death. Diabetes does not appear to play a role in the development of RAS, although little investigation has been performed on this outcome. Interestingly, diabetes may have a protective effect on the development of AAA,

possibly because of its association with greater arterial wall stiffness. There is some evidence to support a role for diabetes in development of venous thromboembolic disease, although results are inconsistent and not confirmatory in several large, well-designed epidemiologic studies. The problem of preventing and treating vascular disease will be a continuing challenge to all persons involved in diabetes, research and treatment. Further research is clearly needed, and studies such as the DCCT/EDIC and UKPDS may be poised to contribute to this knowledge base in the near future.

References

1. American Diabetes Association (2003) Peripheral arterial disease in people with diabetes. *Diabetes Care*, **26**, 3333–41.
2. McGee, S.R. and Boyko, E.J. (1998) Physical examination and chronic lower-extremity ischemia: a critical review. *Archives of Internal Medicine*, **158** (12), 1357–64.
3. Boyko, E.J., Ahroni, J.H., Davignon, D. *et al.* (1997) Diagnostic utility of the history and physical examination for peripheral vascular disease among patients with diabetes mellitus. *Journal of Clinical Epidemiology*, **50** (6), 659–68.
4. Atsma, F., Bartelink, M.L., Grobbee, D.E. and van der Schxaouw, Y.T. (2005) Best reproducibility of the ankle–arm index was calculated using Doppler and dividing highest ankle pressure by highest arm pressure. *Journal of Clinical Epidemiology*, **58**, (12), 1282–8.
5. Halperin, J.L. (2002) Evaluation of patients with peripheral vascular disease. *Thrombosis Research*, **106** (6), V303–11.
6. Boyko, E.J., Ahroni, J.H., Stensel, V.L. *et al.* (1996) Predictors of transcutaneous oxygen tension in the lower limbs of diabetic subjects. *Diabetes Medicine*, **13** (6), 549–54.
7. Pecoraro, R.E., Ahroni, J.H., Boyko, E.J. and Stensel, V.L. (1991) Chronology and determinants of tissue repair in diabetic lower-extremity ulcers. *Diabetes*, **40** (10), 1305–13.
8. Gregg, E.W., Sorlie, P., Paulose-Ram, R., *et al.* (2004) Prevalence of lower-extremity disease in the U.S. adult population >40 years of age with and without diabetes. *Diabetes Care*, **27**, 1591–7.
9. Heiserman, J.E. (2005) Measurement error of percent diameter carotid stenosis determined by conventional angiography: implications for noninvasive evaluation. *American Journal of Neuroradiology*, **26** (8), 2102–7.

10. Boyko, E.J., Alderman, B.W. and Baron, A.E. (1988) Reference test errors bias the evaluation of diagnostic tests for ischemic heart disease. *Journal of General Internal Medicine*, **3**, 476–81.

11. Roeren, T., LeVeen, R.F. and Knecht, L.B. (1988) Sources of error in arterial morphometric measurements. *Investigative Radiology*, **23** (9), 672–6.

12. Stenstrom, H., Knutsson, A. and Smedby, O. (2005) Vessel size estimation in peripheral artery interventions: are angiographic measurements reliable? *Acta Radiologica*, **46** (2), 163–9.

13. Young, M.J., Adams, J.E., Anderson, G.F., *et al.* (1993) Medial arterial calcification in the feet of diabetic patients and matched non-diabetic control subjects. *Diabetolgia*, **36**, 615–21.

14. Rothman, K.J. and Greenland, S. (1998) *Modern Epidemiology*, Lippincott-Raven, Philadelphia, PA.

15. Nathan, D.M., Lachin, J., Cleary, P. *et al.* (2003) Intensive diabetes therapy and carotid intima-media thickness in type 1 diabetes mellitus. *The New England Journal of Medicine* **348** (23), 2294–303.

16. Leng, G.C. and Fowkes, F.G. (1992) The Edinburgh claudication questionnaire: an improved version of the WHO/Rose Questionnaire for use in epidemiological surveys. *Journal of Clinical Epidemiology*, **45**, 1101–9.

17. Criqui, M.H., Fronek, A., Barrett-Connor, E., *et al.* (1985) The prevalence of peripheral arterial disease in a defined population. *Circulation*, **71** (3), 510–15.

18. Fowkes, F.G., Housley, E., Cawood, E.H., *et al.* (1991) Edinburgh Artery Study: prevalence of asymptomatic and symptomatic peripheral arterial disease in the general population. *International Journal of Epidemiology*, **20** (2), 384–92.

19. Fowkes, F.G. (1997) Epidemiology of peripheral vascular disease. *Atherosclerosis*, **131** (Suppl 1), S29–31.

20. Hiatt, W.R., Hoag, S. and Hamman, R.F. (1995) Effect of diagnostic criteria on the prevalence of peripheral arterial disease. The San Luis Valley Diabetes Study. *Circulation*, **91**, 1472–9.

21. Meijer, W.T., Hoes, A.W., Rutgers, D., *et al.* (1998) Peripheral arterial disease in the elderly: the Rotterdam Study. *Arteriosclerosis, Thrombosis, and Vascular Biology*, **18**, 185–92.

22. Hirsch, A.T., Criqui, M.H., Treat-Jacobson, D., *et al.* (2001) Peripheral arterial disease detection, awareness, and treatment in primary care. *Journal of the American Medical Association*, **286**, 1317–24.

23. Orchard, T.J., Dorman, J.S., Maser, R.E., *et al.* (1990) Prevalence of complications in IDDM by sex and duration. Pittsburgh Epidemiology of Diabetes Complications Study II. *Diabetes*, **39** (9), 1116–24.

24. Newman, A.B., Siscovick, D.S., Monolio, T.A., *et al.* (1993) Ankle–arm index as a marker of atherosclerosis in the Cardiovascular Health Study. *Circulation*, **88**, 837–45.

25. Beks, P.J., Mackaay, A.J., de Neeling, J.N., *et al.* (1995) Peripheral arterial disease in relation to glycaemic level in an elderly Caucasian population: the Hoorn Study. *Diabetolgia*, **38**, 86–96.

26. Curb, J.D., Masaki, K. and Rodriguez, B.L. (1996) *et al.* Peripheral artery disease and cardiovascular risk factors in the elderly. The Honolulu Heart Program. *Arteriosclerosis, Thrombosis, and Vascular Biology*, **16** (12), 1495–500.

27. Zheng, Z.-J., Sharrett, A.R., Chambless, L.E., *et al.* (1997) Associations of ankle–brachial index with clinical coronary heart disease, stroke and preclinical carotid and popliteal atherosclerosis: the Atherosclerosis in Communities (ARIC) Study. *Atherosclerosis*, **131**, 115–25.

28. Murabito, J.M., Evans, J.C., Nieto, K., *et al.* (2002) Prevalence and clinical correlates of peripheral arterial disease in the Framingham Offspring Study. *American Heart Journal*, **143**, 961–5.

29. Munter, P., Wildman, R.P., Reynolds, K. *et al.* (2005) Relationship between HbA1c level and peripheral arterial disease. *Diabetes Care*, **28**, 1981–87.

30. Halperin, J.L. and Creager, M.A. (1992) Arterial obstructive diseases of the extremities, in *Vascular Medicine* (eds J. Loscalzo, M.A. Creager and V.J. Dzau), Little Brown, Boston, MA.

31. LoGerfo, F.W. and Coffman, J.D. (1984) Vascular and microvascular disease of the foot in diabetes. Implications in foot care. *New England Journal of Medicine*, **311**, 1615–19.

32. Jude, E.B., Oyibo, S.O., Chalmers, N. and Boulton, A.J.M. (2001) Peripheral arterial disease in diabetic and nondiabetic patients. *Diabetes Care*, **24** (8), 1433–7.

33. Uusitupa, M.I., Niskanen, L.K., Siitonen, O. *et al.* (1990) 5-year incidence of atherosclerotic vascular disease in relation to general risk factors, insulin level, and abnormalities in lipoprotein composition in non-insulin-dependent diabetic and nondiabetic subjects. *Circulation*, **82**, 27–36.

34. Criqui, M.H., Langer, R.D., Fronek, A. *et al.* (1992) Mortality over a period of 10 years in patients with peripheral arterial disease. *New England Journal of Medicine*, **326**, 381–6.

35. Lee, A.J., Price, J.F., Russell, M.J. *et al.* (2004) Improved prediction of fatal myocardial infarction using the ankle brachial index in addition to conventional risk factors. The Edinburgh Artery Study. *Circulation*, **110**, 3075–80.

36. Feringa, H.H., Bax, J.J., van Waning, V.H. *et al.* (2006) The long-term prognostic value of the resting and postexercise ankle–brachial index. *Archives of Internal Medicine*, **166**, 529–35.

37. Kannel, W.B., McGee, D., and Gordon, T. (1976) A general cardiovascular risk profile: the Framingham Study. *American Journal of Cardiology*, **38**, 46–51.

38. Fowkes, F.G., Housley, E., Riemersma, R.A. *et al.* (1992) Smoking, lipids, glucose intolerance, and blood pressure as risk factors for peripheral atherosclerosis compared with ischemic heart disease in the Edinburgh Artery Study. *American Journal of Epidemiology*, **135**, 331–40.

39. Lee, A.J., MacGregor, A.S., Hau, C.M. *et al.* (1999) The role of haematological factors in diabetic peripheral arterial disease: the Edinburgh artery study. *British Journal of Haematology*, **105**, 648–54.

40. Newman, A.B., Rutan, G.H., Sutton-Tyrrell, K. *et al.* (1990) Lower extremity arterial disease in elderly subjects with systolic hypertension. *Journal of Clinical Epidemiology*, **44** (1), 15–20.

41. Adler, A.I., Stevens, R.J., Neil, A. *et al.* (2002) UKPDS 59: Hyperglycemia and other potentially modifiable risk factors for peripheral vascular disease in type 2 diabetes. *Diabetes Care*, **25**, 894–99.

42. Kannel, W.B. and McGee, D.L. (1985) Update on some epidemiologic features of intermittent claudication: the Framingham Study. *Journal of the American Geriatrics Society*, **33**, 13–18.

43. Ogren, M., Hedblad, B., Isacsson, S.O. *et al.* (1993) Non-invasively detected carotid stenosis and ischaemic heart disease in men with leg arteriosclerosis. *Lancet*, **342**, 1138–41.

44. Adler, A.I., Stratton, I.M., Neil, H.A. *et al.* (2000) Association of systolic blood pressure with macrovascular and microvascular complications of type 2 diabetes (UKPDS 36): prospective observational study. *British Medical Journal*, **321**, 412–19.

45. Aschoff, L. (1932) Observations concerning the relationship between cholesterol metabolism and vascular disease. *British Medical Journal*, **2**, 1121.

46. Malinow, M.R., Kang, S.S., Taylor, L.M. *et al.* (1989) Prevalence of hyperhomocyst(e)inemia in patients with peripheral occlusive disease. *Circulation*, **79**, 1180–88.

47. Robinson, K., Arheart, K. and Refsum, H. *et al.* (1998) Low circulating folate and vitamin B6 concentrations: risk factors for stroke, peripheral vascular disease, and coronary artery disease. [See comments]. *Circulation*, **97** (5), 437–43.

48. Schnyder, G., Roffi, M., Flammer, Y. *et al.* (2002) Effect of homocysteine-lowering therapy with folic acid, vitamin B12, vitamin B6 on clinical outcome after percutaneous coronary intervention. *Journal of the American Medical Association*, **288** (8), 973–9.

49. Lowe, G.D., Fowkes, F.G., Dawes, J. *et al.* (1993) Blood viscosity, fibrinogen, and activation of coagulation and leukocytes in peripheral arterial disease and the normal population in the Edinburgh Artery Study. *Circulation*, **87**, 1915–20.

50. Lee, A.J., Fowkes, F.G., Lowe, G.D. and Rumley, A. (1995) Fibrin D-dimer, haemostatic factors and peripheral arterial disease. *Thrombosis and Haemostasis*, **74**, 828–32.

51. Cook, P.J. and Lip, G.Y. (1996) Infectious agents and atherosclerotic vascular disease. *QJM–Monthly Journal of the Association of Physicians*, **89** (10), 727–35.

52. Gibbs, R.G., Carey, N. and Davies, A.H. (1998) *Chlamydia pneumoniae* and vascular disease. *British Journal of Surgery*, **85** (9), 1191–7.

53. Martyn, C.N., Gale, C.R., Jespersen, S. and Sherriff, S.B. (1998) Impaired fetal growth and atherosclerosis of carotid and peripheral arteries. *Lancet*, **352** (9123), 173–8.

54. Hales, C.N., Desai, M. and Ozanne, S.E. (1997) The thrifty phenotype hypothesis: how does it look after 5 years? *Diabetes Medicine*, **14**, 189–95.

55. Sawicki, P.T., Kaiser, S., Heinemann, L. *et al.* (1991) Prevalence of renal artery stenosis in diabetes mellitus – an autopsy study. *Journal of Internal Medicine*, **229** (6), 489–92.

56. Hansen, K.J., Edwards, M.S. and Craven, T.E. *et al.* (2002) Prevalence of renovascular disease in the elderly: a population-based study. *Journal of Vascular Surgery*, **36** (3), 443–51.

57. Munichoodappa, C., D'Elia, J.A., Libertino, J.A. *et al.* (1979) Renal artery stenosis in hypertensive diabetics. *Journal of Urology*, **121** (5), 555–8.

58. Park, S., Jung, J.H. and Seo, H.S. *et al.* (2004) The prevalence and clinical predictors of atherosclerotic renal artery stenosis in patients undergoing coronary angiography. *Heart and Vessels*, **19** (6), 275–9.

59. Liu, B.C., Tang, R.N., Feng, Y. *et al.* (2004) A single Chinese center investigation of renal artery stenosis in 141 consecutive cases with coronary angiography. *American Journal of Nephrology*, **24** (6), 630–4.

60. Ritchie, C.M., McIlrath, E., Hadden, D.R. *et al.* (1988) Renal artery stenosis in hypertensive diabetic patients. *Diabetes Medicine*, **5** (3), 265–7.

61. Courreges, J.P., Bacha, J., Aboud, E. and Pradier, P. (2000) Prevalence of renal artery stenosis in type 2 diabetes. *Diabetes and Metabolism*, **26** (Suppl 4), 90–6.

62. Myers, D.I., Poole, L.J., Imam, K. *et al.* (2003) Renal artery stenosis by three-dimensional magnetic resonance angiography in type 2 diabetics

with uncontrolled hypertension and chronic renal insufficiency: prevalence and effect on renal function. *American Journal of Kidney Diseases*, **41** (2), 351–9.

63. Coen, G., Calabria, S. and Lai, S. *et al.* (2003) Atherosclerotic ischemic renal disease. Diagnosis and prevalence in an hypertensive and/or uremic elderly population. *BMC Nephrology*, **4**, 2.

64. Krohn, C.D., Kullmann, G., Kvernebo, K. *et al.* (1992) Ultrasonographic screening for abdominal aortic aneurysm. *European Journal of Surgery*, **158** (10), 527–30.

65. Smith, F.C., Grimshaw, G.M., Paterson, I.S. *et al.* (1993) Ultrasonographic screening for abdominal aortic aneurysm in an urban community. *British Journal of Surgery*, **80** (11), 1406–9.

66. Pleumeekers, H.J., Hoes, A.W. and van der Does, E. *et al.* (1995) Aneurysms of the abdominal aorta in older adults. The Rotterdam Study. *American Journal of Epidemiology*, **142** (12), 1291–9.

67. Scott, R.A., Wilson, N.M., Ashton, H.A. and Kay, D.N. (1995) Influence of screening on the incidence of ruptured abdominal aortic aneurysm: 5-year results of a randomized controlled study. *British Journal of Surgery*, **82** (8), 1066–70.

68. Kanagasabay, R., Gajraj, H., Pointon, L. and Scott, R.A. (1996) Co-morbidity in patients with abdominal aortic aneurysm. *Journal of Medical Screening*, **3** (4), 208–10.

69. Simoni, G., Pastorino, C. and Perrone, R. *et al.* (1995) Screening for abdominal aortic aneurysms and associated risk factors in a general population. *European Journal of Vascular and Endovascular Surgery*, **10** (2), 207–10.

70. Mattes, E., Davis, T.M., Yang, D. *et al.* (1997) Prevalence of abdominal aortic aneurysms in men with diabetes. *Medical Journal of Australia*, **166** (12), 630–3.

71. Lederle, F.A., Johnson, G.R. and Wilson, S.E. *et al.* (1997) Prevalence and associations of abdominal aortic aneurysm detected through screening. Aneurysm Detection and Management (ADAM) Veterans Affairs Cooperative Study Group. *Annals of Internal Medicine*, **126** (6), 441–9.

72. Lederle, F.A., Johnson, G.R. and Wilson, S.E. *et al.* (2000) The aneurysm detection and management study screening program: validation cohort and final results. *Archives of Internal Medicine*, **160** (10), 1425–30.

73. Blanchard, J.F., Armenian, H.K. and Friesen, P.P. (2000) Risk factors for abdominal aortic aneurysm: results of a case-control study. *American Journal of Epidemiology*, **151** (6), 575–83.

74. Wanhainen, A., Bergqvist, D., Boman, K. *et al.* (2005) Risk factors associated with abdominal aortic aneurysm: a population-based study with historical and current data. *Journal of Vascular Surgery*, **41** (3), 390–6.

75. Wanhainen, A., Bjorck, M., Boman, K. *et al.* (2001) Influence of diagnostic criteria on the prevalence of abdominal aortic aneurysm. *Journal of Vascular Surgery*, **34** (2), 229–35.

76. Eren, M., Gorgulu, S., Uslu, N. *et al.* (2004) Relation between aortic stiffness and left ventricular diastolic function in patients with hypertension, diabetes, or both. *Heart*, **90** (1), 37–43.

77. Schram, M.T., Henry, R.M. and van Dijk, R.A. *et al.* (2004) Increased central artery stiffness in impaired glucose metabolism and type 2 diabetes: the Hoorn Study. *Hypertension*, **43** (2), 176–81.

78. Reddy, G.K. (2004) AGE-related cross-linking of collagen is associated with aortic wall matrix stiffness in the pathogenesis of drug-induced diabetes in rats. *Microvascular Research*, **68** (2), 132–42.

79. Blanchard, J.F. (1999) Epidemiology of abdominal aortic aneurysms. *Epidemiologic Reviews*, **21** (2), 207–21.

80. Goldhaber, S.Z., Grodstein, F. and Stampfer, M.J. *et al.* (1997) A prospective study of risk factors for pulmonary embolism in women. *Journal of the American Medical Association*, **277** (8), 642–5.

81. Goldhaber, S.Z., Savage, D.D. and Garrison, R.J. *et al.* (1983) Risk factors for pulmonary embolism. The Framingham Study. *American Journal of Medicine*, **74** (6), 1023–8.

82. Tsai, A.W., Cushman, M., Rosamond, W.D. *et al.* (2002) Cardiovascular risk factors and venous thromboembolism incidence: the longitudinal investigation of thromboembolism etiology. *Archives of Internal Medicine*, **162** (10), 1182–9.

83. Bergqvist, D., Bergentz, S.E., Bornmyr, S. *et al.* (1985) Deep vein thrombosis after renal transplantation: a prospective analysis of frequency and risk factors. *European Surgical Research*, **17** (2), 69–74.

84. Humar, A., Johnson, E.M. and Gillingham, K.J. *et al.* (1998) Venous thromboembolic complications after kidney and kidney–pancreas transplantation: a multivariate analysis. *Transplantation*, **65** (2), 229–34.

85. Russell, M.W., Taylor, D.C., Cummins, G. and Huse, D.M. (2002) Use of managed care claims data in the risk assessment of venous thromboembolism

in outpatients. *American Journal of Managed Care*, **8** (1 Suppl), S3–9.

86. Petrauskiene, V., Falk, M., Waernbaum, I. *et al.* (2005) The risk of venous thromboembolism is markedly elevated in patients with diabetes. *Diabetologia*, **48** (5), 1017–21.

87. Carr, M.E. (2001) Diabetes mellitus: a hypercoagulable state. *Journal of Diabetes and its Complications*, **15** (1), 44–54.

88. Sobel, B.E. and Schneider, D.J. (2004) Platelet function, coagulopathy, and impaired fibrinolysis in diabetes. *Cardiology Clinics*, **22** (4), 511–26.

34

Epidemiology of Diabetic Neuropathy

Andrew J. M. Boulton

Department of Medicine, Manchester Royal Infirmary, Manchester, UK

34.1 INTRODUCTION

The neuropathies are among the most common of the long-term complications of diabetes, affecting up to 50% of patients. They are heterogonous, affecting different parts of the nervous system and may present with diverse clinical manifestations: they may be focal or diffuse. The first clinical description of peripheral diabetic neuropathy is usually attributed to Dr John Rollo of London, who described pain and paresthesiae in the legs of a diabetic patient in 1798 [1]. The clinical features vary immensely and patients may present to a wide spectrum of specialties, from dermatology to podiatry for example, or from urology to cardiology. Neuropathy is characterized by a progressive loss of nerve fiber that may affect both principle divisions of the peripheral nervous system; that is, somatic and autonomic. The early recognition and appropriate management of neuropathy in patients with diabetes is important for a number of reasons:

(a) It must be remembered that not all neuropathy in diabetes is secondary to the disease itself: nondiabetic neuropathies may also be present.

(b) A number of treatment options exist for symptomatic diabetic neuropathy that are confirmed in multiple, randomized control trials.

(c) Up to 50% of the commonest variety of diabetic neuropathy, sensorimotor neuropathy, may be asymptomatic and patients in this group are at risk of insensate injury to their feet. As >80% of amputations follow a foot ulcer or injury, early recognition of at risk individuals and appropriate interventions is essential.

(d) Autonomic neuropathy may involve any system of the body.

Although there have been numerous publications on the epidemiology of diabetic neuropathy, this area has been beset by numerous problems relating to a lack of agreement as to which diagnostic tests should be used and, in addition, major differences in population selection [2]. First, as diabetic neuropathy may affect different sets of nerve fibers in different patients, then a large fiber test, such as measuring vibration perception, might be completely normal in someone with small-fiber neuropathy. The measurement of nerve function is further complicated by the fact that quantitative assessment of sensation requires the use of complex psychophysical tests which rely on patient response; hence, such tests are subject to poor reproducibility.

Second, determining the true prevalence of neuropathy is difficult, as most studies differ in the populations that have been assessed. Many studies have been hospital or clinic based; such studies are likely to be biased toward more severe neuropathy and, thus, are likely to result in an overestimation of the prevalence. Moreover, as symptomatic neuropathy might be present in the background nondiabetic population, this should be taken into account; however, few studies have attended to this problem [3, 4].

This chapter will first consider definitions and classifications of the diabetic neuropathies; this

The Epidemiology of Diabetes Mellitus, second edition   Edited by Jean-Marie Ekoé, Marian Rewers, Rhys Williams and Paul Zimmet
© 2008 John Wiley & Sons, Ltd

will be followed by a discussion of the etiology and epidemiology of diabetic neuropathy. As neuropathy is a major contributory factor to diabetic foot problems [5], similar data on etiology and epidemiology will be presented for diabetic foot ulceration and amputation.

34.2 CLASSIFICATION OF THE DIABETIC NEUROPATHIES

There have been a number of consensus statements regarding the diagnosis, staging, measurements and assessment of diabetic neuropathy. The 1988 San Antonio Conference considered definition and measurement; a definition was agreed [6]:

> Diabetic neuropathy is a descriptive term meaning a demonstrable disorder, either clinically evident or sub-clinical, that occurs in the setting of diabetes mellitus without other causes for peripheral neuropathy. The neuropathic disorder includes manifestations in the somatic and/or autonomic parts of the peripheral nervous system.

It was recommended that, for full classification, at least one measure should be made from each of five categories: symptoms, neurological examination, quantitative sensory testing (QST), electrodiagnostic studies and autonomic function tests. Whereas such a strict definition is useful for clinical trials, it is clearly not feasible for day-to-day clinical practice. A subsequent international meeting considered the definition, staging and management of diabetic peripheral neuropathy (DPN) for practicing clinicians: neuropathy was defined as 'the presence of symptoms and/or signs of peripheral nerve dysfunction in people with diabetes after exclusion of other causes' [7]. Moreover, it was agreed that 'the diagnosis cannot be made without a careful clinical examination.' Thus, as many patients are asymptomatic, absence of symptoms can never be equated with absence of neuropathy. The importance of excluding nondiabetic causes of neuropathy was emphasized previously in the Rochester Diabetic Neuropathy Study, in which up to 10% of peripheral neuropathy in diabetic patients was deemed to be of nondiabetic causation [8]. A recent position statement on diabetic neuropathies by the American Diabetes Association [9] agreed with the previous international meeting that the diagnosis of chronic

diabetic neuropathy is a clinical one requiring a history, examination and the exclusion of nondiabetic causes.

Numerous classifications of the variety of syndromes affecting the peripheral nervous system in diabetes have been proposed in recent years. Some have been based upon presumed causation, topographical features or pathological involvement. However, those classifications based upon clinical manifestations are most commonly used. Three examples of slightly different clinical classifications are presented in **Table 34.1**. **Table 34.1**(A) describes a purely clinical classification [1], whereas **Table 34.1**(B) bases its classification on a mixture of clinical and anatomical findings [10]. The classification proposed by Thomas [11, 12] will mainly be used in this review. This is based upon the premise that neuropathy results from a number of disturbances in the peripheral nervous system as a consequence of hyperglycemia. A brief description of these subgroups is now provided.

34.2.1 Focal and Multifocal Neuropathies

Focal and multifocal neuropathies are confined to the distribution of a single or multiple peripheral nerves, and their involvement is referred to as *mononeuropathy* or *mononeuritis multiplex*. It is important to differentiate between mononeuritis and nerve entrapment syndromes: whereas mononeuropathies are of sudden onset and are generally due to vasculitis and subsequent ischemia/infarction of nerves, entrapment neuropathies occur when a peripheral nerve is entrapped in a narrow area, such as in carpal tunnel syndrome when the median nerve is compressed under the transverse carpal ligament. Other common entrapment syndromes involve the ulnar, radial and common peroneal nerves. Carpal tunnel syndrome is by far the commonest of these and occurs three times more commonly in people with diabetes than in the healthy population [13]. Common mononeuropathies involve the cranial nerves 3, 6 and 7 and the thoracic and peripheral nerves. It should be easy to differentiate between a mononeuropathy and an entrapment neuropathy, as the latter is gradual in onset and occurs in the distribution of single nerves that are prone to be exposed to trauma. In contrast, the mononeuropathies are of sudden onset, are not progressive

Table 34.1 Three classification systems for diabetic neuropathy.

A: Clinical classification of diabetic neuropathy

Polyneuropathy

Sensory
- Acute sensory
- Chronic sensorimotor

Autonomic
- Cardiovascular
- Gastrointestinal
- Genitourinary
- Other

Proximal motor (amyotrophy)

Truncal

Adapted from Boulton and Malik [1].

Mononeuropathy

Isolated peripheral

Mononeuritis multiplex

Isolated peripheral

Truncal

B: Patterns of neuropathy in diabetes

Length-dependent diabetic polyneuropathy
- Distal symmetrical sensory polyneuropathy
- Large fiber neuropathy
- Painful symmetrical polyneuropathy
- Autonomic neuropathies

Focal and multifocal neuropathies
- Cranial neuropathies
- Limb neuropathies
- Proximal DN of the lower limbs
- Truncal neuropathies

Nondiabetic neuropathies more common in diabetes
- Pressure palsies
- Acquired inflammatory demyelinating polyneuropathy

Adapted from Said [10].

C: Classification of diabetic neuropathy

Rapidly reversible
- Hyperglycemic neuropathy

Generalized symmetrical polyneuropathiescr
- Sensorimotor (chronic)
- Acute sensory
- Autonomic

Focal and multifocal neuropathies
- Cranial
- Thoracolumbar radiculoneuropathy
- Focal limb
- Proximal motor (amyotrophy)

Superimposed chronic inflammatory demyelinating neuropathy

Adapted from Thomas [11, 12]

and do tend to result spontaneously [13]. There are few good studies of the incidence and prevalence of these neuropathies, and with the exception of carpal tunnel syndrome, which may occur in up to 14% of diabetic subjects, other mononeuropathies and entrapment neuropathies are relatively rare.

34.2.2   Chronic Diabetic Peripheral Sensory Polyneuropathy (DPN)

This is by far the commonest subgroup of the diabetic neuropathies that is usually of insidious onset, and may indeed be present at the diagnosis of type 2 diabetes in >10% of subjects [14, 15]. Whereas up to 50% of patients may be asymptomatic, 10–20% may experience troublesome sensory symptoms, particularly in the feet, which require specific treatment. Late sequelae of neuropathy include insensitive foot ulceration, Charcot (neuropathic) arthropathy and occasionally amputation [16].

34.2.3   Diabetic Autonomic Neuropathy

Diabetic autonomic neuropathy (DAN) results in significant morbidity and may lead to mortality in some patients with diabetes [17]. Although any area receiving autonomic innovation may be involved in DAN, the major clinical manifestations of DAN include resting tachycardia, exercise intolerance, orthostatic hypotension, constipation, gastroparesis, erectile dysfunction (ED), abnormalities of sweating and impaired neurovascular function [9, 17].

34.2.4   The Diabetic Foot

The late sequalae of both DPN and DAN include foot ulceration, Charcot's neuroarthropathy and even on occasions amputation [18]. The epidemiology of diabetic foot problems, particularly foot ulceration, will be discussed further at the end of this chapter.

34.3   ETIOLOGY OF DIABETIC NEUROPATHIES

The diabetic polyneuropathies (DPN and DAN) are clearly of multifactorial etiology, and a number of metabolic and vascular defects have now been implicated in their pathogenesis [19]. The strength of the associations of a number of risk factors and the development of neuropathy will now be discussed.

34.3.1   Hyperglycemia

Of all the potential contributory factors that result in the development of DPN and DAN, chronic persistent hyperglycemia is the strongest. The Diabetes Control and Complications Trial (DCCT) study has provided definitive evidence of the importance of preceding hyperglycemia in the pathogenesis of neuropathy in type 1 diabetes [20]: intensive insulin therapy reduced the subsequent development of clinical neuropathy by over 60% in this study. At the end of the first stage of the DCCT, significant reductions in electrophysiological studies were observed in those patients receiving conventional therapy; similarly, at the end of the DCCT trial, 9% of those on conventional therapy had abnormal autonomic function tests compared with 4% on those with intensive treatment [21]. The Epidemiology of Diabetes Intervention and Complications (EDIC) study, which is a follow-up of DCCT, recently reported that the benefits of intensive therapy on neuropathy status extended for at least 8 years beyond the end of the DCCT, which was similar to those findings described for both retinopathy and nephropathy [22].

For type 2 diabetes, data from the longitudinal assessment of the Rochester Diabetic Neuropathic Study cohort demonstrate that duration and severity of exposure to hyperglycemia are related to the severity of neuropathy [23]. The UK Prospective Diabetes Study represents the largest interventional study in type 2 diabetes that has assessed the effects of improved glycemic control to date and preliminary data suggests that deterioration in nerve function as assessed by vibration perception is less in those randomized to intensive control [15]. However, at the time of writing, the detailed results of neuropathy assessments are about to be submitted for publication and should by now be available.

Further support for the relationship between hyperglycemia and the development of neuropathy comes from recent studies in patients with idiopathic neuropathy and would suggest that up to 40% of subjects with neuropathy of previously undiagnosed causation actually have impaired glucose tolerance [24]. Such observations support the hypothesis that impaired glucose tolerance-related neuropathy may actually represent the earlier stage of diabetic neuropathy which is characterized by damage to small nerve fibers. In a recent study of lifestyle intervention in patients with this impaired glucose tolerance neuropathy, it is most interesting to observe that the improvement in metabolic parameters was also associated with significant improvement in measures of small-fiber nerve function [25].

In summary, there are strong longitudinal data to support the major contributions that chronic hyperglycemia has in the pathogenesis of diabetic neuropathy in both type 1 and type 2 diabetes.

34.3.2 Other Metabolic Consequences of Hyperglycemia

Considerable evidence implicates the involvement of the downstream consequences of hyperglycemia in the genesis of diabetic neuropathies. Although most would accept that neuropathy is of multifactorial etiology involving vascular and metabolic factors, the reported severe neuropathy in a patient with Mendenhall's syndrome in the absence of any significant micro- or macro-angiopathy suggests that hyperglycemia alone (and its metabolic consequences) can lead to neuropathy [26].

Considerable evidence implicates the involvement of one of the metabolic consequences of hyperglycemia, namely increased activity in the polyol pathway in the development of neuropathy [19]. Sorbitol levels are increased in peripheral nerves in both experimental diabetic animals and also in man, and inhibition of the rate-limiting enzyme of this pathway, aldose reductase, can prevent the development of experimental neuropathy and improve nerve function in DPN. Hyperglycemia also results in the formation of advanced glycation end-products (AGEs), which in turn act on specific receptors, inducing monocytes and endothelial cells to increase the production of cytokines and adhesion molecules [27]. Although inhibitors of AGE have been under investigation in microvascular complications, no trial data are currently available for human DPN.

An increasing body of data supports the role of oxidative stress in the pathogenesis of diabetic neuropathy in animal models. Antioxidants, such as α-lipoic acid, have been shown to be helpful in symptomatic diabetic neuropathy in large randomized trials [28].

34.3.3 Vascular Factors

A number of observations support the contribution of vascular factors in the pathogenesis of DPN.

Studies have suggested that improving tissue blood flow after large-vessel revascularization may lead to an improvement in electrophysiological measures and also that the use of angiotensin-converting enzyme (ACE) inhibitors might lead to improvement in nerve function [19]. Most recently, further support for vascular factors has been provided by the follow-up of the multinational EURODIAB Prospective Complications Study [29]. The cumulative incidence of neuropathy in this study, as well as being related to glycemic control, was significantly associated with higher levels of total and low-density lipoprotein cholesterol and triglycerides, hypertension and cigarette smoking [30]. This important long-term study of over 1000 patients indicates that the incidence of neuropathy is strongly associated with potentially modifiable cardiovascular risk factors [30].

34.3.4 Age and Diabetes Duration

Two large studies from the United Kingdom and Spain [31, 32] have clearly shown a relationship between advancing age and diabetes duration with the prevalence of DPN. In the Spanish study, for example, the prevalence rose from 14% at under 5 years' duration to 44% at a duration of more than 30 years of diabetes [32].

34.3.5 Genetic Factors

Although clear ethnic and racial differences have been described in other long-term diabetic complications, including nephropathy and macrovascular disease, only limited data are available for DPN. Data from the large community-based North-West Diabetes Foot Care Study [33] suggest that there are ethnic differences in DPN between Europid, Asian and African-Caribbean patients. Among 15 692 diabetic patients examined in this study, 85% were European, 12% Asian ($n = 1866$) and 2% African-Caribbean ($n = 371$). Neuropathy, as assessed by vibration perception, was present in 23% of the Europeans, 14% of the Asians and 13% of the African-Caribbeans ($p < 0.001$ [34]). Other studies have looked at potential genetic predictors: in one case–control study [35], increased susceptibility to DPN was shown in those type 1 patients with a polymorphism at the 5' end of the aldose reductase gene. Although there have been other small studies, there is at present only a low level of evidence for the role of any particular candidate gene in the etiology of neuropathy.

34.4 HOW COMMON IS DIABETIC NEUROPATHY?

34.4.1 Diabetic Peripheral Symmetrical Polyneuropathy (DPN)

In view of the above-mentioned comments in Section 34.1, it is difficult to determine accurately the true prevalence of diabetic neuropathy. However, several large clinic-based studies have attempted to assess the prevalence (e.g. [31, 32]). More recent studies have tended to assess the prevalence of neuropathy in defined populations or large community studies [33–37]. In general, the large clinical-based studies tend to report higher prevalences than population-based studies, although one population-based study in older type 2 diabetic patients suggested that 42% of a sample of 811 subjects had signs of peripheral diabetic neuropathy [37]. Some published studies on the prevalence of DPN in the last 20 years are presented in **Table 34.2**;

as can be seen, methodology is far from uniform, although overall differences in prevalences are not great.

The population-based study from the Liverpool area of northwest England [4] has the advantage that the nondiabetic population was also screened for evidence of peripheral neuropathy; the finding of nearly 5% of neuropathy in nondiabetic individuals in this population is an important observation, suggesting that future studies should also contain a nondiabetic control group.

34.4.2 DAN

The difficulties in studying the epidemiology of diabetic neuropathy are even greater for DAN because of a large variety of nonspecific clinical manifestations with often multiple factors contributing to any particular condition. A good example of the difficulties that might be experienced is the study of the prevalence of ED, which is usually of multifactorial etiology of which DAN is only one. Limited data for the prevalences of ED and cardiovascular DAN will be presented.

Table 34.2 Epidemiological data for DPN.[a]

Reference	Country	Pop- or clinic-based	Total diabetic population	Type of diabetes	Criteria for diagnosis	Prevalence (%)
Maser et al. [38]	USA	Pop	400	1	Sy + signs	34
Franklin et al. [39]	USA	Pop	279	2	Sy + signs	26
Dyck et al. [8]	USA	Pop	380	1 + 2	Sy + signs + EP	48
Kumar et al. [37]	England	Pop	811	2	Signs	42
Young et al. [31]	UK	Clinics (n = 118)	6487	1 + 2	Sy + signs	29
Partanen et al. [14]	Finland	Pop	133	2	Sy + signs + EP	Diagnosis = 8 10 years = 42
Tesfaye et al. [29]	Europe	Clinics (n = 31)	1819	1	Sy + signs + QST	28
Cabezas-Cerrato [32]	Spain	Clinic	2644	1 + 2	Sy + signs	23
Abbott et al. [33]	England	Pop	9710	1 + 2	Signs	22
Daousi et al. [4]	England	Pop	350	1 + 2	Sy + signs	16
Davies et al. [36]	Scotland	Pop	326	2	Sy + signs	19

[a]Sy: symptoms; Pop: population-based study; EP: electrophysiology; QST: quantitative sensory testing; clinic: clinic-based study.

34.4.2.1 ED

It is estimated that over 10% of the nondiabetic population in the United States has ED, and that one-in-three men will experience the problem at some time. Longitudinal data from the Massachusetts Male Aging Study showed significant changes in erection frequency, sexual intercourse, desire and satisfaction in middle-aged men during a 9-year follow-up [40]. The within-person change in all three of these outcomes strongly related to age, with decline in sexual function becoming more pronounced with increasing age. In diabetes, this process appears to be exaggerated. Overall prevalence of ED amongst diabetic men in hospital clinic populations is probably between 30 and 50% [41, 42]. As in those without diabetes, the prevalence increases with age, but is generally lower in those with type 1 diabetes at about 20% [43]. Data from primary care are similar, with one study reporting a prevalence of 55% amongst diabetic men, of whom nearly 40% reported that the problem was persistent [44].

The same primary care study reported on the impact of ED on quality of life (QOL): nearly half of ED sufferers frequently thought about their ED, with a significant majority reporting that ED severely impacted on their QOL [44]. More recently, de Berardis et al. [45] showed that males with type 2 diabetes and ED are prone to poor QOL, worsening physical function, social functioning and general health, as well as an increase in depressive symptoms.

34.4.2.2 Cardiovascular Autonomic Neuropathy

Cardiovascular DAN has attracted much attention, as it can be associated with significant morbidity and mortality [17], and can be detected easily in its earlier stages by a number of noninvasive and validated autonomic function tests. As expected, considerable variability exists among the many prevalence studies that have assessed cardiovascular autonomic function tests; another major problem is the lack of any standard accepted definition of what constitutes DAN. Thus, the prevalence rates in a recent review for cardiovascular DAN varied from 7.7% in newly diagnosed type 1 patients to a high of 90% in patients listed for potential pancreas transplantation [17].

There have been studies that are community based, including one from Oxford, England, where the prevalence of DAN as defined by one or more abnormal tests of cardiovascular autonomic function was reported to be 16.7% [46]. In a larger multicenter study from Germany, Ziegler et al. [47] reported that 25.3% of patients with type 1 diabetes and 34.3% of patients with type 2 diabetes had abnormal findings in more than two of six autonomic function tests. In the DCCT [48], abnormalities of heart rate variation were reported in between 1.6 and 6.2% of patients; any cardiovascular abnormality was found in up to 23% of patients.

In summary, it is clear that cardiovascular DAN cannot generally be regarded as simply a late complication of diabetes: subclinical cardiovascular autonomic dysfunction may be detected early in the natural history of even type 1 diabetes. Another problem, not only in cardiovascular, but also other areas of DAN, is that clinical symptoms and signs do not correlate well with quantitative tests. Thus, for example, whereas diarrhea and constipation may be symptoms of gastrointestinal DAN, they are much more likely to result from causes other than DAN; for example, by taking medications such as metformin. Such problems have confounded and will continue to confound studies as a true prevalence of DAN.

34.5   THE DIABETIC FOOT

The loss of a limb or foot remains one of the most feared complications of diabetes, and yet foot problems remain the commonest reason for diabetic patients to be hospitalized in the Western world [5, 16]. As foot ulceration and amputation are closely interrelated in diabetes [5], they will be considered together in a section of the chapter, especially as >85% of amputations are preceded by an active foot ulcer. The term diabetic foot will be taken to encompass any foot lesion occurring as a result of diabetes or its complications. The financial cost of diabetic foot disease is staggering. The average inpatient costs for lower limb complications in 1997 were: foot ulcers $16 580; toe or toe and other distal amputations $25 241; major amputations $31 436 [49]. The average outpatient costs for one diabetic foot ulcer episode was estimated to be $28 000 over a 2-year period in 1999 [50]. The combination of diabetic foot ulceration and amputations was estimated to cost US health care payers $10.9

billion in 2001 [5]. Using the same methodology, the corresponding UK estimates were that 5% of the total National Health Service expenditure in 2001 ($3 billion) was attributable to diabetes. The total annual cost of diabetes-related foot complications was estimated to be $252 million [5].

In addition to the obvious social, economic and personal consequences of foot ulceration and amputation, the reason for the increased interest in this area in recent years is because the majority of foot ulcers and, thus, amputations are preventable [51]. Therefore, a thorough understanding of the risk factors for foot lesions is essential if a reduction in the late sequalae of neuropathy and peripheral vascular disease (PVD) is going to be achieved [52].

34.6 RISK FACTORS FOR THE DIABETIC FOOT

The breakdown of the diabetic foot has traditionally been considered to result from an interaction of PVD, DPN and trauma; more recently, psychosocial factors and abnormalities of pressures and loads under the feet have also been implicated.

34.6.1 PVD

A large number of studies have confirmed the frequency of PVD in diabetes. Most recently, the Diabetes Audit and Research in Tayside, Scotland (DARTS) study reported that the annual incidence for the development of PVD in diabetic patients is 5.5 per 1000 patients in those with type 1 diabetes and 13.6 per 1000 in type 2 diabetes [53]. PVD tends to occur at an earlier age in people with diabetes and is more likely to involve distal vessels. In the pathogenesis of ulceration, PVD itself, in isolation, rarely causes ulceration: as will be discussed for neuropathy, it is the combination of risk factors with minor trauma that inevitably leads to ulceration.

34.6.2 Peripheral Neuropathy

Both DPN and DAN (sympathetic neuropathy in the lower extremity) have been confirmed as independent risk factors for foot ulceration [16]. Patients can progress to the degree of insensitivity necessary for trophic ulceration without ever having experienced neuropathic symptoms (an important point in terms of the identification of the 'high-risk' foot), whereas others develop the

'painless–painful foot' with positive symptoms, but insensitivity on examination rendering the foot at high risk of ulceration [18]. The link between DPN and ulceration has now been confirmed in two prospective studies [54, 55]. Finally, special mention is made here of the motor component of DPN: small muscle wasting in the feet is common in neuropathy, and atrophy of the foot muscles is closely related to the severity of neuropathy [56].

34.6.3 Ethnicity and Sex

The male sex has been associated with a 1.6-fold increased risk of ulcers [33] and an even higher risk of amputation [57]. Data from cross-sectional studies across Europe suggest that foot ulceration is commoner in Europid subjects than in groups of other racial origins. Recent data from the North-West Diabetes Foot Care Study showed that the age-adjusted prevalence of diabetic foot ulcers (past or present) for Europeans, South Asians and African-Caribbeans was 5.5%, 1.8% and 2.7% respectively [34]. The reasons for these ethnic differences certainly warrant further investigation. In contrast, in the southern United States, ulceration was much more common in Hispanic Americans and Native Americans than in non-Hispanic Whites [58]. However, there is no suggestion that within Europe the risk is related to any geographical differences: Veves et al. [59], for example, showed no differences in risk factors for ulceration according to location in different European centers.

34.6.4 Other Risk Factors

One of the strongest risk factors for foot ulceration is past history of a similar lesion or an amputation. Other recognized risk factors include the presence of peripheral edema [51] and foot deformities [33]. In one study, the presence of plantar callus, especially in the neuropathic foot, was associated with an increased risk of ulceration that was 77-fold higher [60].

34.7 EPIDEMIOLOGICAL DATA ON DIABETIC FOOT PROBLEMS

A selection of epidemiological data for foot ulceration and amputation, originating from population-based studies from a number of

Table 34.3 Epidemiology of foot ulceration and amputation.

Reference	Country	Year	n	Prevalence (%)		Incidence (%)		Risk factors for foot ulcers (%)
				Ulcers	Amputations	Ulcers	Amputations	
Abbott et al. [33]	UK	2002	9710	1.7	1.3	2.2	—	>50
Manes et al. [61]	Greece	2002	821	4.8	—	—	—	>50
Muller et al. [62]	Netherlands	2002	665	—	—	2.1	0.6	—
Ramsey et al. [50]	USA	1999	8965	—	—	5.8[a]	0.9[a]	—
Vozar et al. [63]	Slovakia	1997	1205	2.5	0.9	0.6	0.6	—
Kumar et al. [37]	UK	1994	821	1.4[b]	—	—	—	42
Moss et al. [64]	USA	1992	2900	—	—	10.1[c]	2.1[c]	—

[a] Incidence figures over 3 years.

[b] Active ulcers: 5.4% past or current ulcers.

[c] Incidence figures over 4 years.

different countries, is provided in **Table 34.3**. Globally, the diabetic foot remains a major medical, social and economic problem that is seen in every country [5]. However, the reported frequencies of amputation and ulceration do vary considerably as a consequence of varying diagnostic criteria used, as well as regional differences. It was recently estimated [65] that up to 25% of patients with diabetes will develop a foot ulcer sometime during their lives and, as can be seen from **Table 34.3**, approximately 1% have already undergone amputation. Diabetes remains the major cause of nontraumatic amputation in most Western countries: rates are as much as 15 times higher than in the nondiabetic population.

Although many of the studies referred to and listed in **Table 34.3** were well conducted, several methodological issues remain which make it difficult to do direct comparison between studies. First, the definition as to what constitutes a foot ulcer differs between studies. Second, surveys invariably include only patients with previously diagnosed diabetes, whereas foot problems in type 2 diabetes may be the presenting feature. In one study from the United Kingdom, for example, 15% of patients undergoing amputation were first diagnosed with diabetes on that hospital admission [66]. Finally, reported foot ulcers were not always confirmed by direct examination by the investigators involved in the studies.

As can be seen from **Table 34.3**, in those population-based studies that assessed the percentage of the population that had risk factors for foot ulceration, it was invariably reported that between 40 and 70% of patients fell into the high-risk category [33, 36, 61]. Such observations clearly indicate the need for all diabetes services to have a regular screening program to identify such high-risk individuals.

34.8 PREVENTION OF ULCERATION AND AMPUTATION IN DIABETIC PATIENTS

Although it is usually recommended that people with diabetes and risk factors for ulceration should be offered education about preventative foot care and this should be repeated at intervals, the evidence base for this is still lacking. Valk et al. [67] for example, in a systematic review, reported that whereas education might have a short-term positive effect on foot care knowledge and behaviors, whether it can prevent foot ulcers and amputations remained uncertain. Despite this, it is still recommended that those diagnosed with risk factors for foot ulceration should receive education designed to change their behavior. It is also clear that further research needs to be undertaken to define with greater precision the extent to which any educational program is actually accompanied by behavioral change and, therefore, reduced incidence of the late complications. However, it is not only the patients that require education: sometime ago it was reported that up to 50% of heel ulcers resulted from poor preventative measures by health care professionals, and heel ulcers remain all too common in diabetic patients admitted to hospital for surgical procedures [68]. For further details of recommended strategies to diagnose the high-risk diabetic foot and on the provision of appropriate education, the reader is directed to publications from the International Working Group on the Diabetic Foot: www.iwgdf.org [69].

It is hoped that the existence of international collaborations, such as the International Working Group on the Diabetic Foot and the Global Lower Extremity Amputation Study [70, 71] group will improve our understanding of not only the etiopathogenesis of these conditions, but also steps that might be taken to reduce the all too high incidence of foot ulceration and amputations among those with diabetes.

References

1. Boulton, A.J.M. and Malik, R.A. (1998) Diabetic neuropathy. *The Medical Clinics of North America*, **82**, 909–29.

2. Shaw, J.E., Zimmett, P.Z., Gries, F.A. and Ziegler, D. (2003) Epidemiology of diabetic neuropathy, in *Textbook of Diabetic Neuropathy* (eds F.A. Gries, N.A. Cameron, P. Low and D. Ziegler), Thieme, Stuttgart, pp. 64–82.

3. Garrow, A.P., Silman, A.J. and MacFarlane, G. (2004) The Cheshire foot pain and disability survey: a population-based study assessing prevalence and association. *Pain*, **110**, 378–84.

4. Daousi, C., MacFarlane, I.A., Woodward, A. *et al.* (2004) Chronic painful peripheral neuropathy in an urban community controlled comparison of people with and without diabetes. *Diabetic Medicine*, **21**, 976–82.

5. Boulton, A.J.M., Vileikyte, L., Ragnarson-Tennvall, G. and Apelqvist, J. (2005) The global burden of diabetic foot disease. *Lancet*, **366**, 1719–24.

6. American Diabetes Association and American Academy of Neurology (1988) Report and recommendations of the San Antonio Conference on Diabetic Neuropathy. Consensus statement. *Diabetes*, **37**, 1000–4.

7. Boulton, A.J.M., Gries, F.A. and Jervell, J.A. (1998) Guidelines for the diagnosis and outpatient management of diabetic peripheral neuropathy. *Diabetic Medicine*, **15**, 508–14.

8. Dyck, P.J., Katz, K.M., Karnes, J.L. *et al.* (1993) The prevalence by staged severity of various types of diabetic neuropathy, retinopathy and nephropathy in a population-based cohort: the Rochester Diabetic Neuropathy Study. *Neurology*, **43**, 817–24.

9. Boulton, A.J.M., Vinik, A.I., Arezzo, J.C. *et al.* (2005) Diabetic neuropathies: a statement by the American Diabetes Association. *Diabetes Care*, **28**, 956–62.

10. Said, G. (2001) Different patterns of neuropathies in diabetic patients, in *Diabetic Neuropathy* (ed A.J.M. Boulton), Aventis/Academy Press, Cologne, pp. 16–41.

11. Thomas, P.K. (1997) Classification, differential diagnosis and staging of diabetic peripheral neuropathy. *Diabetes*, **46** (Suppl 2), S54–7.

12. Thomas, P.K. (2003) Classification of the diabetic neuropathies, in *Textbook of Diabetic Neuropathy* (eds F.A. Gries, N.E. Cameron, P.A. Low and D. Ziegler), Thieme, Stuttgart, pp. 175–7.

13. Vinik, A.I., Mehrabyan, A., Colen, L. and Boulton, A.J.M. (2004) Focal entrapment neuropathies in diabetes. *Diabetes Care*, **27**, 1783–8.

14. Partanen, J., Niskanen, L., Lehtinen, J. *et al.* (1995) Natural history of peripheral neuropathy in patients with non-insulin dependent diabetes. *The New England Journal of Medicine*, **333**, 39–84.

15. UKPDS (1998) Intensive blood glucose with sulphonylureas or insulin compared with conventional treatment and risk of complications in patients with type 2 diabetes. *Lancet*, **352**, 837–53.

16. Boulton, A.J.M., Kirsner, R.S. and Vileikyte, L. (2004) Neuropathic diabetic foot ulceration. *The New England Journal of Medicine*, **351**, 48–55.

17. Vinik, A.I., Maser, R.E., Mitchell, B.D. and Freeman, R. (2003) Diabetic autonomic neuropathy. *Diabetes Care*, **26**, 1553–79.

18. Boulton, A.J.M. (2004) The diabetic foot – from art to science. *Diabetologia*, **47**, 1343–53.

19. Boulton, A.J.M., Malik, R.A., Arezzo, J.C. and Sosenko, J.M. (2004) Diabetic somatic neuropathies. *Diabetes Care*, **27**, 1458–76.

20. Diabetes Control and Complications Trial Research Group (1993) The effect of intensive treatment of diabetes on the development and progression of long-term complications in insulin dependent diabetes mellitus. *The New England Journal of Medicine*, **329**, 977–86.

21. DCCT Research Group (1995) The effect of intensive diabetes therapy on the development and progression of diabetic neuropathy. *Annals of Internal Medicine*, **122**, 561–8.

22. Martin, C.L., Albers, J., Herman, W.H. *et al.* (2006) Neuropathy among the Diabetes Control

and Complications Trial cohort 8 years after trial completion. *Diabetes Care*, **29**, 340–45.

23. Dyck, P.J., Davies, J.L., Wilson, D.M. *et al.* (1999) Risk factors for severity of diabetic polyneuropathy: intensive longitudinal assessment of the Rochester Diabetic Neuropathy Study cohort. *Diabetes Care*, **22**, 1479–86.

24. Smith, A.G. and Singleton, J.R. (2006) Idiopathic neuropathy pre-diabetes and the metabolic syndrome. *Journal of the Neurological Sciences*, **242**, 9–14.

25. Smith, A.G., Hamwi, J., Russe, J. *et al.* (2006) Lifestyle intervention for pre-diabetic neuropathy. *Diabetes Care*, **29**, 1294–9.

26. Malik, R.A., Kumar, S. and Boulton, A.J.M. (1995) Mendenhall's syndrome: clues to the aetiology of human diabetic neuropathy. *Journal of Neurology, Neurosurgery, and Psychiatry*, **58**, 493–5.

27. King, R.H. (2001) The role of glycation in the pathogenesis of diabetic polyneuropathy. *Molecular Pathology*, **54**, 400–8.

28. Ametov, A.S., Barinov, A., Dyck, P.J. *et al.* (2003) The sensory symptoms of diabetic polyneuropathy are improved with alpha-lipoic acid: the SYDNEY Trial. *Diabetes Care*, **26**, 770–6.

29. Tesfaye, S., Stevens, L.K., Stephenson, J.M. *et al.* (1996) Prevalence of diabetic neuropathy and its relation to glycaemic control and potential risk factors: the EURODIAB IDDM complications study. *Diabetologia*, **39**, 1377–84.

30. Tesfaye, S., Chaturvedi, N., Eaton, S.E.M. *et al.* (2005) Vascular risk factors and diabetic neuropathy. *The New England Journal of Medicine*, **352**, 348–50.

31. Young, M.J., Boulton, A.J.M., Mcleod, A.F. *et al.* (1993) A multicentre study of the prevalence of diabetic neuropathy in the UK hospital clinic population. *Diabetologia*, **36**, 150–4.

32. Cabezas-Cerrato, J. (1998) The prevalence of clinical diabetic polyneuropathy in Spain. *Diabetologia*, **41**, 1263–9.

33. Abbott, C.A., Carrington, A.L., Ashe, H. *et al.* (2002) The North-West Diabetes Foot Care Study: incidence of, and risk factors for new diabetic foot ulceration in a community-based patient cohort. *Diabetic Medicine*, **19**, 377–84.

34. Abbott, C.A., Garrow, A.P., Carrington, A.L. *et al.* (2005) Foot ulcer risk is lower in South-Asian and African-Caribbean compared with European diabetic patients in the UK. *Diabetes Care*, **28**, 1869–75.

35. Heesom, A.E., Millward, A. and Demaine, A.G. (1998) Susceptibility to diabetic neuropathy in patients with type 1 diabetes is associated with a polymorphism at the 5′ end of the aldose reductase

gene. *Journal of Neurology, Neurosurgery, and Psychiatry*, **64**, 213–16.

36. Davies, M., Brophy, S., Williams, R. and Taylor, A. (2006) The prevalence, severity and impact of painful diabetic neuropathy in type 2 diabetes. *Diabetes Care*, **29**, 1518–22.

37. Kumar, S., Ashe, H.A., Parnell, L.N. *et al.* (1994) The prevalence of foot ulceration and its correlates in type 2 diabetic patients: a population-based study. *Diabetic Medicine*, **11**, 480–4.

38. Maser, R.E., Steenkiste, A.R., Dorman, J.S. *et al.* (1989) Epidemiological correlation of diabetic neuropathy: report from the Pittsburgh Epidemiology of Diabetes Complications Study. *Diabetes*, **38**, 1456–61.

39. Franklin, G.M., Kahn, L.B., Baxter, J. *et al.* (1990) Sensory neuropathy in non-insulin dependent diabetes mellitus. *American Journal of Epidemiology*, **131**, 633–43.

40. Araujo, A.B., Mohr, B.A. and McKinlay, J.B. (2004) Changes in sexual function in middle-aged and older men: longitudinal data from the Massachusetts Male Aging Study. *Journal of the American Geriatrics Society*, **52**, 1502–9.

41. McCulloch, D.K., Campbell, I.W., Wu, F.C. *et al.* (1980) The prevalence of diabetic impotence. *Diabetologia*, **18**, 279–83.

42. Fedele, D., Coscelli, C., Santeusanio, F. *et al.* (1998) Erectile dysfunction in diabetic subjects in Italy. *Diabetes Care*, **21**, 1973–7.

43. Klein, R., Klein, B.E., Lee, K.E. *et al.* (1996) Prevalence of self-reported erectile dysfunction in people with long-term IDDM. *Diabetes Care*, **19**, 135–41.

44. Hackett, G. (1995) Impotence – the neglected complication of diabetes. *Diabetes Research*, **1**, 1–9.

45. De Berardis, G., Pellegrini, F., Franciosi, M. *et al.* (2005) Longitudinal assessment of quality of life in patients with type 2 diabetes and self-reported erectile dysfunction. *Diabetes Care*, **28**, 1637–41.

46. Neil, H.A., Thompson, A.V., John, S. *et al.* (1989) Diabetic autonomic neuropathy: the prevalence of impaired heart rate variability in a geographically defined population. *Diabetic Medicine*, **6**, 20–4.

47. Ziegler, D., Gries, F.A., Spuler, M. and Lessmann, F. (1992) The epidemiology of diabetic neuropathy. Diabetic Cardiovascular Autonomic Neuropathy Multicentre Study Group. *Journal of Diabetes and its Complications*, **6**, 49–57.

48. DCCT Research Group (1998) The effect of intensive diabetes therapy on measures of autonomic nervous system function in the Diabetes Control and Complications Trial (DCCT). *Diabetologia*, **41**, 416–23.

49. Assal, J.P., Mebnert, H., Tritschler, H. *et al.* (2002) 'On your feet': workshop on the diabetic foot. *The Journal of Diabetic Complications*, **16**, 183–94.

50. Ramsey, S.D., Newton, K., Blough, D. *et al.* (1999) Incidence, outcomes and costs of foot ulcers in patients with diabetes. *Diabetes Care*, **22**, 382–7.

51. Reiber, G.E., Vileikyte, L., Boyko, E.J. *et al.* (1999) Causal pathways for incident lower-extremity ulcers in patients with diabetes from two settings. *Diabetes Care*, **22**, 157–62.

52. Boulton, A.J.M., Cavanagh, P.R. and Rayman, G. (2006) *The Foot in Diabetes*, 4th edn, John Wiley & Sons, Ltd, Chichester.

53. McAlpine, R.R., Morris, A.D., Emslie-Smith, A. *et al.* (2005) The annual incidence of diabetic complications in a population of patients with type 1 and type 2 diabetes. *Diabetic Medicine*, **22**, 348–52.

54. Young, M.J., Veves, A., Breddy, J.L. and Boulton, A.J.M. (1994) The prediction of diabetic neuropathic foot ulceration using vibration perception threshold: a prospective study. *Diabetes Care*, **17**, 557–60.

55. Abbott, C.A., Vileikyte, L., Williamson, S. *et al.* (1998) Multicentre study of the incidence of and predictive factors for diabetic foot ulceration. *Diabetes Care*, **21**, 1071–8.

56. Anderson, H., Gjerstad, M.D. and Jakobsen, J. (2004) Atrophy of foot muscles: a measure of diabetic neuropathy. *Diabetes Care*, **27**, 2382–5.

57. Mayfield, J.A., Reiber, G.E., Sanders, L.J. *et al.* (1998) Preventative foot care in people with diabetes. *Diabetes Care*, **12**, 2161–78.

58. Lavery, L.A., Armstrong, D.G., Wunderlich, R.P. *et al.* (2003) Diabetic foot syndrome: evaluating the prevalence and incidence of foot pathology in Mexican-Americans and non-Hispanic Whites from a diabetes management cohort. *Diabetes Care*, **26**, 1435–8.

59. Veves, A., Uccioli, L., Manes, C. *et al.* (1996) Comparison of risk factors for foot ulceration in diabetic patients attending teaching hospital out-patients clinics in four different European states. *Diabetic Medicine*, **11**, 709–11.

60. Murray, H.J., Young, M.J. and Boulton, A.J.M. (1996) The relationship between callus formation, high foot pressures and neuropathy in diabetic foot ulceration. *Diabetic Medicine*, **16**, 979–82.

61. Manes, C., Papazoglou, N., Sassidou, E. *et al.* (2002) Prevalence of diabetic neuropathy and foot ulceration: a population-based study. *Wounds*, **14**, 11–15.

62. Muller, I.S., de Grauw, W.J., van Gerwen, W.H. *et al.* (2002) Foot ulceration and lower limb amputation in type 2 diabetic patients in Dutch primary health care. *Diabetes Care*, **25**, 570–6.

63. Vozar, J., Adamka, J., Holeczy, P. *et al.* (1997) Diabetics with foot lesions and amputations in the region of Horny Zitmy Ostrov 1993–1995. *Diabetologia*, **40** (Suppl 1), A46J.

64. Moss, S., Klein, R. and Klein, B. (1992) The prevalence and incidence of lower extremity amputation in a diabetic population. *Archives of Internal Medicine*, **152**, 510–616.

65. Singh, N., Armstrong, D.G. and Lipsky, B.A. (2005) Preventing foot ulcers in patients with diabetes. *The Journal of the American Medical Association*, **293**, 217–28.

66. Deerochanawong, C., Home, P.D. and Alberti, K.G. (1992) A survey of lower limb amputations in diabetic patients. *Diabetic Medicine*, **9**, 942–6.

67. Valk, G.D., Kriegsman, D.M. and Assendelft, W.J. (2002) Patient education for preventing diabetic foot ulceration: a systematic review. *Endocrinology and Metabolism Clinics of North America*, **31**, 633–58.

68. Fletcher, E.M. and Jeffcoate, W.J. (1994) Footcare education and the diabetes specialist nurse, in *The Foot in Diabetes*, 2nd edn (eds A.J.M. Boulton, H. Connor and P.R. Cavanagh), John Wiley & Sons, Ltd, Chichester, pp. 69–75.

69. Bakker, K., van Houtum, W.H. and Riley, P.C. (2006) World Diabetes Day 2005 on Diabetes Foot Care: what did we achieve and where do we go from here. *International Diabetes Monitor*, **19**, (1).

70. LEA Study Group (1995) Comparing the incidence of lower extremity amputations across the world: the Global Lower Extremity Amputation Group. *Diabetic Medicine*, **12**, 14–18.

71. Renzi, R., Unwin, N., Jubelirer, R. and Haag, L. (2006) An international comparison of lower extremity amputation rates. *Annals of Vascular Surgery*, **20**, 346–50.

35

Epidemiology of Acute Complications: Diabetic Ketoacidosis, Hyperglycemic Hyperosmolar State and Hypoglycemia

Alberta B. Rewers

Department of Pediatrics, University of Colorado at Denver and Health Sciences Center, Denver, CO, USA

35.1 DIABETIC KETOACIDOSIS

35.1.1 Pathogenesis

Diabetic ketoacidosis (DKA) results from very low levels of effective circulating insulin and a concomitant increase in counterregulatory hormones levels, such as glucagon, catecholamines, cortisol and growth hormone. This combination causes catabolic changes in the metabolism of carbohydrates, fat and protein. Hyperglycemia develops due to impaired glucose utilization and increased glucose production by the liver and kidneys. Lipolysis leads to increased production of ketones, especially β-hydroxybutyrate (B-OHB), ketonemia and metabolic acidosis. Most common underlying mechanisms of DKA include progressive β-cell failure in previously undiagnosed patients and omission or inadequate insulin dosing in established patients. Elevation of counterregulatory hormones during infection, gastrointestinal illness, trauma and stress may also precipitate DKA in the absence of increase in insulin dosing. The clinical picture of DKA includes polyuria, polydipsia, dehydration, Kussmaul respiration (rapid, deep and sighing) and progressive worsening of mental status from somnolence to coma.

35.1.2 Definition

The incidence of DKA varies with the definition; therefore, it is important to standardize criteria for comparative epidemiological studies. The American Diabetes Association (ADA) [1, 2], the International Society for Pediatric and Adolescent Diabetes (ISPAD) [3] as well as jointly the European Society for Paediatric Endocrinology (ESPE) and the Lawson Wilkins Pediatric Endocrine Society (LWPES) [4] agreed to define DKA as:

1. hyperglycemia; that is, plasma glucose higher than 250 mg dl^{-1} or $\sim$14 mmol l^{-1}; and
2. venous pH < 7.25 (arterial pH < 7.30) and/or bicarbonate <15 mmol l^{-1};
3. moderate or large ketones level in urine or blood.

The caveats are:

1. Pediatric experts agree that the lower level of hyperglycemia (>200 mg dl^{-1} or >11 mmol l^{-1}) meets criteria for DKA. Pregnant adolescents, young or partially treated children [5] and those fasting during a period of insulin deficiency [6] may have near-normal glucose levels and ketoacidosis ('euglycemic ketoacidosis').
2. DKA is generally categorized by the severity of acidosis. In most laboratories, the normal range for arterial pH is 7.35–7.45 and for venous pH it is 7.32–7.42 in adults and children older than 2 years. Currently recommended severity categories differ between adults and children

The Epidemiology of Diabetes Mellitus, second edition   Edited by Jean-Marie Ekoé, Marian Rewers, Rhys Williams and Paul Zimmet
© 2008 John Wiley & Sons, Ltd

Table 35.1 Classification of DKA severity: current inconsistent guidelines.

Severity of DKA	ADA adults [2]	ADA children [1]	ESPE/LWPES and ISPAD children [3, 4]
Severe	Arterial pH < 7.0 Bicarbonate < 10	Venous pH < 7.1	Venous pH < 7.1 Bicarbonate < 5
Moderate	$7.0 \leq$ arterial pH < 7.25 $10 \leq$ bicarbonate < 15	Venous pH 7.1–7.2	Venous pH < 7.2 Bicarbonate < 10
Mild	Arterial pH 7.25–7.30 Bicarbonate 15–18	Venous pH 7.2–7.3	Venous pH < 7.3 Bicarbonate < 15

(**Table 35.1**), with little evidence to support these differences.

3. While large or moderate ketonuria is sufficient for confirmation of DKA diagnosis, measurement of B-OHB is more helpful in making treatment decisions [7, 8]. Whole-blood B-OHB levels of >1.5 mmol l^{-1} obtained using the Precision Xtra™ meter (MediSense/Abbott) combined with blood glucose >250 mg dl^{-1} ($\sim$14 mmol l^{-1}) indicate probable DKA. With increasing use of B-OHB in home/outpatient diabetes management, more data are needed to define the role of B-OHB measurement in diagnosing milder cases of DKA, now under-diagnosed and treated at home.

In the World Health Organization's International Classification of Diseases ICD-9 codes, DKA is usually coded as 250.1x (250.10–250.13). However, the code 250.3 (diabetes with other coma) is used for DKA coma as well as for coma caused by severe hypoglycemia. In the ICD-10, categories for diabetes (E10–E14), subdivision E1x.1 denotes DKA, while E1x.0 denotes coma with or without ketoacidosis, hyperosmolar or hypoglycemic (x digit is used to define type of diabetes).

35.1.3 Prevalence and Predictors of DKA at the Diagnosis of Diabetes

35.1.3.1 Prevalence of DKA at the Diagnosis of Type 1 Diabetes

Examples of reports concerning the prevalence and predictors of DKA at diagnosis around the world are presented in **Table 35.2**. The largest population-based study to date, Search for Diabetes in Youth Study (SEARCH) in the United States, reported that 29% of patients with type 1 diabetes younger than 20 years at diagnosis presented in DKA [9]. This estimate was lower similar than rates previously reported from hospital series [10, 11]. In European countries, the prevalence varied from 15 to 67% [12–17]. DKA prevalence at diagnosis is generally higher in populations with lower incidence of type 1 diabetes [14, 18]. DKA incidence at the time of diagnosis in Asian and African populations is less clear because of the paucity of metabolic and clinical data. However, 42–85% of type 1 diabetes children in Arab countries presented in DKA [19–21]. Among newly diagnosed patients of all ages in tropical Africa, 22% had diabetes requiring insulin and 23% of those patients presented in DKA [22].

Studies in the United States and elsewhere suggest that the clinical severity at diagnosis of type 1 diabetes in youth may be decreasing. In Colorado, the proportion of children with type 1 diabetes who presented with DKA at the time of diagnosis has significantly decreased, from 38% in 1978–1982 to 29% in 1998–2001 [24, 25]. Similarly, the prevalence of DKA at onset decreased in Finnish children from 30% in 1982–1991 to 19% in 1992–2002 [17]. On the other hand, admission rates for any DKA, at onset or later in the course of disease, have remained unchanged and high (over 20 per 100 000 per year) in Canadian youth between 1991 and 1999, but severity seems to be decreasing [26, 27].

Table 35.2 Prevalence of DKA at Diagnosis of Diabetes.

Country (Ref.)	Age	N	Completeness of record review	Study period	Definition of DKA	Prevalence of DKA (%)	Predictors
USA [9]	0–19	2824	77% population-based	2002–2004	pH <7.3 (venous) or pH <7.25 (arterial) bicarbonate <15 or ICD-9 250.1 or medical record diagnosis	29 type 1 10 type 2	Younger age, lower family income, under insurance, lower parental education
USA [10]	0–18	139	68% hospital series	1995–1998	pH <7.3	38	Younger age, lack of insurance
USA [11]	0–5	247	Hospital series	1990–1999	pH <7.3 or bicarbonate <15	44	—
Europe [14] (11 countries)	0–14	1260	91% varied by center	1989–1994	pH <7.3	26–67 (42 on average)	Area of low incidence of type 1 diabetes
Germany [15]	0–14	2121	97% population-based	1987–1997	pH <7.3 or bicarbonate <15	26	Lower socioeconomic status
Finland [17]	0–14	585	Hospital series	1982–2001	pH <7.3 or bicarbonate $\leq$15	18	Younger age
UK [23]	0–15	328	Hospital series	1987–1996	pH $\leq$7.25 (arterial) or bicarbonate $\leq$15	27	Asian minority Age less than 5 years
UK [12]	0–20	230	Population-based	1985–1986	pH <7.36 or bicarbonate <21	26	Younger age
		97				26	
Ireland [16]	0–14	283	72% population-based	1997–1998	pH <7.3	31	—
Kuwait [21]	0–12	103	Hospital series	2000–2003	pH <7.3	84.5	—

35.1.3.2 Predictors of DKA at the Diagnosis of Type 1 Diabetes

The prevalence of DKA at the diagnosis is significantly higher among younger children [9, 12, 27], reaching over 50% in those aged less than 2 years [28, 29]. Lower socioeconomic status–lower family income, parental education and less favorable health insurance creating barriers in access to care–is a powerful independent risk factor [9, 10, 15, 30]. Low societal awareness of diabetes symptoms, such as in populations with low incidence of type 1 diabetes, adds to the risk, while programs or centers promoting community awareness may decrease the risk (see Section 35.1.10). In addition, high-dose glucocorticoids, atypical antipsychotics, diazoxide and immunosuppresive drugs have been reported to precipitate DKA in individuals not previously diagnosed with diabetes [31, 32].

35.1.3.3 Prevalence of DKA at the Diagnosis of Type 2 Diabetes

Few population-based epidemiologic data exist concerning the prevalence of DKA at the time of presentation of type 2 diabetes in youth. The SEARCH study of youth with type 2 diabetes from six geographic areas in the United States found that 10% of 507 patients presented in DKA [9]. As many as 19% of Thai children and adolescents had DKA at diagnosis of type 2 diabetes [33].

While the conventional belief is that DKA is an uncommon presentation of type 2 diabetes in adults, population-based data are lacking. In the United States, an estimated 20–50% of adult patients with DKA at diagnosis are believed to have type 2 diabetes [34, 35]. Clinical course postdiagnosis may suggest even higher rates: 39–60% [36, 37]. A similar proportion (42–64%) of ketosis-prone type 2 diabetes has been reported among African patients [38], but it seems to be lower in Asian patients. In conclusion, DKA at the diagnosis does not help to distinguish type 1 from type 2 diabetes; with improving understanding of heterogeneity of type 2 diabetes, it is likely that specific types of ketosis-prone disease will be identified.

35.1.4 Incidence of DKA in Established Type 1 Diabetes

The overall incidence of DKA in patients with established type 1 diabetes varies from 1 per 100 to 12 per 100 person-years [12, 39, 47] (**Table 35.3**). The incidence of DKA increases significantly with age in females (4 per 100, 8 per 100 and 12 per 100 person-years in those <7 years, 7–12 years and ≥13 years respectively), but not in males (7 per 100, 5 per 100 and 8 per 100 person-years) (**Figure 35.1**) [39]. There are no comparable population-based data for adults.

Most episodes of DKA beyond diagnosis are associated with insulin omission or treatment error [45, 46]. Children whose insulin treatment

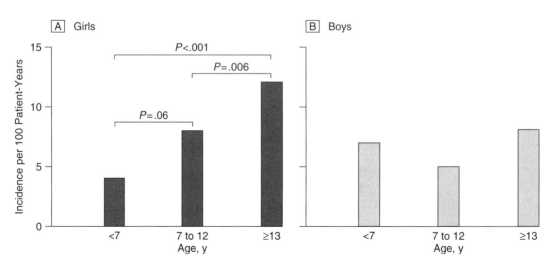

Figure 35.1 Incidence of diabetic ketoacidosis by age and gender, Colorado, 1996–2001. (Reproduced from [39], Copyright © 2002, The American Medical Association.)

Table 35.3 Incidence of DKA in Children and Adolescent with Established Type 1 Diabetes.

Country (ref)	Age group	N	Study design	Length of study	Definition of DKA	Incidence per 100 person-years	Predictors
USA [39]	0–19	1243	Prospective cohort	3.5 years	DKA leading to ED visit or hospital admission	8	Female gender, age, higher HbA$_{1c}$, higher insulin dose, underinsurance, psychiatric disorders
USA [40]	7–16	300	Prospective cohort	1 year	DKA leading to ED visit or hospital admission	15	Higher HbA$_{1c}$
USA [41]	13–17	195	Clinical trial	7.4 years	BG > 250, ketonuria, pH <7.3 or bicarbonate <15	4.7 conventional 2.8 intensive	NA
Sweden [42]	0–18	139	Prospective cohort	3 years	Acidosis	1.5	NA
UK [43]	1–17	135	Retrospective	6 years	pH < 7.3 or bicarbonate <18	10	Female gender, family and school problems
Australia [44]	1–19	268	Retrospective	3 months	pH < 7.2 or bicarbonate <10	12	NA

BG: blood glucose; ED: emergency department.

is supervised by a responsible adult rarely have episodes of DKA [47]. However, inadequate adjustment of insulin therapy during intercurrent illness may cause DKA [12, 47, 48]. Patients with a history of previous episodes of DKA are at higher risk for recurrent DKA. In one study, 60% of all DKA episodes occurred in 5% of patients with recurrent events [39].

While continuous subcutaneous insulin infusion (CSII) is effective and safe in both adults and adolescents with type 1 diabetes [49], CSII interruption can lead to DKA [50]. The incidence of DKA appears to be unchanged during long-term (4 years) follow-up after introduction of CSII in children and youth [51].

Incidence data are not available for adults with type 1 diabetes; however, DKA affects about 8% of the hospitalized patients. Similar to children, main precipitant factors are noncompliance with treatment and infections [52, 53]. DKA due to noncompliance may be associated with drug abuse and cigarette smoking [54].

35.1.5   Incidence of DKA in Established Type 2 Diabetes

Patients with type 2 diabetes may develop DKA or hyperglycemic hyperosmolar syndrome (HHS) and require hospitalization. Hospitalization for other medical or surgical conditions is clearly a risk factor for the development of metabolic deterioration hospitalization [55]. The number of hospitalizations for any DKA among persons younger than 45 years estimated by the US National Diabetes Surveillance System increased from 37 000 (24 per 100 000) in 1980 to 87 000 (47 per 100 000) in 2003 and the number of hospital discharges in United States with DKA diagnosis almost doubled between 1980 and 2003, from 62 000 discharges in 1980 to 115 000 in 2003. While the rates have nearly doubled, average length of hospital stay in this group has decreased from 6.4 days to 3.4 days (http://www.cdc.gov/diabetes/statistics/dkafirst/index.htm, last accessed December 2006).

35.1.6   Risk Factors for Recurrent DKA

Patients from low-income families have higher rates of DKA, and it is frequently more severe [10]. Lack of insurance and less favorable health insurance are

also associated with more severe onset of diabetes in youth [30, 56]. It is unlikely that the risk of DKA differs by race or ethnicity independent of socioeconomic factors and access to care. While young Asian children in the United Kingdom were eight times more likely to present in DKA than non-Asian children of the same age (unadjusted risk ratio) [23], the prevalence of DKA at onset [9] and the recurrence of DKA [39] did not differ by race/ethnicity in the US youth with type 1 diabetes.

The risk of recurrent DKA is higher in patients with poor metabolic control [14, 39, 40]. Lower socioeconomic status and insufficient access to outpatient diabetes care are often the primary mechanism; however, major psychiatric disorders (depression, bipolar disorder, schizophrenia) also play a significant role [39]. Eating disorders, prevalent in adolescent girls [12], contribute to the highest risk for DKA in this group reaching 12 per 100 person-years [39, 43, 57]. This is probably related to issues of body image, as diabetic adolescent girls often omit insulin injections to lose weight [58, 59]. Girls with recurrent ketoacidosis have also been shown to exhibit more behavioral problems, lower social competence and higher levels of family conflict [60]. The patterns of recurrent DKA vary by age (**Figure 35.2**). In children younger than 13 years of age, the risk increases with higher HbA_{1c} and with higher reported insulin dose. In older children, the risk increases with higher HbA_{1c}, higher reported insulin dose, inadequate insurance and the presence of psychiatric disorders [39].

35.1.7   Morbidity and Mortality

DKA is the most common cause of death in children with type 1 diabetes [61, 62]. Mortality and morbidity in DKA is mostly due to cerebral edema, which accounts for most hospital deaths in young diabetic children. The incidence of cerebral edema is 0.3–3.0% [63–65]. Less frequent causes of mortality include hypokalemia, hyperkalemia, thrombosis [53], other neurological complications [66, 67], stroke [68, 69], sepsis and other infections such as rhinocerebral mucormycosis [70, 71], aspiration pneumonia and pulmonary edema [72, 73].

Death rates among adults with diabetes were estimated using national mortality data and the National Health Interview Survey as the denominator for persons with diabetes [74]. Between 1985 and

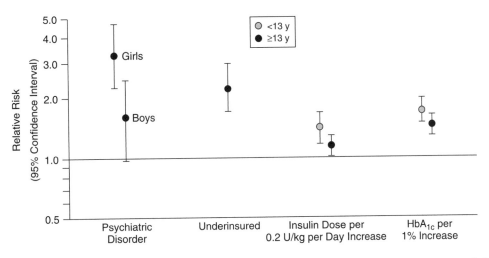

Figure 35.2 Predictors of diabetic ketoacidosis in children with established diabetes, Colorado, 1996–2001. (Reproduced from [39], Copyright © 2002, The American Medical Association.)

2002, annual age-adjusted death rates due to hyperglycemic crisis, which include both DKA and HHS, declined in the United States from 42 per 100 000 to 24 per 100 000 adults with diabetes (on average 4.4% per year). The death rates fell for all race–sex subgroups, with Black men experiencing the smallest decline and the greatest decrease occurring among persons older than 65 years. Comparable statistics for children and adolescents are lacking.

35.1.8 Cost

Direct medical care charges associated with DKA episodes represent 28% of the direct medical care charges for all patients, and 56% for those with recurrent DKAs [75]. Acute complications in children with type 1 diabetes also increase directly and indirectly [76] the costs of care.

The National Hospital Ambulatory Medical Care Survey has shown that, between 1993 and 2003, DKA accounted for ~753 000 visits (95% confidence interval (CI) 610 000–895 000) or an average 68 000 visits per year. Most DKA visits were evenly distributed among patients aged 10–50 years. Most DKA patients (87%) were admitted, with most admissions to a non-intensive care unit setting. The rate of emergency department visits for DKA per 10 000 US population with diabetes was 64 (95% CI 52–76). There was an increase in number of visits for DKA during 1999–2003 compared with 1993–1998 [77].

During 2004, there were approximately 5.2 million hospitalizations in the United States with diagnostic coding indicative of diabetes [78]. Among these, 120 000 admissions were primarily due to DKA, 15 000 to HHS and an additional 5000 were coded as 'diabetic coma.' Based on the Diagnostic Related Group codes in the inpatient records, the total hospital cost for DKA was estimated at $1.4–1.8 billion. An independent analysis also arrived at an estimate of the annual hospital cost of DKA in the United States in excess of $1 billion [79]. The authors based their estimate on an annual average of over 100 000 hospitalizations for DKA, with an average cost of $13 000 per patient. Newly diagnosed patients may account for approximately 25% of this cost [56].

35.1.9 Prevention

Prevention of DKA should be a major goal of diabetes care and a growing body of evidence suggests that primary prevention of DKA in newly diagnosed children should be possible. In the United States, the Diabetes Autoimmunity Study in the Youth, an observational study following children at genetically high risk for type 1 diabetes by periodic testing for diabetes autoantibodies, HbA_{1c} and random blood glucose, demonstrated that the clinical course of diabetes is milder in youth diagnosed without DKA [80]. An intensive community intervention to raise awareness of the signs and symptoms of childhood diabetes among school teachers and primary care providers in a region of Italy was found to reduce the prevalence of DKA at diagnosis of type 1 disease from 83% to 13% [81]. A follow-up study has shown that the campaign for DKA prevention is still effective in Parma's province 8 years later, but there is also an indication that the campaign should be periodically renewed [82].

In the Diabetes Prevention Trial (DPT-1), nearly three-quarters of the subjects in whom diabetes developed were asymptomatic at the time of diagnosis. Awareness of increased level of risk and close biochemical monitoring increases the likelihood of early diagnosis and prevents DKA [83]. Public awareness of signs and symptoms of diabetes also helps earlier diagnosis. If health care providers always consider the possibility of diabetes in ill children and urgently check urine or blood for glucose, then early diagnosis will be likely. If confirmation is rapid, and children are promptly referred to an appropriate center, then development of DKA will be less common. Although these strategies are intuitive, programs to decrease DKA at onset need to be designed and evaluated in diverse populations and age groups. These should include approaches that target both the public at large and health care providers.

Studies to date also suggest that most, if not all, episodes of DKA beyond disease diagnosis are preventable. Studies of the effect of a comprehensive diabetes program and telephone help line reported a reduction in the rates of DKA from 15–60 per 100 to 5–6 per 100 patient-years [84–86]. In the adolescent cohort of the Diabetes Control and Complications Trial (DCCT), intensive diabetes management was associated with less DKA (conventional and intensive treatment groups: 4.7 per 100 and 2.8 per 100 patient-years respectively [41]. In patients treated with insulin pumps, episodes of DKA can be reduced with introduction of educational algorithms. Therefore, it is likely that most episodes of DKA after diagnosis could be avoided if all children with diabetes received comprehensive diabetes health care and education, and had access to a 24 h diabetes telephone help line [39, 84, 87]. The extent to which home measurement of B-OHB may assist in the prevention of hospitalization needs to be further assessed [7].

35.2 HHS

35.2.1 Pathogenesis

Reduction in the net effective action of circulating insulin coupled with a concomitant elevation of counterregulatory hormones is the underlying mechanism for both HHS and DKA. These alterations lead to increased hepatic and renal glucose production and impaired glucose utilization in peripheral tissues, which result in hyperglycemia and parallel changes in osmolality of the extracellular space [88]. Both DKA and HHS are associated with glycosuria, leading to osmotic diuresis, with loss of water, sodium, potassium and other electrolytes. In DKA, release of free fatty acids from adipose tissue and their unrestrained oxidation to ketone bodies (B-OHB and acetoacetate) result in ketonemia and metabolic acidosis. In HHS, on the other hand, insulin levels are inadequate for glucose utilization by insulin-sensitive tissues, but sufficient (as determined by residual C-peptide) to prevent lipolysis and ketogenesis [88].

35.2.2 Definition

HHS is defined as blood glucose >600 mg dl^{-1} (33.3 mmol l^{-1}), venous pH >7.30, bicarbonate >15 mmol l^{-1} and serum osmolality >320. A small amount of ketones may be present in blood and urine. In the ICD-9, HHS is usually coded as 250.2–diabetes with hyperosmolarity or hyperosmolar (nonketotic) coma. In the ICD-10, HHS does not appear to have a specific code; E1x.0 denotes coma with or without ketoacidosis, hyperosmolar or hypoglycemic (x digit is used to define type of diabetes).

35.2.3 Incidence

HHS incidence appears to increase, but it is unclear if this is a real increase or artifact of improving detection. Approximately one-third of adult patients experiencing acute hyperglycemic crisis have mixed DKA and HHS; the frequency of isolated HHS varies from 15 to 45% depending on the selection criteria [89, 90]. HHS may occur at any age, but it is more often in elderly patients who have other comorbidity. Presence of other conditions may be responsible for higher mortality associated with HHS, compared with DKA [90].

The incidence of HHS is difficult to determine because of the lack of population-based studies and multiple comorbidities often found in these patients. It is estimated that the rates of hospital admissions for HHS are lower than those for DKA and account for less than 1% of all primary diabetic admissions, but may affect up to 4% of new type 2 diabetes patients [88].

While HHS is rare in children, more than 50 cases have been described in the literature in small case series not larger than seven patients each [9, 91–94]. Most of the patients were adolescents with newly diagnosed type 2 diabetes and many were of African-American descent. Fatality rate of pediatric HHS apparently exceeds that in adult HHS. Reported complications include rhabdomyolysis and hypovolemic shock.

35.2.4 Risk Factors

The most common precipitating factor in the development of HHS is infection. Other precipitating factors include cerebrovascular accident, alcohol abuse, pancreatitis, myocardial infarction, trauma and drugs. Elderly individuals with new-onset diabetes (particularly residents of chronic care facilities) or individuals with known diabetes who become hyperglycemic and are unaware of it, or who are unable to take fluids when necessary, are at risk for HHS. Drugs that affect carbohydrate metabolism, such as corticosteroids, thiazides and sympathomimetic agents (e.g. dobutamine and terbutaline), may also precipitate the development of HHS. In one of the earliest systematic studies of HHS, female gender (71% in HHS cases versus 53% in diabetic controls), newly diagnosed diabetes (36% versus 7%) and acute infection (39% versus 19%) were independently associated with the presence of HHS [95]. Nursing home residence, dementia and other functionally debilitating diseases, acute illnesses or medications that may impair glucose tolerance had no independent effect. Among 200 HHS patients in Rhode Island, nursing home residents accounted for 18% of the cases [89].

35.2.5 Mortality

In adults, HHS is associated with significant mortality ranging from 4 to 25% [89, 90, 96, 97]. An Australian study of 312 adult patients with hyperglycemic crises has reported overall mortality rate of 4.8% [90]. The mortality increased sharply with age from none in patients aged <35 years, 1.2% in those aged 35–55 years to 15.0% for patients aged >55 years. In this population, mortality in patients with isolated DKA (1.2%) was lower that that in patients with mixed DKA–HHS (5.3%) or with isolated HHS (17%). A US study of 613 adult patients hospitalized for hyperglycemic crises reported similar findings [89]. Fatality rates for DKA, mixed DKA–HHS and isolated HHS alone were, respectively, 4%, 9% and 12%. Both studies agreed that age and the degree of hyperosmolarity were the most powerful predictors of a fatal outcome. In particular, patients aged >65 years presenting with a serum osmolarity >375 mOsmol l^{-1} were at the greatest risk [90].

According to the National Health Interview Survey, deaths due to hyperglycemic crisis in adults with diabetes dropped from 2989 in 1985 to 2459 in 2002. During the time period, age-adjusted death rates decreased from 42 per 100 000 to 24 per 100 000 adults with diabetes [74] (**Figure 35.3**).

In a Taiwanese case series of 119 patients with HHS aged 68 ± 12 years and with male predominance, the mortality rate was as high as of 24% [96]. While the age range of this population was relatively narrow, no association was found between mortality and age or osmolarity. However, nearly 60% of the patients had infection and 42% had stroke. Septic shock was the most frequent cause of death (31%) and fatality was higher in patients with acute myocardial infarction or stroke as the HHS precipitating factor in a Spanish study of 132 HHS events with mortality rate of 17% [97]. While high urea plasma levels were the best predictor of fatality, the authors concluded that the hemodynamic state of the patients, rather than hyperosmolarity itself, was the most influential prognostic factor.

35.2.6 Cost

There are no reliable data concerning the cost of HHS, due to the weakness of the incidence data. However, on an individual basis, cost per event is several times higher than that for uncomplicated DKA.

35.2.7 Prevention

Diabetes management education, adequate treatment and self-monitoring of blood glucose can

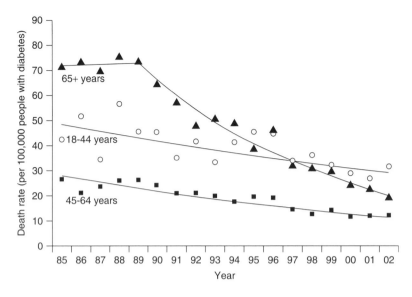

Figure 35.3 Age-specific death rates for hyperglycemic crisis, United States, 1985–2002 [74]. (Copyright © 2006 The American Diabetes Association. From *Diabetes Care*®, vol. 29, 2006; 2018–22. Reproduced with permission from The American Diabetes Association.)

help to prevent HHS in patients with known diabetes. HHS can be precipitated by dehydration and medications such as corticosteroids, thiazides and sympathomimetic agents. Careful use of these medications is indicated in vulnerable patients; for example, in elderly cared for in nursing homes at risk of dehydration and unable to communicate their medical problems promptly.

35.3 HYPOGLYCEMIA

35.3.1 *Pathogenesis*

Hypoglycemia is the most common life-threatening complication of diabetes treatment. It is characterized by multiple risk factors and complex pathophysiology [98]. Hypoglycemia is more common in young children and adolescents and causes a spectrum of acute complications from mild cognitive impairment to coma, seizure and sudden death. The brain depends on a continuous supply of glucose for energy, although it can also utilize ketone bodies.

In insulin-treated patients, common causes of hypoglycemia include missed meals, inadvertent insulin dosing error and rapid insulin absorption due to intramuscular injection or hot shower/bath shortly after injection. Rarely, secondary-gain ideation or suicidal attempt may lead to insulin

overdose. In all these situations, insulin overdose reduces hepatic glucose output. Physical activity increases glucose utilization and may lead to hypoglycemia if not matched by lowering of insulin dose and increased carbohydrate intake. Oral hypoglycemic agents may cause hypoglycemia by either decreasing hepatic glucose output (metformin) or increasing insulin levels (sulfonylureas and metiglinides). In contrast, enhancers of peripheral glucose utilization (thiazolidenediones) do not cause hypoglycemia in patients with residual insulin and glucagon secretion. Release of glucagon–the major counterregulatory response to hypoglycemia in nondiabetic persons–is progressively lost within a few years after diagnosis of type 1 diabetes. Catecholamine release, the other powerful counterregulatory mechanism, is also impaired in diabetic patients, especially type 1 and in those on beta-blocker treatment [99].

35.3.2 *Definition*

Hypoglycemia is usually defined as a blood glucose level below 2.8 mmol l^{-1} (50 mg dl^{-1}). In the DCCT, severe hypoglycemia was defined as an episode in which the patient required assistance with treatment from another person to recover, blood glucose level had to be documented as <50 mg dl^{-1} and/or the clinical manifestations had to be reversed by oral carbohydrate, subcutaneous glucagon or intravenous glucose [100]. This definition is not very practical in children, particularly the youngest, because they require assistance from others even for mild episodes of hypoglycemia. Other studies have limited the definition of severe hypoglycemia in children to episodes leading to unconsciousness or seizure [101, 102]. We have previously proposed [39] the following categories:

- **Severe hypoglycemia:** Loss of consciousness or seizure; definite if confirmed by blood glucose level below 2.8 mmol l^{-1} (50 mg dl^{-1}) or probable, if such a confirmation is lacking.
- **Moderate hypoglycemia:** Episode associated with typical signs and symptoms requiring assistance of another person (including administration of glucagon or intravenous glucose) but not leading to complete loss of consciousness or seizure; definite if confirmed by blood glucose level below 3.3 mmol l^{-1} (60 mg dl^{-1}) or probable, if such a confirmation is lacking.
- **Mild hypoglycemia:** Episode associated with typical signs and symptoms that objectively do not require assistance of another person (beyond simply making oral fluids or food available to the patient) and not leading to loss of consciousness or seizure; definite, if confirmed by blood glucose level below 3.9 mmol l^{-1} (70 mg dl^{-1}) or probable, if such a confirmation is lacking.

In addition, *asymptomatic hypoglycemia* (*biochemical*) is defined as a blood glucose level of 50 mg dl^{-1} or less without any recognizable symptoms.

In the ICD-9, hypoglycemic coma secondary to diabetes treatment is coded 250.3; however, this code is also used for coma with DKA. Other forms of diabetic hypoglycemia are coded 250.8. An additional E code is recommended to identify the drug that induced hypoglycemia. In the ICD-10, E1x.0 denotes coma with or without ketoacidosis, hyperosmolar or hypoglycemic (x digit is used to define type of diabetes) while E16.0 denotes diabetic drug-induced hypoglycemia without coma.

35.3.3 Incidence in Type 1 Diabetic Patients

The true incidence of moderate or mild hypoglycemia is difficult to ascertain; therefore, this

review is limited to studies of severe hypoglycemia, unless noted otherwise. Studies completed before the DCCT [103–107] reported rates of severe hypoglycemia ranging from 3 per 100 to 86 per 100 patient-years. The studies differed in event definition, patient age, duration of diabetes and treatment modalities.

In the DCCT, intensive insulin treatment increased the incidence of hypoglycemia three times compared with that observed with conventional therapy: for hypoglycemia requiring assistance, 61 per 100 versus 19 per 100 patient-years respectively; for coma or seizure, 16 per 100 versus 5 per 100 patient-years respectively [100]. Most (55%) of the episodes occurred during sleep. Of the episodes that occurred while subjects were awake, 36% were not accompanied by warning symptoms [108]. Among 195 adolescent participants, the incidence of hypoglycemia requiring assistance was 86 per 100 patient-years in intensively treated and 28 per 100 patient-years in those conventionally treated [41]. The incidence of coma or seizure in the adolescents was 27 per 100 and 10 per 100 patient-years respectively.

Post-DCCT studies of severe hypoglycemia and its predictors in children are summarized in **Table 35.4**. Few used a prospective design or were population based. A cohort study of 1243 type 1 diabetic children, aged 0–19 years, residing in the six-county Denver Metropolitan Area between 1996 and 2000, reported incidence of severe hypoglycemia of 19 per 100 person-years [39]. The rates decreased significantly with age in females, but not in males (**Figure 35.4**).

A Joslin Clinic study used a similar definition in a cohort of older children, aged 7–16 years, and found a lower rate of 8 per 100 person-years [40]; however, high-risk children with documented psychiatric disorders and unstable living conditions were excluded. The rates were comparable in Europe and Australia, with a notable exception of very low incidence (<4 per 100 person-years) in a Finnish study [111].

35.3.4 Incidence in Type 2 Diabetic Patients

Severe hypoglycemia does not occur in patients with type 2 diabetes treated with diet and exercise and is uncommon in those treated with oral hypoglycemic agents. However, the risk of hyperglycemia increases with transition to insulin

Table 35.4 Incidence of Severe Hypoglycemia in Children and Adolescents in the Post-DCCT Era.

Country (ref)	Age group	N	Study design	Length of study	Definition of hypoglycemia	Incidence per 100 person-years	Predictors
USA [39]	0–19	1243	Prospective cohort	3.5 years	Coma, seizure or admission	19	Male gender, younger age, lower HbA_{1c}, higher insulin dose underinsurance, psychiatric disorders
USA [40]	7–16	300	Prospective cohort	1 year	Coma, seizure, glucagon injection or iv dextrose	8	Higher HbA_{1c}
Sweden [109]	1–18	146	Prospective cohort	3 years	Coma or seizure	15–19	Lower HbA_{1c} higher insulin dose
France [110]	1–19	2579	Cross-sectional	6 mo	Coma, seizure or glucagon injection	45	Lower HbA_{1c} more exercise, number of BG measurements/day
Finland [111]	1–24	287	Prospective cohort	2 years	Coma, seizure or glucagon injection	3.1	Lower HbA_{1c} level higher insulin dose
		329	Retrospective	4 years		3.6	
Australia [102]	0–18	709	Prospective cohort	4 years	Coma or seizure	8	Younger age lower HbA_{1c}
Australia [44]	1–19	268	Retrospective	3 months	Coma or seizure	25	Age, lower HbA_{1c} number of visits
USA, Europe, Japan [112]	1–18	2873	Cross-sectional	5 months	Coma or seizure	22	Younger age lower HbA_{1c}
Canada, Europe, Japan [113]	0–18	2780	Cross-sectional	5–6 months	Coma or seizure	7–20	Poor glycemic control

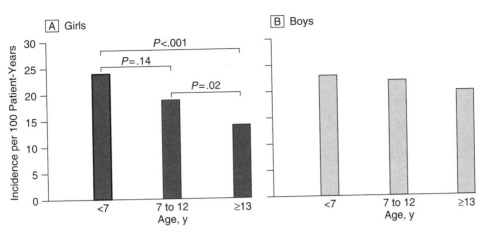

Figure 35.4 Incidence of severe hypoglycemia by age and gender, Colorado, 1996–2001. (Reproduced from [39], Copyright © 2002, The American Medical Association)

dependence. In the UK Prospective Diabetes Study (UKPDS) Group, the risk of severe hypoglycemia was 1.0 per 100 person-years in those intensively treated with chlorpropamide, 1.4 per 100 person-years with glibenclamide and 1.8 per 100 person-years with insulin [114]. Long-acting sulfonylureas confer higher risk than shorter acting ones [115]. Additional risk factors include older age, longer duration of diabetes, polypragmasia and recent hospitalization [116]. Reports of an increased risk of hypoglycemia in patients treated with sulfonylurea and angiotensin-converting enzyme inhibitors [117] have not been confirmed by a recent large trial [118].

35.3.5 Risk Factors

35.3.5.1 Demographic Predictors

Some of the commonly reported predictors of severe hypoglycemia are not modifiable: age (infancy and adolescence) [112, 119], male gender [39] or increased duration of diabetes [110]. Longer duration of diabetes predicts hypoglycemia regardless of age [39, 108].

35.3.5.2 Human Leukocyte Antigen Genotype, Islet Autoantibodies at Onset of Diabetes and Subsequent Risk of Hypoglycemia

The risk of hypoglycemia increases with duration of diabetes, partially due to progressive blunting of α-cell glucagon response to hypoglycemia [120]. This process is inversely related to preservation

of β-cells that often leads to partial remission at 1–12 months after diagnosis [120]. In the DCCT, presence of residual endogenous insulin secretion predicted 65% lower risk of severe hypoglycemia [121]. Abrupt loss of endogenous insulin production is more frequent in patients with the HLA-DR3/4 genotype [122–124] and those positive for multiple islet autoantibodies [123, 125].

35.3.5.3 Imperfect Insulin Replacement

The relation between severe hypoglycemia and tight glycemic control had been extensively explored [126], especially in children [40, 42, 112]. The DCCT showed clearly that the level of metabolic control needed to prevent development and progression of diabetic microvascular complications increases significantly the risk of hypoglycemia (**Figure 35.5**) [41]. As many as 63% of the intensively treated adolescents (ages 13–17 years) participating in the trial, had coma or seizure during the trial, compared with 25% of those treated conventionally [41]. Over the past several years, intensive treatment strategies, with the emphasis on improving glycemic control, have been extended to younger children and may have led to hypoglycemia risk even higher than that reported by the DCCT [40]. When the DCCT definition of hypoglycemia was applied to a large clinic patient population in Colorado, the incidence of severe hypoglycemia increased from 28 per 100 person-years in 1993 to an average of 43 per 100 person-years in 1995–1998,

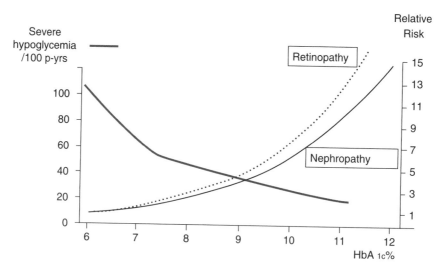

Figure 35.5 Inverse relationship between the risk of microvascular complications and hypoglycemia. DCCT Study. (Reproduced from [197], Copyright © 1996, Elsevier)

reflecting the intensification of diabetes control in the post-DCCT era [127].

35.3.5.4 Hypoglycemia Unawareness

Inability to recognize symptoms of hypoglycemia is seen in approximately one in ten patients and is more common in those who keep blood glucose generally low [128, 129]. A single hypoglycemic episode can lead to significant decrease in neuro-hormonal counterregulatory responses and cause unawareness of hypoglycemia [130]. The syndrome is usually associated with decreased glucagon or epinephrine output [128, 131] and autonomic neuropathy [132]. There is evidence that loss of awareness of hypoglycemia can be reversed by avoiding hypoglycemia for 2–3 weeks [126, 133].

35.3.5.5 Recurrent Severe Hypoglycemia

Unfortunately, severe hypoglycemia is a recurrent problem in some diabetic patients. In our experience, nearly 80% of severe hypoglycemic episodes occur in a relatively small group (14%) of children with recurrent event [39]. While lack of awareness of symptoms is a major factor, we showed that poor medical insurance doubles the risk of recurrence.

35.3.5.6 Exercise

Acute blood glucose lowering effect of physical activity may result in hypoglycemia, if not matched

by decreased insulin delivery and increased ingestion of carbohydrates [134]. Higher habitual physical activity is associated with higher insulin sensitivity. While a large body of evidence suggests that exercise is an important trigger of many events of severe hypoglycemia, there is a paucity of epidemiological data to quantitate the magnitude of the problem.

35.3.5.7 Alcohol Consumption

Alcohol suppresses gluconeogenesis and glycogenolysis [135] and may induce hypoglycemia unawareness [136]. In addition, alcohol ingestion acutely improves insulin sensitivity [137]. In combination with exercise, drinking can lead to severe hypoglycemia, often delayed for 10–12 h [138]. Despite anecdotal reports of severe hypoglycemic events in the morning after drinking and dancing, this phenomenon has not yet been documented in epidemiological studies.

35.3.5.8 Family Dynamics, Behavioral and Psychiatric Factors

The DCCT analyses indicated that conventional risk factors explained only 8.5% of the variance in occurrence of severe hypoglycemia [108]. The majority of severe hypoglycemic events may be attributable not as much to intensive insulin treatment, but rather to insufficient diabetes education,

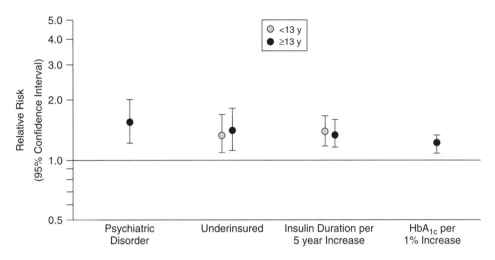

Figure 35.6 Predictors of severe hypoglycemia, Colorado, 1996–2001. (Reproduced from [39], Copyright © 2002, The American Medical Association.)

low socioeconomic status, inability to pay for standard care, unstable living conditions, behavioral factors and psychiatric disorders affecting patients and their families. These factors have a significant influence on glycemic control and the rate of acute complications, as reviewed above in the context of DKA. Family relationship and personality type have a significant effect on adaptation to illness and metabolic control among persons with diabetes. It seems possible that chronic illness points out and fixes perhaps pathological characteristics already present [139]. Initial maternal psychopathology, particularly maternal depression, increases the risk of psychiatric disorder in children with type 1 diabetes [140]. Monitoring of the psychological status of the patients and their mothers may help to identify children at risk for psychiatric disorder and facilitate prevention or treatment efforts. Monitoring may be particularly beneficial during the first year of diabetes [140].

Reported prevalence of psychiatric disorders among patients with type 1 diabetes is high, up to 48% by 10 years of diabetes duration and age 20 years [140, 141]. The most prevalent are major depressive (28%), conduct and generalized anxiety disorders [140]. In addition, diabetic youths have propensity for more suicidal thoughts [142], protracted depressions and the higher risk of recurrence of major depression [139]. There are indications of lower self-esteem in the type 1 diabetes patients that could predispose them

for future depression or difficulties in adaptation [143]. The presence of psychiatric disorders is associated with poor diabetic metabolic control [144, 145] and with noncompliance with the medical regimen [142].

It is not clear whether increased risk of hypoglycemia is caused by noncompliance due to psychiatric illness itself or if it is a side effect of the medications leading to hypoglycemia unawareness. Hypoglycemia unawareness has been reported in patients treated with serotonin reuptake inhibitors commonly prescribed for treatment of psychiatric conditions [146]. More information regarding the relationship between psychiatric disorders, medications, family dynamics and the incidence of hypoglycemic events is needed.

In Colorado children and adolescents with type 1 diabetes, the presence of psychiatric disorders increased the risk of hypoglycemia by 60% in children aged 13 years and older [39] (**Figure 35.6**).

35.3.5.9 Health Insurance and Access to Care
In the Colorado study mentioned above (**Figure 35.6**), lack of adequate health insurance was an independent predictor of severe hypoglycemia in children of any age, increasing the risk by approximately 40% [39]. A study from Wisconsin found similar associations [147].

Studies from countries with nationalized health care systems have shown that socioeconomic status did not appear to play a major role in the risk of hypoglycemia [144]. However, in countries with privatized, largely for profit health care, major economic inequities become barriers in access to care and compliance. In the United States, the cost containment of escalating health care expenditures has left more than a quarter of people with no health insurance and has shifted the others toward managed care organizations. Coverage provided by these plans is similar between the diabetes-affected families and the general population, but out-of-pocket expenses (co-pays, deductibles and uncovered expenses) have been shown to be 56% higher in the diabetes-affected families. Seventeen percent of the diabetes-affected families had expenses over 10% of their household income [148]. Further investigation is needed to clarify the extent of barriers to care, economic decisions regarding health insurance, the use of health care and health outcomes in relation to the risk of acute complications among patient with diabetes.

35.3.5.10   Coexisting Autoimmune Conditions

Autoimmune thyroid, celiac and Addison's disease affect up to 30% of patients with type 1 diabetes and increase, through different mechanisms, the risk of hypoglycemia. Thyroid autoimmune disease is the most common of the above, affecting 6–18% of the patients [149–151]. The clinical presentation of hypothyroidism is associated with increased frequency of severe hypoglycemia [150]. Biopsy-confirmed celiac disease is present in 4–10% of patients with type 1 diabetes [152]. Untreated celiac disease is associated with increased risk of hypoglycemia due to malabsorption. The introduction of a gluten-free diet may reduce the frequency of hypoglycemia [153, 154]. Primary adrenal insufficiency (Addison's disease) is a rare disorder, although it is more common in type 1 diabetes mellitus, affecting nearly 1% of the patients [155]. Recurrent severe hypoglycemia, despite a reduction in insulin dose, and severe hypoglycemia unawareness has been reported in patients with type 1 diabetes and undiagnosed Addison's disease [156, 157].

35.3.6   Mortality

Hypoglycemia contributes significantly to excess mortality in patients with diabetes [158]. Despite recent improvements in therapy, diabetes-related mortality among children has not declined for 14 years [159]. Sudden nocturnal death in young persons with type 1 diabetes has been described, and is known as the *dead in bed* syndrome [160]. It appears to be responsible for about 6% of deaths in diabetic patients below age 40 years [161]. In these cases, nocturnal hypoglycemia is a likely precipitant consistent with demonstrated impairment of counterregulatory hormone response during sleep [162], high frequency of nocturnal hypoglycemia reported by the DCCT [108] and more recent studies using continuous glucose monitoring (CGM) (see Section 35.1.10).

35.3.7   Consequences of Hypoglycemia

The consequences of hypoglycemia range from mild neurogenic symptoms to coma and seizures. Previous studies have shown an association between hypoglycemia and a decrease in cognitive functioning in children with type 1 diabetes [163–165], particularly those diagnosed before the age of 5–6 years [165, 166]. Hypoglycemic seizures lead to significant declines in verbal abilities [167], memory skills [168] and ability to organize and recall information [169], even after mild hypoglycemia [170]. Severe hypoglycemia in children may result in persistent electroencephalographic (EEG) changes [171–174]. EEG abnormalities were found in 80% of diabetic children with a history of severe hypoglycemia, compared with only 30% of those without and 24% of healthy control children [174]. Clearly, severe hypoglycemia is not good for the brain of young children. Interestingly, intensive insulin treatment in the DCCT cohort (age 13–39 at the baseline), while increasing the incidence of hypoglycemia, has not led to a significant worsening of neuropsychological or cognitive functioning during the trial [175, 176], as well as 18 years after entry into the trial [177]. This observation may be further evidence that the effect of severe hypoglycemia on long-term neuropsychological functioning is age dependent.

35.3.8   Quality of Life

Hypoglycemic episodes have a significant influence on the patient's and family life [126]. One-third of the events require assistance of people other than parents, and many are associated with patient school or work absence, parent absence from work, increased need for extra transport and telephone calls [76]. Severe hypoglycemia can lead to increased worry, poor sleep, hospital visits and hospitalizations, excessive lowering of daily insulin dose and worsening of subsequent glycemic control [178]. Patients with severe hypoglycemia also reported lower global quality of life; on the other hand, some patients may inappropriately deny or disregard warning signs of hypoglycemia [179].

35.3.9 Cost

In 1999, a Swedish study estimated the direct health care cost of severe hypoglycemic events at €17 400 per 100 patients per year [42]. Using the incidence rate reported for severe hypoglycemia from Colorado [39] and the average annual cost of severe hypoglycemia estimated at $174 per person [40], the direct medical cost of severe hypoglycemia in the United States children was at least $26 million per year, in the late 1990s. Reliable data are not available concerning the cost of hypoglycemia in adults with diabetes.

The personal, family, and societal cost of trauma of loss of consciousness, seizure, long-term disability and fears are harder to measure. Further studies are needed to update these figures and to estimate, in addition, indirect cost (e.g. lost productivity and diminished quality of life).

35.3.10 Prevention

35.3.10.1 Improved Insulin Delivery

While technological advances provide new opportunities to improve glycemic control without undue risk of severe hypoglycemia, it is important to bear in mind that these modalities have limited use without intensified patient education and compliance [110, 180, 181]. Intensive insulin therapy using insulin pumps, multiple daily injections (MDIs) and new insulin analogues has been found effective in lowering HbA$_{1c}$ levels, but there has been less evidence for a beneficial effect on the risk of hypoglycemia. Insulin pump treatment may lower HbA$_{1c}$ levels and improve quality of life, compared with MDI of insulin and, of importance, reduce the rate of severe hypoglycemia [182, 183].

The introduction of Humalog has made insulin treatment easier and safer. An ecologic analysis explored the effects of the DCCT report in 1993 and that of the introduction of rapid-acting insulin

analogue (lispro) in 1996 on the risk of severe hypoglycemia in type 1 diabetic patients [127]. The HbA$_{1c}$ levels declined significantly during 1993–1996 ($p < 0.001$), following the DCCT report, but the number of severe hypoglycemic events increased ($p < 0.001$) during that time frame. A further decline in HbA$_{1c}$ levels was observed after the introduction of Humalog insulin in 1996 ($p < 0.001$), however, without a concomitant change in the incidence of severe hypoglycemia. The introduction of a long-lasting insulin analogues also suggest a potential for improving glycemic control without an increased risk of hypoglycemia [184–186].

35.3.10.2 CGM

Frequent self-monitoring of blood glucose has been found to be an important factor in attaining better glucose control for the intensively treated participants in the DCCT and in the UKPDS. However, many patients do not accept frequent blood glucose monitoring, mainly because of pain and inconvenience. The results also give data valid for only a few seconds, without any information on glucose trends before or after the glucose value. In addition, patients infrequently measure blood glucose levels during the night, although over 50% of severe hypoglycemic events occur during sleep [102, 106].

CGM holds great promise for prevention of hypoglycemia. Clinical trials of CGM have given reason to believe that tighter glycemic control may not necessarily lead to increased risk of hypoglycemia [187–193]. The ultimate goal remains to be development of a noninvasive sensor or an implantable sensor with long lifetime and capability to control automatic 'closed-loop' insulin delivery system [194].

35.3.10.3 Behavioral Interventions

Interventions integrating intensive medical care, increased access to care and increased level of psychosocial support, including treatment of psychiatric disorders, should be considered to lower the risk of hypoglycemia. There are preliminary indications suggesting the efficacy of this approach [195, 196].

References

1. Wolfsdorf, J., Glaser, N. and Sperling, M.A. (2006) Diabetic ketoacidosis in infants, children,

and adolescents: a consensus statement from the American Diabetes Association. *Diabetes Care*, **29** (5), 1150–9.

2. Kitabchi, A.E., Umpierrez, G.E., Murphy, M.B. and Kreisberg, R.A. (2006) Hyperglycemic crises in adult patients with diabetes: a consensus statement from the American Diabetes Association. *Diabetes Care*, **29** (12), 2739–48.

3. Wolfsdorf, J., Craig, M.E., Daneman, D. *et al.* (2007) Diabetic ketoacidosis. *Pediatric Diabetes*, **8** (1), 28–43.

4. Dunger, D.B., Sperling, M.A., Acerini, C.L. *et al.* (2004) ESPE/LWPES consensus statement on diabetic ketoacidosis in children and adolescents. *Archives of Disease in Childhood*, **89** (2), 188–94.

5. Ireland, J.T. and Thomson, W.S. (1973) Euglycemic diabetic ketoacidosis. *British Medical Journal*, **3** (5871), 107.

6. Burge, M.R., Hardy, K.J. and Schade, D.S. (1993) Short-term fasting is a mechanism for the development of euglycemic ketoacidosis during periods of insulin deficiency. *The Journal of Clinical Endocrinology and Metabolism*, **76** (5), 1192–8.

7. Laffel, L.M., Wentzell, K., Loughlin, C. *et al.* (2006) Sick day management using blood 3-hydroxybutyrate (3-OHB) compared with urine ketone monitoring reduces hospital visits in young people with T1DM: a randomized clinical trial. *Diabetic Medicine: A Journal of the British Diabetic Association*, **23** (3), 278–84.

8. Rewers, A., McFann, K. and Chase, H.P. (2006) Bedside monitoring of blood beta-hydroxybutyrate levels in the management of diabetic ketoacidosis in children. *Diabetes Technology and Therapeutics*, **8** (6), 671–6.

9. Rewers, A., Klingensmith, G., Davis, C. *et al.* (2007) Diabetes ketoacidosis at onset of diabetes: the SEARCH for diabetes in Youth Study (Abstract). *Diabetes*, **54** (Suppl 1), A63–4.

10. Mallare, J.T., Cordice, C.C., Ryan, B.A. *et al.* (2003) Identifying risk factors for the development of diabetic ketoacidosis in new onset type 1 diabetes mellitus. *Clinical Pediatrics*, **42** (7), 591–7.

11. Quinn, M., Fleischman, A., Rosner, B. *et al.* (2006) Characteristics at diagnosis of type 1 diabetes in children younger than 6 years. *The Journal of Pediatrics*, **148** (3), 366–71.

12. Pinkey, J.H., Bingley, P.J., Sawtell, P.A. *et al.* (1994) Presentation and progress of childhood diabetes mellitus: a prospective population-based study. The Bart's–Oxford Study Group. *Diabetologia*, **37** (1), 70–4.

13. Komulainen, J., Lounamaa, R., Knip, M. *et al.* (1996) Ketoacidosis at the diagnosis of type 1 (insulin dependent) diabetes mellitus is related to poor residual beta cell function. Childhood Diabetes in Finland Study Group. *Archives of Disease in Childhood*, **75** (5), 410–15.

14. Lévy-Marchal, C., Patterson, C.C. and Green, A. (2001) Geographical variation of presentation at diagnosis of type I diabetes in children: the EURODIAB study. *Diabetologia*, **44** (Suppl 3), B75–80.

15. Neu, A., Willasch, A., Ehehalt, S. *et al.* (2003) Ketoacidosis at onset of type 1 diabetes mellitus in children – frequency and clinical presentation. *Pediatric Diabetes*, **4** (2), 77–81.

16. Roche, E.F., Menon, A., Gill, D. and Hoey, H. (2005) Clinical presentation of type 1 diabetes. *Pediatric Diabetes*, **6** (2), 75–8.

17. Hekkala, A., Knip, M. and Veijola, R. (2007) Ketoacidosis at diagnosis of type 1 diabetes in children in northern Finland: temporal changes over 20 years. *Diabetes Care*, **30** (4), 861–6.

18. Daneman, D., Knip, M., Kaar, M.L. and Sochett, E. (1990) Comparison of children with type 1 (insulin-dependent) diabetes in northern Finland and southern Ontario: differences at disease onset. *Diabetes Research (Edinburgh, Lothian)*, **14** (3), 123–6.

19. Soliman, A.T., Al Salmi, I. and Asfour, M. (1997) Mode of presentation and progress of childhood diabetes mellitus in the Sultanate of Oman. *Journal of Tropical Pediatrics*, **43** (3), 128–32.

20. Al-Khawari, M., Shaltout, A., Qabazard, M. *et al.* (1997) Incidence and severity of ketoacidosis in childhood-onset diabetes in Kuwait. Kuwait Diabetes Study Group. *Diabetes Research and Clinical Practice*, **35** (2–3), 123–8.

21. Abdul-Rasoul, M., Habib, H. and Al-Khouly, M. (2006) 'The honeymoon phase' in children with type 1 diabetes mellitus: frequency, duration, and influential factors. *Pediatric Diabetes*, **7** (2), 101–7.

22. Swai, A.B., Lutale, J. and McLarty, D.G. (1990) Diabetes in tropical Africa: a prospective study, 1981–7. I. Characteristics of newly presenting patients in Dar es Salaam, Tanzania, 1981–7. *British Medical Journal*, **300** (6732), 1103–6.

23. Alvi, N.S., Davies, P., Kirk, J.M. and Shaw, N.J. (2001) Diabetic ketoacidosis in Asian children. *Archives of Disease in Childhood*, **85** (1), 60–1.

24. Hamman, R.F., Cook, M., Keefer, S. *et al.* (1985) Medical care patterns at the onset of insulin-dependent diabetes mellitus: association with severity and subsequent complications. *Diabetes Care*, **8** (Suppl 1), 94–100.

25. Rewers, A., Chase, P., Bothner, J. *et al.* (2003) Medical care patterns at the onset of type I diabetes in Colorado children, 1978–2001. *Diabetes*, **52** (Suppl 1), A62.

26. Curtis, J.R., To, T., Muirhead, S. *et al.* (2002) Recent trends in hospitalization for diabetic ketoacidosis in ontario children. *Diabetes Care*, **25** (9), 1591–6.

27. HiraSing, R.A., Reeser, H.M., de Groot, R.R. *et al.* (1996) Trends in hospital admissions among children aged 0–19 years with type I diabetes in The Netherlands. *Diabetes Care*, **19** (5), 431–4.

28. Lévy-Marchal, C., Papoz, L., de Beaufort, C. *et al.* (1992) Clinical and laboratory features of type 1 diabetic children at the time of diagnosis. *Diabetic Medicine: A Journal of the British Diabetic Association*, **9** (3), 279–84.

29. Komulainen, J., Kulmala, P., Savola, K. *et al.* (1999) Clinical, autoimmune, and genetic characteristics of very young children with type 1 diabetes. Childhood Diabetes in Finland (DiMe) Study Group. *Diabetes Care*, **22** (12), 1950–5.

30. Maniatis, A.K., Goehrig, S.H., Gao, D. *et al.* (2005) Increased incidence and severity of diabetic ketoacidosis among uninsured children with newly diagnosed type 1 diabetes mellitus. *Pediatric Diabetes*, **6** (2), 79–83.

31. Alavi, I.A., Sharma, B.K. and Pillay, V.K. (1971) Steroid-induced diabetic ketoacidosis. *The American Journal of the Medical Sciences*, **262** (1), 15–23.

32. Wilson, D.R., D'Souza, L., Sarkar, N. *et al.* (2003) New-onset diabetes and ketoacidosis with atypical antipsychotics. *Schizophrenia Research*, **59** (1), 1–6.

33. Likitmaskul, S., Santiprabhob, J., Sawathiparnich, P. *et al.* (2005) Clinical pictures of type 2 diabetes in Thai children and adolescents is highly related to features of metabolic syndrome. *Journal of the Medical Association of Thailand = Chotmaihet Thangphaet*, **88** (Suppl 8), S169–75.

34. Westphal, S.A. (1996) The occurrence of diabetic ketoacidosis in non-insulin-dependent diabetes and newly diagnosed diabetic adults. *The American Journal of Medicine*, **101** (1), 19–24.

35. Umpierrez, G.E., Kelly, J.P., Navarrete, J.E. *et al.* (1997) Hyperglycemic crises in urban blacks. *Archives of Internal Medicine*, **157** (6), 669–75.

36. Balasubramanyam, A., Zern, J.W., Hyman, D.J. and Pavlik, V. (1999) New profiles of diabetic ketoacidosis: type 1 vs type 2 diabetes and the effect of ethnicity. *Archives of Internal Medicine*, **159** (19), 2317–22.

37. Pinero-Pilona, A. and Raskin, P. (2001) Idiopathic Type 1 diabetes. *Journal of Diabetes and its Complications*, **15** (6), 328–35.

38. Mauvais-Jarvis, F., Sobngwi, E., Porcher, R. *et al.* (2004) Ketosis-prone type 2 diabetes in patients of sub-Saharan African origin: clinical pathophysiology and natural history of beta-cell dysfunction and insulin resistance. *Diabetes*, **53** (3), 645–53.

39. Rewers, A., Chase, H.P., Mackenzie, T. *et al.* (2002) Predictors of acute complications in children with type 1 diabetes. *The Journal of the American Medical Association*, **287** (19), 2511–18.

40. Levine, B.S., Anderson, B.J., Butler, D.A. *et al.* (2001) Predictors of glycemic control and short-term adverse outcomes in youth with type 1 diabetes. *The Journal of Pediatrics*, **139** (2), 197–203.

41. The Diabetes Control and Complications Trial Research Group (1994) Effect of intensive diabetes treatment on the development and progression of long-term complications in adolescents with insulin- dependent diabetes mellitus: Diabetes Control and Complications Trial. Diabetes Control and Complications Trial Research Group. *The Journal of Pediatrics*, **125** (2), 177–88.

42. Nordfeldt, S. and Ludvigsson, J. (1999) Adverse events in intensively treated children and adolescents with type 1 diabetes. *Acta Paediatrica*, **88** (11), 1184–93.

43. Smith, C.P., Firth, D., Bennett, S. *et al.* (1998) Ketoacidosis occurring in newly diagnosed and established diabetic children. *Acta Paediatrica*, **87** (5), 537–41.

44. Thomsett, M., Shield, G., Batch, J. and Cotterill, A. (1999) How well are we doing? Metabolic control in patients with diabetes. *Journal of Paediatrics and Child Health*, **35** (5), 479–82.

45. Reda, E., Von Reitzenstein, A. and Dunn, P. (2007) Metabolic control with insulin pump therapy: the Waikato experience. *The New Zealand Medical Journal*, **120** (1248), U2401.

46. Mbugua, P.K., Otieno, C.F., Kayima, J.K. *et al.* (2005) Diabetic ketoacidosis: clinical presentation and precipitating factors at Kenyatta National Hospital, Nairobi. *East African Medical Journal*, **82** (Suppl 12), S191–6.

47. Golden, M.P., Herrold, A.J. and Orr, D.P. (1985) An approach to prevention of recurrent diabetic ketoacidosis in the pediatric population. *The Journal of Pediatrics*, **107** (2), 195–200.

48. Flood, R.G. and Chiang, V.W. (2001) Rate and prediction of infection in children with diabetic ketoacidosis. *The American Journal of Emergency Medicine*, **19** (4), 270–3.

49. Kaufman, F.R., Halvorson, M., Miller, D. *et al.* (1999) Insulin pump therapy in type 1 pediatric patients: now and into the year 2000. *Diabetes/Metabolism Research and Reviews*, **15** (5), 338–52.

50. Hanas, R. and Ludvigsson, J. (2006) Hypoglycemia and ketoacidosis with insulin pump therapy in children and adolescents. *Pediatric Diabetes*, **7** (Suppl 4), 32–8.

51. Sulli, N. and Shashaj, B. (2006) Long-term benefits of continuous subcutaneous insulin infusion in children with type 1 diabetes: a 4-year follow-up. *Diabetic Medicine: A Journal of the British Diabetic Association*, **23** (8), 900–6.

52. Umpierrez, G.E. and Kitabchi, A.E. (2003) Diabetic ketoacidosis: risk factors and management strategies. *Treatments in Endocrinology*, **2** (2), 95–108.

53. Gutierrez, J.A., Bagatell, R., Samson, M.P. *et al.* (2003) Femoral central venous catheter-associated deep venous thrombosis in children with diabetic ketoacidosis. *Critical Care Medicine*, **31** (1), 80–3.

54. Nyenwe, E.A., Loganathan, R.S., Blum, S. *et al.* (2007) Active use of cocaine: an independent risk factor for recurrent diabetic ketoacidosis in a city hospital. *Endocrine Practice: Official Journal of the American College of Endocrinology and the American Association of Clinical Endocrinologists*, **13** (1), 22–9.

55. Quinn, L. (2001) Diabetes emergencies in the patient with type 2 diabetes. *The Nursing Clinics of North America*, **36** (2), 341–60, viii.

56. Maldonado, M.R., Chong, E.R., Oehl, M.A. and Balasubramanyam, A. (2003) Economic impact of diabetic ketoacidosis in a multiethnic indigent population: analysis of costs based on the precipitating cause. *Diabetes Care*, **26** (4), 1265–9.

57. Snorgaard, O., Eskildsen, P.C., Vadstrup, S. and Nerup, J. (1989) Diabetic ketoacidosis in Denmark: epidemiology, incidence rates, precipitating factors and mortality rates. *Journal of Internal Medicine*, **226** (4), 223–8.

58. Polonsky, W.H., Anderson, B.J., Lohrer, P.A. *et al.* (1994) Insulin omission in women with IDDM. *Diabetes Care*, **17** (10), 1178–85.

59. Meltzer, L.J., Johnson, S.B., Prine, J.M. *et al.* (2001) Disordered eating, body mass, and glycemic control in adolescents with type 1 diabetes. *Diabetes Care*, **24** (4), 678–82.

60. Dumont, R.H., Jacobson, A.M., Cole, C. *et al.* (1995) Psychosocial predictors of acute complications of diabetes in youth. *Diabetic Medicine: A Journal of the British Diabetic Association*, **12** (7), 612–18.

61. Edge, J.A., Ford-Adams, M.E. and Dunger, D.B. (1999) Causes of death in children with insulin dependent diabetes 1990–96. *Archives of Disease in Childhood*, **81** (4), 318–23.

62. Podar, T., Solntsev, A., Reunanen, A. *et al.* (2000) Mortality in patients with childhood-onset type 1 diabetes in Finland, Estonia, and Lithuania: follow-up of nationwide cohorts. *Diabetes Care*, **23** (3), 290–4.

63. Edge, J.A., Hawkins, M.M., Winter, D.L. and Dunger, D.B. (2001) The risk and outcome of cerebral oedema developing during diabetic ketoacidosis. *Archives of Disease in Childhood*, **85** (1), 16–22.

64. Lawrence, S.E., Cummings, E.A., Gaboury, I. and Daneman, D. (2005) Population-based study of incidence and risk factors for cerebral edema in pediatric diabetic ketoacidosis. *The Journal of Pediatrics*, **146** (5), 688–92.

65. Glaser, N., Barnett, P., McCaslin, I. *et al.* (2001) Risk factors for cerebral edema in children with diabetic ketoacidosis. The Pediatric Emergency Medicine Collaborative Research Committee of the American Academy of Pediatrics. *The New England Journal of Medicine*, **344** (4), 264–9.

66. Roberts, M.D., Slover, R.H. and Chase, H.P. (2001) Diabetic ketoacidosis with intracerebral complications. *Pediatric Diabetes*, **2** (3), 109–14.

67. Atluru, V.L. (1986) Spontaneous intracerebral hematomas in juvenile diabetic ketoacidosis. *Pediatric Neurology*, **2** (3), 9.

68. Ho, J., Mah, J.K., Hill, M.D. and Pacaud, D. (2006) Pediatric stroke associated with new onset type 1 diabetes mellitus: case reports and review of the literature. *Pediatric Diabetes*, **7** (2), 116–21.

69. Kanter, R.K., Oliphant, M., Zimmerman, J.J. and Stuart, M.J. (1987) Arterial thrombosis causing cerebral edema in association with diabetic ketoacidosis. *Critical Care Medicine*, **15** (2), 175–6.

70. Kameh, D.S., Gonzalez, O.R., Pearl, G.S. *et al.* (1997) Fatal rhino-orbital-cerebral zygomycosis. *Southern Medical Journal*, **90** (11), 1133–5.

71. Gessesse, M., Chali, D., Wolde-Tensai, B. and Ergete, W. (2001) Rhinocerebral mucormycosis in an 11-year-old boy. *Ethiopian Medical Journal*, **39** (4), 341–8.

72. Dixon, A.N., Jude, E.B., Banerjee, A.K. and Bain, S.C. (2006) Simultaneous pulmonary and cerebral oedema, and multiple CNS infarctions as complications of diabetic ketoacidosis: a case report. *Diabetic Medicine: A Journal of the British Diabetic Association*, **23** (5), 571–3.

73. Young, M.C. (1995) Simultaneous acute cerebral and pulmonary edema complicating diabetic ketoacidosis. *Diabetes Care*, **18** (9), 1288–90.

74. Wang, J., Williams, D.E., Narayan, K.M. and Geiss, L.S. (2006) Declining death rates from hyperglycemic crisis among adults with diabetes, U.S., 1985–2002. *Diabetes Care*, **29** (9), 2018–22.

75. Javor, K.A., Kotsanos, J.G., McDonald, R.C. *et al.* (1997) Diabetic ketoacidosis charges relative to medical charges of adult patients with type I diabetes. *Diabetes Care*, **20** (3), 349–54.

76. Nordfeldt, S. and Jonsson, D. (2001) Short-term effects of severe hypoglycaemia in children and adolescents with type 1 diabetes. A cost-of-illness study. *Acta Paediatrica*, **90** (2), 137–42.

77. Ginde, A.A., Pelletier, A.J. and Camargo, C.A. Jr (2006) National study of U.S. emergency department visits with diabetic ketoacidosis, 1993–2003. *Diabetes Care*, **29** (9), 2117–19.

78. Kim, S. (2007) Burden of hospitalizations primarily due to uncontrolled diabetes: implications of inadequate primary health care in the United States. *Diabetes Care*, **30** (5), 1281–2.

79. Kitabchi, A.E., Umpierrez, G.E., Murphy, M.B. *et al.* (2001) Management of hyperglycemic crises in patients with diabetes. *Diabetes Care*, **24** (1), 131–53.

80. Barker, J.M., Goehrig, S.H., Barriga, K. *et al.* (2004) Clinical characteristics of children diagnosed with type 1 diabetes through intensive screening and follow-up. *Diabetes Care*, **27** (6), 1399–404.

81. Vanelli, M., Chiari, G., Ghizzoni, L. *et al.* (1999) Effectiveness of a prevention program for diabetic ketoacidosis in children. An 8-year study in schools and private practices. *Diabetes Care*, **22** (1), 7–9.

82. Vanelli, M., Chiari, G., Lacava, S. and Iovane, B. (2007) Campaign for diabetic ketoacidosis prevention still effective 8 years later. *Diabetes Care*, **30** (4), e12.

83. Diabetes Prevention Trial–Type 1 Diabetes Study Group (2002) Effects of insulin in relatives of patients with type 1 diabetes mellitus. *The New England Journal of Medicine*, **346** (22), 1685–91.

84. Hoffman, W.H., O'Neill, P., Khoury, C. and Bernstein, S.S. (1978) Service and education for the insulin-dependent child. *Diabetes Care*, **1** (5), 285–8.

85. Drozda, D.J., Dawson, V.A., Long, D.J. *et al.* (1990) Assessment of the effect of a comprehensive diabetes management program on hospital admission rates of children with diabetes mellitus. *The Diabetes Educator*, **16** (5), 389–93.

86. Grey, M., Boland, E.A., Davidson, M. *et al.* (2000) Coping skills training for youth with diabetes mellitus has long-lasting effects on metabolic control and quality of life. *The Journal of Pediatrics*, **137** (1), 107–13.

87. Svoren, B.M., Butler, D., Levine, B.S. *et al.* (2003) Reducing acute adverse outcomes in youths with type 1 diabetes: a randomized, controlled trial. *Pediatrics*, **112** (4), 914–22.

88. American Diabetes Association (2001) Hyperglycemic crises in patients with diabetes mellitus. *Diabetes Care*, **24** (11), 1988–96.

89. Wachtel, T.J., Tetu-Mouradjian, L.M., Goldman, D.L. *et al.* (1991) Hyperosmolarity and acidosis in diabetes mellitus: a three-year experience in Rhode Island. *Journal of General Internal Medicine: Official Journal of the Society for Research and Education in Primary Care Internal Medicine*, **6** (6), 495–502.

90. MacIsaac, R.J., Lee, L.Y., McNeil, K.J. *et al.* (2002) Influence of age on the presentation and outcome of acidotic and hyperosmolar diabetic emergencies. *Internal Medicine Journal*, **32** (8), 379–85.

91. Morales, A.E. and Rosenbloom, A.L. (2004) Death caused by hyperglycemic hyperosmolar state at the onset of type 2 diabetes. *The Journal of Pediatrics*, **144** (2), 270–3.

92. Fourtner, S.H., Weinzimer, S.A. and Levitt Katz, L.E. (2005) Hyperglycemic hyperosmolar non-ketotic syndrome in children with type 2 diabetes. *Pediatric Diabetes*, **6** (3), 129–35.

93. Carchman, R.M., Dechert-Zeger, M., Calikoglu, A.S. and Harris, B.D. (2005) A new challenge in pediatric obesity: pediatric hyperglycemic hyperosmolar syndrome. *Pediatric Critical Care Medicine: A Journal of the Society of Critical Care Medicine and the World Federation of Pediatric Intensive and Critical Care Societies*, **6** (1), 20–4.

94. Kershaw, M.J., Newton, T., Barrett, T.G. *et al.* (2005) Childhood diabetes presenting with hyperosmolar dehydration but without ketoacidosis: a report of three cases. *Diabetic Medicine: A Journal of the British Diabetic Association*, **22** (5), 645–7.

95. Wachtel, T.J., Silliman, R.A. and Lamberton, P. (1987) Predisposing factors for the diabetic hyperosmolar state. *Archives of Internal Medicine*, **147** (3), 499–501.

96. Chu, C.H., Lee, J.K., Lam, H.C. and Lu, C.C. (2001) Prognostic factors of hyperglycemic hyperosmolar nonketotic state. *Chang Gung Medical Journal*, **24** (6), 345–51.

97. Pinies, J.A., Cairo, G., Gaztambide, S. and Vazquez, J.A. (1994) Course and prognosis of 132 patients with diabetic non ketotic hyperosmolar state. *Diabete and Metabolisme*, **20** (1), 43–8.

98. Cryer, P.E. (2006) Hypoglycemia in diabetes: pathophysiological mechanisms and diurnal variation. *Progress in Brain Research*, **153**, 361–5.

99. Kerr, D., Macdonald, I.A., Heller, S.R. and Tattersall, R.B. (1990) Beta-adrenoceptor blockade and hypoglycaemia. A randomised, double-blind, placebo controlled comparison of metoprolol CR, atenolol and propranolol LA in normal subjects. *British Journal of Clinical Pharmacology*, **29** (6), 685–93.

100. The Diabetes Control and Complications Trial Research Group (1995) Adverse events and their association with treatment regimens in the diabetes control and complications trial. *Diabetes Care*, **18** (11), 1415–27.

101. Becker, D.J. and Ryan, C.M. (2000) Hypoglycemia: a complication of diabetes therapy in children. *Trends in Endocrinology and Metabolism*, **11** (5), 198–202.

102. Davis, E.A., Keating, B., Byrne, G.C. *et al.* (1998) Impact of improved glycaemic control on rates of hypoglycaemia in insulin dependent diabetes mellitus. *Archives of Disease in Childhood*, **78** (2), 111–15.

103. Bhatia, V. and Wolfsdorf, J.I. (1991) Severe hypoglycemia in youth with insulin-dependent diabetes mellitus: frequency and causative factors. *Pediatrics*, **88** (6), 1187–93.

104. Bergada, I., Suissa, S., Dufresne, J. and Schiffrin, A. (1989) Severe hypoglycemia in IDDM children. *Diabetes Care*, **12** (4), 239–44.

105. Daneman, D., Frank, M., Perlman, K. *et al.* (1989) Severe hypoglycemia in children with insulin-dependent diabetes mellitus: frequency and predisposing factors [see comments]. *The Journal of Pediatrics*, **115**, 681–5.

106. Aman, J., Karlsson, I. and Wranne, L. (1989) Symptomatic hypoglycaemia in childhood diabetes: a population-based questionnaire study. *Diabetic Medicine: A Journal of the British Diabetic Association*, **6** (3), 257–61.

107. Egger, M., Gschwend, S., Smith, G.D. and Zuppinger, K. (1991) Increasing incidence of hypoglycemic coma in children with IDDM. *Diabetes Care*, **14** (11), 1001–5.

108. DCCT (1991) Epidemiology of severe hypoglycemia in the diabetes control and complications trial. The DCCT Research Group. *The American Journal of Medicine*, **90** (4), 450–9.

109. Nordfeldt, S. and Ludvigsson, J. (1997) Severe hypoglycemia in children with IDDM. A prospective population study, 1992–1994. *Diabetes Care*, **20** (4), 497–503.

110. Rosilio, M., Cotton, J.B., Wieliczko, M.C. *et al.* (1998) Factors associated with glycemic control. A cross-sectional nationwide study in 2,579 French children with type 1 diabetes. The French Pediatric Diabetes Group. *Diabetes Care*, **21** (7), 1146–53.

111. Tupola, S., Rajantie, J. and Maenpaa, J. (1998) Severe hypoglycaemia in children and adolescents during multiple-dose insulin therapy. *Diabetic Medicine: A Journal of the British Diabetic Association*, **15** (8), 695–9.

112. Mortensen, H.B. and Hougaard, P. (1997) Comparison of metabolic control in a cross-sectional study of 2,873 children and adolescents with IDDM from 18 countries. The Hvidore Study Group on Childhood Diabetes. *Diabetes Care*, **20** (5), 714–20.

113. Danne, T., Mortensen, H.B., Hougaard, P. *et al.* (2001) Persistent differences among centers over 3 years in glycemic control and hypoglycemia in a study of 3,805 children and adolescents with type 1 diabetes from the Hvidore Study Group. *Diabetes Care*, **24** (8), 1342–7.

114. UK Prospective Diabetes Study (UKPDS) Group (1998) Intensive blood-glucose control with sulphonylureas or insulin compared with conventional treatment and risk of complications in patients with type 2 diabetes (UKPDS 33). *Lancet*, **352** (9131), 837–53.

115. Shorr, R.I., Ray, W.A., Daugherty, J.R. and Griffin, M.R. (1996) Individual sulfonylureas and serious hypoglycemia in older people. *Journal of the American Geriatrics Society*, **44** (7), 751–5.

116. Shorr, R.I., Ray, W.A., Daugherty, J.R. and Griffin, M.R. (1997) Incidence and risk factors for serious hypoglycemia in older persons using insulin or sulfonylureas. *Archives of Internal Medicine*, **157** (15), 1681–6.

117. Shorr, R.I., Ray, W.A., Daugherty, J.R. and Griffin, M.R. (1997) Antihypertensives and the risk of serious hypoglycemia in older persons using insulin or sulfonylureas. *The Journal of the American Medical Association*, **278** (1), 40–3.

118. Heart Outcomes Prevention Evaluation Study Investigators (2000) Effects of ramipril on cardiovascular and microvascular outcomes in people with diabetes mellitus: results of the HOP E study and MICRO-HOPE substudy. *Lancet*, **355** (9200), 253–9.

119. Jones, T.W., Boulware, S.D., Kraemer, D.T. *et al.* (1991) Independent effects of youth and poor diabetes control on responses to hypoglycemia in children. *Diabetes*, **40**, 358–63.

120. Fukuda, M., Tanaka, A., Tahara, Y. *et al.* (1988) Correlation between minimal secretory capacity of pancreatic beta-cells and stability of diabetic control. *Diabetes*, **37** (1), 81–8.

121. The Diabetes Control and Complications Trial Research Group (1998) Effect of intensive therapy on residual beta-cell function in patients with type 1 diabetes in the diabetes control and complications trial. A randomized, controlled trial. *Annals of Internal Medicine*, **128** (7), 517–23.

122. Knip, M., Llonen, J., Mustonen, A. and Akerblom, H.K. (1986) Evidence of an accelerated B-cell destruction in HLA-Dw3/Dw4 heterozygous children with type I (insulin-dependent) diabetes. *Diabetologia*, **29**, 347–51.

123. Dahlquist, G., Blom, L., Persson, B. *et al.* (1988) The epidemiology of lost residual beta-cell function in short term diabetic children. *Acta Paediatrica Scandinavica*, **77**, 852–9.

124. Petersen, J.S., Dyrberg, T., Karlsen, A.E. *et al.* (1994) Glutamic acid decarboxylase (GAD65) autoantibodies in prediction of B-cell function and remission in recent-onset IDDM after cyclosporin treatment. *Diabetes*, **43** (11), 1291–6.

125. Lteif, A.N. and Schwenk, W.F. (1999) Type 1 diabetes mellitus in early childhood: glycemic control and associated risk of hypoglycemic reactions. *Mayo Clinic Proceedings*, **74** (3), 211–16.

126. Cryer, P.E., Fisher, J.N. and Shamoon, H. (1994) Hypoglycemia. *Diabetes Care*, **17** (7), 734–55.

127. Chase, H.P., Lockspeiser, T., Peery, B. *et al.* (2001) The impact of the diabetes control and complications trial and humalog insulin on glycohemoglobin levels and severe hypoglycemia in type 1 diabetes. *Diabetes Care*, **24** (3), 430–4.

128. Simonson, D.C., Tamborlane, W.V., DeFronzo, R.A. and Sherwin, R.S. (1985) Intensive insulin therapy reduces counterregulatory hormone responses to hypoglycemia in patients with type I diabetes. *Annals of Internal Medicine*, **103** (2), 184–90.

129. Jones, T.W., Borg, W.P., Borg, M.A. *et al.* (1997) Resistance to neuroglycopenia: an adaptive response during intensive insulin treatment of diabetes. *The Journal of Clinical Endocrinology and Metabolism*, **82** (6), 1713–18.

130. Heller, S.R. and Cryer, P.E. (1991) Reduced neuroendocrine and symptomatic responses to subsequent hypoglycemia after 1 episode of hypoglycemia in nondiabetic humans. *Diabetes*, **40** (2), 223–6.

131. Amiel, S.A., Simonson, D.C., Sherwin, R.S. *et al.* (1987) Exaggerated epinephrine responses to hypoglycemia in normal and insulin-dependent diabetic children. *The Journal of Pediatrics*, **110** (6), 832–7.

132. Hepburn, D.A., Patrick, A.W., Eadington, D.W. *et al.* (1990) Unawareness of hypoglycemia in insulin-treated diabetic patients: prevalence and relationship to autonomic neuropathy. *Diabetic Medicine: A Journal of the British Diabetic Association*, **7** (8), 711–17.

133. Cranston, I., Lomas, J., Maran, A. *et al.* (1994) Restoration of hypoglycaemia awareness in patients with long-duration insulin-dependent diabetes. *Lancet*, **344** (8918), 283–7.

134. Tsalikian, E., Kollman, C., Tamborlane, W.B. *et al.* (2006) Prevention of hypoglycemia during exercise in children with type 1 diabetes by suspending basal insulin. *Diabetes Care*, **29** (10), 2200–4.

135. van de Wiel, A. (2004) Diabetes mellitus and alcohol. *Diabetes/Metabolism Research and Reviews*, **20** (4), 263–7.

136. Kerr, D., Macdonald, I.A., Heller, S.R. and Tattersall, R.B. (1990) Alcohol causes hypoglycaemic unawareness in healthy volunteers and patients with type 1 (insulin-dependent) diabetes. *Diabetologia*, **33** (4), 216–21.

137. Avogaro, A., Watanabe, R.M., Dall'Arche, A. *et al.* (2004) Acute alcohol consumption improves insulin action without affecting insulin secretion in type 2 diabetic subjects. *Diabetes Care*, **27** (6), 1369–74.

138. Ismail, D., Gebert, R., Vuillermin, P.J. *et al.* (2006) Social consumption of alcohol in adolescents with type 1 diabetes is associated with increased glucose lability, but not hypoglycaemia. *Diabetic Medicine: A Journal of the British Diabetic Association*, **23** (8), 830–3.

139. Bargagna, S., Tosi, B., Calisti, L. and Crespin, L. (1997) Psychopathological aspects in a group of children and adolescent with insulin-dependent diabetes mellitus. *Minerva Pediatrica*, **49** (3), 71–7.

140. Kovacs, M., Goldston, D., Obrosky, D.S. and Bonar, L.K. (1997) Psychiatric disorders in youths with IDDM: rates and risk factors. *Diabetes Care*, **20** (1), 36–44.

141. Blanz, B.J., Rensch-Riemann, B.S., Fritz-Sigmund, D.I. and Schmidt, M.H. (1993) IDDM is a risk factor for adolescent psychiatric disorders. *Diabetes Care*, **16** (12), 1579–87.

142. Goldston, D.B., Kovacs, M., Ho, V.Y. *et al.* (1994) Suicidal ideation and suicide attempts among youth with insulin-dependent diabetes mellitus. *Journal of the American Academy of Child and Adolescent Psychiatry*, **33** (2), 240–6.

143. Jacobson, A.M., Hauser, S.T., Willett, J.B. *et al.* (1997) Psychological adjustment to IDDM: 10-year follow-up of an onset cohort of child

and adolescent patients. *Diabetes Care*, **20** (5), 811–18.

144. Nakazato, M., Kodama, K., Miyamoto, S. *et al.* (2000) Psychiatric disorders in juvenile patients with insulin-dependent diabetes mellitus. *Diabetes Research and Clinical Practice*, **48** (3), 177–83.

145. Kovacs, M., Mukerji, P., Iyengar, S. and Drash, A. (1996) Psychiatric disorder and metabolic control among youths with IDDM. A longitudinal study. *Diabetes Care*, **19** (4), 318–23.

146. Sawka, A.M., Burgart, V. and Zimmerman, D. (2000) Loss of hypoglycemia awareness in an adolescent with type 1 diabetes mellitus during treatment with fluoxetine hydrochloride. *The Journal of Pediatrics*, **136** (3), 394–6.

147. Allen, C., LeCaire, T., Palta, M. *et al.* (2001) Risk factors for frequent and severe hypoglycemia in type 1 diabetes. *Diabetes Care*, **24** (11), 1878–81.

148. Songer, T.J., LaPorte, R., Lave, J.R. *et al.* (1997) Health insurance and the financial impact of IDDM in families with a child with IDDM. *Diabetes Care*, **20** (4), 577–84.

149. Kontiainen, S., Schlenzka, A., Koskimies, S. *et al.* (1990) Autoantibodies and autoimmune diseases in young diabetics. *Diabetes Research (Edinburgh, Lothian)*, **13** (4), 151–6.

150. Leong, K.S., Wallymahmed, M., Wilding, J. and MacFarlane, I. (1999) Clinical presentation of thyroid dysfunction and Addison's disease in young adults with type 1 diabetes. *Postgraduate Medical Journal*, **75** (886), 467–70.

151. Roldan, M.B., Alonso, M. and Barrio, R. (1999) Thyroid autoimmunity in children and adolescents with type 1 diabetes mellitus. *Diabetes, Nutrition and Metabolism*, **12** (1), 27–31.

152. Rewers, M., Liu, E., Simmons, J. *et al.* (2004) Celiac disease associated with type 1 diabetes mellitus. *Endocrinology and Metabolism Clinics of North America*, **33** (1), 197–214, xi.

153. Mohn, A., Cerruto, M., Lafusco, D. *et al.* (2001) Celiac disease in children and adolescents with type I diabetes: importance of hypoglycemia. *Journal of Pediatric Gastroenterology and Nutrition*, **32** (1), 37–40.

154. Iafusco, D., Rea, F. and Prisco, F. (1998) Hypoglycemia and reduction of the insulin requirement as a sign of celiac disease in children with IDDM. *Diabetes Care*, **21** (8), 1379–81.

155. Yu, L., Brewer, K.W., Gates, S. *et al.* (1999) DRB1*04 and DQ alleles: expression of 21-hydroxylase autoantibodies and risk of progression to Addison's disease. *The Journal of Clinical Endocrinology and Metabolism*, **84** (1), 328–35.

156. McAulay, V. and Frier, B.M. (2000) Addison's disease in type 1 diabetes presenting with recurrent hypoglycaemia. *Postgraduate Medical Journal*, **76** (894), 230–2.

157. Phornphutkul, C., Boney, C.M. and Gruppuso, P.A. (1998) A novel presentation of Addison disease: hypoglycemia unawareness in an adolescent with insulin-dependent diabetes mellitus. *The Journal of Pediatrics*, **132** (5), 882–4.

158. Nishimura, R., Laporte, R.E., Dorman, J.S. *et al.* (2001) Mortality trends in type 1 diabetes. The Allegheny County (Pennsylvania) Registry 1965–1999. *Diabetes Care*, **24** (5), 823–7.

159. DiLiberti, J.H. and Lorenz, R.A. (2001) Long-term trends in childhood diabetes mortality: 1968–1998. *Diabetes Care*, **24** (8), 1348–52.

160. Weston, P.J. and Gill, G.V. (1999) Is undetected autonomic dysfunction responsible for sudden death in type 1 diabetes mellitus? The 'dead in bed' syndrome revisited. *Diabetic Medicine: A Journal of the British Diabetic Association*, **16** (8), 626–31.

161. Sovik, O. and Thordarson, H. (1999) Dead-in-bed syndrome in young diabetic patients. *Diabetes Care*, **22** (Suppl 2), B40–2.

162. Jones, T.W., Porter, P., Sherwin, R.S. *et al.* (1998) Decreased epinephrine responses to hypoglycemia during sleep. *The New England Journal of Medicine*, **338** (23), 1657–62.

163. Golden, M.P., Ingersoll, G.M., Brack, C.J. *et al.* (1989) Longitudinal relationship of asymptomatic hypoglycemia to cognitive function in IDDM. *Diabetes Care*, **12**, 89–93.

164. Rovet, J.F., Ehrlich, R.M. and Hoppe, M. (1988) Specific intellectual deficits in children with early onset diabetes mellitus. *Child Development*, **59** (1), 226–34.

165. Rovet, J.F., Ehrlich, R.M. and Czuchta, D. (1990) Intellectual characteristics of diabetic children at diagnosis and one year later. *Journal of Pediatric Psychology*, **15**, 775–88.

166. Ryan, C., Vega, A. and Drash, A. (1985) Cognitive deficits in adolescents who developed diabetes early in life. *Pediatrics*, **75** (5), 921–7.

167. Rovet, J.F. and Ehrlich, R.M. (1999) The effect of hypoglycemic seizures on cognitive function in children with diabetes: a 7-year prospective study. *The Journal of Pediatrics*, **134** (4), 503–6.

168. Kaufman, F.R., Epport, K., Engilman, R. and Halvorson, M. (1999) Neurocognitive functioning in children diagnosed with diabetes before age 10 years. *Journal of Diabetes and its Complications*, **13** (1), 31–8.

169. Hagen, J.W., Barclay, C.R., Anderson, B.J. *et al.* (1990) Intellective functioning and strategy use in

children with insulin-dependent diabetes mellitus. *Child Development*, **61** (6), 1714–27.

170. Ryan, C.M., Williams, T.M., Finegold, D.N. and Orchard, T.J. (1993) Cognitive dysfunction in adults with type 1 (insulin-dependent) diabetes mellitus of long duration: effects of recurrent hypoglycaemia and other chronic complications. *Diabetologia*, **36**, 329–34.

171. Eeg-Olofsson, O. and Petersen, I. (2001) Childhood diabetic neuropathy. A clinical and neurophysiological study (Generic). *Acta Paediatrica Scandinavica*, **55**, 163–76.

172. Schlack, H., Palm, D. and Jochmus, I. (1969) Influence of recurrent hypoglycemia on the EEG of the diabetic child. *Monatsschrift fur Kinderheilkunde*, **117** (4), 251–3.

173. Gilhaus, K.H., Daweke, H., Lulsdorf, H.G. *et al.* (1973) EEG changes in diabetic children. *Deutsche Medizinische Wochenschrift*, **98** (31), 1449–54.

174. Soltesz, G. and Acsadi, G. (1989) Association between diabetes, severe hypoglycaemia, and electroencephalographic abnormalities. *Archives of Disease in Childhood*, **64**, 992–6.

175. DCCT (1996) Effects of intensive diabetes therapy on neuropsychological function in adults in the diabetes control and complications trial. *Annals of Internal Medicine*, **124** (4), 379–88.

176. Austin, E.J. and Deary, I.J. (1999) Effects of repeated hypoglycemia on cognitive function: a psychometrically validated reanalysis of the Diabetes Control and Complications Trial data. *Diabetes Care*, **22** (8), 1273–7.

177. Jacobson, A.M., Musen, G., Ryan, C.M. *et al.* (2007) Long-term effect of diabetes and its treatment on cognitive function. *The New England Journal of Medicine*, **356** (18), 1842–52.

178. Tupola, S., Rajantie, J. and Akerblom, H.K. (1998) Experience of severe hypoglycaemia may influence both patient's and physician's subsequent treatment policy of insulin-dependent diabetes mellitus. *European Journal of Pediatrics*, **157** (8), 625–7.

179. Cox, D.J., Irvine, A., Gonder-Frederick, L. *et al.* (1987) Fear of hypoglycemia: quantification, validation, and utilization. *Diabetes Care*, **10** (5), 617–21.

180. Karter, A.J., Ackerson, L.M., Darbinian, J.A. *et al.* (2001) Self-monitoring of blood glucose levels and glycemic control: the Northern California Kaiser Permanente Diabetes registry. *The American Journal of Medicine*, **111** (1), 1–9.

181. Kubiak, T., Hermanns, N., Schreckling, H.J. *et al.* (2006) Evaluation of a self-management-based patient education program for the treatment and

prevention of hypoglycemia-related problems in type 1 diabetes. *Patient Education and Counseling*, **60** (2), 228–34.

182. Boland, E.A., Grey, M., Oesterle, A. *et al.* (1999) Continuous subcutaneous insulin infusion. A new way to lower risk of severe hypoglycemia, improve metabolic control, and enhance coping in adolescents with type 1 diabetes. *Diabetes Care*, **22** (11), 1779–84.

183. Maniatis, A.K., Klingensmith, G.J., Slover, R.H. *et al.* (2001) Continuous subcutaneous insulin infusion therapy for children and adolescents: an option for routine diabetes care. *Pediatrics*, **107** (2), 351–6.

184. Ratner, R.E., Hirsch, I.B., Neifing, J.L. *et al.* (2000) Less hypoglycemia with insulin glargine in intensive insulin therapy for type 1 diabetes. U.S. Study Group of Insulin Glargine in Type 1 Diabetes. *Diabetes Care*, **23** (5), 639–43.

185. Raskin, P., Klaff, L., Bergenstal, R. *et al.* (2000) A 16-week comparison of the novel insulin analog insulin glargine (HOE 901) and NPH human insulin used with insulin lispro in patients with type 1 diabetes. *Diabetes Care*, **23** (11), 1666–71.

186. Mohn, A., Strang, S., Wernicke-Panten, K. *et al.* (2000) Nocturnal glucose control and free insulin levels in children with type 1 diabetes by use of the long-acting insulin HOE 901 as part of a three-injection regimen. *Diabetes Care*, **23** (4), 557–9.

187. Boland, E., Monsod, T., Delucia, M. *et al.* (2001) Limitations of conventional methods of self-monitoring of blood glucose: lessons learned from 3 days of continuous glucose sensing in pediatric patients with type 1 diabetes. *Diabetes Care*, **24** (11), 1858–62.

188. Chase, H.P., Kim, L.M., Owen, S.L. *et al.* (2001) Continuous subcutaneous glucose monitoring in children with type 1 diabetes. *Pediatrics*, **107** (2), 222–6.

189. UK Hypoglycaemia Study Group (2007) Risk of hypoglycaemia in types 1 and 2 diabetes: effects of treatment modalities and their duration. *Diabetologia*, **50** (6), 1140–7.

190. Clarke, W.L., Anderson, S., Farhy, L. *et al.* (2005) Evaluating the clinical accuracy of two continuous glucose sensors using continuous glucose-error grid analysis. *Diabetes Care*, **28** (10), 2412–17.

191. Fayolle, C., Brun, J.F., Bringer, J. *et al.* (2006) Accuracy of continuous subcutaneous glucose monitoring with the GlucoDay in type 1 diabetic patients treated by subcutaneous insulin infusion during exercise of low versus high intensity. *Diabetes and Metabolism*, **32** (4), 313–20.

192. Maia, F.F. and Araujo, L.R. (2005) Efficacy of continuous glucose monitoring system to

detect unrecognized hypoglycemia in children and adolescents with type 1 diabetes. *Arquivos Brasileiros de Endocrinologia e Metabologia*, **49** (4), 569–74.

193. Streja, D. (2005) Can continuous glucose monitoring provide objective documentation of hypoglycemia unawareness? *Endocrine Practice: Official Journal of the American College of Endocrinology and the American Association of Clinical Endocrinologists*, **11** (2), 83–90.

194. Renard, E., Costalat, G., Chevassus, H. and Bringer, J. (2006) Artificial beta-cell: clinical experience toward an implantable closed-loop insulin delivery system. *Diabetes and Metabolism*, **32** (5 Pt 2), 497–502.

195. Halvorson, M., Carpenter, S., Kaiserman, K. and Kaufman, F.R. (2007) A pilot trial in pediatrics with the sensor-augmented pump: combining real-time continuous glucose monitoring with the insulin pump. *The Journal of Pediatrics*, **150** (1), 103–5.

196. Svoren, B.M., Volkening, L.K., Butler, D.A. *et al.* (2007) Temporal trends in the treatment of pediatric type 1 diabetes and impact on acute outcomes. *The Journal of Pediatrics*, **150** (3), 279–85.

197. Skyler, J., (1996) *Endocrinology and Metabolism Clinics of North America*, **25**, 243–54.

36

Mortality and Life Expectancy Associated with Diabetes

Elizabeth L. M. Barr, Paul Z. Zimmet and Jonathan E. Shaw

International Diabetes Institute, Caulfield, Victoria, Australia

36.1 INTRODUCTION

At the beginning of the twenty-first century it was estimated that 5.2% of all deaths globally were attributable to diabetes mellitus. This ranks diabetes as the fifth leading cause of death after communicable disease, cardiovascular disease (CVD), cancer and injury [1]. For centuries diabetes has been responsible for substantial morbidity and mortality, and although significant treatment advances have been made, mortality rates are still considerably greater in people with diabetes than with the general population [2, 3]. Higher mortality rates among those with diabetes have led to shorter life expectancy, which is approximately 8 years lower in middle-aged people with diabetes [4, 5]. West [6] (p. xi) a pioneering epidemiologist in diabetes research, stated in 1978 that diabetes "has become one of the most important of human problems. It is a significant cause of disease and death in all countries and races. In the past quarter century diabetes has killed more people than all wars combined." It has even been suggested that diabetes could be responsible for attenuating the recent declines in population mortality rates [7].

Well-documented mortality data on diabetes can improve our understanding of the natural history of the disease and of the relationships between risk factors and disease. Higher mortality rates in one population than in another population may indicate that certain factors predominate which increase the likelihood of the disease. Prevention and treatment strategies that target these factors can, therefore,

be developed, with the aim of improving the life expectancy for people with diabetes.

36.2 METHODOLOGICAL ISSUES ASSOCIATED WITH MORTALITY DATA

Diabetes mortality data are often derived from information collected from death certificates. Death certificate data can be useful for monitoring diabetes-related mortality, and is often the only practical way of collecting information on a large enough population to make meaningful conclusions. Moreover, by using documentation of other associated causes of death, researchers are able to investigate whether certain diseases, such as CVD, are more frequently reported causes of death among people with diabetes than those without diabetes. National mortality statistics can also be used to study trends over time.

However, several limitations need to be considered when interpreting mortality data based on death certificates. The greatest limitations apply to those studies that are simple 'surveys' of death certificates (e.g. national mortality data). Because individuals are not identified for these studies prior to death, the ascertainment of diabetes status depends solely on whether or not diabetes is reported on the death certificate. Several studies have reported that diabetes is often underreported as a cause of death, resulting in a large proportion of diabetes deaths not being identified [8–11]. Underreporting of diabetes on death certificates has been attributed to

The Epidemiology of Diabetes Mellitus, second edition   Edited by Jean-Marie Ekoé, Marian Rewers, Rhys Williams and Paul Zimmet
© 2008 John Wiley & Sons, Ltd

several factors, including (i) undiagnosed diabetes, (ii) physician misclassification or misinterpretation of the causes of death [10, 12, 13] and (iii) the increasing likelihood of several competing chronic conditions being related to the death. Often, the contribution of diabetes to the events leading to death is not well understood or is difficult to determine. Indeed, McEwen *et al.* [11] found that having fewer comorbidities increased the likelihood of reporting diabetes on the death certificate. Consequently, national mortality databases which rely upon death certificate information often underreport the impact of diabetes on population health [2].

The methods used for completing and coding death certificates can also vary, which can affect the way in which death certificate data are interpreted and compared. Jougla *et al.* [14] compared death certificate data from nine European countries and found that there were substantial coding practice differences between countries. Another study that compared death certificate reporting methods in Taiwan, Australia and Sweden found that age-adjusted diabetes mortality rates based on the underlying cause of death differed markedly among the three countries, whereas differences were not as striking when rates were based on diabetes being mentioned anywhere on the death certificate. These discrepancies were attributed to differences in physician death certificate recording practices among the three countries [13]. Similar findings were apparent in a study examining death certificate data over a 21-year period in the United Kingdom [15]. Thus, diabetes mortality rates based solely on the underlying cause of death may be significantly influenced by death certificate coding protocols.

Cohort studies provide better information on the mortality attributable to diabetes, because (i) mortality information for all people with diabetes can be examined, rather than only those who have diabetes listed as a cause of death on the death certificate, (ii) the temporal relationship between risk factors and outcomes can be explored and (iii) the excess risk of mortality in people with diabetes compared with those without diabetes can be investigated in relation to other risk factors. It is essential that cohort studies include a representative group from the population of interest, and that the follow-up is complete, otherwise it will be difficult to generalize the findings from the study to the broader community [2]. However, while cohort studies are

able to identify all of those with diabetes, many cohort studies still rely on death certificate data to determine the causes of death. This is problematic for two reasons. First, as death certificates are often completed by relatively inexperienced doctors, their accuracy may be questionable. Second, the single cause of death is taken as being the *underlying* disease causing the terminal event, with other concomitant diseases listed as *contributory* causes on the death certificate. Thus, a typical vascular death might be recorded as myocardial infarction due to ischemic heart disease, with diabetes listed as a contributory disease. In this case, ischemic heart disease would be used as the underlying cause of death, and the death would be considered to be a vascular death. However, if the doctor completing the certificate chose to indicate that ischemic heart disease was due to diabetes, the death would be classified as being due to an endocrine disorder. Such decisions may lead to an underestimate of the CVD burden associated with diabetes.

36.3 MORTALITY TRENDS OF TYPE 1 DIABETES

It is difficult to evaluate the mortality associated with type 1 diabetes, as (i) many studies on diabetic mortality do not distinguish between type 1 and type 2 diabetes, (ii) the prevalence of type 1 diabetes in the general population is considerably lower than the prevalence of type 2 diabetes, making it more difficult to conduct representative population-based studies and (iii) the classification and nomenclature of diabetes has changed over time. The majority of studies on type 1 diabetes mortality are based on patient registries. Unlike type 2 diabetes, which can be asymptomatic for some time prior to diagnosis, type 1 diabetes is usually symptomatic and requires more immediate medical care, as people with the disease are dependent on insulin therapy for survival. Therefore, providing all patients with type 1 diabetes are enrolled on the registry, these cohorts are likely to be largely representative of people with type 1 diabetes in the general community.

Prior to the introduction of insulin in 1922, the mortality rate in those with type 1 diabetes was extremely high, with the majority of people dying as a result of diabetic ketoacidosis [3]. Data from the Joslin Clinic in Boston, US, estimated the annual mortality rate for 1897–1914 to be 824 per 1000 diabetic children aged <10 years, and 600 per 1000 diabetic children aged 10–20 years. These rates had declined for the period 1914–1922, but still remained very high at just under 400 per 1000 diabetic children [16]. The implementation of insulin therapy led to improved metabolic control, and this had a significant impact on type 1 diabetes mortality. Joslin Clinic data revealed an ongoing decline in mortality rates for both males and females aged 5–24 years between the years 1930 and 1958 [17] (**Figure 36.1**). The Pittsburgh Epidemiology of Diabetes Complications Study Experience reported that 20-year cumulative mortality had reduced from 22% in 1950–1959 to 3.5% in 1975–1980 for patients with type 1 diabetes [18]. Moreover, Nishimura *et al.* [19] evaluated the mortality rates for people diagnosed with type 1 diabetes at age <18 years who were listed on a US population-based registry and reported that people diagnosed during 1975–1979 showed significantly improved survival compared with people diagnosed 10 years earlier. Similar mortality trends over the twentieth century have also been reported for Denmark [20] and Australia [21]. Since the 1980s, mortality rates appear to have stabilized [3, 18, 21].

In addition to the dramatic changes in total mortality, the causes of death in type 1 diabetes have also changed. Before the widespread use of insulin, deaths were mainly the result of infections and acute metabolic complications, such as diabetic ketoacidosis. Improved treatment translated into increased survival, which led to the emergence of deaths due to chronic complications, such as renal disease and CVD [3]. Cause of death data in people with insulin-dependent diabetes (this study did not differentiate between type 1 and type 2 diabetes) attending the Joslin Clinic revealed that, in 1887–1914, 17.5% of deaths were due to CVD (including cardiac-, renal-, cerebrovascular- and gangrene-related deaths). The proportion of CVD deaths had increased to 24.6% in 1914–1922 and 76.6% in 1960–1968. Moreover, the rate of diabetes deaths due to diabetic coma fell from 63.8% in 1887–1914 to about 1% in 1960–1968 [22] (**Figure 36.2**).

Although mortality rates for type 1 diabetes in Western developed nations have reduced substantially since the introduction of insulin, similar improvements have not necessarily been achieved in poorer developing countries [23]. Limited data from some countries indicate that mortality rates remain high and that people are more likely to die from acute complications, such as ketoacidosis and infections [24]. While poorer health outcomes and higher mortality rates may be due to a range of factors, it is suggested that the inadequate supply of insulin is the most important factor [23].

36.4 MORTALITY TRENDS OF TYPE 2 DIABETES

Several studies have reported mortality trends associated with diabetes [2, 15, 21, 25–28]; however, the findings are inconsistent, and many have

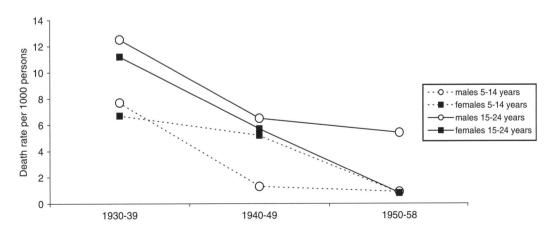

Figure 36.1 Death rates (per 1000) in younger people with diabetes attending the Joslin Clinic, Boston, US between 1930 and 1958. (Adapted from Entmacher *et al.* [17].)

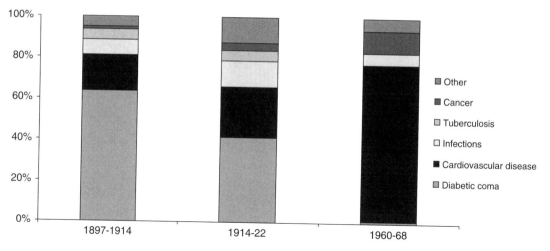

Figure 36.2 Causes of death for people with diabetes attending the Joslin Clinic, Boston, US, over three time periods between 1897 and 1968. (Adapted from Marble [22].)

not distinguished between type 1 and type 2 diabetes. It can be assumed, however, that mortality rates derived from the total diabetic population relate predominantly to type 2 diabetes, as it is much more prevalent than type 1 diabetes. Differences between studies may reflect different population health experiences across differing time periods. However, as these studies have only relied on death certificate data, it is difficult to determine the extent to which the observed mortality trends were influenced by methodological changes relating to death certificate reporting and coding.

Some studies have attempted to evaluate mortality patterns for type 2 diabetes by utilizing cohort data. In Denmark, Støvring *et al.* [29] evaluated mortality trends in people listed on a population-based drug registry. The authors reported that, between 1993 and 1999, mortality rates for people taking diabetic medications had declined. Similarly, McBean *et al.* [30] showed that the overall mortality rates from 1994 to 2001 decreased by approximately 5% for Medicare beneficiaries with diagnosed diabetes aged ≥67 years living in the US, compared with no change in overall mortality rates in the nondiabetic population. Longer survival could be attributed to many factors, including improvements in the underlying life expectancy of the general population, better access to medical care, earlier diagnosis (which leads to an apparent improvement in survival by identifying more people

at an earlier stage of their disease, who then have longer to live) and better treatment.

In contrast to the findings reported by the above-mentioned studies, Leibson *et al.* [31] in a retrospective analysis of medical and laboratory reports for people residing in Rochester, US, reported that, compared with the general population, 10-year survival among people aged >45 years detected to have diabetes in 1980 was not different to the 10-year survival in those detected to have diabetes in 1970. In fact, the 10-year survival experience for women was worse in 1980 than in 1970, whereas mortality rates remained stable for men across this time period. In a more recent study of the same US population, Thomas *et al.* [7] showed that although people with diabetes exhibited improved survival between 1970–1974 and 1990–1994 (mortality rate reduction of 13.8%), they did not experience the same overall improvements observed for people without diabetes (mortality rate reduction 21.4%). In addition, this study revealed that mortality trends for those with diagnosed diabetes during this 20-year period differed according to sex and age. Increasing mortality rates were observed for diabetic women aged 85 years and older, and the improved survival rates observed for men with diabetes diminished with older age.

Several studies which have used complex modeling techniques of population mortality data have revealed that diabetes may be having an increasing impact upon CVD mortality rates [32–34]. In Western countries, it appears that diabetes and related risk factors, such as obesity and inactivity, could even be attenuating the recent gains in reduced CVD mortality [33, 34].

Other population-based cohort studies have investigated this further to determine the impact of diabetes on mortality trends associated with CVD. Utilizing US data collected in the First National Health and Nutrition Examination Survey (NHANES 1), Gu *et al.* [35] demonstrated that although mortality from heart disease had declined in the general population between 1971–1975 and 1982–1984, the decline was less substantial for men with self-reported diabetes, and increasing heart disease mortality was observed for women with self-reported diabetes. In US Pima Indians identified to have diabetes on a glucose tolerance test, Hoehner *et al.* [36] reported that ischemic heart disease mortality rates increased nearly twofold between 1965 and 1998, while ischemic heart disease death rates among those without diabetes remained unchanged. In another US study conducted in Rochester, Thomas *et al.* [7] found that, although heart disease mortality rates declined significantly between 1970–1974 and 1990–1994 for people with and without diagnosed diabetes, there was a trend for increasing cerebrovascular disease mortality rates among those with diabetes, whereas it declined significantly among those without diabetes. In contrast to these studies, Fox *et al.* [37] using data from the Framingham Heart Study and Offspring Cohorts, found that, compared to those without diabetes, people with diabetes had a greater but not statistically significant CVD (fatal and nonfatal) event rate reduction (35% versus 49%) between the 1950–1960s and 1980–1990s time periods. It is difficult to determine from this study whether the findings were driven by the fatal or nonfatal events, as these were combined as the main outcome measure. Furthermore, the contrasting findings of Fox *et al.* [37] and the Rochester [7] and NHANES 1 [4] cohorts may be explained by different cohort characteristics and varying follow-up periods [38]. More recently, Booth *et al.* [39] evaluated the impact of diabetes on the mortality trends associated with both fatal and nonfatal CVD events in Canada between 1992 and 1999. The results indicated that, although patients with diabetes had a significantly greater reduction in nonfatal myocardial infarction

and stroke event rates than nondiabetic patients, similar improvements in all-cause mortality and case-fatality rates for myocardial infarction and stroke were observed for both groups. However, mortality rates were still higher in diabetic patients than in nondiabetic patients for all years.

Overall, although mortality rates may be declining for people with diabetes, these observational studies suggest that the rate of reduction may be less than in the general population. Moreover, diabetes is continuing to have an adverse effect on CVD mortality, with some studies suggesting that this impact could be increasing in some populations. However, as most of these studies have been conducted on Western populations, it is not possible to evaluate the impact of diabetes on mortality trends in other population groups, where temporal mortality patterns may be substantially different.

36.5 TYPE 1 DIABETES AND MORTALITY

36.5.1 Excess Risk of Total Mortality among Those with Type 1 Diabetes

Despite considerable improvements in survival over the past century, people with type 1 diabetes still die at a greater rate than people without the disease. Data from US diabetic patients indicate that life expectancy in those with type 1 diabetes aged <20 years at diagnosis is reduced by approximately 15 years, with the probability of survival among those diagnosed with childhood-onset diabetes reducing from 88% at 20 years of disease duration to 83% after having diabetes for 25 years [3]. Moreover, the mean reduction in life expectancy appears to be greater for younger children than for older children, and in those diagnosed with type 1 diabetes at a younger age than in those diagnosed at an older age (**Table 36.1**) [40, 41]. The estimated relative risks for total mortality vary considerably, with reported risks being 2- to 15-fold in people with type 1 diabetes [3, 5, 42–53]. It should be noted that these estimates may actually underestimate the relative risk of mortality, because most studies rely upon standardized mortality ratios (SMRs), which are calculated by comparing the mortality rates observed in type 1 patients to mortality rates in the general population, which includes people with diabetes. Furthermore, although differences in risk of mortality may be partly related to study design

Table 36.1 Age-related reduction in life expectancy (mean of years lost) for people with diabetes compared with the general population: summary of published data.[a]

Age group (years)	<15	15–19	20–29	30–39	40–49	50–59	60–69	≥70	≥85
Joslin clinic patients, US, 1965 and 1975 (type 1 diabetes mellitus)[b]	17	17	15	—	—	—	—	—	—
Marks and Krall 1971[c, d]	17	16–17	12–14	10–11	8–9	6–7	4–5	—	—
Goodkin 1975[c, e]	27	23	16	11	10	6	5	—	—
Panzram and Zabel-Langhennig[c, e]	—	—	—	—	7–8	5–6	3–4	3	—
Knuiman et al. [54] (type 2 diabetes mellitus)[f]									
Males[d]	—	—	—	—	3.5[g]	3.1[g]	2.5[g]	1.9[h]	—
Females[d]	—	—	—	—	11.4[g]	7.4[g]	3.8[g]	2.9[h]	—
Gu et al. [4]	—	—	—	—	—	8	4	—	—
Morgan et al. [55][e, i, j]									
Males	—	—	24	16	11	6	4	3	2
Females	—	—	27	21	12	10	6	3	2
Roper et al. [5] (type 2 diabetes mellitus)[e, i]									
Males	—	—	—	—	8[g]	5[g]	3[g]	2[h]	—
Females	—	—	—	—	8[g]	7[g]	5[g]	3[h]	—

[a] Data source: [2–5, 40, 54, 55]. Comparison between studies is limited by different study populations, study design and methods.
[b] Data sourced from Portuese and Orchard [3].
[c] Data reproduced from Panzram [40].
[d] Data is based on attained age.
[e] Data is based on age of onset.
[f] Data reproduced from Geiss et al. [2].
[g] Data for mid-point of age range.
[h] Data for age 75 years.
[i] Data estimated from graphed data, and rounded to whole numbers.
[j] Age groups for Morgan et al. [55] differ from table categories, and are according to the following age groups (years): <35, 35–44, 45–54, 55–64, 65–74, 75–84, ≥85.

limitations (such as inadequate sample size), these divergent results could reflect different survival experiences among people with type 1 diabetes, according to country of residence, sex, age at diagnosis and disease duration.

Few studies have compared type 1 diabetes mortality in different countries. The Diabetes Epidemiology Research International (DERI) Mortality Study was established to investigate type 1 diabetes mortality patterns in Finland, Japan, Israel and the US. Patients diagnosed between 1965 and 1979 at age <18 years with insulin-requiring diabetes were included in the cohort and were followed up until 1 January 1985. This study revealed that Japan and the US had much higher age-specific all-cause mortality rates than did Finland and Israel [56]. In another study, Podar et al. [46] reported that, compared with Estonia and Lithuania, people with childhood-onset type 1 diabetes in Finland had much better 10-year survival. The World Health Organization Multinational Study of Vascular Disease in Diabetes also reported variations in intercountry mortality rates. Seven centers contributed data on type 1 diabetes mortality, and the SMRs for men ranged from 188 (95% confidence interval (CI) 133–294) in London to 685 (95% CI 406–1082) in Havana and for women ranged from 336 (95% CI 109–784) in Zagreb to 790 (95% CI 379–1453) in Havana [48] (**Figure 36.3**). These studies suggest that mortality rates vary substantially across countries, which may reflect differences in access to health care. Indeed, frequent contact with specialist diabetes health service providers has been shown to improve health outcomes for people with diabetes [57].

Men have higher absolute all-cause mortality rates than women, and this is true of both the diabetic and nondiabetic populations, and for type 1 and type 2 diabetes. However, when comparing men with type 1 diabetes to nondiabetic men, and women with type 1 diabetes with nondiabetic women, many studies [5, 19, 48, 51, 58], but not all [52, 53], report higher relative mortality risks for type 1 diabetes in women than in men. Overall, type 1 diabetes appears to diminish the protective effects of female sex observed in nondiabetic populations.

Several studies have shown that, for all age groups, all-cause mortality rates are consistently higher in those with type 1 diabetes than the rates observed in the general population. However, differences between the mortality rates observed in those with type 1 diabetes and those observed in the general population tend to diminish in the older age groups [51, 53, 58]. The age of onset may also influence mortality risk among those with type 1 diabetes. One study from Norway that investigated all-cause mortality from 1973 to 2002 in childhood-onset (<15 years) type 1 diabetes found that children diagnosed with diabetes prior to puberty had better survival than children diagnosed during puberty [52]. However, a Swedish study evaluating deaths over a similar time period (1977–2000) in those with type 1 diabetes aged <15 years did not find this. Instead, SMRs were highest in children aged ≤2 years (SMR = 4.66) and were lower in children aged 3–7 years (SMR = 2.00) and 8–15 years (SMR = 2.01) [51].

An early (1933–1972) evaluation of data from the Steno Memorial Hospital in Denmark revealed a 'bell-shaped' association between diabetes duration and mortality in patients diagnosed with type 1 diabetes aged <31 years. The risk of mortality peaked at 15–20 years duration [20]. However, this bell-shaped relationship was only observed in type 1 diabetic patients with proteinuria. Diabetic patients without proteinuria displayed a constant linear relationship between diabetes duration and mortality [59]. A population-based Swedish study on those with type 1 diabetes aged <15 years

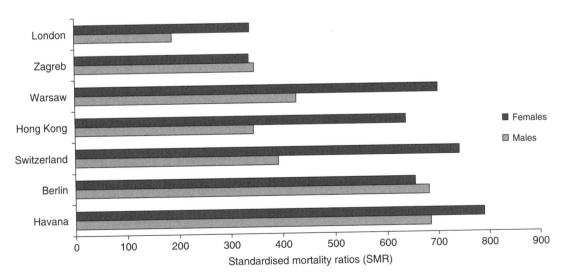

Figure 36.3 International variations in risk of all-cause mortality for people with type 1 diabetes, according to sex. SMR is the ratio of the number of deaths observed in the diabetic population to the number of deaths expected in the background population, multiplied by 100 (Adapted from Morrish et al. [48].)

also found that mortality rates peaked at 10–12 years' duration of diabetes [51]. In contrast, a Norwegian study that evaluated mortality among those with childhood-onset type 1 diabetes found that cumulative survival progressively reduced with increasing duration of diabetes [52]. Furthermore, a study from the UK did not find a strong relationship between diabetes duration and all-cause mortality independent of age, because age and duration were highly correlated [53]. Therefore, although the literature suggests that the excess mortality over the general population appears to decrease with ageing, there are conflicting findings on the relationships between age of onset and disease duration with risk of mortality in people with type 1 diabetes.

Few studies have compared the mortality rates of type 1 diabetes with type 2 diabetes. The World Health Organization Multinational Study of Vascular Disease in Diabetes, which collected mortality data on type 1 and type 2 diabetes from 10 centers throughout the world, found that SMRs tended to be higher for type 1 diabetes than for type 2 diabetes [48]. Similarly, a more recent UK study, based on mortality data collected between 1994 and 1999 from a population-based diabetes register, reported that, compared with type 2 diabetes, SMRs were higher for type 1 diabetes [5].

36.5.2 Causes of Death among Those with Type 1 Diabetes

The causes of death for people with type 1 diabetes differ according to age and duration of the disease. In general, metabolic disturbances account for a large proportion of deaths in younger people and among those who have had diabetes for a shorter time, whereas deaths in older people or people who have had type 1 diabetes for longer are more likely a result of renal disease or CVD [3, 52, 60]. Few studies have sought to investigate whether type 1 diabetes is associated with an increased risk of non-CVD mortality. To date, data from large population-based studies suggest that the risk of death from cancer is not significantly higher among people with type 1 diabetes than in the general population [50, 60, 61].

In childhood-onset type 1 diabetes, some studies have revealed that a large proportion of deaths in childhood could be due to neglected treatment of the disease. Edge *et al.* [45] found a high proportion

(~70%) of deaths among those with type 1 diabetes aged 10–19 years to be due to diabetic ketoacidosis, hypoglycemia or an unknown cause–found 'dead in bed'. Moreover, a Swedish study [51] also reported 'a very large proportion of unexplained deaths in bed' (p. 2384).

Several studies have shown that people with type 1 diabetes have a considerably increased risk of death from renal disease [3, 50, 60]. Compared to type 1 diabetic patients without nephropathy, those with nephropathy are more likely to die [62–64]. It appears that the mortality risk associated with renal disease is particularly elevated in the intermediate stages of type 1 diabetes (between 10 and 30 years' duration) [3]. Furthermore, elevated albumin excretion increases the risk of CVD mortality in people with type 1 diabetes [3, 65].

In many developed countries, improvements in health care have led to increased survival for people with type 1 diabetes. However, as people are living longer with the disease, their risk of CVD mortality has increased. Few large population-based studies have specifically evaluated CVD mortality in people with type 1 diabetes. However, a recent UK study based on general practice data reported mortality rates for over 7000 type 1 diabetic patients with mean disease duration of 15 years in comparison with age- and sex-matched control patients. This study found that the age- and sex-adjusted hazard ratios for fatal CVD were 5.8 (95% CI 3.9–8.6) for men and 11.6 (95% CI 6.7–20.1) for women. Furthermore, the 10-year fatal CVD risk for men and women with type 1 diabetes increased according to age, with significantly greater risk observed for people aged over 45 years. The authors note that there was no association between duration of disease and CVD mortality after accounting for age [66]. Similar patterns were found for coronary heart disease (CHD) mortality in the Diabetes UK Cohort, another large UK study of nearly 24 000 patients with insulin-treated diabetes who were diagnosed at <30 years in 1972–1993 and followed for 28 years. SMRs of ischemic heart disease were particularly high for young women, where SMRs were 44.8 (95% CI 20.5–85.0) and 41.6 (95% CI 26.7–61.9) for women aged 20–29 years and 30–39 years respectively [67]. One limitation of both these studies relates to inadequate risk factor evaluation. Neither study was able to account for the influence of other risk factors, such as hypertension or smoking, as details regarding these factors were not routinely entered into the databases. Hence, the relative mortality risks observed among the patients with type 1 diabetes may have been overestimated.

36.5.3 Modifiable Risk Factors in Type 1 Diabetes

Several risk factors for mortality in type 1 diabetes have been identified, and these include hyperglycemia, hypertension, microalbuminuria, cholesterol, smoking and other psychosocial characteristics [3]. However, apart from the Diabetes Control and Complications Trial (DCCT)/Epidemiology of Diabetes Interventions and Complications (EDIC) study on intensive glycemic therapy versus usual glycemic therapy, no large-scale intervention studies have been conducted to evaluate whether modifying these factors reduces the risk of mortality for people with type 1 diabetes. Even the DCCT/EDIC study was not sufficiently powered to evaluate the impact of intensive therapy on mortality alone.

36.5.4 Glycemic Control

Mortality data from the Steno Memorial Hospital in Denmark indicated that metabolic regulation was strongly associated with survival in type 1 diabetes (insulin-dependent diabetes diagnosed <31 years) [68]. The observational follow-up of the DCCT was able to investigate whether intensive glycemic control over 6.5 years affected the long-term incidence of CVD. Over 17 years, the cumulative incidence of nonfatal myocardial infarction, stroke or death from CVD was significantly less in the group initially randomized to intensive therapy than in the control group [69]. The improvement in glycemic control during the initial 6.5 years of intervention was strongly associated with the reduction in CVD, indicating that intensive glycemic control in people with type 1 diabetes has long-term effects on CVD outcomes, even if the same level of control is not maintained over a longer period of time [69].

36.5.5 Blood Pressure

Few studies have evaluated the mortality risk associated with hypertension in people with type 1 diabetes. Hypertension may increase the risk of death in people with type 1 diabetes, as it has been shown to be associated with other microvascular complications, such as nephropathy [65] and

retinopathy [70], which are independent risk factors for death [62, 64, 71–73]. However, some studies have reported that hypertension is associated with an increased risk of mortality independent of these complications. Klein *et al.* [72], using data from the Wisconsin Epidemiologic Study of Diabetic Retinopathy, reported that in people with type 1 diabetes (insulin-dependent diabetes diagnosed <30 years), high blood pressure was a risk factor for 6-year all-cause mortality, independent of age, glaucoma, smoking, diuretic use and the presence of proteinuria. In another cohort study of Danish hospital outpatients aged >18 years with type 1 diabetes (insulin-dependent diabetes diagnosed <40 years), hypertension was associated with a 60% increased risk for 10-year all-cause mortality and a twofold risk for CVD mortality, independent of age, sex, diabetes duration, microalbuminuria and other risk factors [65]. Similar findings were also reported for an African-American cohort of hospital patients with type 1 diabetes. Diastolic blood pressure remained independently associated with all-cause mortality after it was included in a multivariate model with age and other markers of microvascular disease [74].

36.5.6 Lipids

Some studies have shown that abnormal lipoprotein metabolism is associated with microalbuminuria [75–77] and the development of renal insufficiency [78] in people with type 1 diabetes. Because renal disease significantly increases the risk of mortality, abnormal lipoprotein metabolism may have a role in increasing this risk. However, few studies have evaluated whether abnormal lipoprotein metabolism is a risk factor for mortality in type 1 diabetes. A nested case-control analysis of data from the Epidemiology of Diabetes Complications Study showed that increased low-density lipoprotein (LDL)-cholesterol was associated with CVD, independent of nephropathy [79]. A more recent large cohort study that followed 3674 type 1 diabetic patients for 10 years found a weak independent association between elevated serum cholesterol and total mortality (hazard ratio 1.1, 95% CI 1.0–1.2), after adjusting for age, sex and other risk factors. However, it is difficult to generalize these findings to the wider type 1 diabetes population, as this study enrolled patients who underwent intensified insulin therapy [63]. In another study, which followed

147 patients with type 1 diabetes, characteristics of abnormal lipoprotein metabolism were found to be significantly associated with CVD morbidity or CVD death, but not associated with all-cause mortality. However, multivariate analyses that included diabetes duration and serum creatinine revealed that these factors were not independent predictors of CVD morbidity or CVD death [64].

36.5.7 Psychosocial Factors

Psychosocial factors such as education level [80–82], smoking [63, 65, 79, 83], social class [63, 65] and unemployment [82] have been implicated in increasing the risk of total mortality in people with type 1 diabetes. Furthermore, a recent nested case–control study by Laing *et al.* [84] investigated risk factors for mortality in younger onset (<15 years) type 1 diabetic patients according to (i) acute events, such as hypoglycemia, diabetic coma, accidents and violent death, and (ii) chronic events, such as renal disease and CVD. The study revealed that living alone, drug abuse and psychiatric referral were all significantly associated with death from acute events, but not death from chronic disease. In contrast, hypertension, retinopathy, renal disease and neuropathy were all significantly associated with chronic disease mortality, but not related to acute deaths.

36.6 TYPE 2 DIABETES AND MORTALITY

36.6.1 Excess Risk of Total Mortality among Those with Type 2 Diabetes

It is well established that type 2 diabetes is associated with an increased risk for all-cause mortality. Although most studies have not differentiated between type 1 and type 2 diabetes, one can assume that the findings reported by these studies predominately relate to type 2, as this accounts for approximately 90% of all cases of diabetes [85]. Geiss *et al.* [2] summarized the findings from cohort studies published between 1970 and 1993, and concluded that there was a twofold mortality risk for people with type 2 diabetes compared to those without diabetes, even after adjusting for the older age of people with diabetes. The findings from more recent studies support this estimate [4, 86–96]. A few studies on predominantly Asian populations

have reported a threefold relative risk of all-cause mortality for people with previously diagnosed diabetes compared to those people without diabetes [97–99], suggesting that the risk for all-cause mortality may be greater in these populations. However, the higher risk observed in these studies may have been influenced by inadequate sample size. Another study that conducted a meta-analysis on data from several Asian-Pacific studies found that there was no significant difference between Asian studies and Australian/New Zealand studies for risk of all-cause mortality [100]. Findings from the US NHANES 1 study revealed that, among those with diabetes, non-Hispanic Blacks had an age-adjusted mortality rate that was 27% higher than the rate observed for non-Hispanic Whites [4]. The differences in mortality risks between these different ethnic groups living in the US may reflect the overall poorer health experiences of non-Hispanic Blacks.

It is estimated that middle-aged people with type 2 diabetes experience a 5–10 year reduction in life expectancy [2, 4, 5, 40, 54, 55]. The findings from several studies indicate that the reduction in life expectancy associated with diabetes is greater in younger people than older people (**Table 36.1**) [2, 40, 55]. Mortality data from the US NHANES 1 study (1971–1993) suggested that median life expectancy was 8 years shorter for people with self-reported diabetes aged 55–64 years, and 4 years shorter for those aged 65–74 years [4]. Similarly, a UK study revealed that the reduction in life expectancy diminished with age, whereby life expectancy was reduced by 8 years in people diagnosed with type 2 diabetes at age 40 years, but was reduced by less than 2 years in people diagnosed at 80 years. These authors also found that, for people diagnosed with type 2 diabetes after 50 years of age, women showed significantly shorter life expectancy than men, but the differences according to sex reduced with increasing age at diagnosis [5] (**Figure 36.4**). This concurs with an earlier study by Knuiman *et al.* [54], which also reported that the reduction in life expectancy for women with type 2 diabetes was greater than that observed for men with type 2 diabetes. Moreover, for women, the reduction in life expectancy was greater at both younger age of disease onset and younger current age, whereas the reduction in life expectancy for males only varied according to current age, not according to the age of disease onset.

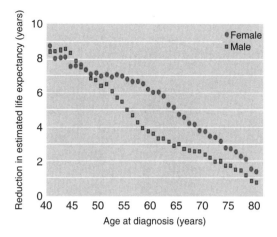

Figure 36.4 Reductions in estimated life expectancy according to age at diagnosis for those with type 2 diabetes compared with the South Tees UK general population. (Reproduced from Roper *et al*. [5] by permission of the BMJ Publishing Group Ltd.)

Several studies have also shown that the excess mortality risk observed in people with diabetes remains significant after controlling for the influence of other risk factors, such as hypertension, dyslipidemia and smoking [2, 86, 87, 89–95, 99]. This suggests that the coexistence of other known risk factors does not fully explain the increased mortality risk observed in people with diabetes. Other factors, either directly or indirectly associated with diabetes, must also be contributing to the unfavorable risk profile.

The excess risk attributable to diabetes varies according to age, sex, duration of disease and age at diagnosis. Many studies [2, 55, 87, 94, 101], but not all [4, 91, 102, 103], report that the excess risk for total mortality is greater for women than for men. Although several studies have reported that diabetes confers an excess risk for total mortality among older people, the risk tends to attenuate with increasing age [2, 4, 55, 94, 101, 102, 104, 105]. The smaller excess risk of mortality in older people with diabetes is due to the increasing risk of death among people without diabetes at these ages. It is important to point out that, although the relative risk for mortality in those with diabetes compared to those without diabetes generally decreases with age, the overall burden of mortality is still much greater among older people than

younger people because the prevalence of diabetes increases with age. Saydah *et al*. [94] illustrated this for the US population by showing that the population attributable risk, which takes the prevalence of diabetes into account, increased from 3.1% in those aged 30–49 years to 6.9% in those aged 65–74 years (**Figure 36.5**). Several studies have shown a positive relationship between increasing diabetes duration and risk of mortality [2, 4, 102, 104, 106]. The excess mortality risk associated with diabetes also increases with earlier age of diagnosis [2, 102, 104]. Interestingly, Barnett *et al*. [107] demonstrated in a meta-analysis of 14 studies published between 1974 and 2004 that there was no excess mortality risk associated with diabetes in people diagnosed at age 70 years or older. The increased risk of mortality in those who have had diabetes for longer is attributed to the longer exposure of chronic hyperglycemia and associated CVD risk factors.

36.6.2 Causes of Death among Those with Type 2 Diabetes

A significant proportion of the excess risk for death among those with type 2 diabetes is due to CVD. Geiss *et al*. [2] combined data from four US cohort studies published in the 1980s and found that there was substantial agreement between each of the studies on the leading causes of death listed on death certificates for those with type 2 diabetes. Ischemic heart disease (40%) was the most common, with the other leading causes of death being other heart disease, diabetes, malignant neoplasms, cerebrovascular disease and pneumonia/influenza (**Figure 36.6**). However, findings from The World Health Organization Multinational Study of Vascular Disease in Diabetics suggest that the mortality rate from circulatory diseases might vary substantially between different countries. For example, this study showed a preponderance of stroke rather than ischemic heart disease in diabetic patients from Hong Kong and Tokyo [108].

36.6.3 Cardiovascular Disease Mortality among Those with Type 2 Diabetes

Prospective cohort studies indicate that people with diabetes have a two- to four-fold risk for CVD mortality [2, 91, 94, 99, 109, 110]. Furthermore, the risk of in-hospital [111] and out-of-hospital

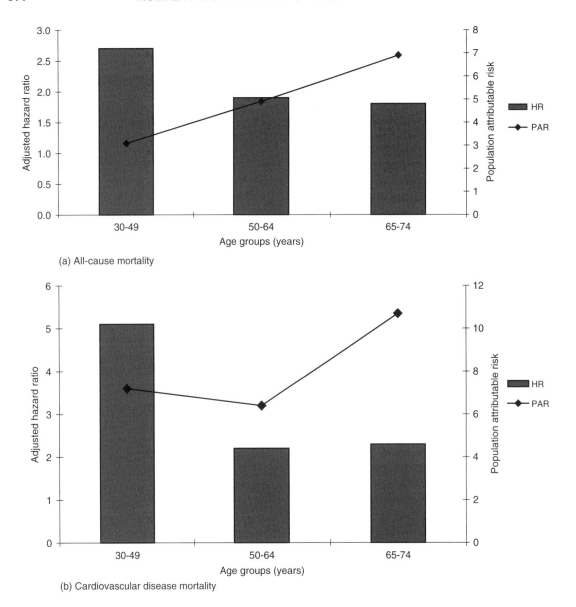

(a) All-cause mortality

(b) Cardiovascular disease mortality

Figure 36.5 The relative risk and population attributable risk of all-cause and cardiovascular disease mortality in people with diabetes, according to age (US NHANES II). (a) All-cause mortality. (b) Cardiovascular disease mortality. HR: hazard ratio adjusted for age, sex, education, smoking, physical activity, total cholesterol, body mass index, and systolic blood pressure; PAR: population attributable risk of diabetes for all-cause mortality. (Adapted from Saydah *et al.* [94].)

mortality [111–116] in people with diabetes who suffer myocardial infarction is significantly increased compared with nondiabetic patients. Some population-based studies have also indicated that there is a twofold risk of fatal cerebrovascular disease among those with diabetes compared with those without diabetes [2, 4, 100, 117]. The

excess risk of CVD mortality is higher than the risk observed for all-cause mortality and remains significant despite adjustment for age and other CVD risk factors [2, 91, 94, 99, 109, 110]. This suggests that physiological mechanisms associated with diabetes must play a role in the pathophysiology and development of CVD [118, 119].

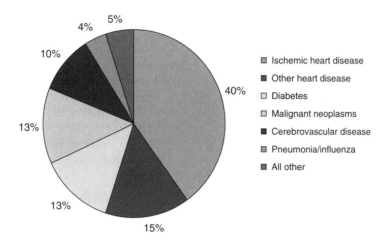

Figure 36.6 Causes of death in people with type 2 diabetes. (Adapted from Geiss *et al.* [2].)

Further evidence suggests that the risk of CVD mortality is already elevated prior to the diagnosis of diabetes. A retrospective analysis of the Nurses Health Study revealed that women who developed diabetes had a threefold risk for myocardial infarction prior to their diagnosis compared with women who did not develop diabetes [120]. Other studies have shown that the risk for CVD mortality is already elevated in those with newly diagnosed diabetes [2, 121] and among those with impaired glucose tolerance, a condition whereby blood glucose levels are above normal but not to the threshold to diagnose diabetes [122].

Most studies report that the relative risk of CVD mortality reduces for those who are older or diagnosed at an older age than those who are younger or diagnosed at a younger age [2]. Moreover, longer duration [2, 123, 124] and insulin use [2] (which may be a marker for more severe disease) have also been associated with excess risk of CVD mortality. Several studies [91, 94, 105, 114, 125–130], but not all [2], have found that the relative risk of CVD mortality is greater in women than in men, suggesting that the usual protective factors for CVD which are afforded by the female sex may be lost or diminished in those with diabetes.

These findings confirm that diabetes confers a greater risk for CVD mortality, in particular CHD death. However, there is still considerable uncertainty about how this diabetes-related risk compares with the risk associated with prior myocardial infarction. One of the first studies to investigate this used data from a Finnish population-based study

and found that, after adjusting for other risk factors, the risk of fatal CHD among men and women with diabetes and no prior myocardial infarction was not significantly different to the risk observed in those without diabetes who had prior myocardial infarction, suggesting that both conditions conferred the same risk for subsequent CHD mortality [131]. In a follow-up study, Juutilainen *et al.* [132] reported that the findings from the original cohort persisted during 18 years of follow-up. Some observational studies [124, 128, 133] have supported the results from the Finnish study, whereas others have not [123, 130, 134–136].

The discrepancies observed between these studies may have been attributable to a number of factors, including different cohort characteristics. The Nurses Health Study revealed that the risk of CVD mortality in women with diabetes increased according to the duration of the disease. In this study, women with diabetes without prior myocardial infarction who had a long duration of diabetes (≥20 years) demonstrated a similar risk for fatal CHD or CVD to nondiabetic women with prior myocardial infarction. However, the mortality risk associated with diabetes diminished and became substantially smaller than the nondiabetic group who had prior myocardial infarction, once women with both newly diagnosed diabetes and shorter duration diabetes were included in the diabetic group without prior myocardial infarction [123]. Furthermore, Howard *et al.* [130] found that the risk of CHD depended on an individual's risk factor profile. Diabetic American Indians with no previous

CHD who had few concurrent risk factors for CHD were less likely to experience a fatal or nonfatal CHD event. Therefore, diabetes does not necessarily pose the same risk for subsequent CHD that prior CHD does in the nondiabetic population, so it may be important to evaluate the entire risk factor profile of people with diabetes to assess the likelihood of future CHD events. Nevertheless, it should be highlighted that most diabetic patients do possess many other CVD risk factors, indicating that the vast majority of people with diabetes are in fact at high risk for CHD [137].

36.6.4 Noncardiovascular Mortality among Those with Type 2 Diabetes

It is more difficult to evaluate the associations between diabetes and non-CVD mortality, as these events do not occur as frequently as CVD fatal events. Hence, most population-based studies are not sufficiently large to capture enough data on noncardiovascular mortality to draw statistically meaningful conclusions. Cancer is the most common noncardiovascular event, and although some studies have shown that people with diabetes have a moderately increased risk of mortality from some types of cancer [138–145], other studies have found that the risk of cancer mortality in people with diabetes is not significantly different to the risk observed in the nondiabetic population [2, 117, 146–148]. These conflicting results may partly be due to differing study characteristics, inadequate sample size and incomplete adjustment for the influence of other confounding factors.

It is postulated that the relationship between diabetes and cancer mortality may be mediated by hyperinsulinemia and/or peripheral insulin resistance. One study revealed that having a postload blood glucose ≥ 11.1 mmol l^{-1} and normal fasting blood glucose significantly elevated the risk of cancer death in men [98]. Furthermore, it has been shown that even in people without diagnosed diabetes, elevated postload glycemia is a risk factor for cancer-related mortality [148–150]. In contrast, others have not found a positive relationship between asymptomatic postload glycemia and cancer mortality [151]. It has been suggested that diabetic medication that increases insulin activity could increase the risk of cancer-related mortality among those with diabetes, as the findings from a recent

study revealed that, compared with metformin, sulfonylureas or exogenous insulin increased the risk of death from cancer in people with type 2 diabetes. However, the authors also point out that this association between diabetes and cancer mortality could have been related to the potentially protective effects of metformin or may be due to other unknown confounders [152]. Therefore, at this stage, it is unclear as to whether people with type 2 diabetes are at increased risk for cancer-related mortality.

36.6.5 Modifiable Risk Factors in People with Type 2 Diabetes

Risk factors associated with diabetes-related CVD and mortality include hyperglycemia, hypertension, obesity, dyslipidemia and insulin resistance. People with diabetes often have more than one of these risk factors, suggesting that they may be physiologically related [119, 153]. The 'common soil' hypothesis proposes that there may be common genetic and environmental conditions that give rise to the development of these risk factors and, hence, CVD [154]. Some intervention studies have evaluated whether modification of these risk factors reduces the risk of CVD and mortality in people with diabetes. In addition to these physiological factors, the psychosocial environment can also influence the risk of mortality [155].

36.6.6 Glycemic Control

Diabetes is characterized by the abnormal regulation of glucose. Experimental studies suggest that hyperglycemia increases the risk of CVD by altering the normal mechanisms of vascular cell function [118]. As outlined throughout this chapter, epidemiological studies provide additional support that hyperglycemia plays a significant role in increasing the risk of CVD and mortality. The United Kingdom Prospective Diabetes Study (UKPDS) is the largest intervention study to investigate whether improved glycemic control reduces microvascular and macrovascular disease in patients with newly diagnosed type 2 diabetes. The outcomes of this study revealed that, although intensive glycemic control (median HbA_{1c} achieved was 7%) with either sulfonylureas or insulin significantly reduced the development of microvascular disease (relative risk 0.75, 95% CI 0.60–0.93), there was no significant reduction in either diabetes-related deaths (relative risk 0.90, 95% CI 0.73–1.11) or all-cause mortality (relative risk 0.94; 95% CI 0.80–1.10) [156]. The nonsignificant reduction in macrovascular disease could be a result of inadequate glucose control in the intervention group. Much greater reductions in glucose levels may be required to achieve macrovascular disease prevention. This would concur with the findings from observational studies that have shown that even moderately elevated blood glucose below the threshold to diagnose diabetes are associated with macrovascular disease [122].

36.6.7 Blood Pressure Control

The UKPDS also investigated whether tighter blood pressure control (<150/85 mmHg) with either captopril (an angiotensin-converting enzyme inhibitor) or atenolol (a β-blocker), compared with less tight control (<180/105 mmHg), would reduce the risk of CVD and mortality in people with type 2 diabetes. This study found that, compared with less tight blood pressure control (mean 154/87 mmHg), intensive blood pressure control (mean 144/82 mmHg) resulted in a significant 32% risk reduction (relative risk 0.68, 95% CI 0.49–0.94) for diabetes-related mortality and a nonsignificant 17% risk reduction (relative risk 0.82, 95% CI 0.63–1.08) in all-cause mortality [157]. The Heart Outcomes Prevention Evaluation (HOPE) study investigated the effects of another angiotensin-converting enzyme inhibitor, ramipril, to reduce CVD in 9297 people at high risk for CVD. This study included 3577 people with diabetes (98% had type 2 diabetes) who were aged ≥55 years, and analysis of this subgroup revealed that there was a 37% relative risk reduction (95% CI 21–51%) in CVD death and a 24% relative risk reduction (95% CI 8–37%) in total mortality in the ramipril group. Risk reduction for diabetes-related mortality and total mortality occurred despite there being no significant reduction in blood pressure control in the ramipril group (2.2 mmHg and 1.4 mmHg reductions for systolic and diastolic blood pressure respectively). The authors suggested that the benefits of ramipril may be related to its effects on improving endothelial function through its action on lowering angiotensin II [158]. Furthermore, the Hypertension Optimal Treatment (HOT) trial demonstrated that aggressive lowering of diastolic blood pressure significantly reduced the risk of CVD mortality. Compared

to people with a diastolic blood pressure treated to a target of ≤90 mmHg, people treated to a target of ≤85 mmHg had a significantly lower risk of CVD mortality, as did people treated to a target of ≤80 mmHg. There was no significant difference between these groups for total mortality [159]. These studies provide supportive evidence that antihypertensive therapy reduces the risk of mortality in both those with newly diagnosed type 2 diabetes and in those with type 2 diabetes who are at high risk for CVD.

36.6.8 Lipid Control

The benefits of statin therapy to lower LDL-cholesterol in people with type 2 diabetes who have varying risk for CVD has been demonstrated by a number of large clinical trials showing reductions in CVD with statins [160–162]. However, diabetes is often characterized by high triglycerides and low high-density lipoprotein, and although statin treatment can reduce the risk of CVD and mortality in people with type 2 diabetes by lowering LDL-cholesterol, statins have less impact on other abnormalities of lipid metabolism. Recently, the Fenofibrate Intervention and Event Lowering in Diabetes (FIELD) study sought to investigate the impact of fenofibrate on lowering CVD in 9795 people with and without prior CVD aged 55–75 years who had type 2 diabetes. However, there was a nonsignificant 19% (hazard ratio 1.19, 95% CI 0.90–1.57) increase in CHD mortality and a nonsignificant 11% (hazard ratio 1.11, 95% CI 0.95–1.29) increase in total mortality for the fenofibrate group compared with the control [163]. Therefore, although convincing trial data exist on the benefits of lowering LDL-cholesterol in people with type 2 diabetes to prevent CVD events and mortality, more research is required to investigate whether treatment of other forms of dyslipidemia has additional benefits on CVD prevention and survival.

These studies demonstrate that many of the risk factors for CVD and mortality in type 2 diabetes can be managed with various medications. The Steno-2 study demonstrated that interventions targeting several of these risk factors are beneficial in lowering CVD risk in middle-aged people (mean age 55.1 years) with newly diagnosed type 2 diabetes and microalbuminuria. This open-label randomized parallel trial found that a combination of intensified therapies which incorporated a reduction in dietary fat intake, an increase in exercise, smoking cessation, aspirin use and medications to lower blood pressure, lipids and blood glucose were able to achieve a 50% reduction (hazard ratio 0.47, 95% CI 0.24–0.73) in nonfatal and fatal CVD over 8 years [164].

36.7 CONCLUSIONS

During the last 100 years there has been a dramatic reduction in mortality from diabetes, largely due to the introduction of insulin. However, compared to those without diabetes, people with both type 1 and type 2 diabetes still experience an excess risk of both CVD mortality and total mortality. Recent clinical interventions have shown that risk factor modification can effectively reduce the threat of CVD and mortality, especially in type 2 diabetes. However, further progress in the management of diabetes is required to improve the life expectancy of people with this disease.

References

1. Roglic, G., Unwin, N., Bennett, P.H. *et al.* (2005) The burden of mortality attributable to diabetes: realistic estimates for the year 2000. *Diabetes Care*, **28**, 2130–5.

2. Geiss, L.S., Herman, W.H. and Smith, P.J. (1995) Mortality in non-insulin-dependent diabetes, in *Diabetes in America*, NIH Publication 95–1468, National Diabetes Data Group, National Institutes of Health, Bethesda, MD, pp. 233–57.

3. Portuese, E. and Orchard, T. (1995) Mortality in insulin-dependent diabetes, in *Diabetes in America*, NIH Publication 95–1468, National Diabetes Data Group, National Institutes of Health, Bethesda, MD, pp. 221–32.

4. Gu, K., Cowie, C.C. and Harris, M.I. (1998) Mortality in adults with and without diabetes in a national cohort of the U.S. population, 1971–1993. *Diabetes Care*, **21**, 1138–45.

5. Roper, N.A., Bilous, R.W., Kelly, W.F. *et al.* (2001) Excess mortality in a population with diabetes and the impact of material deprivation: longitudinal, population based study. *British Medical Journal*, **322**, 1389–93.

6. West, K.M. (1978) *Epidemiology of Diabetes and its Vascular Lesions*, Elsevier Press, New York.

7. Thomas, R.J., Palumbo, P.J., Melton, L.J. III. *et al.* (2003) Trends in the mortality burden associated with diabetes mellitus: a population-based study in Rochester, Minn, 1970–1994. *Archives of Internal Medicine*, **163**, 445–51.

8. Whittall, D.E., Glatthaar, C., Knuiman, M.W. and Welborn, T.A. (1990) Deaths from diabetes are under-reported in national mortality statistics. *The Medical Journal of Australia*, **152**, 598–600.

9. Will, J.C., Vinicor, F. and Stevenson, J. (2001) Recording of diabetes on death certificates. Has it improved? *Journal of Clinical Epidemiology*, **54**, 239–44.

10. Thomason, M.J., Biddulph, J.P., Cull, C.A. and Holman, R.R. (2005) Reporting of diabetes on death certificates using data from the UK Prospective Diabetes Study. *Diabetic Medicine*, **22**, 1031–6.

11. McEwen, L.N., Kim, C., Haan, M. *et al.* (2006) Diabetes reporting as a cause of death: results from the Translating Research Into Action for Diabetes (TRIAD) study. *Diabetes Care*, **29**, 247–53.

12. Messite, J. and Stellman, S.D. (1996) Accuracy of death certificate completion: the need for formalized physician training. *The Journal of the American Medical Association*, **275**, 794–6.

13. Lu, T.H., Walker, S., Johansson, L.A. and Huang, C.N. (2005) An international comparison study indicated physicians' habits in reporting diabetes in part I of death certificate affected reported national diabetes mortality. *Journal of Clinical Epidemiology*, **58**, 1150–7.

14. Jougla, E., Papoz, L., Balkau, B. *et al.* (1992) Death certificate coding practices related to diabetes in European countries–the 'EURODIAB Subarea C' Study. *International Journal of Epidemiology*, **21**, 343–51.

15. Goldacre, M.J., Duncan, M.E., Cook-Mozaffari, P. and Neil, H.A. (2004) Trends in mortality rates for death-certificate-coded diabetes mellitus in an English population 1979–1999. *Diabetic Medicine*, **21**, 936–9.

16. White, P. (1932) *Diabetes in Childhood and Adolescence*, Lea & Febiger, Philadelphia, PA.

17. Entmacher, P.S., Root, H.F. and Marks, H.H. (1964) Longevity of diabetic patients in recent years. *Diabetes*, **13**, 373–7.

18. Pambianco, G., Costacou, T., Ellis, D. *et al.* (2006) The 30-year natural history of type 1 diabetes complications: the Pittsburgh Epidemiology of Diabetes Complications Study Experience. *Diabetes*, **55**, 1463–9.

19. Nishimura, R., LaPorte, R.E., Dorman, J.S. *et al.* (2001) Mortality trends in type 1 diabetes. The Allegheny County (Pennsylvania) Registry 1965–1999. *Diabetes Care*, **24**, 823–7.

20. Borch-Johnsen, K., Kreiner, S. and Deckert, T. (1986) Mortality of type 1 (insulin-dependent)

diabetes mellitus in Denmark: a study of relative mortality in 2930 Danish type 1 diabetic patients diagnosed from 1933 to 1972. *Diabetologia*, **29**, 767–72.

21. Bi, P., Parton, K.A. and Donald, K. (2005) Secular trends in mortality rates for diabetes in Australia, 1907–1998. *Diabetes Research and Clinical Practice*, **70**, 270–7.

22. Marble, A. (1972) Insulin–clinical aspects: the first fifty years. *Diabetes*, **21** (Suppl 2), 632–6.

23. Alberti, K.G. (1994) Insulin dependent diabetes mellitus: a lethal disease in the developing world. *British Medical Journal*, **309**, 754–5.

24. McLarty, D.G., Kinabo, L. and Swai, A.B. (1990) Diabetes in tropical Africa: a prospective study, 1981–1987. II. Course and prognosis. *British Medical Journal*, **300**, 1107–10.

25. Barquera, S., Tovar-Guzman, V., Campos-Nonato, I. *et al.* (2003) Geography of diabetes mellitus mortality in Mexico: an epidemiologic transition analysis. *Archives of Medical Research*, **34**, 407–14.

26. Hu, J., Robbins, G., Ugnat, A.M. and Waters, C. (2005) Trends in mortality from diabetes mellitus in Canada, 1986–2000. *Chronic Diseases in Canada*, **26**, 25–9.

27. Choi, Y.J., Cho, Y.M., Park, C.K. *et al.* (2006) Rapidly increasing diabetes-related mortality with socio-environmental changes in South Korea during the last two decades. *Diabetes Research and Clinical Practice*, **74** (3), 295–300.

28. Thomas, D.P., Condon, J.R., Anderson, I.P. *et al.* (2006) Long-term trends in indigenous deaths from chronic diseases in the Northern Territory: a foot on the brake, a foot on the accelerator. *The Medical Journal of Australia*, **185**, 145–9.

29. Støvring, H., Andersen, M., Beck-Nielsen, H. *et al.* (2003) Rising prevalence of diabetes: evidence from a Danish pharmaco-epidemiological database. *Lancet*, **362**, 537–8.

30. McBean, A.M., Li, S., Gilbertson, D.T. and Collins, A.J. (2004) Differences in diabetes prevalence, incidence, and mortality among the elderly of four racial/ethnic groups: Whites, Blacks, Hispanics, and Asians. *Diabetes Care*, **27**, 2317–24.

31. Leibson, C.L., O'Brien, P.C., Atkinson, E. III. *et al.* (1997) Relative contributions of incidence and survival to increasing prevalence of adult-onset diabetes mellitus: a population-based study. *American Journal of Epidemiology*, **146**, 12–22.

32. Critchley, J., Liu, J., Zhao, D. *et al.* (2004) Explaining the increase in coronary heart disease mortality in Beijing between 1984 and 1999. *Circulation*, **110**, 1236–44.

33. Unal, B., Critchley, J.A. and Capewell, S. (2004) Explaining the decline in coronary heart disease mortality in England and Wales between 1981 and 2000. *Circulation*, **109**, 1101–7.

34. Bennett, K., Kabir, Z., Unal, B. *et al.* (2006) Explaining the recent decrease in coronary heart disease mortality rates in Ireland, 1985–2000. *Journal of Epidemiology and Community Health*, **60**, 322–7.

35. Gu, K., Cowie, C.C. and Harris, M.I. (1999) Diabetes and decline in heart disease mortality in US adults. *The Journal of the American Medical Association*, **281**, 1291–7.

36. Hoehner, C.M., Williams, D.E., Sievers, M.L. *et al.* (2006) Trends in heart disease death rates in diabetic and nondiabetic Pima Indians. *Journal of Diabetes and its Complications*, **20**, 8–13.

37. Fox, C.S., Coady, S., Sorlie, P.D. *et al.* (2004) Trends in cardiovascular complications of diabetes. *The Journal of the American Medical Association*, **292**, 2495–9.

38. Leibson, C.L. and Narayan, K.M. (2006) Trends in cardiovascular complications of diabetes (letter). *The Journal of the American Medical Association*, **293**, 1723–4.

39. Booth, G.L., Kapral, M.K., Fung, K. and Tu, J.V. (2006) Recent trends in cardiovascular complications among men and women with and without diabetes. *Diabetes Care*, **29**, 32–7.

40. Panzram, G. (1987) Mortality and survival in type 2 (non-insulin-dependent) diabetes mellitus. *Diabetologia*, **30**, 123–31.

41. Panzram, G. (1984) Epidemiologic data on excess mortality and life expectancy in insulin-dependent diabetes mellitus–critical review. *Experimental and Clinical Endocrinology*, **83**, 93–100.

42. Riley, M.D., McCarty, D.J., Couper, D.J. *et al.* (1995) The 1984 Tasmanian insulin treated diabetes mellitus prevalence cohort: an eight and a half year mortality follow-up investigation. *Diabetes Research and Clinical Practice*, **29**, 27–35.

43. Swerdlow, A.J. and Jones, M.E. (1996) Mortality during 25 years of follow-up of a cohort with diabetes. *International Journal of Epidemiology*, **25**, 1250–61.

44. Warner, D.P., McKinney, P.A., Law, G.R. and Bodansky, H.J. (1998) Mortality and diabetes from a population based register in Yorkshire 1978–1993. *Archives of Disease in Childhood*, **78**, 435–8.

45. Edge, J.A., Ford-Adams, M.E. and Dunger, D.B. (1999) Causes of death in children with insulin

dependent diabetes 1990–1996. *Archives of Disease in Childhood*, **81**, 318–23.

46. Podar, T., Solntsev, A., Reunanen, A. *et al.* (2000) Mortality in patients with childhood-onset type 1 diabetes in Finland, Estonia, and Lithuania: follow-up of nationwide cohorts. *Diabetes Care*, **23**, 290–4.

47. Laron-Kenet, T., Shamis, I., Weitzman, S. *et al.* (2001) Mortality of patients with childhood onset (0–17 years) type I diabetes in Israel: a population-based study. *Diabetologia*, **44** (Suppl 3), B81–6.

48. Morrish, N.J., Wang, S.L., Stevens, L.K. *et al.* (2001) Mortality and causes of death in the WHO Multinational Study of Vascular Disease in Diabetes. *Diabetologia*, **44** (Suppl 2), S14–21.

49. Wibell, L., Nystrom, L., Ostman, J. *et al.* (2001) Increased mortality in diabetes during the first 10 years of the disease. A population-based study (DISS) in Swedish adults 15–34 years old at diagnosis. *Journal of Internal Medicine*, **249**, 263–70.

50. Florkowski, C.M., Scott, R.S., Graham, P.J. *et al.* (2003) Cause-specific and total mortality in the Canterbury (New Zealand) insulin-treated Diabetic Registry population: a 15-year follow-up study. *Diabetic Medicine*, **20**, 191–7.

51. Dahlquist, G. and Kallen, B. (2005) Mortality in childhood-onset type 1 diabetes: a population-based study. *Diabetes Care*, **28**, 2384–7.

52. Skrivarhaug, T., Bangstad, H.J., Stene, L.C. *et al.* (2006) Long-term mortality in a nationwide cohort of childhood-onset type 1 diabetic patients in Norway. *Diabetologia*, **49**, 298–305.

53. Soedamah-Muthu, S.S., Fuller, J.H., Mulnier, H.E. *et al.* (2006) All-cause mortality rates in patients with type 1 diabetes mellitus compared with a non-diabetic population from the UK general practice research database, 1992–1999. *Diabetologia*, **49**, 660–6.

54. Knuiman, M.W., Welborn, T.A. and Whittall, D.E. (1992) An analysis of excess mortality rates for persons with non-insulin-dependent diabetes mellitus in Western Australia using the Cox proportional hazards regression model. *American Journal of Epidemiology*, **135**, 638–48.

55. Morgan, C.L., Currie, C.J. and Peters, J.R. (2000) Relationship between diabetes and mortality: a population study using record linkage. *Diabetes Care*, **23**, 1103–7.

56. Diabetes Epidemiology Research International Mortality Study Group (1991) Major cross-country differences in risk of dying for people with IDDM. *Diabetes Care*, **14**, 49–54.

57. Nicolucci, A., Cavaliere, D., Scorpiglione, N. *et al.* (1996) A comprehensive assessment of the avoidability of long-term complications of diabetes. A case–control study. SID-AMD Italian Study Group for the Implementation of the St. Vincent Declaration. *Diabetes Care*, **19**, 927–33.

58. Laing, S.P., Swerdlow, A.J., Slater, S.D. *et al.* (1999) The British Diabetic Association Cohort Study, I: all-cause mortality in patients with insulin-treated diabetes mellitus. *Diabetic Medicine*, **16**, 459–65.

59. Borch-Johnsen, K., Andersen, P.K. and Deckert, T. (1985) The effect of proteinuria on relative mortality in type 1 (insulin-dependent) diabetes mellitus. *Diabetologia*, **28**, 590–6.

60. Laing, S.P., Swerdlow, A.J., Slater, S.D. *et al.* (1999) The British Diabetic Association Cohort Study, II: cause-specific mortality in patients with insulin-treated diabetes mellitus. *Diabetic Medicine*, **16**, 466–71.

61. Green, A. and Jensen, O.M. (1985) Frequency of cancer among insulin-treated diabetic patients in Denmark. *Diabetologia*, **28**, 128–30.

62. Stephenson, J.M., Kenny, S., Stevens, L.K. *et al.* (1995) Proteinuria and mortality in diabetes: the WHO Multinational Study of Vascular Disease in Diabetes. *Diabetic Medicine*, **12**, 149–55.

63. Muhlhauser, I., Overmann, H., Bender, R. *et al.* (2000) Predictors of mortality and end-stage diabetic complications in patients with type 1 diabetes mellitus on intensified insulin therapy. *Diabetic Medicine*, **17**, 727–34.

64. Weis, U., Turner, B., Gibney, J. *et al.* (2001) Long-term predictors of coronary artery disease and mortality in type 1 diabetes. *QJM Monthly Journal of the Association of Physicians*, **94**, 623–30.

65. Rossing, P., Hougaard, P., Borch-Johnsen, K. and Parving, H.H. (1996) Predictors of mortality in insulin dependent diabetes: 10 year observational follow up study. *British Medical Journal*, **313**, 779–84.

66. Soedamah-Muthu, S.S., Fuller, J.H., Mulnier, H.E. *et al.* (2006) High risk of cardiovascular disease in patients with type 1 diabetes in the U.K.: a cohort study using the general practice research database. *Diabetes Care*, **29**, 798–804.

67. Laing, S.P., Swerdlow, A.J., Slater, S.D. *et al.* (2003) Mortality from heart disease in a cohort of 23,000 patients with insulin-treated diabetes. *Diabetologia*, **46**, 760–5.

68. Borch-Johnsen, K., Nissen, H., Salling, N. *et al.* (1987) The natural history of insulin-dependent diabetes in Denmark: 2. Long-term survival–who and why. *Diabetic Medicine*, **4**, 211–16.

69. Nathan, D.M., Cleary, P.A., Backlund, J.Y. *et al.* (2005) Intensive diabetes treatment and cardiovascular disease in patients with type 1 diabetes. *The New England Journal of Medicine*, **353**, 2643–53.

70. Klein, B.E., Klein, R., Moss, S.E. and Palta, M. (1995) A cohort study of the relationship of diabetic retinopathy to blood pressure. *Archives of Ophthalmology*, **113**, 601–6.

71. Borch-Johnsen, K. and Kreiner, S. (1987) Proteinuria: value as predictor of cardiovascular mortality in insulin dependent diabetes mellitus. *British Medical Journal*, **294**, 1651–4.

72. Klein, R., Moss, S.E., Klein, B.E. and DeMets, D.L. (1989) Relation of ocular and systemic factors to survival in diabetes. *Archives of Internal Medicine*, **149**, 266–72.

73. Van Hecke, M.V., Dekker, J.M., Stehouwer, C.D. *et al.* (2005) Diabetic retinopathy is associated with mortality and cardiovascular disease incidence: the EURODIAB Prospective Complications Study. *Diabetes Care*, **28**, 1383–89.

74. Roy, M., Rendas-Baum, R. and Skurnick, J. (2006) Mortality in African-Americans with type 1 diabetes: The New Jersey 725. *Diabetic Medicine*, **23**, 698–706.

75. Jensen, T., Stender, S. and Deckert, T. (1988) Abnormalities in plasmas concentrations of lipoproteins and fibrinogen in type 1 (insulin-dependent) diabetic patients with increased urinary albumin excretion. *Diabetologia*, **31**, 142–5.

76. Dullaart, R.P., Dikkeschei, L.D. and Doorenbos, H. (1989) Alterations in serum lipids and apolipoproteins in male type 1 (insulin-dependent) diabetic patients with microalbuminuria. *Diabetologia*, **32**, 685–9.

77. Kapelrud, H., Bangstad, H.J., Dahl-Jorgensen, K. *et al.* (1991) Serum Lp(a) lipoprotein concentrations in insulin dependent diabetic patients with microalbuminuria. *British Medical Journal*, **303**, 675–8.

78. Klein, R., Klein, B.E., Moss, S.E. *et al.* (1999) The 10-year incidence of renal insufficiency in people with type 1 diabetes. *Diabetes Care*, **22**, 743–51.

79. Portuese, E.I., Kuller, L., Becker, D. *et al.* (1995) High mortality from unidentified CVD in IDDM: time to start screening? *Diabetes Research and Clinical Practice*, **30**, 223–31.

80. Dorman, J.S., Tajima, N., LaPorte, R.E. *et al.* (1985) The Pittsburgh Insulin-Dependent Diabetes Mellitus (IDDM) Morbidity and Mortality Study: case-control analyses of risk factors for mortality. *Diabetes Care*, **8** (Suppl 1), 54–60.

81. Matsushima, M., Shimizu, K., Maruyama, M. *et al.* (1996) Socioeconomic and behavioural risk factors for mortality of individuals with IDDM in Japan: population-based case-control study. Diabetes Epidemiology Research International (DERI) US–Japan Mortality Study Group. *Diabetologia*, **39**, 710–16.

82. Robinson, N., Lloyd, C.E. and Stevens, L.K. (1998) Social deprivation and mortality in adults with diabetes mellitus. *Diabetic Medicine*, **15**, 205–12.

83. Moy, C.S., LaPorte, R.E., Dorman, J.S. *et al.* (1990) Insulin-dependent diabetes mellitus mortality. The risk of cigarette smoking. *Circulation*, **82**, 37–43.

84. Laing, S.P., Jones, M.E., Swerdlow, A.J. *et al.* (2005) Psychosocial and socioeconomic risk factors for premature death in young people with type 1 diabetes. *Diabetes Care*, **28**, 1618–23.

85. Gan, D. (ed) (2003) *Diabetes Atlas*, 2nd edn, International Diabetes Federation, Brussels.

86. Lowe, L.P., Liu, K., Greenland, P. *et al.* (1997) Diabetes, asymptomatic hyperglycemia, and 22-year mortality in black and white men. The Chicago Heart Association Detection Project in Industry Study. *Diabetes Care*, **20**, 163–9.

87. Wei, M., Gaskill, S.P., Haffner, S.M. and Stern, M.P. (1998) Effects of diabetes and level of glycemia on all-cause and cardiovascular mortality. The San Antonio Heart Study. *Diabetes Care*, **21**, 1167–72.

88. The DECODE study group on behalf of the European Diabetes Epidemiology Group (1999) Glucose tolerance and mortality: comparison of WHO and American Diabetes Association diagnostic criteria. The DECODE study group. European Diabetes Epidemiology Group. Diabetes Epidemiology: Collaborative analysis Of Diagnostic criteria in Europe. *Lancet*, **354**, 617–21.

89. Rodriguez, B.L., Lau, N., Burchfiel, C.M. *et al.* (1999) Glucose intolerance and 23-year risk of coronary heart disease and total mortality: the Honolulu Heart Program. *Diabetes Care*, **22**, 1262–5.

90. Gillum, R.F., Mussolino, M.E. and Madans, J.H. (2000) Diabetes mellitus, coronary heart disease incidence, and death from all causes in African American and European American women: the NHANES I epidemiologic follow-up study. *Journal of Clinical Epidemiology*, **53**, 511–18.

91. The DECODE study group on behalf of the European Diabetes Epidemiology Group (2001) Glucose tolerance and cardiovascular mortality: comparison of fasting and 2-hour diagnostic criteria. *Archives of Internal Medicine*, **161**, 397–405.

92. Khaw, K.T., Wareham, N., Luben, R. *et al.* (2001) Glycated haemoglobin, diabetes, and mortality in men in Norfolk cohort of European Prospective Investigation of Cancer and Nutrition (EPIC-Norfolk). *British Medical Journal*, **322**, 15–18.

93. Saydah, S.H., Loria, C.M., Eberhardt, M.S. and Brancati, F.L. (2001) Subclinical states of glucose intolerance and risk of death in the U.S. *Diabetes Care*, **24**, 447–53.

94. Saydah, S.H., Eberhardt, M.S., Loria, C.M. and Brancati, F.L. (2002) Age and the burden of death attributable to diabetes in the United States. *American Journal of Epidemiology*, **156**, 714–19.

95. Simons, L.A., Simons, J., McCallum, J. and Friedlander, Y. (2005) Impact of smoking, diabetes and hypertension on survival time in the elderly: the Dubbo Study. *The Medical Journal of Australia*, **182**, 219–22.

96. Meisinger, C., Wolke, G., Brasche, S. *et al.* (2006) Postload plasma glucose and 30-year mortality among nondiabetic middle-aged men from the general population: the ERFORT Study. *Annals of Epidemiology*, **16**, 534–9.

97. Collins, V.R., Dowse, G.K., Ram, P. *et al.* (1996) Non-insulin-dependent diabetes and 11-year mortality in Asian Indian and Melanesian Fijians. *Diabetic Medicine*, **13**, 125–32.

98. Shaw, J.E., Hodge, A.M., de Courten, M. *et al.* (1999) Isolated post-challenge hyperglycaemia confirmed as a risk factor for mortality. *Diabetologia*, **42**, 1050–4.

99. Nakagami, T. (2004) Hyperglycaemia and mortality from all causes and from cardiovascular disease in five populations of Asian origin. *Diabetologia*, **47**, 385–94.

100. Woodward, M., Zhang, X., Barzi, F. *et al.* (2003) The effects of diabetes on the risks of major cardiovascular diseases and death in the Asia-Pacific region. *Diabetes Care*, **26**, 360–6.

101. Bertoni, A.G., Krop, J.S., Anderson, G.F. and Brancati, F.L. (2002) Diabetes-related morbidity and mortality in a national sample of U.S. elders. *Diabetes Care*, **25**, 471–5.

102. Muggeo, M., Verlato, G., Bonora, E. *et al.* (1995) The Verona Diabetes Study: a population-based survey on known diabetes mellitus prevalence and 5-year all-cause mortality. *Diabetologia*, **38**, 318–25.

103. The DECODE Study Group on behalf of the European Diabetes Epidemiology Group (1999) Consequences of the new diagnostic criteria for diabetes in older men and women. DECODE Study (Diabetes Epidemiology: Collaborative Analysis Of Diagnostic criteria in Europe). *Diabetes Care*, **22**, 1667–71.

104. Berger, B., Stenstrom, G. and Sundkvist, G. (1999) Incidence, prevalence, and mortality of diabetes in a large population. A report from the Skaraborg Diabetes Registry. *Diabetes Care*, **22**, 773–8.

105. Roper, N.A., Bilous, R.W., Kelly, W.F. *et al.* (2002) Cause-specific mortality in a population with diabetes: South Tees Diabetes Mortality Study. *Diabetes Care*, **25**, 43–8.

106. Spijkerman, A.M., Dekker, J.M., Nijpels, G. *et al.* (2002) Impact of diabetes duration and cardiovascular risk factors on mortality in type 2 diabetes: the Hoorn Study. *European Journal of Clinical Investigation*, **32**, 924–30.

107. Barnett, K.N., McMurdo, M.E., Ogston, S.A. *et al.* (2006) Mortality in people diagnosed with type 2 diabetes at an older age: a systematic review. *Age and Ageing*, **35**, 463–8.

108. Head, J. and Fuller, J.H. (1990) International variations in mortality among diabetic patients: the WHO Multinational Study of Vascular Disease in Diabetics. *Diabetologia*, **33**, 477–81.

109. Stamler, J., Vaccaro, O., Neaton, J.D. and Wentworth, D. (1993) Diabetes, other risk factors, and 12-yr cardiovascular mortality for men screened in the Multiple Risk Factor Intervention Trial. *Diabetes Care*, **16**, 434–44.

110. Knuiman, M.W., Vu, H.T. and Bartholomew, H.C. (1998) Multivariate risk estimation for coronary heart disease: the Busselton Health Study. *Australian and New Zealand Journal of Public Health*, **22**, 747–53.

111. Miettinen, H., Lehto, S., Salomaa, V. *et al.* (1998) Impact of diabetes on mortality after the first myocardial infarction. The FINMONICA Myocardial Infarction Register Study Group. *Diabetes Care*, **21**, 69–75.

112. Sprafka, J.M., Burke, G.L., Folsom, A.R. *et al.* (1991) Trends in prevalence of diabetes mellitus in patients with myocardial infarction and effect of diabetes on survival. The Minnesota Heart Survey. *Diabetes Care*, **14**, 537–43.

113. Behar, S., Boyko, V., Reicher-Reiss, H. and Goldbourt, U. (1997) Ten-year survival after acute myocardial infarction: comparison of patients with and without diabetes. SPRINT Study Group. Secondary Prevention Reinfarction Israeli Nifedipine Trial. *American Heart Journal*, **133**, 290–6.

114. Benderly, M., Behar, S., Reicher-Reiss, H. *et al.* (1997) Long-term prognosis of women after myocardial infarction. SPRINT Study Group. Secondary Prevention Reinfarction Israeli Nifedipine Trial. *American Journal of Epidemiology*, **146**, 153–60.

115. Chun, B.Y., Dobson, A.J. and Heller, R.F. (1997) The impact of diabetes on survival among patients with first myocardial infarction. *Diabetes Care*, **20**, 704–8.

116. Gandhi, G.Y., Roger, V.L., Bailey, K.R. *et al.* (2006) Temporal trends in prevalence of diabetes mellitus in a population-based cohort of incident myocardial infarction and impact of diabetes on survival. *Mayo Clinic Proceedings*, **81**, 1034–40.

117. De Marco, R., Locatelli, F., Zoppini, G. *et al.* (1999) Cause-specific mortality in type 2 diabetes. The Verona Diabetes Study. *Diabetes Care*, **22**, 756–61.

118. King, G.L. and Wakasaki, H. (1999) Theoretical mechanisms by which hyperglycemia and insulin resistance could cause cardiovascular diseases in diabetes. *Diabetes Care*, **22** (Suppl 3), C31–7.

119. Tuomilehto, J., Rastenyte, D., Qiao, Q. and Jakovljevic, D. (2004) Epidemiology of macrovascular disease and hypertension in diabetes mellitus, in *International Textbook of Diabetes Mellitus*, 3rd edn, John Wiley & Sons, Ltd, Chichester, pp. 1345–70.

120. Hu, F.B., Stampfer, M.J., Haffner, S.M. *et al.* (2002) Elevated risk of cardiovascular disease prior to clinical diagnosis of type 2 diabetes. *Diabetes Care*, **25**, 1129–34.

121. Smith, N.L., Barzilay, J.I., Kronmal, R. *et al.* (2006) New-onset diabetes and risk of all-cause and cardiovascular mortality: the Cardiovascular Health Study. *Diabetes Care*, **29**, 2012–17.

122. Unwin, N., Shaw, J., Zimmet, P. and Alberti, K.G. (2002) Impaired glucose tolerance and impaired fasting glycaemia: the current status on definition and intervention. *Diabetic Medicine*, **19**, 708–23.

123. Hu, F.B., Stampfer, M.J., Solomon, C.G. *et al.* (2001) The impact of diabetes mellitus on mortality from all causes and coronary heart disease in women: 20 years of follow-up. *Archives of Internal Medicine*, **161**, 1717–23.

124. Cho, E., Rimm, E.B., Stampfer, M.J. *et al.* (2002) The impact of diabetes mellitus and prior myocardial infarction on mortality from all causes and from coronary heart disease in men. *Journal of the American College of Cardiology*, **40**, 954–60.

125. Barrett-Connor, E.L., Cohn, B.A., Wingard, D.L. and Edelstein, S.L. (1991) Why is diabetes mellitus a stronger risk factor for fatal ischemic heart disease in women than in men? The Rancho Bernardo Study. *The Journal of the American Medical Association*, **265**, 627–31.

126. Folsom, A.R., Szklo, M., Stevens, J. *et al.* (1997) A prospective study of coronary heart disease in relation to fasting insulin, glucose, and diabetes. The Atherosclerosis Risk in Communities (ARIC) Study. *Diabetes Care*, **20**, 935–42.

127. Lee, W.L., Cheung, A.M., Cape, D. and Zinman, B. (2000) Impact of diabetes on coronary artery disease in women and men: a meta-analysis of prospective studies. *Diabetes Care*, **23**, 962–8.

128. Malmberg, K., Yusuf, S., Gerstein, H.C. *et al.* (2000) Impact of diabetes on long-term prognosis in patients with unstable angina and non-Q-wave myocardial infarction: results of the OASIS (Organization to Assess Strategies for Ischemic Syndromes) Registry. *Circulation*, **102**, 1014–19.

129. Juutilainen, A., Kortelainen, S., Lehto, S. *et al.* (2004) Gender difference in the impact of type 2 diabetes on coronary heart disease risk. *Diabetes Care*, **27**, 2898–904.

130. Howard, B.V., Best, L.G., Galloway, J.M. *et al.* (2006) Coronary heart disease risk equivalence in diabetes depends on concomitant risk factors. *Diabetes Care*, **29**, 391–7.

131. Haffner, S.M., Lehto, S., Ronnemaa, T. *et al.* (1998) Mortality from coronary heart disease in subjects with type 2 diabetes and in nondiabetic subjects with and without prior myocardial infarction. *The New England Journal of Medicine*, **339**, 229–34.

132. Juutilainen, A., Lehto, S., Ronnemaa, T. *et al.* (2005) Type 2 diabetes as a 'coronary heart disease equivalent': an 18-year prospective population-based study in Finnish subjects. *Diabetes Care*, **28**, 2901–7.

133. Whiteley, L., Padmanabhan, S., Hole, D. and Isles, C. (2005) Should diabetes be considered a coronary heart disease risk equivalent? Results from 25 years of follow-up in the Renfrew and Paisley survey. *Diabetes Care*, **28**, 1588–93.

134. Evans, J.M., Wang, J. and Morris, A.D. (2002) Comparison of cardiovascular risk between patients with type 2 diabetes and those who had had a myocardial infarction: cross sectional and cohort studies. *British Medical Journal*, **324**, 939–42.

135. Lotufo, P.A., Gaziano, J.M., Chae, C.U. *et al.* (2001) Diabetes and all-cause and coronary heart disease mortality among US male physicians. *Archives of Internal Medicine*, **161**, 242–7.

136. Eberly, L.E., Cohen, J.D., Prineas, R. and Yang, L. (2003) Impact of incident diabetes and incident nonfatal cardiovascular disease on 18-year mortality: the multiple risk factor intervention trial experience. *Diabetes Care*, **26**, 848–54.

137. Grundy, S.M. (2006) Diabetes and coronary risk equivalency: what does it mean? *Diabetes Care*, **29**, 457–60.

138. Balkau, B., Barrett-Connor, E., Eschwege, E. *et al.* (1993) Diabetes and pancreatic carcinoma. *Diabetes and Metabolism*, **19**, 458–62.

139. Everhart, J. and Wright, D. (1995) Diabetes mellitus as a risk factor for pancreatic cancer. A meta-analysis. *The Journal of the American Medical Association*, **273**, 1605–9.

140. Koskinen, S.V., Reunanen, A.R., Martelin, T.P. and Valkonen, T. (1998) Mortality in a large population-based cohort of patients with drug-treated diabetes mellitus. *American Journal of Public Health*, **88**, 765–70.

141. Hu, F.B., Manson, J.E., Liu, S. *et al.* (1999) Prospective study of adult onset diabetes mellitus (type 2) and risk of colorectal cancer in women. *Journal of the National Cancer Institute*, **91**, 542–7.

142. Lai, M.S., Hsieh, M.S., Chiu, Y.H. and Chen, T.H. (2006) Type 2 diabetes and hepatocellular carcinoma: a cohort study in high prevalence area of hepatitis virus infection. *Hepatology (Baltimore, Md)*, **43**, 1295–302.

143. Michels, K.B., Solomon, C.G., Hu, F.B. *et al.* (2003) Type 2 diabetes and subsequent incidence of breast cancer in the Nurses' Health Study. *Diabetes Care*, **26**, 1752–8.

144. Batty, G.D., Shipley, M.J., Marmot, M. and Smith, G.D. (2004) Diabetes status and post-load plasma glucose concentration in relation to site-specific cancer mortality: findings from the original Whitehall Study. *Cancer Causes and Control*, **15**, 873–81.

145. Coughlin, S.S., Calle, E.E., Teras, L.R. *et al.* (2004) Diabetes mellitus as a predictor of cancer mortality in a large cohort of US adults. *American Journal of Epidemiology*, **159**, 1160–7.

146. Moss, S.E., Klein, R., Klein, B.E. and Meuer, S.M. (1994) The association of glycemia and cause-specific mortality in a diabetic population. *Archives of Internal Medicine*, **154**, 2473–9.

147. Adlerberth, A.M., Rosengren, A. and Wilhelmsen, L. (1998) Diabetes and long-term risk of mortality from coronary and other causes in middle-aged Swedish men. A general population study. *Diabetes Care*, **21**, 539–45.

148. Saydah, S.H., Loria, C.M., Eberhardt, M.S. and Brancati, F.L. (2003) Abnormal glucose tolerance and the risk of cancer death in the United States. *American Journal of Epidemiology*, **157**, 1092–100.

149. Levine, W., Dyer, A.R., Shekelle, R.B. *et al.* (1990) Post-load plasma glucose and cancer mortality in middle-aged men and women. 12-year follow-up findings of the Chicago Heart Association Detection Project in Industry. *American Journal of Epidemiology*, **131**, 254–62.

150. Balkau, B., Shipley, M., Jarrett, R.J. *et al.* (1998) High blood glucose concentration is a risk factor for mortality in middle-aged non-diabetic men. 20-year follow-up in the Whitehall Study, the Paris Prospective Study, and the Helsinki Policemen Study. *Diabetes Care*, **21**, 360–7.

151. Smith, G.D., Egger, M., Shipley, M.J. and Marmot, M.G. (1992) Post-challenge glucose concentration, impaired glucose tolerance, diabetes, and cancer mortality in men. *American Journal of Epidemiology*, **136**, 1110–14.

152. Bowker, S.L., Majumdar, S.R., Veugelers, P. and Johnson, J.A. (2006) Increased cancer-related mortality for patients with type 2 diabetes who use sulfonylureas or insulin. *Diabetes Care*, **29**, 254–8.

153. Laakso, M. and Lehto, S. (1998) Epidemiology of risk factors for cardiovascular disease in diabetes and impaired glucose tolerance. *Atherosclerosis*, **137** (Suppl 1), S65–73.

154. Stern, M.P. (1995) Diabetes and cardiovascular disease. The 'common soil' hypothesis. *Diabetes*, **44**, 369–74.

155. Wilkinson, R. and Marmot, M. (2003) *The Social Determinants of Health: the Solid Facts*, 2nd edn, World Health Organization, Denmark

156. UK Prospective Diabetes Study (UKPDS) Group (1998) Intensive blood-glucose control with sulphonylureas or insulin compared with conventional treatment and risk of complications in patients with type 2 diabetes (UKPDS 33). UK Prospective Diabetes Study (UKPDS) Group. *Lancet*, **352**, 837–53.

157. UK Prospective Diabetes Study (UKPDS) Group (1998) Tight blood pressure control and risk of macrovascular and microvascular complications in type 2 diabetes: UKPDS 38. *British Medical Journal*, **317**, 703–13.

158. Heart Outcomes Prevention Evaluation Study Investigators (2000) Effects of ramipril on cardiovascular and microvascular outcomes in people with diabetes mellitus: results of the HOPE study and MICRO-HOPE substudy. *Lancet*, **355**, 253–9.

159. Hansson, L., Zanchetti, A., Carruthers, S.G. *et al.* (1998) Effects of intensive blood-pressure lowering and low-dose aspirin in patients with hypertension: principal results of the Hypertension Optimal Treatment (HOT) randomised trial. HOT Study Group. *Lancet*, **351**, 1755–62.

160. Kjekshus, J. and Pedersen, T.R. (1995) Reducing the risk of coronary events: evidence from the Scandinavian Simvastatin Survival Study (4S). *The American Journal of Cardiology*, **76**, 64C–68C.

161. Collins, R., Armitage, J., Parish, S. *et al.* (2003) MRC/BHF Heart Protection Study of cholesterol-lowering with simvastatin in 5963 people with diabetes: a randomised placebo-controlled trial. *Lancet*, **361**, 2005–16.

162. Colhoun, H.M., Betteridge, D.J., Durrington, P.N. *et al.* (2004) Primary prevention of cardiovascular disease with atorvastatin in type 2 diabetes in the Collaborative Atorvastatin Diabetes Study (CARDS): multicentre randomised placebo-controlled trial. *Lancet*, **364**, 685–96.

163. Keech, A., Simes, R.J., Barter, P. *et al.* (2005) Effects of long-term fenofibrate therapy on cardiovascular events in 9795 people with type 2 diabetes mellitus (the FIELD study): randomised controlled trial. *Lancet*, **366**, 1849–61.

164. Gæde, P., Vedel, P., Larsen, N. *et al.* (2003) Multifactorial intervention and cardiovascular disease in patients with type 2 diabetes. *The New England Journal of Medicine*, **348**, 383–93.

37

Economic Costs

Rhys Williams[1] and Thomas J. Songer[2]

[1] Clinical Epidemiology at the School of Medicine, University of Swansea, Swansea, UK

[2] Department of Epidemiology, University of Pittsburgh, Pittsburgh, PA, USA

37.1 INTRODUCTION

A common question posed throughout the world for the previous two decades relates to the costs associated with diabetes. Cost and other forms of economic data are important contributors to the decisions made by health departments, health care providers and health insurers regarding diabetes. Decision makers need reliable economic information to determine equitably which health services should be funded (e.g. diabetic care versus the control of communicable disease). They need information for decisions regarding payment for insulin, syringes, oral hypoglycemic agents and blood glucose testing supplies, and for decisions on the number and nature of facilities for people with diabetes and the number and type of health personnel trained to treat and care for them. Decision makers also need information on the relative 'value for money' of health care treatments and programs to determine the relative merits of apparently costly treatments in diabetes, such as intensive control of blood glucose, blood pressure and dyslipidemia, screening programs (such as those for diabetic retinopathy), educational interventions and many others.

How did we get to this point? Several factors have contributed to the current situation. First, health care is a dynamic process. Medical advances and new therapies require us to adapt and change our approaches to health care. Many new advances, though, are costly technologies, surgeries or drugs. Second, health care provision has, in many circumstances, been a political process. In many areas, an oversupply of physicians and a redundancy in some facilities (such as hospitals) exist. Third, the life expectancy of the world's population is increasing. With aging populations comes an increased need for the long-term treatments that are required for chronic conditions.

The above features have all played a role in the current reality that faces many health systems. In particular:

1. The costs of health care are rising at a significant rate. Over the last 40 years, expenditures for medical care have risen extensively throughout the world [1–4]. Indeed, health care expenditures have risen much faster than the cost increase reported in other sectors of the economy.
2. There are limited resources available for health care and, often, an inability to obtain more.
3. Health care coverage is often not available to all individuals in a population, and many governments are unable to provide it.
4. There is a large variation in health care use by geographical area and health care setting. This variation exists with no apparent difference in a patient's health.

As a result of the above, fundamental changes are taking place in health care systems throughout the world. There is now an expanding focus being placed on the economic aspects of health care. The underlying issue throughout most of the discussions on health care reform and the appropriateness of

---

The Epidemiology of Diabetes Mellitus, second edition   Edited by Jean-Marie Ekoé, Marian Rewers, Rhys Williams and Paul Zimmet

health care is that of costs. Are we spending health care resources wisely? How much does it cost to provide treatment? What benefits are obtained with that treatment? Which treatments provide benefits and at what cost? With limited resources, health care decision-makers must make choices about the direction to pursue in health care and the intensity with which to pursue it.

37.2 HEALTH ECONOMICS

Health economics is a discipline involved with the study of health care costs, the rational use of limited resources and the subsequent choices made regarding health care and health care costs. Health economic studies provide information which can help to guide decisions regarding health care funding, planning, provision and evaluation. Common economic issues that are examined include:

1. The costs related to disease or illness, such as the money that we spend to treat patients. These costs involve the expenditures for medical care and the treatment of a disease and its complications (hospital care, physician services, long-term care, drugs, facilities and overheads, etc.)
2. The indirect costs associated with disease, such as the impact of a disability or premature mortality. These costs relate to lost productivity, an inability to continue working, or from interference with usual activities.
3. The costs of disease that directly affect the patient. Persons with severe illnesses face several economic decisions. These include the out-of-pocket payments for health care and the sacrifices in time (opportunity costs) made in searching for medical care, employment and insurance.
4. The costs of using resources devoted to a specific disease or treatment inappropriately, or the costs of pursuing inappropriate priorities.
5. The influence of excesses or shortages in the number (supply) of medical technologies and drugs, and the demand for health care.

There are several reasons why it is important to understand these issues as they apply to diabetes care. First and foremost is that governments increasingly have little money to spend on the health of the public. In this environment, it is important that appropriate levels of resources are directed to

diabetes, and that the money available for diabetes is used to its greatest benefit.

37.3 IDENTIFYING THE COSTS OF DIABETES

What are the costs of diabetes? As outlined above, there are a number of different approaches that one can take to examine the costs associated with diabetes. The types of economic costs related to the diabetes mellitus include the medical costs of treating people with diabetes, the indirect costs related to early disability or early death, the costs that individuals with diabetes face personally when they forgo spending money in one area to help pay for treating diabetes (opportunity costs), the costs of using resources available inappropriately and the costs of having too few diabetes services (not everyone gets care) or too many diabetes services.

37.4 DIRECT MEDICAL COSTS

Studies of the medical costs of treating diabetes are the most common form of diabetes economic analysis in the literature. Direct medical costs of disease include the expenditure for medical care and the treatment of the illness (hospital care, physician services, related laboratory tests, nursing home care, drugs and the cost of daily diabetes management (insulin, syringes, oral hypoglycemic agents, blood testing supplies) among other items). The monetary costs of medical treatment are often easily measured by services and studies of medical or billing records.

37.5 INDIRECT MORBIDITY AND MORTALITY COSTS

Indirect economic costs include the consequences of morbidity, disability and premature mortality resulting from diabetes. These nonmedical costs are not easily measured or calculated, but are commonly associated with detrimental changes in activity among persons with diabetes. For instance, the degree to which an individual must stop or decrease the amount of time spent in usual activities. One example is with work. People with the complications of diabetes often have to stop working. There is a cost incurred here related to the lost productivity of that individual. These types of costs are also found for people who die prematurely or for people with higher rates of absenteeism from work than the general population.

Estimates of the monetary costs of these effects are usually based on the human capital approach, whereby costs from the illness are valued in terms of lost earnings and production of the patient. This allows for the estimates to be applied as monetary units. However, there has been some controversy over the most appropriate method to value losses from premature disability and mortality [5–7]. Other methods exist, such as the willingness-to-pay approach, that value lost opportunities from an estimate that patients provide of the monetary figure that they would be willing to pay to avoid illness, disability or premature death. The human capital approach has been the most common method used in the cost of diabetes studies. However, there is now at least an attempt to use the 'frictional costs' approach to this problem [8, 9]. The frictional cost approach measures the marginal costs of recruiting and training individuals to make good any deficiency in the workforce created by sickness absence, disability and premature death caused in other workers by a given disease or condition. This is a much more realistic scenario in industry compared with the work remaining undone. It does not, as does the human capital approach, rely on complete employment–an unrealistic assumption for any economy.

37.6 DIRECT COST ESTIMATES

The availability of direct cost estimates for the care of diabetes in individual countries has been transformed by the publication, in the second [10] and third [11] editions of the International Diabetes Federation's (IDF's) *Diabetes Atlas*, of calculated costs based on the formula first advocated by Jönsson [12]. Hitherto, estimates had been calculated under the framework of cost of illness studies pioneered by Dorothy Rice in the 1960s [13]. Specific details of these methods are discussed more thoroughly elsewhere[14–17].

Many of these reports were specific to the United States' experience, with a few from other countries. Examples of the latter are Barcelo *et al*.'s [18] work on Latin American and Caribbean countries, Koster *et al*.'s [19] estimate for Germany and Colagiuri *et al*.'s [20] estimate for Australia. The most recent estimate for the United States is that of the American Diabetes Association (ADA) [21]. All of these

reports show that the economic burden of diabetes care is considerable and that the largest component of direct medical costs is generally the cost of hospital care related to diabetes.

The CODE-2 study [22], the first diabetes cost of illness study to employ the same protocol in more than one country simultaneously, quantified the influence of diabetes complications on hospital costs. The presence of both microvascular and macrovascular complications in the same patient increased hospital expenditure fivefold compared with average cost of hospitalizations of patients without either type of complication.

These individual studies of direct costs have, as mentioned above, been complemented by the *Diabetes Atlas* calculations. The most recent set [11] contains estimates (for 2007) and projections (for 2025) of the direct health care costs of diabetes for individual countries and for IDF regions. These are calculated according to Jönsson's formula [12], which requires knowledge of the prevalence of the condition, the total expenditure on health in each country and the ratio R of the costs of care for people with diabetes compared with the costs of care for those without diabetes. The prevalence estimates and projections used are set out elsewhere in the *Diabetes Atlas* [23].

Direct costs to the state are presented both in terms of the US dollar (USD) and the International dollar (ID). The ID is a common currency unit that takes into account differences in the relative purchasing power of various currencies. Figures expressed in ID are calculated using purchasing power parities purchasing power parity (PPPs), which are rates of currency conversion constructed to account for differences in price level (particularly of labor) between countries. Thus, for the United States 1 ID = 1 USD, but for a low resource country, such as Somalia, where labor is low cost, 2.17 ID = 1 USD. It is estimated that expenditures on diabetes and its complications worldwide in 2007 have reached 286 billion ID (232 billion USD) and that, by 2025, the prediction is that this will have risen to at least 381 billion ID (302 billion USD).

Although India and China are the countries with the largest number of people with diabetes, expenditure on diabetes in the United States far outstrips that of any other country. Expenditures in Europe and North America together are far more than the rest of the world combined, even though, in 2007, these two IDF regions are estimated to contribute only a third (81.5 million) to the total (246.1 million) people, aged 20–79 years, with diabetes globally [11]. A summary of these data, for IDF regions and for selected countries within these regions is given in **Table 37.1**.

The countries selected in **Table 37.1** are, for each of the IDF regions, the countries with the most and least estimated mean per person (state) expenditures on diabetes in 2007 (at $R = 2$ and expressed in ID). Comparison of national health expenditures is complicated by differences in diabetes prevalence and in total national health care expenditures. Comparisons of per person expenditures, however, are valid and demonstrate considerable disparities. Thus, for Africa, the countries at the extremes of per person expenditure, Somalia and South Africa, differ by a factor of 42.5 (25 ID and 1064 ID respectively); in the eastern Mediterranean and Middle East, Afghanistan and Qatar by 21.3 (56 ID and 1198 ID); in Europe, Monaco and Tajikistan by 52.0 (4212 ID and 81 ID); in North America, Trinidad and Tobago and the United States by 11.1 (559 ID and 6231 ID); in South and Central America, Argentina and Honduras by 4.9 (1326 ID and 271 ID); in South East Asia, Maldives and Bangladesh by 5.7 (540 ID and 94 ID); and in the Western Pacific Region, Australia and the Democratic People's Republic of Korea by 40.0 (3205 ID and 80 ID). The global disparity in this respect is that individuals in the United States have almost 250 times the per person expenditure on diabetes as individuals in Somalia.

As a validation of this approach to the estimation of diabetes health care expenditures, Brown *et al.* [11] cite examples of direct studies of diabetes expenditures which concur with these calculated estimates and support the assumption that $R \approx 2$. These include Koster *et al.* [19] for Germany and Colaguiri *et al.* [20] for Australia. As they point out [11], the ADA's 2002 estimate for the United States [21] is rather lower than the calculated value for 2007, a discrepancy which may be explained by the rise in prevalence in the United States from 2002 to 2007 and the fact that the formula calculation includes expenditures on diabetes that may not be captured by the ADA. Detailed work on the relationship between values of R and age [11] confirm that, as expected, the ratio of health expenditure for people with diabetes to that of

people without diabetes decreases with age, though health expenditure, in absolute terms, rises with age.

There are few satisfactory publications of time trends in the direct costs of diabetes in specific countries. A recently published report [24] includes time trends (from 2004 to 2007) for Denmark, India, the United Kingdom and the United States. Although time trends for indirect costs (productivity losses) are also presented for these countries and for the People's Republic of China, no data for direct costs in China were given in this report [24]. Such data are expected from the current World Health Organization (WHO)/IDF study–'Diabetes Action Now' http://www.who.int/diabetes/actionnow/en/ (accessed 23 December 2007)–sponsored by the International Diabetes Foundation. As shown in **Table 37.3**, even over this short period of study, direct costs of diabetes increased by 40% in Denmark, 24% in India, by 16% in the United Kingdom and by 28% in the United States. Direct comparison of these estimates with those listed in **Table 37.1** is rendered difficult by the differing methodologies employed. However, those for the United States in 2007 are within around 10% of each other (119.3 billion USD (**Table 37.1**) versus 134.8 billion USD (**Table 37.3**)).

Often, cost estimates have been used to highlight the importance of diabetes to health care systems and health care insurers. Diabetes organizations commonly use these data as evidence of the need to devote more resources to diabetes care. One of the first of these was the Juvenile Diabetes Federation in their document 'The Economics of Medical Research' [25], which used the direct cost estimate by Rubin *et al.* [26], to advance the argument that investing in diabetes research is worthwhile.

Is this argument true? Not necessarily. While cost of illness studies can estimate the monetary burden of diabetes, they cannot provide an answer to the question of whether the money is being spent wisely, nor whether investment in research or clinical practices is worthwhile. These issues are best addressed with another type of economic analysis: a cost–benefit, cost–effectiveness or cost–utility study.

Thus, there are limits to the interpretation of estimates of direct costs as there are limits to their comparability because of differing methodologies and differing frameworks for analysis. Nevertheless, carefully constructed estimates of direct costs

Table 37.1 Health expenditures for diabetes, estimates for 2007 and projections for 2025, for IDF regions and selected countries.[a]

IDF region	Country	Health expenditures (2007) USD (ID) ('000)		Health expenditures (2025) USD (ID)	
		R = 2	R = 3	R = 2	R = 3
Africa		710 180 (2 137 027)	1 270 784 (3 824 368)	922 542 (2 754 377)	1 672 591 (5 001 165)
	Somalia	1 061 (2 299)	1 928 (4 178)	1 897 (4 111)	3 465 (7 507)
	South Africa	385 824 (1 290 449)	688 013 (2 301 169)	424 815 (1 420 861)	778 004 (2 602 157)
Eastern Mediterranean and Middle East		3 195 799 (7 511 656)	5 349 671 (12 787 425)	6 191 714 (13 982 139)	10 366 100 (23 825 035)
	Afghanistan	25 602 (62 175)	43 089 (104 644)	45 913 (111 502)	77 162 (187 393)
	Qatar	99 205 (94 854)	152 287 (145 609)	180 143 (172 243)	280 008 (267 730)
Europe		63 987 133 (82 158 649)	119 090 727 (152 427 546)	76 258 302 (97 909 474)	143 136 315 (183 064 381)
	Monaco	6 954 (8 100)	12 964 (15 098)	8 882 (10 344)	16 752 (19 510)
	Tajikistan	1 198 (9 381)	2 157 (16 900)	2 345 (18 373)	4 184 (32 777)
North America		128 691 947 (132 163 097)	230 344 260 (236 460 803)	174 485 018 (179 903 410)	319 487 464 (329 140 328)
	Trinidad and Tobago	35 377 (57 354)	58 701 (95 167)	47 849 (77 573)	80 752 (130 916)

(continued overleaf)

Table 37.1 (*continued*)

IDF region	Country	Health expenditures (2007) USD (ID) ('000)		Health expenditures (2025) USD (ID)	
		R = 2	R = 3	R = 2	R = 3
	United States	119 358 449 (119 358 449)	213 817 522 (213 817522)	160 155 467 (160 155 467)	293 787 319 (293 787 319)
South and Central America		4 503 248 (12 555 309)	8 049 217 (22 511 523)	71 196 796 (19 969 324)	13 007 973 (36 192 479)
	Argentina	490 972 (1 972 140)	894 039 (3 591 181)	657 474 (2 640 944)	1 201 380 (4 825 712)
	Honduras	27 957 (72 687)	48 646 (126 481)	52 423 (136 301)	91 158 (237 010)
South East Asia		2 067 942 (6 811 580)	3 664 551 (12 070 481)	3 239 120 (10 676 508)	5 790 771 (19 087 682)
	Maldives	2 187 (5 594)	3 803 (9 731)	4 121 (10 542)	7 167 (18 336)
	Bangladesh	73 321 (359 941)	129 815 (637 275)	122 269 (600 227)	218 683 (1 073 534)
Western Pacific		28 811 441 (42 729 935)	53 886 502 (78 832 195)	34 187 702 (55 857 411)	65 105 388 (104 880 442)
	Australia	2 193 190 (2 967 127)	4 135 956 (5 595 461)	3 178 633 (4 300 317)	6 130 269 (8 293 532)
	Korea (Democratic People's Republic of)	338 (2 277 727)	606 (4 017 903)	438 (3 182 402)	788 (5 732 761)
Global total		**231 967 689 (286 067 252)**	**421 655 708 (518 914 340)**	**302 481 194 (381 052 643)**	**558 566 601 (701 191 512)**

[a] Adapted from Ref. 11.

Table 37.2 Time trends in direct and indirect costs of diabetes in the People's Republic of China, India, the United Kingdom and the United States from 2004 to 2007 (in billions of USD).[a]

Country	Cost	2004	2005	2006	2007
China	Direct health care cost of diabetes (with percentage increase over 2004 estimate)	N/G[b]	N/G	N/G	N/G
Denmark		0.5	0.6	0.6	0.7 (40%)
India		2.1	2.3	2.3	2.6 (24%)
United Kingdom		6.3	6.8	7.0	7.3 (16%)
United States		105.5	115.5	125.4	134.8 (28%)
China	Productivity loss (indirect costs) resulting from diabetes (as percentage of total cost)	12.4	14.4	17.0	20.5 (N/A)
Denmark		1.2 (70%)	1.2 (67%)	1.3 (68%)	1.3 (65%
India		16.1 (88%)	17.7 (89%)	18.8 (89%)	20.4 (89%)
United Kingdom		2.6 (29%)	2.7 (28%)	2.9 (29%)	3.3 (31%)
United States		37.7 (26%)	38.8 (25%)	40.1 (24%)	41.4 (23%)

[a] Adapted from Ref. 24.
[b] N/G: not given in this publication.

are a useful adjunct to incidence and prevalence as surrogates for measuring the impact of conditions on health services. Indeed, the argument may be advanced that costs are more meaningful, in this particular context, than either incidence or prevalence taken alone, since cost estimates embrace the impact both of newly diagnosed disease (incidence) and that of caring for established disease (prevalence)–both of which are distinct and important in diabetes.

37.7 ESTIMATES OF COSTS FACED BY PEOPLE WITH DIABETES

Few reports have examined the economic impact of diabetes in the daily lives of individuals living with the condition. In the United States, however, there is evidence that individuals living with diabetes face an increased personal health care cost burden. Health care in the United States is the most expensive in the world. Access to this expensive system is dictated by the presence of health insurance, both public-based and private. Health insurance coverage varies widely, and marked inequities exist in access to health care. About 17% of the general population under age 65 has no health insurance coverage [18]. Young people and those without work or in low-paying jobs are the individuals most likely to be without coverage. It has been estimated [27] that at least 3 million people with diabetes in the United States, probably more, 'have either insufficient cover for reasonable healthcare or none at all.'

Around 15% of families who have a child with type 1 diabetes have difficulty in obtaining coverage because of pre-existing illness clauses in the insurance policies [28]. It has long been known that most people with diabetes use health services more frequently than the general population [29] and that the out-of-pocket payments for diabetes care are roughly twice as high for a person with diabetes than for a person without diabetes under the age of 65 years [30].

Nearly one-third of the families with a child with diabetes spent more than $1000 (1996 prices) of their own money on health care compared with 16% in the families having no diabetic children [28]. The burden of out-of-pocket medical expenses was more profound among the lowest income families. The out-of-pocket health care expenses for the poorest (annual income 0–19 999 USD) families with a child with type 1 diabetes was over twice that of families in the same income bracket but with no child with diabetes. In the wealthiest families (annual income 60 000 USD or more), the out-of-pocket expenses, although greater overall than in the poorest families, were the same whether or not there was a child with diabetes.

More recently, exactly the same pattern, of a considerable financial burden to families with a diabetic member and a greater proportional burden on the poor, has been found in a country with an economic climate very different to that of the United States, namely India. Shobhana *et al.* [31] estimated that, in 1998, a considerable proportion of family income was devoted to the payment for treatment at a chosen location outside the public sector. In their diabetes centre in Chennai, families in the poorest section of the population spent as much as 25% of their income in order to obtain the care of their choice. While these out-of-pocket costs were high in all income categories, it was this poorest section which devoted the greatest proportion of their income to this end. When this same methodology was repeated, in the same centre, 6 years later [32], the proportion of family income devoted to diabetes by the poorest families had risen to over a third.

37.8 EVALUATIVE STUDIES IN DIABETES HEALTH ECONOMICS

Current practice in diabetes health economics has been the use of evaluative studies to examine the economic efficiency of diabetes treatments and programs. Evaluative studies consider the cost of a treatment or intervention relative to the health outcomes produced. As health care costs are continuing to rise worldwide, these evaluations provide important information that can inform decisions about the proper allocation of limited resources. Comparisons of the costs and outcomes of a new treatment will help in determining whether

it is an efficient and effective use of resources compared with other approaches. The principles of these methodologies are well established [33] and widely used.

Evaluative designs include cost–benefit, cost–effectiveness and cost–utility analyses. All three designs evaluate the costs and benefits of one intervention to determine whether resources might be used more efficiently with a change in clinical practice. Cost–benefit, cost–effectiveness and cost–utility studies are generally similar in the ways in which they estimate costs. These are almost always expressed in monetary terms. The three forms of analyses, though, differ in how they assess the outcomes of a program or treatment. Cost–benefit analyses compare the costs and benefits in monetary terms. Cost–effectiveness studies usually summarize health outcomes in physical units (such as the number of lives saved) and express these outcomes relative to the costs of the interventions required to produce them. Cost–utility studies generally summarize health outcomes in terms of quality of life gained as well as quantity of life gained. These two parameters are frequently amalgamated into the cost per quality adjusted life year (QALY) (gained). One cost-effectiveness index being used with increasing frequency in such studies is the incremental cost–effectiveness ratio (ICER)–the additional cost of a new intervention (compared with its alternative) for each additional unit of effectiveness (such as a QALY gained).

Differences in the assessment of health outcomes between these three studies can also affect the manner in which they are used in policy decisions. Cost–benefit analyses often seek to determine if an objective (like reducing the impact of diabetes complications) is worthwhile from an economic perspective. Since cost–benefit studies value outcomes in monetary terms, the results can be compared directly with other programs (both inside and outside of the health sector). It is then possible to examine whether such a program is worth pursuing and to what degree resources might be committed to it.

In contrast, cost–effectiveness and cost–utility analyses already assume that the objective is worth pursuing. The decision here is determining whether one type of intervention or another is better able to meet the intent of the objective. For example, one may find that the objective of reducing blindness from diabetic retinopathy is economically efficient. The task of cost–effectiveness and cost–utility analyses, then, is to evaluate which intervention in retinopathy is the most efficient. In general, cost–effectiveness and cost–utility studies are favored over cost–benefit studies in the health-care sector.

Undertaking a cost–effectiveness study can be complex, as data are needed from a variety of areas. The appropriate data and endpoints to consider in an evaluation will vary according to the intervention taking place. Most evaluations, however, consider the costs of starting and operating an intervention, the additional direct and indirect costs involved to improve health outcomes, the savings in direct and indirect costs when disorders are prevented or delayed and the costs associated with any side-effects of the intervention. Other basic principles include stating the perspective in which the evaluation is being conducted, discounting costs that occur in future years, testing the results to consider the impact of uncertainty and providing a summary measure of the efficiency of an intervention, such as a ratio of costs to effects. These principles are critically analyzed elsewhere [34], and several authoritative publications (e.g. [35, 36]) suggest standards that all cost–effectiveness analyses should follow and point out common flaws in existing studies.

37.9 ESTIMATES FROM EVALUATION STUDIES

Evaluation studies differ substantially from cost of illness studies. They usually consider the costs of a diabetes program or treatment relative to the benefits obtained. In this design, comparisons are often made with an existing standard in an attempt to prioritize the direction of future resources and treatments.

The first studies in the literature dealing with the economic benefits of new treatments primarily examined diabetes education programs. Kaplan and Davis [37] critically discussed a large portion of the then available literature on this topic in their benchmark publication. They pointed out that many of the early studies neglected significant issues, such as accounting for the costs of starting and operating the education program. Most focused instead on the benefits of the program and, thus, the results give an unbalanced perspective. The

majority of studies also did not include control groups for comparative purposes in their evaluations. Kaplan and Davies also point out the danger of evaluating programs simply on the basis of a reduction of medical costs, since health care costs can be influenced by a variety of factors, including simple changes in how services are paid for.

Many of the reports examined by Kaplan and Davies were completed in the 1970s and early 1980s. Since that time, there has been an explosion in the number of reports that address economic issues in diabetes from an evaluation perspective. **Table 23.5** of the first edition of this chapter [38] and the 'Resources related to diabetes health economics' website (http://www.google.co.uk/search?hl = en&q = Health+economics+of+diabetes&meta = (accessed 27 December 2007)) outline the majority of these studies up until 2005 while the 'Diabetes Health Economics Resource' website of the UK Yorkshire and Humberside Public Health Observatory (http://www.york.ac.uk/yhpho/cfm/dhedbform.cfm (accessed 27 December 2007)) brings this database up to date. Brown *et al.* [11] cites a number of estimates provided by the World Bank which expand the previously rather restricted focus of evaluative studies to include developing countries.

Findings from this developing database strongly suggest that screening for and treating diabetes retinopathy is extremely cost-effective. Javitt *et al.* [39], reporting in 1990, found that it saved 62–109 million USD for an annual incidence cohort of patients with type 1 diabetes (when compared with not screening). Further reports [40, 41], from the same group, confirmed these findings, adding that additional savings of 9500 USD occurred with each new type 1 diabetes person enrolled in a screening program (over the number already being screened). More recent work confirms these findings in general, but is becoming more discerning in that the cost-effectiveness of annual screening in people with well-controlled type 2 diabetes is being questioned [42], a finding similar to that previously described by Dasbach *et al.* [43], who in 1991 found that the costs of screening and subsequent treatment were recovered for persons using insulin (both young and old), but not in people diagnosed with diabetes at a later age and not on insulin. The underlying message is that the economic benefits of different screening strategies (and interventions in general) are likely to vary depending upon the characteristics of the population, the availability of equipment and the therapies required, as well as the goals of the program relative to the resources available to carry it out. In the developing regions of the world, estimates of the cost per QALY for annual eye examination vary from 320 to 700 USD (2001 prices) [44] cited by [11]. Such an investment would be regarded, in virtually every country, as 'good value for money.'

The cost-effectiveness of treatments for diabetic foot ulcers was described in the first edition of this chapter [38] as 'muddled.' In support of this, a paper by Eckman et al. [45] was cited. That review examined treatment strategies for foot ulcers with suspected osteomyelitis. The underlying message emerged that treatment with a long course of antibiotics is more cost-efficient in most situations than amputation. The authors, however, examined several treatment alternatives in their analysis and, as such, only general conclusions could be drawn form the work rather than specific recommendations. Since then, the field has been clarified by simulation studies, such as that of Ortegon et al. [46] and systematic reviews such as Matricali et al. [47]. The former has established that guideline-based care for the diabetic foot results in a gain in QALYs at a cost acceptable in most developed countries (<25 000 USD over a lifetime) with an indication that such care, in those at high risk, is actually cost saving. This latter result is supported by the World Bank report for all developing regions with the added advantage of being feasible even in low-resource areas. An important observation from the review by Matricali et al. [47] is that, while all the studies they reviewed showed 'acceptable cost-effectiveness,' this was present in the long term, rather than short term, since benefits took years to accrue.

Herein lies the crux of most economic analyses. Evaluations are most useful when they elicit specific recommendations regarding the pursuit of a treatment, technology or program. Such recommendations can be readily put to use by decision makers in health care. Clear recommendations, though, are not apparent for many of the issues pertaining to diabetes care.

The evolution of the evidence base relating to the cost-effectiveness of intensive glycemic control is illustrative of at least three important lessons for

the interpretation of economic data: the need to examine costs and benefits in the widest possible way; the need to consider data specific to clearly defined patient groups; and the need to consider costs and benefits not only from the perspective of the state or health care payer, but from that of the individual. An early examination of the cost of intensive insulin treatments among people with type 1 diabetes, by Stern and Levy [48], found that, over 35 years, the cost of intensive treatment was far greater than the cost of standard forms of treatment, even after accounting for the greater costs of treating complications in the standard treatment group. Their report, however, did not consider indirect costs or the relative benefit of improved health associated with intensive treatment. As evidence from the Diabetes Control and Complications Trial (DCCT) became available [49], simulation studies were able to reveal that intensive treatment, though considerably more costly than standard treatment, reduced complications and improved the quality and length of life sufficiently to represent good value for money. This was true for people with onset of diabetes before age 50 years, but considerable doubts remained as to its economic value in those with onset at 65 years or above [50]. A detailed study of the costs and benefits of intensive glycemic control in older (≥65 years of age) patients [51] revealed the high degree of sensitivity of the results in relation to not only the form of treatment used to achieve such control, but also to the perspective from which quality of life was assessed. Intensive control with oral medication (but not insulin) was deemed cost-effective (ICER ≤ 100 000 USD) only when patient-derived utilities (quality of life weights) were incorporated both for complications and for treatments.

Economic analysis of the United Kingdom Prospective Diabetes Study (UKPDS) has widened consideration from solely blood glucose control to blood glucose and blood pressure control, this time in people with type 2 diabetes [52]. Considering three different policies (intensive blood glucose control with insulin or sulfonylurea, intensive blood glucose control with metformin for those also overweight and tight blood pressure control in those with hypertension, in addition to their type 2 diabetes), the authors described acceptable ICER estimates for the first and third of these policies (6028 GB pounds (GBP) and 369 GBP per QALY gained (2004 UK prices)) and cost saving (i.e. negative cost per QALY gained for treatment with metformin in the overweight). The World Bank's analysis [44] suggests that, for all developing regions, cost savings for both tight glycemic control (in those with an HbA_{1c} of over 9%) and effective blood pressure control (in those with blood pressures over 160/95 mmHg).

The logical step from these trials focusing solely on blood glucose intervention (DCCT) and blood glucose and blood pressure interventions (UKPDS) is to trials which evaluate multiple simultaneous interventions dealing with all of the main components of metabolic syndrome: hyperglycemia, hypertension and dyslipidemia. The Steno 2 trial [53] is such a study which has convincingly shown the effectiveness of multiple intervention and which also suggests cost-effectiveness. As these authors state, the challenge is now to move from intensive interventions within the realm of randomized controlled trials (RCTs) into everyday practice (and to confirm the effectiveness and cost-effectiveness of such policies in pragmatic RCTs).

Similar observations could be made about the effectiveness and cost-effectiveness of primary prevention interventions in the hyperglycemic precursors of type 2 diabetes (impaired glucose tolerance and impaired fasting glycemia). The cost-effectiveness of early interventions, particularly those directed at weight loss and increased physical activity, within the confines of RCTs (the Finish Diabetes Prevention Study, the US Diabetes Prevention Program (DPP) and the Indian DPP) has been described (e.g. [54]). The challenges now are to investigate the economic consequences of these interventions in the 'real-life' situation and to implement those preventive strategies which are found to be cost-effective and which are feasible on a regional or national basis. Not to do so is unacceptable. As has been stated [55]:

> In economic terms, the consequences of inaction are likely to be disastrous–disastrous for national economic well-being, for public health and social services, and for individuals and families. As with most phenomena such as these, the blow will fall particularly heavily on developing countries, on the poor in these countries in particular, and on the poorer sections of the developed countries.

37.10 INDIRECT COST ESTIMATES

To a certain extent, indirect costs (also known as the costs of lost production or productivity losses) are the 'poor relation' in diabetes cost of illness studies. The methods for estimating direct health care and individual costs are, in concept if not in execution, simple and are largely standard. Methods for estimating benefits (e.g. QALYs gained) are somewhat more sophisticated but, where data on utilities exist, accepted. The methodologies for measuring indirect costs, however, have had somewhat less attention and are polarized into two main conceptual areas, namely the human capital and frictional cost approaches, both already mentioned above. The former, which, strictly speaking, is valid only in the theoretical state of full employment, tends to overestimate indirect costs. The latter, which is a more realistic concept, is much more difficult to calculate and results in a considerably lower estimate [8].

As Brown *et al.* [11] point out, many studies have set out to estimate this social impact of diabetes. The ADA 2002 estimate [21] of the value of productivity lost to the US economy as a result of diabetes was 39.8 billion USD or 3290 USD per person per year. The WHO [56] has estimated that diabetes, heart disease and stroke together will cost 558 billion USD in lost income to China between 2005 and 2015, and even in a low-income country like Tanzania the cost is 2.5 billion USD. These estimates take into account premature mortality only and ignore the costs of lost production resulting from disability and sickness absence.

Early studies which included both direct and indirect costs (e.g. [26]) concluded that they were both of similar magnitude. This has not been confirmed by more recent studies, and that of the Economist Intelligence Unit [24] finds a very different (and unexplained) pattern of costs in the United Kingdom and United States from that of Denmark and India (**Table 37.3**). In the former, indirect costs are just over a quarter of total costs, whereas in the latter they are around 70% (Denmark) or almost 90% (India) of total costs. Further work is clearly necessary to clarify the balance between direct and indirect costs and to resolve the methodological uncertainties surrounding the latter.

37.11 CONCLUSIONS

An understanding of the economic issues that both individuals and society face in preventing, detecting and treating diabetes is vitally important. Health care choices are a reality of life throughout the world, and health care payers and providers must make decisions that affect not just diabetes, but also other noncommunicable and communicable diseases.

Although the estimation of costs has many difficulties (particularly that of indirect costs), these difficulties should not be an excuse for disinterest. Estimates of direct health care costs are a useful indication of the totality of the impact of diabetes on health systems and on families–an index superior to incidence, prevalence, hospital admission rates or lengths of hospital stay, each taken alone. The global disparity between annual public health expenditure per person with diabetes is enormous. Estimates of indirect costs, though currently inexact, are an important indication of the extent to which a region, a country or indeed the world forgoes wealth because of our currently inadequate attempts at preventing diabetes and its complications.

Cost of illness studies are the descriptive epidemiology of economics. Alone, they are barren. Evaluative studies are necessary to inform us of what we should do in terms of interventions. Cost-effective interventions that are feasible in context and which at least do not increase inequities are the target for preventive and therapeutic health services. Economics is one of the contributors to deciding how important and difficult choices can be made in the field of diabetes.

References

1. Simanis, J.G. (1987) Health care expenditures: international comparisons, 1970–80. *Social Security Bulletin*, **50**, 19–24.
2. Simanis, J.G. and Coleman, J.R. (1980) Health care expenditures in nine industrialized countries, 1960–76. *Social Security Bulletin*, **43**, 3–8.
3. Organization for Economic Cooperation and Development (1990) *Health Care Systems in Transition: The Search for Efficiency*, OECD Social Policy Studies No. 7, Organization for Economic Cooperation and Development, Paris, pp. 129–35.
4. Poullier, J.-P., Hernandez, P., Kawasata, K. and Savedoff, W.D. (2002) Patterns of Global Health Expenitures: Results for 199 Countries, EIP/HFS /FAR Discussion Paper No. 51, World Health Organization, Geneva.
5. Cohen, D.R. and Henderson, J.B. (1991) *Health, Prevention and Economics*, Oxford University Press, Oxford.
6. Hodgson, T.A. (1983) The state of the art of cost of illness estimates. *Advances in Health Economics and Health Services Research*, **4**, 129–64.
7. Lubeck, D.P. and Yelin, E.H. (1988) A question of value: measuring the impact of chronic disease. *The Milbank Quarterly*, **66**, 444–64.
8. Koopmanschap, M.A., Rutten, F.F.H., Ineveld, B.M. and Roijen, L. (1995) The friction cost method for measuring indirect costs of disease. *Journal of Health Economics*, **14**, 171–89.
9. Stukken, O. (2000) Gedetailleerde raming van de maatschappelijke kosten van diabetes mellitus. *Nederlands Tijdschrift voor Geneeskunde*, **144**, 842–6.
10. Williams, R. (2003) The economic impact of diabetes, in *Diabetes Atlas*, 2nd edn (ed D. Gan), International Diabetes Federation, Brussels.
11. Brown, B.B., Vistisen, D., Sicree, R. *et al.* (2006) The economic impacts of diabetes, in *Diabetes Atlas*, 3rd edn, International Diabetes Federation, Brussels, pp. 237–65.
12. Jönsson, B. (1998) The economic impact of diabetes. *Diabetes Care*, **21** (Suppl 3), C7–10.
13. Rice, D.P. (1966) *Estimating the Cost of Illness*, Health Economic Series No. 6, PHS Publication No. 947–6, US Government Printing Office, Washington, DC.
14. Cooper, B.S. and Rice, D.P. (1976) The economic cost of illness revisited. *Social Security Bulletin*, **39** (2), 21–6.
15. Rice, D.P., Hodgson, T.A. and Kopstein, A.N. (1985) The economic cost of illness; a replication and update. *Health Care Financing Review*, **7**, 61–80.
16. Hodgson, T.A. and Meiners, M.R. (1982) Cost of illness methodology, a guide to current practices and procedures. *The Milbank Memorial Fund Quarterly*, **60**, 463–91.
17. Scitovsky, A.A. (1982) Estimating the direct cost of illness. *The Milbank Memorial Fund Quarterly*, **60**, 429–62.
18. Barcelo, A., Aedo, C., Rajpathak, S. and Robles, S. (2003) The cost of diabetes in Latin America and the Caribbean. *Bulletin of the World Health Organization*, **81** (1), 19–27.
19. Koster, I., von Ferber, L., Ihle, P. *et al.* (2006) The cost burden of diabetes mellitus: the evidence from Germany–the CoDiM Study. *Diabetologia*, **49**, 1498–504.

20. Colagiuri, S., Colagiuri, R., Conway, B. *et al.* (2003) *DiabCost Australia: Assessing the Burden of Type 2 Diabetes in Australia*, Diabetes Australia, Canberra.

21. American Diabetes Association (2003) Economic costs of diabetes in the U.S. in 2002. *Diabetes Care*, **26**, 917–32.

22. Williams, R., Van Gaal, L. and Lucioni, C. (2002) Assessing the impact of complications on the costs of type 2 diabetes. *Diabetologia*, **45**, S13–17.

23. Sicree, R., Shaw, J. and Zimmet, P. (2006) Diabetes and impaired glucose tolerance, in *Diabetes Atlas*, 3rd edn, International Diabetes Federation, Brussels, pp. 15–109.

24. Economist Intelligence Unit (2007) *The Silent Epidemic: An Economic Study of Diabetes in Developed and Developing Countries. A Report from the Economist Intelligence Unit*, Economist Intelligence Unit, London.

25. Juvenile Diabetes Foundation (1996) The Economics of Medical Research, available at http://www .jdfcure.org/ (accessed May 2008).

26. Rubin, R.J., Altman, W.N. and Medelson, D.N. (1994) Health care expenditures for people with diabetes mellitus, 1992. *The Journal of Clinical Endocrinology and Metabolism*, **78**, 809A–809F.

27. Vinicor, F. and Engelgau, M. (2006) Health insurance for all: the key to improved diabetes management? *Diabetes Voice*, **51**, 34–6.

28. Songer, T.J., LaPorte, R.E., Lave, J.R. *et al.* (1997) Health insurance and the financial impact of IDDM among families with a child with IDDM. *Diabetes Care*, **20**, 577–84.

29. Aubert, R.E., Geiss, L.S., Ballard, D.J. *et al.* (1995) Diabetes-related hospitalization and hospital utilization, in *Diabetes in America*, 2nd edn, (eds M.I. Harris, C.C. Cowie, M.P. Stern *et al.*), National Institute of Health Publication No. 95-1468, US Government Printing Office, Bethesda, MD.

30. Taylor, A.K. (1987) Medical expenditures and insurance coverage for people with diabetes: estimates from the National Medical Care Expenditure Survey. *Diabetes Care*, **10**, 87–94.

31. Shobhana, R., Rao, P.R., Lavanya, A. *et al.* (2000) Expenditure on health care incurred by diabetic subjects in a developing country–a study from southern India. *Diabetes Research and Clinical Practice*, **48**, 37–42.

32. Ramachandran, A., Ramachandran, S., Snehalatha, C. *et al.* (2007) Increasing expenditure on health care incurred by diabetic subjects in a developing country. *Diabetes Care*, **30**, 252–6.

33. Drummond, M.F. and Stoddart, G.L. (1995) Principles of economic evaluation of health programmes. *World Health Statistics Quarterly*, **38**, 335–76.

34. Udvarhelyi, I.S., Colditz, G.A., Rai, A. and Epstein, A.M. (1992) Cost–effectiveness and cost–benefit analyses in the medical literature. Are the methods being used correctly? *Annals of Internal Medicine*, **116**, 238–44.

35. Gold, M.R., Siegel, J.E., Russel, L.B. and Winstein, M.C. (eds) (1996) *Cost-Effectiveness in Health and Medicine*, Oxford University Press, Oxford, pp. 304–12.

36. Drummond, M.F. and Sculpher, M. (2005) Common methodological flaws in economic evaluations. *Medical Care*, **43**, 5–14.

37. Kaplan, R.M. and Davis, W.K. (1986) Evaluating the costs and benefits of outpatient diabetes education and nutrition counselling. *Diabetes Care*, **9**, 81–6.

38. Songer, T. (2001) Economic costs, in *The Epidemiology of Diabetes Mellitus* (eds J.-M. Ekoé, P. Zimmet and R. Williams), John Wiley & Sons, Ltd, Chichester.

39. Javitt, J.C., Canner, J.K., Frank, R.G. *et al.* (1990) Detecting and treating retinopathy in patients with type 1 mellitus: a health policy model. *Ophthalmology*, **97**, 483–95.

40. Javitt, J.C., Ferris, F.L., Aiello, L.P. *et al.* (1994) Preventative eye care in people with diabetes is cost-saving to the federal government; implications for health care-reform. *Diabetes Care*, **17** (8), 909–17.

41. Javitt, J.C. and Aidello, L.P. (1996) Cost-effectiveness of detecting and treating retinopathy. *Annals of Internal Medicine*, **124**, 164–9.

42. Swanson, M. (2005) Retinopathy screening in individuals with type 2 diabetes: who, how, how often, and at what cost–an epidemiologic review. *Optometry*, **76**, 636–46.

43. Dasbach, E.J., Fryback, D.G., Newcomb, P.A. *et al.* (1991) Cost-effectiveness of strategies for detecting diabetic retinopathy in patients with type 1 diabetes mellitus; savings associated with improved implementation of current guidelines. *Ophthalmology*, **98**, 1565–74.

44. World Bank (2008) *Disease Control Priorities in Developing Countries*, 2nd edn, World Bank, Chapter 30, available at http://www.dcp2.org /pubs/DCP/30/FullText (accessed 4 January 2008).

45. Eckman, M.H., Greenfield, S., Mackey, W.C. *et al.* (1995) Foot infections in diabetic patients: decision and cost-effectiveness analyses. *Journal of the American Medical Association*, **273** (9), 712–20.

46. Ortegon, M.M., Redekap, W.K. and Niesen, L.W. (2004) Cost-effectiveness of prevention and

treatment of the diabetic foot: a Markov analysis. *Diabetes care*, **27**, 901–7.

47. Matricali, G.A., Dereymaeker, G., Muls, E. *et al.* (2007) Economic aspects of diabetic foot care in a multi-disciplinary setting: a review. *Diabetes/Metabolism Research and Reviews*, **23**, 339–47.

48. Stern, Z. and Levy, R. (1996) Analysis of direct cost of standard compared with intensive insulin treatment of insulin-dependent diabetes mellitus and costs of complications. *Diabetologia*, **33**, 48–52.

49. The DCCT Research Group (1997) Lifetime benefits and costs of intensive therapy as practiced in the Diabetes Control and Complications Trial: an economic evaluation. *Journal of the American Medical Association*, **278**, 1409–15.

50. Eastman, R.C., Javitt, J.C., Herman, W.H. *et al.* (1997) Model of complications of NIDDM II: analysis of the health benefits and cost-effectiveness of treating NIDDM with the goal of normoglycaemia. *Diabetes Care*, **20**, 735–44.

51. Huang, E., Shook, M., Jin, L. *et al.* (2006) The impact of patient preferences on the cost-effectiveness of intensive glucose control in older patients with new-onset diabetes. *Diabetes Care*, **29**, 259–64.

52. Clarke, P.M., Gray, A.M., Briggs, A. *et al.* (2005) Cost–utility of intensive blood glucose and tight blood pressure control in type 2 diabetes (UKPDS 72). *Diabetologia*, **48**, 868–77.

53. Pedersen, O. and Gaede, P. (2003) Intensified multifactorial intervention and cardiovascular outcome in type 2 diabetes: the Steno-2 study. *Metabolism*, **52**, 19–23.

54. Herman, W.H., Hoerger, T.J., Brandle, M. *et al.* (2005) The cost-effectiveness of lifestyle modification or metformin in preventing type 2 diabetes in adults with impaired glucose tolerance. *Annals of Internal Medicine*, **142**, 323–32.

55. Williams, R. and Shaw, J. (2006) Prevention and diabetes: possibilities for success and consequences of inaction, in *Diabetes Atlas*, 3rd edn, International Diabetes Federation, Brussels, pp. 317–25.

56. World Health Organization (2005) *Preventing Chronic Disease: A Vital Investment*, World Health Organization, Geneva.

Further Reading

Schroeder, S. (2001) Prospects for expanding health insurance coverage. *The New England Journal of Medicine*, **344**, 847–52.

38

Clinical Practice Guidelines: A Global Perspective

Barbara Currie, Ehud Ur and Thomas Ransom

Division of Endocrinology, QEII Health Sciences Centre, Halifax, Nova Scotia, Canada

38.1 HISTORY OF CLINICAL PRACTICE GUIDELINES

Clinical practice guidelines (CPGs) have been developed internationally to assist with the translation of research into everyday practice for the purpose of improving care for persons with diabetes. Whereas the prevalence of type 1 diabetes mellitus (T1DM) remains relatively constant, the global rise in the prevalence of type 2 diabetes mellitus (T2DM) is reaching epidemic proportions and most developed countries are presented with staggering increases in the economic burden of diabetes and its related complications. The total number of persons worldwide with diabetes is projected to rise from 171 million in 2000 to 366 million in 2030, with the most striking global demographic change occurring in persons greater than 65 years of age [1]. According to the World Health Organization (WHO), most of the new cases of T2DM diagnosed over the next decade will occur in Asia and other parts of the developing world, where Western cultural influences and improved living standards are producing an increase in physical inactivity and obesity, both important risk factors for T2DM. As a result, the population with diabetes in these countries will grow at a much faster rate than the overall population. By the year 2010, Asia is expected to have over 60% of the world's diabetes cases. In Canada, diabetes is now being recognized as a public health problem of enormous proportions. Over 1 million Canadians are currently living with diabetes, and

age-standardized rates of diabetes among Aboriginal peoples are triple those found in the general population [2].

Over the past 20 years, guidelines have emerged as popular tools for the synthesis and dissemination of medical research with the goal of influencing health outcomes for a particular disease by reducing the delivery of inappropriate care and supporting the dissemination of new knowledge into clinical practice [3]. Given the increasing concerns over quality of care, marked variation in practice and increasing health care costs, many believe that guidelines could be the vehicle to address the growing demand for disease management, especially chronic disease management, and population health worldwide. In 1992, the Canadian Diabetes Advisory Board produced the first Canadian CPGs to address the educational needs of primary care physicians and other members of the diabetes health care teams involved in the management of persons with diabetes [4]. Without the benefit of evidence from the United Kingdom Prospective Diabetes Study (UKPDS) and Diabetes Control and Complications Trial (DCCT) data, formation of these guidelines relied heavily on expert opinion. With the emergence of the landmark UKPDS and DCCT data, the 1992 guidelines were revised in 1998 by the Clinical and Scientific Section of the Canadian Diabetes Association (CDA) to reflect advances in diagnosis and outpatient management of diabetes [5]. These were amongst the first practice guidelines in diabetes to identify and assess the

The Epidemiology of Diabetes Mellitus, second edition   Edited by Jean-Marie Ekoé, Marian Rewers, Rhys Williams and Paul Zimmet
© 2008 John Wiley & Sons, Ltd

scientific literature supporting the recommendations systematically. Major changes from the 1992 document included the reclassification of the types of diabetes based on pathogenesis, increased sensitivity of criteria for diagnosis, recommendations for screening and tighter metabolic control, and improved delivery of care; and optimal methods were identified for screening, prevention and treatment of diabetes-related complications. With the increasing number of guidelines being developed for specific diseases, the process of developing guidelines became a rigorous science in and of itself. In 2003, the third Canadian CPGs were released in Canada and represented a more thorough scientific approach [6]. The guidelines were formalized with documentation of the literature search, grading of the evidence and grading of each recommendation.

There has been a proliferation of practice guidelines for the treatment of diabetes worldwide, with many countries generating guidelines for the prevention, management and treatment of diabetes and its related complications that best reflect their unique demographics and economic means. In general, there has been a greater emphasis on creating guidelines that pertain to T2DM given that T2DM has a much higher prevalence and is more complex than T1DM in terms of diagnosis, management and associated metabolic disturbances. As multiple guidelines are developed utilizing the same clinical research, one can only assume that there would be natural convergence of recommendations and management strategies. In an attempt to standardize care and reduce the diabetes-related burden of disease, many countries and organizations have made great efforts and committed significant amounts of resources in the development of practice guidelines. Despite tremendous efforts to develop sound guidelines objectively and scientifically, there exists some disparity between individual guidelines that has subsequently generated questions around possible intrinsic bias and conflict of interest of the developers. As the chapter authors discovered, there is debate ensuing within the health care literature on the credibility of CPGs and their ability to affect meaningful health outcomes for a variety of identified diseases.

Any given recommendation may impact significantly an individual patient and/or a health care system, with this concept being most obvious as it

pertains to the economic burden of diabetes. The cost of diabetes to an individual can be staggering, with the impact of a single recommendation resulting in marked financial stress. A recommendation that applies to millions of patients can have profound economic implications. There is much money to be made in the diabetic industry from the individual health care provider to the pharmaceutical and device industries. Direct costs for medications and supplies for a person with diabetes in Canada can range from $1000 to $15 000 a year and diabetes with its associated complications costs the Canadian health care system approximately $13.2 billion every year, with this value expected to rise to $15.6 billion a year by 2010 and to $19.2 billion a year by 2020 [7]. In general, disease-specific guidelines are written by experts who represent the various stakeholders pertaining to the disease in question. Often, the experts who write the guidelines have been involved in the creation of the evidence upon which the specific guideline is based and this calls into question the potential for bias or conflict of interest:

> Conflict of interest exists when an author (or the author's institution), reviewer, or editor has financial or personal relationships that inappropriately influence (bias) his or her actions (such relationships are also known as dual commitments, competing interests, or competing loyalties) [8].

Increasingly, the methods by which guidelines are developed and the processes taken to ensure their validity are being scrutinized not only by their end users, but also by researchers in general. To address the issue of conflict of interest, the Appraisal of Guidelines Research and Evaluation (AGREE) Collaboration has created validated tools for users to rate guidelines according to the rigor of the developmental process and editorial independence so as to judge the potential for bias [9]. The evaluation of the guideline development process asks questions such as: Was the literature search thorough and systematic? Was the search well documented? Is there explicit evidence linked to a given recommendation? Was the evidence graded? When considering editorial independence, the AGREE instrument allows the users to assess and grade issues such as industry sponsorship of the guideline development and authors' declarations of potential conflicts of interest.

When asked to write this chapter on the world-wide daily fight against diabetes focusing on CPGs from Canada and comparing them with those from the United States, Europe and New Zealand, we first set out to compare and contrast the various guidelines utilizing a standardized evaluative approach. However, as we progressed in our own review of the literature, a predominant theme emerged that was both surprising and enlightening, namely the global concern over the actual validity of disease-specific practice guidelines and the quest for a standardized development instrument. This concern has manifested itself in the quest for research supporting the development of unbiased guidelines that are able to demonstrate measurable differences in the outcomes of disease management from the perspective of health economics.

38.2 GUIDELINES FOR GUIDELINES

CPGs are defined as 'systematically developed statements to assist practitioner and patient decisions the massive volumes of medical about appropriate health care for specific clinical circumstances' [10]. Given research generated within the last 20 years, CPGs have emerged as the cornerstone of evidence-based best practice for a variety of chronic diseases of which diabetes is no exception. CPGs serve the purpose of collecting, deciphering and making sense of the plethora of research that has inundated health care professionals' daily existence, and to provide an evidence-based reference source for practicing clinicians. However, there is a shared opinion that the benefits will not be realized until well-developed and valid guidelines are implemented by clinicians and policy-makers worldwide [11–17].

Within the medical literature over the last 10–15 years, there has been an increase in the published work on how to appraise primary research critically [18–21]. However, the application of a critical appraisal approach to guidelines is not as developed. In 1992 the Institute of Medicine (IOM) developed a provisional appraisal instrument based on a number of 'desirable attributes' of good guidelines [22]. Since this time, a number of studies have examined the methods used to develop guidelines and found the majority did not meet established standards. For example, in a study to determine whether practice guidelines published in the peer-reviewed medical literature between 1985 and 1997 adhered to established methodological standards, Shaneyfelt *et al.* [16] examined 279 guidelines and found that the mean adherence to standards by each guideline was only 43%, but that the methodological quality of guideline development was improving over time. The authors identified the areas of CPGs requiring the greatest improvements were identification, evaluation and synthesis of the scientific evidence. Likewise, Grilli *et al.* [17], in a survey of 431 guidelines produced by specialty societies between 1988 and 1998, found that 67% did not report any description of the type of stakeholders involved in the development, 88% gave no information on how the published evidence was identified (i.e. search methods) and 82% did not give any explicit grading of the strength of the recommendations. Despite these disturbing statistics, the authors did acknowledge that there was improvement over time for search methods (from 2% to 18%, $p < 0.001$) and explicit grading of evidence (from 6% to 27%, $p < 0.001$). The authors recommended that explicit methodological criteria for the development of guidelines be established and shared among public agencies, scientific societies and patients' associations. Similarly, in an attempt to address the growing global problem of guideline development validity, Cluzeau *et al.* [12] developed an appraisal instrument to assess whether developers of 60 guidelines published between 1991 and 1996 took appropriate actions to minimize the biases inherent in creating guidelines, and identified requirements for effective implementation. The instrument is comprised of 37 items describing suggested predictors of guideline quality grouped into three dimensions that address rigor of development, clarity of presentation (including context and content) and implementation issues. In a similar fashion, under the auspices of the AGREE Collaboration, an international collaborative team in the United Kingdom, the AGREE Instrument [9] was developed. The AGREE Instrument was designed to serve as a generic tool to assist guideline developers and to aid guideline users in assessing the methodological quality of CPGs. This instrument addresses the internal and external validity of the CPGs, and assesses their feasibility for practice. The process takes into account the benefits, harms and costs of the specific recommendations, as well as the practical issues attached to the guidelines. By virtue of the instrument design, it requires judgments about the methods used for guideline development, the content of the final recommendations and the factors linked to their uptake. Cluzeau *et al.*'s Appraisal Instrument for Clinical Guidelines and the AGREE Instrument for the evaluation of guideline development are the most frequently cited tools in the medical literature on guideline appraisal.

In a Canadian study by Graham *et al.* [11], three independent appraisers utilizing the 'Appraisal Instrument for Clinical Guidelines' evaluated 217 drug therapy guidelines produced or reviewed from 1994 to 1998 on rigor of guideline development, context and content and application. Of the 217 guidelines, only 14.7% met half or more of the 20 items that assessed rigor of development, 61.8% met half or more of the 12 items assessing guideline context and content and, surprisingly, not one met half or more of the five items assessing guideline application. The authors concluded that the quality of guidelines assessed varied considerably depending on the developer, publication status and degree of drug company involvement/sponsorship and showed little improvement in quality over the 5-year study period.

An international study by Burgers *et al.* [23] compared 15 T2DM guidelines from 13 countries for the purpose of examining whether differences in recommendations could be explained by the incorporation of different research evidence throughout the guideline development process. Using the AGREE Instrument, the clinical guidelines were evaluated by comparing the recommendations and specific bibliometric methods in an effort to measure the extent of overlap in citations used by the various guidelines. Overall, there was a high degree of international agreement in recommendations made with respect to the clinical management of T2DM; however, only 18% (185/1033) of citations were shared with at least one other guideline, and only 1% (10 studies) appeared in six or more guidelines. When reviews and multiple publications from the same study were taken into account, the measurable overlap in evidence between guidelines increased. Forty percent of the research originated in the United States; however, 91% (11/12) of guidelines were more likely to cite evidence originating from their own country. Despite the globalization of research evidence through easily accessible bibliographic databases, there is still not international consensus on the evidence chosen to strengthen the management of T2DM. Many of the differences in the dissemination and implementation of guidelines are secondary to differences in health care systems and political and cultural factors unique to the country of origin. As a result, globalization of recommended diabetes management continues to be a challenge and international collaboration is required to improve guideline methodology and analyses of the burgeoning medical literature [24]. Grilli *et al.* [17] suggest that

> guidelines developed by specialty societies fall short of the desirable infomativeness since practice guidelines are meant to inform and guide choices in health care and, as such, should be explicit and transparent.

38.3 COMPARISON OF INTERNATIONAL GUIDELINES

On comparison of the actual recommendations in the different CPGs there is considerable agreement, with most differences being minor. Such comparisons are limited, given that not all CPGs address the same issues; for example, many CPGs are written for T2DM only, with no recommendations for T1DM. Also, each national set of CPGs may have unique recommendations applicable to its special populations only. On review of specific recommendations that are universally addressed there are occasionally few small differences. For example, the recommended low-density lipoprotein targets may differ by a few percent, but this may represent a lag time between publications, with the more recent CPGs having access to pertinent data not previously available, or the difference may simply represent the rounding up or down of a number as it is converted from imperial to metric units or vice versa. In general, as the amount and level of evidence increases pertaining to a specific recommendation, the greater the agreement and the higher the grade of the recommendation, if there is a grading system, as is seen with blood pressure and lipid recommendations. As the level of evidence decreases, the differences in recommendations increase, with an example being the slightly more aggressive recommendations for screening in the CDA guidelines compared with those in the American Diabetes Association (ADA) guidelines (**Figure 38.1**).

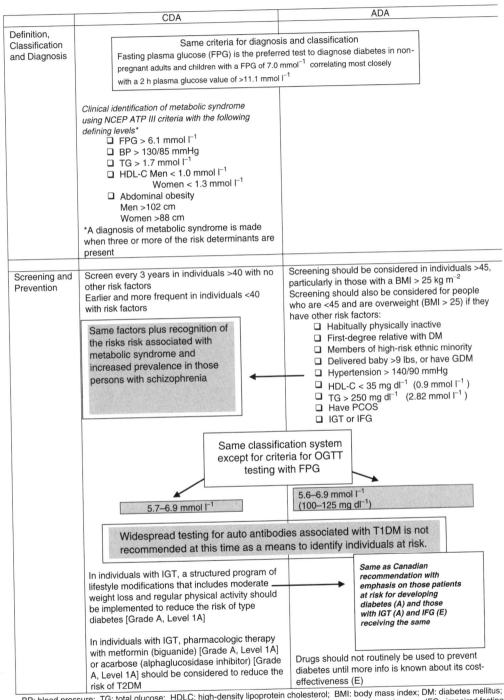

	CDA	ADA
Definition, Classification and Diagnosis	Same criteria for diagnosis and classification Fasting plasma glucose (FPG) is the preferred test to diagnose diabetes in non-pregnant adults and children with a FPG of 7.0 mmol^{-1} correlating most closely with a 2 h plasma glucose value of >11.1 mmol l^{-1}	

	Clinical identification of metabolic syndrome using NCEP ATP III criteria with the following defining levels*
	❏ FPG > 6.1 mmol l^{-1}
	❏ BP > 130/85 mmHg
	❏ TG > 1.7 mmol l^{-1}
	❏ HDL-C Men < 1.0 mmol l^{-1}
	         Women < 1.3 mmol l^{-1}
	❏ Abdominal obesity
	         Men >102 cm
	         Women >88 cm
	*A diagnosis of metabolic syndrome is made when three or more of the risk determinants are present	

The figure content reads:

Screening and Prevention

CDA: Screen every 3 years in individuals >40 with no other risk factors. Earlier and more frequent in individuals <40 with risk factors

Same factors plus recognition of the risks risk associated with metabolic syndrome and increased prevalence in those persons with schizophrenia

ADA: Screening should be considered in individuals >45, particularly in those with a BMI > 25 kg m^{-2}. Screening should also be considered for people who are <45 and are overweight (BMI > 25) if they have other risk factors:
❏ Habitually physically inactive
❏ First-degree relative with DM
❏ Members of high-risk ethnic minority
❏ Delivered baby >9 lbs, or have GDM
❏ Hypertension > 140/90 mmHg
❏ HDL-C < 35 mg dl^{-1} (0.9 mmol l^{-1})
❏ TG > 250 mg dl^{-1} (2.82 mmol l^{-1})
❏ Have PCOS
❏ IGT or IFG

Same classification system except for criteria for OGTT testing with FPG

5.7–6.9 mmol l^{-1}

5.6–6.9 mmol l^{-1} (100–125 mg dl^{-1})

Widespread testing for auto antibodies associated with T1DM is not recommended at this time as a means to identify individuals at risk.

In individuals with IGT, a structured program of lifestyle modifications that includes moderate weight loss and regular physical activity should be implemented to reduce the risk of type diabetes [Grade A, Level 1A]

Same as Canadian recommendation with emphasis on those patients at risk for developing diabetes (A) and those with IGT (A) and IFG (E) receiving the same

In individuals with IGT, pharmacologic therapy with metformin (biguanide) [Grade A, Level 1A] or acarbose (alphaglucosidase inhibitor) [Grade A, Level 1A] should be considered to reduce the risk of T2DM

Drugs should not routinely be used to prevent diabetes until more info is known about its cost-effectiveness (E)

BP: blood pressure; TG: total glucose; HDLC: high-density lipoprotein cholesterol; BMI: body mass index; DM: diabetes mellitus; GDM: gestational diabetes mellitus; PCOS: polycystic ovarian syndrome; IGT: impaired glucose tolerance; IFG: impaired fasting glucose; OGTT: oral glucose tolerance test. New Zealand: T2DM only, does not cover diagnosis and the user is referred to the national guidelines for assessment and management of cardiovascular risk where screening for T2DM is addressed. IDF: uses the same diagnostic criteria. The issue of screening is discussed with no specific strategy being recommend; however, the authors suggest that the decision by a health care service to screen or not should be based on the prevalence of undiagnosed T2DM, the population's willingness to be screened, the health system's capacity to do the screening and manage those who test positive, and the cost to both the individual and the health care system.

Figure 38.1 Sample recommendation comparisons.

Table 38.1 Criteria for assigning levels of evidence to the published studies (CDA).

Level	Criteria
Studies of diagnosis	
Level 1	(i) Independent interpretation of test results (without knowledge of the result of the diagnostic or gold standard)
	(ii) Independent interpretation of the diagnostic standard (without knowledge of the test result)
	(iii) Selection of people suspected (but not known) to have the disorder
	(iv) Reproducible description of both the test and diagnostic standard
	(v) At least 50 patients with and 50 without the disorder
Level 2	Meets four of the Level 1 criteria
Level 3	Meets three of the Level 1 criteria
Level 4	Meets one or two of the Level 1 criteria
Studies of treatment and prevention	
Level 1A	Systematic overview or meta-analysis of high quality randomized, controlled trials Appropriately designed randomized, controlled trial with adequate power to answer the question posed by the investigators
Level 1B	Nonrandomized clinical trial or cohort study with indisputable results
Level 2	Randomized, controlled trial or systematic overview that does not meet Level 1 criteria
Level 3	Nonrandomized clinical trial or cohort study
Level 4	Other
Studies of prognosis	
Level 1	(a) Inception cohort of patients with the condition of interest, but free of the outcome of interest
	(b) Reproducible inclusion/exclusion criteria
	(c) Follow-up of at least 80% of subjects
	(d) Statistical adjustment for extraneous prognostic factors (confounders)
	(e) Reproducible description of outcome measures
Level 2	Meets criterion (a) above, plus three of the other four criteria
Level 3	Meets criterion (a) above, plus two of the other criteria
Level 4	Meets criterion (a) above, plus one of the other criteria

In the context of comparing CPGs and their specific recommendations it is important not only to know what literature was reviewed, but also how it was evaluated and how the evaluation in turn affected the grade or level of confidence in the given recommendation. **Table 38.1** illustrates the criteria used to grade evidence and **Table 38.2** gives the criteria for assigning grades to the recommendations by the CDA.

Similarly, the ADA developed a classification system to grade quality of scientific evidence

Table 38.2 Criteria for assigning grades of recommendations for clinical practice (CDA).

Grade	Criteria
A	The best evidence was at Level 1
B	The best evidence was at Level 2
C	The best evidence was at Level 3
D	The best evidence was at Level 4 or consensus

supporting their recommendations. The ADA recommendations were assigned ratings of A, B or C, depending on the quality of the study being reviewed. Expert opinion (E) was assigned to recommendations in which there was no evidence existent from clinical trials or in the case where trials may have been impractical, or in which there was conflicting evidence (**Table 38.3**).

The CPGs from New Zealand are a modified composite of a few preexisting CPGs from other international organizations. For the evaluation of the evidence the New Zealand authors honored the grading systems of the parent CPGs from which the individual recommendations came. For the grading of the individual recommendations, one grading system was chosen as the standard, with

adjustments being made and noted when a recommendation came from a guideline using a different grading system. The International Diabetes Federation (IDF) CPGs did not include formal grading of the literature or the recommendations.

Comparing CPGs using a formalized grading instrument is conceptually easy but practically very difficult. The four CPGs chosen represent significantly different approaches to the development of their specific guideline, and the tools to evaluate them are not universally applicable. Each set of guidelines has its unique purpose and each CPG development team had access to different resources. Direct comparison of the four CPGs is not entirely appropriate. Despite the limitations of the grading tools, we elected to use Cluzeau *et al.*'s

Table 38.3 ADA evidence grading system for clinical practice recommendations.

Level of evidence	Description
A	Clear evidence from well-controlled, generalizable, randomized controlled trials that are adequately powered, including: • evidence from a well-conducted multicenter trial • evidence from a meta-analysis that incorporated quality ratings in the analysis • compelling nonexperimental evidence; that is, 'all or none' rule developed by the Centre for Evidence Based Medicine at Oxford[a] Supportive evidence from well-conducted randomized controlled trials that are adequately powered, including: • evidence from a well-conducted trial at one or more institutions • evidence from a meta-analysis that incorporated quality ratings in the analysis
B	Supportive evidence from well-conducted cohort studies, including: • evidence from a well-conducted prospective cohort study or registry • evidence from a well-conducted meta-analysis of cohort studies Supportive evidence from a well-conducted case–control study
C	Supportive evidence from poorly controlled or uncontrolled studies, including: • evidence from randomized clinical trials with one or more major or three or more minor methodological flaws that could invalidate the results • evidence from observational studies with high potential for bias (such as case series with comparison with historical controls) • evidence from case series or case reports Conflicting evidence with the weight of evidence supporting recommendations
E	Expert consensus or clinical experience

Either all patients died before therapy and at least some survived with therapy, or some patients died without therapy and none died with therapy. Example: use of insulin in the treatment of diabetic ketoacidosis.

Appraisal Instrument for Clinical Guidelines as a guide for commenting on the CPGs from Canada [6], the United States [25–32], Europe [33] and New Zealand [34], highlighting commonalities and differences in guideline development. Recognizing that we are not formally trained critical appraisers of guideline development, we followed the user's guide that accompanies the appraisal instrument and present to the reader a modest objective evaluation of the four above-mentioned guidelines (**Table 38.4**).

The Canadian CPGs represent an all-encompassing set of guidelines in a single document developed by a national team of experts under the CDA and are updated every 5 years. Resources allow for a rigorous developmental process for each recommendation. The ADA's CPG is a compilation of position statements (official points of view or beliefs of the ADA), technical reviews (reviews and analysis of the literature that provides scientific rational for position statements) and consensus statements (developed by panels of experts after comprehensive examinations of medical issues pertaining to diabetes). Position statements are updated as necessary according to new relevant literature. This approach results in a cumulative body of recommendations that is as up to date as possible, with summary statements highlighting changes being published on a routine basis. The New Zealand CPGs were created in the context of not having the resources of the ADA and CDA. The approach of the developers was to adopt recommendations from a few agreed-upon existing CPGs, with one being the principal CPG, and make adjustments when deemed appropriate. This approach is cost-effective and appropriate for many nations. The IDF has developed a 'Levels of care approach' in the context of most published national guidelines coming from relatively resource-rich countries, which may not be applicable in countries with limited resources. They have proposed three levels of care as follows:

Standard care: Evidence-based care, cost-effective in most nations with a well developed service base and with health care funding systems consuming a significant part of their national wealth.
Minimal care: Care that seeks to achieve the major objectives of diabetes management, but is provided in health care settings with very limited resources – drugs, personnel, technologies and procedures.
Comprehensive care: Care with some evidence-base that is provided in health care settings with considerable resources.

The recommendations in the IDF guidelines are based on recent existing international CPGs considered to be of high quality, and section authors considered data published since the release of the CPGs so as to be as up to date as possible. Each set of recommendations in a given section of the guidelines is accompanied by documentation of the rationale and evidence supporting the recommendations, and mention is made about strategies for implementation and evaluation.

38.4   THE FUTURE OF GUIDELINES

Guidelines from around the globe are expected to converge in the context of standardization of methodology and evaluation of evidence. Tools to guide and evaluate guideline development will continue to evolve and become increasingly more important in ensuring adherence to rigorous developmental processes, appropriateness of content and avoidance of bias. Future CPGs will likely resemble a composite of the four guidelines reviewed in this chapter with the rigor of the Canadians' developmental process, the Americans' method to keep the guidelines current, the approach of the IDF's levels of care so as to be appropriate according to a population's resources and New Zealand's method of adopting preexisting recommendations and modifying them to fit their unique population.

The next important stages pertaining to CPGs will be implementation and evaluation of impact. We must all ask ourselves whether guidelines have made a difference in delivery of care and clinical outcomes. CPGs may outline recommendations that, if followed, would result in optimal health but which without effective implementation strategies their effectiveness is diminished. Currently, little is known about the impact of CPGs for diabetes. Some clinicians and researchers may argue that perhaps it is too soon to measure the success or failure of the 'new' guidelines in view of the fact that only since the advent of the UKPDS data have diabetes professionals truly appreciated the

Table 38.4 Comparison of the CDA, ADA, IDF and New Zealand (NZ) clinical practice guidelines.

Clinical practice guidelines	CDA	ADA	IDF	NZ
Dimension 1: Rigor of development				
Responsibility of guideline development				
1. Is the agency responsible for the development of the guidelines clearly identified?	Yes – Clinical and Scientific Section of the Canadian Diabetes Association	Yes – American Diabetes Association	Yes – International Diabetes Federation (IDF)	Yes – New Zealand Guideline group
2. Was external funding or other support received for developing the guidelines?	Yes	Explicit funding sources not identified in the 2006 Supplement issued in *Diabetes Care*, **29**, (Suppl 1)	Yes – industry sponsorship acknowledged. Industry did not take part in development but were able to comment on draft versions	No – funding from Ministry of Health
3. If external funding or support was received, is there evidence that the potential biases of the funding body(ies) were taken into account?	Yes			
Guideline development group				
4. Is there a description of the individuals (e.g. professionals, interest groups – including patients) who were involved in the guidelines development group?	Good representation from all relevant disciplines – no mention of patient representation	Good representation from all relevant disciplines – no mention of patient representation	Broad-based group including people with diabetes, health-care professionals from diverse disciplines, and people from non-governmental organizations	Good representation from all relevant disciplines with both aboriginal (Māori) and non-aboriginal consumer representation
5. If so, did the group contain representatives of all key disciplines?				
Identification and interpretation of evidence				
6. Is there a description of the sources of information used to select the evidence on which the recommendations are based?	Inclusion criteria are not explicit (i.e. search tools not identified)	Literature search used to select the evidence not explicit. Grading system identified (Table 38.2)	Recommendations were taken from existing international guidelines published over the preceding 5 years and used as a 'base' with revisions based on an	Recommendations from three existing international guidelines were used as a 'base' with revisions based on regional particularities and an updated literature
7. If so, are the sources of information adequate?	Exclusion criteria clearly stated	ADA Clinical practice recommendations consist		

(continued overleaf)

Table 38.4 (*continued*)

Clinical practice guidelines	CDA	ADA	IDF	NZ
8. Is there a description of the methods(s) used to interpret and assess the strength of the evidence?	Clear description of methods used to assess strength of evidence. Each recommendation graded (Table X) and accompanied by the corresponding research citation	of position statements that represent official ADA opinion as denoted by formal review and approval by the Professional Practice Committee and the Executive Committee of the Board of Directors	updated literature searches The authors state that their methodology is not described in detail in the document but follows principles of guideline development. No grading of the evidence or guidelines is made. Each recommendation is supported by brief rationale and evidence sections	search. Literature search methodology not explicit. One grading system was chosen as the standard – adjustments were made and noted when a recommendation came from a guideline using a different grading system. Each recommendation graded and accompanied by the corresponding research citation
9. Is so, is (are) the method(s) for rating the evidence satisfactory?				
Formulation of recommendations				
10. Is there a description of the methods used to formulate the recommendations?		ADA statements, consensus statements and technical review are not official ADA recommendations; however invited guests produce them under the auspices of the Association		
11. If so, are the methods satisfactory?				
12. Is there an indication of how the views of interested parties not on the panel were taken into account?				
13. Is there an explicit link between the major recommendations and the supporting evidence?				
Peer review				
14. Were the guidelines independently reviewed prior to their publication/release?	Yes	Yes	Good explanation of the review process and how recommendations were incorporated	Reviewed externally using AGREE instrument.
15. If so, is explicit information given about methods and how comments were addressed?	Feedback was 'incorporated' from stakeholders; however, no description of the major revisions is mentioned	Feedback was 'incorporated' from stakeholders; however, no description of the major revisions is mentioned		Feedback solicited from a variety of stakeholders and a draft made available on a governmental website for comment. Not stated explicitly how comments were addressed
16. Were the guidelines piloted?	Guidelines were not piloted	Guidelines were not piloted	Guidelines were not piloted	Guidelines were not piloted

	Guideline 1	Guideline 2	Guideline 3	Guideline 4
17. If the guidelines were piloted, is explicit information given about the methods used and the results adopted?				
Updating				
18. Is there a mention of a date for reviewing or updating the guidelines?	Guidelines are reviewed every 5 years; however, no explicit statement of this process is provided	Position statements are updated as necessary according to new relevant literature	IDF will consider updating in 3 to 5 years. Reviewers and process not explicitly stated	Planned section updates
19. Is the body responsible for the reviewing and updating clearly identified?				Reviewers not identified
Overall assessment of development process				
20. Overall, have the potential biases of guideline development been adequately dealt with?	Transparent process with the exception of clear identification of the sources of evidence selected for review	The different position statements, consensus statements and technical reviews vary in their degree of documentation pertaining to development and potential bias	Well-documented 'hands off' industry funding of guideline development but lacking in disclosers of the individual section authors	Documented declarations of competing interests
Dimension 2: Context and Content				
Objectives				
21. Are the reasons for the development of the guidelines clearly stated?	Purpose of guidelines clearly stated along with target population. The overall goal is to translate evidence into practice and help to shape health care policy. Minority populations are addressed including separate sections for the treatment and management of type 1 DM, aboriginal people and the elderly. Individual patient preferences are taken into account whenever recommendations have associated risks	Purpose of guidelines is stated with limited background information on the significant US health care burden associated with the disease. 'Standards of Care' are intended to provide clinicians, patients, researchers, payors and other interested individuals with the components of diabetes care, treatment goals and tools to evaluate the quality of care	Clear rationale for the creation of 'global' guidelines and the reasoning behind the different levels of care	Reasons and objectives clear and well defined. Goals are to close the 'practice gap'
22. Are the objectives of the guidelines clearly defined?				
Content				
23. Is there a satisfactory description of the patients to which the guidelines are meant to apply?			Implicit to the levels of care feature of the guidelines is the ability to apply the recommendations to most individuals worldwide	Although scope is limited it is well defined, e.g. not for children or patients with gestational diabetes
24. Is there a description of the circumstances (clinical or nonclinical) in which exceptions might be made in using the guidelines?				
25. Is there an explicit statement of how the patient's preferences should be taken into account in applying the guidelines?			Mention is given to both population and individual preferences	No explicit mention of approach to exceptions or accommodating patient preferences

(continued overleaf)

Table 38.4 (*continued*)

Clinical practice guidelines	CDA	ADA	IDF	NZ
Clarity				
26. Do the guidelines describe the condition to be detected, treated, or prevented in unambiguous terms?	Classification and diagnostic criteria for: DM, prediabetes and metabolic syndrome	Classification and diagnosis of type 1, type 2 DM and GDM and other specific types of diabetes due to other causes (genetic, exocrine diseases etc.)	Diagnostic criteria clearly stated. Different options clearly stated according to levels of care	Graded diagnostic criteria are stated clearly in table form
27. Are the different possible options for management of the condition clearly stated in the guidelines?	Recommendations are clearly presented in tables with relevant research citations assigned to each recommendation for ease of reference			Graded management algorithms with options are easy to follow
28. Are the recommendations clearly presented?		Recommendations for management and/or treatment are presented at the beginning of each subsection, however they are not easily distinguishable from the rest of the document in the form of tables. Recommendations are not cited with corresponding evidence		
Likely costs and benefits				
29. Is there an adequate description of the health benefits that are likely to be gained from the recommended management?	Risks and benefits of recommendations noted with importance of individualized goals addressed throughout document		Likely benefits are mentioned and referenced	The body of the guidelines addresses potential benefits and harm along with cost with referenced estimates for each
30. Is there an adequate description of the potential harms or risks that may occur as a result of the recommended management?			Limited mention of potential risks	

	Col 1	Col 2	Col 3	Col 4
31. Is there an estimate of the costs or expenditures likely to incur from the recommended management?			Given the global nature of the guidelines difficult to estimate cost but cost is emphasized throughout document	
32. Are the recommendations supported by the estimate benefits, harms and costs of the intervention?	Projected costs of recommendations not addressed	Projected costs of recommendations not addressed		
Dimension 3: Application				
Guideline dissemination and implementation				
33. Does the guideline document suggest possible methods for dissemination and implementation?	Dissemination strategy was developed simultaneously with the guidelines with appendices and clinical and patient tools and identified resources to help clinicians adopt and implement evidence-based recommendations	Strategies for improving diabetes care are included as a subtitle at the end of the guideline with a review of successful programs reported in the literature	No global dissemination plan but guidelines are available at www.idf.org and versions will be available in multiple languages	All individuals in New Zealand with the diagnosis of diabetes are entitled to one free annual health check which will facilitate implementation
Monitoring of guidelines/clinical audit				
34. Does the guideline document specify criteria for monitoring compliance?			Treatment goals are specific according to level of care	Treatment goals are specific
35. Does the guideline document identify clear standards or targets?		No specific recommendations or strategies to disseminate the actual CPG were found	Aside from assessing for treatment target attainment no explicit measures of compliance	Aside from assessing for treatment target attainment no explicit measures of compliance
36. Does the guideline document define measurable outcomes that can be monitored?	Clinical parameters are provided for the purposes of outcome measurement of specific recommendations (i.e. BP, lipid, A1C targets)			
National guidelines only				
1. Does the guideline document identify key elements, which need to be considered by local guideline groups?	A searchable web-based version of the guidelines is available at: www.diabetes.ca			Considerable effort to be applicable to the Māori population

long-term benefits of the new glycemic targets on the reduction of microvascular and macrovascular complications. Formal evaluation will provide the necessary feedback to guide the evolution of CPGs. One can speculate that, as the science of CPGs is refined, they will become integral to the everyday management of diabetes worldwide.

References

1. Wild, S., Roglic, G., Green, A. *et al.* (2004) Global prevalence of diabetes. *Diabetes Care*, **27** (5), 1047–53.
2. Public Health Agency of Canada (1999) available at: www.phac-aspc.gc.ca/publicat/dic-dac99 (accessed 3 March 2007).
3. Shiffman, R., Shekelle, P. Overhage, J.M. *et al.* (2003) Standardized reporting of clinical practice guidelines: a proposal from the Conference on Guideline Standardization. *Academia and Clinic*, **139** (6), 493–500.
4. Expert Committee of the Canadian Diabetes Advisory Board (1992) Clinical practice guidelines for treatment of diabetes mellitus. *Canadian Medical Association Journal*, **147** (5), 697–712.
5. Meltzer, S., Leiter, L.M., Daneman, D. *et al.* (1998) Clinical practice guidelines for the management of diabetes of Canada. *Canadian Medical Association Journal*, **159** (Suppl 8), S1–9.
6. Canadian Diabetes Association Clinical Practice Guidelines Expert Committee (2003) Canadian Diabetes Association 2003 Clinical Practice Guidelines for the Prevention and Management of Diabetes in Canada. *Canadian Journal of Diabetes*, **27** (Suppl 2), S10–13.
7. Canadian Diabetes Association (2007) The Prevalence and Costs of Diabetes, available at www.diabetes.ca (accessed 22 March 2007).
8. International Committee of Medical Journal Editors (ICMJE) (2007) Uniform Requirements for Manuscripts Submitted to Biomedical Journals: Writing and Editing for Biomedical Publication, available at www.icmje.org/aboutur, (accessed 9 January 2007).
9. AGREE Collaboration (2001) Appraisal of Guidelines, Research, and Evaluation, available at www.agreecollaboration.org (accessed 9 January 2007).
10. Field, M. and Lohr, K.N. (1990) Attributes of good practice guidelines, in *Clinical Practice Guidelines: Directions for a New Program* (eds M. Field and K.N. Lohr), National Academy Press, Washington, DC, pp. 53–77.
11. Graham, I.D., Berdall, S., Carter, A.O. *et al.* (2001) What is the quality of drug therapy clinical

12. Cluzeau, F.A., Littlejohns, P., Grimshaw, J.M. *et al.* (1999) Development and application of a generic methodology to assess the quality of clinical guidelines. *International Journal for Quality in Health Care*, **11**, 21–8.
13. Sudlow, M. and Thomson, R. (1997) Clinical guidelines: quantity without quality. *Quality in Health Care*, **6**, 60–1.
14. Varonen, H. and Makela, M. (1997) Practice guidelines in Finland: availability and quality. *Quality in Health Care*, **6**, 75–9.
15. Ward, J. and Grieco, V. (1996) Why we need guidelines for guidelines: a study of the quality of clinical practice guidelines in Australia. *The Medical Journal of Australia*, **165**, 574–6.
16. Shaneyfelt, T.M., Mayo-Smith, M.F. and Rothwangl, J. (1999) Are guidelines following guidelines? The methodological quality of clinical practice guidelines in the peer-reviewed medical literature. *The Journal of the American Medical Association*, **281** (20), 1900–5.
17. Grilli, R., Magrini, N., Penna, A. *et al.* (2000) Practice guidelines developed by specialty societies: the need for a critical appraisal. *Lancet*, **355**, 103–6.
18. Downs, S.H. and Black, N. (1998) The feasibility of creating a checklist for the assessment of the methodological quality both of randomized and non-randomized studies of health care interventions. *Journal of Epidemiology and Community Health*, **52**, 377–84.
19. Moher, D., Pham, B., Jones, A. *et al.* (1998) Does quality of reports of randomized trials effect estimates of intervention efficacy reported in meta-analyses? *Lancet*, **352**, 609–13.
20. Moher, D., Jadad, A.R., Nichol, G. *et al.* (1995) Assessing the quality of randomized controlled trials: an annotated bibliography of scales and checklists. *Controlled Clinical Trials*, **16**, 62–73.
21. Chalmers, I. and Haynes, B. (1994) Reporting, updating, and correcting systematic reviews of the effects of health care. *British Medical Journal*, **309**, 862–5.
22. Lohr, K.N. and Field, M.J. (1992) A provisional instrument for assessing clinical practice guidelines, in *Guidelines for Clinical Practice. From Development to Use*, (eds M.J. Field and K. Lohr), National Academy Press, Washington, DC, (Appendix B).
23. Burgers, J.S., Grol, R., Van Der Bij, A.K. *et al.* (2002) Comparative analysis of recommendations and evidence in diabetes guidelines from 13 countries. *Diabetes Care*, **25** (11), 1933–9.
24. Burgers, J.S., Grol, R., Klazinga, N.S. *et al.* (2003) Towards evidence-based clinical practice:

an international survey of 18 clinical guideline programs. *Quality in Health Care*, **15** (1), 31–45.

25. American Diabetes Association (2006) Committee reports and consensus statements. *Diabetes Care*, **29** (Suppl 1), S73–4.

26. American Diabetes Association (2006) Diabetes care at diabetes camps. *Diabetes Care*, **29** (Suppl 1), S56–8.

27. American Diabetes Association (2006) Hypo-glycemia and employment/licensure. *Diabetes Care*, **29** (Suppl 1), S67.

28. American Diabetes Association (2006) Introduction. *Diabetes Care*, **29** (Suppl 1), S1–2.

29. American Diabetes Association (2006) Position statements and ADA statements. *Diabetes Care*, **29** (Suppl 1), S75–7.

30. American Diabetes Association (2006) Standards of medical care in diabetes – 2006. *Diabetes Care*, **29** (Suppl 1), S4–42.

31. American Diabetes Association (2006) Summary of revisions for the 2006 clinical practice recommendations. *Diabetes Care*, **29** (Suppl 1), S3.

32. American Diabetes Association (2006) Technical reviews. *Diabetes Care*, **29** (Suppl 1), S70–2.

33. IDF Clinical Guidelines Task Force (2005) *Global Guidelines for Type 2 Diabetes*, International Diabetes Federation, Brussels.

34. New Zealand Guidelines Group (2003) Management of Type 2 Diabetes, available at www.nzgg.org.nz (accessed 10 October 2006).

39

Antipsychotic Therapies and Glucose Dysregulation in the Mental Illness Population

Gilbert L'Italien[1,3] and John Newcomer[2]

[1]Global Epidemiology and Outcomes Research Bristol Myers Squibb Pharmaceutical Research Institute, 5 Research Parkway, Wallingford, CT, USA; Yale University Medical School, New Haven CT, USA

[2]Department of Psychiatry,Washington University School of Medicine, 660 S. Euclid, St Louis, MO 63110, USA

[3]Yale University Medical School, 333 Cedar Street, New Haven, CT, USA

39.1 INTRODUCTION

The advent of the so-called second-generation antipsychotic (SGA) agents has resulted in a marked improvement in the management of patients suffering from mental illness. These agents impart both superior efficacy and improved safety and tolerability compared with previously existing therapies [1–6].

As use of these agents increased over time, one ominous development has been the observation of increasing metabolic risk deemed to be associated with SGAs. Metabolic adverse events ranging from weight gain (specifically visceral adiposity), and dyslipidemia to the more clinically relevant metabolic syndrome and frank diabetes have been reported somewhat extensively in the literature [7–12]. This occurrence is particularly problematic since it coincides with both the reaffirmation of the relevant prognostic impact of these factors in the literature [13–18] and their elevated prevalence and incidence in the mentally ill relative to general populations [19–22].

All this attention has prompted the psychiatric and medical community to raise concerns that address the overall health of those entrusted to their care. Despite initial resistance driven by the concept of efficacy primacy and a 'silo' mentality which separated psychiatric from medical care, this community of practitioners has responded to this issue with great concern for patient well-being. The recent American Diabetes Association (ADA) consensus statement on the risk of metabolic events associated with SGAs offers further guidance to practitioners that not all such therapies are alike in terms of metabolic risks [23]. Further, recent studies posit that monitoring of metabolic adverse events is crucial to proper patient care and consequent changes to therapy may be required. These positions have being codified into guidances which have and will pervade the forthcoming literature [24–26]. Although their application by the medical community has been slow in coming [27], their importance cannot be minimized.

The purpose of this chapter is first to illustrate the epidemiology of metabolic symptoms and their diabetogenic and cardiovascular impact in general populations, then to document their elevated risk status of the mentally ill. Lastly, evidence in support of a differential risk for these events among the major SGAs will be presented, coupled with

The Epidemiology of Diabetes Mellitus, second edition Edited by Jean-Marie Ekoé, Marian Rewers, Rhys Williams and Paul Zimmet
© 2008 John Wiley & Sons, Ltd

data demonstrating the benefit of early intervention or alteration in therapeutic regimen.

39.2   THE EPIDEMIOLOGY OF METABOLIC SYNDROME IN THE MENTALLY ILL

In order to fully understand the impact of SGAs on metabolic and cardiovascular events, it is important to characterize the disease status of this population without regard to antipsychotic treatment. A recent study by Enger et al. [19] provides a compelling perspective on the psychiatric population risk status relative to the general population. A matched cohort of schizophrenia and general patients was compared on the person-time incidence of both cardiovascular disease (e.g. myocardial infarction and cardiovascular mortality) and diabetes. Among treated patients, the person-time incidence rates for cardiovascular disease and diabetes are two- and three-fold higher respectively in the schizophrenia population. These findings have been partly corroborated by Goff et al. [20], who reported a doubling of the risk for coronary heart disease among Clinical Antipsychotic Trials of Intervention Effectiveness Study patients compared with a general population (i.e. National Health and Nutrition Examination Survey (NHANES)) referent group.

Both the Enger et al. and Goff et al. studies provide compelling evidence as to the elevated risk status of this patient group. One limitation to these analyses is that all patients in the studies are treated with antipsychotic medications (both SGAs and first-generation). Nevertheless, it may be inferred that much of the incident disease is attributable to elevations in risk factor levels, including those which constitute the so-called metabolic syndrome. The extent to which these factors are exacerbated by the antipsychotic medications is unclear.

Metabolic syndrome as defined by both the Adult Treatment Panel (ATP)-III and the International Diabetes Federation conventions poses a great concern to the mentally ill. A recent systematic review [7] described the prevalence of metabolic syndrome among patients with schizophrenia, which suggested that the prevalence of metabolic syndrome was approximately doubled in the mentally ill compared with general populations. This observation was corroborated by Corell et al. [28] and De Hert et al. [29].

There are two reasons for concern regarding this higher observed prevalence in the mentally ill, again driven by the epidemiologic evidence. First, the wealth of data on the prognostic significance of metabolic syndrome [13–18] demonstrates that it is a strong independent risk factor for both cardiovascular disease and diabetes. Most of these studies report an effect estimate which has been adjusted for the traditional cardiovascular risk factors, such as total cholesterol, age and smoking status where available. These findings were also replicated in a recent meta-analysis by Ford [30], who demonstrated a nearly twofold elevated risk for cardiovascular events and a threefold higher diabetes rate among patients with metabolic syndrome versus those without it.

The second major concern regarding the elevated prevalence of metabolic syndrome is that four of the five risk factors which constitute the syndrome are exacerbated by certain SGAs. The evidence in support of this assertion is overwhelming [7–12], [31–39]. Both clinical trial data and large-scale observational epidemiologic studies report elevations in plasma lipid levels, clinically significant weight, and plasma glucose levels related to the use of antipsychotic medications. For example, in a recent extensive review, Koro and Meyer [37] reported hyperlipidemia and hypertriglyceridemia related to clozapine, olanzapine and quetiapine use, but not for risperidone use. The newer agents, ziprasidone and aripiprazole were found to be weight and lipid neutral. A recent study of weight gain among patients treated with atypical antipsychotics [9] reported clinically significant weight changes among patients treated with olanzapine, quetiapine and risperidone, but not ziprasidone and aripiprazole. Farwell et al. [38] reported a similar pattern of weight gain for olanzapine, quetiapine and risperidone.

The previously available data on glucose elevations related to atypical antipsychotics is limited. Unlike weight and lipid parameters, hyperglycemic events leading to diabetes do not occur until drug exposures are prolonged, typically in excess of 6 months [39]. A notable exception to this trend is found in the work reported by De Hert and co-workers [40]. Using more sophisticated monitoring techniques, such as the oral glucose tolerance test (OGTT), De Hert and co-workers detected an apparent drug-induced diabetes/glucose dysregulation at 3–6 months following initial exposure to antipsychotics. Importantly, the De Hert and co-workers' findings suggest a differential effect of atypical agent on the incidence of glucose dysregulation, consistent with the patterns seen with weight and dyslipidemia: rates of diabetes/glucose dysregulation were 4% for amisulpride, 0% for aripiprazole, 52% for clozapine, 29% for risperidone, 21% for quetiapine and 29% for olanzapine.

A *post hoc* analysis by L'Italien *et al.* [41] of four clinical trials reporting the incidence of ATP-III-defined metabolic syndrome found that rates among schizophrenia patients treated at 6 months with aripiprazole (19.9%, $n = 267$) were indistinguishable from placebo (25.8%, $n = 155$, $p = 0.466$). In contrast, patients treated with olanzapine experienced metabolic syndrome rates that were double that for aripiprazole (41.6% versus 27.9% for olanzapine versus aripiprazole respectively, $p = 0.0002$). The observed differences in rates appeared to be driven by short-term changes in waist circumference, high-density lipoprotein (HDL) and triglycerides and less by glucose elevations. De Hert *et al.* [29] also reported on metabolic syndrome rates among treated patients, but did not provide treatment specific rates.

In conclusion, epidemiologic studies suggest that the underlying risk for metabolic and cardiovascular events among the mentally ill remains elevated compared with the general population. Both the incidence rate for these events and the underlying prevalence of metabolic syndrome is at least double that of the general population. Lastly, there is considerable evidence that levels of certain metabolic syndrome risk factors (e.g. obesity, lipids, glucose) are exacerbated by particular antipsychotic medications. The rate of change in these component risk factors' parameters with exposure appears to be obesity followed by dyslipidemia. Changes in fasting glucose do not appear until longer exposures (>6 months) are observed.

39.3 ATYPICAL ANTIPSYCHOTICS AND DIABETES

The entire literature describing the relationship between atypical antipsychotic exposure and diabetes is premised exclusively on observational studies. In fact, the American Psychiatric Association (APA)–ADA consensus panel on metabolic risk with atypicals concluded that there was a differential effect and this interpretation was based

entirely upon observational epidemiologic studies. One of the first such studies, by Koro *et al.* [12], suggested that there was a differential relationship between the atypicals clozapine, olanzapine and risperidone. A recent study in Veterans Affairs (VA) patients [39] described this relationship in more detail among patients treated with olanzapine, quetiapine, clozapine and risperidone. The VA study reports rates of diabetes incidence differing by agent, appearing after one full year of exposure. Lastly, a meta-analysis conducted by Newcomer *et al.* [42], which included the two cited studies, found a similar pattern of differential incidence, with highest relative risks for clozapine and olanzapine followed by quetiapine and risperidome. One limitation is that these studies did not include the newer agents, ziprasidone and aripiprazole. Two more recent studies, one by Gianfranscesco *et al.* [43] and the other by Guo *et al.* [11], reported no diabetes association for ziprasidone in contrast to significant associations for olanzapine, quetiapine and risperidol compared with nontreatment or conventional treatment. At present, no data are available on long-term diabetes incidence for aripiprazole.

Intriguing work by van Winkel *et al.* [40] suggests that more intensive, albeit feasible, monitoring detects a short-term glucose dysregulation/diabetes that differs according to prescribed agent. After only 3 months, reported rates were highest for clozapine, followed in order by olanzapine, quetiapine, risperidone, amisulpride and aripiprazole. The investigator employed the OGTT, which is a more sensitive measure of impaired glucose tolerance, impaired fasting glucose or diabetes mellitus than fasting glucose alone. Although this observational study must be interpreted with caution, the findings at minimum highlight the importance of metabolic monitoring in this population.

In conclusion, the preponderance of evidence, albeit from observational studies, suggests that atypical antipsychotics differ in terms of risk for diabetes. However, reported variations in the rates from different published studies render it difficult to ascribe a particular effect to a particular agent. The trend suggested by the literature ascribes the highest rates to clozapine and olanzapine, followed by either risperidone or quetiapine, with the lowest rate for ziprasidone, admittedly with little data. The De Hert and co-workers' [44] results present a similar pattern based upon short-term (<6 months) diabetes/glucose dysregulation incidence, with the lowest rates for amisulpride and aripiprazole.

39.4 REVERSAL OF METABOLIC SYNDROME AND GLUCOSE DYSREGULATION/DIABETES

The previously cited work and other studies highlight the importance of metabolic monitoring in the mentally ill population. It is apparent that these conditions can appear early in treatment and that some intervention is warranted. Current guidelines recommend lifestyle modification and/or change in antipsychotic regimen among patients who develop metabolic abnormalities [24, 25]. One assumption inherent to the change in regimen is that this will improve the patient's metabolic status. The evidence supporting this contention continues to grow. Independent studies by Casey et al. [44] and Weiden et al. [46] suggest that patients switched from olanzapine to ziprasidone or aripiprazole will experience a 2 kg weight loss within 6 weeks. Patients switched from risperidone exhibited a 1 kg weight loss on average. Case studies by Henderson et al. [47], Littrell et al. [48] and Lin et al. [49] report a normalization of glucose levels, lipids and weight following either switch from olanzapine or risperidone to aripiprazole, or of augmentation of clozapine with aripiprazole. These findings were corroborated by L'Italien et al. [41], who demonstrated reversal of early onset diabetes/glucose dysregulation among 30 patients switched from clozapine, olanzapine, quetiapine or risperidol to either amisulpride or aripiprazole. De Hert [50] also demonstrated normalization of lipid levels, waist circumference and non-HDL cholesterol, an important determinant of coronary heart disease. Rates of metabolic syndrome were halved by switch to aripiprazole or amisulpride. *Post hoc* analyses of active comparator clinical trials by Newcomer et al. [50] and Allison et al. [52] suggest that rates for metabolic syndrome and abnormal levels of non-HDL cholesterol can be reduced significantly by treatment with aripiprazole versus olanzapine.

The finding of a reversal in glucose dysregulation/diabetes and normalization of lipid and weight parameters enforces the need to monitor these patients early and often and to intervene when abnormalities are detected. Of note, the work of Ader et al. [53] may provide the underlying mechanism of diabetes/glucose dysregulation

reversal; they have postulated the mechanism of antipsychotic-induced diabetes to be as follows: neuronal signaling of the pancreatic islet cells to secrete insulin in response to glucose elevation is blocked by certain agents, notably olanzapine. In the short term, reversal of this blockage is achieved by removal of antipsychotic agent. The clinical findings of De Hert *et al.* [50] on reversal of insulin resistance and glucose dysregulation among patients switched from olanzapine to aripiprazole lend support to this postulated mechanism.

39.5 CONCLUSIONS

The wealth of research on the subject of antipsychotic therapies and glucose dysregulation in the mentally ill supports a number of conclusions pertinent to the management of these patients. First and foremost, the mentally ill constitute a population at elevated risk for both metabolic events, such as diabetes, and cardiovascular disease. The level of this risk is substantial: it is typically double that of the general population for metabolic syndrome and coronary heart disease, and three-fold higher for diabetes. Clearly, lifestyle issues, such as the high prevalence of smoking, poor diet and a sedentary lifestyle, explain much of this elevated risk. However, certain SGAs exacerbate this risk above and beyond lifestyle issues. Third, careful (albeit intensive) metabolic monitoring can identify short-term diabetes/glucose dysregulation, as well as dyslipidemias, which increase the risk for coronary heart disease. Current guidelines suggest lifestyle modification and consideration of a change in the therapeutic regimen. Lastly, such changes might actually reverse glucose regulation and normalize levels of glucose, lipids and body weight.

Our current knowledge of the epidemiology of metabolic and cardiovascular risk in the mentally ill, drug-induced or otherwise, is the consequence of a body of evidence that has been accumulating steadily over the past several years. The source of this information has ranged from clinical trials to case series to large-scale epidemiologic studies to basic research. The interpretation and proper utilization of this vast evidence to enhance patient management has relied upon the multidisciplinary expertise of epidemiologists, psychiatrists, endocrinologists, diabetologists and cardiologists. Better management and safeguarding of the overall physical health of the mentally ill should rightly ensue from these endeavors.

References

1. Casey, D.E. (1996) Side effect profiles of new antipsychotic agents (Review). *The Journal of Clinical Psychiatry*, **57** (Suppl 11), 40–45; discussion 46–52.
2. Remington, G. and Chong, S.A. (1999) Conventional versus novel antipsychotics: changing concepts and clinical implications (Review). *Journal of Psychiatry and Neuroscience*, **24** (5), 431–41.
3. Shen, W.W. (1999) A history of antipsychotic drug development (Review). *Comprehensive Psychiatry*, **40** (6), 407–14.
4. Kane, J.M. (1999) Pharmacologic treatment of schizophrenia (Review). *Biological Psychiatry*, **46** (10), 1396–408.
5. Krausz, M. (2002) Efficacy review of antipsychotics (Review). *Current Medical Research and Opinion*, **18** (Suppl 3), S8–12.
6. Lieberman, J.A. (1996) Atypical antipsychotic drugs as a first-line treatment of schizophrenia: a rationale and hypothesis (Review). *The Journal of Clinical Psychiatry*, **57** (Suppl 11), 68–71.
7. Meyer, J., Koro, C.E. and L'Italien, G.J. (2005) The metabolic syndrome and schizophrenia: a review. *International Review of Psychiatry (Abingdon, England)*, **17** (3), 173–80.
8. Koro, C.E. and Meyer, J.M. (2005) Atypical antipsychotic therapy and hyperlipidemia: a review. *Essential Psychopharmacology*, **6** (3), 148–57.
9. Brixner, D.I., Said, Q., Corey-Lisle, P.K. *et al.* (2006) Naturalistic impact of second generation antipsychotics on weight gain. *The Annals of Pharmacotherapy*, **40**, 626–32.
10. Olfson, M., Marcus, S.C., Corey-Lisle, P. *et al.* (2007) Hyperlipidemia following treatment with antipsychotic medications. *The American Journal of Psychiatry* **164** (3), 525–6.
11. Guo, J.J., Keck, P.E., Corey-Lisle, P. *et al.* (2006) Risk of diabetes mellitus associated with atypical antipsychotic use among patients with bipolar disorder: a retrospective, population-based, case-control study. *The Journal of Clinical Psychiatry*, **67**, 1055–61; McNeill, A.M., Rosamond, W.D., Girman, C.J., and Ballantyne, C.M. (2002) A new definition of the metabolic syndrome predicts incident coronary heart disease and stroke [abstract]. *Circulation*, **106** (Suppl II), 765.
12. Koro, C.E., Fedder, D.O., L'Italien, G.J. *et al.* (2002) Assessment of independent effect of olanzapine and risperidone on risk of diabetes among patients with schizophrenia: population-based nested case-control study. *British Medical Journal*, **325**, 243–7.
13. Lakka, H.-M., Laaksonen, D.E., Lakka, T.A. *et al.* (2002) The metabolic syndrome and total and cardiovascular disease mortality in middle-aged men. *The Journal of the American Medical Association*, **288**, 2709–16.
14. Sattar, N., Gaw, A., Scherbakova, O. *et al.* (2003) Metabolic syndrome with and without CRP as a predictor of coronary heart disease and diabetes in the West of Scotland Coronary Prevention Study. *Circulation*, **108**, 414–19.
15. Lorenzo, C., Stern, M.P., Okoloise, M. *et al.* (2003) The metabolic syndrome as a predictor of type 2 diabetes. *Diabetes Care*, **26**, 3153–59.
16. Ninomiya, J.K., L'Italien, G.J., Criqui, M.H. *et al.* (2004) Association of the metabolic syndrome with history of myocardial infarction and stroke in the Third National Health and Nutrition Examination Survey. *Circulation*, **109**, 42–6.
17. Malik, S., Wong, N.D., Franklin, S.S. *et al.* (2004) The impact of the metabolic syndrome and diabetes on mortality from coronary heart disease, cardiovascular disease and all causes in United States adults. *Circulation*, **110**, 1239–44.
18. Hu, G., Qiao, Q., Tuomilehto, J. *et al.* (2004) Prevalence of the metabolic syndrome and its relation to all cause and cardiovascular mortality in non-diabetic European men and women. *Archives of Internal Medicine*, **164**, 1066–76.
19. Enger, C., Weatherby, L., Reynolds, R.F. *et al.* (2004) Serious cardiovascular events and mortality among patients with schizophrenia. *The Journal of Nervous and Mental Disease*, **192**, 19–27.
20. Goff, D.C., Sullivan, L.M., McEvoy, J.P. *et al.* (2005) A comparison of 10-year cardiac risk estimates in schizophrenia patients and matched controls. *Schizophrenia Research*, **80** (1), 45–53.
21. Colton, C.W. and Manderscheid, RW (2006) Congruencies in increased mortality rates, years of potential life lost, and causes of death among public mental health clients in eight states. *Preventing Chronic Disease* **3** (2) [serial online], (April 2006) http://www.cdc.gov/pcd/issues/2006/apr/05_0180 .htm (last access May 2008).
22. Weiss, A.P., Henderson, D.C., Weilburg, J.B. *et al.* (2006) Treatment of cardiac risk factors among patients with schizophrenia and diabetes. *Psychiatric Services (Washington, D.C.)*, **57** (8), 1145–52.
23. American Diabetes Association and American Psychiatric Association (2004) Consensus development conference on antipsychotic drugs and obesity and diabetes. *Diabetes Care*, **27**, 596–601.

24. Marder, S.R., Essock, S.M., Miller, A.L. *et al.* (2004) Physical health monitoring of patients with schizophrenia. *The American Journal of Psychiatry*, **161** (8), 1334–49.

25. Newcomer, J.W. (2005) Second generation (atypical) antipsychotics and metabolic effects; a comprehensive literature review. Drug therapy in neurology and psychiatry. *CNS Drugs*, **19** (Suppl 1), 1–93.

26. De Nayer, A., De Hert, M., Sheen, A. *et al.* (2005) Belgian consensus on metabolic problems associated with atypical antipsychotics. *International Journal of Psychiatry in Clinical Practice*, **9** (2), 130–7.

27. Weiss, A.P., Henderson, D.C., Weilburg, J.B. *et al.* (2006) Treatment of cardiac risk factors among patients with schizophrenia and diabetes. *Psychiatric Services (Washington, D.C.)*, **57** (8), 1145–52.

28. Corell, U.C., Frederickson, A.M., Kane, J.M. and Manu, P. (2006) Metabolic syndrome and the risk of coronary heart disease in 367 patients treated with second generation antipsychotic drugs. *The Journal of Clinical Psychiatry*, **67**, 575–83.

29. De Hert, M., van Winkell, R., Van Eeyk, D. *et al.* (2006) Prevalence of metabolic syndrome in patients with schizophrenia treated with antipsychotic medication. *Schizophrenia Research*, **83**, 87–93.

30. Ford, E.S. (2005) Risks for all-cause mortality, cardiovascular disease and diabetes associated with the metabolic syndrome: a summary of the evidence. *Diabetes Care*, **28** (7), 1769–78.

31. Allison, D.B., Mentore, J.L., Heo, M. *et al.* (1999) Antipsychotic-induced weight gain: a comprehensive research synthesis. *The American Journal of Psychiatry*, **156** (11), 1686–96.

32. Allison, D.B. and Casey, D.E. (2001) Antipsychotic-induced weight gain: a review of the literature. *The Journal of Clinical Psychiatry*, **62** (Suppl 7), 22–31.

33. McIntyre, R.S., McCann, S.M. and Kennedy, S.H. (2001) Antipsychotic metabolic effects: weight gain, diabetes mellitus, and lipid abnormalities. *Canadian Journal of Psychiatry*, **46** (3), 273–81.

34. Sernyak, M.J., Leslie, D.L., Alarcon, R.D. *et al.* (2002) Association of diabetes mellitus with the use of atypical neuroleptics in the treatment of schizophrenia. *The American Journal of Psychiatry*, **159** (4), 561–6.

35. Henderson, D.C. (2002) Atypical antipsychotic-induced diabetes mellitus: how strong is the evidence? *CNS Drugs*, **16** (2), 77–89.

36. Newcomer, J.W. (2001) Metabolic disturbances associated with antipsychotic use. *The Journal of Clinical Psychiatry*, **62** (Suppl 27), 1–42.

37. Koro, C.E. and Meyer, J.M. (2005) Atypical antipsychotic therapy and hyperlipidemia: a review. *Essential Psychopharmacology*, **6** (3), 148–57.

38. Farwell, W.R., Stump, T.E., Wang, J. *et al.* (2004) Weight gain and new onset diabetes associated with olanzapine and risperisone. *Journal of General Internal Medicine*, **19** (12), 1200–5.

39. Leslie, D.L. and Rosenheck, R.A. (2004) Incidence of newly diagnosed diabetes attributable to atypical antipsychotic medications. *The American Journal of Psychiatry*, **161** (9), 1709–11.

40. Van Winkel, R., De Hert, M.A., Van Eyck, D. *et al.* Screening for diabetes and other metabolic abnormalities in patients with schizophrenia and schizoaffective disorder: evaluation of incidence and screening methods. *The Journal of Clinical Psychiatry*, **67** (10), 1493–500.

41. L'Italien, G.J., Kon, H.J., Marcus, R. *et al.* (2007) Comparison of metabolic syndrome incidence among schizophrenia patients treated with aripiprazole versus olanzapine or placebo. *The Journal of Clinical Psychiatry*, **68** (10), 1510–16.

42. Newcomer, J.W., L'Italien, G.J., Pugner, K.M. *et al.* Atypical antipsychotics and incident diabetes mellitus in schizophrenia: a meta-analysis. *The American Journal of Psychiatry* (submitted).

43. Gianfrancesco, F., Pisa, F., Wang, R.H. and Narallah, H. (2006) Assessment of antipsychotic-related risk of diabetes mellitus in a Medicaid psychosis population: sensitivity to study design. *American Journal of Health-System Pharmacy*, **63** (5), 431–41.

44. De, H.M., Schreurs, V., Sweers, K. *et al.* (2008) Typical and atypical antipsychotics differentially affect long-term incidence rates of the metabolic syndrome in first-episode patients with schizophrenia: A retrospective chart review. *Schizophr Res*, **101** (1-3), 295–303. Epub 2008 Mar 4. PMID: 18299188 (in- process)

45. Casey, D.E., Carson, W.H., Saha, A.R. *et al.* (2003) Switching patients to aripiprazole from other antipsychotic agents: a multicenter randomized study. *Psychopharmacology*, **166** (4), 391–9.

46. Weiden, P.J., Daniel, D.G., Simpson, G. and Romano, S.J. (2003) Improvement in indices of health status in outpatients with schizophrenia switched to ziprasidone. *Journal of Clinical Psychopharmacology*, **23** (6), 595–600.

47. Henderson, D.C., Kunkel, L., Nguyen, D.D. *et al.* (2006) An exploratory open-label trial of aripiprazole as an adjuvant to clozapine therapy in chronic schizophrenia. *Acta Psychiatrica Scandinavica*, **113** (2), 142–7.

48. Littrell, K.H., Petty, R.G., Hillgose, N.M. *et al.* (2004). The effect of aripiprazole on insulin

resistance in schizophrenia. Presented at the Annual Meeting of the American Psychiatric Association, New York, May.

49. Lin, S.K. and Chen, C.K. (2006) Reversal of antipsychotic induced hyperprolactinemia, weight gain and dyslipidemia by aripiprazole: a case report. *The Journal of Clinical Psychiatry*, **67** (8), 1307.

50. van, W.R., De, H.M., Wampers, M. *et al.* (2008) Major changes in glucose metabolism, including new-onset diabetes, within 3 months after initiation of or switch to atypical antipsychotic medication in patients with schizophrenia and schizoaffective disorder. *J Clin Psychiatry*, **69** (3), 472–479. PMID: 18348593 [PubMed-indexed for MEDLINE]

51. Newcomer, J.W., L'Italien, G.J., Vester-Blokland, E. *et al.* (2006) Improvement of non-HDL cholesterol levels among patients randomized to aripiprazole versus olanzapine. Presented at the Annual Meeting of the American Psychiatric Association, Toronto, Canada, May.

52. Allison, D.B., L'Italien, G.J., Vester-Blokland, E. *et al.* (2006) Metabolic syndrome rates among patients with schizophrenia treated with aripiprazole, placebo, or olanzapine. Presented at the Annual Meeting of the American Psychiatric Association, Toronto, Canada, May.

53. Ader, M., Catalano, K.J., Ionut, V. *et al.* (2005) Metabolic dysregulation with atypical antipsychotics occurs in the absence of underlying disease: a placebo-controlled study of olanzapine and risperidone in dogs. *Diabetes*, **54** (3), 862–71.

Further Reading

De, H.M., Hanssens, L., van W.R. *et al.* (2006) Reversibility of antipsychotic treatment-related diabetes in patients with schizophrenia: a case series of switching to aripiprazole.. *Diabetes Care*, (10), 2329–30. PMID: 17003321 [PubMed-indexed for MEDLINE]

40

Diabetes, Insulin Resistance and Glucose Metabolism in HIV Infection and its Treatment

Kathy Samaras and Don J. Chisholm

Diabetes and Obesity Program, Garvan Institute of Medical Research, Darlinghurst, New South Wales, Australia

40.1 INTRODUCTION

Treatment of human immunodeficiency virus-1 (HIV-1) infection with highly active antiretroviral therapy (HAART) has become increasingly effective in controlling this life-threatening condition, but it increases the risk of type 2 diabetes through disturbances in adipocyte function, body fat partitioning (lipodystrophy) and lipid homeostasis. Effects on insulin resistance, impaired mitochondrial function and insulin secretion result in a high prevalence of disorders of glucose metabolism, in addition to concomitant dyslipidemia and other metabolic risks. This chapter will review the documented prevalence and pathogenesis of disorders of glucose metabolism in treated HIV infection, within the wider framework of metabolic disorders induced by HAART.

40.2 PREVALENCE

Diabetes in HIV infection was relatively uncommon in the era prior to HAART. One US study published in 1998 found a prevalence of hyperglycemia (>11.0 mmol 1^{-1}) of only 2% in approximately 1400 HIV patients [1]. Where hyperglycemia was found, causative drug factors were readily identifiable, such as pancreatic β-cell injury secondary to

pentamidine therapy and characterized by insulin deficiency and ketoacidosis [2–4].

Since HAART has become the treatment standard in HIV infection, the prevalence of type 2 diabetes has increased substantially in this patient population, due to their impact on adipocyte and lipid metabolism. The first description of insulin resistance in association with protease inhibitors found only 2% of patients had diabetes after a mean of 14 months of therapy, though lipodystrophy affected 64% of protease inhibitor recipients [5]. A subsequent prospective, observational study of the natural history of lipodystrophy found progression of body fat partitioning disorders (peripheral fat wasting and central fat accumulation). documented by dual-energy X-ray absorptiometry, with duration of protease inhibitor therapy. Baseline and current triglyceride levels and C-peptide were predictive of the disorder [6]. In this study, the prevalence of disturbances in glucose homeostasis were greater than previously reported: impaired glucose tolerance 16% and diabetes 7% [6]. Concomitant hyperlipidemia was found, affecting 74% of protease inhibitor recipients, versus 28% of protease inhibitor-naive patients [6]. Insulin resistance (by homeostasis model assessment (HOMA)) was doubled [6].

The Epidemiology of Diabetes Mellitus, second edition Edited by Jean-Marie Ekoé, Marian Rewers, Rhys Williams and Paul Zimmet
© 2008 John Wiley & Sons, Ltd

Since these initial reports of disordered glucose metabolism in association with wider metabolic derangements (peripheral lipoatophy, central fat accumulation, hyperpidemia), there have been numerous other reports of insulin resistance, impaired glucose tolerance and diabetes.

40.2.1   Insulin Resistance

The study of insulin resistance presents challenges in clinical research, since accurate assessment of insulin sensitivity relies upon the resource- and staff-intensive hyperinsulinemic euglycemic clamp. Few studies in HIV-infected subjects have utilized this methodology. A further challenge in understanding this area is the need for careful phenotyping and categorizing of subjects; for example, allowing separation of effects of HIV infection *per se*, differences in body composition and, finally, drug-induced effects.

Several studies have documented diminished insulin sensitivity in HIV-infected HAART recipients [5–7]. Insulin sensitivity determined by glucose infusion rate during a hyperinsulinemic euglycemic clamp demonstrated a doubling of insulin resistance in HIV-infected HAART recipients compared with age- and body mass index (BMI)-matched HIV-infected HAART-naïve controls [7]. Studies using HOMA have found insulin resistance was greater in protease inhibitor recipients than protease inhibitor-naïve HIV-infected subjects [5, 6]. A further study using HOMA found that, in HIV-infected subjects with lipodystrophy, treatment with rosiglitazone induced significant improvements in insulin sensitivity without altering body fat [8].

40.2.2   Lipodystrophy

Disturbances in body fat partitioning (limb and facial lipoatrophy, buffalo hump, abdominal obesity) have been documented in a large number of studies [5, 69–11]. In the first description of this syndrome, 64% of protease inhibitor recipients were found to have clinically evident lipodystrophy [5]. Subsequent studies have shown 40–50% of all HIV-infected subjects have body fat partitioning abnormalities; the proportions are greater amongst those receiving HAART [12]. Prospective studies indicate that lipodystrophy progresses over time, with evidence of a mean fat loss of 0.13 kg per month over 8 months measured by

dual-energy X-ray absorptiometry [6]. The contribution of HAART drugs other than protease inhibitors to the syndrome of lipodystrophy is now recognized. Nucleosidase analogues contribute to lactic acidemia that can be associated with lipodystrophy [9]. Lactic acidemia, indicative of impaired mitochondrial function, may underlie or accompany the cellular derangements that result in lipodystrophy. Prospective studies of untreated HIV-infected patients commencing HAART show an initial increase (presumably due to viral load control) and then progressive loss of peripheral fat stores (limb fat) over 3 years [13]. This study estimated fat loss to be 14% per year of therapy in patients receiving combination therapy with a nucleosidase reverse-transcriptase inhibitor and either a protease inhibitor or nonnucleosidase reverse-transcriptase inhibitor [13]. A large, international case–control study from the HIV Lipodystrophy Case Definition Cohort ($n = 1081$) defined a model with a sensitivity and specificity of 80% for diagnosis of lipodystrophy [14]. Parameters included age, duration of HIV infection, HIV disease stage, waist/hip ratio, anion gap, high-density lipoprotein (HDL)-cholesterol, trunk/peripheral fat ratio and intraabdominal/extraabdominal fat ratio (**Table 40.1**) [14]. Detection of early parameters of lipodystrophy in HIV-infected HAART recipients (such as an objective definition or simple parameters such as fasting triglycerides) identifies individuals with increased risk for diabetes for preventative strategies, earlier identification and treatment.

Clinical acumen remains the tool of choice in detecting body fat partitioning changes in HIV-infected HAART recipients. Studies show clinical detection of increased central adiposity and peripheral lipoatrophy within 12–24 months of commencement of combination HAART [15, 16].

40.2.3   Diabetes Mellitus

The prevalence of diabetes in HIV infection can be expected to vary from one population to another, modified by factors such as genetic risk and obesity. Reported diabetes prevalence rates in HIV-infected subjects that are treatment naïve differ widely. A study of 419 treatment-naïve HIV-infected subjects found 2.6% had diabetes [17]. In a further large study of HIV-negative subjects ($n = 710$), HIV-infected HAART recipients

Table 40.1 Summary of the studies documenting the prevalence of type 2 diabetes mellitus in HIV infection.

Authors	No.	Population	Males (%)	Age (years)	Assessment[a]	Diabetes prevalence (%)		
						HIV−	HIV+ no HAART	HIV+ HAART
El-Sadr et al. [17]	419	African American (60%) Latino (10%)	79	38	FGL	—	2.6	—
Brown et al. [18]	1278	White (85%)	100	48	FGL	5	7	14
Carr et al. [6]	113	White	98	41	OGTT	—	0	7
Howard et al. [19]	221	Hispanic (44%) Black (41%)	0	45	OGTT	13	—	12
Justman et al. [20][b]	1785		0			1.4	1.2	2.8
Salehian et al. [21]	101					—		12
Mehta et al. [22]	1230	African American (76–87%) Hepatitis C+ (53%)	70	29–43	RBG	—	—	3.3–5.9

[a]FGL: fasting glucose level; OGTT: oral glucose tolerance test; RBG: random blood glucose on two occasions.

[b]Incidence (not prevalence) rates are tabled.

($n = 411$) and HIV-infected treatment-naïve subjects ($n = 157$), BMI in the overweight range, and matched for abdominal obesity (by waist/hip ratio), fasting glucose was significantly greater in those receiving HAART, compared with HIV-infected treatment-naïve subjects [18]. In that same study, the prevalence of diabetes (by fasting glucose) in HIV-negative subjects was 5%, in HIV-infected treatment-naïve subjects 7%, but 14% in HAART recipients [18]. Based on the prevalence of diabetes in the HIV-negative population studied, HIV infection per se increased the relative risk of diabetes to 2.21 (95% confidence interval 1.12–4.38) and the combination of HIV infection and HAART increased the relative risk to 4.64 (95% confidence interval 3.03–7.1) [18]. Over the 4-year follow-up in this study, 10% of HIV-positive HAART-recipients developed diabetes, compared with 3% in HIV-negative subjects [18].

In another prospective study of lipodystrophy progression, the prevalence of diabetes (by oral glucose tolerance test) was 7% and impaired glucose tolerance 16% after a mean duration of protease inhibitor therapy of 21 months [6]. Importantly, this study illustrated the need for the oral glucose tolerance test to establish the diagnosis of diabetes: 72% of subjects shown to be diabetic by oral glucose tolerance test had nondiabetic fasting glucose levels [6]. Therefore, studies of diabetes prevalence where glucose metabolism assessment was limited to fasting glucose may underestimate the real prevalence of diabetes.

There may be ethnicity sensitivity to the development of diabetes. A prospective study of HIV-infected patients in the Los Angeles area found a prevalence of 12% amongst protease inhibitor recipients at baseline [21]. After 3 years, the incidence of new cases of diabetes was 7%; all were African Americans [21].

A further consideration is the impact of obesity on diabetes prevalence in HIV infection.

A study from Philadelphia, USA, found the prevalences of overweight and obesity were 31% and 14% respectively in their HIV-infected patients ($n = 1669$), similar to that found in their general population [23]. In contrast, HIV wasting was present in only 9% [23]. As obesity has a promoting effect on insulin resistance and diabetes, it can be expected that HIV-infected patients with coexisting obesity will have higher prevalences of diabetes than that reported thus far. Few studies have examined the prevalence of disorders of glucose metabolism in HIV-infected women. One study, using oral glucose tolerance tests, found a prevalence of 12% in HIV-positive HAART recipients, compared with 13% in HIV-negative women [19]. Important confounders in this study were the differences in BMI and waist/hip circumferences between the two groups: 86% of HIV-negative women were overweight or obese compared with 67% in HIV-infected subjects and waist/hip ratio was significantly less in the HIV-positive groups [19]. The lower total and central obesity in the HIV-positive group may have resulted in lower diabetes prevalence.

A further study of 1785 HIV-infected women using self-reported diabetes or use of diabetic medications at annual interview has reported the incidence of diabetes as 2.8% among protease inhibitor recipients, versus 1.2% in those who were HAART naïve and 1.4% in the HIV-negative controls over a median follow up of 2.9 years [20]. Despite the lower incidence of diabetes, the HIV-negative women had higher rates of overweight/obesity at 33% versus 23% in the HIV-infected women [20]. Coexistence of HIV and hepatitis C infection appears to increase diabetes risk. Hepatitis C infection *per se* is associated with increased insulin resistance [24]. One study of 1230 HIV-infected patients (50% coinfected with hepatitis C virus) found the prevalence of diabetes was almost double in those with coinfection (5.9%), compared with HIV alone (3.3%); all were HAART recipients [22]. This retrospective study also found incident cases of diabetes to be higher in those with HIV–hepatitis C coinfection: 5.8% versus 2.8%, with analyses showing the incidence of hyperglycemia per 100 person-years to be 4.9 in those with coinfection (95% confidence interval 3.4–7.1) versus 2.3 in those with HIV infection alone (95% confidence interval 1.4–3.7) [22]. Most of the published studies on diabetes in HIV infection arise from the United States and Australia, where HAART is generally available. Very little published data exist for diabetes in HIV infection from other continents, such as Africa and Asia, where HAART may not be readily available. Statistical models predicting diabetes in South Africa have suggested the prevalence may decrease, due to the devastating effect of untreated HIV infection on the number of adults who survive into middle age [25]. A further statistical model has suggested that, with wider use of HAART in South Africa, the incidence of diabetes may increase from 1% to 11% [26]. Long-term follow-up studies of diabetes prevalence are lacking and of particular importance, since some of these drugs have now been in use for over a decade and the effects on body fat partitioning appear progressive. Little is also known about the natural history of diabetic complications in HIV infection. For example, do the immunological or inflammatory disturbances of HIV modify progression of complications? Are there interactions between hyperglycemia and the documented effects of HIV infection or its treatment (e.g. neuropathy, renal dysfunction, retinal disease) and, if so, are these additive or multiplicative? What is the interaction between the known high cardiovascular risks of diabetes and the impact of HAART metabolic complications on atherosclerosis? Careful and long-term prospective observational studies are required to answer these important questions.

40.3 PATHOGENESIS

40.3.1 β-cell Dysfunction

Hyperglycemia in HIV-infected HAART recipients occurs when pancreatic β-cell secretion of insulin is inadequate to serve increased peripheral requirements. The β-cell may fail as a consequence of programmed (genetic) limitations (suggested by family history of type 2 diabetes) or due to β-cell lipotoxicity, due to the presence of elevated circulating free fatty acids and triglycerides in lipodystrophy [6, 27, 28]. Elevated circulating lipids interfere with the islet cells' ability to secrete insulin [29]. Mitochondrial effects within

β-cells impairing glucose sensing and insulin secretion are mechanisms postulated to contribute to eventual insulin secretory failure in type 2 diabetes [30]. There is little evidence that this mechanism contributes to eventual β-cell failure in the specific setting of HAART in HIV infection; however, given that one form of HAART, nucleosidase reverse-transcriptase inhibitors, impair mitochondrial function, drug-induced β-cell mitochondrial dysfunction is a potential contributor to eventual insulin secretory failure. Insulin resistance increases the β-cell's secretory demand in the prodrome to diabetes in HAART. The β-cell's subsequent functional decline may then be partly genetically inherited [31], with additive insults as a consequence of lipodystrophy and associated hypertriglyceridemia (**Figure 40.1**).

40.3.2 *Insulin Resistance in HIV-infected Patients*

Insulin resistance in HIV lipodystrophy is associated with features typically found in other insulin-resistant states: increased intramyocellular triglyceride has been demonstrated by nuclear magnetic resonance in insulin-resistant patients with lipodystrophy, compared with age and BMI-matched HIV-infected patients who were protease-inhibitor naïve [7] (**Figure 40.2**). This study utilized gold standard measures of insulin resistance (hyperinsulinemic, euglycemic clamp), visceral obesity (magnetic resonance) and body fat distribution (dual-energy X-ray absorptiometry). Increased intramyocellular lipid was associated with lower insulin-stimulated glucose disposal and greater visceral adiposity and circulating triglycerides [7]. The finding of a doubling of intramyocellular lipid deserves some discussion, as this is considered a pivotal component of the insulin resistance [32, 33]. Intramyocellular lipid contributes, probably by active moieties such as diacylglycerides and ceramides, to lipotoxicity and impairment of insulin signaling pathways that promote glucose uptake. Mitochondrial dysfunction may also contribute to intramyocellular lipid accumulation and impaired glucose uptake in muscle and is discussed below in considering the effects of HAART on adipocyte metabolism. A further, smaller study has also utilized clamps to measure insulin sensitivity, using HIV-negative subjects as controls, and reported that visceral fat predicted insulin resistance [34]. This study utilized positron-emission tomography to quantitate basal and insulin-stimulated glucose uptake into muscle and subcutaneous and visceral adipose tissue, finding that uptake in subcutaneous

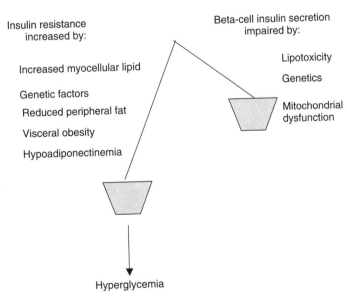

Figure 40.1 Events leading to hyperglycemia in diabetes associated with highly active antiretroviral therapy in HIV-infected patients. Hyperglycemia develops when insulin resistance outweighs insulin secretion.

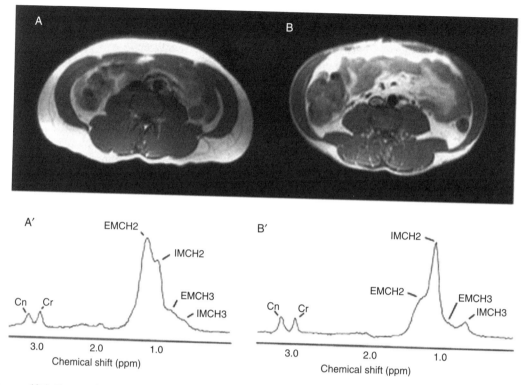

Figure 40.2 Intra-abdominal fat is increased in HIV-infected subjects with lipodystrophy and associated with increased intramyocellular fat and insulin resistance, compared with BMI- and age-matched HIV-infected, protease-inhibitor-naïve subjects. Subjects shown were matched for abdominal fat by magnetic resonance imaging and dual-energy X-ray absorptiometry. Image B shows the subject with lipodystrophy, who has less subcutaneous and greater intraabdominal fat than the control (A). Muscle lipid partitioning differed substantially, as shown by the ^{1}H magnetic resonance spectroscopy soleus muscle spectra below (A', B'). There was increased intra- and reduced extra-cellular lipid in the lipodystrophic subject (B') compared with the control subject (A'). (Chemical shift indicated in parts per million.) Cn: carnitine; Cr: creatine [7]. (Copyright © 2002 American Diabetes Association. From *Diabetes*, Vol.51, 2002; 3163–3169. Adapted with permission from The American Diabetes Association.)

fat was increased in lipoatrophic subjects [34]. The authors postulate this is compensatory for demonstrated reductions in muscle glucose uptake [34]. HAART effects on lipid and glucose metabolism resulting in insulin resistance do not appear to be solely dependent on the presence of lipodystrophy. *In vitro* studies show protease inhibitors reduce glucose transport in isolated skeletal muscle [35]. Studies of noninfected volunteers with 4 weeks of indinavir produced insulin resistance without disturbance in circulating fatty acids [36]. Generalized peripheral lipoatrophy and increased visceral adiposity obviously contribute to insulin resistance but are also an end product of a chain

of adipocyte events which impact separately on insulin resistance. The lack of functional peripheral adipose promotes fatty acid spill into the circulation (thereby worsening lipotoxicity). *In vitro* studies in the adipocyte cell line 3T3-L1 have shown that protease inhibitors decrease insulin-stimulated glucose uptake into this particular model, by effects on glucose transporter 4 action, without effects on post-receptor insulin signaling pathways [37]. Whether the findings in this cell line can be extrapolated to muscle, the key organ for glucose uptake and insulin resistance, is questionable.

Adiponectin, an insulin-sensitizing molecule, has been shown to be reduced in HIV-infected subjects with lipodystrophy, compared with HIV-infected subjects with no body fat disturbances and HIV-negative controls [38]. Adiponectin levels increase with rosiglitazone with improvement in insulin sensitivity, without any change in body fat partitioning [8]. Therefore, the hypoadiponectinemia found in lipodystrophy may affect insulin-mediated glucose disposal independent of changes in adipocyte mass or functionality. Differential regulation of adiponectin discrete of adipose mass has already been raised [38] and may again reflect the functionality of adipocyte tissue, rather than quantity. A study of hypertriglyceridemic HAART recipients found increased ghrelin, a promoter of hepatic triglyceride deposition and regulator of adiponectin action [39].

Further studies have also implicated disturbances in glucose metabolism beyond muscle tissue. In metabolic studies using tritiated glucose infused during hyperinsulinemic euglycemic clamp, HAART recipients with lipodystrophy had markedly reduced hepatic and muscle insulin sensitivity, peripheral glucose storage and glucose oxidation than BMI- and fat mass-matched non-lipodystrophic HAART recipients and HIV-infected HAART-naïve subjects did [40].

Mitochondrial dysfunction is a recognized player in the pathogenesis of insulin resistance and diabetes. The intramyocellular lipid accumulation found in insulin-resistant offspring of probands with type 2 diabetes is attributed, in part, to mitochondrial dysfunction [41], which may be due to genetic effects on mitochondrial oxidative phosphorylation. The contribution of mitochondrial dysfunction to insulin resistance in HAART is receiving wider attention, since one form of HAART, the nucleoside reverse-transcriptase inhibitors (NRTIs), inhibit mitochondrial DNA polymerase gamma, impairing synthesis of mitochondrial enzymes that generate adenosine-5apos-triphosphate. This produces lactic acidemia and appears related to lipoatrophy [9]. In a study of HIV-infected subjects treated with NRTIs, higher lactate levels independently predicted higher insulin resistance (by HOMA) [42]. Additional mitochondrial events occur within adipocytes with putative adverse metabolic effects (discussed below). Therefore, specific drug-induced mitochrondrial dysfunction in HAART may exert additional deleterious effects promoting insulin resistance due to lipotoxicity.

40.3.3 Adipocyte Function

HAART has been shown to exert potentially multiple effects on adipocyte function, which may produce peripheral lipoatrophy, increased central adiposity and circulatory lipid spill. Initial hypotheses suggested homology of protease inhibitors to retinoic acid binding protein interfering with activation of the retinoid X receptor (RXR) and peroxisome proliferator-activated receptor type gamma (PPAR-gamma) heterodimer, a key step in peripheral adipocyte differentiation, inducing apoptosis [27]. A study testing this hypothesis used rosiglitazone in subjects with HIV lipodystrophy to increase signaling down this pathway of adipocyte differentiation [8]. No increase in adipocyte mass was found after 12 months of therapy, though there were significant increases in insulin sensitivity and adiponectin [8]. A large volume of subsequent work indicates the great complexity of HAART action on adipocytes. Effects upstream of PPAR-gamma have been suggested to play a causative role in lipoatrophy, with evidence of reduced expression of the adipogenic factor sterol regulatory enhancer-binding protein-1 (SREBP-1) [43] or inhibition of the SREBP-1 activation of the RXR–PPAR-gamma heterodimer [44] in adipocytes derived from HIV-infected subjects. Inhibitory effects of protease inhibitors on lipogenesis through suppression of preadipocyte differentiation and apoptosis have been demonstrated in vitro [45]. Other in vitro studies have shown that protease inhibitors block adipogenesis but also stimulate lipolysis [46], providing a mechanism beyond apoptosis for adipocyte lipid spill. Protease inhibitors have also been shown in vitro to impair SREBP-1 localization within the adipocyte nucleus and promote defects in lamin maturation, organization and stability [47].

In vitro studies of protease inhibitors and nucleosidase reverse-transcriptase inhibitors suggest diverse effects in differentiating and differentiated adipocyte cell lines, with marked alteration in the expression and secretion of the adipokines IL-6, TNFalpha, IL-1beta and adiponectin in differentiating adipocyte cell lines and little or less marked effect in differentiated cell lines [48]. In mature adipocyte lines, selected protease inhibitors did not alter adipokine secretion and expression [48]. In vivo studies of the effects of

NRTIs on adipocyte gene expression in seronegative humans implicate effects on the functionality of the adipocyte mitochondrium, with decreased transcription of mitochondrial RNA and concomitant upregulation of nuclear genes involved in its transcriptional regulation and fatty acid oxidation [49]. Importantly, this study also found down regulation of PPAR-gamma and that changes in nuclear gene expression corresponded to changes in peroxisome proliferator-activated receptor-gamma coactivator-1 (PGC1), which may play a pivotal role in the nuclear responses to mitochondrial dysfunction within the adipocyte [49]. The study of seronegative human subjects permits ascertainment of HAART effects independent of HIV infection. HIV infection *per se* may compound or exacerbate drug effects through its effects on inflammatory cytokines. In summary, the contribution of HAART to the pathogenesis of hyperglycemia in HIV infection is multifactorial, influencing numerous important pathways, including glucose transport, intramyocellular lipid partitioning and metabolism, adiponectin metabolism, mitochondrial function, adipocyte function, differentiation and apoptosis, β-cell function and lipotoxicity.

40.4 LIPODYSTROPHY TREATMENT CONSIDERATIONS

The enigma of deterring or ameliorating lipoatrophy in HIV-infected HAART recipients remains unsolved. As already mentioned above, a large, randomized, placebo-controlled 48-week study of rosiglitazone did not increase peripheral body fat stores measured by dual-energy X-ray absorptiometry [8]. A smaller study of 12 weeks found an increase in subcutaneous leg fat measured by computed tomography [50]. Both studies reported improvements in insulin sensitivity and increased adiponectin [8, 50].

More recently, a study of the cholesterol-lowering drug pravastatin showed increased peripheral fat [51]. Studies of gemfibrozil have shown no effect on body fat distribution [52]. Moreover, the lipid lowering effects of these agents in HIV lipodystrophy are probably less than in the general population.

Metformin therapy for 3 months reduced both visceral and subcutaneous abdominal fat by computed tomography, but in the context of metformin-induced weight loss [53]. Use of metformin with an aerobic and resistance training program of 3 months' duration reduced waist/hip ratio [54] and thigh muscle adiposity and subcutaneous thigh fat [55], compared with metformin alone.

Studies suggest that cessation of protease inhibitors has little effect on reversing lipodystrophy [56–58]; however, alteration of nucleosidase reverse-transcriptase inhibitors may have some benefit. The large, prospective, randomized controlled Mitochondrial Toxicity Study changes subjects from a thymidine NRTI (zidovudine or stavudine) to abacavir or continued thymidine-NRTI-containing HAART regimen and found that, after 24 weeks, limb fat improved by 11% (or 0.4 kg) in the switched group [59]. After 2 years, there was a 35% increase in limb fat (1.3 kg) in the switched group [60]. These and other reversibility studies suggest a central role for thymidine analogue nucleosidase reverse-transcriptase inhibitors in the pathogenesis of lipoatrophy [61, 62]. Alteration to a patient's HAART regimen must be considered against potential toxicities of new drugs and the possibility of destabilizing viral control.

A major concern regarding the dyslipidemia and metabolic complications associated with HAART has been the likely increased risk of cardiovascular disease in a relatively young group. There have been a number of anecdotal reports of 'premature' cardiovascular events, and the Data Collection on Adverse Events of Anti-HIV Drugs Study indicated a 26% increase in the risk of myocardial infarction (95% confidence interval 1.12–1.41) per additional year of antiretroviral therapy, an increase statistically predicted from the lipid levels and other risk factors measured in the cohort [63].

40.5 SUMMARY

Advances in treatment of HIV infection have conferred virological benefits, but at the cost of metabolic complications that include lipodystrophy, insulin resistance and high rates of type 2 diabetes mellitus. Few strategies have substantially ameliorated body fat partitioning changes, and the cellular mechanisms that result in lipodystrophy are incompletely understood.

References

1. Kilby, J.M. and Tabereaux, P.B. (1998) Severe hyperglycemia in an HIV clinic: preexisting versus drug-associated diabetes mellitus. *Journal of Acquired Immune Deficiency Syndromes and Human Retrovirology*, **17**, 46–50.

2. Coyle, P., Carr, A.D., Depczynski, B.B. and Chisholm, D.J. (1996) Diabetes mellitus associated with pentamidine use in HIV-infected patients. *The Medical Journal of Australia*, **165**, 587–8.

3. Ubukata, E., Mokuda, O., Nagata, M. *et al.* (1997) A pentamidine-treated acquired immunodeficiency syndrome patient associated with sudden onset diabetes mellitus and high tumor necrosis factor alpha level. *Journal of Diabetes and its Complications*, **11**, 256–8.

4. Lu, C.P., Wu, H.P., Chuang, L.M. *et al.* (1995) Pentamidine-induced hyperglycemia and ketosis in acquired immunodeficiency syndrome. *Pancreas*, **11**, 315–16.

5. Carr, A., Samaras, K., Burton, S. *et al.* (1998) A syndrome of peripheral lipodystrophy, hyperlipidaemia and insulin resistance due to HIV protease inhibitors. *AIDS*, **12**, F51–8.

6. Carr, A., Samaras, K., Thorisdottir, A. *et al.* (1999) Natural history, diagnosis and prediction of HIV protease inhibitor-induced lipodystrophy, hyperlipidaemia and diabetes mellitus. *Lancet*, **353**, 2094–9.

7. Gan, S.K., Samaras, K., Thompson, C.H. *et al.* (2002) Altered myocellular and abdominal fat partitioning predict disturbance in insulin action in HIV protease inhibitor-related lipodystrophy. *Diabetes*, **51**, 3163–9.

8. Carr, A., Workman, C., Carey, D. *et al.* (2004) Rosiglitazone for the treatment of HIV lipoatrophy: a randomised, double-blind, placebo-controlled trial. *Lancet*, **363**, 429–38.

9. Carr, A., Miller, J., Law, M. and Cooper, D.A. (2000) A syndrome of lipoatrophy, lactic acidaemia and liver dysfunction associated with HIV nucleoside analogue therapy: contribution to protease inhibitor-related lipodystrophy syndrome. *AIDS*, **14**, F25–32.

10. Thiebaut, R., Daucourt, V., Mercie, P. *et al.* (2000) Lipodystrophy, metabolic disorders, and human immunodeficiency virus infection: Aquitaine Cohort, France, 1999. *Clinical Infectious Diseases*, **31**, 1482–7.

11. Mallal, S.A., John, M., Moore, C.B. *et al.* (2000) Contribution of nucleoside analogue reverse transcriptase inhibitors to subcutaneous fat wasting in patients with HIV infection. *AIDS*, **14**, 1309–16.

12. Grinspoon, S. and Carr, A. (2005) Cardiovascular risk and body-fat abnormalities in HIV-infected adults. *The New England Journal of Medicine*, **352**, 48–62.

13. Mallon, P.W., Miller, J., Cooper, D.A. and Carr, A. (2003) Prospective evaluation of the effects of antiretroviral therapy on body composition in HIV-1-infected men starting therapy. *AIDS*, **17**, 971–9.

14. HIV Lipodystrophy Case Definition Study Group (2003) An objective case definition of lipodystrophy in HIV-infected adults: a case control study. *Lancet*, **361**, 726–35.

15. Martinez, E., Mocroft, A., Garcia-Viejo, M.A. *et al.* (2001) Risk of lipodystrophy in HIV-1-infected patients treated with protease inhibitors: a prospective cohort study. *Lancet*, **357**, 592–8.

16. Heath, K.V., Hogg, R.S., Singer, J. *et al.* (2002) Antiretroviral treatment patterns and incident HIV-associated morphologic and lipid abnormalities in a population-based chort. *Journal of Acquired Immune Deficiency Syndromes*, **30**, 440–7.

17. El-Sadr, W.M., Mullin, C.M., Carr, A. *et al.* (2005) Effects of HIV disease on lipid, glucose and insulin levels: results from a large antiretroviral-naive cohort. *HIV Medicine*, **6**, 114–21.

18. Brown, T.T., Cole, S.R., Li, X. *et al.* (200) Antiretroviral therapy and the prevalence and incidence of diabetes mellitus in the multicenter AIDS cohort study. *Archives of Internal Medicine*, **165**, 1179–84.

19. Howard, A.A., Floris-Moore, M., Arnsten, J.H. *et al.* (2005) Disorders of glucose metabolism among HIV-infected women. *Clinical Infectious Diseases*, **40**, 1492–9.

20. Justman, J.E., Benning, L., Danoff, A. *et al.* (2003) Protease inhibitor use and the incidence of diabetes mellitus in a large cohort of HIV-infected women. *Journal of Acquired Immune Deficiency Syndromes*, **32**, 298–302.

21. Salehian, B., Bilas, J., Bazargan, M. and Abbasian, M. (2005) Prevalence and incidence of diabetes in HIV-infected minority patients on protease inhibitors. *Journal of the National Medical Association*, **97**, 1088–92.

22. Mehta, S.H., Moore, R.D., Thomas, D.L. *et al.* (2003) The effect of HAART and HCV infection on the development of hyperglycemia among HIV-infected persons. *Journal of Acquired Immune Deficiency Syndromes*, **33**, 577–84.

23. Amorosa, V., Synnestvedt, M., Gross, R. *et al.* (2005) A tale of 2 epidemics: the intersection between obesity and HIV infection in Philadelphia. *Journal of Acquired Immune Deficiency Syndromes*, **39**, 557–61.

24. Yazicioglu, G., Isitan, F., Altunbas, H. *et al.* (2004) Insulin resistance in chronic hepatitis C.

International Journal of Clinical Practice, **58**, 1020–2.

25. Panz, V.R. and Joffe, B.I. (1999) Impact of HIV infection and AIDS on prevalence of type 2 diabetes in South Africa in 2010 (Letter). *British Medical Journal*, **318**, 1351A.

26. Levitt, N.S. and Bradshaw, D. (2006) The impact of HIV/AIDS on type 2 diabetes prevalence and diabetes healthcare needs in South Africa: projections for 2010 (Letter). *Diabetic Medicine*, **23**, 103–4.

27. Carr, A., Samaras, K., Chisholm, D.J. and Cooper, D.A. (1998) Pathogenesis of protease-inhibitor-associated syndrome of peripheral lipodystrophy, hyperlipidaemia and insulin resistance. *Lancet*, **351**, 1881–3.

28. Gan, S.K., Samaras, K., Carr, A. and Chisholm, D.J. (2001) Antiretroviral therapy, insulin resistance and lipodystrophy. *Diabetes, Metabolism and Obesity*, **3**, 67–71.

29. McGarry, J.D. (2002) Banting Lecture 2001: Dysregulation of fatty acid metabolism in the etiology of type 2 diabetes. *Diabetes*, **51**, 7–18.

30. Wollheim, C.B. (2000) Beta-cell mitochondria in the regulation of insulin secretion: a new culprit in type II diabetes. *Diabetologia*, **43**, 265–77.

31. Samaras, K., Nguyen, T.V., Jenkins, A.B. *et al.* (1999) Clustering of insulin resistance, total and central abdominal fat: are the relationships due to same genes or same environment? *Twin Research*, **2**, 218–25.

32. Pan, D.A., Lillioja, S., Kriketos, A.D. *et al.* (1997) Skeletal muscle triglyceride levels are inversely related to insulin action. *Diabetes*, **46**, 983–8.

33. Perseghin, G., Scifo, P., De Cobelli, F. *et al.* (1999) Intramyocellular triglyceride content is a determinant of *in vivo* insulin resistance in humans: a ^{1}H–^{13}C nuclear magnetic resonance spectroscopy assessment in offspring of type 2 diabetic parents. *Diabetes*, **48**, 1600–6.

34. Hadigan, C., Kamin, D., Liebau, J. *et al.* (2006) Depot-specific regulation of glucose uptake and insulin sensitivity in HIV-lipodystrophy. *American Journal of Physiology. Endocrinology and Metabolism*, **290**, E289–98.

35. Nolte, L.A., Yarasheski, K.E., Kawanaka, K. *et al.* (2001) The HIV protease inhibitor indinavir decreases insulin- and contraction-stimulated glucose transport in skeletal muscle. *Diabetes*, **50**, 1397–401.

36. Noor, M.A., Lo, J.C., Mulligan, K. *et al.* (2001) Metabolic effects of indinavir in healthy HIV-seronegative men. *AIDS*, **15**, F11–18.

37. Murata, H., Hruz, P.W. and Mueckler, M. (2002) Indinavir inhibits the glucose transporter isoform Glut4 at physiologic concentrations. *AIDS*, **16**, 859–63.

38. Tong, Q., Sankale, J.L., Hadigan, C.M. *et al.* (2003) Regulation of adiponectin in human immunodeficiency virus-infected patients: relationship to body composition and metabolic indices. *The Journal of Clinical Endocrinology and Metabolism*, **88**, 1559–64.

39. Falasca, K., Manigrasso, M.R., Racciatti, D. *et al.* (2006) Associations between hypertriglyceridemia and serum ghrelin, adiponectin, and IL-18 levels in HIV-infected patients. *Annals of Clinical and Laboratory Science*, **36**, 59–66.

40. Haugaard, S.B., Andersen, O., Dela, F. *et al.* (2005) Defective glucose and lipid metabolism in human immunodeficiency virus-infected patients with lipodystrophy involve liver, muscle tissue and pancreatic beta-cells. *European Journal of Endocrinology*, **152**, 103–12.

41. Petersen, K.F., Dufour, S., Befroy, D. *et al.* (2004) Impaired mitochondrial activity in the insulin-resistant offspring of patients with type 2 diabetes. *The New England Journal of Medicine*, **350**, 664–71.

42. Lo, J.C., Kazemi, M.R., Hsue, P.Y. *et al.* (2005) The relationship between nucleoside analogue treatment duration, insulin resistance, and fasting arterialized lactate level in patients with HIV infection. *Clinical Infectious Diseases*, **41**, 1335–40.

43. Bastard, J.P., Caron, M., Vidal, H. *et al.* (2002) Association between altered expression of adipogenic factor SREBP1 in lipoatrophic adipose tissue from HIV-1-infected patients and abnormal adipocyte differentiation and insulin resistance. *Lancet*, **359**, 1026–31.

44. Caron, M., Auclair, M., Vigouroux, C. *et al.* (2001) The HIV protease inhibitor indinavir impairs sterol regulatory element-binding protein-1 intranuclear localization, inhibits preadipocyte differentiation, and induces insulin resistance. *Diabetes*, **50**, 1378–88.

45. Dowell, P., Flexner, C., Kwiterovich, P.O. and Lane, M.D. (2000) Suppression of preadipocyte differentiation and promotion of adipocyte death by HIV protease inhibitors. *The Journal of Biological Chemistry*, **275**, 41325–32.

46. Lenhard, J.M., Furfine, E.S., Jain, R.G. *et al.* (2000) HIV protease inhibitors block adipogenesis and increase lipolysis *in vitro*. *Antiviral Research*, **47**, 121–9.

47. Caron, M., Auclair, M., Sterlingot, H. *et al.* (2003) Some HIV protease inhibitors alter lamin A/C maturation and stability, SREBP-1 nuclear localization and adipocyte differentiation. *AIDS*, **17**, 2437–44.

48. Lagathu, C., Bastard, J.P., Auclair, M. *et al.* (2004) Antiretroviral drugs with adverse effects on adipocyte lipid metabolism and survival alter the expression and secretion of proinflammatory cytokines and adiponectin *in vitro*. *Antiviral Therapy*, **9**, 911–20.

49. Mallon, P.W.G., Unemori, P., Sedwell, R. *et al.* (2005) *In vivo*, nucleoside reverse transcriptase inhibitors alter expression of both mitochondrial and lipid metabolism genes in the absence of mitochondrial DNA depletion. *Journal of Infectious Diseases*, **191**, 1686–96.

50. Hadigan, C., Yawetz, S., Thomas, A. *et al.* (2004) Metabolic effects of rosiglitazone in HIV lipodystrophy: a randomized, controlled trial. *Annals of Internal Medicine*, **140**, 786–94.

51. Mallon, P.W.G., Miller, J., Kovacic, J. *et al.* (2006) Changes in body composition and surrogate markers of cardiovascular disease in hypercholesterolaemic HIV-infected men treated with pravastatin – a randomised, placebo-controlled study. *AIDS*, **20**, 1003–10.

52. Miller, J., Brown, D., Amin, J. *et al.* (2002) A randomized, double-blind study of gemfibrozil for the treatment of protease inhibitorsassociated hypertriglyceridaemia. *AIDS*, **16**, 2195–200.

53. Hadigan, C., Corcoran, C., Basgoz, N. *et al.* (2000) Metformin in the treatment of HIV lipodystrophy syndrome: a randomized controlled trial. *The Journal of the American Medical Association*, **284**, 472–7.

54. Driscoll, S.D., Meininger, G.E., Lareau, M.T. *et al.* (2004) Effects of exercise training and metformin on body composition and cardiovascular indices in HIV-infected patients. *AIDS*, **18**, 465–73.

55. Driscoll, S.D., Meininger, G.E., Ljungquist, K. *et al.* (2004) Differential effects of metformin and exercise on muscle adiposity and metabolic indices in human immunodeficiency virus-infected patients. *The Journal of Clinical Endocrinology and Metabolism*, **89**, 2171–8.

56. Martinez, E., Conget, I., Lozano, L. *et al.* (1999) Reversion of metabolic abnormalities after switching from HIV-1 protease inhibitors to nevirapine. *AIDS*, **13**, 805–10.

57. Carr, A., Hudson, J., Chuah, J. *et al.* (2001) HIV protease inhibitor substitution in patients with lipodystrophy: a randomised, controlled, open-label, multicentre study. *AIDS*, **15**, 1811–22.

58. Martin, A., Smith, D., Carr, A. *et al.* (2004) Progression of lipodystrophy (LD) with continued thymidine analogue usage: long-term follow-up from a randomised clinical trial (The PIILR Study). *HIV Clinical Trials*, **5**, 192–200.

59. Carr, A., Workman, C., Smith, D.E. *et al.* (2002) Mitochondrial Toxicity (MITOX) Study Group. Abacavir substitution for nucleoside analogs in patients with HIV lipoatrophy: a randomised trial. *The Journal of the American Medical Association*, **288**, 207–15.

60. Martin, A., Smith, D.E., Carr, A. *et al.* (2004) Mitochondrial Toxicity Study Group. Reversibility of lipoatrophy in HIV-infected patients 2 years after switching from a thymidine analogue to abacavir: the MITOX Extension Study. *AIDS*, **18**, 1029–36.

61. Moyle, G.J., Baldwin, C., Langroudi, B. *et al.* (2003) A 48-week, randomized, open-label comparison of three abacavir-based substitution approaches in the management of dyslipidemia and peripheral lipoatrophy. *Journal of Acquired Immune Deficiency Syndromes*, **33**, 22–8.

62. John, M., McKinnon, E.J., James, I.R. *et al.* (2003) Randomized, controlled, 48-week study of switching stavudine and/or protease inhibitors to combivir/abacavir to prevent or reverse lipoatrophy in HIV-infected patients. *Journal of Acquired Immune Deficiency Syndromes*, **33**, 29–33.

63. Friis-Moller, N., Sabin, C.A., Weber, R. *et al.* (2003) Data Collection on Adverse Events of Anti-HIV Drugs (DAD) Study Group. Combination antiretroviral therapy and the risk of myocardial infarction. *The New England Journal of Medicine*, **349**, 1993–2003.

Index

Note: Figures and Tables are indicated by *italic page numbers*; abbreviations: DM = diabetes mellitus, IFG = impaired fasting glycemia, IGT = impaired glucose tolerance, T1D = type 1 diabetes, T2D = type 2 diabetes

The Epidemiology of Diabetes Mellitus, second edition   Edited by Jean-Marie Ekoé, Marian Rewers, Rhys Williams and Paul Zimmet
© 2008 John Wiley & Sons, Ltd